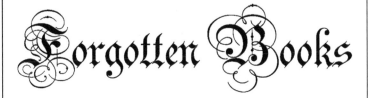
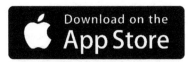
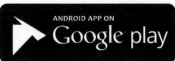

ISBN 978-1-330-29169-6
PIBN 10015772

1 MONTH OF
FREE
READING

at

www.ForgottenBooks.com

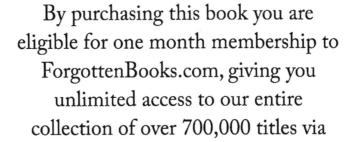

By purchasing this book you are eligible for one month membership to ForgottenBooks.com, giving you unlimited access to our entire collection of over 700,000 titles via our web site and mobile apps.

To claim your free month visit:
www.forgottenbooks.com/free15772

English
Français
Deutsche
Italiano
Español
Português

www.forgottenbooks.com

Mythology Photography **Fiction**
Fishing Christianity **Art** Cooking
Essays Buddhism Freemasonry
Medicine **Biology** Music **Ancient
Egypt** Evolution Carpentry Physics
Dance Geology **Mathematics** Fitness
Shakespeare **Folklore** Yoga Marketing
Confidence Immortality Biographies
Poetry **Psychology** Witchcraft
Electronics Chemistry History **Law**
Accounting **Philosophy** Anthropology
Alchemy Drama Quantum Mechanics
Atheism Sexual Health **Ancient History**
Entrepreneurship Languages Sport
Paleontology Needlework Islam
Metaphysics Investment Archaeology
Parenting Statistics Criminology
Motivational

THE

MEDICAL AND SURGICAL

REPORTER

EDITED BY

CHARLES W. DULLES, M.D.

JANUARY–JUNE, 1889.

VOL. LX.

PHILADELPHIA:
N. E. CORNER THIRTEENTH AND WALNUT STREETS.
1889.

CONTRIBUTORS.

ADLER, LEWIS H. Jr., M.D., Philadelphia.
ALLYN, HERMAN B., M.D., Philadelphia.
ANDERS, JAMES M., M.D., Philadelphia.
ASHHURST, JOHN Jr., M.D., Philadelphia.

BALDY, J. M., M.D., Philadelphia.
BALLOU, WILLIAM R., M.D., New York City.
BARR, G. WALTER, M.D., Bridgeport, Ill.
BARTON, J. M., M.D., Philadelphia.
BAUM, CHARLES, M.D., Philadelphia.
BEALL, E. J., M.D., Fort Worth, Texas.
BENEDICT, A. L., Philadelphia, Pa.
BENJAMIN, D., M D., Camden, N. J.
BOUCHARD, PROFESSOR, Paris, France.
BRUEN, EDWARD T., M.D., Philadelphia.
BUCKLIN, C. A., M.D., New York City.
BURR, WILLIAM H., M.D., Wilmington, Delaware.

CARRELL, J. B., M.D., Hatboro, Pa.
CARY, WILLIAM S., Gothenburg, Nebraska.
CATES, B. BRABSON, M.D., Maryville, Tenn.
CHARCOT, PROFESSOR J. M., Paris, France.
CHRISTINE, G. W., M.D., Philadelphia.
COHEN, SOLOMON SOLIS, M.D., Philadelphia.
COLVIN, D., Clyde, New York.
CONSTABLE, HERBERT L., M.D., New York City.
CROTHERS, T. D., M.D., Hartford, Conn.
CURRIER, JOHN M., M.D., Newport, Vermont.
CURWEN, JOHN, M.D., Warren, Pennsylvania.

DABNEY, WILLIAM C., M.D., Charlottesville, Va.
DA COSTA, J. M., M.D., LL.D., Philadelphia.
DAVIS, EDWARD P., A.M., M.D., Philadelphia.
DEAN, GEORGE R., M.D., Spartansburg, N. C.
DEEKENS, A. HAMILTON, Philadelphia.
DERCUM, F. X., M.D., Philadelphia.
DILLER, THEODORE, M.D., Danville, Pa.
DUNDORE, CLAUDE A., M.D., Ashland, Pa.

EDWARDS, C. P., M.D., Graniteville, S. C.
ELIOT, LLEWELLYN, M.D., Washington, D. C.
ELLIS, J. C., M.D., Philadelphia.
EUSTIS, W. C., M.D., Farmington, Minn.

FIELDE, ADELE M., M.D., Swatow, China.
FLICK, LAWRENCE, M.D., Philadelphia.
FORBES, WILLIAM S., M.D., Philadelphia.
FOX, L. WEBSTER, M.D., Philadelphia.

GLEASON, E. BALDWIN, M.D., Philadelphia.
GOODELL, WILLIAM, M.D., Philadelphia.
GOODYEAR, MILES D., M.D., Groton, N.Y.
GOULD, GEORGE M., M.D., Philadelphia.
GRAHAM, JAMES, M.D., Philadelphia.
GRAY, JOHN, M.D., Mystic River, Conn.
GREEN, TRAILL, M.D., Easton, Pennsylvania.

HAPPEL, T. J., A.M., M.D., Trenton, Tenn.
HARDCASTLE, JEROME, M.D., Cecilton, Md.
HARE, HOBART A., M.D., Philadelphia.
HARRIS, R. P., M.D., Philadelphia.
HARVEY, THOMAS W., M.D., Orange, N. J.
HELM, ERNEST C., M.D., Beloit, Wis.
HENGST, D. A., M.D., Pittsburgh, Pa.
HENRY, FREDERIK P., M.D., Philadelphia.
HODGES, FRED. JENNER, B.Sc., M.D., Chicago, Illinois.
HOUGH, ORSON, M.D., Conneautville, Pa.
HUBER, L., M.D., Rocky Ford, Colorado.
HUNTER, S. M., M.D., Hope, Kansas.

JACKSON, EDWARD, A.M., M.D., Philadelphia.
JOHNSON, J. B., M.D., Washington, D. C.

KAUFFMANN, VALENTINE, M.D., Catorce, Mexico.
KEATING, JOHN M., M.D., Philadelphia.
KEMPER, G. W. H., M.D., Muncie, Indiana.

LEUF, A. H. P., M.D., Philadelphia.
LONG, J. A., M.D., Long's Mills, Tenn.
LONG, J. W. M.D., Randleman, N.C.
LYMAN, HENRY M., M.D., Chicago, Ill.

MARTIN, W. L., M.D., Rancocas, New Jersey.
MAXWELL, GEORGE TROUP, M.D., Jacksonville, Fla.
McCLELLAN, GEORGE, M.D., Philadelphia.
McDUFFIE, M. V. Rev., Brunswick, N. J.
McGUIRE, C. F., M.D., Brooklyn, N. Y.
MILNER, J. C., M.D., Comanche, Texas.
MINICH, J. A., M.D., Worthington, Ind.
MOLLENHAUER, R., M.D., New York City.
MORRIS, G. G., M.D., Washington, D.C.
MUSGROVE, CHARLES W., M.D., Austinville, Pa.
MUSSER, J. H., M.D., Philadelphia.

NOBLE, CHARLES P., M.D., Philadelphia.

PACKARD, FREDERICK A., M.D., Philadelphia.
PARKER E. H., M.D., Poughkeepsie, N. Y.
PARVIN, THEOPHILUS, M.D., Philadelphia.
PENROSE, CHARLES B., Ph.D., M.D., Philadelphia.
PEPPER, WILLIAM, M.D., Philadelphia.
PERSINGER, E. I., M.D., Campti, Louisiana.
PETER, PROF. M., Paris, France.
PRICE, MORDECAI, M.D., Philadelphia.

RANSLEY, A. W., M.D., Philadelphia.
RECORDS, B. F., M.D., Smithville, Mo.
REID, JOHN J., M.D., New York City.
RIDLON, JOHN, M.D., New York City.
ROBBINS, HONORA A., M.D., Bloomsburg, Pa.
ROBERTS, A. SYDNEY, M.D., Philadelphia.
ROBERTS, JOHN B., M.D., Philadelphia.
RORER, Mrs. S. T., Philadelphia.
RUNNALLS, H. B., M.R.C.S. Eng., Bedford Springs, Pa.

SCOTT, T. Y., M.D., Bentleyville, Pa.
SEGNITZ, B. H., M.D., New York City.
SHEPARD, C. S., M.D., La Porte City, Iowa.
SCHMIDT, JOSEPH, M.D., Berlin, Germany.
SCHÜLLER, MAX, PROF., Berlin, Germany.
SCHWARTZ, N. F., M.D., Shanesville, Ohio.
SHARPLES, CASPAR W., M.D., Philadelphia.
SHIVERS, C. H., M.D., Haddonfield, New Jersey.
SHOEMAKER, GEORGE ERETY, M.D., Philadelphia.
SHULTZ, R. C., M.D., New York City.
SMITH, B. M. Jr., M.D., Parsons, West Va.
STUBBS, H. J., M.D., Wilmington, Del.
SWAN, J. M., M.D., Canton, China.

TODD, WILLIAM C., M.D., Roxborough, Pa.
TOWLER, S. S., M.D., Marienville, Pa.
TRENT, I. N. M.D., Columbus, Ohio.
TULL, M. GRAHAM, A.M., M.D., Philadelphia.

VANDERBECK, C. C., M.D., San Francisco, California.
VANDERPOEL, E., M.D., New York City.

WALKER, JAMES B., M.D., Philadelphia.
WARD, STANLEY M., M.D., Scranton, Pa.
WHITE, J. WILLIAM, M.D., Philadelphia, Pa.
WILLARD, De FOREST, M.D., Ph.D., Philadelphia.
WILLIAMS, CHARLES B., M.D., Philadelphia.
WILLIS, H. F., M.D., Preston, Md.
WILSON, JAMES C., M.D., Philadelphia.
WOOD, H. C., M.D., Philadelphia.
WOODRING, CHARLES P., M. D., Meadville, Pa.

YOUNG, JAMES K., M.D., Philadelphia.

INDEX.

Parvin, Theophilus.—Tait's operation for partial rupture of the perineum, 673.
Pathogeny, practical value of a knowledge of, 617.
Pathological specimens, rare, 81.
Pelvic inflammation, massage in, 409.
Pelvic (intra-) injury corrected by laparotomy, 479.
Pelvis, justo-minor, 486.
Penis, amputation of, 525.
Pennsylvania State Medical Society, 411.
Pennsylvania, University of, commencement of Medical and Dental Departments, 559.
Penrose, Charles B.—Secretion of milk following ovariotomy, 326; trismus following dog-bite of the finger; recovery after amputation, 544; Tuberculosis of the testicle in a child nine months old, 706.
Pepper, William.—Duodenal ulcer; sudden enormous hemorrhage; death, 471.
Pericarditis, purulent, 84.
Perineum, new procedure in anticipated complete rupture, 460; laceration, and rectocele, 634; Tait's operation for partial rupture, 673.
Peritonitis, pelvic, 47; tubercular, laparotomy for, 447; tubercular, surgical intervention in, 628; operative treatment of perforating, 688; tubercular, diagnosis and treatment, 697.
Peru balsam in buccal leucoplakia, 285.
Pessaries, 309.
Peter, Prof. M.—Rheumatism with articular, cerebral and visceral symptoms, 193.
Petroleum fuel, solidified, 154.
Pharmacopœia of the United States, convention for revision and publication of, 440.
Pharmacy, welfare of, 250.
Phenacetin, 158; and antipyrin, 615.
Philadelphia Hospital, 159.
Philadelphia, two months in hospitals of, 707.
Phosphorus, danger of white, 124.
Phthisical habit, anatomical basis of, 668.
Phthisis (see also "Consumption"), creasote in, 31; 274; prevention of, 369; pulmonary, 502; relation of dusty occupations to, 604; treatment by inhalations of hot air, 635; nightsweats of, ice bags in, 752.
Physical education, 705.
Physician, White Caps attack on, 31; advertisement of a, 151.
Physicians and Surgeons, New York, College of, 770.
Physicians, clergyman's charges against, 29.
Physicians, protection for American, 93.
Pilocarpine, in itching of jaundice, 586.
Placenta previa, abortion with, 376.
Placenta, retained, due to spasmodic contraction of uterus, 197; retained; removal, 439.
Pleurisy with effusion, 457.
"Pneumatic cabinet," European view of, 222.
Pneumonia, lobar, a new study of, 18; treatment of, 202; lobar; pericarditis, 273; fibrinous, etiology, 454; croupous, infectiousness of, 577.
Pneumothorax, recurrent, 239.
Poison, death by, expert testimony, 698; arrow, Mr. Stanley on, 744.
Poisoning, septic, in early life, 175; lead, 202; mercury, 286.
Polyclinic, Philadelphia, 149.
Polyuria, with localizing symptoms, 85.
Porro-Cæsarean method of Mr. Tait, historically considered, 57.
Post-mortem examinations upon infants, method of conducting, 391.

Potassium, iodide of, example of great tolerance of, 766.
Potato, dried, 528.
Potter railroad hospital, 614.
Pott's disease, 236; 393; 394; successfully treated by suspension, 513.
Pregnancy, albuminuria of, and puerperal eclampsia, 206; remains of extra-uterine, 307; and pulmonary tuberculosis, 485; Hegar's sign of, 713; severe vomiting of, 742.
Presbyterian Hospital, munificent gift to, 286.
Prescription, a fatal, 379.
Price, Mordecai.—Amputations of thigh and leg, 135.
Prize, three thousand dollar, 159.
Procreation, relative age in, 254.
Prostate, electrolysis for the results of gonorrhœal disease of, 92.
Prostatectomy, suprapubic, 366.
Prostatitis, diagnosis and therapeutics, 662.
Protection for American physicians, 93.
Pruritus senilis, salicylates in, 755.
Psoriasis, cases and treatment, 573.
Ptomaines, newly discovered, 688.
Public Health Association, American, 721.
Puerperal eclampsia, albuminuria of pregnancy and, 206.
Puerperal eclampsia, observations on, 474.
Puerperal endometritis, treatment of with the curette, 45.
Purpura, from iodide of potash, 222; relation to malignant disease, 368.
Pylorus, digital dilatation of, 443; stricture, dilatation, 629; diagnosis of and operation for, 687.
Pyosalpinx, ovariotomy for, 275; 365; and pelvic abscess, 634.
Pyuria, 561.

Quacks, German laws to prevent deception by, 660.
Quadriceps extensor femoris, rupture of, 48.
Quarantine station, new, at entrance to Delaware Bay, 726.
Quinine idiosyncrasy, sodium bromide for, 614.
Quinine rash, 751.
Quinine, so-called tasteless, 586.

Railway Surgeons, National Association of, 411.
Ransley, A. W.—Report of a death under ether, 653.
Records, B. F.—Observations on puerperal eclampsia, 474.
Rectum, stricture of, 757.
Reid, John J.—Anchylosis of laryngeal articulations from cancer; relief by intubation, 572.
REVIEWS:
  Acton, William.—Functions and disorders of the reproductive organs, 216.
  Allingham, William.—Diseases of the rectum, 523.
  Andrews, Edmund.—Rectal and anal surgery, 523.
  Ashton, W. E.—Essentials of obstetrics, 121.
  Bashore, H. B.—Clinical chart, 121.
  Biddle, John B.—Materia medica and therapeutics, 584.
  Binet, Alfred.—Psychic life of micro-organisms, 750.
  Bowditch, H. P.—Hints for teachers of physiology, 523.
  Bowen, Cuthbert.—Handbook of materia medica, pharmacy and therapeutics, 345.

THE

MEDICAL AND SURGICAL

REPORTER

No. 1662.   PHILADELPHIA, JANUARY 5, 1889.   VOL. LX.—No. 1.

CONTENTS:

COMMUNICATIONS.

FIBRO-CYSTIC TUMOR OF THE UTERUS; UNUSUAL TREATMENT; CURE.[1]

BY E. J. BEALL, M.D.,
FORT WORTH, TEXAS.

At the April, 1887, meeting of the Texas State Medical Association, I presented a paper upon uterine fibro-myomata complicating delivery. In that paper I strongly urged enucleation in lieu of other measures, and gave the history of a case in which I enucleated a fibroid weighing three pounds,

[1] Read at the meeting of the Southern Surgical and Gynecological Association, Birmingham, Ala., Dec. 7, 1888.

that completely blocked the pelvis, having incarcerated behind it a male child weighing fully ten pounds. The case was successful in every particular—mother and child both well at the present time.

Twelve weeks ago I was called in consultation with one of the most intelligent physicians of this section to see Mrs. S., aged 37 years; married one year; had never conceived. Her mother, a sister, and a maternal aunt died of "malignant disease" within the abdominal cavity. Upon her cousin I had performed laparotomy for intra-peritoneal abscess that followed childbirth. She had suffered from metrorrhagia for several years. Some time prior to marriage her abdomen had begun to enlarge, and at the time of my visit the fundus uteri reached a point somewhat above the umbilicus. She was anæmic from profuse and protracted hemorrhage, and had more or less abdominal pain.

A few days before I visited the case, an electrical trocar had been introduced into a fibro-cystic tumor that extended into and very much distended the vagina. As a result an ulcerative gangrenous process had arisen, attended with slight flow and odor. To the above procedure, though strict antisepsis had been observed, I attributed the elevated temperature and increased frequency of pulse I found present at my visit. Yet, some days prior to the elevation of temperature there had existed fever, which readily responded to quinine, and the patient lived in a malarious locality. The abdomen presented a symmetrical contour; the enlarged and elevated uterus inclined only slightly toward the right side.

An examination disclosed a hard, slightly elastic tumor, filling a very much dilated and elongated vagina, extending to and slightly bulging the labia and just within a firmly closed and rigid ostium. The finger could be swept around the mass; the edges of the cervix uteri could be made out, but it was widely dilated and occupied by the growth.

As the tumor gradually developed, the uterus was both dilated and elevated, and the vagina dilated and lengthened. A sound could be introduced into the uterus on one side to a considerable depth; but the sound movement was quite limited, and indicated a very lengthened and narrow cavity unoccupied by the attachments of the growth. This led me to infer that I had a tumor to deal with, the attachments of which, to the internal surface of the uterus, were quite extensive. Palpation and percussion also indicated a large, firm, very slightly elastic tumor, doubtless fibro-cystic, filling the vagina and elevating and enlarging the uterus to the dimensions already indicated.

These facts of the case well in mind, what course should be pursued which would prove safest for a patient whose life is in the balance, to be turned for weal or woe by the act needed to be carried out by the physician for relief?

It may be well to review some of the measures hitherto suggested for the treatment of uterine fibroids that the hearer may be prepared for comparison when I present the plan adopted, and which terminated so happily in this case.

Palliative treatment, while applicable to minor and less severe cases, promised little in the one under consideration. Correcting displacement of the uterus was not indicated. Arresting hemorrhage by hæmostatics, tampon, rest, etc., could only put off the inevitable day for action of a decisive character. The medical treatment by alterative agents, whose office, it is thought, is to induce fatty degeneration; the use of ergot, which in some cases has produced good results, when tumors were decidedly interstitial or perhaps subserous, more particularly the former, when muscular contractility (the result of ergotism) would induce compression by muscular fibre—this method was not, to my mind applicable; at least it would be fraught with danger, by reason of the delay needed before radical results could be expected.

From reading and experience I could not expect that electrolysis, so strongly urged by Apostoli, could effect changes in the growth with sufficient rapidity and thoroughness, nor sufficiently exempt from danger, to commend it to this case, which I thoroughly believed, required prompt, immediate measures.

To the art of surgery and its ready application I now turned for a remedy.

1st. Was abdominal section advisable? I believe there are those who would have resorted to the measure. That road has many a warning post, to one of limited experience, at every crook and fork; like a boatman slowly and gently descending some placid winding stream; suddenly and unexpectedly he encounters unforeseen rocks or falls, while just before, everything was merrily well. The abdomen opened, an enlarged uterus and fibro-cystic contents turned over the pubes; the broad ligaments ligated off; a large dilated and filled cervix to be cobble-stitched around, secured and tied, disengaging a mass from its circular grasp; that cervix as large as the calf of one's leg—all this is pretty to read about in books and journals; it is exciting, and does well when one has the ægis of a metropolitan hospital, with its reports fingered only by the actor, and has leisure for study of results at a dead-house, the janitor his vigil; but not upon the living woman, at a farm-house; the laity his audience; the husband, the mother, the sister hard by the operating-table, urging the surgeon to seek a safer, less formidable plan of treatment, if his conscience will allow and his judgment devise such.

2d. As the tumor could be drawn downward, should I attempt to cut it away with scissors? This is sometimes practicable, and has been done often.

3d. After traction with volsellum, should

I endeavor to encircle the mass with the écraseur and sever it as near as practicable to its fibrous attachments?

4th. Should I endeavor to remove the tumor with Dr. Thomas's serrated spoon, as has been done rapidly, safely, and surely, so often, by that brilliant man and his followers?

5th. Should I enucleate, as I had done in former cases—a notable instance of which I have heretofore brought before the profession?

The high opinion I entertain of this last measure induced me to preface this paper with a reference to a case in which I put that plan into successful execution. It is, in many instances, easily done, and attended with little danger. I urge the method when practicable, which it is in very many interstitial, submucous, and mixed tumors. My first effort in this case was to institute the enucleation process. At several places I essayed the plan, but signally failed: the capsule could not be peeled from the growth.

To have incised the capsule and endeavored to force a gradual extrusion of the intracapsular fibro-cystic growth by ergot, would have involved much time, besides subjecting the patient to further systemic infection.

To the first proposition: Disinclination, by reason of inexperience, and fear of shock, etc., prevented its adoption.

To the second and third: I could not consent for various reasons: pertinently, portions of the mass would have been left, presenting a surface through which poisons could readily reach the uterine sinuses and lymphatics, and thus originate a process of systemic infection fraught with great danger.

To the fourth: The objections urged against the second and third are of equal import here. Additionally, in the hands of one whose experience with the Thomas serrated spoon is limited, uterine tissue might be injured—even the peritoneal cavity might be invaded.

Having referred to the more prominent measures relied upon for the removal of growths connected with the uterus, it must not be inferred that cases do not occur to which these various plans are applicable. But to tumors with a broad and extensive intra-uterine attachment, the sawing process, the *écrasement*, or the incision must be followed by a digging-out of tumor remains: a harsh usage of the uterus, accompanied by the danger that belongs to shock, hemorrhage, etc. Even after much digging, tumor elements will be left which may develop again at a future time, entailing perhaps, if nothing more, a hemorrhagic condition of a new endometrium, great risk of infection, etc.

I do not claim that the manner in which I treated the case, the technique of which I am about to relate, is without precedent. But the plan has no advocates; and if such cases are known to others of the profession they may have had similar management accidentally, not intentionally. This, however, is not so in my own case. What I did was not an accident growing out of an effort to do otherwise; but was the outcome of premeditation.

If I am to be criticized for the method pursued it must not be ascribed to rashness, but to sober thought and conscientious conclusions. At all events, the patient lives; the interested ones are of a good family and happy; and I have the knowledge that they have applauded and appreciated the services rendered in this most interesting case.

The patient was placed in the dorsal position, the hips elevated, and chloroform administered. Sawyer's forceps were introduced as high as the cervix and caused to embrace the tumor; gentle traction with slight to and fro movement was exercised. Very soon the labia and perineum were being bulged outward by the tumor upon which traction was being made. The left hand was held upon the enlarged abdomen, and the uterus could be felt descending *pari passu* with the advance of the tumor within the grasp of the forceps. At this stage of the operation I intended doing an epicistotomy to avoid an irregular laceration of the perineum, which was becoming pronouncedly distended. I did not do so, however, but elevated the handle of the forceps and endeavored to keep apace with the perineal tension. By external palpation and intra-vaginal examination I watched the lowering of the uterus and condition of parts as delivery progressed. Just here, notwithstanding the traction was cautiously and gently done, I discovered that the thinned perineum was giving away. I had now withdrawn at least a pound of the seven-pound growth beyond the external genitalia, and at once instituted search for cysts, upon finding which I opened and relieved of viscid colloidal material, thus reducing the mass I was endeavoring to remove. I then enlarged the perineum; made further traction, and further reduction by disposing of other small cysts. Pursuing this plan I was soon enabled to introduce my hand (having removed the forceps) by the side of the tumor, grasp it and make more intelligent traction. A few minutes later I could insinuate my hand into the uterus, grasp the tumor more firmly, and determine that the attachments were very general. Instead of removing large portions of the tumor and allowing fragments to remain, I determined gently to *invert the uterus,* which I did, and bring in view the attachments of the growth, in order more thoroughly to separate it from the uterine wall, and better stanch the bleeding with hæmostatic forceps and hot sublimate water. The tumor now being entirely removed by aseptic fingers and scissors; a hypodermic of ergot having been given; the bleeding all stopped, I *returned the uterus* to its normal position with great ease. The perineum was neatly stitched with number three gut ligature, and patient put to bed, knees tied together.

Doing what I did, I could observe strict antisepsis. I left nothing within the uterus, nor returned anything for septic mischief. Little or no shock supervened, and but little hemorrhage. The patient was soon comfortable. No fever or other untoward circumstance retarded a rapid restoration to health.

The perineum was primarily united; menstruation is occurring normally; health is re-established; and a happy husband has a happy housewife, in every way qualified for her duties, domestic and marital.

TRAUMATIC TETANUS.

BY WILLIAM C. TODD, M.D.,
ROXBOROUGH, PA.

I have just treated a case of traumatic tetanus, which terminated in recovery, and it occurred to me that a short account of some cases which have happened recently in my practice may be of interest.

Case I.—J. B., a lad 13 years old, in running barefoot along some rough boards, had a splinter about three inches long enter the foot under the toes, and penetrate deeply into the centre of the foot. Nothing was done for several days, until symptoms became serious. When called in, I found tetanus fully developed; the jaws being locked and the whole body bent forcibly backward, with occasional spasms in which the tongue was bitten. The foot was much inflamed, swollen, and very painful. An anæsthetic was given, the part laid freely open, and the splinter removed; warm emollient poultices were then constantly applied, and the room was kept at a warm and even temperature. He was kept under the influence of full doses of chloral and bromide of potash, with belladonna applications along the spine. Liquid food was given at regular intervals, and special attention was given to the proper action of the bowels and kidneys. The result in this case was recovery in four weeks.

Case II.—M. P., a young man 15 years old, received an injury of the foot on the railroad, by which the great toe and metatarsal bone of one foot were partly crushed. In a few days tetanus set in. He was treated in much the same way as the patient just mentioned, and recovered in three weeks.

Case III.—A. H., a boy 13 years old, received a wound in the hand with a toy pistol. About a week afterward tetanus set in very violently. Various remedies were tried without any apparent benefit, death taking place on the third day.

Case IV.—W. T. A., 14 years old. In this case the great toe was crushed by being run over with a wagon-wheel. When recovery had nearly taken place he contracted a cold. The result was a chill followed by tetanus. Treatment in this case was the same as in the first case, with recovery in four weeks.

Case V.—R. B., a painter, 34 years old, had a fall from the second story of a house, and suffered a compound fracture of the forearm. On the fifth day after the injury tetanus set in. Treatment in this case was the same as in the first case at the beginning; but his temperature going up to 104° Fahr. a few doses of antipyrin were given, with the effect of reducing the temperature. Tincture of Calabar bean was given in gradually increased doses in this case, but without the slightest benefit, death taking place on the fourth day.

Case VI.—C. McA., a young man 16 years old. The thumb was crushed in a mortising machine. About a week afterward he was exposed to a cold, which was followed by an attack of tetanus. Treatment in this case was that already described, the result being recovery in four weeks.

In the cases that recovered there was very much prostration for some time afterward, and all the patients required tonics, nourishing diet, and careful nursing.

I am indebted to my friend Dr. W. W. Keen for valuable services, in consultation, in several of the above cases.

It will be observed that in six cases of traumatic tetanus, there were four recoveries and two deaths.

SOME OBSTETRIC CASES.

BY A. H. P. LEUF, M.D.,
OF THE UNIVERSITY OF PENNSYLVANIA, PHILA-
DELPHIA.

The following cases were put together after the reading of those reported by Dr. Charles P. Noble, in the REPORTER for August 25, 1888. My only object in publishing them is that they may prove instructive in a practical way to some of those readers whose gaze they may encounter. It is also supposed that some of them might gladden the heart of the ever-searching statistician. I have purposely omitted detailed accounts because they seldom have any value, but should anyone desire additional information, I promise gladly to forward it.

Case I.—Abortion; High Fever; Peritonitis; Rapid Digital Dilatation of Os and Removal of Putrid Placenta.—In the summer of 1882, I was called to see a young woman, who was the mistress of a medical student who has since died, and upon whom he had performed an abortion at the fourth month of gestation. He had at first called in another physician who gave the patient repeated small doses of ergot, opium, brandy, and chloral, with a little quinine; but these did her no good, and when I saw her on the fifth or sixth day, her temperature was 106° F.; she was delirious, the pulse was very rapid, the abdomen was much distended and extremely tender, there was a very fœtid vaginal discharge, the uterus felt soft, and the edge of a small placenta could be felt projecting from the os. I ordered a half-ounce of fluid extract of ergot, a half-drachm of hydrate of chloral, and asked that the attending physician meet me there in four hours. He was a graduate of only two months' standing, though a practitioner of many years. Upon my return, he was afraid to do anything, believing that the patient would die. The student began to give chloroform by dropping it from a bottle stoppered with a grooved cork. Instead of letting it fall on the towel over the patient's mouth and nose, he was so excited that he squirted it into her eye. I had to give it to her myself, and when fully under its influence, I rapidly dilated the os, seized the putrefying placenta with my index and middle fingers, and extracted it. The nozzle of a fountain syringe was passed up against the fundus and one quart of hot carbolic water allowed to pass through. The patient was then cleansed, put to rest, and given a hypodermic injection of gr. i

of the sulphate of morphia, though the same amount had been given her a little over four hours previously in two doses to control excessive pain. In forty-five minutes I gave another half-grain, and after this she was relieved; the temperature fell rapidly and she was much improved in a few hours. Her improvement continued until the sixth day, when she insisted upon getting out of bed. The result was renewed peritonitis, but this was rapidly controlled by the prompt use of hot applications to the hypogastrium, and the injection of morphine.

Remarks.—The object in giving the ergot was to insure a tonic condition of the uterus and a diminution of its circulation before dilatation, and the chloral was given to insure a rest to the goaded nervous system before subjecting it to the additional strain of dilatation. The advisability of at once giving large doses of morphine for the arrest of the pain of peritonitis was well demonstrated in this case; smaller amounts would have been ineffectual and the pain would have caused additional weakness. The efficiency, expediency, and good effect of rapid digital dilatation in these cases cannot be questioned. The relief is prompt and immediate. I have had a number of such cases, and all have recovered promptly. I shall relate several more, and also a counter case. Unless a patient is already moribund, I see no reason why a case of abortion should die if rapid digital dilatation is resorted to as a means of relief. It seems to me that the thorough removal of the placenta in such cases is the most positive indication, and that it should be done without a moment's loss of time. It is a very prompt procedure, as it can almost always be completed without the additional use of an anæsthetic after the patient is once completely unconscious—at least, such has been my experience.

Case II.—Abortion; Rapid Digital Dilatation and Removal of Fœtus and Placenta.—In the summer of 1881, Mrs. X——, U. S., 18 years old, was a little over three months pregnant. She had pains in the back and a bloody discharge from the vagina. I gave her minimum doses of ergot and digitalis to control hemorrhage, and ordered the patient to bed; but her pains and hemorrhage became worse. On the second day she became feverish, and the pains had to be controlled with morphine. The membranes had ruptured, the os hardly admitted the index finger, and what appeared to be a foot occasionally presented at the uterine orifice. I sent for assistance, gave chloroform, inserted my finger into the os, and dilated it with considerable difficulty, but in less than ten minutes, so as to be able readily to pass the index and middle fingers into the uterus, seize and thoroughly remove a dead fœtus and a quite firmly adherent putrescent placenta. The fever rapidly subsided and the patient made a perfect recovery in a little over one week.

Case III.—Abortion; Rapid Digital Dilatation; Removal of Uterine Contents. —In the fall of 1883, Dr. N. called me to see with him a case of abortion at three and a half months which had been self-induced by a young married woman, the mother of one child. He had attended her for several days and treated her with ergot, poultices, quinine and opium. She had considerable pain, due in part to peritonitis and in part to excessive uterine contractions. The vagina was hot and emitted the characteristic putrescent odor of these cases. The fetus had come away, but the placenta was still there and could plainly be felt. I also gave her an anæsthetic (ether in this case) and then turned it over to Dr. N., while I rapidly dilated this, extracted the placenta which was in pieces, washed out the uterus with one quart of hot carbolic water, and made the patient clean and comfortable. Her recovery was prompt, rapid and uninterrupted. A hypodermic injection of morphine was given after the operation to insure freedom from pain and undisturbed sleep for several hours.

Case IV.—Abortion; Rapid Digital Dilatation; Removal of Fetus and Placenta; Chronic Myocarditis and the Harmless Use of Chloroform; Subsequent Death and Autopsy.—Mrs. H., U. S., mother of two children, thought herself pregnant and several times took the liberty of requesting of me an abortifacient, which was refused. She was a very good patient, a most devoted mother, having at the time of her last request just ended a two weeks' vigil over her small child, a girl of 3 years, during her suffering with, and recovery from, a double pneumonitis. I was called to see her at midnight, for the purpose of relieving her suffering in "miscarriage." I found her with a vigorously contracting uterus, a very small os, ruptured membranes, and a foot or hand presenting at the uterine mouth. She was a strong, well-built, and beautifully formed woman. The former physician, Dr. J., had told her that he feared she had some cardiac disease. I never had heard anything peculiar in listening to her heart, though she was very easily "winded." At all events I hazarded an anæsthetic, using chloroform myself with nitrite of amyl, and, instructing the husband how to keep it up, permitted him to continue it for a few moments while I rapidly dilated with my fingers and removed the dead fetus of 3 months and its placenta. I gave her a hypodermic injection of the fluid extract of ergot in the hypogastrium, and left her in good condition for the rest of the night. Her recovery was as prompt and satisfactory as that of any of the others, but on the fourth day she developed a dry pleuritis in the right infra-mammary region. This was treated with counter-irritation and small amounts of opium. She remained in bed. On the ninth or tenth day I left her in the evening almost well and anxious to sit up next day. I discontinued all medicine and promised her that she could consider herself my patient no longer after the next day. When I left her, her pulse was full, strong, and regular. At 5 A.M. the next day I was called to see her, and before I could leave I received a second summons. When I arrived she was dead. I sent for a student at my house and began artificial respiration and continued it with his aid till *post-mortem* lividity and slight rigor mortis began to set in, at the end of more than one hour. In addition to the artificial respiration, I tried cardipuncture but without any positive result. Then I tried a digitalis injection into the heart muscle or substance, but also without avail. She died just after awaking and asking for some medicine. When it was held to her mouth she refused it, saying that she would rest a moment before taking it, and she rested from that time on until I saw her dead. At the autopsy, I found a localized dry pleuritis at the diagnosed site over an area as large as the palm of the hand. The heart was pale, soft, fatty, and gave undoubted evidence of chronic interstitial myocarditis. The death was due to sudden heart failure; the heart was found filled with blood. The uterus showed a very slight remnant of red and softened endometrium, besides being somewhat enlarged.

Remarks.—The central point of interest in this case is the indifference with which the chloroform was borne, and the fortunate escape I had in not having my patient die during its administration. This case also certainly demonstrates that very serious disease of the heart does not absolutely contra indicate the use of chloroform, though I would prefer the safe side.

Case V.—Abortion; Retention of Placenta; and its Spontaneous Removal in 9 or 10 Weeks Without Bad Symptoms Except Menorrhagia.—In the summer of 1886, I attended Mrs. R., about 29 years old, U. S., and the mother of several children. She first came to my office to learn if she was pregnant, and I told her that she was. She did not want to go to full term, but failed in getting from me anything but the advice to let matters take their natural course. As is customary in most such instances, she tinkered with herself till she miscarried during the fourth month of gestation. She consulted me soon afterward for a menorrhagia which was due to the retention of all or part of the placenta. I gave fifteen minim doses of the fluid extract of ergot daily. This relieved the bleeding for a time, but it returned. The placenta was still in place. She objected to its removal, because it was still partly attached. Two or three hemorrhages followed, but they were not very copious. During the last one I was called to her and was still refused permission to remove the offending body. At last, about ten days later, she "flooded" quite freely and passed the cause of all the trouble, and soon recovered.

Remarks.—This case shows that retention of a placenta in a case of abortion is not necessarily dangerous, and that it may be carried for a long time, as in this instance, when it did not come away till nine or ten weeks after the loss of the fetus. Nevertheless, there is always some danger of more or less severe sudden hemorrhage in all cases in which it is retained and kept from putrefaction because of vascular union to the uterine wall.

Case VI.—Laceration of Vagina and Cervix during Labor; Peritonitis; Version; Death; Autopsy.—Mrs. O., 37 years old, married, Swede, mother of seven children, and about to be delivered of her eighth child. A midwife was in attendance during the present confinement and had been during the first three, but a regular physician had been employed for the last four. The patient had been in labor over twenty-four hours when Dr. R. was summoned. He found a transverse presentation with the child's left arm in the vagina and the head in the left iliac fossa (L. D. P.). The uterus was firmly contracted and the child apparently dead. The mother complained of intense pain in both iliac fossæ, but more especially on the left side. The midwife had been giving large doses of ergot at frequent intervals during almost the entire labor. Dr. M. was summoned to assist in the delivery. Podalic version was performed and a dead child extracted. Before anything could be done, the mother died of collapse.

Autopsy.—Feb. 27, 1883, I examined the body twenty-four hours after death. Body of average height, thin; yellow skin, light complexion. Both lungs were markedly congested, and the heart was flaccid, fatty and almost empty. The liver was fatty and the spleen soft and slightly enlarged. Both kidneys were fatty. There was marked injection of the vessels of the gastro-intestinal peritoneum, but without any disturbance of the mucous membrane. The uterus was well contracted, almost filled the pelvic cavity, and hardly projected above the true pelvic brim. There was a large laceration of the left side of the vagina from the utero-vaginal juncture almost to the vulva; its margins were widely separated. The portio vaginalis of the cervix was also lacerated as far as the junction. The margins of the tear were dark and sloughy. Considerable dark, grumous-looking malodorous fluid had passed into the abdominal cavity through this rent. Similar fluid had dissected its way up behind the peritoneum in the extra-peritoneal connective tissue of the left iliac and lumbar regions. The peritonitis was general; there was no lymph; and the vascular injection was most marked in the broad ligaments and both iliac fossæ, but especially in the left.

Remarks.—The large amount of ergot administered by the midwife had induced powerful tonic uterine contractions, which forced the child's head firmly against the left side of the cervix and vagina, compressing them between the head and pelvis for a long enough time to cause sloughing of the cervix and vagina of that side and eventual rupture. After this, it was easy for the liquor amnii remaining above the child and blood to find their way into the abdominal cavity and set up peritonitis. Thus the laceration and the strain of the continuous uterine contractions so exhausted the mother that, with her fatty heart, kidneys, and liver, she had a fatal collapse. She had been a moderate beer-drinker. The midwife was indicted by the coroner's jury, but the case never went to trial, so far as I can remember. This case shows the danger of using too much ergot.

Case VII.—Puerperal Peritonitis and Septicæmia Treated by a Midwife as "After-pains."—Mrs. ——, married, German, multipara, was confined on the morning of

April 3, 1882. The next morning she had a pronounced chill, lasting fully one hour. There was also hypogastric pain, which increased in severity and became diffused over the whole abdomen. The patient was treated by the midwife for ordinary "after-pains." The pain being worse on the next day, a drug-store remedy was tried but gave no relief. Two bottles of citrate of magnesia were then taken and caused free evacuations. Dr. D. was called in two days later, the fifth since the labor. He found the patient in a state of extreme collapse. She was semi-conscious, and with a tongue so dry and swollen that her articulation was too indistinct to be understood. She also had subsultus tendinum. The pulse was 140, and the axillary temperature 105½° F. The abdomen was much distended, extremely tender, and tympanitic. There was persistent vomiting of dark gruelly matter. Death took place on the next day. There were, then, well-marked chills—the first on the second day after delivery, lasting fully one hour; the second on the morning of the fourth day, lasting one hour; and the third and last on the evening of the same day, lasting a half-hour.

Autopsy.—The examination of the body was made by me about fifty or sixty hours after death. The body was 5 ft. 6 in. long, emaciated, and of dark complexion. Markedly distended veins were visible all over the abdomen as high as the ensiform cartilage and around both thighs as far down as the knees. There was an extra-vulvar prolapse of the posterior vaginal wall (a rectocele), and slight reddening and vascular injection of the peritoneum of the hypogastrium. The gastro-intestinal tract appeared normal. The liver and kidneys were exceedingly soft, flabby, and pale. Both kidneys were so soft that they could be pressed longitudinally so that the fingertips were but one inch apart. Both were granular. The bladder was 1½ inches above the pubic symphisis. The uterus extended half-way up to the umbilicus and was very relaxed and flabby.

Remarks.—This case serves to show how expensive it may be to employ midwives. A little care on the part of a competent obstetrician, or an early diagnosis, would probably have saved life.

Case VIII.—Post-Partum Hemorrhage Controlled by Prolonged Manual Pressure.—Mrs. D., 24 years old, a tall, stout and healthy multipara, was in her fourth labor in May, 1882. I was in attendance; the position was L. O. A.; the labor was normal, except the third stage. A severe and continuous hemorrhage set in soon after the delivery of the child and placenta, and all efforts to arrest it were unavailing. I tried hypodermic injections of ergot, amounting in all to one and one-half fluid drachms, in the hypogastrium; intra-uterine digital irritation (scratching); lemon-juice, vinegar, hot and cold water injections and external applications, and the external and internal use of ice. A clot as large as a fist had formed in the uterus, and still there was some oozing. Much to my immediate sorrow, I turned out this clot, not being satisfied to leave well enough alone. Thereupon the bleeding became more profuse than ever. My patient's surface was exceedingly pale, and she was cold even inside the vulva, in the axilla, and at the lips. The pallor of the lips was so marked that it was difficult to distinguish clearly between the mucous membrane and the integument. The uterus could not be identified by palpation, and per vaginam the cervix felt like a large, soft, flaccid, ragged rim. I pressed my flat open hand against the belly just below the umbilicus, and against the sacral promontory and pelvic outlet. The other hand was in the vagina, and could feel the blood slowly but steadily trickling from the mouth of the uterus. The patient by this time was unconscious and taking deep breaths, and sighing at intervals. Her head was lowered and her feet elevated, while rubber bags filled with hot water were applied to her lower extremities. No cardiac stimulant was given for fear that it would increase the hemorrhage. At last, after more than one hour's continuous manual compression, the bleeding ceased and the uterus could be felt as a large soft mass. It again contained a clot as large as a fist, and this I gladly permitted to remain. While making manual pressure, I occasionally stopped to see if it was any longer necessary, but only for an instant, for any slight relaxation would increase the flow of blood decidedly. My arms, especially the right, were weak and tremulous for days afterward from the continuous severe exertion, so as seriously to interfere with writing. Well-marked after-pains developed because, as I supposed, of the intra-uterine clot. Much to my surprise at that time, injections of hot water into the cervix, and for aught I know into the body, of the uterus caused an entire cessation of the pains at once and for four or five hours. The patient rapidly recovered without a bad symptom.

Remarks.—This case shows how difficult it sometimes is to account for, prevent, or control a post-partum hemorrhage, besides demonstrating the value of manual pressure when other means fail. Brandy or other cardiac stimulants were not given while the bleeding continued, and the fainting of the patient was looked upon with no little relief, as it was hoped that the weakened heart would be unable to force out much more blood from the open vessels, and so it happened. Again, this case teaches the value of hot water injections for the relief of after-pains. I have often had the same results since that time in preventing the same pains in my own cases and in those of others with whom I happened to be associated in the treatment of a case. I have also met with the same result in treating the pains of leucorrhœa and the vaginal catarrh itself by simple hot water injections, three or four times a day, each of at least 20 minutes' duration.

Case IX.—Contracted Pelvis; Post-partum Hemorrhage; Hour-Glass Contraction; Laceration of Cervix and Vagina; Retention of Urine; Recovery.—Mrs. H., about 24 years of age, married, German, stout and healthy, had had one miscarriage. Her uterine contractions were strong, the position of the child was L. O. A. She had a contracted pelvis and the child was full size. I called in Dr. H., at that time a hospital interne. Chloroform was given (chloroform f ℥ i and nitrite of amyl gtt. ii), and the forceps applied. It seemed almost impossible to effect delivery. The forceps were handed to Dr. H. for trial as he had never used any. Too much traction was made, and I renewed work with them. At no time did I pull with a force of more than about from ten to twelve pounds. The child was born in half an hour, but did not breathe, and could not be resuscitated. The mother was lying across the bed with her buttocks at the edge. I heard a dripping and noticed that she was bleeding freely. Examination discovered that there was a rent of the cervix almost to the cervico-vaginal junction. In passing my hand up into the uterus to liberate the placenta, it encountered a constriction of the womb at its middle, compressing the placenta at this point and preventing its descent and expulsion. I passed my fingers into the upper chamber, scratched the fundus, causing contraction of the upper chamber, expulsion of the placenta, and, in a very short time, even contraction of the entire uterus. The hemorrhage continued, and digital examination satisfied me that it came from the rent of the cervix. The nozzle of a syringe was pressed into the angle of the laceration and hot water made to flow against the bleeding surface until the bleeding was arrested. The patient was prepared for the night. She slept well and had no bad symptoms except retention of urine for five days. She was catheterized several times a day. On the second day I noticed that just within the introitus vaginæ there had been torn away a piece of mucous membrane of triangular shape and measuring about ¾ inch by 1¼ inches. Except the retention of urine, there was nothing abnormal after the first night. She was up on the tenth day. Her husband opposed the sewing of the cervical laceration on the grounds of a probable rupture at the next childbirth, and the extra expense for doctor's fees. His wife believed his view of the case, and nothing could change their opinion.

Remarks.—This patient did well in spite of an uncommonly severe and complicated labor, recovered in a short time, suffered no distress but that of a retention of urine, which was always relieved in time to prevent any annoyance, and all this without any medication internally or locally except ordinary warm hydrant-water injections to remove the discharges consequent upon the cervical-vaginal rents.

Case X.—Post-partum Hemorrhage due to Adherent Fibrous Placenta; Rapid Removal.—Mrs. H., married, German, multipara, was attended by me in her confinement. All went well. The nurse was holding the child as I sat by the bedside with my hand on the mother's belly, making pressure upon the well-contracted uterus and gently moving the belly wall over the fundus. The mother sighed; I gently reminded her that all would soon be over and she could then rest as long as she pleased. Very soon she yawned and I thought she would be sound asleep in a short time. Then I looked at her and noticed the "whites" of her eyes through her half-open lids; she had very pale lips, in fact they had been red a moment ago; and her face was very pallid. Then she sighed and yawned again and looked frightened, while I became suddenly alarmed for her welfare. Passing my hand to her wrist I found it quite cold. The uterus under my watchful hand was all that could be desired. The other hand found between her thighs a wedge-shaped clot filling the hollow formed by the buttocks, thighs and bed. It seemed fully one and a half inches thick just below the vulva. Then I found that the placenta was entirely within the uterus; that it was stiff; that it and its membranes were adherent; and that the hemorrhage came from the uterine wall near the edge of the os, from which the placenta had become detached. By this time the patient was alive to her danger. I called her husband to my aid, having him crowd my hand down toward the pelvic floor so as to help force out the placenta while I loosened it from within. After about forty seconds' most vigorous clawing, I had loosened the placenta, and with his help and the uterine contractions, it was expelled. The pain to the patient must have been agonizing, for it caused her to shriek in a way that perfectly astounded me—it was almost deafening. It only lasted during the removal of the placenta. She had no further trouble except that due to loss of blood, and she left her bed in less than two weeks. The placenta was very firm and dark-gray in color, having undergone a marked fibrous degeneration. At its lower edge was a surface about as large as a silver dollar, and circular in shape, that had a normal placental appearance, and this spot was the source of the hemorrhage

Remarks.—This case proves that a well-contracted uterus containing a placenta is not an absolute indication that all is safe. If hemorrhage occur in a dark, windowless room, as this one was, it is best to keep one hand at the vulva, or at least pass it there at short intervals, to guard against sudden surprises. It is always well to watch your patient's pulse and the color of her lips until she can be left for the next call.

—The appointment to the vacant chair of Medicine at the University of Vienna has not yet been made. The names mentioned in connection with it, in addition to that of Professor Schrötter, are Professor Riegel of Giessen, Dr. Mossler of Greifswald, Dr. Quincke of Kiel, and Professor Rembold of Vienna.

—The *British Med. Journal,* Dec. 8, 1888, says that chocolates, confectionery, dried fruits, cheeses, and other food products are very often wrapped in what appears to be, and is described as, tin foil, but it is really an alloy, containing a good deal of lead. This dangerous practice is now prohibited in France, and the tin foil destined for wrapping food-stuffs and confectionery must be composed of "fine tin," that is, an alloy containing at least 90 per cent. of tin.

THE CONJUGAL QUESTION.

BY W. C. EUSTIS, M.D.,

FARMINGTON, MINN.

Almost every sane person with rare exceptions expects to enter the married state sooner or later, and the question naturally arises: what are the impelling motives to seek a life union with one of the opposite sex?

It is generally conceded that the sexes were intended to contribute through conjugal oneness to each other's happiness as well as to the multiplication of their own species. If the wedded state were always entered with correct views of what it implies, and with a sincere purpose to live afterward properly and naturally, all would be well; but when it is once entered, disappointment often arises in unexpected ways. One or both of the contracting parties find that the new relation has cares and responsibilities which were, perhaps, not even thought of. If both are disposed to be just and reasonable, all may yet be well; but a fretful, fault-finding spirit too often invades the household and paves the way for multiplied troubles. Sometimes the wife finds herself unable to meet the demands of her husband for the sexual act; while on his part, regarding the act as one of his marital rights, he may fail to apprehend the damage it may do to his wife, and, if he is not morally well balanced, he may grieve her by neglect or even obtain sexual gratification in the arms of a courtezan or a mistress. He may know that such infidelity is both wrong and debasing, and yet excuse himself on the ground that he has a sexual nature imperious in its demands, and that, since the woman whom he married can not fully satisfy it, nothing is left him but to seek elsewhere for what is wanting in his own home.

A partial remedy for marital infelicities is to be found in marrying stronger and healthier women. No mother ought to be ignorant of the natural demands that will be made on her daughter, and mothers, of all persons, ought to object to their daughters' marrying, unless confident that they are capable of meeting the sexual requirements of the married state. Unfortunately, instead of this being the case, there is apparently no attention paid to the matter, but delicate girls and feeble women marry without hesitation men of powerful physique and men whose very physiognomy bespeaks the strong sexual passion of their natures. So long as people continue to wed those who are not their sexual equals, so long will trouble arise from these unequal unions. It is of little use to demand of men that they shall limit the gratification of their sexual appetite to the strength of the weaker vessel; for few men are reasonable and just enough to do this, and husbands who are married to sexually weak women feel as though they had been defrauded to some extent, and this feeling often makes them less considerate than they ought to be of the comfort of those who have disappointed them.

Look at it as we may, unless a woman is fully able to satisfy the sexual appetite of her husband, she had far better never take part in the conjugal relation. It is only too true that men often regard women merely as a natural means of gratifying the sexual appetite, and on the other hand women of respectability often encourage this view in ways calculated to appeal to the animal passions of man : forgetting apparently, that men rarely place women on a higher plane than they place themselves upon. It is notoriously true that man is more particular before the world in regard to his female society than is woman of male society. It is no uncommon event for a woman of refinement to wed a man who is suspected or even known to be unchaste. If women made good character an invariable condition of marriage, they would do more for themselves than men have ever done or ever will do in their behalf.

On the other hand, the ills that many women suffer in the married state are not wholly due to man. They ought to bear in mind that men have to be taken as they are, and if they do not like them so, they should not take them at all. No wife dreads anything on the part of her husband more than his marital infidelity, yet how little wives sometimes appear to think of some of the causes which lead to it. There are few husbands who do not like to be petted by their wives; and, while many do not deserve it, still there are others who do, but too often meet with fault-finding or indifference which gradually leads them to care little for, if not actually to hate, the real or prospective mothers of their own children.

Fallen women study the weak side of man's nature, and meet him with sexual gratification, petting and caressing to his heart's content. What wonder, then, that morally weak husbands sometimes grow weary of the conjugal yoke, and seek abroad what their own homes fail to yield them? A wife's imperfections are a poor excuse for a husband to prove false to his marriage vows; but in every age they have led to the fall of excellent men, and thus we may expect it will ever be. Should the time ever come when from childhood both sexes shall be properly trained for the relations and duties of mature years, then and then only may we expect the millennium of married life. The conjugal relation is a complex one, and its problems can only be satisfactorily solved by a proper training of both sexes for their respective stations in life The artificial state of the world socially is largely to blame for much of the married wretchedness that exists in every community. Too many wives look upon motherhood beyond two or three children with aversion if not with positive hatred. They declare openly that they prefer to sacrifice themselves on the altar of fashion or of some other god of this world than on the altar of maternity and of home. As a natural consequence of this condition of too many wives' minds, a large number of husbands find themselves joined to women who shirk in every possible way their maternal and housewifely duties, leaving to hirelings many of the sacred obligations that belong to them only, and cannot properly or successfully be assumed by any other. It can not be that such a state of things should exist without much domestic clashing. A quiet well-ordered home is an earthly heaven to a husband, even though he is possessed of no more than an average appreciation of the good and the beautiful, while the opposite can only exert a baneful influence.

Let woman take her proper place in the word's economy and keep it; let her ever insist on sound morals and a sound body in her future husband, and the conjugal question will be practically solved. But let no man or woman expect to violate natural laws and escape their penalty, for all such are surely doomed to disappointment.

—Dr. Joseph J. Kenyoun, in his report on the use of phosphorus as a disinfectant, made at the laboratory of the United States Marine-Hospital Service at New York, says that the conclusions from his experiments are that phosphoric pentoxide is a disinfectant to surfaces only; that it has no penetrating power, and is altogether unfit for fumigation of anything where penetration of the agent is desirable. He did not deem it worth while to pursue the subject further when it promised so little; therefore no observation on the spores of different microörganisms was made.

SOCIETY REPORTS.

OBSTETRICAL SOCIETY OF PHILA-
DELPHIA.

Thursday, Dec. 6, 1888.

DR. T. M. DRYSDALE in the chair.

DR. WM. GOODELL showed a

Recurrent Intraligamentary Cyst,

removed without entrance into the peritoneal cavity.

The patient, a woman 31 years old, at the age of eighteen had an ovarian cyst removed by Dr. Joseph Schnetter, of N. Y., who, in answer to a letter of inquiry, was kind enough to write the following description of his operation : "The cyst had no pedicle and was attached with a very thick mass of fibrous tissue to the right side of the uterus. This attachment being very vascular, it was necessary to ligature in several portions the parts representing the pedicle and to sew them into the incision of the abdominal integuments for the purpose of being able to control the secondary hemorrhage, if any should occur—which, in fact, soon took place, several days after the operation."

"Mrs. ——, after recovery, menstruated regularly through the cicatrix, and had an attack in New York similar to the one for which you are attending her at present. My opinion is that a piece of the lining membrane of the cyst may still be left in the cicatrix, causing an accumulation from time to time and opening the cicatrix."

"I should have mentioned that after the opening of the abdomen, the large omentum was found rolled up, forming a large tumor, including an abscess containing almost a pint of purulent matter. This was probably the sequence of two or three tappings of the cyst, preceding laparotomy."

On the 25th of last Nov., Dr. Goodell was called to see the patient by Dr. Thomas C. Potter, of Germantown. She was hectic, much emaciated, and bed-ridden, and was daily losing strength from a free discharge of pus, which escaped through a fistulous opening in the abdominal cicatrix. This he probed, but the instrument ran upward and inward, more in the direction of the kidney, than in that of the pelvis. So much blood followed the use of the probe that its use was not pushed very far. Under the cicatrix lay a tumor of some kind, which in front was hard and unyielding, but by bi-manual palpation it gave the sense of a very large pelvic abscess. Into this tumor the probe did not enter. The womb was fixed, the fundus being pushed over to the right. The fistula had opened early in 1885, and has lasted ever since. In Dec. 1886, the patient had a very severe attack of peritonitis, which kept her two months in bed, and it was after this attack that the tumor first appeared. The hardness of that part of the tumor which lay under the cicatrix, and the sense of fluctuation by vaginal palpation, so perplexed me that I wrote to Dr. Schnetter for further particulars, and his reply, which he courteously placed at my disposal, I have just read to you. On Dec. 1, I operated on her at my private hospital, and I must confess that no case ever puzzled me so much. The fistula was first enlarged so as to admit the finger. As this gave no satisfactory information the incision was lengthened in the old cicatrix to about four inches. This revealed a solid colloid tumor about as large as a cocoanut. It was firmly adherent to the cicatrix, and to the abdominal wall in front and to the left side. When the lateral adhesions were severed, a very large amount of pus escaped from the wound, and the hand now entered into a capacious cavity wholly shut off from the peritoneal cavity by walls of thick pyogenic membrane, which at the navel looked like a false diaphragm. Into this cavity the colloid tumor hung as if it were suspended ; that is to say, while its upper and right lateral surfaces were firmly and closely adherent to the abdominal wall, its under or lower surface, free from adhesions, projected into the fluid of the abscess cavity. A short and slender pedicle running from the lower end of the tumor was lost in the pelvic floor of pyogenic membrane. Where this pedicle ended it was impossible to discover, as not a pelvic organ could be felt through the thick membrane ; but it was closely adherent to the lower abdominal wall, from which it was detached before being tied and cut. The tumor was now cut open and its size lessened by digging out its contents with the finger-nail. When it was removed, free hemorrhage occurred from the broken adhesions. This was checked by Monsel's solution and by the free application of vinegar, a pint of the latter being poured into the cavity and plashed about the bleeding surfaces. This large cavity was then treated by the capillary drainage of Mikulicz—viz., by packing it with iodoform gauze. Since the operation the patient has done unexceptionably well, the temperature being always normal and the pulse not more frequent than it would be in a patient as reduced as she is.

In reviewing this curious case it seems to me that the original tumor removed by Dr. S. was an intraligamentary cyst of the right ovary ; that, as he suspected,. a small piece of the cyst wall was left in that portion of the broad ligament which was made the pedicle, and sewed into the abdominal incision ; and that, *pari passu* with the growth of this fragment of the cyst, an abscess had formed between it and its capsule of broad ligament, which formed the walls of the abscess. The four-inch incision into the abdominal wall did not open into the peritoneal cavity, but merely into a vast pus-sac. The tumor was therefore a recurrent intraligamentary cyst and wholly extra-peritoneal. The wonder to me is that this patient bore for so long a time so large an abscess without losing her life.

DR. GOODELL also showed an

Ovarian Cyst

which he had removed a few hours before, in which the characteristic green hue of necrosis was marked.   Torsion of the pedicle occurred one month ago, and was characterized by severe abdominal pains and excessive vomiting.   After this the woman gradually failed in health and lost flesh from chronic blood-poisoning. A few hours before the operation another attack of pain and vomiting took place. The cyst was universally adherent to the abdominal wall, intestines, and omentum. The pedicle, a very slender and short one, was so twisted as to stop all circulation, the cyst being nourished merely by its adhesions.

DR. GOODELL showed a specimen of what he deemed to be an

Extra-Uterine Fœtation.

A healthy woman, 33 years old, had been married 13 years without conceiving. Her catamenia had always been regular up to two months before Dr. Goodell saw her, when they were delayed for over two weeks. A few days before they reappeared, she was seized with a violent pain, "like cramps," in the pelvis, "shooting upward like knives." This was followed by syncope. Hypodermics of morphia were resorted to and she was left with a pelvic soreness that kept her in bed for several days. During the flow of this delayed period a second attack of pain occurred, analogous to the first, but not quite so severe. In about a week another hemorrhage came on. A few

days later she had a third attack of pain and of syncope, which took place at night. A third hemorrhage now occurred, which was also followed three days later by a severe pelvic colic. This seized her as she was in the act of getting out of bed. The last attack took place on Nov. 18, and she was left for several days very weak and nervous. On the 25th, she consulted Dr. Goodell about the pelvic colics, irregular hemorrhages, painful defecation, and occasional pains running down the left leg. He found a small womb pushed forward and to the right by a boggy tumor, lying to the left in Douglas's pouch. The diagnosis of extrauterine fœtation was made, its dangers explained, and an early operation insisted upon. Both the patient and her husband were so shocked by this discovery, and seemed to be so incredulous, that Dr. Goodell deemed it best for them to get the opinion of another physician. He sent them to Dr. Joseph Price, who confirmed the diagnosis. Very early in the morning of Nov. 29, while she was in his private hospital, a fifth attack of pain, with a "bursting feeling," aroused her out of a sleep. This was followed by faintness.   At nine o'clock, about six hours after this attack, laparotomy was performed. As soon as the cavity of the abdomen was opened a large amount of black blood, of the consistency of thin molasses, welled out of the incision. Several knuckles of intestine were also forced out, which could not be wholly kept back during the operation. The right ovary was found, but the left could not be discovered.   In its place was found an irregular cavity, within which was found a tumor about the size of an egg, containing within its sac layers of coagulated blood. It was attached to the broad ligament, which was tied and cut off. A very large number of old clots and shreds of fibrin were flushed out of the abdominal cavity by means of a syringe, six quarts of water being used for this purpose. A drainage tube was put in and the wound dressed with iodoform gauze. So much hemorrhage occurred later through the tube, that he spent several hours by the side of his patient, fearing it would be needful to reopen the wound. But, by dint of keeping the blood from collecting in the tube, the bleeding points were kept dry and the hemorrhage ceased spontaneously. The tube was removed on Dec. 3, and the patient has thus far had an uninterrupted convalescence. Dr. Goodell had not been able to examine the specimens carefully, but Dr. Baldy, who was present at the operation, had cut it open and he would like him to describe it.

Dr. BALDY said that the history of the case had been rather typical of extra-uterine pregnancy, and the escape of dark-colored blood from the abdominal incision at the operation seemed to confirm this opinion. The mass, which had been shown, was brought to the surface and cut away, after being tied. This was apparently all there was to come away, there being nothing left except a sac filled with old blood-clots, which sac was formed by adherent intestines and uterus and pelvic walls. The mass itself contained a semi-fluctuating tumor the size of a small egg, which he felt confident contained the fœtus, before it was opened. On being laid open it appeared like a large blood-clot, parts of which had undergone degeneration, presenting a mottled appearance. A small portion of normal tube seemed to run directly into this mass, and, as it reached it, spread its coats out over the mass. The ovary was nowhere to be found. He believed that the mass was blood-clot; but could not explain its occurrence. The fœtus was not found.

On motion of Dr. Baer, the specimen was referred to the committee on morbid growths.

Dr. JOSEPH PRICE read a paper on

Tubal Disease a Primary Cause of Intestinal Obstruction.

In reporting cases I have repeatedly called attention to the frequency of adhesions occurring between the uterine appendages and some part of the intestines, and my purpose in this brief note is to emphasize the importance of recognizing the danger of obstruction of the intestine arising from inflammatory conditions of the pelvic viscera. In glancing over the cases I have operated on during the past year, I find that in more than 15 per cent. there were noted "dense firm adhesions" between the intestines and uterus and appendages, malignant cases not included. In every case, with one single exception, as far as I could determine from the history, symptoms, and operative developments, the inflammatory conditions causing the adhesions originated in the uterine appendages. I do not intend to discuss the pathology of inflammations in the pelvis, nor to present statistic evidence, nor to cite numerous authors who have recognized these lesions, as Greig Smith and others, for the few general observations I desire to make. And first as to the form or kind of obstruction likely to occur. The inflamed serous surface of the diseased tube or ovary coming in contact with a loop of intestine or an edge of omentum, provokes inflammation there, and with characteristic promptitude these surfaces cohere. If the process is not severe and is of slight duration, these adhesions may disappear as promptly as they occurred. This is accomplished by the enormous absorptive power of the peritoneum and is hastened by the mild influence of the peristalsis of the bowel. If however the inflammation is severe, or assumes a chronic condition, these adhesions gain in extent and strength, and give rise to all the variety of conditions classified by Treves as "strangulations by bands." In most cases where these adhesions occur there is a history of constipation. The latter is probably due as much to the pain caused by defecation as to interference from the condition. Again, the pain is often so great as to mislead the physician into thinking that a more virulent inflammation exists than is actually present. But the pain is not always proportionate to the amount of mischief. I have seen cases in which a mere omental adhesion has caused most agonizing pain. For instance, I recently saw a case in consultation—a woman had had the appendages removed for backache, sometime before, and suffered excruciating pain especially on defecation. In this case the only lesion found was the omentum firmly adherent to the original incision. The omentum here was much elongated and the transverse colon was dragged below the level of the umbilicus. In like manner I have seen the omentum adherent over the entire pelvis, dragging the transverse colon so out of place that a twist or kink of the bowel could be very easily found. It is not at all rare to find the vermiform appendix glued fast to the uterine appendages, while almost any loop of the small intestine may become adherent to the inflamed pelvic viscera. As I have said, these adhesions vary in extent and density from those that will tear like wet tissue-paper to those so well organized that it requires the scissors to release them; and it is not rare in pus-cases for the bowel to be almost gangrenous about these points of adhesion, and, in fact, to tear through. That adhesions do not cause complete occlusion at the time of their formation oftener than they appear to is no reason for regarding them lightly, for Mr. Treves tells us that in the series of cases he studied the average duration of the interval between the causation and the obstruction was three years; the shortest period being five weeks and the longest 21 years. In view of these general considerations it is hardly necessary to insist upon the release of the intestine wherever and to whatsoever extent adhesions exist. For, if the surgeon leaves adhesions when he closes the abdomen, he leaves a probable cause of future serious trouble. Louis reports a case in which an ovarian cyst when emptied by the trocar so dragged upon an adherent bowel that intestinal obstruction developed. I am inclined to believe that some of the deaths from intestinal obstruction after operation are due to leaving old bowel adhesions undisturbed.

Dr. WM. GOODELL said that his experience in ovariotomy led him to say that it is a mistake to postpone the opening of the bowels to a late period. He used to follow the old plan of not giving a cathartic until the eighth day, but he was confident that he had had death result from this practice in consequence of the formation of intestinal kinks from adhesions, making it impossible for the bowels to be moved. He now almost always gives an aperient or an enema on the fourth day, and earlier if any symptoms, such as vomiting and tympanites, present themselves.

Dr. B. F. BAER said that up to a few years ago he also had followed the plan of keeping the bowels confined after laparotomy, but now he had them moved on the second or third day—rarely as late as the fourth day. That good plan of quenching the thirst by allowing a pint of warm water to flow into the rectum, facilitates the passage of flatus and feces. He thinks it a mistake to give opium, as was formerly done. Intestinal obstruction is likely to result, as well as adhesions. But this question must be settled by the requirements of each case. He had a case four years ago in which very serious collapse occurred at the end of the second day. Stercoraceous vomiting occurred and large quantities of flatus were passed by the mouth, but none by the anus. These symptoms were thought to be due to obstruction, and reopening was considered but not done. The patient recovered, although she did not pass flatus for five days. Should such a case occur again he would open the wound, and he would have the endorsement of most operators in so doing. Large doses of salines are advised in such cases, but he wondered if there was not some danger of rupture of the bowel in these cases of adhesion after serious operations, and he related the following case: An ovarian cyst was closely adherent to the large intestine for a considerable distance:

On the evening of the 3d day after operation, symptoms of a septic peritonitis developed. A large dose of Epsom salt was given. The next morning the general condition was better, but he found that liquid feces were flowing from the wound. He reopened the wound and tried to find the point of rupture and close it with sutures. Even after having enlarged the original opening, the ruptured point could not be found on account of its depth in the pelvis and the amount of lymph thrown out. He then closed the wound, without drainage, but freshened the surface of the drainage tube-tract and closed it, hoping that the freshened edges would unite. In two days fecal matter again appeared, symptoms of collapse developed and she was expected to die. She, however, finally recovered. The fistula has entirely closed. The lesson he learned from the case was, that when rupture of the bowel occurs under similar circumstances the best plan is to let it alone. Dr. Price had referred to two cases in which he reopened the abdomen for pain and found the omentum adherent to the line of incision. It is unfortunate that we do not know of some means to prevent these adhesions, but it is a wonder that they do not more frequently occur in the line of the incision and to the raw surfaces left after separating adhesions. He knew of no better way to prevent this accident than by the early use of laxatives. Probably much of the pain complained of after operations is due to adhesions, and it is unfortunate that we should be called upon to reopen the abdomen in order to release them. Would it not be wise to give nature time to adjust matters, since there is danger of the formation of other adhesions from the second operation?

Dr. WM. L. TAYLOR read a paper on

Fixed Uteri.

In looking over my case-book I find the remark "uterus fixed" so often noted, so often helplessly, but I trust not hopelessly, underscored, as much as to say "there again," that I fain would ask, how many of these cases were in their inception recognized as cases of peritoneal inflammation? In a number the note is made: "patient had attack of inflammation of bladder." "Inflammations of the bowels" has been of alarming frequency, whilst "congestions of the liver," makes me wonder at the special degree of sensibility of that organ in women. In one case in which there was eventually a fatal relighting of a former peritonitis, the original trouble was noted as an attack of "wind colic of the bladder." If these attacks of peritonitis with their resultant lymph deposits are so grossly misnamed, is it not more than likely.that the abortion, or at least the curative treatment, is as far afield? In a series of cases in which the lymph deposit seemed to be the most diffused a positive history of an active and acute inflammatory trouble could not be obtained. There was only the history of a continued abdominal pain and tenderness, dating from an abortion, from heavy lifting,' seldom from normal labors, and presumably never from gonorrhœal infection : seldom— I might say never—have I had perfect success in my efforts to trace the cause to this infection. The history of the husbands, as to the existence of a gonorrhœa or gleet, at the time of commencement of pelvic trouble, is in the vast majority of cases worse than uncertain. In several of the subacute cases the only ascribable cause appeared to be, indirectly if not directly, the effort to prevent conception. Freedom from the possibility of at least paternal cares, leads to an amiable weakness, and coition follows coition in quicker succession than the law of conservatism would recognize, and, in addition to the menstrual congestions, which now even occur sooner than is normal, without the restful periods of pregnancy and lactation, congestion and inflammation of the peri-uterine tissues follow. I am inclined to believe that this is as immediately the cause of the fixed uteri, the thickened and enlarged ligaments and tubes and tender ovaries, as is gonorrhœal infection, even in prostitutes. Where the deposit of lymph was more localized or larger in quantity, seeming as if it had been poured out quickly and had by gravity centered itself around the uterus, there were the histories of acute, well-marked attacks of cellulitis or peritonitis. The causes were difficult labors, with badly lacerated cervices, these lacerations extending through into the cellular tissue, and also criminal abortions. In these cases it is impossible to say how often traumatism and ·how often septic poisoning was the exciting cause. Catching cold while menstruating, falls and various other accidental causes were among the number.

The average physician, as soon as the patient is up out of bed, shakes himself by the hand and says : "I have cured my patient." But he has not. There is still the important sequel to deal with—the lymph deposit. In fully three-fourths of all the cases the body of the uterus has become fixed in retroflexion, even in multipara. Just as soon as the uterus feels the stimulus of congestion or inflammation of surrounding tissue, it becomes turgid and heavy, and sinks decidedly lower in the pelvis until the cervix is near the vulvar orifice ; and following the curve of Carus, the fundus is retro-displaced. Here it is, as it were, frozen in, fixed immovably. All around it is a mass of inflammatory lymph becoming more dense and resisting as organization advances. In the centre of this the sound probably indicates the uterine body, with a measurement of $3\frac{1}{2}$ inches. The cavity is tender and the cervix softened, congested with venous blood. Now this deposit varies greatly in quantity as the inflammation has been limited by judicious treatment or by nature alone, or has been allowed to involve a great extent of peritoneal surface. The possibility of determining the amount of lymph deposit and the degree of fixation by bi-manual examination seems to me to be one of the few certainties in gynecological practice. A uterus which is low in the pelvis and which cannot be raised to the normal line, and a fundus which is retroflexed and cannot be reposited, with the other evidences bi-manually of thickening and deposit, cannot but point to the certainty of previous inflammation. A sterile uterus and a fixed uterus seem to be almost synonymous. The ovaries and Fallopian tubes have become merely painful spots and useless for the purpose of conception ; and should the patient conceive, the uterus seems unable to enlarge, and expels the fœtus for want of growing-room. When I find a young married woman with evidences of a former peritonitic inflammation, I am very guarded in my promises for her future fertility. Backache, ovarian pains, and headache, metrorrhagia or menorrhagia, profuse leucorrhœa, bladder and bowel irritation, and a . thousand and one nervous phenomena mark a very unenviable period in the patient's life. Hysterical, fretty and worrisome, she is a burden to herself. The ovaries have prolapsed with the uterus and are imbedded in and virtually strangulated by surrounding lymph Menstruation, which before was painless, now gives place to severe dysmenorrhœa. The pain is different and more wearing than that due to simple stenosis. It begins several days before the menstrual flow as a more or less steady, throbbing, sickening pelvic pain, extending down the inside of the thighs. As soon as the flow is established this pain gradually gives way to the never-ending backache and pelvic dragging. Sometimes there is pre-menstrual nausea and vomiting, due undoubtedly to ovarian pressure.

In nearly all the cases there is fungoid endometritis as a result of the continued uterine congestion ; hence the metrorrhagia or menorrhagia, notwithstanding which the uterus seems to become more congested and more tender.

The need of shortening these attacks of pelvic peritonitis, aborting them if possible, can only be appreciated by those called upon frequently to treat the sequelæ. In traumatic cases, where there is no reason to suspect septic. influence, as soon as the usual symptoms of peritoneal trouble present themselves, the lower bowel is thoroughly moved by an enema of sweet-oil and turpentine ; the patient's hips are then decidedly elevated by pillows or by elevating the foot of the bed, so as to drain off the pelvis as much as possible, and also to keep the pelvic organs from prolapsing. From 20 to 30 grains of chloral by the bowel, and from $\frac{1}{8}$ to $\frac{1}{4}$ grain of morphia hypodermically are given. A thin flannel binder is applied loosely, and on that, over the abdomen, an ice-bag is placed and kept there, not one hour, but for hours. A febrifuge is given, and the ice-cap with antifebrin if the temperature reaches 102°. Where there is evidence of septicæmia, with the clammy skin, the sunken eyes, the central heat, I have the bowels thoroughly evacuated by divided doses of calomel and soda, and administer quinine in 10 grain doses every four hours, until my patient complains of tinnitus. To the abdomen I apply a large turpentine stupe, followed by a light poultice. The hips are elevated and if there is positive need for an opiate a vaginal suppository of aqueous extract of opium, grains 3, extract of belladonna, grains 1½, is used. If these attacks are thoroughly treated the amount of lymph thrown out is small and probably will be absorbed almost as rapidly as it was thrown out. But we meet a case which was treated by "the other doctor around the corner," and the uterus and its appendages are, as before described, imbedded and immovable. Now what are we to do ? The great object is to get rid of as much of this effused matter as we possibly can. The older and more thoroughly organized this becomes, the less chance there is of rapid and complete absorption. So the moral is, Commence early ! It is going to do one of three things : undergo absorption, break down and form a pelvic abscess, or become organized, acquiring an adventitious circulation. When I meet a case of recent or comparatively recent deposit, in which I can have my directions enforced, I am confident of success. I commence treatment by correcting the digestive tract, getting the stomach, liver and bowels in better condition, and surface circulation stimulated by warm baths and frictions. I then give the corrosive chloride of mercury with the iodide of potash, commencing with small doses frequently repeated and gradually increasing the dose and lengthening the interval. In the use of the bichloride and iodide I have had marked success, much greater than in cases treated with iron and bitter tonics, the same local treatment being used in both. Locally, I rely upon the abdomino-vaginal galvanic current and gentle or more decided uterine massage, as there is great or little tenderness. I prefer uterine massage in cases of long standing, in which the tenderness has disappeared, but I still use it carefully when there is tenderness ; I find it beneficial. Every other day, or twice a week, I make steady pressure upon the fundus of the uterus with the index finger of my left hand in the rectum, and upon the cervix and body of the uterus with the right index finger in the vagina. This pressure I keep up for two or three minutes, gradually trying to force the body upward and forward. Then efforts at lateral movement are made for the same length of time. This massage I follow with the continued galvanic current, using the abdomino-vaginal method. For the breaking down of pelvic lymph, I have not used electropuncture, preferring the slower and as certain absorption by the stimulation of pelvic circulation. Where there is tenderness I use the positive pole in the vagina and the negative over the abdomen for the first three or four applications, and it is marvelous how speedily this tenderness disappears. I then reverse the poles, using the negative with a ball or small crescent-shaped electrode in the vagina. These seances, including the massage, last for about fifteen or twenty minutes. The strength of current averages about twenty-five to thirty milliamperes. After this is over I frequently pack the fornix with wool, introducing a small ring pessary to keep the wool as much as possible in position. After I gain a certain amount of mobility I introduce a Smith-Hodge pessary, small at first, increasing to a more suitable size as the uterus rises to the normal line. Tincture of iodine to the fundus of the vagina, flying blisters and the hot water douche I have tried faithfully, with uncertain success, but I have not tried them so often since I have found such positive relief from galvanism. In the cases of much longer standing, I acknowledge that all I can get from galvanism sometimes is the relief from pelvic pain. Can we get anything more from other treatment? Out of a series of 20 cases, in which galvanism and massage were employed for the purpose of relieving pelvic soreness and pain and inducing mobility of the uterus, twelve patients were discharged after an average of twenty applications, each sufficiently improved to need no after-treatment. Four are improving under treatment, and four disappeared after one to five applications. In over one-half of these total cases, prior treatment had been faithfully tried before galvanism was resorted to.

NEW YORK ACADEMY OF MEDICINE.

Stated Meeting, December 20, 1888.

The President, A. JACOBI, M.D., in the Chair.

DR. THOMAS E. SATTERTHWAITE read a paper entitled:

A New Study of Lobar Pneumonia, with Deductions from an Analysis of 56 Fatal Cases.

Epidemic pneumonia, he said, does not prevail to any great extent at the present time, yet a certain number of facts sustain the theory that the disease is occasionally epidemic.

His paper treated of lobar pneumonia in its primary and secondary forms; the first form he called acute lobar pneumonia, and the other, secondary pneumonia.

But to avoid obscurity he mentioned the principal types of pneumonia, which are acute lobar pneumonia; secondary lobar pneumonia; embolic lobar pneumonia; bronchial lobular pneumonia; and the interstitial pneumonia of heart disease.

Acute lobar or croupous pneumonia is the most common form. In 100 fatal cases, taken from his hospital and private records, the several varieties were represented as follows: Acute lobar, 36 per cent.; secondary lobar, 19 per cent.; bronchial-lobular, 20 per cent.; interstitial of heart disease, 7 per cent. He has found it most common in males. It is for the most part a disease of middle life, and occurs almost altogether in northern and middle latitudes. When it originates in one lung it usually selects the right, and in his cases commenced in a lower lobe.

In the stage of engorgement the whole lung tissue is increased in volume, infiltrated with a serous fluid, with more or less transudation of blood from the vessels. In the second stage, or stage of red hepatization, the lung is of a deep red color, unyielding to the touch, and difficult to distinguish from an inflamed liver. It contains little if any air, and almost no fluid. Its cut surface has a granular and dull aspect, each speck corresponding to an air vesicle or cut bronchiole filled with a firm pellet consisting of blood cells and epithelium mixed with fibrine, which hold all firmly together. In the third stage, that of gray hepatization, the reddish tint yields to a dirty gray, at first tinged with brown, and then with yellow; the tissue is softer, and on pressure exudes a small amount of fluid; the walls of the blood vessels are studded with leucocytes; in many cases there is dark pigmentation of the interlobular spaces. The lung may weigh sixty ounces.

In Dr. Satterthwaite's experience the order of the symptoms is as follows: One, pain, prostration, and cough; two, a severe chill; three, nausea; four, rise of temperature. Chilly sensations may take the place of a severe chill. Within a few hours the temperature commonly reaches 103° or 104°. An early sign, though seldom the earliest, is fine crepitation heard only during inspiration. Occasionally this sign lasts the full course of the disease. As soon as the second stage begins there is dulness on percussion, with bronchial breathing and bronchophony, and also increased vocal fremitus. In the fourth stage, that of resolution, the returning crepitant rale is heard.

The author is inclined to think that the locality of the affection, whether in the upper or lower lobe, does not influence the production of cough or affect its character. In old people cough may be absent. The expectoration is peculiarly tenacious and variously colored. The characteristic prune-juice color is sometimes absent, and is replaced by a red, black, or green color; or the expectoration may be colorless. The characteristic sputum of pneumonia has three qualities: color, consistence, and coalescence. It may appear on the first day, or not until the third or fourth. It is not always present, and may occur occasionally when no pneumonia exists, as in nasal or pharyngeal catarrh with hemorrhage, or in acute laryngitis.

Diarrhœa is often present, and so are

nausea and vomiting. The urine is often scanty. Albuminuria is common, and is usually most marked at the height of the disease. There was kidney trouble in 41 per cent. of his cases ; in 5 per cent. of these chronic kidney trouble of long standing existed ; in only 8 per cent. was it shown by clinical and post-mortem evidence that there was no urinary implication. The greatest danger occurs in an exacerbation of an old kidney affection.

Little has been added to our knowledge of the clinical aspects of pneumonia since the studies of Laennec. In the stage of engorgement we may expect to find dulness, but we do not. Grisolle found in this stage loss of elasticity in the chest walls, especially when percussed in the supra- and infra-spinous fossæ. The crepitant rale was regarded by Laennec as the first pathognomonic sign. It is produced by fluid matter passing into the vesicles of the lung. In some seasons it is rarely heard ; in old people it may be replaced by a coarse crepitant rale. Fine crepitation may be heard in other types of pneumonia, in pulmonary phthisis and syphilis, and even in bronchitis.

Prolonged expiration precedes tubular or bronchial breathing. Bronchophony and metallic voice, when considerable area of dulness exists, are also signs.

Pain is most frequent in the region of the nipple ; next, at the base of the lung. It may be felt at any part of the chest. It is due to pleurisy. The pulse is usually 100 or more, and may reach 160. Jaundice is not very infrequent, delirium is common. Coma occurred in three per cent. of his cases ; it is often uræmic. At first the respiration rises from 22 to 36 per minute, but within two days it may reach 40, 50, or 60.

Inflammation of the lower lobe seems to produce more oppression than inflammation of the upper.

In children the temperature reaches a greater height than in adults. It rises one or two degrees at night, and falls in the morning. The highest temperature in his cases was 108°, the lowest, 100.2° ; in ten cases the highest average temperature was 104.3°. The crisis usually occurs between the fifth and seventh days. Unless there are unusual complications or sequelæ it never occurs later than the fourteenth day. The immediate cause of death is usually heart failure from prolonged and exhaustive work, or from the influence of poisoned blood on the nerve centers.

In speaking of the etiology, Dr. Satterthwaite quoted Sturges's opinion that it was produced by cold, dry, penetrating winds ; some later writers, however, think cold an infrequent cause. Twenty-two per cent. of his own cases were ascribed to exposure to cold. The disease seldom occurs during the warmer months. Occupation has little bearing on the causation. Regarding the influence of microörganisms, it would be necessary, to prove that they are a cause, to show that a pure culture inoculated in the blood remote from the lungs would produce lobar pneumonia ; but experiments have almost always failed in this respect, and when the lung itself has been inoculated lobular, not lobar, pneumonia has commonly resulted.

The pleura is always involved except in the rare instances when the inflammation remains central. A comparatively frequent complication is pericarditis ; a more important complication is disease of the kidneys. The spleen is apt to be enlarged, and there is catarrh of the intestinal tract. True abscess of the lung is rare. Gangrene was noted in his cases. He does not believe phthisis could ever develop from acute lobar pneumonia.

The question of mortality, he said, has given rise to much dispute, largely because of indefinite statistics. Its discussion, to be of value, requires a knowledge of the variety ; the patient's age ; the general character of the attack. At some seasons the mortality is greater than at others, notwithstanding the same general treatment. Statistics before the middle of the present century give a mortality of from 16 to 55 per cent. Just before the middle of this century Skoda published statistics tending to prove that pneumonia is a self-limited disease. About 1842 Fleischmann, a homœopath, had a mortality of less than 6 per cent., which set other physicians thinking, and gradually led to less heroic treatment. The fact that the mortality varies in the hands of the same physicians shows that each case stands by itself. Dr. Satterthwaite's own experience shows that the expectant plan of treatment is best   The causes of death show what should be the direction of treatment. It should not be the reduction of temperature so much as the sustaining of the heart and obviating renal complications. The author has been led to believe by post-mortem studies that antipyretics not only weaken the heart's action, but also have some unfavorable action on the kidneys. Every case of acute lobar pneumonia should be treated by itself, and the indications met as they arise. He has often seen benefit from copious repeated cuppings in sthenic cases. In less vigorous persons relief often follows cold water applications. In defective hepatic action relief has come from large doses of mercurials. In weak heart patients have been carried through with alcoholic stimulants. In renal complications marked relief of pulmonary symptoms has followed remedies directed chiefly to the kidneys.

The author then passed to the consideration of secondary lobar pneumonia. This subdivision had been recognized by the old French school. His views of it are based upon 19 of his recorded cases. Without committing himself to an opinion as to their etiological value, he has found the antecedent conditions as follows: nephritis in 5; alcoholism in 2; phthisis in 2; burns in 2; rheumatism in 1; fracture of the ribs in 1; hypertrophy of the heart in 1.; pleurisy with effusion in 1; pericardial effusion in 1. Contemporaneous affections were present as follows: abdominal dropsy in 1; pericardial effusion in 1; gangrene of the extremities in 1; aneurism of the aorta in 1; bronchitis in 2; syphilis in 2; endocarditis in 2; hydrothorax in 1. Cases in which there was a suspicion of phthisis or syphilis were not included.

Secondary pneumonia is usually insidious. Chill is frequently absent, and when present is not severe. Difficulty in breathing may not be marked. The crepitant rale is heard as a rule. The temperature rises rapidly, as in acute lobar pneumonia, but averages somewhat lower in range. The pulse often rises sharply at the outset, but averages lower than in the acute form. Bronchial breathing and dulness may be the most decided symptoms, and in his experience they have been the most common. The expectoration is apt to be scanty and afford little help in diagnosis. Renal symptoms are likely to be more prominent than in the acute disease. There is a decided tendency to suppuration. The duration is about the same as in acute pneumonia, but the crisis is likely to come earlier. The causes of death are about as in acute lobar pneumonia, and indicate the treatment.

—Dr. Guerra Y. Estape, according to the *New Orleans Medical and Surgical Journal,* Dec., 1888, regards the local application to the larynx and pharynx of a 10 per cent. solution of resorcin as the best treatment of whooping-cough at present known.

PHILADELPHIA COUNTY MEDICAL SOCIETY.

Stated Meeting, December 12, 1888.

The President, J. SOLIS-COHEN, M.D., in the Chair.

DR. JOHN H. PACKARD read a paper on

Notes of a Successful Case of Laparotomy for Injury by a Circular Saw.

Charles Brown, aged twelve years, was brought to the Pennsylvania Hospital, September 24, 1888, having fallen against a circular saw in rapid motion. The accident occurred about one mile from the hospital.

On his admission, the ascending colon and about two feet of the small intestine were protruding from a wound four inches or more in length, nearly vertical, on the right side of the belly, some two inches from the middle line. The mass was tightly grasped in the wound, so that access of air to the peritoneal cavity was prevented. The boy was in a condition of marked but not excessive collapse.

He was etherized, and the parts antiseptically cleansed. The bowel was then carefully examined. Three wounds of the intestinal wall were detected; one involving the entire thickness, the other two the peritoneal coat only. At several points the omentum had been wounded, and the mesentery was cut in two places. The boy's woolen clothing had been torn by the teeth of the saw, and a great many minute shreds of the stuff deposited on the surface of the protruded mass.

The three intestinal wounds were carefully sutured with very fine silk, after the method of Lembert. All the bleeding points were secured with fine carbolized catgut. Some ragged portions of omentum were similarly tied and cut off. Attention was next given to the cleansing of the peritoneal surface from all the bits of woolen threads deposited on it; a very tedious process, occupying more time than any other part of the operation.

In order to return the protruded mass it was necessary to enlarge the wound somewhat; after which reduction was accomplished without difficulty. After irrigation of the peritoneal cavity, the edges of the wound were brought together with silkworm-gut sutures, secured by shot. A glass drainage tube with a closed and rounded end was inserted, and the usual antiseptic dressings applied, with a flannel over all.

Every two hours the cotton rope filling the tube was removed, and suction was made with a hard-rubber syringe with a long nozzle, so as to prevent any accumulation of secretions.

Reaction took place very favorably; the boy had only very slight pain, but some nausea and vomiting.

The nausea and vomiting continued all next day, subsiding toward evening. A free movement of the bowels occurred, and I learned later that an attendant, just after the boy's admission, had given him by mistake ten grains of blue mass, intended for another patient. As soon as the stomach became quiet, the administration of prepared milk and beef-tea, alternately every two hours, was begun.

On the 28th (the fourth day) there was only a slight yellowish discharge from the tube.

29th. The glass tube was removed, and a soft rubber one substituted for it. Solid food (milk toast) was given.

30th. He ate an egg and some chicken-broth.

A day or two after this the tube was removed, and a few days later the sutures.

For some two weeks after this the boy was kept in bed; he was allowed first to sit up in bed, and then to get up and walk about.

On October 31, thirty-seven days after the injury, he walked into the clinic-room; and on November 12 he was discharged, with directions to wear a binder for some time, and to report to us before dispensing with it.

1 should have mentioned that, after the spontaneous movement of the bowels on the second day, an enema of turpentine and sweet oil was administered about every third day until his dismissal.

Certain features of this case may be briefly commented upon. The boy's youth was, of course, in his favor. He was stout and healthy, although his surroundings had not been, by any means, hygienic. But there was one circumstance of special advantage—the fact that the protruded mass quite filled up and plugged the wound in the abdominal wall. Besides this, the wounds were all of small extent, and no large vessels were divided. The presence of the almost innumerable shreds of soiled woolen clothing on the peritoneal surface was of course an element of danger, only to be set aside by the utmost care and patience in their detection and removal.

It would scarcely be fair to conclude this report without acknowledging the assiduous care and attention, and the skill in manipulation bestowed upon the case by Dr. Walter D. Green, the resident surgeon, who first had charge of it, as well as by his successor, Dr. Harvey Shoemaker. Much of the credit of the favorable result attained belongs fairly to these gentlemen.

[The patient was shown to the Society and examined by the members.]

DR. JOSEPH PRICE, in opening the discussion, said: The fact that the protruding intestine completely closed the wound had a great deal to do with the successful result in this case. We know that undue manipulation and prolonged and needless exposure of intestine are frequent causes of shock and death; this fact is beautifully illustrated in needlessly prolonged operations. I never could understand the vicious do-nothing policy of ambulance surgeons in these cases of abdominal incised wounds. The ambulance surgeon should be prepared and instructed to act promptly in such accidents. Promptitude is everything. A pitcher of warm water and a few threads might save lives that are lost by carrying the patient untreated, with the intestines exposed, covered by filthy clothing, to the distant hospital, there to wait for the chief to arrive before anything is done. I recently read of a case of a man who was accidentally eviscerated while hunting alone in the backwoods. Someone found him with the intestines protruding and covered with dirt, and carried him to the nearest brook, washed and sewed him up. He was also fortunate in *being away from opium* and from meddlesome nurses and officious residents of a general hospital, and he recovered. The strictest simplicity, absence of opium and of milk, indeed of all food till the patient asks for it, except in greatly exhausted cases demanding early support or stimulation, will give the happiest results.

I give plenty of fluids, toast water, barley water, stimulating enemata of beef-tea, with perhaps a little whiskey if needed, and enemata of water to relieve thirst. We know how difficult it is to prevent hemorrhage in ether nausea. Careful preparation for the operation by the free use of salines will minimize the ether and bowel disturbance. I am satisfied that the free use of the salines is of greater importance *before* operation than after in abdominal work. The unintentional administration of blue mass in this case of Dr. Packard's was a happy accident and helped recovery.

I wish particularly to congratulate Dr. Packard upon the excellence of the toilet, the care to secure perfect cleanliness under such difficult conditions, and the perfect drainage. The careful removal of all foreign material from the bowel, free irrigation, and perfect glass drainage in two desperate cases have given him a triumph in two cases of abdominal work.

DR. PACKARD: I must say a word in reply to Dr. Price in defense of "my friend opium." You remove a tumor; all goes well until water is injected into the abdomen. Pain ensues immediately. You give a grain of the extract of opium by the rectum, when the pain disappears, the patient goes to sleep and wakes in comfort. Are you not justified in attributing this to the opium, and relying upon the same measure in similar cases?

Of course it would be a great mistake to treat all cases of peritonitis with opium. The saline treatment is proper in suitable cases, and saves many lives. So may we say of opium in suitable cases. The error is in exclusiveness, whether in the one direction or the other. We must use our judgment in individual cases, and prescribe in view of all the conditions present.

In this case I think nothing would have served my patient as the one grain of the extract of opium did. It was not a case of peritonitis, however, and I did not so regard it. But suppose some enthusiast in salines had ticketed the case peritonitis and immediately administered purges? I hardly think such prompt relief would have been afforded.

I would like, while on this subject, to mention a measure which I have employed for many years, and which has repeatedly seemed to me to avert threatened peritonitis, and that is the application of a dozen leeches to the abdomen. After operation for stone especially, as well as in other cases of traumatism, marked benefit has been derived from the adoption of this plan.

DR. JOHN H. PACKARD read a paper on

Tumor Probably of Uterine Origin, Attached to the Small Intestine; Removed by Laparotomy.

For the following notes I am indebted to the kindness of Dr. L. I. Blake, resident surgeon to the hospital. It is due to him also that I should acknowledge his skill and attention in dressing and caring for this patient.

Kate M., native of Ireland, aged twenty-six, domestic, single. Admitted to St. Joseph's Hospital November 13, 1888. Family history good. Personal history also good, with the exception of an ill-defined

attack she suffered from three years ago, probably resembling in some points the present one, and which was pronounced by her physician at that time to be intestinal inflammation of some sort.

She had been examined by two physicians before admission into the hospital. The first stated that she had inflammation of the womb, while the second led her friends to believe that she was pregnant.

On admission, she stated that she had been suffering for three weeks, getting worse gradually. On examination her abdomen was found to be enormously distended, and exquisitely tender to the touch. Constant pain was felt throughout the greater portion of the trunk. Temperature 101° F.; pulse 100 and moderately strong. There being neither history of traumatism nor marks of violence, a vaginal examination was made, but no abnormalities noted. Her menstruation was established at fifteen, and has always been regular. When pain was sufficiently relieved to permit manipulation of the abdomen, distinct fluctuation was elicited, and in the left ovarian region was an area of dulness, which, though slightly variable, was not obliterated when the patient was turned on the left side. Deep pressure on this spot detected a hard mass which receded from the touch, but returned, the hand being kept in position. Owing to the extreme tension of the abdominal walls it was impossible to ascertain anything as to its nature or attachments.

The tympanites and ascites failing to respond to medicinal agents, the patient growing weaker, and at the end of three weeks the respiration being interfered with, an exploratory incision was decided upon.

The patient being in tolerably fair condition, the operation was performed by Dr. Packard on Saturday, December 8th.

The peritoneum was found to be very much thickened and congested, its appearance being scarcely distinguishable from that of intestine.

After removing five or six quarts of clear serum from the peritoneal cavity, the incision was enlarged, revealing a growth attached to a knuckle of intestine in the lower segment of the abdominal cavity to the left of the median line. This tumor, a little larger than a fœtal head, was hard and dense in structure, weighing one and a half pounds; encapsulated and attached by a narrow pedicle, little more than an inch in breadth, which seemed to be a redundant portion of the capsule thrown around almost the entire circumference of the intestine. This was carefully dissected away from the intestine, and all bleeding points ligatured.

The peritoneal cavity was irrigated thoroughly with a solution of the bichloride of mercury, 1 part to 15,000 of distilled water. The peritoneum and abdominal walls were sutured separately, the former with catgut, the latter with silkworm-gut. A glass drainage tube, perforated and closed at the bottom, was placed in Douglas's pouch, and the wound closed and dressed.

The operation was done under full antiseptic precautions. The patient showed considerable shock after the operation, from which she rallied slowly. It was accompanied by persistent vomiting, which was relieved by one drop of creasote every two hours, administered in syrup of vanilla. A peculiar temperature was exhibited during this period, the same thermometer registering successively in the mouth 96⅘°, in the axilla 97⅘°, in the rectum 101°. During the first twenty-four hours there was not sufficient discomfort or restlessness to call for anodynes. Up to this time, about six ounces of bloody serum had been drained from the cavity. Four ounces of warm distilled water were then injected through the tube, and allowed to remain four or five minutes. Since that time, during the last seventy-two hours, not more than three ounces of serum have been removed, and scarcely tinged with blood. A short time after the warm water was removed, the patient complained of sharp, shooting pains, with marked tenderness over the abdomen. These became so severe as to require a suppository of opium (one grain), which soon induced a quiet sleep, with no return of pain on waking.

Thirty-six hours after the operation a slight but persistent cough was developed, probably due to hypostatic congestion, since change of position gave relief.

During the last three days the temperature taken in the mouth has not risen above 100⅔°, the pulse varying from 90 to 100.

Ever since the operation the patient has evinced a strong craving for food, giving milk the preference above anything else.

[The subsequent progress of this case has been very favorable. On the 11th of December (the sixth day) the glass tube was removed, and a soft-rubber one substituted, until the 17th, when it was dispensed with. On this day she had a spontaneous and quite natural movement of the bowels.

Suppuration occurred in the suture tracks, probably from insufficient preparation of the silkworm-gut used. On the 24th of December (the sixteenth day) she was allowed to sit up in bed, the wound being quite healed.—P.]

DR. OSLER said: I agree with Dr. Packard as to the pathological nature of the growth, and the possibility which he mentions is quite well recognized. An interesting feature of the case is the association of peritoneal effusion with solid growths in the abdomen. I have on several occasions been asked to see cases of ascites which depended upon the presence of tumors of ovaries or uterus.

PERISCOPE.

Lacerated Wound of Brain.

At the meeting of the Medical Society of London, Oct. 22, 1888, Dr. Fletcher Beach read the notes of a case in which a boy was injured on July 20 by a window-pole being pushed into the cranium, 2¼ inches above and 1 inch to the left of the occipital protuberance, penetrating to the depth of an inch. There was some rise of temperature, with bad temper, and even delirium. The pulse too remained high, and on August 16 a cerebral abscess broke through the wound, and a quantity of greenish pus escaped. The patient was enabled to leave the hospital well on September 5. The treatment, apart from local antiseptics, was confined to tincture of opium, chloral, and bromide of sodium. Mr. Knowsley Thornton quoted a case related to him by Dr. Image, of Bury St. Edmunds. A boy, 7 years old, was struck by a sort of pitchfork, the prong of which entered the cranial cavity, carrying with it a quantity of filth. No treatment was adopted beyond the application of some carbolic lotion, but the lad made a perfect recovery. He suggested that children recovered from such injuries more easily than adults. Dr. Symes Thompson agreed with the remark as to the recovery of children, and mentioned that a month ago he saw a case brought before a medical society at Capetown in which Dr. Beck had trephined for suspected abscess of the brain. He, however, only alighted on the abscess after plunging the trocar three times for two inches into the brain substance. A good recovery resulted. Dr. Beevor asked if the sight had been affected in Dr. Fletcher's case. He recollected the case of a boy, who had been kicked by a horse on the head, but recovered. Dr. Money asked if any relationship had been found to exist between the hernia cerebri and the frequency of the pulse. Dr. Fletcher Beach, in reply, said that he did not know of any symptoms having occurred subsequently. There were no visual troubles.—*British Med. Journal*, Oct. 27, 1888.

Inoculation of Syphilis by Tattooing.

At the meeting of the South-East Hants Medical Society, Oct. 11, 1888, Surgeon F. R. Barker read a paper on syphilis communicated by tattooing. The patients, three of whom were exhibited, were all soldiers of a regiment stationed at Portsmouth, and they were all tattooed by the same man, a discharged soldier. They were tattooed at various dates during the present year, and the periods of incubation varied from eighty-seven to thirteen days. In the first case admitted, the lesion appeared like a poisoned wound; but, two days after, two more men of the same regiment appeared with similar ulcers with hardened bases, caused by tattooing. The next day another patient was admitted with three inflamed patches on the arm, presenting well-marked rupial crusts. The fifth case was admitted a few days after the others, and from this patient a clue was obtained to the man who had performed the tattooing. This man was asked to come to the hospital, where he stated that he had tattooed about fifteen men of the regiment since its arrival at Portsmouth in April last. He at first denied, but afterward admitted, that he mixed his paints with his saliva, and wetted his finger and applied it to the part tattooed: he had also put the needles into his mouth. He used four ordinary needles on a piece of stick, quite as close together as he could get them. He used vermilion and India ink. He had never had a sore on his penis, but had had gonorrhœa. Whilst talking to him, Dr. Barker noticed a slight sore at the left angle of his mouth, and, on looking into it, the greater part of the buccal mucous membrane and soft palate was found studded with mucous tubercles. There was a coppery rash on his chest. On the glans penis there was a dark-colored scar the size of a shilling. This, the man said, had come a year before; he had had no treatment for it, and it went away of its own accord. He had also condylomata about the anus, and suffered from alopecia. The inguinal and cervical glands were enlarged. Of the fifteen men he had tattooed, eleven contracted the disease. Dr. Ward Cousins remarked upon the very unusual appearance of well-marked rupial crusts at the points of inoculation. He had never seen rupial prominences before, except during the secondary or tertiary stages of the disease. There was no previous history of syphilis in this case. All the patients were most certainly inoculated from the same source, and yet they presented very different forms of local inflammation and widely different skin disease.—*British Med. Journal*, Oct. 27, 1888.

Anthrax in Swine.

The *Lancet*, Nov. 3, 1888, says: Since among veterinarians some difference of opinion exists as to whether or not swine are capable of suffering from anthrax, or if cases described as anthrax may not be instances of septic poisoning, Professor Crookshank, at the request of Professor Brown, of the Agricultural Department of the Privy Council, carried out some experiments to ascertain the nature of the disease induced in swine by the ingestion of the offal of animals that have died of anthrax. He communicated his results to the Glasgow meeting of the British Medical Association. Professor Crookshank proved that the disease produced in swine by experimentally feeding them with anthrax offal was anthrax, which could also be produced in swine by injection of the blood of a bullock which died of anthrax, or transmitted to swine by injection of the blood of the spleen of a guinea-pig inoculated with the disease; and, lastly, produced in swine by direct injection of a pure cultivation of the anthrax bacillus. He was enabled to isolate the anthrax bacillus from cases occurring in the practice of Mr. Wilson of Berkhampstead, and concludes that anthrax can be communicated to swine, both young and old. A yellowish jelly-like œdema of the subcutaneous areolar tissue extends from the point of entrance of the virus, and, if the "disease is induced by ingestion of anthrax offal, the tonsils are found to be ulcerated, and constitute the point of access of the bacilli to the blood. In such cases the characteristic symptom is enormous swelling around the throat." The anthrax bacilli are very scantily present in the blood, due probably to the septic organisms which may readily have gained entrance at the same time from the offal consumed. As the anthrax bacillus rapidly disappears in presence of putrefactive organisms, failure to produce anthrax by inoculating guinea-pigs or mice from swine during an outbreak must not, if septicæmia is present, be held as conclusive against the outbreak being anthrax.

THE
MEDICAL AND SURGICAL
REPORTER.

ISSUED EVERY SATURDAY.

CHARLES W. DULLES, M.D.,
EDITOR AND PUBLISHER.

The Terms of Subscription to the serial publications of this office are as follows, payable in advance:

Med. and Surg. Reporter (weekly), a year,	**$5.00**
Quarterly Compendium of Med. Science, -	2.50
Reporter and Compendium, - - - -	6.00
Physician's Daily Pocket Record, - -	1.00
Reporter and Pocket Record, - - - -	6.00
Reporter, Compendium, and Pocket Record,	7.00

All checks and postal orders should be drawn to order of

CHARLES W. DULLES,

N. E. Cor. 13th and Walnut Streets,

P. O. Box 843.   Philadelphia, Pa.

☞SUGGESTIONS TO SUBSCRIBERS:
See that your address-label gives the date to which your subscription is paid.
In requesting a change of address, give the old address as well as the new one.
If your REPORTER does not reach you promptly and regularly, notify the publisher *at once*, so that the cause may be discovered and corrected.

☞SUGGESTIONS TO CONTRIBUTORS AND CORRESPONDENTS:
Write in ink.
Write on one side of paper only.
Write on paper of the size usually used for letters.
Make as few paragraphs as possible. Punctuate carefully. Do not abbreviate, or omit words like "the," and "a," or "an."
Make communications as short as possible.
NEVER ROLL A MANUSCRIPT! Try to get an envelope or wrapper which will fit it.
When it is desired to call our attention to something in a newspaper, mark the passage boldly with a colored pencil, and write on the wrapper "Marked copy." Unless this is done, newspapers are not looked at.
The Editor will be glad to get medical news, but it is important that brevity and actual interest shall characterize communications intended for publication.

AN ACCUSATION AGAINST PHYSICIANS.

Our attention has been called by a subscriber in Wisconsin to an item, said to be going the rounds of the Western papers, and copied from the New York *Herald,* which attributes to a clergyman in New Brunswick, N. J., the following language: "Judging from statements I have heard there are five hundred infantile murders committed in this city by physicians every year. The people need to be taught not only that this destruction of life is contrary to nature, ruinous to health and the cause of disease, but that it is murder and a sin against God. There are physicians who, knowing the penalty of the law upon those who thus destroy life, use their knowledge to make whatever demand they choose upon the guilty parties. The married women are said to be as bad in this respect as the unmarried." After this, the clergyman in question is said to have read a letter from the superintendent of the Florence Mission, in New York—an institution intended for the reclaiming of fallen women. The letter stated that the majority of the inmates, by their own confession, were first corrupted and influenced to lead a life of shame by their family physicians.

The item from which we copy these charges states that they had created a profound sensation; and our correspondent asks us to call the clergyman who made them to account. Before doing this we thought it proper to give him an opportunity to explain himself; and so we addressed him a letter, enclosing the slip and asking him if he had any comment to make on it. This brought a prompt reply, which is published in our Correspondence columns. This reply shows that the report in the *Herald* was incorrect, and did injustice to the clergyman as well as to physicians.

In considering the whole matter we think the Rev. Mr. McDuffie might have made a little clearer—if he did not—the distinction between the few physicians who practice criminal abortion and the great mass who regard this as a heinous crime. And we think he might have made a more guarded use of the accusation, coming from prostitutes, against family physicians. All who are familiar with the characteristics of such women as find shelter in the Florence Mission know that they not rarely seek to screen themselves behind the basest accusations of others. The Florence Mission itself has furnished a charge reflecting as severely against the clergy as the one above quoted against family physicians. Both charges may have some small foundation in fact; but neither deserves any consideration, as bearing upon the reputation of the classes accused.

Physicians, so far from deserving such criticism as the Rev. Mr. McDuffie was reported to have made, are, as a rule, remarkably pure in the face of temptations such as surround no other set of men in the world. It is for this very reason that they enjoy the implicit confidence of maids and matrons, of husbands and fathers all over the world, and nowhere more than in the United States.

THE YELLOW FEVER PANIC.

More than once last year have we in these columns expressed our sympathy with those who, in various parts of the United States, have raised a voice against the unreasonable panic created by the recent outbreak of yellow fever at Jacksonville, Florida. Some of the events connected with the epidemic have suggested nothing so much as the ignorance and superstition of the Middle Ages. For the belief in horrible spiritual agents we have had substituted a belief in a germ endowed by the imagination with almost equally mysterious and improbable powers; and methods of combating it have been adopted which, in some respects, were as senseless as ever were practised. The worst of it all has been that some of these senseless practices had the real or apparent sanction of men who were chosen to direct the means of limiting the spread of the epidemic.

In a recently issued pamphlet by Dr. J. C. LeHardy, of Savannah, Georgia, entitled "The Yellow Fever Panic," there is a vigorous argument against the opinion that yellow fever is a contagious disease, and against the absurd methods adopted to prevent its spread, and the general neglect of efforts to prevent its outbreak.

Dr LeHardy has had a large experience with yellow fever, having lived through the epidemics of 1854, 1858, and 1876, besides attending numbers of cases in the intervening years. Dr. LeHardy attributes the pro-duction of yellow fever to a germ, but believes that the germ requires certain conditions of extreme heat and of moisture in order that it shall produce an epidemic. He points out the inefficiency of quarantine and the value of local sanitary measures to prevent the conditions which favor endemics of the disease, and especially condemns the way in which the authority delegated to the Surgeon-General of the Marine Hospital service has been used.

In the last received report of the Illinois State Board of Health, Dr. Rauch also protests vigorously against the ignorance and inhumanity brought to the surface in the recent epidemic, and especially against the senseless quarantine methods adopted.

In this we think he and Dr. LeHardy are entirely right. We have been anxiously hoping that this epidemic would furnish some valuable addition to our knowledge of the nature of yellow fever and the best method of preventing its outbreak and spread; but so far we have seen nothing of the kind—unless it be such protests as we have cited. It seems as if the learned and conclusive studies of yellow fever by Bache and others had been forgotten or ignored by those who have been dealing with the last epidemic, and we have little expectation of improvement until the health authorities return to the point reached by careful observers fifty years ago.

TRIBUTE TO DR. LEIDY.

The Philadelphia *Ledger*, Dec. 15, 1888, says: "Dr. Joseph Leidy, President of the Academy of Natural Sciences and Professor of Anatomy at the University of Pennsylvania, has had another honor added to the many he has had conferred upon him. A recent letter from the distinguished French naturalist, Milne Edwards, brings the information that the Cuvier prize of the French Academy of Sciences has been unanimously voted to him. The letter goes on to state that this prize has never been conferred except to the most distinguished scientists, such as Agassiz, Owen, von Baer and Ehrenburg. The award is therefore all the more a great distinction. Dr. Leidy, though he receives honors from the ends of the earth, may have the gratification to know that his learning is nowhere more highly prized than in his native city, where those who know him best honor him most."

The Nation, December 20, 1888, says: "It will be gratifying to students of science in this country to know that the Cuvier Prize of the French Academy of Sciences, which is awarded triennially for the most important researches in the domain of general natural history and geology, and which has associated with it, among others, the names of Von Baer, Ehrenberg, Richard Owen, Agassiz, and Heer, has been this year decreed to the distinguished president of the Academy of Natural Sciences of Philadelphia, Professor Joseph Leidy. Following closely upon the award to the same scientist of the Lyell Medal of the Geological Society of London, and of the Walker Grand Prize of the Boston Society of Natural History, this recognition is a just tribute to the worth of one who has, with a degree of modesty uncommon to men of such eminence, kept himself well in the background among aspirants for fame and honors. There are probably few among the distinguished naturalists of this country who are less generally known than Professor Leidy, yet it is safe to say that during the last quarter of a century he has had no peer among the native-born, nor any co-laborer whose works have been held in higher repute by the savants of both Europe and America. As a comparative anatomist and microscopist, he easily leads the field; and if in the department of vertebrate palæontology he has seen rivals grow about him, it can yet be said that Dr. Leidy was the founder of the science in this country, and that to his pen belong the records of the first important researches made into the extinct life of the Western Territories. To Dr. Leidy, likewise, humanity is indebted in great part for the determination of the nature of trichina."

To these appreciative notices of the honor done to Dr. Leidy little can be added, except that those who know him best know that they are sincere and just.

NOT CRUELTY, BUT NOT SPORT.

The eminent physiologists to be found in all the petit juries in Queens County, New York, have now for the second time decided that rabbit coursing is not cruel. Certain persons, judging solely by appearances and guided by unreasonable prejudice, had assumed that rabbits suffered in mind and body when taken out, given a short start, and made to run for their lives from a pack of dogs. But Mr. August Belmont, Jr., and other like-minded sportsmen, maintained the contrary, and two juries of Queens County have supported them, intimating that rabbits rather like this kind of diversion, and that it would be a pity to interfere with their enjoyment. Unfortunately, however, for the prospective pleasure of the rabbits, the authorities of the Jersey City Kennel Club have announced that rabbit coursing, as carried out in this country, should be condemned by all true sportsmen, as it is condemned in England, where only people of low degree ever indulge in it. It seems too bad that the bright expectations of the rabbits should be thus dashed to the ground; but their friends will be pleased to learn that their existence will not be wholly monotonous; for they still have the excitements of the physiological laboratories left them, where very lately certain French investigators have subjected them to violent and prolonged shakings and other commotions, in order to get at the philosophy of sea-sickness.

—While heating a platinum point at a lamp, in the Cincinnati Hospital, Dec. 13, the lamp exploded and Dr. Hoppe was dangerously burned. The clothes of the patient on whom the doctor was to have operated caught fire and he ran out of the room.

BOOK REVIEWS.

MEDICAL DIAGNOSIS. A MANUAL OF CLIN-ICAL METHODS. BY J. GRAHAM BROWN, M.D., F.R.C.P. Edinburgh, etc. Second edition, illustrated. 8vo, pp. 285. New York: E. B. Treat, 1888. Price, $2.75.

Dr. Brown's treatise on Medical Diagnosis is well and favorably known; but this particular edition has not much to commend it to professional esteem. If it is not an example of what is often called literary piracy, there is nothing in the book to correct the suspicion that it is. As a piece of book-making, it is what may be called pretentious. The paper is stiff and bulky, and the binding is showy but unsubstantial. The printing is very fair; but the illustrations are poor, and so few as scarcely to justify the use of the word "illustrated" on the title-page.

A MANUAL OF DIETETICS FOR PHYSI-CIANS, MOTHERS AND NURSES. BY W. B. PRITCHARD, M.D. 8vo, pp. 88. Published by the Dietetic Publishing Co., New York. Price, 50 cents.

This little book contains a great deal of useful information in regard to the care of infants and invalids, and especially in regard to their food. The author considers first the care and feeding of infants, and then passes on to discuss the feeding of invalids in a variety of diseases. His views are in the main correct, and are founded partly on his own experience and partly on the writings of well-known medical men. A noticeable feature of the book is its enthusiastic praise of a certain food preparation. This is so enthusiastic as to excite suspicion; although the suspicion may do the author injustice. Be this as it may, the book before us has much to recommend it to the attention of medical men, and its moderate price places it within easy reach of all of them.

THE LIFE INSURANCE EXAMINER. A PRACTICAL TREATISE UPON MEDICAL EXAMINATIONS FOR LIFE INSURANCE. BY CHARLES F. STILLMAN, M.S., M.D., ETC. Large 8vo, pp. 188 and appendix. New York: The Spectator Co., 1888.

The title of the book indicates the class of medical men for whom it is especially intended; but the volume contains much of great interest and value for all studious physicians. The opinions which guide insurance companies in accepting or rejecting applications for life insurance represent quite accurately the mature opinion of careful students as to the conditions which conduce to life and health or to death or disease. These opinions are, of course, valuable in other relations; and the careful reader of the book before us will find much in it which bears upon questions arising constantly in his professional relations with his patients. Matters of local and racial hygiene are discussed here with an acuteness sharpened by commercial interests of great importance; and the laws which restrain or protect life insurance companies are touched upon in a way which would interest everyone who wishes to be insured or who is concerned in the insurance of others.

PAMPHLET NOTICES.

169. ACUTE INFECTIOUS PHARYNGITIS. BY E. M. HEWISH, M.D., Philadelphia. From the *Medical News*, Sept. 8, 1888. 5 pages.

170. XERODERMA PIGMENTOSUM. BY BUCHANAN KLOPHEL, M.D., Memphis, Tenn. From the New York *Medical Record*, June 2, 1888. 8 pages.

171. OCCURRENCE OF THE MAMMARY SECRETION ACCOMPANIED BY CERTAIN RATIONAL SIGNS OF PREGNANCY IN TWO NON-PREGNANT WOMEN. BY GEORGE WOODRUFF JOHNSTON, M.D., Washington, D. C. From the *American Journal of Obstetrics*, August, 1888. 6 pages.

172. CONTRIBUTIONS TO ABDOMINAL SURGERY. BY ROSWELL PARK, M.D., Buffalo, N. Y. From the *Medical Press of Western New York*, August, 1888. 7 pages.

169. Dr. Hewish gives the history of a curious case marked by inflammation and swelling of the soft parts surrounding the fauces, and afterward by diffuse swelling of the neck. In spite of the treatment, which included laryngotomy, the patient died on the ninth day of the disease. The history of this case is followed by a brief sketch of the pathology of the disease.

170. Dr. Klophel, who says he has never seen a case of xeroderma pigmentosum, gives in this pamphlet his views as to the pathology of the disorder, and recommends treating it with ignipuncture, using for this purpose the galvano-cautery.

171. Dr. Johnston gives an account of observations made upon two non-pregnant women who presented the phenomena of a milky secretion in the breasts, and sensations like those experienced by many women when pregnant. The cases are well described, and a brief study of the cause of the condition follows.

172. Dr. Park reports two cases: one a gastrostomy on a woman 47 years old, with stricture of the œsophagus, done under cocaine anæsthesia; the other a successful resection of the intestine for the relief of a fecal fistula.

The latter of these operations was of exceptional interest, and proved perfectly successful. Both are valuable contributions to the literature of abdominal surgery. The report would be better if the writer did not speak of operations being "made," and if he gave linear measures in English instead of in metric terms.

LITERARY NOTES.

—The publisher of *The Writer*, Boston, Mass., announces the intended appearance of a companion periodical, to be called *The Author*, which will be issued on the fifteenth of each month, at one dollar a year, and contains original and selected matter of interest to literary workers. In calling attention to this publication, it is pleasant to be able to say that, if it is at all what the excellent character of *The Writer* would lead one to expect, we would be glad to know that every subscriber to the REPORTER was also a subscriber to both these periodicals.

CORRESPONDENCE.

A Clergyman's Charges Against Physicians.

To the Editor.

Sir: Your note, inclosing me a slip cut from some newspaper referring to the *Herald's* report of a sermon preached by me in September last, has been received, and I thank you for your request and the opportunity which you give me to do justice to the medical profession and to myself by correcting the false statements made in the *Herald.* I attempted to correct the mistake by promptly writing to the *Herald*, denying the truthfulness of the report and specifying the points wherein it terribly exaggerated and perverted the statements which I made ; but my letter to the *Herald* was never published, though duly received. It is very often utterly impossible to get some newspapers to correct the false reports which they make, without going to law : this I never do. I will try to give you in a few words the truth of the whole matter.

(1) I did not say that the infantile murders were committed *by the physicians* as a general thing, though they sometimes give the drugs and use the instruments for this purpose. On the authority of four of the most reputable physicians of this city I stated that the sin named was and is shamefully common in this city, and making a rough estimate I supposed that from three hundred to five hundred natural births were prevented every year in this city of 20,000 people. I am still of this opinion; and the further I investigate, by conversation with physicians and druggists and by reading medical books, the more I am convinced of the fact that this is "a great American sin." As for the physicians of this city, I distinctly stated that they would compare favorably with the other physicians of the United States both as to intelligence and moral character. I am still of this opinion notwithstanding the fact that I know some of them whose record is not clean. My remarks were not confined to the physicians of this city. I happened at the time to know of some disreputable work which was being arranged for by physicians outside of this city, and it was in connection with an effort to defeat wicked plans that I came into a knowledge of the terrible crimes constantly being committed here and elsewhere. You may rest assured of the fact that I did not make a false alarm. I knew what I was talking about and have seen no reason to change my mind.

(2) I read no letter from the Florence Mission in New York, nor did I pretend to read any such letter. I read a letter from a brother minister who gave me some facts to the effect that many of the fallen women who have been reclaimed by that mission attributed their ruin to their family physicians.

I did all I could to strengthen the hands and multiply the legitimate practice of worthy men, and all I could to warn my people against immoral physicians. In this I believe I have the sympathy and prayers of the best men in the medical profession. I have a higher respect and more tender feeling for men in this profession than for the men of any other profession, and I would not for any consideration injure their position in the estimation of the world. The man who reported for the *Herald* did not hear the sermon or read it, but got his points from others and fixed up his article so as to create a sensation, not realizing or intending to do the mischief which resulted. I feel that I am the most injured of all by the report, but freely forgive the reporter, as he did it ignorantly. Good will doubtless come of it. Sin needs to be exposed, and even if the enormity of it should by accident be exaggerated it is better than if nothing had been said. Please publish this statement and do me the kindness to send me a printed copy.

Yours truly,
M. V. McDuffie,
Pastor Remsen Avenue Baptist Church, New Brunswick, N. J., December 17, 1888.

Velpeau's Compound.

To the Editor.

Sir: In answer to question 3 of Dr. G. M. Foskett (Med. and Surg. Reporter, Dec. 22, 1888, p. 789) allow me to inform you of Velpeau's formulas.

℞ Camphoræ,
Potassii nitratis . . . . āā 5 parts
Pulv. radicis ipecac. . . . . . . 2.5 "
M. ft. pilulæ No. L.
Sig. One pill every three hours.

This is used in delirious states after operations, also in erysipelas of the face.

℞ Aceti rosæ . . . . f℥ss
Aquæ destillat. . . . . f℥xx
M. Sig. For injection.

This is used in cases of granulations of the neck of the uterus, and also in leucorrhœa.

Yours truly,
B. Segnitz, M.D.
149 East 63d St., New York,
Dec. 22, 1888.

NOTES AND COMMENTS.

Amputation of the Pregnant Uterus.

Mr. Lawson Tait, in a paper published in the *Sacramento Med. Times*, Dec., 1888, says: This operation, I venture to predict, will revolutionize the obstetric art, and in two years we shall hear no more of craniotomy and eviscerations, for this new method will save more lives than these proceedings do, and it is far easier of performance. It is the easiest operation in abdominal surgery, and every country practitioner ought to be able and always prepared to perform it. No special instruments are required—nothing but a knife, some artery forceps, a piece of rubber drainage tube, two or three knitting-needles, and a little perchloride of iron.

My method of operating is to make an incision through the middle line large enough to admit my hand, and then I pass a piece of rubber drainage-tube (without any holes in it) as a loop over the fundus uteri, and bring it down so as to encircle the cervix, taking care that it does not include a loop of intestine. I then make a single hitch and draw it tight around the cervix, so as completely to stop the circulation. I give the ends of the tube to an assistant, who keeps them well on the strain, so as to prevent the loose knot from slipping; the reason for this being that should there be any bleeding and any necessity for further constriction, I could secure this in a moment, without undoing any knot; the simplicity of this method greatly commends it. I then make a small opening in the uterus, and enlarge it by tearing with my two forefingers, seize the child by a foot and remove it. I then remove the placenta, and by that time the uterus has completely contracted and is easily drawn through the wound in the abdominal wall. The constricting tube will now probably require to be tightened, and the second hitch of the knot may be put on at the same time, and the work is practically done. Stuff a few sponges into the wound to keep the cavity clear of blood, and pass the knitting-needles through the flattened tube and through the cervix, and in this simple way a clamp of the most efficient kind is at once made; the uterus is removed about three-quarters of an inch above the rubber tube. The usual stitches are put in, the wound closed around the stump, which, of course, is brought to the lower part of the opening, and then the stump is dressed with perchloride of iron in the usual way.

The operation takes far less time to perform than it takes to describe, and as there is hardly any possibility of complications; it is one of the simplest operations that can be undertaken, and must always be pretty much the same; for this reason no one need be in any fear about undertaking it; for, in the absence of variation in the difficulties to be encountered, it differs entirely from any other operation in abdominal surgery. If performed before the patient has been mauled about by ineffectual attempts to deliver, its mortality will be no greater than that of ovariotomy, and the arguments in its favor against all alternative proceedings are: first, that it cannot be more dangerous to the mother than most of these are; that it saves the life of the child; that it prevents the unfortunate mother from again being placed in a similar condition; and it certainly has the great advantage over alternative proceedings having a similar object, that its great simplicity, as contrasted, for instance, with operations proposed by Thomas, Müller and Sänger, will make it possible for the country doctor, less experienced in surgery, to perform it without hesitation. These complicated and difficult proceedings may have their advantages, though I confess I do not see them, but they will be left for the hands of experienced specialists. The operation I have described will be the operation of emergency, when only the resources of general practice are at hand.

Is the Communication of Infection an Assault?

A remarkable judgment was delivered last week by the High Court of Justice in London upon the question whether it is an assault in law to communicate an infective disease to another person. Thirteen judges considered the case, and it was discussed in all its bearings in the course of the delivery of the judgments. The prisoner was charged, under the Offences against the Person Act, 24 and 25 Vict., cap. 100, on two counts, with inflicting grievous bodily harm upon his wife, and with an assault, he having communicated to her a disease (syphilis). He was convicted, but the question of whether he could be properly convicted under the statute was reserved for the consideration of this Court. Mr. Justice Wills was of opinion that the conviction should be quashed. No mention was made in the statute of this class of offences, and the alteration of the criminal law involved, if the conviction were affirmed, would have very widespread consequences. It was clear that what the Act contemplated was personal violence. Justices Smith, Mathew, and Grantham also were in favor of the conviction being quashed. Mr. Justice Stephen said that if the principle involved in a conviction was right, it must apply to women as well as men, and unmarried women as well as wives, and to diseases of any kind communicated by one person to another, and a man who had scarlet fever and shook hands with another might be indicted under these sections. He did not think there was grievous bodily harm or an assault of the nature contemplated by the statute. He was, therefore, of opinion that the conviction should be quashed. Mr. Justice Hawkins did not think the consequences shadowed forth by his learned brothers would follow if the conviction were upheld, and he could not be a party to a judgment which would proclaim to the world that, under the law of England, in the year 1888, a man might maliciously be guilty of such barbarity and not be punished. He thought the conviction should be confirmed. Mr. Justice Day, who was absent, concurred, it was said, in this judgment. Mr. Justice Manisty, Mr. Baron Huddleston, and Mr. Baron Pollock were in favor of quashing the conviction; while Mr. Justice Field thought it should be affirmed, as did also Mr. Justice Charles, who was absent. There being nine judges in favor of quashing the conviction, and four only supporting it, the conviction was quashed, in accordance with the view of the majority. Conviction quashed accordingly.—*Medical Press and Circular*, Nov. 21, 1888.

Creasote in Phthisis.

In a paper on Creasote in Phthisis, contributed to the *N. Y. Med. Journal*, Dec. 8, 1888, Dr. Austin Flint reports ten cases and says that the records of the ten cases reported show that creasote by the stomach and the inhalations (consisting of equal parts creasote, alcohol and spirit of chloroform) in cases of solidification without cavities, effect prompt and decided improvement in all phthisical symptoms, with increase in appetite, weight, and strength, even with surroundings much less favorable than would obtain in many cases in private practice. In cases with small cavities much less improvement is to be looked for, but some benefit may be expected. In cases with large cavities the treatment seems to have little more than a palliative influence. His recorded observations, he says, are defective as regards the influence of the treatment upon the bacilli. In one case, with large cavities, it was noted that the number of bacilli was diminished. No other examinations for bacilli were made during or after treatment.

No estimate was made of the relative value of creasote taken into the stomach. As regards the inhalations, it is assumed that the chief benefit was derived from the creasote, the spirit of chloroform and the alcohol rendering this agent more volatile, and soothing the mucous surfaces. The inhaled vapor undoubtedly penetrated by diffusion as far as the air-cells. It is by diffusion that fresh air, anæsthetic vapors, etc., penetrate the lungs, and cases of pneumonokoniosis illustrate the fact that even solid particles may be carried to the pulmonary vesicles.

Dr. Flint says he has employed the method of inhalation here described, conjoined with other treatment, in private practice, with good results. In a case of irritative cough of several months' standing, with slight bronchitis and emphysema, but no signs of phthisis, which resisted ordinary treatment, three inhalations produced complete relief, and the cough had not reappeared at the end of four weeks.

Fatal Error of a Druggist.

It is reported from Jersey City, N. J., under date of December 27, that a boy four years old had died as the result of having administered to him a medicine intended for another person. A prescription given for the boy was taken to a drug-store and left to be compounded. About that time another prescription was sent to the drug-store with the same instructions as to its being delivered. The two prescriptions were of a widely different nature, one of them being highly poisonous.

White Caps Attack a Physician.

A dispatch from Martin's Ferry, Ohio, dated Dec. 27, 1888, says: At Hopedale, Harrison County, Christmas night, White Caps visited Dr. John Parkhill, a leading physician, and gave him a terrible thrashing. His errand-boy had been intoxicated, and the White Caps accused Parkhill of drugging him.

NEWS.

—Dr. Frederick A. Packard has removed to 259 South Fifteenth Street.

—Prof. Unverricht has accepted the Chair of Internal Medicine in the University of Dorpat.

—The Annual Reunion and Banquet of the Ex-Residents of the Pennsylvania Hospital was held Dec. 27, 1888.

—Dr. Carl Zeiss, of Jena, who is widely known as the maker of the Zeiss microscopes, has just died at the age of seventy-three years.

—Prof. Billroth has been elected President of the Imperial-Royal Society of Physicians of Vienna, in place of the late Prof. von Bamberger.

—The Montfiore Home for Chronic Invalids was opened in New York City Dec. 18. There are accommodations in it for 180 patients. It is non-sectarian.

—At an address delivered in Edinburgh recently by Sir Morell Mackenzie, the more prominent members of the medical profession in Edinburgh were conspicuous by their absence.

—Contagious diseases still prevail to a considerable extent in New York City. During the week ending Dec. 22, there were 241 cases of scarlet fever and 53 deaths; 374 cases of measles and 24 deaths; 144 cases of diphtheria and 49 deaths.

—Dr. Charles W. Drew, in a communication to the *Norwestern Lancet*, Dec., 1888, on food adulteration in the State of Minnesota, states that of 1084 samples of foodstuffs examined by him, 470 were found to be adulterated and 614 of good quality.

—Dr. George Homan, Medical Examiner of the St. Louis Police Department, states that the police of that city are peculiarly liable to pulmonary diseases. Experience justifies the expectation that about half of all who join the St. Louis police force and serve ten years will die of consumption soon after reaching forty years of age.

———————

A New Diathesis.—Dr. W. V. Morgan, of this city, recently attended a case of obstetrics in which there occurred *post-partum* hemorrhage. The nurse, who has picked up a few medical terms though her association with physicians, very innocently inquired of the doctor if he did not think the patient had a *hemorrhoidal diathesis.*—*Indiana Medical Journal.*

HUMOR.

Mrs. J. Browne Stone (who has just returned from Europe, to her daughter, who has staid at home)—"Good gracious, Emma! We must do something at once for your figure; it's getting as bad as the Venus of Milo's!"—*Puck.*

When to Imbibe.—Scene: Pharmacy in rural district. Enter typical "son of toil" hurriedly. Peasant: "Och, dochter, is it pizen oi've taken? Thry! Thry!" Chemist (smelling bottle): "Begor, Pat! it smells strongly of potheen." Pat: "Bedad, mebee it's meself brought yez the wrong cruiskeen." Gives it back. Then, pocketing the bottle, "Shure, Father Burke sez oi mustn't take any spirits, barrin' what I get frum the dochter, and amn't I doin' his biddin' entoirely? Top iv the mornin' t'ye, dochter, an' thank ye koindly."—*Chemist and Druggist.*

A Wide Distinction, Mind You.—Young physician (at a consultation)—"I have no hesitation in pronouncing the disease angina pectoris, complicated with muscular atrophy." Old physician—"You haven't, hey? Young man, when you have been practising forty years, you will have learned how to hesitate, sir. It is important, in a case of this kind, sir, to hesitate, and it is also more professional, sir." Young physician—"May I ask you, sir, what your opinion is of the disease?" Old physician (impressively)—"The disease, sir, is muscular atrophy, complicated with angina pectoris." Young physician (humbly)—"Yes, sir."—*Chicago Tribune.*

———————

OBITUARY.

JOSEPH L. BODINE, M.D.

Dr. Joseph L. Bodine, a well-known physician of Trenton, N. J., died Jan. 2, after an illness of nearly nine weeks. He was about forty-nine years of age. His father, the late Daniel B. Bodine, was Clerk in Chancery from 1851 to 1856, and about ten years ago Mayor of Trenton.

Dr. Bodine was a graduate of Princeton College, and in 1865 was graduated in medicine from the University of Pennsylvania. He subsequently served as resident physician at the Episcopal Hospital, Philadelphia. He was for a time a member of the State Sinking Fund Commission, and ex-Governor Abbett urged him to retain the office, owing to his conspicuous honesty and ability, but the Doctor's professional duties compelled him to insist upon the acceptance of his resignation.

THE

MEDICAL AND SURGICAL

REPORTER

No. 1663.   PHILADELPHIA, JANUARY 12, 1889.   VOL. LX.—No. 2.

CONTENTS:

LECTURE.[1]

FOODS FOR THE SICK.

BY MRS. S. T. RORER,

PRINCIPAL OF THE PHILADELPHIA COOKING SCHOOL.

(Specially reported for the MEDICAL AND SURGICAL
REPORTER.)

Milk is by far the most important food which we have to give to the sick, as it contains all the substances necessary for the support of the human body. No doubt many of the recipes which I shall speak of are well known; still those who attempt to follow them often fail from lack of attention to small details; so I would emphasize the importance of following the directions which I shall give implicitly, and especially of being sure to measure each ingredient used.

A doctor will rarely be called upon to

make these articles; but it is of the greatest importance for him to know exactly how to direct the person in attendance to prepare the food, and when prepared to be able to tell that it is made as desired. Where there is only one sick person to be provided for, it is wise to prepare small quantities of any food at one time, and in serving to be sure to have the food either hot or cold, and never lukewarm. When prepared, the same food should be presented at different times in different dishes, and uneaten food should never be allowed to remain in the sight of the patient.

Barley water.—Barley water is best prepared by taking one ounce of barley and covering it with one quart of boiling water; it is then to be boiled rapidly five minutes, and the water thrown away, as it has an objectionable color. Add a first boiled water—by this I mean water which has just come to the boiling point, and not that which has been drawn from the hot water faucet, or that which has been boiling on the fire for hours at a time. A first boiled water is cold water which has been heated

[1] Delivered at the University of Pennsylvania, November 21, 1888, and provided through the liberality of Dr. George Strawbridge.

rapidly until it boils and has not parted with its gases. Let the pot in which the barley and water have been placed simmer, not boil, gently two hours, strain, and it is ready for use.

Two thirds of milk and one third of barley water prepared in the above manner, make a most acceptable food, especially in typhoid fever, where we desire some starchy food.

Koumiss.—For koumiss mixed milk is the best, Alderney milk being too rich. Put one quart of sweet milk into a farina boiler, and stir constantly (over the fire?) until it has reached blood heat. Dissolve one quarter of a cake of compressed yeast in two tablespoonfuls of lukewarm water; stir the yeast until it is thoroughly dissolved. If you are unable to procure compressed yeast, two tablespoonfuls of liquid yeast may be used. Take one ounce of sugar (which is equal to two tablespoonfuls of sugar level to the brim) and dissolve it in two tablespoonfuls of water; stir over the fire until it boils, and then allow it to boil ten seconds; when you should have a perfectly clear syrup. Put the yeast into the milk and then add the syrup, stirring backward and forward, until they are thoroughly mixed.

Fill a quart bottle up to the neck with the mixture, and put in a tight fitting cork, which must be fastened down by means of a string; and keep the bottle in an upright position at a temperature of 70° F. for twelve hours; then in a temperature of 55° F., the bottle being placed on its side. The koumiss is ready for use in twenty-four hours; but patients often prefer it after standing forty-eight hours, as the taste is then slightly more acid.

Scalded milk.—There is a great difference between scalded and boiled milk. If we place milk in a farina boiler, no matter how hard we may boil the water underneath, the milk in the upper kettle will only be raised to a temperature of about 204° F., and this is not enough to boil milk. Scalded milk is often much more acceptable to a patient and not nearly as constipating as ordinary boiled milk. Put a quart of milk in a farina boiler and as soon as a scum of coagulated albumen floats on the surface the milk is scalded. In boiling milk the caseine which sinks to the bottom is apt to be burnt. I have known patients, who would become disgusted with boiled milk in a few days, to relish milk prepared in this way for months at a time.

Carrageen.—Take two pieces of Irish moss, thoroughly cleaned from any adherent sand and dirt, add some cold water, and let them soak five minutes; then wash, and allow to soak five minutes more in cold water, when the moss will have a soft, white look, and, having absorbed water, will be considerably increased in size. Scald one half pint of milk, and, after shaking any adherent water from the moss, drop it into the farina boiler. Stir well, and then cook, with the lid on the pot, for five minutes. Add one ounce of sugar. No flavoring extract is to be added unless especially ordered; but vanilla, wine, etc., may be added, or a sauce may be made and added to the jelly when cold. Strain through a sieve, and put into small moulds, which have been washed with cold water so as to prevent the jelly from adhering to the sides; then it is taken from the moulds and placed immediately on ice, or in a very cool place, and it will be ready for use in about one hour. It must be served very cold, or it will have a fishy taste. The quicker it is made, the better it is.

Milk punch.—Milk punch is made by taking two thirds of a tumbler full of milk and one half-ounce of sugar, and adding the amount of spirits ordered. The whole must be thoroughly shaken, with or without ice, in a wide mouthed bottle or a tin shaker; and then served in a clean tumbler. A little nutmeg grated on the top, makes the flavor more acceptable to some palates.

Egg-nog.—Egg-nog may be prepared with the whole egg, or with the yolk, or the white of the egg alone. If the whole egg is to be used, separate the white from the yolk and beat the white until it is light—not to so dry a froth, that it would stand alone. Then beat the yolk, and slowly add one half-cup of milk to it; put in some ice—not cracked too fine; add the white of the egg and one half an ounce of sugar, and beat until well mixed. Then add whiskey or brandy in quantities required, mix again, and serve at once.

If the white alone be used, mix as if making milk punch, but add from one to one-half ounce sherry, as this removes the taste of the white of the egg better than brandy or whiskey. Shake the whole as for milk punch. If correctly made there will be but little froth, the whole being of a light consistency. If the yolk alone be used, beat the yolk and add the milk slowly, beating all the time. Then add the sugar, ice, and spirits; and shake well.

Milk gruel.—Scald one half-pint of milk; add six good-sized raisins; and allow to stand five minutes. Take a table-spoonful of corn-starch and thoroughly mix with two tablespoonfuls of cold milk. Add this mixture to the scalded milk quickly, stirring backward and forward over the fire in a farina boiler, until it begins to thicken; then add one ounce of sugar, and let it cook one minute. Strain, and place in moulds in a cool place.

Beef-tea.—Great care must be used in the selecting of meat for beef-tea, and that part of the meat is to be used which contains the greatest amount of nourishment. The piece best adapted for this is the "sticking-piece" (that part of the neck where the knife is thrust through in killing the animal), as here there is the greatest amount of blood in the part. The worst piece is the tenderloin. If the sticking-piece cannot be obtained, take the round. It is indifferent whether you use the upper part, which is the tender part, or the under side.

Take one pound of meat which has been well freed from fat, and chop it as fine as possible; add one pint of *cold* water; stir well; and allow to stand in a cool place for two hours. The cold water is added to soften the fibres and extract the juices. If boiling water is added a film is coagulated on the outside, and no amount of boiling will make it tender or extract all the juices. Stir the beef-tea, as it is soaking, every little while. Put in a farina boiler; but do not let it boil. For seasoning, it is better to add six whole peppers than the ordinary ground pepper. A bay-leaf imparts an agreeable flavor, and may often be added with no harm to the patient. Salt is to be added just before taking from the fire, because if it be added sooner the fibres are hardened and the juices are prevented from coming out. The fat that rises to the surface is to be removed with small pieces of white blotting paper. Keep stirring till the red color is changed to a slight white tinge, which will occur in about fifteen minutes. Then cover the kettle for a few moments and strain, pressing hard to get all the juices out.

It is wise to prepare beef-tea fresh every day, and never to hurry its preparation. Beef-tea is to be served icy cold or very hot; and to prevent the tea from cooling in being carried from the fire to the sickroom, it is wise to serve it in a metal tea pot, pouring the beef-tea into a cup only when the room is reached. Never warm up more than you intend to use, and any quantity left over must not be poured back into the remainder of the tea. The fibrin settles to the bottom, therefore before re-warming, be sure that the vessel in which the beef-tea is kept, is well shaken When properly prepared, beef-tea should not have a cooked taste, like a soup, but should taste more like rare meat.

Clarified Beef-tea.—Take the shell of one egg and crush it in small pieces; add the white and a little water and beat until well mixed. Allow the beef-tea, prepared in the manner stated above, to come to a boil, and then add the shell and white of the egg. Allow the mixture to boil in a covered vessel for two minutes; and strain, and the dark colored beef-tea has given place to a clear light straw-colored liquid. This liquid is very stimulating and should not be given in more than two ounce doses at a time, or it may lead to dangerous symptoms from over stimulation.

Mutton Broth.—Mutton is less nutritious than beef, but is more easily digested, and can often be given when the latter should not be introduced into the system. The sticking-piece is the best part to use. Take one and one-half pounds of meat and one and one-half pints of water, and two tablespoonfuls of previously washed rice (if necessary the rice may be omitted) put on a slow fire, and allow to come to the boiling point; then remove any fat that may come to the surface, and allow to simmer for three hours. Keep the pan covered so as to prevent the evaporation of the water; strain; and re-warm as needed. Celery salt can often be added, and this imparts a nice flavor. The milky color is due to the rice.

Chicken Stock.—The legs and wing of the chicken make the best stock, as the sinews and bone in them contain gelatinous materials. The breast of the same fowl can often be saved and cooked for the patient in some other way. Take a one-pound chicken, which has been cut in large pieces and the bones cracked, and one pint of water, and allow it to soak three-quarters of an hour. Then simmer in a closed pot for two hours. Salt and pepper are then to be added, and the whole strained, and removed at once to a cold place. The fat is to be removed when cold, by a spoon. The solid stock as thus prepared can be used for food, or by adding water and heating, and afterward cooling, it may be served as a drink, or it may be given warm, in the form of soup. with or without rice.

Wine Whey.—The caseine can be removed from milk by acids, such as lemon juice, tamarind juice, wine, etc. Take one half-pint of milk; raise it just to the boiling point; add one-half as much sherry or madeira;

and remove it from the fire. Strain through a fine sieve or several thicknesses of cheese cloth. Do not squeeze, as all the curd must be removed—otherwise, it would be more indigestible than plain milk. Wine whey must not have too white a color, as this is a sign that the milk has boiled. Serve warm or cold, slightly seasoned.

Beef-tea with Yolk of an Egg.—Take one gill of clarified beef-tea, scalding hot, and thoroughly mix the yolk of an egg with a small amount of the liquid; pour quickly back into the pot; stir; and serve at once.

Cream Beef-tea.—One of the nicest and most nutritious dishes for the sick that I know of is prepared as follows: To one ounce of well made beef-tea, add an equal volume of barley-water; then heat, but do not boil the mixture. Add the whole to a half ounce of cream or to the yolk of one egg, stirring well. Heat for a minute, and serve at once.

Boiled Eggs.—To boil eggs so that they can be most easily digested, bring some water to the boiling point, drop the eggs in, and remove the vessel from the fire. Allow to stand five minutes, and when served the whites will be found cooked, but as soft as the yolk.

Scraped Beef.—Prepare two ounces of scraped beef by scraping a piece of beef in the direction of the fibres, and not across them. Put on a piece of bread one inch square, being sure that the meat is well pressed into the pores of the bread. Dust with salt, and toast both sides for a minute over a hot fire.

COMMUNICATIONS.

IDENTITY OF SCARLATINA AND DIPHTHERIA.

BY I. N. TRENT, M.D.,
COLUMBUS, O.

A few years ago the medical journals were teeming with arguments for and against the identity of diphtheria and croup. While the argument in favor of this doctrine seemed inconclusive to me, I wondered at the silence of the profession on the present subject. And while I wondered and waited the arguments and evidence kept piling up till the conclusion was irresistible.

The fact that they have so long been considered two diseases is no reason why the truth of it should not be questioned. Error may exist for centuries and when it is detected it is hard for us to believe we could have been deceived so long. For example, Galen taught that the blood passed directly from the right side to the left side of the heart through the pits he observed between the columnæ carnæ, which pits he supposed were the openings of foramina. This idea no one dared deny and "it stood undisputed for a thousand years and three centuries more." How strange it seems to us now that such a glaring error could be undetected under the eye of the medical profession for those thirteen hundred years.

Diphtheria meaning "a skin or membrane" is named from its gross pathological lesion. *Scarlatina*—"a deep red," is named from its prominent symptom. But these names signify nothing, for we have diseases named from the progress they make, as *cancer* referring to the movements of an animal; or from the actions of a patient as *chorea*—"a dance," and so on with no rule for the names we use. This is wrong and no doubt in time will be so changed that from the name of a disease its pathological lesion may be known. But what's in a name? "A rose by any other name would smell as sweet."

Thus, with no rule to guide in the application of names, it is not strange that one disease should receive two or more names as different observers were impressed by different pathological lesions, or different conditions, or symptoms.

So with the two diseases under consideration; one is named as we have seen from its pathological lesion, the other from its prominent symptom; but this difference of name does not prove that the diseases are *two*.

If, on the other hand, it can be shown that they are alike in etiology, pathology, symptoms and sequelæ, and then cases cited where one disease is generated from exposure to the other, it must be conceded that their identity is highly probable.

This I shall attempt to do by a careful research of the literature of the subject, and by the report of a few cases from the records of a private country practice, where every facility is present for knowing the source of infection. And what we have to say as to pathology, cause, symptoms, or sequela, is substantiated by these works and again by the cases recorded.

As to *Pathology.*—Both are infectious. Both are but slightly contagious. Both are diseases of the glandular structure, affecting regularly the adenoid tissue; the adenitis being a part of the disease and not a complication. Both present a croupous inflammation of the mucous membrane of the tonsils and pharynx, often extending to that of the stomach and bowels. And, according to Drs. Delafield and Prudden, "such a croupous inflammation in diphtheria is anatomically identical with croupous inflammation due to trauma and *other* causes."

Admitting then on their authority that the throat trouble is the same, it behooves us to show that the causes are the same. This we can not do, but far less can it be proved that they are different. And as to their etiology, we know nothing positive of their real cause, but judging from its effects and mode of behavior, it is generally conceded to be a micro-organism. The micro-organism of these diseases has not yet been subjected to the crucial tests of always finding it present in the lesion, of isolating it by a series of pure cultures, and, lastly, of reproducing the disease by inoculation with these isolated cultures. Prof. Palmer says: "The specific character of diphtheria, its dependence on a poison, cannot be doubted. But the positive character of that poison has not been demonstrated, and its mode of action in producing such serious results is unknown." The same may be said of scarlatina. While acknowledging the want of knowledge as to the exact germ, we must all have been impressed by the similarity of its workings in the two diseases.

In both it acts best. or the susceptibility is greatest, between the ages of two and seven years. In both the period of incubation varies from a few hours to seven or eight days, with an average of four days. In both the micro-organism clings to life with great tenacity, each disease having been contracted by persons occupying rooms where many months before there had been patients affected by one or the other disease. In both it is often impossible to trace the source of infection. Hence we say both are sporadic, if not spontaneous. In both the contagium not only is carried directly from the sick to the well, but it may also be communicated through a third party, or through fomites in which it may lie dormant but preserve its vitality. Both attack and complicate wounds. In both one attack produces immunity against future attacks as a rule, while recurrent attacks in either are not very infrequent.

In symptoms both vary from the mildest to the most malignant type. Both have a common seat of croupous inflammation, namely, the mucous membrane of the fauces and nasal passages. Both agree in the profound toxæmia and prostration in graver cases. In both there is an eruption.

In *sequelæ* they agree by both having the adenitis and nephritis, which are considered as a regular part of the disease, but which some consider as complications. J. Solis Cohen calls especial attention to the physical resemblance between the pseudo-membranous casts in diphtheria and the desquamated epidermis of scarlatina. In both we have paralysis of the muscles of the throat.

Now, having shown these striking similarities as conceded by the authors quoted above, I present a few cases in which most of the points of identity are illustrated. I well know I am likely to meet the thought, whether expressed or not, that I have been mistaken in my diagnosis, and that the cases I called diphtheria were simply scarlatina without the eruption.

While I claim to have ordinary observing powers, and to be capable of making a differential diagnosis, as it is generally called, I must fortify my position by stating that every case but one was seen by one or two other good practitioners of many years' standing, practitioners whose opinions stand unquestioned where they are known.

Case I.—Myrtle H.—After complaining a few hours the patient was seized with a general convulsion. I saw her in half an hour and found her in a state of great prostration, with the twitching of muscles and the rolling of the eye-balls so characteristic of approaching convulsions Her temperature was 104°, which steadily increased to 106½° just before death, which occurred in twenty-four hours from the time of first convulsion. When she was first seen there was a croupous membrane on both the tonsils and on the posterior wall of pharynx. At this time considerable swelling of the glands of the neck was present, which steadily increased. An eruption was to be seen, dim but sufficiently distinct, when taken with the other symptoms, to warrant a diagnosis of scarlatina. a diagnosis which was confirmed by Dr. Clarke, who saw her shortly before her death.

No history of contagion nor of infection could be obtained; her two brothers and her sister did not take the disease, though they were in the room during her sickness.

No other case occurred for 10 days, when I was called to see

Case II, Bert W., 12 years old, who lived three miles from the first patient. I saw the patient on the second day of his sickness, and was informed that a diagnosis of diphtheria had been made the day before by another physician. The throat did look like it, but a further examination revealed a typical scarlatinal eruption on the body and limbs. The case ran a favorable course, ending in profuse desquamation followed by general œdema. The only source of infection was association with the man who held Case I in his arms while the patient was in her first convulsion, ten days before.

Case III.—In five days after Bert was attacked, Worden K., who was living in the family with Bert, was stricken down and had a typical case of scarlet fever.

Case IV.—Mrs W., the mother of Bert, in a week from the beginning of the latter's sickness was attacked by fever and sore throat, with a deposit on both tonsils and pharynx, and every symptom to make a case of diphtheria. No eruption was present at any time.

Case V.—Clint W., the brother of Bert, in two weeks after the latter's illness was attacked by chill, vomiting, fever, and all premonitory symptoms of scarlatina, which subsequently developed.

Case VI.—Lanie W. was a playmate of Bert whom Lanie had visited a week before he was attacked, and while Bert was in the midst of his fever. When first seen he had a temperature of 102½°, and a typical diphtheritic deposit in the throat. No eruption was then to be seen, nor did any appear afterward. He was said to have had scarlatina nine years before.

Case VII.—In five days after Lanie was taken sick his sister, Bessie W., was taken with a chill, and in eighteen hours was thoroughly covered with a scarlatinous eruption, with a diffuse mottled redness of the throat, but no deposit. In due time desquamation came on and the muscles of the throat were partly paralyzed for several months, to such a degree that she swallowed with difficulty, and articulation was at first impossible. Both gradually improved.

Case VIII.—Charles R., a neighbor to W.'s family, where Bert, Clint, and others lived, did not himself come in contact with the sick, but from the beginning of sickness in this family his wife visited them often. In eight days from the beginning of Bert's attack this patient was stricken down with what I pronounced diphtheria, a diagnosis confirmed by Dr. Clarke.

The next group of patients was three miles distant from the first group just reported, and had no communication with them whatever.

Case I.—While visiting Myrtle (Case I of the first group) a messenger came hurriedly saying that his child had croup. I had seen the patient, Opal W., two days before, at which time she had a temperature of 100°, with a slight deposit confined to the tonsils. At that time she had a dull, listless expression, which I was informed had existed for a week. Knowing this much about the case I at once concluded the croup was due to extension downward of the false membrane I had seen two days before. Upon visiting her I found her very hoarse, with a pseudo-membrane covering both tonsils, the pharynx, and extending high up on the soft palate and as low down as I could see. I at once made a diagnosis of diphtheria, with a fatal prognosis. Dr. Franks saw her with me in the evening of the same day, and confirmed the diagnosis. At this evening visit the hoarseness was nearly gone, but in no other respect was she better. Next morning her temperature was 104°, and she was fast sinking. Diarrhœa had set in during the night. Fluids regurgitated through the nostrils when she attempted to swallow, showing paralysis of the muscles of the throat.

The source of infection in this case could not be found, but may be conjectured as follows: The patient and Myrtle—the first patient of the first group—had been taken to a large funeral three weeks before. As both were attacked about the same time, and as this had been the only place at which either had been from home, it seems probable that both were infected at this funeral, though one died of scarlatina and the other of diphtheria.

Case II.—Five days after Opal died her brother, Claude, was seen with a characteristic diphtheritic deposit in the throat, and all the symptoms which go to make up a case of diphtheria. No eruption appeared and he made a good recovery.

Case III.—The night before Opal died, Mrs. C. attended her, holding her in her lap. Without changing her clothes she went home among her own children. In a week Ed. C. was attacked. In twenty-four hours he was thoroughly covered with the eruption of scarlet fever, which ran a severe course, but ended in recovery after an abscess had formed on each side of the neck.

Case IV.—A week after Ed. was attacked his sister Alma was attacked with a sore throat which looked like that of diphtheria; no eruption was ever seen.

In another family consisting of father, mother, and five children, the five children had well-marked scarlet fever, while the mother had as severe and as well-marked an attack of diphtheria as I ever saw recovered from. The false membrane covered the tonsils and pharynx and extended up over the soft palate and out on the hard palate to near the incisor teeth. She was exposed to no infection except from her children with scarlet fever.

This family had no communication with either group of patients reported above.

In addition to my own cases, I offer a few from Dr. Mendenhall, of Woodford Co , Ill. He says: " A young man who had been West came home sick. I saw him the day after his arrival and found him suffering with diphtheria. He had been boarding in a family in which one child had died of this disease. This young man recovered, and his sister, two years younger, was then attacked with diphtheria and had a very hard struggle with the disease. Before she recovered her two younger sisters, five and seven years old respectively, were attacked with scarlatina, the younger one dying. There had been neither scarlatina nor diphtheria in the neighborhood up to that time. Immediately afterward I treated in that neighborhood four cases of scarlatina and nine of diphtheria. The original case was one of diphtheria, and the first two patients with scarlatina were in the house with it. Undoubtedly the scarlatina was developed from contagion of diphtheria."

Dr. J. B. Clarke, of Economy, Ind., to whom I referred as seeing some of my patients, writes: " I am quite willing to be quoted as confirming your diagnosis in the cases to which you refer. I have observed for many years the close relation between diphtheria and scarlatina, and believe them to be identical. A number of times when scarlatina was prevailing epidemically, I have had in the same family well-marked cases of scarlatina and of diphtheria. I have never known an epidemic of scarlatina without quite a good deal of diphtheria in the same locality. I have no doubt of the identity of the two diseases."

In the transactions of the Chicago Medical Society, Nov. 16, 1885, I find the following: Dr. Carter mentions the fact that simple cases of tonsillitis are often accompanied or followed by diphtheria or scarlatina among other members of the same family. Dr. Quine says: " Often one member of a family, probably the first one attacked, exhibits plainly-marked features of simple follicular tonsillitis, and those who sicken afterward exhibit the phenomena of diphtheria or, less frequently, those of scarlatina."

Dr. Stevenson relates a case in which a child took scarlatina from its mother who had tonsillitis. The child died and the Doctor says: "This is the first case in which I ever suspected that a benign form of tonsillitis might reproduce a malignant form."

Dr. Angear, at the same meeting, comes nearer advocating the doctrine of identity when he says: "We can readily imagine a robust, healthy child, with strong resistance to morbid influences, and especially that of diphtheria, on exposure would have simple tonsillitis; but suppose his brother, with strong susceptibility, is exposed to the same morbid influence; he will develop a case of undoubted diphtheria.

"In this house we have tonsillitis and our neighbor severe diphtheria. By remembering these facts, we shall see that it is, or may be, all the same morbid influence here and yonder—here, recovery in a few days; there, death in a few hours."

I have shown by the case of Bert that scarlatina may be conveyed by a third party from one with scarlatina ; and by Charles R. that diphtheria was carried from scarlatina ; and by Ed. C., that scarlatina may be carried from diphtheria.

From Bert, who had scarlatina, two cases of scarlatina and three of diphtheria developed ; from Lanie, with diphtheria, his sister contracted scarlatina; from Opal, with diphtheria, her brother contracted diphtheria, and Ed. C., scarlatina; from Ed., his sister contracted diphtheria. Opal, with diphtheria, had paralysis of the muscles of the throat, which also occurred in the case of Bessie, sick with scarlatina.

Let me insist that when I say diphtheria I mean this dreaded disease, and not every affection of the throat in which there is an exudation ; and that I rule out all cases of simple and follicular tonsillitis, which are so often classed as diphtheria by a class of practitioners who desire the reputation of curing all cases of diphtheria. Another thing I wish to emphasize is the inability to trace the source of infection in city patients, and the reliability of an investigation of this matter by a country practitioner. For parents in the country can tell every place to which the child has been for six months, and also who has been at the house, and almost everyone who has been within a mile of the patient for the same length of time.

Knowing this and having my diagnoses confirmed by such reputable physicians, and my ideas corroborated by such careful country practitioners as I have mentioned, and the, to me, unanswerable argument presented by the cases recorded, I am forced to the conclusion that scarlatina and diphtheria are very, very similar, if not identical.

503 Oak Street.

TYPHOID FEVER.

BY J. A. LONG, M.D.,
LONG'S MILLS, TENN.

Since Feb. 4, 1888—the date of my short article on typhoid fever in the REPORTER— I have witnessed a remarkable endemic of typhoid fever, in Polk County, Tennessee. In seeing, diagnosticating, and treating fevers for more than forty years, I never met with so puzzling a group of symptoms before in my practice.

The fever district was about six miles long, by three wide — lying between the Hiwassee River (a tributary of the Tennessee) and Chilhowee Mountain, a part of the Allegheny range. This section of country is mainly level or slightly undulating, and interspersed with basins of water in wet seasons, like the latter part of the past summer and fall. The soil is poor and sandy, and is mainly drained by three small streams which take their rise at the base of the mountains, running a little south of west across the fever-stricken section, and emptying into the Hiwassee River. The streams are quite subject to overflow, spreading over a considerable amount of low lands, depositing a quantity of filth and mixed soils, in various portions of this particular section of country; in wet seasons this part of the country is mainly cultivated in cotton by renters, some of whom are colored people, nearly all of them living in old, dilapidated log-houses, with a great many small out-houses, in a filthy condition. Near the river there are some large, well-ventilated, and comfortable dwellings; in which also the fever prevailed to a considerable extent. The water supply comes mostly from shallow wells, not in the best condition.

The disease was confined to persons in the prime of life—none, I believe, under ten, or over thirty or thirty-five years of age. The onset of the disease was invariably slow, insidious, and tedious; the patients moped around for some days, or even weeks, before being confined to their beds, complaining of nothing but weakness, and indisposed to mental or physical exertion. One of the first symptoms worthy of note after the patients were confined to bed, was sick stomach and vomiting of bilious matter. This latter symptom, in some cases, was quite troublesome and intractable—fully as much so as in bilious remitting fever—and was accompanied with a bilious diarrhœa. The morning remissions were pretty well defined, and seemed to be controlled by the use of quinine ; but this drug had little or no influence upon the regular course of the disease. The coat on the tongue would peel off, and again reappear, as in typical cases of typhoid fever. The tongue was not so pointed, nor its edges and tip so clean and red as is usual in typhoid fever. The pulse was quick and small, with a well-marked reacting beat, even when the patient was perspiring well from the use of quinine. It would range from 90 to 100 beats in a minute in mild cases, and from 100 to 120 in grave cases.

The range of temperature in all cases that came under my observation, was in proportion to the gravity of the case. The duration of the disease was from four to ten weeks in cases of recovery ; and the fatal cases were from three to five weeks in duration.

Abdominal symptoms.—A tympanitic state of the bowels was not common, in the cases I saw ; the bowels seemed flat, and rather hard, very sore on pressure, and especially if pressure was made over the right iliac region. The bowels had to be controlled throughout the entire course of the disease ; the color of the evacuations was yellow, and dark, and they had a strong bilious odor. Epistaxis and hemorrhage from the bowels were seen in many cases. The latter symptom was probably induced in some of the cases by the use of too frequent, or strong purgatives, as there were several physicians in the fever-stricken district entertaining very different views of diagnosis and treatment.

The disease was diagnosticated, by the various practitioners who saw it, to be nearly every kind of fever known to the medical profession. I think most practitioners, seeing one of these cases early in its onset, would have been inclined to call the disease grave bilious remittent fever, and more especially if they ignored, or paid little or no attention to, the tediousness of the onset. The impression made upon my mind, in seeing the first case, was that I had a grave case of bilious remittent fever to contend with, strongly marked with a *typhoid type :* and I remained twenty-four hours with the patient watching the action of medicine, and left undecided as to the real nature of the case, and impatiently waited the further developing of symptoms.

On my next visit I saw plainly I had a case of typhoid fever in a person with a malarial diathesis—what some practitioners call "*typho-malarial fever.*"

I stated in an article on typhoid fever, published in the *Augusta Medical and Surgical Journal*, about the year 1854 or 1855, when the late lamented Dr. Eve was its Editor, that where typhoid fever prevailed, malarial fevers were uncommon, and *vice versâ;* and I have had no cause to change my opinion until the present endemic occurred. This is the first time I ever witnessed a typhoid fever endemic or epidemic, or even sporadic cases in a district in which malarial fevers were prevalent. Others I have no doubt have a different experience; especially in malarial districts of old settled countries. There can be little doubt that the poisons of malarial and typhoid fevers are as essentially different as are the poisons of small-pox and typhoid fever, or of any one of the specific diseases. I have examined as faithfully as I could, with the limited means at my command, into the cause or causes of typhoid fever; and in this section of country have certainly traced them to *filth;* such as is found in old, damp cellars, filthy drinking-water, cesspools, old filthy out-houses, and accumulated about old farm-houses and outbuildings. I could illustrate these facts by the recital of many cases. I think the facts are as well established as that so-called malaria produces periodical fevers. It is well known by all observing medical practitioners who have many years' experience, that the home of periodical fevers is in newly settled countries; and that of typhoid fever is in old settled places. This view of the subject does not limit malarial fevers to new settled districts or typhoid fever to old settled ones; but as a rule what I have stated is the case.

The belief that different kinds of microbes in malarial and typhoid fevers, develope different groups of symptoms and require altogether different medicines, as germicides, seems to have brought us no nearer to successful treatment in either form of fever; nor do I think it ever will. While I am willing to admit the fact, of the finding of different kinds of micro-organisms in the various diseases of the human body, I cannot believe that they are the cause of disease, but look upon them rather as its *product.*

My reason for diagnosticating the fever of this endemic as typhoid is this: that the remarkable group of symptoms which makes up the picture of typhoid fever was clearly seen throughout its entire course. Notwithstanding the sick stomach, the vomiting of bile, the bilious stools, the absence of tympanites in many cases, the fact that the tongue was not very characteristic, and that there were pretty well defined morning remissions in the fever apparently yielding to quinine, obscured the diagnosis. We had the tedious and insidious onset, bleeding from the bowels, epistaxis, constant diarrhœa throughout the entire course, soreness of the bowels, especially over the right iliac region, attended with a gurgling sound on pressure, a quick nervous reacting pulse, even when sweating was free; and the length of time in running its course even in those cases that progressed to a favorable termination. The muttering delirium so characteristic of typhoid fever was not well marked; the mind as a rule was clearer but slow and dull. This feature was so striking that I made it a practice to inquire after the natural turn of mind, and speech, when the patient was well.

I have said nothing about the *rose spots,* because I saw none of the patients before the end of the third week, and I found only what I took to be a faded eruption, but was not positive as to its existence.

I have but little to say on the subject of treatment, as I saw no patients but such as were far advanced in the disease—one of them, a negro girl, died from hemorrhage of the bowels. I saw one patient, who had been sick for seven weeks; who had had but little attention or treatment; she was treated in a mild conservative way with a proper course of diet, and stimulants, and she got up at the end of ten weeks. Others that I saw were slowly convalescing. I saw the last patient about November 30. I failed to meet the family physician, and, as the patient was doing well enough, I only advised following the direction given by his regular medical attendant, and that the patient should not be in too great a hurry about leaving his bed.

The fact that these attacks have extended into the winter months is confirmatory of the diagnosis of typhoid fever.

Finally, I would like to say that it seems to me we ought to have more help from our fellow-practitioners in regard to the matter of fevers, and less on gynecology. I cannot see why a practitioner is not entitled to as much credit for diagnosticating, and successfully treating a grave case of fever of any kind, as if he had performed a successful laparotomy.

JABORANDI.

BY J. B. CARRELL, M.D.,

HATBORO, PA.

In conversation with physicians, I find that the great value of this drug in the cure of disease is not fully appreciated, and for this reason I wish to speak of it.

The plant is found in Brazil, and its botanical name is *Pilocarpus pennatifolius*. The only alkaloid of value so far found in it is pilocarpine; others have been found, but they are of little use to the therapeutist.

As an introduction I shall state that the more the drug is employed the better it will be liked; at least such is my experience. The class of diseases in which it should be used is of the active or sthenic type, such as congestion of the lungs, pleura, and of other organs, in which are found great dryness of the skin and a high grade of fever. Its value in the early stages of high inflammatory conditions is very marked, and justly deserves a place in every physician's list of medicines. If an infusion of from sixty to ninety grains of jaborandi, or an equivalent of its active alkaloid, pilocarpine, be given to an adult, profuse perspiration will be produced in from thirty minutes to an hour, and will continue for several hours. The salivary glands will act quite freely, and if the saliva is swallowed, nausea and vomiting will in all probability be produced. This nausea, according to the observations of some, seems to be due to the irritating character of the saliva coming in contact with the stomach. Dr. Bruen, of Philadelphia, asserts that the dialysate of pilocarpine will not produce sickness of the stomach. The pulse and respiration are usually quickened and the temperature for a time may be slightly increased, but will soon begin to fall; at least it has done so in my experience. After the sweating has ceased, the patient is more or less exhausted, and should on no account be allowed to leave the bed unless he is well covered, in order to prevent chill and the syncope which may result there-·from.

The nasal and lachrymal secretions are very generally increased, and Gubler has noted diarrhœa. Ringer and other experimenters have not found this present. There is sometimes contraction of the pupils and even disturbance of vision. Ringer found children very insusceptible, but such has not been my experience either in children or in adults; the dose is not always constant,

that is, free diaphoresis may be produced in one person with ten drops of the fluid extract given every hour, for three or four hours, while in another double this amount may be required, or even quadruple to produce the same effect. The sweat produced by jaborandi is often enormous in quantity. In cases of nephritis the loss by weight after injections of pilocarpine, according to Dr. Zelentski, of St. Petersburg, was 514 grammes or more than one pound; 306 grammes were lost by perspiration and 208 by salivation. The elimination of urea is said to be especially marked. For this reason the drug is valuable especially in destructive kidney diseases. The cause of the excessive secretion is a direct action upon either the gland-cells or the peripheral nerve endings, more probably the former. On account of its certain and powerful action as a diaphoretic it has taken rank as the most reliable remedy of its class, and has greatly extended the use of diaphoretics. It will be well now to take up its use in the various diseases.

In the early stages of pneumonia, that is, in the congestive stage—characterized by sudden rise of temperature, throbbing pulse, dryness of the skin, hurried and difficult respiration, chilliness, etc.—where my esteemed friend, Dr. Hiram Corson, would employ the lance and cold pack, I will, with equal confidence, put my patient to bed and produce free diaphoresis by the administration of jaborandi. With the appearance of free sweating there will be an amelioration of all the violent symptoms and a speedy and perfect cure within three or four days. A temperature of 105° in congestion of the lungs has, time and time again in my practice, been reduced to 99.5° in twenty-four hours.

While my friend, Dr. Corson, applies the lance to relieve the active congestion, I can produce as decided an effect with the drug under consideration. What has been said of congestion of the lungs can be said also of pleurisy. I am not writing from fancy but from experience.

Dr. J. M. Da Costa says that the pilocarpine treatment of erysipelas grows upon him, and, in thus speaking, my own views are expressed. It may be well to narrate one or two cases described by this eminent physician: "In a case of erysipelas of the face and leg the patient was given one-sixth of a grain of pilocarpine by hypodermic injection; two hours later he was given one-eighth of a grain and was purged with a mercurial pill. He was then ordered twenty drops of the fluid extract of jaborandi every two hours, when he *did* sweat, and the disease was checked in twelve hours after the first hypodermic ; the temperature went down to normal and he made a rapid convalescence from that time. He is now taking twenty drops of the fluid extract thrice daily ; he still sweats, and his urine has increased from two and one-half to three and one-half pints in the twenty-four hours. The drug did not have sialogogue effects, nor did it seem to have any action on the heart. The second case is one of erysipelas of the nose. On admission the temperature was 103.5°. After the injection of pilocarpine it fell to 100°, later to 99°, and has never since been up to the fever temperature.''

A week ago I was called to see a young man with erysipelas of the hand and arm, which were much swollen and very hot and painful. The temperature was 104°, pulse 120, with chilliness and general febrile symptoms. I gave him twenty drops of fluid extract of jaborandi every hour and a half alternately with three drops of tincture of aconite and one-half drop of extract of ipecac. In twenty-four hours the temperature had fallen to 99.5°, and all the unpleasant symptoms had disappeared. Locally warm flaxseed poultices and laudanum were applied. The treatment was completed by giving five drops of tincture of iron and two drops of Fowler's solution three times daily. I could mention many similar cases, but they would make needless repetition. If there is a tendency to exhaustion it is well to combine nux vomica and digitalis as heart tonics. By this course exhaustion will be obviated and the good effects of the drug secured.

Jaborandi has been largely employed for the relief of dropsies, especially the dropsies resulting from the destruction of kidney substance. In uræmic poisoning it is the most efficient remedy at our command. It is certainly of great value in either acute or chronic Bright's disease. The œdematous collections formed in this disease can be relieved by the use of jaborandi. It is asserted confidently by some 'that it acts in a special manner upon the kidneys, helping to free the tubes when they are obstructed with epithelial or fibrous *débris.* In the acute cases, in conjunction with proper diet, it may bring about a cure. The word ''cure,'' says a writer, should be used in this connection in the same sense in which we apply the word cure to any other disease in which organic changes have taken place ;

or, in other words, the cure would consist in assisting nature to stop a morbid process by throwing off effete material, and by placing a barrier between diseased and healthy structure. The principle upon which we base our action is the benefit to be derived from *rest* in the relief and cure of inflammations. By the use of jaborandi the skin performs double duty—its own work and also that of its co-laborer, the kidneys. The latter are rested and inflammatory action is suspended. Wherever and whenever we can, we should place inflamed tissue at rest. That which cannot be cured with medication may without medicine be cured by rest.

In scarlatina, jaborandi is a most valuable remedy. It can do valiant service. Its well-known action upon the skin makes it of especial use in all of the exanthematous diseases. I have used it in a great many cases of scarlatina with the happiest results, and cannot help thinking that many cases of nephritis might be obviated by its use.

Little has been said of the value of jaborandi as a galactagogue. The mammary glands in many respects resemble the action of sudoriferous glands, and in cases in which the milk supply has failed, or is failing, it can be increased and redeveloped by the administration of jaborandi. This has been conclusively proved by numerous experiments. To obtain the galactagogue effect jaborandi should not be given in sufficient doses to effect free diaphoresis. In case of scanty supply, daily doses are required for ten or twelve days. If there is complete cessation of the milk secretion, it will be necessary to administer the drug every three or four hours, until gentle diaphoresis is established, and then keep up daily doses until the secretion is fully established. The patient, as is usually the case, will be run down, and should be built up with tonics and a generous diet. On January 5, 1885, I delivered a multipara of a fine boy baby. I saw her on the 6th, 7th, and 9th. At the last date the milk secretion was established and the temperature was normal. On the 11th, I was summoned and found her temperature 105°, pulse 130, severe headache, chilliness, coated tongue, dry burning skin ; secretion of milk stopped, and breasts extremely sensitive and inflamed. The symptoms were as bad as one could wish if a test were needed for a drug-trial. I ordered free doses of jaborandi every two hours until free sweating had taken place. In three or four hours the dry hot skin was moist and in six hours she was in a dripping sweat. Small doses of quinine were given every four hours and also five drop doses of extract of jaborandi. Twenty-four hours after the first dose of jaborandi the temperature had fallen to 99.5°, the milk was re-established and every unfavorable symptom had become favorable. This is one of several cases I have treated in this manner, and the result has been highly satisfactory.

The action of pilocarpine and atropine are directly antagonistic, so that in cases of belladonna poisoning jaborandi should be employed as the physiological antidote I have not had the opportunity of testing their antidotal effects, but others have had, and in the cases I have seen reported the results have been favorable.

Dr. H. C. Yarrow, of Washington, D. C., has been recently experimenting with the view of determining the value of certain reputed antidotes to serpent venom. All of them in his hands have thus far proved useless with the exception of the fluid extract of jaborandi, which seems to possess antidotal powers—at least in the case of mammals; but upon fowls it appears to have no such effect. He has given hypodermically to rabbits fourfold lethal doses of crotalus venom, and then by the administration of thirty-five drops of the fluid extract of jaborandi he has prevented any serious results. Dr. Josso, of Paris, reports a case of viper bite cured with an infusion of jaborandi leaves.

While much more could be written on the subject, I think what I have already said will awaken an interest in this very valuable drug, and am sure that its powers and uses will be appreciated if they are fully tested.

—Dr. Ira Russell, of Winchendon, Mass., died December 19, of pneumonia, at the age of 74 years. He was graduated from the Medical Department of the New York University in 1844.

—The Tennessee *State Board of Health Bulletin* for November, says: The number of localities reporting the existence of typhoid fever each month in Tennessee demands of the local health authorities immediate and careful investigation. No water or soil contamination, no typhoid fever, is the axiomatic teaching of sanitary science, and consequently no weary weeks of suffering and prostration, no long nights of anxious watching by friends, and no untimely deaths, whereas hundreds are now annually consigned to premature graves by this preventable scourge.

ODD COURSE OF A MISSILE.

BY E. H. PARKER, M.D.,

POUGHKEEPSIE, N. Y.

Very few persons practise surgery many years without meeting with instances in which missiles, such as bullets, pieces of shells and so on, take curious and often inexplicable courses after striking the bodies of living animals. In the following instance I was as much surprised as in any case with which I have met. In preparing for a frolic, a young man made a cannon by taking the long axle-box from the worn-out wheel of a horse-rake, plugging one end thoroughly, and boring a touch-hole. After loading this cannon, he fired it, and it being made of cast iron, and only one-fourth of an inch thick, it naturally blew to pieces. One of the fragments struck him. When I was called to see him, some thirteen hours later, it was evident that the missile was just underneath the skin of his neck, its upper end just touching the left mastoid process, and the only "solution of continuity" to be found was over the sternum, three-fourths of an inch below the upper end of that bone, and extending a little to the left of the median line. This wound was parallel to the upper margin of the sternum, was three-fourths of an inch long, and one-sixteenth of an inch wide. There was no discoloration of the skin at any point except that of entrance, which was a little bloody.

Making my preparations to meet any possible injury to the blood-vessels of the neck, I cut down upon, and removed, the fragment. Some bits of clothing were found just above the missile. There was no bleeding, and the patient recovered entirely in a few days.

The piece of iron weighs nearly two ounces (twenty-one grains short), is three inches long, one-fourth of an inch thick, and from three-fourths to seven-eighths of an inch on its convex surface for half its length, and then tapers to three-eighths of an inch. The other end, which was against the mastoid process, is broken almost square off, and is three-fourths of an inch across. All the edges of the fracture-lines are sharp and cutting. The convex surface of the fragment was next the skin. It has always puzzled me to understand how this piece of iron got through the small wound over the sternum, and from that point to the mastoid process, without breaking the clavicle and without doing any serious damage.

SOCIETY REPORTS.

MEDICAL SOCIETY OF THE COUNTY OF NEW YORK.

Stated Meeting, December 24, 1888.

The President, ALEXANDER S. HUNTER, M.D., in the chair.

DR. RALPH L. PARSONS read the history of

A Case of Cerebral Syphilis,

more for the purpose, he said, of emphasizing the importance of early and long-continued anti-syphilitic treatment than because of special interest in the case itself. The man, forty-five years old, of good constitution, married, came under his care with symptoms of loss of appetite, sleeplessness, depressed physical and mental condition, worry about business affairs, and fear of softening of the brain. His friends attributed his condition to worry over the sickness of his children. He began to have attacks of impending fainting, during which his ideas became confused, and he had difficulty of expressing his ideas. Before the attacks he was irritable. In spite of anti-syphilitic treatment, under which he improved for a time, he became worse, had attacks first of *petit mal*, later of *grand mal*, and finally died of symptoms due to syphilis of the brain. There had been no history of impure connection. But before Dr. Parsons saw him there had been a suspicious intractable ulcer of the lip. There was also evidence of syphilis, in sores on the scalp and in an eruption on the arm. It seemed probable that the cerebral symptoms might have been averted by early and long continued treatment.

DR. NATHAN S. ROBERTS read a paper on the

Treatment of Diseases of the Nose by the General Practitioner,

in which he called attention to some of the more common affections of the nose which when neglected were of great local annoyance, and frequently gave rise to reflex conditions which could only be cured by treatment directed to the nose. Among these reflex conditions which have been well established by both European and American authorities are: asthma, hay fever, vertigo, headache, disturbances of vision and of hearing. It is not necessary that the general practitioner should devote as much time to special training as is required of the rhinologist in the treatment of nasal affections; but

with a moderate amount of clinical experience at the dispensary or medical school he will readily learn to do minor operations, to use the nasal speculum and mirror, to make applications of astringents and caustics if necessary, and to resort to those cleansing measures which are of so marked benefit in catarrhal affections. Speaking of chronic nasal catarrh, he said it is not only liable to invade the Eustachian tube, but to extend and involve the larynx and pharynx. The constant flow from the nasal passages into the stomach is a source of much disturbance to that organ. If the same care and discrimination were bestowed on these cases as are commonly given, for instance, to uterine diseases, the result would be at least equally successful. The author dwelt somewhat on the liability to loss of smell and its attendant dangers from long continued nasal disease, and sometimes from wrong treatment, such as the use of too strong astringents, or of mild ones too long continued.

DR. EGBERT H. GRANDIN then read the principal paper of the evening, entitled

A Plea for the Active Treatment of Puerperal Endometritis by Means of the Curette.

The profession, he said, accepts novelties in many other branches of medicine with much less conservatism than in obstetrics. While it is desirable not to manifest undue haste in the acceptance of new things, lest it appear like meddlesome midwifery, yet the author thought we should not reject good things because they had not been practised by our forefathers. Every day adds to the knowledge of the obstetrician who carefully watches his cases, and sooner or later facts show him that his early training in some respects has been faulty, and he may attain to that stage when he will admit that judicious meddlesomeness is good.

After delivery, the interior of the womb resembles a large surgical wound, except that the condition is physiological and not the result of disease. During a physiological puerperium the vast degenerative and regenerative changes going on in the womb and genital tract take place without disturbance of health; but if the normal process is arrested the fatty metamorphosis becomes checked or is replaced by necrosis; the cellular elements, the thrombi, etc., take on so-called puerperal degeneration. This process may start from any point in the endometrium, but usually from the placental site, and it extends progressively until it involves the whole surface. The surface, often extending down to the muscularis, becomes converted into a mass of pus cells and a vast cicatrix. A part of the degenerative material becomes absorbed into the circulatory fluid, and gives rise to constitutional symptoms. If the surgeon found such a condition after amputation of a limb he would get rid of the slough as soon as possible. He would not rest satisfied with simply washing the wound and sprinkling on iodoform. He would remove decaying matter with the forceps and seek to establish healthy granulations.

The theory of to-day is that puerperal endometritis or septicæmia is a septic process arising from the introduction of germs into the genital tract. Without stopping to inquire whether this theory is well established, Dr. Grandin said it served his purpose to state that in the vast majority of instances the septic process is localized at the outset. The cases which constitute exceptions are those to which the French have applied the term *septicæmie foudroyante.*

The necessity for attacking the septic process while it is local, and before the poison has thoroughly invaded the general system, becomes evident to all. The symptomatology gives a very early clew to puerperal endometritis, yet the obstetrician requires the use of all his senses. Before the pulse, or the general aspect of the patient or of the lochia indicates danger, the physician will frequently find reason for suspicion in the odor imparted to his finger on examination of the cervix.

Prophylactic measures are of the greatest importance. As far as possible, asepsis should be observed during the lying-in period. Dr. Grandin does not approve of the routine use of the intra-uterine douche after delivery. If the accoucheur has reason to believe a part of the placenta or membranes is left behind, he should remove it, otherwise there will be great risk of puerperal endometritis. If it is good practice to keep out germs, it is better practice to leave nothing in the uterus which will prove a fertile soil for their development. If, however, endometritis has developed, what shall we do?

The practice of to-day seems to be to use the intra-uterine douche. As a rule, the fluid now employed is a solution of bichloride of mercury in water, and the douching is repeated once in three hours by some, by others as often as once in two hours or every hour, and it is continued sometimes a full week. The object of the douche is to stop the septic process. There are objections to this method. That the douche is not always effectual, but that eventually an adjuvant has to be resorted to, is the experience of all. The difficulty, if not the impossibility, of douching decomposing shreds out of the uterus has been demonstrated by experiments in washing shreds out of a bag. Then the danger of the toxic effect, even of death, from the agent commonly employed has to be considered. In certain maternities in Europe this danger is thoroughly recognized, and the use of a solution of corrosive sublimate is prohibited. Dr. Grandin had not used it in the intra-uterine douche for two years. There is the further objection to this mode of treatment, that it is often repeated and causes disturbance of the patient. There is also some danger of re-introducing septic matter, when the injections are continued at intervals for days.

It is the author's belief that we possess in the dull curette an instrument which will often replace the douche and at the same time answer all the indications. The indications are: to remove from the uterus the products of decomposition, whether free in the cavity, partly adherent, limited to the superficies, or extending to the muscularis. Timely action is important, for at the outset the septic process is limited to the cavity of the organ. Soon it goes beyond local measures. The dull curette is harmless if used with care, as every instrument should be. The practitioner should be as competent to use it understandingly as to use the forceps or insert an irrigation tube.

The method which Dr. Grandin prefers to the repeated douche, and the value of which he has in a number of instances established to his own satisfaction, is the following: As soon as fetor of the lochia appears he proceeds carefully to differentiate its source, and without going into the details of the differential diagnosis it is sufficient to say that a thorough vaginal douching with boiled water or antiseptic solution will cause this fetor to disappear, in case it is due to decomposition in the vagina. If the fetor soon returns, also after the intra-uterine douche, it may be regarded as an indication for active treatment. He then places the patient in Sims's position, introduces the speculum, seizes the cervix with the tenaculum, inserts the curette, and thoroughly scrapes out the interior of the uterus. Finally he gives another douche, and then confidently expects to see a marked change for the better within twenty-four hours. Thus will be accomplished at once by the curette all that the douche can do if continued days. He deprecates as much as anyone unnecessary interference with the genital tract after labor, but when the necessity arises he believes in speedy action. It will be observed that he does not advocate the radical measure until the milder ones have been tried and failed. The use of the dull curette is attended with no more danger than the use of the irrigation tube, but if anyone fears it, he may resort to Doléris's brush.

The paper was discussed by Drs. Janvrin, Currier, R. A. Murray, Jacobus, and others, who agreed in the main with the author.

PERISCOPE.

Pelvic Peritonitis.

In the *American Journal of Obstetrics,* September, 1888, Dr. Joseph Eastman states that from his experience in the past year he feels warranted in emphasizing the importance of pelvic peritonitis—a disease often overlooked, yet the most common disease of the female pelvis. According to the text-books, pelvic cellulitis more frequently follows labor than pelvic peritonitis. Post-mortem examinations, and, within the past few years, abdominal sections, are demonstrating that without some pre-existing peritonitis, the trauma of child-birth, and other causes heretofore related, would less frequently result in cellulitis. He refers to the autopsies (for all diseases) made by Winckel—well-marked pelvic peritonitis was found in one-third of the cases. The same authority found pronounced disease of the Fallopian tubes in 182 cases, out of a total of 575, which were examined *post-mortem*. These instructive statements should lead to the early medical treatment of salpingitis, which so frequently causes inflammation of structures contiguous to the tubes owing to their movements and periodical engorgement.

The sharp stitch-like pains felt by young women before, during and after menstruation are, as in the chest, significant of more or less inflammatory adhesion of some portions of the serous covering of the pelvic structure. The term pelvic peritonitis may be applied to a circumscribed spot of inflammation, or signify coexistence of perimetritis, perisalpingitis, perioöphoritis, pericystitis, and periproctitis. The delicate silky membrane at first becomes opaque, then adheres to the fold of peritoneum nearest in contact. Thus the uterus, rectum, tubes and bladder may become adherent one to the other, or all together: and each recurring attack of inflammation strengthens the adhesions. The serum poured out may become purulent, forming abscesses in the broad ligament, or between coils of intestines; these seriously impair various functions, sometimes causing intestinal obstruction. Should they discharge into the bowel or bladder the ultimate cure is seriously complicated.

Congenital defects in the sexual organs may favor the development of peritonitis. The brain-cramming of our school systems is also a predisposing cause, since it interferes with the normal development of the pelvic organs in young girls. Allusion is made to the observation of Tait that disease of the tubes is at times due to the exanthemata, which probably act by causing catarrh of the tubes, or by interfering with the proper development of the epithelial lining of these organs. Dr. Eastman has removed diseased tubes from several cases in which the history clearly showed that scarlet fever was the cause of the disease. While gonorrhœa is admitted to be a frequent cause of pelvic peritonitis, the extreme views of Noeggerath and Saenger are not accepted. Still there is reason to shudder at the fate of marriageable young ladies when it is remembered that a large percentage of marriageable young men have suffered from gonorrhœa, and have been imperfectly cured, or rather, not cured at all. The teaching, heretofore extant, that gonorrhœa in the female is less serious than in the male is wrong, *and must be rewritten.* The statement of Van Buren and Keyes that "gonorrhœa sends more to the tomb than syphilis" is quoted with commendation, and it is added that the same foul virus sends twice as many women to the grave as men. While serious lesions in the urethra (resulting from gonorrhœa) are less common in the female than in the male, the Fallopian tube and ovaries furnish a secret lurking-place for the gonorrhœal virus, where its work of destruction is beyond the reach of remedial agents. Means used to prevent conception, especially cold water injections used after coition, cause many cases of tubal and ovarian inflammation. Induced abortion is a prolific cause of peritonitis from which many deaths result.

The treatment given refers more particularly to advanced stages of the disease, in which operative treatment alone offers a prospect of benefit or cure. Opium is still accorded the first place in the treatment of acute peritonitis; but we are warned against its use in chronic cases, lest the "opium habit" be induced. Hot applications to the hypogastrium, combined with hot antiseptic vaginal douches, given with the Hildebrandt douche (which instrument allows the use of water ten or fifteen degrees hotter than can be borne by the external parts) are also regarded with favor.

In case that each recurring menstrual period rekindles the inflammation, removal of the uterine appendages, to relieve the pelvis of its periodical congestion, is undoubtedly a warrantable operation if all other methods of treatment have failed. [Are not the appendages removed as the *fons et origo mali* rather than to bring on the menopause, and when peritonitis is caused by pyo-salpinx is it not warrantable to remove the appendages before employing all other methods of treatment?—ED.] In answer to the claim that the uterine appendages are being removed without sufficient cause, Eastman states that from his limited experience he believes that for every case in which these structures have been removed, unnecessarily, ten women have gone to the grave whose lives could have been saved by timely removal of the appendages by skilful hands.

The attention of those who condemn salpingo-oöphorectomy is called to the following propositions, and they are requested to use anatomical, physiological, pathological, and therapeutical common sense in the consideration. Could the ovaries and Fallopian tubes, like the testicle and epididymis, descend during early life and remain within reach of poultices, iodine, suspensory bandages, etc., and if they could remain free from monthly engorgement, they also might be relieved of congenital defects, physiological abuses, the destructive sequelæ of mumps, the fevers of childhood, and the pernicious gonorrhœa virus, before disorganization had so far advanced as to necessitate their removal. After suppuration has occurred, whether the pus is discharging by the rectum, vagina or not, the treatment instituted by Tait—to open the abdomen, drain the abscess from its fountain source (whether in the broad ligament or between coils of intestines) by stitching the peritoneal margins of the abscess to the abdominal wound and using the drainage tube—is considered the safest and most satisfactory method of treatment. It is preferred to opening the abscess *per vaginam* with the trocar or bistoury; also to enlarging sinuses communicating with the vagina and rectum when such exist. Martin's method of drainage through Douglas's pouch may be more suitable in some cases.

Rupture of the Quadriceps Extensor Femoris.

Dr. W. R. Cluness, in a letter to the *Sacramento Medical Times*, Nov., 1888, says: The subcutaneous rupture of muscles or tendons is a comparatively common occurrence, the rupture usually taking place at the junction of the muscular with the tendinous tissue. Erichsen says that it occurs more frequently from the muscular contraction, which must necessarily precede it, than from direct violence. Gross, Ashhurst, and indeed all of the authorities I have found it convenient to consult upon the subject, convey the idea that much force is always necessary to cause this kind of injury, especially when a muscle or tendon of considerable size becomes ruptured. The few cases that have heretofore come under my observation confirm this view, or indicate that sudden and unexpected tension is necessary, even when not accompanied by very great strain. When therefore the complete rupture of so powerful a muscle as the quadriceps femoris takes place during the ordinary efforts of walking, and without stepping upon a pebble or other similar substance, or in any manner encountering an obstruction which would in the slightest degree impede locomotion, it is deemed worthy of permanent record. The history of such a case is briefly as follows: G. W. D., 75 years old, 5 feet 8 inches in height, and weighing 188 pounds, a well-preserved and robust man, apparently ten years younger than he really is, and of good habits, while returning from a few hours' recreation at fishing in the Sacramento River on the 20th of last month, and while carrying a small string of fish in his left hand as he was slowly wending his way homeward, distinctly heard a snap, as if his thigh bone had been broken. Falling backward instantly, he endeavored to prevent himself from sustaining injury by quickly throwing his arms behind him for support, but so sudden and unexpected was the seizure that he fell to the earth before he could realize what had occurred. He says: "I first heard a crack, and away I went, heels over head, turning a complete somersault; I then flopped around on my face and tried to get up, but could not; I tried again and failed.

By this time I realized that my leg was paralyzed, and I called for the assistance of the Yard-Master of the S. P. Co., who soon placed me in a hack and sent me home." Upon reaching his home I was immediately summoned, and readily diagnosticated a rupture of the quadriceps femoris at its insertion into the patella, the separation being complete and the detached end being distinctly felt fully two inches above the upper border of that bone. Treatment for the first two weeks consisted in the relaxation of the ruptured muscle, by position, and the application of an evaporating lotion to subdue what inflammation might ensue. There having been but little pain at any time, no anodynes were required. He is now, just a month after the accident, able to move about in his room upon crutches, the limb being properly bandaged, and the joint rendered immovable by suitable appliances.

Resins used by the Ancient Egyptians.

A small jar of resin was recently submitted to Mr. E. M. Holmes for identification by Mr. Flinders Petrie, of the Egypt Exploration Exhibition. This jar, which was in a perfect state, was disinterred from a heap of rubbish found among the ruins of Naucratis and dates from the sixth century B.C. Naucratis was at this time the only Greek colony in Egypt, and it was through this town alone that trade with Greece was permitted. Mr. Holmes states in the *Pharmaceutical Journal* that the jar contained Chian turpentine. According to Flückiger there is no evidence that the old Egyptians were acquainted with the resin. The discovery of this pot of resin carries the history of the commerce of the drug two hundred years further back. The other resin was found on a mummy cloth on the body of a person to all appearance of some rank. It was found in Hawara Cemetery, in the Fayum province of Lower Egypt, and it dates from a period not earlier than the second century A.D. On heating some of the resin in a flame, the vapors of benzoic acid were given off, and a decided vanilla odor was recognized. This points to the conclusion that the resin must be a Siam benzoin. The authors of the Pharmacographia state that there is no evidence that the Greeks and Romans, or even the earlier Arabian physicians, had any acquaintance with benzoin.—*Lancet,* Nov. 24, 1888.

Value of Salicylic Acid in Dermatology.

At the meeting of the American Dermatological Association, at Washington, Sept. 18, 1888, Dr. C. Heitzman, of New York, read a paper on the value of salicylic acid in dermatology, in which he said that he had been using the remedy for the last three years. It has two well-marked properties. The first is the peculiarity of acting on the horny layers of the epidermis. There is no agent so active in softening, and at last destroying, the epidermal formations as salicylic acid. Its other action is as a parasiticide. These two properties open a large field for research. We should be careful not to include cases in which we have merely impressions as to its value ; but there are many cases in which there can be no question as to its utility, and in some of these it has never been used before. The remedy may be used as a powder, as a plaster, or in the alcoholic solution. It has the advantages that it does not discolor the skin or linen, and has no odor. It is used in twenty-four kinds of cases. In hyperidrosis its action is well known. The German soldiers use it in a one per cent. salve, made with tallow, applied to the feet when upon the march. In seborrhœa, especially when combined with acne, it has given brilliant results. One per cent. of the acid with six to eight per cent. of sulphur, is an excellent application for dandruff. A prescription with tar Dr. Heitzman likes better, but it is less agreeable to the patients. In urticaria it is an excellent means of allaying the itching. In furunculosis an ointment of six to ten per cent. has prevented an outbreak and checked the disease. But, to be sure of results, the quality of the acid must be guaranteed. In two cases in which the prescription had been filled at random there had been no good result, but when Scheering's salicylic acid was substituted the effect was immediate.

In one case of dermatitis herpetiformis a lotion of the acid proved the best thing the patient had tried, although it was not capable of smothering the disease or preventing recurrences. In psoriasis, after chrysarobin and tar, it is the very thing to be applied, though the peeling off of the scales is not so rapid as with other remedies. In lichen planus salicylic acid is far superior to carbolic acid or corrosive sublimate. It can also be applied over a larger area with safety. It allays the itching, removes the scales, and flattens down the papules. The author has prescribed three per cent. solutions, which are to be diluted at the beginning of treatment. Six cases were treated, and all did uniformly well without the administration of arsenic.

In all varieties of eczema the results were satisfactory. Ninety-six cases were treated, generally with one per cent. of the acid, with equal parts of zinc-powder and starch, in two parts of ointment. In eczema madidans, one-half per cent. is better. Sometimes it may be used as strong as ten per cent. where there is great thickening in the very chronic cases. As the acid does not attack the connective tissue, there can be no caustic effect. In acne a three per cent. solution removes pigment patches, assists in removing comedones, and renders the skin soft. In acne rosacea the results were good, but in sycosis less good. The remedy does not seem to penetrate deep enough between the furrows. In impetigo contagiosa it cures the disease in ten or twelve days. If combined with the liquor gutta-perchæ and some oil to make an emulsion, it adheres to the skin. In keratitis senilis, callosity, clavus, and verruca its action in removing the thickened portions is well known. In ichthyosis it is easy to remove the scales, but they return. In lupus erythematosus and lupus vulgaris the results were brilliant at first, the excrescences flattening down rapidly at first, but not a case was cured. For pruritus, in the shape of a lotion, it is excellent. In tinea the solution with gutta-percha is better than Taylor's remedy. But generally the disease will not be cured by any one remedy, and we are only too glad to have more than one. In tinea versicolor a one per cent. solution is effective.

Dr. Pye Smith, of London, spoke of his use of the remedy in the hypertrophic inflammations in the soles of the feet and the palms of the hands where there were fissures; here the effects of the remedy are wonderful. He corroborated what Dr. Heitzman said in reference to the use of the remedy in furunculosis, especially as it occurs in youths or school-boys, sometimes for months together. He believes that the contagion is carried from one point to another in the dressing. In the treatment of the individual pustules he always hardens the surrounding skin by bathing it in lead lotion, thus giving less opportunity for the invasion of the micro-organisms than does the old method of poulticing, which makes the skin sodden and readily permeable. In lichen planus he has tried the salicylic acid with some success, but has found it difficult to follow the cases closely enough to be sure of his ground. He prefers to wait till more material has been

collected. In general, he said he felt that there were not enough cases to warrant definite conclusions.

Dr. L. D. Bulkley, of New York, said he had used the remedy largely in many of the cases referred to, and mentioned particularly hyperidrosis of the axilla in women. He uses with great confidence a ten per cent. powder, with one drachm of oxide of zinc and the rest starch. In eczema care must be used. He has seen acute attacks started up by it. He also mentioned favus of the scalp, in which he considers salicylic acid very valuable in the form of a strong lotion. He has had several cases under observation for several months, and the disease has not yet returned. It is good in seborrhœa, but, if it is too strong, even when mixed with oil, the patients come back and say it is too drying.

Dr. A. Van Harlingen, of Philadelphia, uses it in the treatment of chronic eczema of the legs in a paste with glycerine and zinc oxide, made into a paste with five per cent. of the acid. If it is carefully applied, the patients go for from three days to a week without redressing.

Dr. E. B. Bronson, of New York, thinks that in most cases we use the remedy as a preliminary measure, as it prepares the surface for other remedies. This is true especially where there is an enormous accumulation of the epidermis, as in cases of seborrhœa. In these cases he has generally been obliged to resort afterward to some other remedies.

Dr. Heitzman, in closing the discussion, said that the field of the remedy in hyperidrosis extends to any portion of the body which is affected, especially the folds of the groin and the genital regions.—*N. Y. Med. Journal*, Dec. 1, 1888.

Formula for Chronic Cystitis.

At the meeting of the Sacramento Society for Medical Improvement, Oct. 16, 1888 (*Sacramento Med. Times*, Dec., 1888), Dr. Mary J. Magill read a paper on the treatment of cystic disease in women, in the course of which she said that the following formula had proved very serviceable:

℞ Ol. cubebæ,
   Ol. santali,
   Ol. copaibæ . . . . āā f℥ iii
   Liq. potassæ . . . . f℥ iss
   Syr. acaciæ,
   Aquæ anisi . . . . āā f℥ iiiss

M. Sig. Two teaspoonfuls every 4 hours.

THE

MEDICAL AND SURGICAL
REPORTER.

ISSUED EVERY SATURDAY.

CHARLES W. DULLES, M.D.,
EDITOR AND PUBLISHER.

The Terms of Subscription to the serial publications of this office are as follows, payable in advance:

Med. and Surg. Reporter (weekly), a year,	$5.00
Quarterly Compendium of Med. Science, -	2.50
Reporter and Compendium, - - -	6.00
Physician's Daily Pocket Record, - -	1.00
Reporter and Pocket Record, - - -	6.00
Reporter, Compendium, and Pocket Record,	7.00

All checks and postal orders should be drawn to order of

CHARLES W. DULLES,

N. E. Cor. 13th and Walnut Streets,

P. O. Box 843.   Philadelphia, Pa.

☞SUGGESTIONS TO SUBSCRIBERS:

See that your address-label gives the date to which your subscription is paid.

In requesting a change of address, give the old address as well as the new one.

If your REPORTER does not reach you promptly and regularly, notify the publisher *at once,* so that the cause may be discovered and corrected.

☞SUGGESTIONS TO CONTRIBUTORS AND CORRESPONDENTS:

Write in ink.

Write on one side of paper only.

Write on paper of the size usually used for letters.

Make as few paragraphs as possible. Punctuate carefully. Do not abbreviate, or omit words like "the," and "a," or "an."

Make communications as short as possible.

NEVER ROLL A MANUSCRIPT! Try to get an envelope or wrapper which will fit it.

When it is desired to call our attention to something in a newspaper, mark the passage boldly with a colored pencil, and write on the wrapper "Marked copy." Unless this is done, newspapers are not looked at.

The Editor will be glad to get medical news, but it is important that brevity and actual interest shall characterize communications intended for publication.

REGULATING VETERINARY MEDICINE.

A committee of well-known practitioners of veterinary medicine in Philadelphia and other parts of Pennsylvania has recently drawn up an address to the Legislature, recommending to its attention the importance of adopting some measure to regulate the practice of veterinary medicine in the State. The address recites the value of the cattle in Pennsylvania, which is put at about one hundred and twenty-five million dollars. In addition to this, the committee dwells upon the danger of communication of tuberculosis from animals to man.

In doing this they have fallen into an exaggeration which may do their cause harm. This is to be regretted, because their cause is a good one, and could be maintained on its merits. There can be no serious question of the importance of legal regulation of the practice of veterinary medicine, as all enlightened communities ought to regulate the practice of medicine among human beings.

At present a large part of the practice of veterinary medicine in this country is in the hands of uneducated and even ignorant men; and animals are often subjected to medication, and other treatment, which is barbarous and worse than useless. To remedy this condition of affairs, the State should use its influence and authority to compel those who wish to enter this calling to prepare themselves by study in some of the excellent schools to be found in this country or abroad; and it is plainly its duty to protect its citizens against the malpractice of those who have no right to assume the responsibilities of veterinary medicine.

With some modifications, the bill proposed by the Committee we have referred to would do a great deal to this end, and it would also furnish a much-needed stimulus to the study of veterinary medicine, by making the title of veterinary surgeon more honorable than it is now. There is, we believe, a great opportunity in this country for the ambition of first-rate men in the study of the nature and treatment of diseases of the lower animals. So far, few men of ability and promise in the United States have cared to devote themselves to this pursuit; but more will do so whenever it is understood that such a course opens up a most inviting field for scientific investigation and an excellent one for financial success.

The bill proposed will tend to elevate the standing of veterinarians in the community, and to encourage the kind of men to study veterinary medicine who are most needed in this department of science, for the good of the community and for the credit of their calling.

THE PROGNOSIS OF CARCINOMA AFTER OPERATION.

No one who is familiar with the recent advances in surgery can fail to appreciate the change which has taken place during the last ten or fifteen years in the attitude of surgeons toward the treatment of patients suffering with cancer. The time was, and not so long ago, when surgeons regarded the removal of a carcinoma as an operation involving great danger to the life of the patient, and as furnishing but a temporary and brief freedom from active manifestations of the disease. Nowadays the methods of wound treatment have been so perfected that the danger to life is reduced to a minimum, and it hardly enters into the calculation of results, except when the cancer occupies some peculiarly dangerous position.

The final result of an operation for cancer falls under one of three heads: first, perfect success, when a patient recovers from the operation and lives for years without any local or remote recurrence; second, partial success, when the patient recovers from the operation and lives for a period of months before recurrence takes place; and, third, failure, when the patient dies soon after the operation, or suffers with local or distant recurrence of the growth within a very short period.

In looking over the whole field, using statistics in a legitimate way, and giving due weight to what is of equal worth, namely, the opinions of skilful and experienced surgeons, it appears that the modern method of early and complete removal of cancerous growths has very much improved the chances of those who suffer with them.

The number of those who seem to be absolutely cured, and who prove this by freedom from disease for ten or more years, is exceedingly small; and there seems to be no period of freedom long enough to be a sure sign of cure; but the number of those who are freed from active manifestations of carcinoma for months is relatively very great. In an address before the Seventeenth Congress of German Surgeons, Professor König, of Göttingen, estimated the proportion of patients temporarily cured as high as thirty per cent.

This large percentage of comparative cures is not found in operations for cancer of the mucous passages, such as the larynx or the rectum, because in these situations a cancer is sometimes very hard to approach and hard to extirpate thoroughly, and its removal causes functional defects which are in themselves very dangerous to life. Besides this, cancers in the breathing passages, or the digestive tract, are not, as a rule, brought to the notice of the surgeon until they have already assumed formidable proportions. But, even in the case of cancers of the rectum, it is encouraging to note that the mortality has within the last ten years fallen to nearly one-half what it was formerly.

In view of these facts, the outlook for persons afflicted with cancer is very much more hopeful than it was a decade or two ago. The methods of operating are much less immediately dangerous to life, and the prospect of temporary relief from the distress and horror of a cancer is much greater.

It is very important, in estimating the value of operations for cancer, to measure, not only the months or years of life which can be credited to them, but also the amount of peace and comfort which they secure for the patient, the hope—even though it last but a comparatively short time —which succeeds to the hopeless despair of one who denies himself, or who is denied, the chances of an operation.

When all these factors are taken into consideration, we may regard with great satisfaction the attainments of the last ten or fifteen years in this field, and entertain a reasonable hope that the future may develop more accurate methods of diagnosis of carcinoma and more successful methods of operating for its relief, with a corresponding improvement in the prospects of those who are the victims of its ravages.

FLUORINE AS A REMEDIAL AGENT.

The recent active search for new remedial agents has led to the introduction into medical practice of a number of new remedies, some of which have proved of real value, while others have only seemed for a time to be of service, and on more extended experience have proved of little worth. One of these agents is fluorine, an element which is well calculated to attract attention on account of its remarkable chemical properties.

In a temperate and thoughtful article in the *Deutsch-Amerikanische Apotheker Zeitung*, November 1, 1888, Dr. Theodor W. Schaefer, of Kansas City, Missouri, calls attention to the characteristics of fluorine and its compounds, and discusses its use as a medicament. He refers to the experiments of Dr. Eduard Wernigk, of Alhambra, California, who used it with satisfaction in the treatment of epilepsy, and, by subcutaneous injection, in a variety of tumors. The form which he found most serviceable was the fluoride of potassium, half-grain doses of which in solution proved of decided value in the treatment of an osteoma of the lower maxillary bone, in a fibrous tumor of the face, and in a lupoid growth of the hand. Dr. Schaefer himself used hypodermic injections of fluoride of potassium in a case of goitre, with encouraging results, and applied the remedy by pencilling and by gargling in a case of diphtheria, which ended in recovery. These cases cover the ground in which Dr. Schaefer has so far found the compounds of fluorine to be useful.

As a remedy for internal administration, the salts of fluorine have not yet given any specially good results. It has been used in certain affections of the heart, but without much success. Dr. Da Costa, of Philadelphia—whom Dr. Schaefer erroneously locates in New York—some years ago made a number of interesting experiments in the use of certain fluorides internally, and published the result of his investigations in a very instructive paper in the *Archives of Medicine*, June, 1881. This paper was a report of the first systematic attempt to use the salts of fluorine in medical practice. The salts Dr. Da Costa chiefly made use of were the fluorides of potassium and of sodium, and the ferrous and ferric fluorides. His observations led him to the conclusion that the preparations of fluorine are too irritating to the stomach to be of much value, and—as we have ascertained by personal inquiry—he does not now have a high opinion of their availability in therapeusis.

From all this it appears that the investigation of the effects of fluorine upon the animal economy has not yet led to any very important developments, and yet it certainly invites to further study. Theoretically one would expect that an agent which has such marked chemical peculiarities must have effects upon physiological and pathological processes not less marked. If heretofore it has not proved of much service in the treatment of disease, this may be because it has not been studied carefully enough or generally enough, and Dr. Schaefer has done a good thing in calling attention anew to what has been done in this direction, and in inviting the profession to pursue the investigation further.

ACCOUNTS RENDERED QUARTERLY.

There was a time when the services of physicians were not considered as an article of merchandise, with a fairly definite price, but rather as acts of benevolence and humanity, and then grateful patients signified their appreciation of these services by gifts in the nature of an honorarium. But this time has passed away, and now every medical man is compelled to keep accounts, and periodically to try to collect what he believes is due him by the unromantic method of sending out bills.

No physician need be told how troublesome and often how disagreeable a part of his work this is. The question of what he shall charge is not rarely a trying one; for he cannot always figure out so many visits at a certain price and put this down on his bill. There are many circumstances which may compel him to make his charge less than he thinks it might properly be; and when he has fixed it, he is sometimes troubled to think it may be more—or, alas! less—than his debtor has estimated it at.

In addition to this source of distress there is the question as to the periods at which a physician shall render his accounts. In many parts of this country it has become a custom for physicians to send out bills every six months; and some men send out their bills only once a year. There are advantages in this plan for men of means and of large and lucrative practice; but it has very great disadvantages for the great majority of medical men. It is especially hard on physicians in the earlier years of their practice, because then they usually need speedy returns for their work, and treat a class of persons that requires pretty close watching. But almost all physicians lose by sending out bills only at long intervals. Patients treated with such indulgence sometimes become careless about paying, because from this very fact they imagine the doctor does not need money as they do, and some patients deliberately impose on their physicians as long as they can, and, when called upon to pay what they owe, simply transfer their patronage to someone else until his endurance is exhausted.

These and other reasons which will occur to our readers make it desirable that medical men should—except in rare cases— render bills more frequently than once or twice a year. The proper interval in most cases appears to be three months. This was the conclusion arrived at by the West Philadelphia Medical Society at a recent meeting, when the following was adopted :

"Realizing that the time has arrived when, in order to keep pace with the increasing business sentiments of the world, it is necessary to insist more strongly on the strictly business aspect of our professional services; and, believing that this will be ensured by the rendering of our accounts more frequently than has been the general custom;

"It is resolved, that the West Philadelphia Medical Society deems it to the best interests of its members, and of the profession generally in West Philadelphia, that they shall render their accounts for services quarterly or more frequently, and hereby urges upon them concerted action in this matter, reserving to them discretion to make exceptions in cases in which they may deem it to their best interests or those of their fellow-practitioners."

We fully concur with the sentiment of this resolution and believe it would be a good plan for physicians to render their accounts every three months. There are very few patients who would not approve of such a practice, and it would be a great advantage to medical men if it were generally carried out.

OPERATION FOR STENOSIS OF THE PYLORUS.

Operations for stenosis of the pyloric orifice of the stomach are no longer very rare, and a variety of methods have been proposed for treating this condition surgically, among the most promising of which was the method of digital dilatation of Loreta. Another method, which has proved of value, was first practised about three years ago by Heincke, and two years later by Mikulicz. A third operation by this method was performed in July, 1888, by Bardeleben, and is reported, with comments by Dr. A. Koehler, in the *Berliner klin. Wochenschrift*, Nov. 12, 1888. The method consists in opening the abdomen, dividing the stricture longitudinally, and then drawing the wound apart vertically so that the horizontal opening is converted into a vertical one, after which the wound is united with a continuous suture. In this way the contracted tissue is made to occupy only the posterior wall of the newly formed canal, while its anterior wall is largely made up of the healthy tissue of the stomach and duodenum.

Bardeleben's operation was performed on a man, thirty-five years old, who a month before had swallowed some strong hydrochloric acid. The time consumed in the operation was only half an hour, and its result was entirely successful.

EXECUTION BY ELECTRICITY.

The law to execute criminals by electricity in the State of New York, which has just gone into effect, has led to some interesting discussion in regard to its merits and demerits. Among others the editor of the *Electrical Review* states his opposition to the law, on the ground that the execution of murderers by electricity is "an unnecessary and an unwarranted debasement of one of the most enlightening elements of the age, and that he does not believe that it is practical from a scientific standpoint." For the sake of the citizens of New York, we would hope that it may be long before they shall have an opportunity to demonstrate either the correctness or incorrectness of this opinion. Our view, however, is that the application of electricity as a means of execution of criminals is objectionable on the score of its difficulties, its uncertainty, and its effect upon the community. As we have stated before —in the REPORTER of February 11, 1888— we are of the belief that humanity no longer requires any modification in the method of executing the death sentence, and that this attempt to substitute electricity for the usual method is not in accordance with the dictates of sound policy nor justified by anything which physiologists know of the sensations connected with death by hanging.

INOCULATION FOR YELLOW FEVER.—Doctor Paul Gibier, a French experimenter, who has been studying yellow fever in Florida, proposes to establish an experimental station for treating this disease. He thinks that a safe method of inoculation will result in the prevention of the disease, and suggests that a laboratory should be established on one of the keys off the Florida coast, and a year spent in experimenting with the inoculations upon monkeys, thus perfecting a method of treatment of the fever.

BURN-BRAE VINDICATED.—Some time ago a patient suffering with acute mania was admitted to Burn-Brae, a private hospital for the insane near Philadelphia. After his dismissal he made complaint of harsh treatment and improper detention against the physicians in charge. The Committee on Lunacy of the State Board of Public Charities has investigated the complaint and has found no justification for it. In concluding his report for the Committee, the chairman, Dr. Thomas G. Morton, said that there was ample evidence to show that the patient's treatment was proper, and his recovery rapid, complete, and satisfactory.

PHOTOGRAPHY OF THE MALE BLADDER.— According to the *British Medical Journal*, Dec. 22, 1888, Mr. Hurry Fenwick, and Mr. Pearson Cooper of the London Camera Club, have been working for some time at photography of the human bladder. Various obstacles were in turn recognized and overcome, and they have now so far perfected their vesical camera and method as to obtain good negatives of the interior of "dummy" and dead bladders. They hope before very long to describe a method of recording the appearances and progress of diseases of the living bladder. The negatives are taken *per urethram* through a tube of 23 French calibre.

—The United States Steamer Yantic, which was recently sent on Government business to Hayti, is on its way home with yellow fever on board.

PAMPHLET NOTICES.

[Any reader of the REPORTER who desires a copy of a pamphlet noticed in these columns will doubtless secure it by addressing the author with a request stating where the notice was seen and *enclosing a postage-stamp.*]

173. THE SIGNIFICANCE OF THE EPIBLASTIC ORIGIN OF THE CENTRAL NERVOUS SYSTEM. BY GEORGE W. JACOBY, M.D., New York. From the *New York Medical Journal*, May 5, 1888. 15 pages.

174. ACCIDENTS INCIDENTAL TO THE USE OF THE EXPLORING NEEDLE FOR DIAGNOSIS. BY HERMANN M. BIGGS, M.D., New York. From the *New York Medical Journal*, August 18, 1888. 12 pages.

175. OSTEOPLASTIC RESECTION OF THE FOOT. BY FERDINAND H. GROSS, M.D., Philadelphia. From the *Medical News*, October 27, 1888. 7 pages.

176. MEMORIAL OF DR. NATHAN LEWIS HATFIELD. BY ROBERT J. HESS, M.D., Philadelphia. 8 pages.

177. ENTEROSTOMY FOR ACUTE INTESTINAL OBSTRUCTION. BY B. FARQUHAR CURTIS, M.D., New York. From the *Medical Record*, September 1, 1888. 12 pages.

178. THE FAILURE OF DR. J. B. THOMAS'S TREATMENT OF URETHRAL STRICTURE BY ELECTROLYSIS. BY ROBERT NEWMAN, M.D., New York. From the *Journal of the Amer. Med. Association*, September 8, 1888. 15 pages.

179. REMARKS ON PELVIC INFLAMMATIONS AND THE MANAGEMENT OF THEIR RESIDUES. BY WILLIAM WARREN POTTER, M.D., Buffalo, N. Y. From the *Buffalo Med. and Surg. Journal*, July, 1888. 16 pages.

173. Dr. Jacoby's pamphlet contains his presidential address before the New York Neurological Society, in May, 1888, and presents an argument in favor of the view that the nervous system of vertebrates, although formed from the epiblast of the embryo, like the skin and surface epithelium, has lost its epithelial character and has returned to a state of indifference in which it is impossible to decide whether a tissue is epithelial, therefore epiblastic, or connective tissue, therefore mesoblastic.

The whole paper is exceedingly interesting, and contains very instructive suggestions as to the development of the organs of sense.

174. Dr. Biggs protests against the indiscriminate use of the exploring needle for diagnosis when other means give more reliable information. The dangers of the use of the exploring needle rest upon the traumatism produced and the risk of septic infection. The cases cited by Dr. Biggs should be used with caution; although it would be going too far to admit that they all illustrate the danger of its use. His warning, however, is timely and may be commended to the attention of our readers.

175. Dr. Gross describes an operation such as has been but rarely performed in this country, and not often in any country, namely that originally done in 1871 by Wladimiroff, of Russia, and independently, in 1880 by Mikulicz, of Vienna. Dr. Gross's operation was successful as far as reported; but it would be interesting to know how good use of his foot the patient has to-day.

176. This is a warm tribute by a personal friend to the virtues of a well-known medical man of Philadelphia, whose life of eighty-four years was full of useful and kindly ministration to his fellow-men, and of pleasant relations with his professional brethren.

177. Dr. Curtis has made a careful study of sixty-two cases of the formation of an artificial anus—for acute intestinal obstruction—all that he has been able to collect from medical literature—and gives the result of his analysis of their various features. It is an interesting statistical study, and of great practical value. It leads the writer of the paper to the conclusion that enterostomy is preferable to laparotomy except when the patient's condition is so good that he can bear the shock of the latter operation, and when the intestines are not so greatly distended as to offer a serious obstacle to a thorough exploration of the abdominal cavity.

178. Dr. Newman defends himself, and the operation which he advocates and practices for the cure of stricture of the urethra, against the criticisms of Dr. J. B. Thomas, of Pittsburgh, who failed to cure a case by electrolysis, and in his report of it discussed Dr. Newman's earlier report of his own experience. The defense is warm and interesting; and it is fair to say that its warmth is warranted by the terms used by Dr. Thomas in discussing Dr. Newman's methods.

179. Dr. Potter's paper presents a temperate and intelligent study of the various views as to the nature of inflammations in the pelvis of women, and a brief review of their proper treatment. The writer cites the opposing opinions of a number of well-known gynecologists, and endeavors to bring out the truth contained in what seems contradictory. The result is a very entertaining and suggestive paper, which may be recommended to the attention of our readers for their careful consideration.

LITERARY NOTES.

—We have received the Catalogue of the Tokyo Medical Library. The library contains 1092 well-selected books and pamphlets.

—After January 1, 1889, Dr. D. A. Hodghead will succeed Dr. William S. Whitwell as Editor of the *Pacific Medical and Surgical Journal.*

—*The United Service* appears in a new series for January, 1889, with the name of L. R. Hamersly & Co. as publishers. It is a handsome large octavo of 116 pages, containing a number of interesting papers by military and naval officers, and the announcements of the editor and of the publishers, short notes, and news of the Loyal Legion. Those of our readers who have served in the army or navy will be interested to know that the publication of this journal has been resumed, and that it promises to be more interesting in the future than it has been in the past.

—From and after the first of January, 1889, *The Canadian Practitioner* is to be published as a semi-monthly, instead of a monthly, as heretofore—twenty-four issues in the year being given, instead of twelve. *The Practitioner* is now about to enter on its fourteenth year, and its history has been one of steady progress and development. At the beginning of 1888 a great improvement was made in the typographical appearance and material make-up of the journal, and its prospectus for the coming year promises still further advances. The subscription price remains what it was formerly: $3 00 a year.

CORRESPONDENCE.

The Porro-Cæsarean Method of Mr. Lawson Tait, historically examined.

To THE EDITOR.

Sir : In the *British Medical Journal* for November 17, 1888 (see also the REPORTER, January 5, p. 30), we find the following from Mr. Tait: "I have now done four operations on the principle laid down by Professor Porro, and all the mothers have recovered, and the children have all lived. The operation I perform is certainly not Porro's operation, for I have altered nearly every detail."

"My own method of operating is to make an incision through the middle line large enough to admit my hand, and then I pass a piece of india rubber drainage tube (without any hole in it) as a loop over the fundus uteri, and bring it down so as to encircle the cervix, taking care that it does not include a loop of intestine. I then make a single hitch and draw it tight round the cervix so as completely to stop the circulation. I give the ends of the tube to an assistant, who keeps them well on the strain, so as to prevent the loose knot from slipping, the reason of this being that should there be any bleeding and any necessity for further constriction, I could secure this in a moment, without undoing any knot, and the simplicity of the method greatly commends it. I then make a small opening in the uterus, and enlarge it by tearing with my two fingers, seize the child by a foot and remove it. I then remove the placenta, and by that time the uterus has completely contracted and is easily drawn through the wound in the abdominal wall. The constricting tube will now probably require to be tightened, and the second hitch of the knot may be put on at the same time, and the work is practically done. Stuff a few sponges into the wound to keep the cavity clear of blood, and pass the knitting needles " (2) " through the flattened tube and through the cervix, and in this simple way a clamp of the most efficient kind is at once made. The uterus is removed about three quarters of an inch above the rubber tube. The usual stitches are put in, the wound closed round the stump, which of course is brought to the lowest part of the opening, and then the stump is dressed with per-chloride of iron in the usual way."

This is certainly in many respects, an excellent way to operate, and Mr. Tait has shown his wisdom by accepting and grouping together a series of alterations made and tested before he ever operated. His altering, does not mean, that he claims to have originated the alterations. The Esmarch tube and transfixing pins are in very frequent use.

The opening of the uterus *in situ*—the delivering of fœtus by the feet—the constriction of the cervix—and securing the stump in the wound after its amputation, are the points of the operation as performed by Prof Porro. The alterations in the details are as follows

1. *The constriction of the cervix, after the manner of Esmarch;* as applied first by Prof. Litzmann of Kiel, now of Berlin, in case 15, in chronological order, on June 14th, 1878. The elastic ligature was used to continue the constriction, instead of the *serre nœud* or clamp. Elastic ligation was also employed in case 71, Dec. 7, 1880, under Dr. J. De Rull of Barcelona, Spain, and in case 72, of the same date, by Prof. Hegar, of Freiburg, Germany.

2. *Opening the uterus by small incision and enlarging the opening by digital laceration;* as introduced by Dr. Clement Godson, of London, on November 27, 1882 ; who says in his report, "I made" . . . "a small incision, large enough to admit the finger" . . . "I immediately inserted the tips of each fore-finger, and tore the womb open transversely." There is no necessity to tear the uterus, where the elastic tube of Esmarch is used.

3. *The transfixing of the cervix by two long pins or knitting needles.* Prof. Chiara of Milan lost a case in December, 1877, by the stump falling in and the bowels protruding, as the result of vomiting : in his next operation, May 22d, 1878, he made use of one transfixing pin as a preventive. Six days later, Prof. Domenico Tibone, of Turin, introduced the plan now in general use, of employing "two long transfixing pins." It is also the custom of some operators to stitch in the cervix with the abdominal wound, to secure an early and intimate union, as a means of safety.

Half-knotting the Esmarch tube, as practised by Mr. Tait, is better than whole knotting it, and then being obliged to untie and retie. Clamping the half-knot by strong pressure-forceps is a common mode of security. Passing the pins through the tube instead of beneath it, belongs to Mr. Tait. As the pins come away with the tube when the stump separates, they will fail of the purpose for which they were originally introduced in Italy, if separation should happen to take place too early. The pins fix the stump, and secure it from being kept in slipping motion excited by vomiting, by respiration, and the dragging upon it from within, all of which have a tendency to delay union. The chief value of the pins is in the first few days, and their office ceases with the union of stump and abdominal wall: hence the additional advantage of cervico-abdominal suturing, through the tissues which are to remain after the pins come away. Much temporary disfiguring of the abdomen in the line of the cicatrix, by its being deeply drawn in, remains in many cases. Where there is extreme antero-posterior pelvic collapse, as in rickets, and the sacro-vertebral angle is so altered as to bring the plane of the superior strait nearer in parallelism with the abdominal wall than normal, there will be the least vagino-cervical tension, and *vice versa*, when the pelvis is normal, as in tumor cases. In time, the stretching of the stump within, relieves the abdominal wall from being deeply indented.

The Porro-Cæsarean operation is much more of a principle, than of a special method devised by the Pavian professor, and departures from the technique of his original plan, do not in the least weaken the claim which associates his name with the operation as a whole. Prof. Porro designed to save life, by giving the uterus a form of wound after a Cæsarean delivery, that might be dressed outside of the abdominal cavity, and by which septic peritonitis could be avoided. The quasi unsexing of the woman was scarcely to be considered; as her living, to become again pregnant, after the old operation was a great rarity in Italy. Her being made sterile is now claimed as an advantage by many operators. Professor Porro by saving five women out of a record of six, has shown, that his own technique has a high capability of securing success. As supra-vaginal hysterectomy existed before Prof. Porro applied it in parturient cases, it is an error to attach his name to any hysterectomy case which is not "completive of the Cæsarean section." To remove an unopened uterus for tumor, and with it a fœtus in the early months, is not strictly a Porro operation, and such cases have no claim to enter into a statistical record of Porro cases, as the fœtal column can have but one result, and that a fatal one: the same may be said of hysterectomy following a rupture of the uterus.

The Porro-Cæsarean section has at this time an additional interest from the fact, that the records of the last four years show a very decided decrease in the percentage of deaths over that of former years. A full record of 1884, shows 28 Porro operations, with 18 women and 10 children lost. This appears to have been the maximum year for cases, with the exception of 1880, when there were 33, with 22 deaths. Since the introduction of the Sänger method, there has been a gradual falling off in the number of Porro operations, and at the same time an increase in the percentage of women saved under each: viz., in 1885 there were 13 Sänger operations with 4 deaths: in 1886, 33 operations with 10 deaths; and in 1887, 47 operations with 10 deaths. In 1885, there were 22 Porro operations with 5 deaths, and in 1886, 22 operations with 4 deaths. There may be possibly a few Porro cases for these two years not yet collected: the record of 1887 is very incomplete as yet, showing twelve cases, with two deaths and one suicide. The reports of 1888 are thus far equally encouraging.

Mr. Tait strongly advocates the Porro operation in preference to the Sänger, but strangely withholds from publication three cases, that might add force to his claimed preference. As we do not know even the years of their performance, they are as yet useless in the comparison.

Since the above was written, I have learned that Mr. Tait, in an operation performed last June, used the Esmarch tube temporarily; then applied his own modification of Kœberlé's *serre nœud;* and secured the stump by a "fixation pin," like a large hair-pin, with trocar points and caps to cover them. This is, then, his proper and last method of operating.

Yours truly,
Robert P. Harris, M.D.
329 S. 12th Street, Philadelphia,
December 24th, 1888.

Typhoid Fever in West Virginia.

To the Editor.

Sir: Since Aug. 1, 1888, we have had an epidemic of typhoid fever here in the mountains. Where it comes from, or what is its prime cause, I am unable to say. The country here I believe to be healthy. We live on a large river—the Clear—in Tucker County, West Virginia, and our drainage is good. There is a new railroad being built through this region, and some believe the typhoid fever is due to the stirring-up of the soil. The water I do not think the best, and there is a great deal of decaying vege-table matter also through this country.

I have had cases in the healthiest localities and cannot understand it except that, as an epidemic, it must be everywhere. All cases, if sent away in time, soon get well; those that stay generally suffer.

I have talked to my brother physicians on the subject and they give me little satis-faction. I write to ask for information. I am young in the profession, and need help, and wish to learn all I can. The REPORTER helps me, and whenever I see anything of typhoid fever, especially, I at once wish to see if I can get what I wish. Now, tell me: what is it that might have started it here? As far as I can learn, the first case was seen by a doctor some eight or ten miles from this point, some time early in May. The epidemic started on the railroad above this place, among some negro railroad hands. Doctors Porter, Harr, Baker, and I had the camps moved to a dryer place, and soon had no return of the trouble there. It is now all over our country and we still fight it. I have advised cleanliness about the houses and yards, have used disinfectants, have begged the people to use lime, both in and about the houses; but still we are kept on the go to see new cases. Let me hear from the readers of the REPORTER. I would like to hear from other physicians on the subject of typhoid fever—giving the means of preventing its spread and their treatment of cases, etc.

Yours truly,
B. M SMITH, JR., M.D.
Parsons, W. Va.,
Dec. 17, 1888.

Long Continued Diabetes Mellitus.

TO THE EDITOR.

Sir: I saw in the REPORTER, November 10, 1888, a short article by Dr. Henry C. Coe, about albuminuria in diabetes mellitus and its conclusions. I have at present a patient, 69 years of age, who had for four-teen years glycosuria, and has now albu-minuria, but no diabetes any more. It is about a year he developed the nephritis; urine, sp. gr. 1.005, albumin 2 per cent., fatty, hyaline casts, with some blood and pus casts; latterly he commenced to have abundant epistaxis; at one time the attacks continued for a whole week, the patient losing sometimes more than a pound of blood daily. Now he loses a few drops of blood once in a while. His heart is rather weak, and he has slight swelling of the extremities; but his appetite is pretty good,

his mind is clear, and he is not at all emaciated. His urine is abundant and acid; and acetone is also present in it. The patient has been formerly a hard drinker. I would not be surprised if he should die of coma. I only cite this as a case of long diabetes, apparently without much harm; but I think this chronic nephritis brought on by the irritation of the kidneys through frequent micturition. Besides, he will not take any medicines nor observe any diet; only when he is much frightened, as in the bleeding from the nose.

Yours truly,
VALENTINE KAUFMANN, M.D.
Catorce, Mexico,
Dec. 7, 1888.

NOTES AND COMMENTS.

Splenectomy.

Mr. G. A. Wright, in a communication on splenectomy in the *Medical Chronicle*, Dec., 1888, says that splenectomy has been performed for the following conditions: painful floating spleen; painful "hyper-trophy" of the spleen; malarial enlarge-ment; cystic enlargement, whether from the presence of hydatids or from the develop-ment of simple cysts of unknown origin; abscess of the spleen; enlargement in leukæmia; tumor of the spleen. He has collected records of 62 cases. Twenty-two cases of leukæmia were operated on with fatal result in every case except one, which is classed, not as an instance of leukæmia, but of hypertrophy, by Thornton, Collier, and Crédé. This case is that of Franzolini. The cause of death in 12 cases was hemor-rhage. In 5 of these the patient did not live more than one hour. Three patients died of shock, one of peritonitis, only one survived for twenty-four hours, and the longest recorded survival was forty-eight hours, except in one doubtful case.

Twenty-three cases are classed as hyper-trophy. He suggests that probably in some of these, as in a case of his, there was chronic perisplenitis. Of the twenty-three, 15 died, the most common recorded cause of death being hemorrhage, which killed four patients. The cause of death is, how-ever, not stated in the majority of the cases. In three of the cases that died of hemor-rhage, including his own patient, the bleeding came from a vessel in the diaphragm. This was also the cause of death in one of the cases of leukæmia. There is not sufficient evidence to show any relation between the weight of the spleen and the mortality of the operation.

In seven malarial cases there were five recoveries, if one is included that lived for 35 days, and then died, apparently of old nephritis and peritonitis. In this series there seems to have been no relation between the size of the spleen and the mortality.

Three patients with cystic disease all recovered. Five of unenlarged, or only slightly enlarged, "floating" spleen all recovered. In two of the successful malarial cases the organ was also "floating," as well as in one of the cases of hypertrophy, in which recovery occurred.

The more recent operations in cases of hypertrophy show a marked improvement over the older records.

In the vast majority of cases in which the sex of the patient is recorded the patients were females.

The conclusions at which he has arrived from a study of these cases, he presents as follows: 1. Splenectomy for leukæmia is inadmissible. 2. Splenectomy for hypertrophy is very dangerous, the chief danger being from hemorrhage and shock, and there being especially danger of bleeding from a vessel that passes between the spleen and the diaphragm. Whether it is altogether an abnormal vessel or merely a dilatation of a small vessel existing there, he says he does not know, but it is responsible for the death of his patient, and for that of three others, including a patient with leukæmia. 3. If malarial patients require removal of the organ there is a good prospect of recovery. 4. Cases of floating spleen and of simple cyst are eminently favorable for operation. 5. From a special consideration of his own case, he says that in a patient with simple hypertrophy or chronic splenitis, whichever it may be, a careful examination of the relations of the organ should be made before dividing any vessel, and if large adhesions to the diaphragm are found, and the spleen is firmly fixed, and the pedicle broad and ill-defined, the operation had better be abandoned. It is, of course, impossible to stop if once there is any laceration of the splenic tissue, since the bleeding can only be arrested by removal of the organ. If removal is found to be impracticable after opening the abdomen, the question of ligature of one or more of the main vessels supplying the spleen, is worth considering. Ligature of the splenic artery was suggested by Lucas, but has, so far as Mr. Wright knows, never been tried.

Successful Gastrostomy.

At the meeting of the Southern Surgical and Gynæcological Association, held at Birmingham, Ala., Dec. 4, 5 and 6, Dr. W. B. Rogers, of Memphis, Tenn., reported a successful case of gastrostomy, which he had performed for relief of a patient with cicatricial stricture of the œsophagus. The patient, a white man, 24 years of age, swallowed a solution of concentrated lye one year before the operation. The contraction was situated seven and a half inches from the incisor teeth. The opening was so small that repeated examinations failed to pass it with the smallest urethral bougies. The patient's flesh and strength were rapidly failing from starvation.

Operation, June 29, 1888. Fenger's incision was made ; the stomach was held in the abdominal wound by means of hare-lip pins, and stitched to the abdomen with silk. Every aseptic precaution was taken, and the patient recovered without any serious symptoms. On the tenth day, the gastric opening was made, and fifteen weeks later the patient was in excellent health, with flesh and strength fully restored ; ability to swallow solid food had gradually returned, and though the opening was not being used, it gave no trouble, the edges having fully cicatrized.

Treatment of Shock.

In some remarks of the treatment of shock, in the *Therapeutic Gazette*, Dec., 1888, Dr. H. C. Wood says that the most characteristic symptoms of shock are the great loss in the force of the pulse, the height of the arterial pressure, and the extraordinary fall of the bodily temperature. He suggests that the unconsciousness which comes very late in shock is due to failure of blood-supply to the brain and the lowering of the temperature of the cerebral mass. The chief cause of the heart failure is the lack of resistance to its contraction caused by the vaso-motor paralysis, which also accounts for the great fall in temperature.

If these physiological views are correct, the two chief indications for the treatment of shock are to overcome the vaso-motor paralysis and to maintain the bodily heat. Stimulation of the heart is, of course, useful, but such stimulation will amount to very little if there is no reawakening of the resistance to the heart action ; and if such resistance is aroused in any individual case, it is almost certain that it in turn will re-excite the heart.

With regard to the propriety of giving liquid food in cases of shock, Dr. Wood points out that in severe shock digestion must be in great part, if not altogether, arrested; and the advisability of putting food into the stomach seems to him very doubtful. Raw meat-juice, or better, beef essence, highly seasoned and given hot, is a stimulant rather than a food, and may achieve good at a time when so simple a true food as milk might be actually dangerous.

He advises for the maintenance of body-heat either the hot bath at 110° Fahr., or the hot-water bed. The latter is almost as powerful, he says, as the former, and is free from its objections. If an ordinary water-bed is filled three-quarters full of water at a temperature of 130° or 140°, and blankets spread over it, and the patient laid thereon, his body will sink down so that it will be almost surrounded by the heated mass. If the bed is well covered with blankets many hours will be required for the cooling of the water, so that the body heat can be kept up for a length of time without the patient being disturbed. Dr. Wood says he has found this method of heating the body in collapse extraordinarily efficacious by practical trial.

With regard to the choice of medicines in surgical collapse, he reiterates his well-known opinion that as the action of ether and of alcohol is practically identical, the use of the latter as a stimulant in collapse from the former is improper.

In shock unconnected with anæsthesia, atropine hypodermically is very valuable by virtue of its action as a vaso-motor stimulant. If ergot is used, it should be in the form of the official aqueous extract, five grains dissolved in ten minims of water with two minims of glycerine and ½ minim of carbolic acid. Digitalis, he says, is strongly indicated in shock, not only on account of its power over the heart, but because it appears to be a powerful vaso-motor stimulant. It might be injected directly into a vein in extreme cases; in this case its effect would be immediate but very temporary. Dr. Wood says that he is not aware that anyone has ever proposed the intravenous use of the drug in collapse or shock, but he commends it for trial as practically free from danger, unless over-doses are given, and says it offers the possibility of a brilliant and novel result. Five minims of the tincture diluted with a drachm of distilled water might be *slowly* injected, and repeated or increased *pro re nata.*

Creolin in Eye Diseases.

Dr. J. H. Thompson, of Kansas City, Mo., in a communication to the *Kansas City Med. Record*, Nov., 1888, says that for many years, in certain diseases of the cornea, he has used powdered iodoform and the ointment, which are introduced into the eye two or three times a day in sufficient quantity to bring the antiseptic in immediate contact with the ulcer. In other cases he has had recourse, sometimes exclusively, sometimes in conjunction with the drug mentioned, to an application to the inverted lids and cornea of a solution of the nitrate of silver (1 to 40). The result of this treatment, prolonged two or three months, has been nearly always satisfactory; but to obtain a radical cure it was often necessary to continue the treatment three or four months. He says he has found cases, however, in which this treatment has given but incomplete results; the inflammation diminishes, the functional troubles disappear almost entirely, and the patient is satisfied, believing himself cured; yet when the cornea is examined through a strong lens, small ulcers are seen on its surface, showing that the epithelium has not been completely reproduced. These ulcers, under certain special conditions, may occasion a relapse. Under these circumstances it is imperative that we should seek other remedies which can more completely and certainly destroy the micro-organisms in the cornea.

It is in these cases that he has tried creolin, and he expresses himself as much pleased with it. At present he only speaks of its healing virtues in two cases.

Creolin is a product of the decomposition of coal-tar. It comes now as a brownish liquid, very complex and very impure. It smells like tar, and it is slightly irritating to the cornea, as all the phenols are, for it is strongly acid and slightly caustic. It is probable that before long it will be purified, when it will be as neutral as vaseline, and will then be of even greater value to the ophthalmologist than it is now. Its antiseptic properties are undoubtedly superior to all other drugs at our command.

Dr. Thompson uses creolin in the following manner. A solution is made of:

R Creolin . . . . gr. iss
    Aquæ destil. . . . . ℥cl

With a brush dipped into this solution he touches the ulcers once or twice a day, after anesthetizing the eye with cocaine. Sometimes he uses a spray of creolin:

℞ Creolin . . . . gr. viii
Aquæ destil. . . . . f ℥ iii

This fluid is sprayed upon the eyeball for
a moment or so five or six times a day.
With this treatment he has generally obtained
rapid healing of the cornea in from one
month to six weeks, while with other
remedies he has had only incomplete
success.

Peripheral Neuritis.

At the meeting of the Nottingham Medico-Chirurgical Society, Nov. 16, 1888, Mr.
T. D. Pryce read a paper on this subject.
Having discussed the chief types of multiple
neuritis, he especially alluded to diabetic
neuritis, stating that this disease might
occur in two forms: (1) one in which the
motor nerve-fibres were chiefly affected,
with consequent paralysis; seen in some
cases of advanced diabetes; (2) a form in
which the sensory, vasomotor, and trophic
nerve-fibres were mostly implicated, with
consequent and corresponding symptoms.
This type closely resembled locomotor
ataxia, and also that form of alcoholic
neuritis described by Dreschfeld as alcoholic ataxia. Mr. Pryce suggested the
term diabetic ataxia or diabetic pseudo-
tabes. He related three cases illustrating
this form of disease, in one of which extensive peripheral neuritis was found after death.
He considered that the diabetic poison was
peculiarly apt to affect the peripheral sensory nerves, and, in support of this view
instanced the comparatively frequent occurrence of symmetrical neuralgia in diabetes.
He further drew attention to a suggestion
made by him, two years before, as to the
nature of the ataxia which so often occurred
in diabetes, and believed that it was in
many cases due to a peripheral sensory
neuritis. A case of peripheral neuritis
associated with phthisis was also related.
The patient was a woman, 57 years old,
and presented most of the typical symptoms
of the disease, namely, pains of varying
character, anæsthesia, impairment of superficial reflexes, loss of knee-jerk, tenderness
of muscles to pressure, together with muscular paralysis and atrophy. The disease
had run an extremely chronic course.
Peripheral neuritis was found after death.
In this case there was no history of alcohol,
syphilis, rheumatism, etc. The paper was
illustrated by drawings, photographs, and
microscopic specimens of alcoholic, diabetic, and idiopathic neuritis. — *British
Med. Journal*, Dec. 8, 1888.

Accidental Rashes in Typhoid Fever.

At the meeting of the Royal Academy of
Medicine in Ireland, Nov. 16, 1888, Dr. J.
W. Moore made a communication on accidental rashes in typhoid fever. He
explained that it was not his intention to
allude to the essential rose-spot rash of
typhoid fever; or to the more common
epiphenomena of the disease connected with
the skin, such as *taches bleuâtres*, purpura
spots, vibices, and sudamina or sweat
vesicles; or, lastly, to the coexistence with
typhoid fever of other specific diseases showing characteristic eruptions, such as scarlatina, measles, variola, and, above all,
typhus. He desired rather to draw attention to certain other accidental or adventitious appearances of the skin, which were of
somewhat rare occurrence, and, from a
diagnostic point of view, of considerable
importance. These were (1) simple hyperæmia; (2) miliary eruptions; (3) erythematous rashes; and (4) urticaria. Dr.
Moore then detailed a series of cases which
exemplified the occurrence of these accidental rashes, and summed up as follows:
1. Not infrequently, in the course of typhoid
fever, an adventitious eruption occurred,
either miliary, urticarious, or erythematous.
2. When this happened, a wrong diagnosis
of typhus, measles, or scarlatina respectively
might be made, if account was not taken of
the absence of the other objective and subjective symptoms of these diseases. 3. The
erythematous rash was the most puzzling of
all; but the prodromata of scarlet fever were
absent, nor was the typical course of that
disease observed. 4. This erythema scar-
latiniforme was most likely to show itself at
the end of the first, or in the third, week of
typhoid fever. 5. In the former case it
probably depended on a reactive inhibition
of the vasomotor system of nerves; in the
latter, on septicæmia, or secondary blood-
poisoning; or both these causes might be
present together. 6. The cases in which
this rash appeared were often severe; but
its development was important rather from
a diagnostic than from a prognostic point
of view. 7. Hence, no special line of
treatment was required beyond that already
employed for the safe conduct of the patient
through the fever.

Dr. Duffey asked if there had been eliminated the possibility of the rash being due
to drugs administered during the course of
the disease. He had himself seen four cases
of profuse miliary eruption following the
administration of antipyrin. So, too, an
erythematous eruption similar to scarlet

fever followed the administration of quinine, while scarlatinal eruption followed the administration of antipyrin, salicylic acid, and other drugs. Rashes occurred in fevers attended with serious blood-changes, and disappeared without any marked effect on the patient.

Dr. Pollock pointed out as remarkable that while most writers observed that the rash occurred in the first week or early stage of the fever, in a case of his the rash did not appear until the third week, although the rose spots had been out for a fortnight before. The pulse was never very high, but on the night of the 18th it suddenly rose to 108, and the rash was then noticed coming out over the back, chest and abdomen. Next day there was a sudden collapse—the temperature fell to 96°, and the pulse was low and very weak. On the following day Dr. Moore saw the patient, and on the day after the rash came out over the extremities. In reference to the medicines administered, he had given two grains of quinine, but, as it made the patient deaf, he stopped, and no more was given until after the erythematous rash disappeared. No antipyrin had been given.

Dr. Walter Smith said there were drug rashes and food rashes; and the explanation given by Dr. Duffey applied to many cases. Most rashes belonged to the erythematous class, and were due to a transitory disturbance of the vascular system of the skin, liable to arise in four different ways: First, direct action on the central nervous system by drugs; secondly, reflex irritation from the intestinal tube, produced by articles of diet; thirdly, direct dilatation of the vessels of the skin caused by such drugs as nitrite of amyl, nitro-glycerine, and alcohol; and, fourthly, the diffuse transudation of irritating drugs through the skin, as the essential oils of copaiba and cubebs, etc.

Dr. John William Moore replied that in Case No. 1, no medicine had been administered for some days, and the only possible cause of the efflorescence was the extreme rise of temperature, followed by sweating. It was not true erythema, but an efflorescence on the skin. In Case No. 2, he understood that the patient had been getting morphine to produce sleep, but only in small quantities; and that drug could scarcely have had anything to do with the development of the miliary eruption. In Dr. Pollock's case, quinine in only two-grain doses had been given several days before the rash appeared, but it disagreed, and was stopped.—*British Med. Journal,* Dec. 1, 1888.

Disinfection of the Air-Passages with Myrthol.

The Vienna correspondent of the *New Orleans Med. and Surg. Journal,* Dec., 1888, says that hitherto inhalations of turpentine in the respiration mask of Curschmann have been used for disinfecting the air-passages, or for combating putrid processes. Aside from the frequent disagreeable after-effects which were produced by this medication, the results also were very little favorable. In spite of the inhalations a patient affected with putrid bronchitis used to infect a whole ward in the hospital. Dr. Eichherst has recommended a medicament which, taken by the mouth, met all these inconveniences, and moreover favorably influenced the appetite and the general condition of the patient. This drug, myrthol, has a rapid and sure effect. It is that part of the myrtle-oil which boils at from 160° to 170° C. (320° to 338° F.), and which represents a clear fluid of an aromatic odor. It had formerly been recommended as a deodorant in bronchial catarrh. According to the present recommendation it is the best medicament for rapidly and surely combating the putrescence, and for removing the bad odor of the breath and the secretions.

When a gelatine capsule containing two and one-half minims of myrthol is taken the breath distinctly smells of myrthol for an hour, and this odor can also be perceived for twenty-four and even forty-eight hours after the administration. In putrid processes much larger doses are required; in most cases two capsules are administered at intervals of two hours. There is no disgust against the drug on the part of the patients.

Though myrthol proves very effectual in combating the putrid process and the bad odor connected therewith it is quite ineffectual for preventing an infection with tubercle bacilli, as tuberculosis developed even when myrthol was in use.

New York Academy of Medicine.

At the meeting of the Academy January 3, 1889, the annual reports of officers and committees were read. The total amount of money in the permanent fund is $120,776.85. The library has received during the year 1888 2,600 volumes, 3,235 pamphlets, 17,452 medical journals. Four thousand dollars was granted to the library for expenses during the current year. The number of members has been increased by 55.

NEWS.

—Dr. Horace Jayne will succeed Prof. E. Otis Kendall as Dean of the College Faculty of the University of Pennsylvania.

—Dr. C. N. Campbell, of Poughkeepsie, N. Y., died December 20. He was graduated from the Medical Department of the New York University in 1848, and was President of the Poughkeepsie Civil Service Board.

—Press dispatches indicate that smallpox exists in widely separated portions of this country. It is reported to be spreading in Albany, N. Y., and the inmates of Auburn State Prison are to be vaccinated. It is also increasing in New Washington, Ohio, to such an extent that business has been interfered with and trains are not allowed to stop. A few cases are reported from Newport, Kentucky.

—The Mills Training School for Male Nurses, in New York, was opened December 19. There were 110 applicants, of whom 22 were admitted to the school. The *Doctor* says: "The old Reign of Terror in many of our hospitals is drawing to a close. The Warden of Bellevue Hospital began discharging the orderlies in the wards for male patients the other day, and filling their places with the students just admitted to the new Mills school for training male nurses. Now the male patients will probably be as skillfully nursed as the female patients have been for some time."

—The New York *Medical Record*, January 5, 1889, says that the statistics of the New York State Board of Charities for the year ending October 1, 1888, show only a little increase in the number of the dependent classes other than the insane, and in the expenditures during the year as compared with last year. The whole number of insane in the institutions of the State on October 1, 1888, was 14,772, as against 14,062 on October 1, 1887, an increase of 710. This is the greatest increase in any year in the history of the State. All of the asylums are full, and many are greatly overcrowded.

———◆◆———

DOUBTFUL CUSTOMER.—"Are these 'ere specs genuine crystal?" Street-stand merchant: "Chenooine? Of you don't mention it, I tell you someding. My bruder Isidore has bought dot Crystal Palace in England and is cutting him up into spectacles—dot makes dem so cheap. One dollar an' a halluf a pair!"—*Puck.*

HUMOR.

A MATCH between two dentists in their art would probably result in a draw.—*Boston Courier.*

WANTED THE FREE LIST EXTENDED.— Big Brother College-Graduate—"Are you in favor of wool being free of all duty?" Undergraduate (with conditions)—"Yes, sheepskins too."—*New Haven News.*

MISS KEANE (to handsome young physician)—"Oh, doctor, how do you do? You look killing this evening!" Young Physician (quietly)—"Thank you, but I'm not; I'm off duty, don't you know."—*Drake's Magazine.*

SOMEONE who has given attention to the subject says that anodynes are laborious in their operation. The discovery lacks the merit of originality, however. It has long been known that anodynes are pains-taking. —*Binghamton Leader.*

THE OTHER WAY ABOUT.—Irate passenger (as train is moving off)—Why the —— didn't you put my baggage in as I told you, you old ——? Porter—Eh, man! yer baggage es na sic a fule as yersel'. Ye-re i' the wrong train.—*London Punch.*

"HOW MUCH WILL A NEW SET of teeth cost?" "Fifty dollars, madam." "Oh, that is much too dear!" "But, madam, think: you will be able to eat with them." "Yes, but if I pay so much as that I will have nothing to eat."—*Fliegende Blätter.*

IT IS SAID that "a Dakota girl ate twenty ears of green corn for supper and then went to a party and danced all night." We should think she would. Eight ears of corn are enough to make some people dance all night—and howl, too.—*Norristown Herald.*

JOHNNY—"Pa, this paper says that Mr. Smith died intestate. What does that mean?" Pa—"It means, my son, that—er, that Mr. Smith had something the matter with his intestines—some sort of inflammation of the bowels, probably." *Boston Transcript.*

A LONG TERM.—Irish guide to American tourist—"And there is no King nor Quane nayther in America, they're tellin' me, sur?" Indifferent Tourist—"No; we've a President there." "And how long have you been havin' a President, moight I ax, sur?" I. T.—"Oh, something over a hundred years!" Irishman, stopping, paralyzed with astonishment — "Howly saints! And do they live that long beyant there?"

MEDICAL AND SURGICAL REPORTER

No. 1664.   .PHILADELPHIA, JANUARY 19, 1889.   VOL. LX.—No. 3.

CONTENTS:

COMMUNICATIONS.

OSTEOTOMY FOR ANTERIOR CURVATURES OF THE LEG.[1]

BY DE FOREST WILLARD, M.D., PH.D.,
PHILADELPHIA.
LECTURER ON ORTHOPÆDIC SURGERY, UNIVERSITY OF
PENNSYLVANIA ; SURGEON TO PRESBYTERIAN
HOSPITAL ; CONSULTING SURGEON TO
THE WHITE AND TO THE
COLORED CRIPPLES'
HOMES.

One of the most frequent deformities produced by rickets is a forward arching of the bones of the leg, which deviation is very often associated with a lateral curve of both tibia and fibula.

Rickets is a constitutional disease, and is so seldom seen in country practice in healthy districts, that physicians frequently overlook the early symptoms, which are manifested by an indisposition of the child to be lifted, by peevishness, and by general symptoms of mal-nutrition. Ordinarily these conditions are attributed to indigestion, and certainly the stomach and intestines are largely at fault in the production of this state of defective digestion, and still more defective assimilation ; but simple indigestion does not give the beaded ribs or "rickety rosary," the softened cranial bones, the cranio-tabes, the lengthened dolicho-cephalic skull, the open fontanelles, the softened bones, the enlarged epiphyses, the excessive head sweatings, the flabby muscles, and the enlarged epiphyses—deformities so characteristic of rachitis. Rickets is essentially a disease of early childhood, is rarely congenital or hereditary, and only occasionally develops at or after puberty. It differs entirely from either tuberculosis or scrofulosis.[1] In small cities it is rare ; in larger ones, it is found in proportion to the exist-

[1] Read before the American Orthopædic Association, September, 1888.

[1] Ashhurst, International Encyclopædia of Surgery, Vol. I; p. 251.

ing amount of filth, squalor, bad air, scanty food and deficient light. When found in the rich, it can be traced to improper food or hygiene. In this country the colored race is more affected than the white, and the results are also more serious.[1]

While it is a constitutional disease affecting all the tissues of the body, yet its worst manifestations are exhibited in deformities of the bones. These deformities are due to the relative preponderance of the organic over the earthy tissues in the bone, and the failure of the formative cartilage cells to produce true bone cells. This is the stage of softening; and during its progress, if the child is allowed out of bed, the osseous tissues are unable to sustain the superincumbent weight and consequently easily yield to a greater or less degree. Not only do the tibia, fibula and femur become bent, but the pelvis is deformed, and either from creeping or from being lifted, the humerus, or the radius and ulna of the patient, may also be distorted. In severe grades even the clavicles are arched.

Upon the resumption of proper assimilation, however, the deposit of earthy salts begins, and then follows the stage of *sclerosis* or hardening, which permanently fixes the distorted bones in their faulty positions.

Among the most frequent of bone deviations are *anterior tibial curves*. These are not produced by contraction of the gastrocnemius; for the calf-muscles are at first flabby and only become shortened at a later stage. The distortion may extend in a long curve from knee to ankle, or it may be abrupt and angular at any portion of the bone, usually the lower third.

The treatment of these anterior curves is accomplished by

I. Manual Straightening and the Use of Apparatus.

In the second and third years of life, if the bones are still either soft or springy, it is possible to correct the deformity by frequent manual straightening, provided the mother or nurse is willing to give the requisite time and patience to the case. The pressure should be as forcible as the integrity of the bone will permit ; this will give the child pain for only a few moments after the force is removed. This pressure should be repeated many times daily. If gentle manual pressure could be constantly

applied it would doubtless, as in club-foot, be perfectly curative. Instrumental pressure, made in the proper direction by spring power or by strap connected with steel uprights, may be employed in connection with manipulation, during this stage.

After the bone has hardened, however, I agree with Gibney[1] in saying that I have never seen a case of anterior curve of the tibia of any magnitude reduced by apparatus. Many surgeons spend months in attempting to straighten the bones in these cases, and then condemn the patient to perpetual cripplehood ; whereas a slight operation will produce a perfect cure. The conditions are mechanically entirely different from those met with in legs bowed laterally.[2]

II. Forcible Fracture.

A. *By the Hands.*
B. *By the Osteoclast.*

A. *Manual Fracture.* — In children under three years of age, by far the safest and best plan to be adopted, is fracture of the two bones at the proper point, if the surgeon possesses the requisite strength. For additional power the knee may be used, or the child may be placed upon its face and a very small sand-bag, or a wide roller bandage, be used as a fulcrum. Frequently it is timidity rather than lack of strength that prevents success. Up to the point compatible with the life of the soft parts, its great advantage lies in the fact that only a simple fracture is produced and speedy union is the result.[3] The objection to the plan lies in the inability of the surgeon to regulate exactly the point of fracture.

The proper dressing after manual fracture is fixation, as described under osteotomy.

B. *Osteoclasis.* — The osteoclast, while a very efficient instrument in the thigh, yet in the leg has the great disadvantage that pressure must be made upon the sharp edge of the tibia covered only by thin skin. It offers the advantages, however, that in the centre of the bone pressure can be applied to a definite point, and that its resultant is a simple fracture, provided sloughing is avoided. When the apex of projection is near to either epiphysis, however, neither

---

[1] Transactions American Surgical Association, 1887, p. 261.

[1] Transactions Academy of Medicine, New York, 1886. Vol. XLV.

[2] MEDICAL AND SURGICAL REPORTER, July 25 and August 1, 1885. *Archives of Pediatrics*, 1885, p. 680.

[3] *Dublin Journal Medical Science.* Vol. LXXIX; p. 483.

the Rizzoli pattern nor any of its modifications is easy of adjustment.[1]

III. Osteotomy.

A. *By chisel:* 1. Simple. 2. Cuneiform.
B. *By saw.*

A. *Chisel.* Both simple and wedge osteotomy necessitate the production of a compound fracture; but in the former the operation is almost subcutaneous, and in the latter there is the absence of contusion and other ordinary accompaniments of such an injury. The results may therefore be expected to be very much better, provided strict asepsis is enforced.

The procedure which I have found most effective is as follows:

On the day previous to the operation the leg should be shaved, then washed with soap

The rubber cloth should be placed on top of the sand-bag, and then covered with a single layer of wet bichloride towels. The region of the operation should be well surrounded with carbolated towels. One of the osteotomes should be both wider and thicker than the other, the latter being used in the deeper portion of the section so as to prevent wedging. I have never been unfortunate enough to break off an instrument in the bone, but this accident has occurred in the practice of experienced surgeons, and a portion of the chisel has been allowed to remain. I should prefer to loosen and remove it by cuts alongside.

The osteotome should taper gradually, not abruptly, and should be driven by light taps of the mallet after the anterior cancellous tissue has been passed, lest a splintering

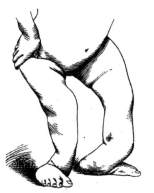

Fig. 1.

Fig. 1 shows only the lower half of the body; but in this case nearly every long bone was curved. Locomotion was impossible except with a waddling gait and with the trunk supported upon the thighs by the hands. When the patient stood, each tibia rested upon the dorsum of the foot. Both legs were "cork-screwed," and the femora bent both outward and forward. All the epiphyses were enlarged, and the elbow articulation was so distorted that the arms could be only partly flexed. Both clavicles were sharply bent forward at their centres.

and water and afterward with ether, after which it is enveloped in towels which have been dipped in sublimate solution (1–2000), and then dried. These will remain *in situ* until the patient is etherized, when the final washing with bichloride (1–1000) is made. Instruments are first to be placed in boiling water, then in carbolic acid solution (1–20).

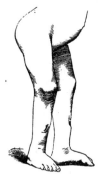

Fig. 2.

Fig 2, from a photograph, shows the result of the osteotomies in case shown in Fig. 1.

or a long oblique fracture be produced. Several times while rapidly demonstrating this operation to a class, I have in the cadaver made a fracture that extended obliquely for many inches. The posterior one-fourth of the bone should always be fractured manually, lest the instrument injure the artery, which, from displacement, may lie directly behind or alongside the bone. Dandridge[1] was unfortunate enough to lose a patient from pyemia, after an injury of the posterior tibial artery and vein, which both lay directly against the tibia.

1. *Linear Osteotomy.*—In simple osteotomy an Esmarch bandage is not desirable,

---

[1] *New York Medical Journal*, 1886, xliii, p. 129.

[1] *Boston Med. and Surg. Journal*, 1885, cxiii, 25.

as the outflowing blood is of advantage in effectually preventing the entrance of air.

In regard to the cases suitable for the simple cut, experience has taught me that even where the angle has been very prominent, there is no necessity for taking out a wedge, as nature is abundantly able, provided no septic influence is introduced, to unite the bones solidly even if they were angularly placed. The incision with the knife should be directly down through the periosteum, and should be no longer than just sufficient to permit the osteotome to turn crosswise without tension. In children the fibula need not be touched, as it can be easily fractured; but in the sclerosed bones of lads or adults, a separate section will be necessary. The larger osteotome should not be removed from the bone until more than one-third of the diameter has been traversed, although it should frequently be moved sidewise to prevent wedging, and to incise different portions of the structures in large bones. The smaller instrument should be carefully inserted in the exact track of its predecessor.

An operator soon learns to distinguish the increased density of the compact tissue when the posterior region is reached, and will withdraw the osteotome before it has penetrated this layer, when fracture will readily complete the solution of continuity.

Rectification being now performed, section of the tendo Achillis is usually done with benefit, as it relieves much of the tension upon the parts, permits better adjustment and reduces the tendency to future displacement. Irrigation with sublimate solution should be frequently practised during the progress of the section, and upon the withdrawal of the instrument an aseptic sponge should at once close the wound, and remain in position.

Without waiting for hemorrhage to cease, unless it be profuse, all tissue is removed from between the edges of the wound, a few strands of cat-gut introduced, and the lips drawn together by cat-gut suture or strip of adhesive plaster—preferably the former. Irrigation should be continued until the sublimate gauze (freshly wet, in children, with 1–2000 solution) is actually in place.

I have abandoned both protective and iodoform. Dry sublimate cotton is now applied as a roller to the leg and foot and is held in position by an antiseptic or flannel bandage.

Plaster-of-Paris rollers soaked in warm salt water are now applied, the limb is extended, and the deformity slightly over-corrected, until fixation is complete. To insure accuracy of position the plaster encasement of the leg should first be completed; an assistant then rests the heel of the patient upon the thumb and finger of one hand and grasps the toes with the other, which position he must maintain during the envelopment of the foot and the setting of the plaster. As a rule, but little morphia will be required, and if no pain or odor is present, and the temperature is good, the surgeon will have little to do for four or five weeks as the case progresses to good union without suppuration.

The temperature chart is not an infallible guide as to the condition of the parts, yet it is one of the best indications; and if no evidences of suppuration exist, the dressing need not be interfered with, as disturbance of any wound, so long as it is sweet, is harmful. Should the cast become loose, it should be sawed open, the leg examined to see that good position is maintained, and the encasement drawn closer together by a bandage.

If other osteotomies are to be performed at the same operation, each fracture as it is produced should be wrapped in a sublimated towel, while a pledget of antiseptic cotton is fastened over the wound. A temporary wooden or paste-board splint should be applied, lest in the manipulations of the subsequent operations the muscles and possibly the bloodvessels should be lacerated by a sharp-pointed fragment.

2. Cuneiform Osteotomy.—The removal of a wedge-shaped piece from the tibia is only necessary when the angle of curvature is very great, and especially when it approaches the right angle. To determine the amount of bone necessary to be excised, one soon learns to judge with sufficient accuracy by his eye. If exactness is desired the sphenometer[1] may be used, or the anterior surface of the limb may be outlined upon a piece of stiff paper. This line paralleled by one at about the supposed anteroposterior diameter of the tibia, will give the size of this bone. When the pattern is cut out as drawn, a rude representation of the tibia will be secured which, when cut through at the point of the curvature, and straightened, will at once show the size of the wedge.

As a cuneiform section is much more serious than simple osteotomy, every aseptic precaution should be used to prevent suppuration. These have already been enumerated. The application of a sterilized

[1] *Therapeutic Gazette*, 1887, p. 154.

Esmarch bandage assists greatly in the proper formation of the wedge, by giving a good view of the cut bone surfaces. A chisel, beveled upon one side, is used instead of an osteotome.

If rigid, and in large children, the fibula should be first divided, but the removal of a wedge from this bone is never necessary. The knife incision over the tibia should be a little larger than the proposed base of the wedge, and the periosteum should be cut not only longitudinally but also laterally, in order that it may be preserved intact without laceration, and that it may be subsequently sutured.

The wedge is not taken away entire, but is made rather by a series of chippings until the proper amount is removed.

The posterior portion of the bone is fractured by manual force as in simple osteotomy. If the instrument is driven too rapidly, or carried too deeply into the bone, a very oblique fracture may result. Tenotomy of the tendo Achillis should always be performed if there is any restraint against rectification.

Many surgeons fasten the ends of the bones with wire,[1] silkworm-gut, kangaroo-tendon, etc.; but I see no necessity in the majority of cases for the delay and for the additional incentive to suppuration. In angular malunion following fracture, however, I always use the inter-osseous suture, as there is ordinarily a tendency to non-union. Upon the removal of the Esmarch bandage the hemorrhage will be very free from the cut surfaces, but hot water or eburnation will usually arrest it. Stuffing the wound with alum gauze is rarely if ever necessary, and if it is used the material should be removed within twenty-four hours. Drainage, while unnecessary in simple osteotomy in which organization of blood-clot will occur, is here of the greatest importance for the prevention of suppuration.

All fragments of bone should be thoroughly removed by irrigation (with 1 to 2000 sublimate solution, in children), and the ends brought closely together *without any pinching of tissues.* A failure to observe this rule will ensure defeat, as will also the retention of any tissue in the lips of the wound when it is closed by cat-gut sutures. Either sterilized horse-hair or cat-gut may be used for drainage; I prefer the former.

When there is an opening at the fibula a roll of horse-hairs is carried into the tibial

wound with a pair of forceps, and made to emerge at the opening of the former; another small bundle is carried directly through from the bottom of the wound to the posterior aspect of the leg through a counter opening. Cat-gut may be allowed to remain permanently, although I prefer to take it away, as I do the hair, in thirty-six hours.

In applying the dressings, the same thorough precautions are necessary to obtain asepsis until the moment that the wound is covered with gauze. The sublimate cotton, plaster bandage, etc., are applied as before, except that the latter is put on as a recurrent longitudinally along the sides of the limb at the seat of operation, in order to give additional strength laterally. In front and behind, at the site of the proposed windows, the cast is made thinner and the ends of the horse-hairs arranged so that they can be withdrawn without interference with the remainder of the dressing.

A slight over-correction of the deformity is advisable while the plaster is setting, and extension should also be made in order to secure good apposition of the fragments. When windows are cut in the cast on the second day, the staining of dressings with blood does not necessitate their removal so long as decomposition has not taken place. A moderate wetting with sublimate solution after the withdrawal of the drain will prevent all odor for a week or ten days, when union of the soft parts will have occurred, and a fresh dressing may be applied through the opening. Care should be taken that pressure should be accurately made upon the tissues beneath the window, lest local œdema and pain ensue. Usually these cases go on to speedy and perfect union. Occasionally, through some fault in the operation or in the dressing, suppuration ensues, in which case the cast about the opening should be coated with shellac, the wound thoroughly washed and antiseptically dressed, when the cessation of pus formation may be soon secured.

In the case from which the accompanying figures were prepared, while one limb healed kindly, the other suppurated, and several particles of bone were discharged; nevertheless, a perfect union and a good leg resulted.

I have never ventured beyond six osteotomies at one time, but as high as ten have been performed.[1] It is my custom to

[1] *St. Bartholomew Hospital Reports*, 1886, xxii, 40; also 1884, vol. xx, p. 59.

[1] *Dublin Jour. Med. Science*, vol. LXXIX, p. 292; MacEwen, Trans. Eighth International Medical Congress, Copenhagen, 1884.

rectify coexistent knock-knee by a simultaneous supra-condyloid osteotomy, Figs. 3 and 4; but I have always left the high curve which so often exists in the femur, intending to do section later. Thus far, however, all my cases have been so greatly improved in locomotive powers that I have hesitated to incur the possible risk of rotation of fragments or of placing the head of the femur after reunion in a new relation to the acetabulum; and have also reasoned that as both pelvic and thigh muscles had for years accommodated themselves to the abnormal positions, more or less disability might occur by throwing them into new mechanical relations.

All my sections at the upper end of the femur have been for hip-joint anchylosis, and in cases in which I did not expect to secure the proper apposition of femoral

be only just large enough to admit the saw. Care should be exercised that neither blood-vessels nor nerves are injured.

Will the deformity return? Doubtless, if too early locomotion is attempted without support, or if a febrile or other exhaustive disease speedily follows the operation. Such a softening of the callus before it is thoroughly ossified is possible after any fracture; but is rare. Should it accidentally occur, the case should be treated as one of mal-union or of delayed union; *i. e.*, first, by reposition and fixation with gypsum; then, secondly, by open osteotomy and wiring of fragments, with long-continued subsequent support.

Conclusions.—1. Anterior tibial curves during the soft and springy stages may be corrected by manual rectification and the use of apparatus.

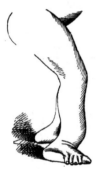

Fig. 3.

Double knock-knee with double anterior curves.

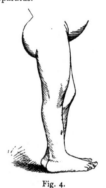

Fig. 4.

After osteotomy.

head and acetabulum, since both had been either greatly altered or already destroyed.

B.—*Section with the Saw.*—Several very oblique fractures which have recently been produced by me in making sections of the bones by the osteotome and chisel, in which very sharp ends of fragments have rendered injury of the soft parts and blood-vessels imminent, have led me to look favorably upon the operation with the saw. I have never practised it upon the leg bones, although frequently employing the·saw on other bones. The section could be performed almost absolutely subcutaneously, and I have never had suppuration follow its use in other cases. The saw should be blunt pointed, should have a short cutting face, and the puncture with the knife should

2. Braces are useless after hardening has occurred.

3. Manual fracture is the best and safest remedial operation in young children.

4. Instrumental fracture, or osteoclasis, is not as safe or effective as osteotomy.

5. Aseptic simple osteotomy, for all moderate degrees of curve, and cuneiform section for very severe grades, give almost uniformly good and speedy results, without suppuration. Subcutaneous section by the saw is also a reliable operation.

6. Plaster of Paris is the simplest and most effective material for securing accurate position and maintaining absolute fixation. By its use the delay and injury incident to suturing the ends of the bones is avoided.

1818 Chestnut St.

TUBERCULAR MENINGITIS.[1]

BY T. J. HAPPEL, A.M., M.D.,
TRENTON, TENN.

PRESIDENT OF THE TENNESSEE STATE MEDICAL
SOCIETY.

Tubercular meningitis is one of the most fatal of diseases. I do not refer in this statement to the total number of deaths from it, but to the fact that there are very few recoveries when the victim is once seized with it.

Definition.—The name itself defines the disease. By tubercular meningitis is meant an inflammation of the meninges, usually at the base of the brain, due to the deposit in these membranes of tuberculous material. The presence of tubercles in the meninges, and inflammation arising therefrom, is the "*sine qua non*" of tubercular meningitis. Post-mortem examination may reveal tubercular deposits throughout the system, as well as in the meninges. In the meninges, we find miliary tubercles—grayish white granules, varying in size from a minute speck to that of a pin-head, which in the aggregate may make a mass as large as a pea. These tubercles are very unevenly distributed, being most commonly found in the pia mater at the base of the brain, though at the same time they are often met with in other locations. The amount of inflammation does not depend upon the number of tubercles.

Etiology.—The causes of the disease may be divided into predisposing and exciting. Among the predisposing causes may be classed any and every thing that tends in any way to impair vitality. Heredity, therefore, becomes a strong predisposing factor. Tuberculosis, scrofula, the so-called scrofulous diathesis, and syphilis are chief among the diseases which when transmitted by either parent to the child may implant in the offspring such a condition of malnutrition as may lead to the production of a state of the body favorable to the development and growth of tubercles. I emphasize the three diseases above named, as I shall have occasion later on in this paper to refer to them again. The eruptive fevers, and whooping-cough in young children, may also be classed as predisposing causes, because in many cases, children, after attacks of those diseases, are left feeble and weak—almost in a condition of marasmus— furnishing pabulum just suited to tubercular deposits and growths.

[1] Read before the Gibson County Medical Society, September, 1888.

Age can be cited as another predisposing cause. We find the disease oftenest in children between two and seven years of age; and next in frequency in young adults, between twenty and thirty years of age. Marriage in close consanguinity, by tending to weaken the offspring of such unions, favors the development of tubercular meningitis. Children of a scrofulous diathesis, however it may have been acquired, and children in whom the nervous system has been developed at the expense of the muscular, are predisposed to the disease. Precocious children, with a pale, flabby skin, soft, relaxed muscles, blue eyes, with a mature general appearance, are prone to the development of the disease. In some cases, however, no predisposing cause can be discovered. One child in a whole family may have the disease, and all the rest, as well as the parents, remain healthy.

Among the exciting causes may be classed, first of all, poor hygienic surroundings. Bad, scanty, and improperly cooked food, close confinement in tenements, and such like influences, as well as sudden changes in temperature, exposure to cold, etc., act as important exciting causes. Hence we find the disease more common among the poor in cities than we do in the country and among the rich; though the latter are by no means exempt. Improper feeding of children, where there is any tendency to tubercle, especially hereditary, is liable to develop tubercular meningitis. Caries may act as an exciting cause; so also may the presence of caseous material anywhere in the system. In many cases, no exciting cause can be discovered. The latest, newest, and therefore the most commonly accepted cause of tubercular meningitis, is a specific cause, the *bacillus tuberculosis*. The disposition of late is to trace all diseases to some micro-organism, animal or vegetable, and we find the disease in question no exception. It is contended that wherever tubercle exists, especially in the lungs, this bacillus can always be found and its presence in the sputum of the patient demonstrated with a powerful microscope, and that it can be differentiated by staining with a strong solution of carbolic fuchsine, which imparts a red color to the bacillus, and then by making "the contrast staining by what is known as Fraenkel's solution, the specific bacillus remaining a deep red, and the other elements in the sputum blue." In my own opinion, this bacillus has not been positively shown to be the cause of the disease, but is more probably a sequence.

Proper pabulum for its development is furnished in systems enfeebled as above described, and the bacillus finds its nidus in this prepared soil and there grows.

The symptoms of the disease may be divided into those pertaining to two periods : the prodromic, and the stage of invasion. The prodromic stage corresponds to and represents the period of the deposit of miliary tubercles, or, as believers in a specific bacillus would say, the time elapsing between the date of the reception of the bacillus into the system, and its multiplication and fixation in sufficient numbers in the pia-mater at the base of the brain to give rise to irritation. This period is of variable duration, from a few days to weeks or perhaps months. During this time changes are noted in the general disposition of the child and in its conduct. The disease rarely appearing before the second year, these changes can be easily noted and studied. As remarked previously, the victims of this disease are usually bright precocious children abounding in life. From being always playful, the child becomes dull and listless, at times apathetic, fretful, peevish, irritable. He cannot be interested long at a time in any way. Whilst playing, he suddenly stops, and wants to be taken up. He becomes a different child in every respect. But the most marked change is in the loss of flesh. The child becomes pale, and his flesh loose, flabby, and progressively diminishes. His features take on an old look. There is a vacant stare about him. His appetite diminishes and he occasionally vomits. He complains at times in a vague way of his head. At night, in his sleep, he is restless, tossing from side to side in his bed, and frequently groaning, and grinding his teeth. According to Pepper, young children often "manifest a strange perversity', or an unusual disobedience, for which they may be punished under the belief that it is intentional." Whilst the foregoing are some of the chief symptoms of the disease in children, they may vary from being so slight as to be overlooked, to being most severe.

The symptoms of the stage of invasion may be subdivided into those of irritation, pressure, and collapse. It is difficult to mark the transition from the prodromic stage to that of irritation. The change is so gradual that it is impossible to say just where one ends, and the other begins. The chief distinguishing feature of this period is the occurrence of fever. The prodromic stage is ordinarily attended by no fever, but in the stage of invasion the temperature rises to 103°, or in some cases higher, though generally lower. The pupils are unequally dilated, and sometimes strabismus is present. Headache increases. There is sensitiveness to light and sound, and sometimes twitching of the muscles. In a few cases violent convulsions occur. The pulse rate in this stage is usually slow, though, exceptionally, it is frequent. The respiration is slow and irregular, and the tongue coated. The bowels are constipated, and the abdominal walls retracted, and vomiting is a prominent symptom. The little patient at times lies in a stupid, comatose condition, from which he arouses with a sharp shrill cry—the hydrocephalic cry. During sleep, delirium is a prominent symptom. There is intolerance of light, the little patient frequently trying to shut out the light by burrowing the head down into the pillows. His somnolence becomes more marked in the latter part of this stage, though he can be roused, and will answer questions rationally, after which he lapses almost at once into a condition of half-sleep. He gradually becomes less and less irritable, allowing examinations to be made without resistance of any kind. The eyes become dull, the cornea takes on a lustreless appearance. Somnolence deepens still more, and it becomes next to impossible to rouse him.

In this stage of the disease symptoms of apparent improvement may occur. The parents flatter themselves that convalescence is about to set in. All symptoms appear better ; but these hopes are soon blasted. The duration of the stage of irritation is from a few days to a week. The transition from this to that of effusion with depression, is not marked except by the gradual deepening of all the foregoing symptoms. The pupils are unequal and respond slowly, if at all, to the light. The muscles of the back of the neck become stiff, and occasionally opisthotonos occurs. The bowels are constipated, and the urine is retained or is passed involuntarily. Deglutition becomes difficult ; the appetite is completely lost The respiration is irregular and sighing—the Cheyne-Stokes form being common. The temperature in children is frequently subnormal, even when there are convulsions. The pulse is slow, irregular, and intermittent, the irregularity being a marked feature. The sudden vomiting ceases. The child at times interrupts this condition of stupor by convulsions, and by giving utterance to the peculiar, sharp, hydrocephalic cry. According to Prof. Loomis, "the ophthalmoscope reveals varicosities of the retinal veins, points of hemorrhage . . . and white, miliary granulations on the retina and choroid." As in the first stage, so in this, there are cases of apparent improvement or even recovery, but in a few hours the child rapidly lapses into a more stupid condition than before. In the stage of collapse, all the symptoms point to a speedy dissolution. The whole system may become relaxed. The paralyses, which up to this point may have been transient, now become permanent. The child is bathed in a cold, sticky perspiration. The pulse becomes very frequent and feeble, varying from 120 to 200 a minute, the heart being released from the inhibitory influence of the *par vagum*. The respiration sympathizes, and becomes frequent, but sighing and very irregular. The pupils are widely dilated. The eyes are rolled upward, showing but little of the cornea, and are insensible to light. The abdomen becomes tympanitic. Involuntary discharges from the bladder and rectum take place. Subsultus is marked. Coma deepens, and death may take place quietly and gradually during this condition, or it may occur from asphyxia in the midst of a convulsion. This stage usually lasts from twenty-four to forty-eight hours, though very rarely the child may linger for an indefinite time in this state of living death.

I have not referred to the condition of the fontanelles in this disease, as it rarely occurs before they have closed ; but in the stage of invasion in very young children they are prominent from distention of the brain with the hydrocephalic fluid, whilst in the state of collapse they are depressed.

There are some distinctive features of this disease which should be carefully studied, in order to diagnosticate it promptly when it is met with. The premonitory stage presents usually a frequent pulse, with possibly some little irregularity ; the respiration is normal and the temperature almost normal. There is loss of flesh, and vomiting. In the irritative stage of invasion, the pulse and respiration become slow and irregular, the latter frequently sighing. The temperature begins to rise, rising and falling irregularly, though rarely going above 103°. It varies many times each day, but the evening temperature averages a little higher than the morning. Loss of flesh continues, so also does

the vomiting. In this stage of the disease, in the majority of cases, the *tache cérébrale* is found—the red mark responding promptly to pressure of the finger on the face ; but general flushes alternating with pallor are met with in nearly all cases.

In the stage of collapse, the pulse and respiration become rapid and more irregular. The Cheyne-Stokes respiration marks the last stage of the disease. The temperature may sometimes rise till just before death, and then it falls rapidly. The peculiarities of circulation and respiration are very easily understood and explained by remembering the fact that both are controlled by the *par vagum*, and that in the prodromic period the disturbance of the roots of the nerve and the medulla oblongata is irregular, producing a frequent, varying pulse and respiration ; but in the first and second stages of invasion, the irritation is continuous and the inhibitory function of the nerve is kept in play, so that both acts are restrained, whilst in the stage of collapse, in the resulting paralysis, the nerve loses all controlling power and both respiration and pulsation are quickened and made irregular. In an analysis of fifty-six consecutive cases, reported by Dr. Wortmann (*Jahrbuch für Kinderheilkunde*, 1884) "retraction of the head was present in all but one case, and commenced when the pulse became irregular." The temperature never rose above 104°. Hyperæsthesia was present in all but one case where the spinal meninges were involved. Vomiting was one of the most characteristic symptoms, and was considered a diagnostic one when it occurred from a comparatively empty stomach and without effort. When food was present, it seemed to be almost a regurgitation of the ingesta.

The duration of the disease, after the prodromic period, ranges on an average from two to two and a half weeks ; but in some few cases the disease has terminated abruptly in a few days. Many circumstances may aid in bringing about a rapidly fatal result. Those cases in which heredity can be traced are more apt to run a rapid course.

Tubercular meningitis is to be distinguished from typhoid fever, which also has a prodromic period, by the fact that epistaxis is very rare in tubercular meningitis ; that in typhoid fever the temperature is more regular, and the pulse grows progressively more rapid, whilst in tubercular meningitis it is first rapid, then slow, then rapid again. Again in typhoid fever the abdomen is, early in the disease, tympanitic and tender, with a tendency to too frequent evacuations from the bowels, whilst in the disease we are considering, up to the stage of collapse, the abdomen is retracted, while there is no tympanites and no tenderness, and constipation is a marked symptom. Vomiting is a prominent symptom in tubercular meningitis, whilst in typhoid fever it is not marked, or it is absent. The acute pain in the head differs in this disease from the dull, heavy headache in typhoid fever. Finally, tubercular meningitis most often occurs in children under six years of age, whilst typhoid fever rarely does. In adults, it would be necessary to keep in mind the whole history of the attack to make a certain diagnosis.

From remittent fever of children, the diagnosis is made by the fact that in the latter disease there are usually no prodromic symptoms, the invasion being abrupt. Whilst there may be vomiting, it is not a marked symptom of the disease. The coated tongue, aching head and back, the enlarged spleen and liver, with the regular rise and fall of temperature, are symptoms distinctive of remittent fever. Especially does the temperature aid much in making the diagnosis. In tubercular meningitis the temperature rarely exceeds 103°; whilst in remittent fever, it frequently reaches 105°, falling during the day to about 100°, these variations taking place regularly, and not as they do in tubercular meningitis. The pulse in remittent fever is quick and full throughout, and frequent in direct proportion to the temperature; whilst in tubercular meningitis it is, up to the period of collapse, slow, feeble, and irregular, frequently intermitting.

From cerebro-spinal meningitis the diagnosis can be made by remembering that in this disease there are no prodromic symptoms. The invasion is sudden and without warning. All of the symptoms are more grave at the very onset. The temperature at first is higher and the pulse more frequent. Cerebro-spinal meningitis in fatal cases does its work quickly. Headache, pyrexia, convulsions in children, and active delirium, are present early in the disease. Unconsciousness ensues in a few days, and the duration of the disease does not usually exceed a week. There are a number of other diseases from which it might be necessary to distinguish tubercular meningitis; but, while none of the symptoms of tubercular meningitis are pathognomonic, yet when grouped together they afford ready means of making a diagnosis.

The prognosis is fatal. There have been a few so-called cases of tubercular meningitis cured; but when careful investigation is made of the history of these cases, the conclusion reached is that they were not cases of tubercular meningitis. Dr. de Gassicourt concludes that most of the alleged cures are "examples of meningitis of a limited extent arising from tubercular tumörs, syphilitic gummata, cerebral scleroses, and neoplasms of various kinds." Loomis says: "Tubercular meningitis is one of the most fatal diseases of childhood." Many authors state that it is always fatal after its characteristic symptoms are developed. Watson claims that there is some chance of saving life, if "the complaint, or tendency to the complaint, is detected early." He cites authorities to prove the cure of some cases. He refers to 76 cases, with 19 recoveries. He closes by saying: "I must confess my own suspicion, that they were, most of them at least, cases of what I have called simple encephalitis." Bartholow says: "Although a very few cases have been reported cured, it is held to be an incurable disease, and the termination fatal."

To the same purport, I might quote Flint, Wood, and others. The German writers are the only ones who claim cures. All my own cases have proved fatal.

The only rational treatment is prophylactic. The surest prophylaxis that could possibly be adopted would be to prevent the begetting of children of a scrofulous or tubercular diathesis. It is wrong, and ought to be made a punishable offense in some way, for persons known to be scrofulous or tuberculous to marry, *especially* to *intermarry*. The offspring of such unions, in far the majority of cases, will be diseased. The "survival of the fittest" in such cases should be substituted for the preservation of the fittest. Syphilis in many cases bears the same relation to tubercular meningitis that scrofula does, and needs to some extent similar legislation. Persons having contracted syphilis should not be allowed to marry before the expiration of not less than three years from the date of the development of the disease, and then only when there exists no trace of the disease. I do not pretend to argue the question of the transmission of the tubercular diathesis as a result of such unions; this fact is admitted by all of the best authorities of the present day. In my opinion, close consanguineous marriages should be forbidden by law. No raiser of fine stock will breed "in and in." The strains of blood must be crossed. He recognizes the fact that the "in and in" breeding produces, as a rule, feeble, delicate, deformed, short-lived offspring; hence such breeding is not done on the best stock farms. If the rule holds good in reference to horses and cows, much more should it hold good in reference to the human family, animals of finer mechanism and more to be guarded. I find on page 339 of "Medical Statistics of the Provost-Marshal General's Bureau," the following statement in reference to a family near Altoona, Pa.: There were "two families of Scotch-Irish birth located there, who were intelligent, healthy, thorough-going people, possessing strong vitality and great endurance. Their children commenced marrying and intermarrying, until now, in the fourth and fifth generations, there is not really a sound adult known in all their extensive connection, proving as far as it goes, the evils of the intermarriage of relatives." In Pepper's System we read as follows: "Consanguineous marriages have been time out of mind held to be very objectionable. . . . My own conclusion is . . . reproduction is most normal, and gives best results when a considerable genetic difference (within the limits of species) exists between parents. . . . Moreover, so few families possess an absolutely faultless health-record, that the chances of increasing existing morbid traits by intermarriages are quite sufficient to justify the commonly held objection against them." It is an admitted fact that everything that tends to deteriorate the vital powers, to that extent aids in producing a tuberculous diathesis, and that when this diathesis exists, then we may have in the children tubercular meningitis. I could cite many authorities to show the injurious effect of consanguinity in the marriage relation. My own observation teaches the same. If I were asked to say where the line should be drawn, I would answer that there should be no intermarrying where the blood relationship was closer than that existing between those in common parlance called "third cousins." Confirmed drunkards should not be allowed to marry, because in many cases the children resulting from such unions are epileptics, or have other cerebral or nervous disorders, besides a general feebleness of constitution.

In the next place, where we have these children inheriting a tuberculous diathesis, what can be done to prevent tubercular meningitis? They should be kept much in the open air, where they can bask in the sun's rays; should be supplied with plenty of nutritious, wholesome, well-cooked food; and should be well clothed so as to be protected against sudden changes of temperature. Sedentary amusements should be prohibited as much as possible School hours for such children should be short. School-rooms, where they attend school, should be well ventilated and the temperature kept uniform, and light should be abundant. They should sleep in well-aired bed-chambers, so that there could be no possible doubt of an abundant supply of pure air at night. They should be bathed daily in cold or tepid water, according to the age of the child or the season of the year. The bowels should be kept regular and open. Cod-liver oil should be administered freely—the more the better—up to the point of toleration. Iron, either in the form of the syrup of the iodide, of the potassio-tartrate, should be prescribed. Visits to the seashore, or some general change of air, should be made once a year at least. Whenever it can possibly be done, all of the children born of such unions as would be expected to produce feeble, delicate offspring, should be cared for as just pointed out.

When tubercular meningitis has once fully begun, since nothing can be done to arrest its progress, all the symptoms should be met as they arise. In the early stage of the disease, the nervous restlessness and irritability must be met with sodium or potassium bromide in full doses. Sometimes it will be necessary to add chloral to induce sleep. If the pain in the head is great, the ice-cap may be applied to relieve it; should that fail, opium in some form will be needed. The bowels should be kept open, but active purgation should be avoided. Liquid diet should be freely given. In the stage of effusion, iodide of potassium will be necessary; shaving the head and anointing it with an ointment of the biniodide of mercury may be resorted to. The iodide of potassium should be given in dose of two grains every four hours to a child three years old, and the ointment should be rubbed on, morning and night. After any treatment patients with tubercular meningitis die—at least that has been my experience with the few cases which have come under my experience. We should, however, prescribe suitable remedies, because it may be possible that simple meningitis (cerebro-spinal) may have been mistaken for tubercular.

In conclusion, I would impress upon you the thought that an early diagnosis should be made, and that the parents of the child should be candidly informed of the hopelessness of the case.

A CASE OF ENCEPHALOCELE.

BY D. A. HENGST, M.D ,
PITTSBURGH, PA.

On September 24, 1888, I was called to attend Mrs. James G., 22 years old, in her second confinement. On my arrival at the house I found that the child had been born for several minutes, and that the labor presented nothing unusual and had lasted only about one hour. On examination it was found that the child had what, upon a superficial examination, seemed to be a large hernial tumor protruding from the posterior part of the cranium ; this tumor was larger than the head of the child, and was covered with hair around its circumference for about one-third of its extent, the covering consisting of a continuation or stretching of the scalp. It was of a soft, doughy feeling, and slightly discolored in several places. The head of the child was almost flat from the eyebrows backward. and consequently appeared much smaller than the ordinary foetal head at full time.

The child, which was a male, had no other malformations, was of the ordinary size and well developed in all its parts. The presentation had evidently been by the vertex position, as the woman who was present stated that the tumor appeared first at the vulva ; the mass being soft and the head otherwise small made the delivery quite easy. The child lived three days, death being apparently due to starvation. It had made no effort to nurse at the breast and it would not swallow when artificial feeding was attempted ; it could open its eyes and cried lustily several times.

On *post-mortem* examination made twelve hours after death, the tumor was found to make its exit from what seemed to be the posterior fontanelle, which was greatly enlarged ; the anterior fontanelle was absent and the sutures united by cartilage, so that the entire cranium seemed to be one. About three-fourths of the cerebrum was found within the tumor, and it was highly injected ; the part of the cerebrum remaining within the cranium was normal in its appearance. The membranes of the brain were normal in appearance and covered the entire mass. The cerebellum was entirely absent, the growth having apparently originated from and underneath the tentorium cerebelli. The cerebral ventricles were found within the tumor and in a normal condition ; the sac also contained about four ounces of serum, no communication existing between the ventricles and the serous fluid, as is commonly found in these cases. In this kind of labor there should be no difficulty in the delivery of the child, inasmuch as the tumor was soft and the bony parts of the head small.

On first examination the tumor might be mistaken for a second head, and podalic version performed, as in a case reported by Tarnier. Should the child present by the breech and delay occur in the delivery of the aftercoming head, the obstacle to

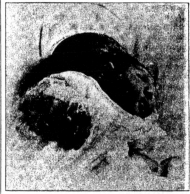

delivery might be overcome by puncturing the head. These cases are exceedingly rare and very interesting ; in an obstetric practice of nearly one thousand cases this was my first of the kind.

The accompanying wood-cut, made from a photograph taken thirty-six hours after the birth of the child, will serve to illustrate the size and appearance of the deformity.

3600 Fifth Ave.

—The *Popular Science News*, Jan., says that the body of a boy drowned at Winchendon, Mass., recently, was found through the use of the electric light, a bulb being fastened to a pole and submerged, illuminating the water for a considerable distance in the neighborhood. The electric light promises to become an important aid in all manner of submarine operations.

SUB-SPINOUS LUXATION OF THE HUMERUS; REPORT OF A CASE.

BY B. BRABSON CATES, M.D. (Univ. Pa.),
MARYVILLE, TENNESSEE.

Whilst sub-glenoid, sub-coracoid and sub-clavicular luxation of the head of the humerus are met with in the practice of almost every physician, systematic writers such as Agnew, Ashhurst, Gross, Erichsen and others are agreed that the backward or sub-spinous dislocation of the head of the humerus is a very rare occurrence; there being, according to Ashhurst, only twenty or thirty cases recorded in the literature of surgery.

Without following compiled statistics, showing the relative frequency with which various parts are dislocated, I trust the report of the following case will merit the attention of the profession.

Mrs. A. White, married, 58 years old, was out driving with her little granddaughter on July 18, 1888, when her horse became frightened and ran away with her. The buggy was dashed against a tree and overturned. In the effort to save her little grandchild from injury, Mrs. A. was thrown forward, striking on her right elbow and on her right shoulder. She was also struck on her head and was rendered unconscious for some time. When first seen by my friend Dr. B. A. Morton she had somewhat recovered from shock, and was able to answer questions. Dr. Morton made her as comfortable as the surroundings would permit and had her taken to her home, where I saw the patient in consultation with him.

When I first saw her she was suffering great pain. On examination I found an ugly gash over the olecranon process of the right elbow, and the shoulder of the right side was very much swollen and contused, and very tender on pressure. She complained bitterly of any attempts to move the arm. I noticed a round tumor beneath the spinous process of the right scapula, which on palpation was firm and unyielding. By pressing my hand firmly into the axilla of the same side and rotating the arm I could not elicit any movements from the head of the humerus, but, on the other hand, I could see the round tumor move beneath the spinous process of the scapula. No other injuries, beyond those of the head, shoulder and elbow, were received.

Dr. Morton and I agreed that our patient had sustained a sub-spinous dislocation of the right humerus, which we set to work to reduce. We reduced the dislocation by extension, and counter-extension, and pressure from behind. I then bound the arm in the Velpeau position, and ordered evaporating lotions to be applied to the injured parts to allay the inflammation and to reduce the swelling; and also ordered morphine to relieve the pain.

A NEW METHOD OF DIAGNOSIS IN OBSCURE CASES OF ENTERO-VESICAL FISTULA—SENN'S HYDROGEN GAS TEST.

BY CHARLES P. NOBLE, M.D.,
SENIOR ASSISTANT PHYSICIAN TO THE PHILADELPHIA
LYING-IN CHARITY.

I was recently asked by Dr. Charles Meigs Wilson, physician in charge of the Philadelphia Lying-in Charity, to see a patient of the institution, supposed to be suffering from fistula. It is not my purpose to report the case in full. Briefly, the woman had what was called an ischio-rectal abscess about five years before she entered the hospital. Some time after this abscess discharged she states that she began to pass, at irregular intervals, wind and small pieces of fecal matter *per urethram.* No symptoms of bladder irritation exist. An extensive cicatrix, following ulceration produced by a pessary, is present in the vagina. It extends along both sides of the vagina and across the posterior fornix (behind the cervix). In view of the absence of bladder irritation, and of the well-known ignorance of anatomy exhibited by the laity, it was thought likely that if the fistula did exist it was a recto-vaginal fistula. A careful examination under anæsthesia by touch and sight made by Drs. Wilson, Hawley, myself and others, failed to demonstrate the existence of any fistula communicating with the vagina. But two conclusions could be drawn; either the patient was right, or else she was a malingerer. The last seemed probable from what was known of her. It was suggested that a careful and extended study of the urine made with the microscope might determine the diagnosis—particles of vegetable fibre, or the seed of small fruits might be found. This plan involved much labor and time.

It occurred to me that the hydrogen gas test would settle the matter quickly and positively, and I suggested that it be employed. The recommendation was accepted and the following day Dr. Wilson forced the gas into the rectum and lighted the gas at the end of a catheter introduced into the bladder. I could not be present at the time, but Dr. Wilson told me that no gurgling sound was heard (caused by gas passing the ileo-cæcal valve), hence it seems plain that communication exists between the bladder and large intestine.

I offer this as a new and valuable method of diagnosis in obscure cases of entero-vesical fistula; or, if you choose, a new application of Senn's hydrogen gas test.

SOCIETY REPORTS.

MASSACHUSETTS MEDICAL SOCIETY, SUFFOLK DISTRICT, SECTION FOR SURGERY.

Stated Meeting, January 2, 1888.

The President, EDWARD H. BRADFORD, M.D., in the chair.

The Treatment of Cleft-Palate.

G. F. Grant, D.D.S., and H. A. Baker, D.D.S., presented the subject of the treatment of cleft-palate, and spoke of the use of artificial appliances in the treatment of the deformity, and exhibited apparatus and patients wearing it. The value of surgical interference was discussed by Charles B. Porter, M.D., and J. Collins Warren, M.D.

DR. G. F. GRANT referred to an experience of 21 years in the treatment of fissures of the palate by means of mechanical appliances, commencing just after the appearance of a paper in 1867 by William Suersen, of Berlin. For several reasons the results of surgical interference have been unsatisfactory: (1) because there is no union of the divided hard palate even under the most favorable conditions; (2) because there is not so much improvement in speech as was expected; and (3) because there is an increased difficulty in the adjustment of mechanical appliances afterward.

In 1873 and 1874 the surgeons of Boston—Bigelow, Warren, Hodges and Cabot—were giving attention to this subject, which they discarded later. It was about this time that Dr. Grant had his first success with a mechanical appliance After the introduction of the plate, there was at once a noticeable improvement in the speech. At first the improvement was slight, but it gradually improved for a year, when the difference was very marked. Since that time, or during the last ten years, the patient has been a teacher in one of the public schools of a large town in Massachusetts. Since 1871 Dr. Grant has treated

115 cases of congenital fissure of the palate, and the results have been such as to warrant the conclusion that there is no reasonable doubt as to the success of the appliance. The mechanism of the appliance has been urged by some as an objection, but the argument has little if any more weight than in the case of spectacles for the eyes. The cases in which adjustment is most difficult are those in which only a portion of the soft palate is absent; here the difficulty is to obtain contact of the appliance with the edge of the remaining portion of the palate. In fissures of the hard palate, on the contrary, an arched plate easily fills up the deficiency.

According to the experience of Dr. Grant, the appliance can be adjusted with success as early as the seventh year of age. It is of great importance that the hare lip, which generally accompanies the cleft palate, should be operated upon in such a way as to secure the greatest amount of mobility, because a short and inflexible lip will interfere with the articulation.

Dr. Grant exhibited a patient for whom he had adjusted an appliance several years before. The patient read from a book handed him by the Secretary of the Society, both with his appliance in position and with it removed. This test, as well as his answers to questions from members of the Society, both with and without the appliance, showed how very decidedly his speech had been improved by the appliance.

DR. H. A. BAKER said that in 1841 Dr. Stearns, a physician, made for himself the first mechanical appliance, which was adjusted and worn successfully in a case of cleft-palate. This apparatus was very complicated, having three wings, and many hinges and springs. Stearns, however, selected soft vulcanized rubber, which is not a permanent material, as it retains its value for only two and one-third or three months to a year.

In 1860, Dr. Norman W. Kingsley simplified Stearns's apparatus. He used only two wings, and he employed metal instead of wooden moulds in its construction, and thus he secured a smoother result with a better finish.

In 1867 William Suersen, of Berlin, introduced permanent materials for the construction of the appliance, thus securing a great advantage. He used hard rubber.

In 1881 Dr. Baker made his first successful appliance, and since then he has had about a hundred cases. The first apparatus was made of hard rubber and it had hinges to aid the levator muscles in bringing it up to the posterior pharyngeal wall. The patient was 12 years of age, and the operation of staphylorraphy had been performed unsuccessfully. The Doctor considers a certain amount of training, as to the proper way of using the lips and tongue in the formation of sounds, to be essential to success after the adjustment of an appliance. In illustration, Dr. Baker exhibited several diagrams and plaster models with the appliances in position, and also two patients who showed a marked improvement in speech when wearing the apparatus.

DR. CHARLES B. PORTER said that he did not appear as an opponent of the views which had been advanced by the dentists; but he believed that the time has come, when it is best to review the operation of staphylorraphy, which is now so rarely performed. He would consider then:

1. Is the operation feasible and in what cases? Trelat says that it should be performed in any case unless the extent of the fissure is too great; unless previous operation has failed; or unless the parents object.

2. At what age? Dr. Porter thinks that it should be done when the child has a sufficient number of teeth to support a diaphragm, in order to keep the pressure of the tongue away from the stitches in the wound. He quoted many authorities, some of which gave the age as early as 16 months, and others at 16 years.

3. The method of operation. This should be comparatively simple. The edges should be freshened. The mucous membrane, together with the periosteum, should be freed from the bone by means of a periosteum elevator. Lateral incisions parallel to the line of union will relieve tension. Stitches should be introduced every quarter of an inch. These sutures may be either of silk or of silver wire. A diaphragm should be inserted to protect the stitches from the tongue.

4. Subsequent training in the formation of sounds is the most important of all things, and without this there can be no success attained.

Dr. Porter spoke of two cases in which he has performed the operation of staphylorraphy. In the first case, a child 14 months old, did well until about the sixth day, when the mother, in the absence of the nurse, gave the child a hard crust of bread, and the stitches were pulled out and the operation was a failure. In the second case, in a girl 16 years old, nine sutures were introduced and these were protected by a gutta-percha diaphragm. This patient did well and was exhibited. There was marked improvement in speech.

DR. J. COLLINS WARREN said that no operations for staphylorraphy were done previous to this century; but in the early part of the century Rue began to do the operation, and later it was done by Drs. Bigelow, John Warren, Cabot, Mason Warren and others. Dr. Mason Warren (the speaker's father) modified the method of operating, and performed a great many operations. He incised the soft parts freely, seized the uvula with a pair of long forceps, and then, having drawn it firmly across the fissure, he divided with a pair of strong curved scissors *all* of the tense tissues of the posterior pillars whether they were muscles or not. After this, the side operated on hung loose, and the same thing was then done on the other side. The edges of the fissure were then pared with a pointed double-edged knife and then the mucous membrane was separated from the parts beneath, almost as far as the alveolar processes, after which it was united by sutures. Dr. Warren performed about 100 operations. In his later operations he did not attempt to unite the fissure in its entire length, believing that the essential thing is the restoration of the arch with enough soft palate united to form a valve.

DR. WARREN exhibited the case of instruments with which his father had performed all of his operations for staphylorraphy. For sutures, he used silk which had been soaked in compound tincture of benzoin, which had the advantage that it prevented the knot from slipping. Some also claimed for it antiseptic qualities, but it is doubtful if this claim has any foundation.

DRS. EDWARD REYNOLDS and ROBERT W. LOVETT read a paper on

Removal of Nasal Obstruction; Results in 112 Cases.

Dr. Robert W. Lovett gave the statistics of the series of cases, which were the ordinary patients that presented themselves for treatment at the Dispensary during three months in the summer. Three conditions were chiefly observed: (1) Chronic folliculitis; (2) congested mucous membrane, with abundant secretion; (3) a dry shining mucous membrane.

The treatment employed involved the destruction of the mucous membrane covering the lower turbinated bones by cauterization with chromic acid. Of the cases, 75 were subjected to this treatment;

33 were kept as check cases and only the ordinary conservative treatment by douches, etc., was employed. The history in the latter showed little if any improvement. In 5 cases there were exostoses or deviations of the septum.

Of the 75 cases in which cauterization with chromic acid was employed, 16 patients were cured; 38 were much improved; 2 were not benefited; the remainder were not heard from.

The method employed to ascertain the result after three months, was to send to each person an addressed postal card with questions to be answered and the card returned. The cards with the questions and replies were exhibited. Of the 75 cases, 16 patients were cauterized only once, and the remainder two, three, or even four times, according to the amount of the hypertrophy.

Of the check cases, two patients were cauterized after a trial without benefit of the conservative treatment for three months, with the final result of a cure.

DR. EDWARD REYNOLDS said that the purpose of the mucous membrane of the nose is to temper the air which is going to the lungs, and thus the nose is the respiratory organ. The air always enters the lungs at a temperature of about 30° C. (86° F.), and saturated with moisture, whatever the external conditions are. The turbinated bones divide the anterior nares into three main compartments, which are normally narrow spaces, and the mucous membrane which envelops the turbinated bones is so richly supplied with blood-vessels, that it is almost an erectile tissue. The operation which was done in these cases is simple and but little apparatus is requisite.

A six per cent. solution of cocaine is first sprayed into the nostril and then deliquesced crystals of chromic acid on a cotton applicator, made of a flattened piece of copper wire, are then applied to the whole surface of the lower turbinated bones, unless it is so large that it is best to make two applications, in which case it is first applied to the inner half. If examined, with the speculum the eschar is at once seen. The application to the other nostril, if this is necessary, should be delayed from three days to a week, and the eschar should come away before a second application is made, if it be necessary. The eschar produced by chromic acid is very superficial and thus the degree of cauterization can be regulated somewhat. After the operation has been performed it is difficult or even impossible to detect any scar.

Dr. Reynolds exhibited a number of preparations of skulls that showed very nicely the swelling of the mucous membrane, the exostoses, and the deviation of the septum.

In the discussion that ensued, DR. VINCENT Y. BOWDITCH said that he had used chromic acid in the treatment of this class of cases for over a year in his office practice. He believes that the nose is the true respiratory organ. Some enthusiasts declare that nasal hypertrophies should be removed for everything, and thus they weaken their cause. Some even assert that asthma can be cured by this means.

DR. THOMAS A. DE BLOIS said: The nasal hypertrophies appear both on the anterior and on the posterior ends of the turbinated bones. The hypertrophies which are anterior are the ones which are chiefly benefited by cauterizations with chromic acid. I prefer to use a round probe rather than a flat one, and I cauterize in lines only. These are made by drawing the end of the probe over the surface where it is desirable. The hypertrophies in the posterior nares are generally large, puffy masses, which shrink up a great deal after removal with the snare.

DR. HENRY L. MORSE said: Many of the cases that have been reported by the speakers were patients sent by me from the Ear Department at the Dispensary to the Throat Department. I believe that a free opening through the nose is very essential in the treatment of the ear. In the case of children, nasal obstruction will increase the ingrowing of the drum of the ear, and unless the nose is taken care of, the benefit to the hearing by treatment is only temporary.

DR. GEORGE A. LELAND said: I have obtained good results from this method of treatment. There is a certain normal erectility to the mucous membrane of the nose, and hence is is not best to cauterize it too much. Dry catarrh may follow. Dr. Bosworth, of New York, applies the chromic acid by fusing a bead on the end of a silver wire. The reduction of the mucous membrane of the turbinated bones has cured the condition known as "hay fever." I saw a patient four years ago who had suffered for twenty-three consecutive years from hay fever. Not having any chromic acid with me, I curetted the mucous membrane from the lower turbinated bone. There was of course much bleeding, but there was no "hay fever" that year, nor any since.

S.

FOREIGN CORRESPONDENCE.

LETTER FROM BERLIN.

The New Ophthalmoscopic Examination.—
Rare Pathological Specimens. — Three
Dermoid Cysts. —Therapeutical Sugges-
tions in Diphtheria.—The Latest Victim of
" the Code."—German Students and their
Habits.

BERLIN, Dec. 21, 1888.

The new ophthalmoscopic examination advocated at a recent meeting of the *Berliner Medicinische Gesellschaft* by Dr. Bellarminow, of St. Petersburg, has attracted universal interest among the profession ; regarding its scientific value and practical utility, however, considerable difference of opinion seems to exist. Your correspondent has interviewed the two greatest ophthalmological authorities in Berlin, Profs. Hirschberg and Schweigger, on the subject in question, and has found to his surprise a very different estimation of Bellarminow's method. Prof. Hirschberg said that "the same method, or one strikingly similar to it," had been described by him in 1882, in the *Archive* of Du Bois Raymond (p. 501). The method then published had reference only to the eye of fish, the pike in particular. As cocaine was not yet known Prof. Hirschberg said he had no great confidence in the new method, and did not expect any great advantages from its application. Prof. Schweigger, on the contrary, spoke rather warmly of the new method, and emphasized especially its ease of application. He stated that he had used the method repeatedly and was prepared to recommend it.

As some of the readers of the REPORTER may not yet be familiar with Bellarminow's method it will not be amiss briefly to enunciate its principles. The cornea is first anæsthetized with a two per cent. solution of cocaine, and a plain glass plate is then brought into contact with and gently pressed against it. The moisture of the cornea will by capillary action develop a layer of fluid between the glass plate and the cornea, and the curvature of the latter in this way will be obliterated—two parallel surfaces being substituted for the convex lens, the normal cornea. In other words, a thin glass plate is pressed on the cocainized cornea and a high grade of hypermetropia is produced, and, consequently, an enlargement of the ophthalmoscopic field. The simplicity and ease of application of the new method are evidently its chief advan-tages, but it is questionable, if delicate structural changes can be observed by its use. The new method will recommend itself to beginners, and for purposes of demonstration, as an examination of the eye may be made through its use by two or three persons at the same time. It may be of interest to mention that Bellarminow's principle has been practically utilized by the Fick contraction-spectacles, which consist of a glass plate ground in accordance with the curvature of the cornea and placed on the latter. The slight interval between the plate and the cornea is filled out by a drop of fluid, which eliminates the influence of the irregular curvature of the cornea.

Berlin is justly termed the pathological centre, for nowhere is pathology cultivated to the same extent as here. The focus of all pathological work is, of course, the *Patologisches Institut*, an integral portion of the Royal Charité, and presided over by Virchow. The collection of pathological specimens in the Institute is a truly grand one, and is supposed to be unsurpassed by any in the world. The latest additions to this collection were made by Virchow last week, and consist of a kidney showing deposits of lime as a result of poisoning with cyanide of mercury. These deposits can be seen with the naked eye in very fine sections on favorable illumination. Microscopically, of course, the lime deposits are very distinctly visible. Another recent addition to the collection is a very rare specimen of idiopathic perichondritis of the arytenoid cartilages. Hitherto it has been usually believed that purulent perichondritis of these cartilages was traceable always to typhoid, syphilitic, or to tubercular infection. The idiopathic nature of the perichondritis in the specimen in question was well established. Dr. Bramann, assistant of Prof. Bergmann, has recently enriched the collection by four dermoid cysts of the nose, which were all taken out by himself. One cyst was from a child four months old.

Dr. Rieck's proposal to treat diphtheria with yeast, though theoretically interesting, will find but little appreciation with the practitioner of medicine. Rieck's treatment is based on the fact that the gastric contents in diphtheria, just as in cholera, scarlet fever and measles is always alkaline. The yeast-cells—cerevisiæ—proliferate only in a neutral or slightly alkaline soil, which at the same time contains sugar. They furnish carbonic, acetic and lactic acids. The latter acid has been extensively used in the treatment of diphtheria, though rarely ever in quantity sufficient to acidify the gastric contents. If lactic acid is pushed that far the proliferation of the yeast-cells stops simultaneously with the reduction power of the micro-organisms, and recovery takes place. The proposal is, in other words, an attempt to combat the specific diphtheria-germs with proliferating hetero-genous cells—a fight between bacillus and cell on a common soil, the blood. The method constitutes, therefore, an experiment the reverse of a pure culture.

Another suggestion regarding the treatment of diphtheria, made by Dr. Gaucher, of Paris, to cauterize the deposits with the Paquelin cautery, will not be received with greater enthusiasm than Rieck's proposal. Gaucher has saved 17 cases by this method, and Dubousquet has treated 81 cases with a mortality of only five per cent. Gaucher's method, by the way, is nothing new, for a German physician proposed the same treatment in 1885. Your correspondent in that year assisted Prof. Henoch, of the Royal Charité, in the cauterization of deposits in a grave case in a girl thirteen years old. The girl recovered and, as Prof. Henoch thought, only as the result of this treatment. Nevertheless, the cauterization treatment has never been adopted by Prof. Henoch nor by any other German pediatrist. It is clear, that this treatment can only be of avail in the initial stage of the affection, before the specific germs have entered the circulation. Besides, the treatment is undoubtedly too heroic ever to become popular.

Adherence to false conceptions of honor and to medieval and barborous usages has again resulted in the death of a human being, this time a youthful medical student of the Berlin University. A mere difference of opinion, and the assertion that academical associations, the chief principles of which consist in antisemitic tendencies, are a disgrace to German Universities, led to a duel with pistols, three rounds at ten paces. Young Blum was shot through the left lung, and died immediately. It is a shame and disgrace that in an enlightened country such as Germany, and among its most intellectual associations, such barbarous and outrageous customs should still exist. Not a year passes that the "code" does not demand its victim or victims at some of the German Universities. I believe that the fault is entirely with the Government, and that severe punishment of the murderers will alone prevent the further perpetration of this atrocious crime.

The great trouble in this matter, however, is the fact that the highest officials of the Government have all been ardent advocates of the code, and that they cannot well condemn in others what they have upheld themselves. Mere fencing, which is the universal custom among all German students, though from an American point of view scarcely commendable, is, nevertheless, regarded in Germany as absolutely necessary to the maintenance of a proper *esprit de corps* among the students. As the result of this view and practice every other student whom you meet at Berlin or any other German University has a more or less lacerated face, of which he feels very proud. He exhibits his facial scars with the same pride and self-consciousness as, for instance, an officer his medals and orders. In some future letter I will write more about the German students and their habits.   J. S.

PERISCOPE.

Poisoning with Cyanide of Mercury.

At the meeting of the Berlin Medical Society, November 21, 1888 (*Deutsche med. Wochenschrift*, Nov. 29, 1888), Virchow demonstrated specimens from a case of poisoning with cyanide of mercury, which presented a series of anatomical changes analogous to those described by him as occurring in poisoning with corrosive sublimate. The patient from whom the specimens were taken was a young man who had poisoned himself, but who survived eight days, so that the changes produced by the poison were very completely shown. The parts of the digestive apparatus above the pylorus, with which the poison came in contact first, presented no noteworthy changes of any kind, and especially no traces of erosion. The more marked changes began in the lowest section of the ileum. In a characteristic manner the affected areas occur at intervals, always on the flexures of the colon, while between these areas are comparatively normal stretches of tissue. The kidneys throughout the cortex, but preferably the convoluted tubules, are filled with lime to a much greater extent than in any of the cases hitherto described: Virchow explains this result by saying that the mercury had acted upon the bones so that the lime salts were set free in the circulation; thence they were carried to the kidneys, which were inflamed by the effort at excretion.

Foreign Body in the Larynx.

At the meeting of the Medico-Chirurgical Society of Glasgow, Oct. 12, 1888 (*Glasgow Med. Journal*, Nov. 1888), Mr. George A. Clark read notes of a case of foreign body in the larynx, and exhibited the patient.

J. H., 9 years old, was admitted on August 16 into Ward 25 of the Royal Infirmary, suffering from what was described as fits, coming on, at irregular intervals, without any warning, and for which no cause could be assigned. Between the attacks, which lasted for variable lengths, the patient seemed in the best of health, was able to run and play about, and in every way enjoy himself; but when seized with a "fit" he became cyanotic, and after the seizure had passed off there was profuse perspiration with exhaustion. As the character of these attacks did not simulate those of epilepsy, and as no history could be obtained, the patient was kept under close observation. It was then noticed that these attacks, which were spasmodic, seemed to come on after the slightest attack of coughing or laughing, during which time the child had to sit up in bed; and although some attacks passed off in a few moments, others would last for some time, and when a constant irritating cough terminated in a severe fit of coughing the child would struggle for breath, and at times become so cyanotic as to be in danger of suffocation. It now became conclusive that the affection was in the larynx, and on inquiry from the parents it was learned that a bean was supposed to have gone down his throat. It seems that on the previous day he was playing with some other boys, during which time he had his mouth full of beans, and a bigger boy having run after him hurled him to the ground on his back and knelt on his chest, when, it was supposed, one of these beans went down his throat. On the morning after admission the throat was carefully examined with the aid of the laryngoscope, but nothing could be detected. During that day he had a few attacks, which, at times, became somewhat serious; but beyond causing great prostration, nothing serious followed. During the night he had attacks also, and on the following morning it was decided to perform tracheotomy; but after making preparations, owing to the absence of any positive proof of the presence of a foreign body, it was postponed, with the understanding that the operation should be done only if an attack should come on so severe as to threaten life. That same afternoon Mr. Clark happened to pass through the ward, when he saw the boy sitting up in bed playing dominoes with two others. A few seconds later he was followed by one of the boys, who said that the child was choking. On returning, the boy was found lying back in bed quite cyanotic, and his breathing short and hurried. Mr. Clark immediately held him up by the legs and smacked his back, but this decidedly made him worse. His breathing became slow and gasping, and he seemed half insensible, so tracheotomy was performed low down. On opening the trachea immediate relief was given, and as the operation was only done as a palliative measure, the tube was introduced. That night little if any spasm took place, and the patient passed a fairly comfortable night. On the following morning the tube was removed and the trachea examined, but nothing could be detected. The tube was again introduced, but the spasms still continued, and at times became so troublesome as to be only checked by the inhalation of a few drops of chloroform. During these attacks Mr. Clark noticed a distinct "click" as of something coming up from below and striking the lower end of the tube; and the patient himself said he could feel something rising and falling. The temperature which had been high had fallen since the operation, and as the spasms were also decreasing the tube was ordered to be removed. No bad effects followed this, and as the throat showed signs of laryngitis it was suggested that only this was the cause of the spasms. Potassium bromide was therefore given; but it was soon noticed that as the wound began to close the temperature began to rise and the spasms to increase in severity. By September 1 the wound had quite healed, and the patient had a very severe spasm during the night, which had to be allayed by the inhalation of chloroform. On the following night Mr. Clark was again called, being told that the child was threatened with convulsions. He again found him in an asphyxiated condition, and resolved to perform tracheotomy again, if possible to satisfy himself that there was nothing present. Accordingly the old wound was opened up and a free opening made in the trachea. The trachea was then opened up well with retractors, which caused a severe spasm of the glottis. Mr. Clark then watched closely, and after some time noticed something occasionally rise and immediately fall. This was dark in color, and at first sight seemed like a clot of blood, but after being successful in touching it, he was satisfied that some solid body was present. He then took a tracheal hook and opened up the trachea with the retractors to cause a spasm, and, watching his opportunity, succeeded when the body rose in placing the hook beneath to prevent its return. He then managed to turn the hook round, and pinning it, withdrew it. The foreign body turned out to be a horse-bean, and its removal gave, of course, immediate relief. The wound was dressed, and healed rapidly. There was no return of spasms. The patient was dismissed September 9.

Inoculation with Leprosy.

The *Lancet*, Nov. 24, 1888, says that Archdeacon Wright lately called public attention in *The* (London) *Times* to the spread of leprosy, and the evidence of its contagiousness. He now furnishes a report from the Board of Health, Honolulu, giving information of the condition of a condemned criminal at Oahu Gaol who was inoculated with leprosy by Dr. Arning on November 5, 1885. Dr. Emerson, the President of the Board of Health, and Dr. Kimball examined this man on September 25, 1888, and reported that he presented marked signs of tubercular leprosy. Archdeacon Wright thinks that this "terrible experiment" goes far to prove the contagiousness of leprosy; and there is no doubt that such an experiment is proof of its inoculability. But we venture to think that the case for contagion is not rendered any stronger than it was already by the facts of the disease and of its nature gathered from various sources of late years; and it is questionable whether the transmission of such a disease by inoculation, even on a condemned criminal, is an experiment that ought rightly to have been made.

On the other hand, in a letter to the *British Med. Journal*, Dec. 15, 1888, H. P. Wright, Rector of Greatham, gives the following important particulars, which were contained in a letter to him from Dr. Arning, who asks a very reasonable question: "The experiment was performed after mature deliberation, and on the authority of the advisers of the Crown and the Privy Council of State; influential foreigners, laymen, and learned judges reporting in committee on the subject. It was done with the condemned criminal's written consent, and with all such due care and exactness as really to advance our knowledge of the obscure disease. Will it not stand as having been done in the interests, not against the laws, of humanity?"

Purulent Pericarditis; Aspiration and Drainage.

At the meeting of the Clinical Society of London, Nov. 23, 1888, Dr. Dickinson related the case of a boy, 10 years old, who was brought to St. George's Hospital, having had symptoms which Dr. Harris and Mr. Noad, both of Norwood, interpreted as pyæmic. A large gluteal abscess was followed by signs of pleural effusion and œdema of the face and chest. On admission, on June 15, 1887, there was evidence of effusion in the left pleura and in the pericardium. The position of the heart was almost indiscoverable amid the dulness, which involved the left pleural and præcordial regions. There was much dyspnœa, blueness, and irregularity of pulse. There was œdema more or less general, but especially marked about the thorax. The liver was enlarged or depressed so as to reach the umbilicus. On the 18th the pleura was aspirated, and thirty-seven ounces of serum were drawn off, which operation was repeated on the 23d, with the removal of thirty-two ounces. The dyspnœa, blueness, and œdema were but slightly and temporarily relieved by each operation, which had to be repeated on the 25th and 28th, so great was the distress and so rapid the reaccumulation. On the 30th the futility of dealing with the pleura having become apparent, the pericardium was aspirated by Mr. Rouse, and one ounce of creamy pus withdrawn; the aspiration was repeated with more success on July 8, twelve ounces of similar fluid being withdrawn, and on the 15th, with the withdrawal of nineteen ounces. The place selected for puncture was on the right side close to the edge of the sternum, in the fifth interspace. The heart before each of these operations had been drawn to the left by a preceding evacuation of the pleura. The lower part of the pericardium where the swing of the heart was greatest, and the right extremity of the cavity, from which the heart was furthest removed, was obviously the part which could be penetrated with the greatest safety. By July 22 the pericardium was again as full as ever, and the general symptoms as distressing. It was clearly necessary to replace aspiration by a tapping opening. Mr. Rouse accordingly made an incision where the punctures had been, and put in a tube. The aspiration was followed by some faintness, but subsequently by great relief. Not to follow the case in further detail, recovery, after some temporary drawbacks and three subsequent aspirations of the pleura, became complete. By the middle of September there was no remnant of the pericardial puncture except a small cicatrix, which moved with each beat of the heart. In the course of less than two months the chest had been punctured sixteen times, the pleura twelve times, with the removal of serous fluid; the pericardium four times—thrice with the aspirator, once with a knife—so as to leave an opening and a constant discharge of pus. A remarkable fact in the history of the case—one, however, not unprecedented in similar circumstances—was the nearly total absence of præcordial friction, which was recognized only on one occasion.—*British Med. Journal*, Dec. 1, 1888.

Meningocele; Ligation and Removal of Sac.

Dr. W. O. Roberts, Professor of the Principles and Practice of Surgery, University of Louisville, in communicating this case to the *American Practitioner and News*, Dec. 1, 1888, says that on March 19, 1888, he saw, with Dr. Milner, of Uniontown, a child five weeks old, who had a pedunculated tumor, about the size and very much the shape of a goose egg, situated just beneath the occipital protuberance. The history of the case was as follows: The growth was first noticed immediately after the birth of the baby. It was then about one-half its present size. When the child slept the tumor was much smaller; and would become suddenly greatly swollen and tense when it cried. The tumor had always been exceedingly sensitive to the touch, and the slightest pressure upon it caused the child to cry violently. In consequence, it had never been able to lie on its back. Dr. Milner was called in a few days before Dr. Roberts saw it, and tapped the growth and drew off a quantity of serous fluid slightly tinged with blood. This diminished the size, of course, but did not lessen the sensitiveness of the growth. He then advised that the child be brought to Louisville, where Dr. Roberts saw it with him. At the time of the latter's visit the child was asleep in its mother's lap, lying on its abdomen. Hanging from the occiput was a flabby tumor. Just as he touched the growth the child awoke, crying violently. There was an immediate and great distension of the tumor. The pedicle or attached portions measured five and the body of the tumor eight inches in circumference. The skin over the tumor was well covered with hair.

Fluctuation was marked. There was no pulsation. The growth was unmistakably a meningocele.

As the growth was increasing rapidly in size, and as the sensitiveness had not diminished a particle after Dr. Milner had partly drawn off the fluid, its removal was advised. The parents, having been fully advised of the nature of the affection and the danger of the operation, decided to have it performed. On the following day Dr. Roberts removed the tumor. An elliptical incision was made through the skin and fascia covering the neck of the sac. This was first carefully dissected, then transfixed and ligated close up to the edge of the opening in the skull with a double stout silk ligature, and the tumor cut through in front of the ligature. As the ligature was tightened the child had a slight convulsion. When the tumor was opened nearly three ounces of a slightly bloody serous fluid escaped. The cyst was sacculated. There were three sacculi connected with the main cavity of the cyst. No brain substance was found in it. The opening in the skull was just below the occipital protuberance, and was about an inch in its vertical and half an inch in its transverse diameter. The ends of the ligature around the neck of the sac were cut short, and the integuments then brought together, provision being made for drainage. The operation was done under strict antiseptic precautions. Recovery took place without an untoward symptom. At the end of ten days the wound had healed, and the child was taken to its home. Three months after the operation the child was reported to be in perfect health, with no recurrence of the tumor.

Case of Polyuria with Localizing Symptoms.

At the meeting of the Pathological Section of the Medico-Chirurgical Society of Glasgow, Oct. 19, 1888 (*Glasgow Med. Journal*, Nov. 1888), Dr. Alexander Robertson read the notes of a case of polyuria.

A patient was shown suffering from diabetes insipidus of about eight months' standing. He was a soldier for some years, and is now about 30 years of age. Careful examination failed to elicit any indications of syphilis, and none were admitted. His illness dates from about six months before admission into the Infirmary, which was on the 2d August last. He had lost about 28 lbs. in weight in the earlier months of his malady. No probable cause could be assigned: The amount of urine ranged from 150 to 190 ounces in 24 hours, though once it had reached 290 ounces. The specific gravity was generally from 1003 to 1006. It was always free from albumin and sugar. Dr. Ritchie had found that the quantity of urea excreted in the 24 hours was 479 grains. There were no general symptoms of renal disease. Though scarcely any appreciable difference existed between the two sides of his face when at rest, movements which called into action the lower facial muscles—*e.g.*, showing his teeth, the articulation of certain words, etc.—showed that the right side was distinctly weak. On many occasions, especially during the last three or four weeks, he had sudden attacks of difficulty in speaking, lasting from 20 minutes to 24 hours. They were preceded in most cases by a feeling of sleepiness. The defect was in articulation—a marked stammering, with special difficulty in the beginning of a sentence; there was no loss of language. Dr. Fergus reported that there was a moderate degree of neuro-retinitis, and that the movements of the right pupil (the sight of the left eye being damaged by an old injury) were restricted, not responding much to light, or accommodation, or cutaneous irritation. The pupil itself was moderately contracted. The pulse ranged between 50 and 60. Without inquiry he stated that he had often a feeling of chilliness, but that sometimes he had only become aware of this fact by the remarks of his friends on his pale, cold aspect. Besides this, several times he had felt the right ear very hot. Dr. Robertson had seen it in this condition, and said that it was scarlet from the injection of the blood-vessels, and that the redness extended to the cheek. The contrast with the other ear was very marked, as it was blanched and chilly. There was no undue secretion from the eye or nose. General sensation and motion had never been affected. Consciousness had not been involved, and his general intelligence was good.

In reviewing the facts of the case, Dr. Robertson said: As you are aware, Claude Bernard induced a glycosuria by puncturing the floor of the fourth ventricle, and by puncturing, a little higher up, a polyuria. Still, there are wanting cases in the human subject corroborating the idea that the lesion is in that part of the brain; but this case clearly supports the indications derived from Claude Bernard's experiments. The speech being affected in the manner described pointed to temporary disorder in the nucleus of the ninth nerve. But there is an organic and more permanent defect of the facial nerve present, the nucleus of which is a little higher up, but not far from the same situation. Also we have temporary irritation and palsy of different parts of the vaso-motor nerves, the centre of which is situated there also. There is probably an important controlling centre of the vaso-motor system in the cortex of the brain, but we also know that there is a centre of great importance in the medulla oblongata. Further, the slowness of the pulse may indicate an inhibitory influence on the pneumogastric nucleus, but the reduction in the number of pulsations did not warrant much stress to be laid on this point. We have, then, these indications of disease independent of the polyuria altogether. The state of the pupil might also suggest some degree of paralysis of the sympathetic. The pupil is generally somewhat contracted, which may no doubt be due to stimulation of the nucleus of the third nerve; but in view of the other indications of vaso-motor paralysis, we may conclude that not improbably this condition of myosis is due to the same cause. With regard to the polyuria, what is it to be ascribed to? Is it due to trophic nerves whose function is impaired, though their existence is still called in question; or is it rather due to a paralysis of the vaso-motor nerves of the kidney? Dr. Robertson held that the latter view was much the more probable, considering the clear indications of general disorder of the sympathetic which were obvious in the case. He thought there was distinct change of nerve-structure present, though scarcely amounting to a definite tumor.

Medicinal treatment, the details of which were mentioned, had not been of much use. It was, however, intended to try galvanism passed through the medulla oblongata.

———◆◆◆———

—Dr. R. Brudenell Carter, of London, according to the *American Lancet*, Jan., 1888, says that when he sees a pamphlet or book purporting to contain an addition to our knowledge, he tries first of all to ask himself: "What do I know of the author? What is his character, in the estimation of those who know him well, for sagacity, dexterity, and truthfulness? What is the extent of his experience? What are his claims to be received as a guide and instructor in the matters with which he attempts to deal?" If these questions are fairly answered, the pamphlet will sometimes be relegated to the waste basket.

THE
MEDICAL AND SURGICAL
REPORTER.

ISSUED EVERY SATURDAY.

CHARLES W. DULLES, M.D.,
EDITOR AND PUBLISHER.

The Terms of Subscription to the serial publications of this office are as follows, payable in advance:

Med. and Surg. Reporter (weekly), a year, **$5.00**
Quarterly Compendium of Med. Science, - 2.50
Reporter and Compendium, - - - - 6.00
Physician's Daily Pocket Record, - - - 1.00
Reporter and Pocket Record, - - - - 6.00
Reporter, Compendium, and Pocket Record, 7.00

All checks and postal orders should be drawn to order of

CHARLES W. DULLES,
N. E. Cor. 13th and Walnut Streets,
P. O. Box 843. Philadelphia, Pa.

☞ SUGGESTIONS TO SUBSCRIBERS:
See that your address-label gives the date to which your subscription is paid.
In requesting a change of address, give the old address as well as the new one.
If your REPORTER does not reach you promptly and regularly, notify the publisher *at once*, so that the cause may be discovered and corrected.

☞ SUGGESTIONS TO CONTRIBUTORS AND CORRESPONDENTS:
Write in ink.
Write on one side of paper only.
Write on paper of the size usually used for letters.
Make as few paragraphs as possible. Punctuate carefully. Do not abbreviate, or omit words like "the," and "a," or "an."
Make communications as short as possible.
NEVER ROLL A MANUSCRIPT! Try to get an envelope or wrapper which will fit it.
When it is desired to call our attention to something in a newspaper, mark the passage boldly with a colored pencil, and write on the wrapper "Marked copy." Unless this is done, newspapers are not looked at.
The Editor will be glad to get medical news, but it is important that brevity and actual interest shall characterize communications intended for publication.

JUDICIOUS MANAGEMENT OF A CASE OF SUPPOSED HYDROPHOBIA.

Near the end of last December Dr. Healy, of Philadelphia, was called to attend a very ill young man who had a history of a dog-bite and certain symptoms of hydrophobia. In conference with Dr. Wirgman, he decided to invite to consultation a medical man who is well known as a specialist in nervous diseases, and another who had made a special study of hydrophobia.

When the consultation was held a very careful and thorough examination of the patient was made, and it was found that he presented clear evidence of disease of the brain. He had some paralysis of one arm and paresis of the muscles of the mouth and throat. He had a most typical difficulty in swallowing liquids, unaccompanied by any real pain. This was exactly like the symptom to which the name "hydrophobia" is most fitly applied. It was wholly due to want of power or of co-ordination in the muscles of the mouth and fauces, and not to any notion of the patient that he was suffering with rabies humana. This fact was ascertained to the entire satisfaction of all of the consultants.

The case was regarded as one of disease at the base of the brain—perhaps in the pons Varolii—and treated accordingly.

The condition of the patient, at the time of the consultation, was so grave that little hope was entertained that he could recover; and, as was anticipated, he died in a few days. The cause of death was not hydrophobia, however, and the case will not go to increase the fear of this disorder. We call attention to it chiefly to applaud the judgment of the physicians immediately in charge, who secured what we regard as an ideal consultation. They themselves were thoroughly competent to judge of the purely general medical aspects of the case, and they secured the counsel of a man familiar with the difficult problems of disease of the brain and spinal cord, and of one who had made hydrophobia a subject of special study for years at the bedside and in medical literature.

We believe that it would be of incalculable value to our science if every case of suspected hydrophobia could be thus studied, carefully and without bias, by men skilful in general diagnosis, who would not fail to recognize any underlying constitutional or local disease which might cause dysphagia, and men trained to detect the evidences of disease of the brain and spinal cord. By such a combination the danger of an error of diagnosis would be reduced to a minimum, and we have no doubt that in many cases the fatal result which usually follows a diagnosis of hydrophobia would be averted.

PROTECTION FOR AMERICAN PHYSICIANS.

A recent editorial in the *Medical Record,* making a plea for the protection of American physicians against the competition of German physicians, who come to this country to practise, has been somewhat misunderstood by the *Press* of Philadelphia, which takes the *Medical Record* to task, and asserts that the community needs protection against incompetent physicians— native as well as foreign. The *Press* editorial will be found in another column.

In this the *Press* is undoubtedly right, and no one, we are sure, will endorse its sentiments more heartily than the *Medical Record.* It is unfortunate that the title and contents of the editorial in the latter journal are misleading, and that it seems to lay more stress upon the nationality of the competing physicians and the cheapness of their charges than upon the imperfection of their medical training. As a matter of fact, American physicians need no legal protection against any class of competitors, except on the ground of unfitness for their work; and our lay contemporaries must not mistake a local wail for a general complaint. In New York the social and professional conditions are peculiar, and largely influenced by its enormous foreign population. It is, in important respects, unlike any other American city, and probably less American than any other. No doubt some of its physicians are inconvenienced by the natural consequences of its peculiar make-up; but this is a purely local matter, and of no interest outside of New York.

All over the United States the members of the medical profession are content to protect themselves, and to secure respect and patronage by deserving it. They are the strongest advocates of a high standard of medical education, and welcome every evidence that the community is awaking to the necessity for exacting this from those who intend to practice medicine. They will not endorse any effort to secure discrimination in their favor for other reasons than those of merit, and the best of them would be glad to have the State take intelligent charge of the regulation of medical practice and abolish all the privileges of the mere title of M.D., requiring a license to practice, which should be issued only to those who pass a satisfactory examination before a Board of Examiners appointed by the State.

This is the kind of protection which every intelligent citizen would approve, and which we hope some day to see established in this country.

ABORTION IN CHICAGO.

The *Chicago Times* has recently been investigating the subject of criminal abortion in Chicago, by means of a decoy, who visited a large number of midwives and physicians, pretending she was pregnant and asking them to help her out of her dilemma. The results of this investigation were published in December, and they show that a woman who is ready to undergo the risks of an abortion in Chicago need not search hard to find a medical man to share them with her for a consideration.

The issue of the paper for Dec. 17 contains a list of midwives and physicians in Chicago who would bring on an abortion— one of the latter being the official surgeon of the Police Department, and a supplementary list of men who declined to commit this crime themselves, but recommended others who would do it.

The same issue contains a letter from Dr. Doering, President of the Chicago Medico-Legal Society, expressing approval of this investigation and promising the support of the Society to its work. This fact may be taken as an index of the attitude of every decent medical man in the United States; for there are no more uncompromising enemies of the crime of abortion for convenience than physicians; and the fact that some men or women, whom the lax laws of most of the States permit to practice medicine, are willing to use the knowledge they have in an infamous way simply illustrates the adage that black sheep are to be found in every flock.

We cannot approve of the sensational way in which the *Chicago Times* has been exploiting its discoveries in regard to the crime of abortion in Chicago, and fear that it may do much harm by advertising the methods of abortionists ; but we trust that this serious disadvantage may be offset by the fact that it is also calling attention in a most striking way to the heinous character of this offense against public morals.

ELECTION OF PROFESSORS AT THE UNIVERSITY OF PENNSYLVANIA.

At the last regular meeting of the Trustees of the University of Pennsylvania, Dr. John Ashhurst, Jr., now Professor of Clinical Surgery, was elected to the chair of general Surgery vacated by the resignation of Dr. Agnew, and Dr. James Tyson, now professor of Morbid Anatomy and General Pathology, to the chair of Clinical Medicine, made vacant by the resignation of Dr. Osler. The title of Emeritus Professor of Surgery and Clinical Surgery was conferred on Dr. Agnew. This action of the Trustees will make two more vacancies: one in the chair of clinical surgery, and one in the chair of morbid anatomy and general pathology. It is commonly believed that the former of these positions will be secured by Dr. J. William White, of Philadelphia, and the latter by Dr. John Guitéras, of Charleston. Dr. White is now Clinical Professor of Genito-Urinary Surgery and Demonstrator of Surgery in the University, and Dr. Guitéras is a graduate of the University, who was formerly one of the Visiting Physicians to the Philadelphia Hospital, and enjoyed an enviable reputation as a diagnostician and clinical lecturer. He is at present Professor of Pathology in the South Carolina Medical College, and a surgeon in the U. S. Marine Hospital Service.

BOOK REVIEWS.

[Any book reviewed in these columns may be obtained upon receipt of price, from the office of the REPORTER.]

DIE GESCHICHTE DER TUBERCULOSE. Von Dr. med. AUGUST PREDÖHL, assistenzarzt am allgemeinen Krankenhause zu Hamburg. 8vo, pp. 502. Hamburg und Leipzig : Verlag von Leopold Voss, 1888.

This is an important contribution to the history of the development of our ideas concerning tuberculosis, showing how they emerged from dimness and gradually assumed a definite form. Even the earliest writers on the subject recognized the presence of nodular bodies in diseases of the lungs, which they called tubercles, but which would hardly come up to the more modern acceptation of that term. All the so-called lung tubercles of that time were contained within the vesicular structures. But here, as in everything else, our knowledge advanced from the simple to the complex, and disease within the air cells was of easier recognition than that without. Stark, in 1785, was the first to realize that the lungs became studded with small nodules, the composition of which he believed to have been coagulated lymph. Both Laennec and Louis, following Bayles, admitted but one kind of phthisis—the tubercular. Rokitansky, in 1845, was the first to distinguish between true and false tubercle; and he termed the first : interstitial tuberculosis, and the second : pneumonia. Engel and Hamernyk agreed with Rokitansky; but Addison, who held that tubercle is due to a proliferation and accumulation of epithelial cells, was probably the first to comprehend the true nature of the intra-vesicular nodule. It was not, however, until 1854 that the illuminating mind of Virchow defined the nature and proper relation of these structures, as follows (a) tubercle, or miliary tuberculosis; (b) hyperplasia (neubildung) of lymphatic tissue; (b) pseudo tubercle—an inflammatory product.

With Villemin began a period of experimental investigation, which, ending with Koch, tends to overturn the exact ideas of the earlier workers in this direction. The criterion of tubercle now is the bacillus, and the nature of a product is judged in relation to the presence or absence of this microorganism. Investigation shows that the bacillus is found in the false as well as in the true tubercle. There is no reason to find fault with this drift of things, if the bacillus theory tends to place our knowledge of tubercular diseases on a more scientific basis than it has heretofore occupied. It is evident, however, that the bacillus is not satisfied with anything short of the whole earth, for just so soon as it became a recognized element in the diagnosis of tubercle, it also began to play the rôle of an etological factor. In the first, it is a success; in the second, it is a failure. Clinical, and not experimental, medicine must render an ultimate decision as to the etiological relation of the bacillus tuberculosis, and this otherwise very valuable work is slightly defective in not giving a more complete history of the clinical statistics which have already been garnered, and which substantially show the worthlessness of the bacillus as a practical cause of tuberculosis. Reference is made especially here to the Brompton Hospital statistics, and to the *Statistical study of the Etiology of Phthisis Pulmonalis*, contributed by Dr. Schnyder to the *Correspondenz-Blatt für Schweizer*

Aertzte, 1886, Nos. 10, 11 and 12; both of which are left unnoticed in the book before us.

The book as a whole is of uncommon interest, and we sincerely trust that it will obtain a large number of readers on this side of the Atlantic.

PAMPHLET NOTICES.

[Any reader of the REPORTER who desires a copy of a pamphlet noticed in these columns will doubtless secure it by addressing the author with a request stating where the notice was seen and *enclosing a postage-stamp.*]

180. MINERAL AND THERMAL SPRINGS OF CALI-FORNIA. BY W. F. McNUTT, M.D., San Francisco, Cal. From the *Transactions of the Ninth International Med. Congress*, vol. v, 9 pages.

181. DOUBLE OVARIOTOMY DURING PREGNANCY; SUBSEQUENT DELIVERY AT TERM. BY WILLIAM WARREN POTTER, M.D., Buffalo, N. Y. From the *American Journal of Obstetrics*, October, 1888. 4 pages.

182. SULFANOL, THE NEW HYPNOTIC. BY B. SACHS, M.D., New York. From the *Medical Record*, October 6, 1888. 8 pages.

183. VALEDICTORY ADDRESS AT THE COMMENCE-MENT OF THE DEPARTMENTS OF MEDICINE AND DENTISTRY OF THE UNIVERSITY OF PENNSYL-VANIA, May 1, 1888. BY JOHN ASHHURST, JR., M.D., Philadelphia. 14 pages.

184. A PECULIAR CASE OF HERPES ZOSTER OPHTHAL-MICUS, SEROUS IRITIS, OR "OPHTHALMO-NEURITIS." BY GEORGE M. GOULD, M.D., Philadelphia. From the *Polyclinic*, October, 1888.. 6 pages.

185. TRANSACTIONS OF THE AMERICAN ASSOCIA-TION OF OBSTETRICIANS AND GYNECOLOGISTS. FIRST ANNUAL MEETING. ABSTRACT. From the *Buffalo Med. and Surg. Journal*.

186. GRADUATED TENOTOMY IN THE TREATMENT OF INSUFFICIENCIES OF THE OCULAR MUSCLES. BY CHARLES HERMON THOMAS, M.D., Philadelphia, From the *Transactions of the Philadelphia County Med. Society*, 1888. 12 pages.

187. REPORT OF PROCEEDINGS OF THE ILLINOIS STATE BOARD OF HEALTH. October, 1888. THE YELLOW FEVER EPIDEMIC OF 1888, ETC. 25 pages.

188. PERI-CÆCAL INFLAMMATION. PATHOLOGY. BY JOHN H. MUSSER, M.D DIAGNOSIS. BY WILLIAM PEPPER, M.D. TREATMENT. BY THOS. G. MORTON, M.D. From the *Transactions of the Philadelphia County Med. Society*, 1887. 19 pages.

180. This pamphlet, as its title indicates, gives an account of the various springs of California which are of value in the treatment of diseased conditions. It contains useful information as to the location of these resorts, and tables of analyses of the constituents of many of the waters.

181. Dr. Potter reports the first case of which he has knowledge in which a double ovariotomy during pregnancy was followed by delivery at term. His patient was in the fourth month of pregnancy. The history of the case is exceedingly interesting.

182. The spelling of the title of this pamphlet is probably chargeable to the Editor of the *Medical Record*, and not to the author, as he could hardly have made such a mistake. The substance of the paper is a report of Dr. Sachs's experience with

sulphonal in eleven cases. He finds—as most men who use it have found—that sulphonal is a good hypnotic in cases of functional insomnia; and that it has very little narcotic influence.

183. Dr. Ashhurst's address contains kindly and valuable advice to those for whom it was prepared, and is of such a character that it is not surprising to find the name of à bishop heading the list of those who asked him for a copy for publication.

184. Dr. Gould gives the history of a case of ophthalmo-neuritis with some peculiar symptoms. His report will interest ophthalmologists on account of the curious features of the case, and its developments under treatment.

185. The contents of this pamphlet are indicated fully by its title. The cover states that it is from the *Buffalo Med. and Surg. Journal;* the first page credits it to the *Amer. Journal of Obstetrics*. The contents are interesting and instructive; and, as might be expected, there is rather a preponderance of gynecology over obstetrics in it.

186. As Dr. Thomas's paper was published in full, with the accompanying plate, in the REPORTER, April 14, 1888, its contents are probably familiar to most of our readers. It advocates and illustrates the advantages of the method of treating insufficiency of the muscles of the eyeball proposed by Dr. Stevens, of New York, to which we have more than once called attention in these pages.

187. This report, prepared by Dr. Rauch, contains some very instructive reading in regard to the history of the recent yellow fever epidemic and the absurd and damaging methods adopted to limit its spread. We can heartily commend it to the attention of our readers, in the hope that it may correct some false notions in regard to yellow fever, which experience teaches are entertained by medical men as well as by the laity.

188. These papers, with the discussion which followed their reading, were published in the REPORTER, Jan. 7, 1888, and they are so valuable that we can recommend those who have become subscribers since that date to endeavor to get a copy of this pamphlet and make themselves acquainted with its contents.

LITERARY NOTES.

—Commencing with the January, 1889, number, the name of the *Sacramento Medical Times* will be changed to the *Occidental Medical Times*. The journal will be enlarged to 56 pages and the subscription will be reduced to $2.00.

—The *Internationales Centralblatt für die Physiologie und Pathologie des Urogenitalsystems* is the title of a new journal about to appear in Germany. Among the members of the editorial staff are Profs. Preyer and Zülzer of Berlin.

—The *Alabama Medical and Surgical Age* began its course in December, 1888, under the editorial management of Dr. John C. Le Grand, at Anniston, Ala. The first number is an octavo of 26 pages, containing a good deal of interesting matter, and an appeal for support in the State of Alabama which deserves a hearty response. The fact that it is the only medical journal now published in a State which has a large and able body of physicians makes its appeal especially worthy of consideration. It is to be issued monthly; subscription price $2.00, payable in advance.

CORRESPONDENCE.

"Grass Bur" in Left Bronchus.

To THE EDITOR.

Sir: I notice in the REPORTER of Dec. 8, an account of a case of "Sand-Bur in the Larynx," which recalls to my mind a somewhat similar case occurring in my practice about five years ago, while practising in Texas, and perhaps it is worthy of recording.

I was called to see the patient, a boy four or five years of age, and found him with a high temperature, severe pain in the left side, rapid breathing, with cough and muco-purulent expectoration. On physical examination I found entire absence of respiratory murmur on the left side, and all the symptoms of pneumonia; and such was my diagnosis. I visited him daily and found no improvement in the lung. On about the sixth day, after examining him—and while I was giving some direction in regard to his medicine, he was seized with a violent fit of coughing, and then began to cry, telling his mother that something was sticking him. The mother, using her handkerchief to clear the mucus from the boy's mouth, brought out something and passed it to me. This on inspection proved to be a "grass-bur"—the name applied to a bur, or ball that is covered with very sharp spines or "stickers," the whole thing being perhaps one-fourth of an inch in diameter, and the product of a species of grass indigenous to Texas. The only information I could get to explain how this foreign body found its way into the lung, was from the mother, who recollected that some weeks before the child, while running and playing in the yard, fell down and began to cry as though severely hurt, but soon seemed all right, and nothing more was thought of the occurrence until the bur was expelled from the lung. The patient began to improve from that time and made a complete recovery.

To those who are familiar with the "grass bur," it will seem strange that such a formidable body could enter the bronchi without causing symptoms of a more violent character.

Yours truly,
T. A. CRAVENS, M.D.

Los Angeles, Cal.,
Dec. 20, 1888.

———————

—The town of Nanticoke, Penna., is alarmed over some cases of small-pox which exist within its limits.

NOTES AND COMMENTS.

Effect of Glycerine on the Quantity of Secretion poured into the Vagina.

At the meeting of the Obstetrical Society of London, Dec. 5, 1888, Dr. Herman read a paper which related observations made to see whether the commonly, but not universally, accepted belief, that the local use of glycerine causes a flow of fluid from the vagina, was correct or not. The observations were made with cotton-wool plugs soaked in glycerine, and with pessaries made of gelatine and glycerine. The amount of glycerine inserted into the vagina was weighed; the discharge from the vagina was weighed, and the amount of vaginal discharge from the same patient when glycerine was not used was also ascertained by weight. The result of the observations was in favor of the following conclusions: 1. That when the secretions poured into the vagina were not abundant, the local use of glycerine increased them. 2. That when the secretions poured into the vagina were already abundant the local use of glycerine did not increase them.

Dr. Champneys asked if Dr. Herman had estimated the loss on the diapers from evaporation. The conditions were favorable for evaporation, and would confirm the conclusions arrived at in the paper.

Dr. Herman, in reply, stated that he thought the loss of weight by the napkins or pads due to evaporation was but slight; on the other hand, the perspiration from the skin with which the napkin was in contact, might cause a slight increase in weight. Dr. Herman had used the words "secretions poured into the vagina," which did not imply any opinion as to their source. Whether the secretion was of uterine or vaginal origin, whether it was produced by glandular activity or simple osmosis, he could not tell. He would be obliged if Dr. Griffith could suggest any method, harmless to the patient, by which the excretions of the uterus could be separated from those of the vagina. Dr. Herman believed that the vagina did secrete mucus. In cases of atresia of the vagina at more than one place, collections of mucous fluid were found between the occlusions. In cases of atresia of the os externum, the vagina was as moist as in most other patients. That under pathological conditions the vagina might pour out fluid in abundance needed no demonstration.—*British Med. Journal*, Dec. 15, 1888.

Electrolysis for Alterations in the Prostate caused by Gonorrhœa.

At the recent meeting of the Southern Surgical and Gynecological Association, held at Birmingham, Ala., Dr. J. D. S. Davis read a paper in which, after establishing the true physiological reason, as he thinks, for the use of electrolysis in hypertrophy of the prostate, based on well-known physiological facts, he gave explicit directions as to the method of its use. He emphasized the great importance of a good galvanometer and rheostat, next to a reliable battery. He recommended the nickel-plated insulated *bougie à boule*. The cutaneous electrode should be large, and applied to the abdomen. In order to obtain the maximum therapeutic effect, the cathode must be introduced into the prostatic urethra, and a very weak current passed through it (to avoid shock, the rheostat should always be used), increasing gradually until the galvanometer registers the required number of milliampères.

The method of *Electrolysis* is simple, and can be executed by the physician without aid; it is painless, requiring no anæsthetic; very little inconvenience is felt after the operation, and anodynes are never required; it is absolutely harmless; it is antiseptic on account of the energy of the low chemical current employed: and electrolysis, which is called galvano-chemical absorption by Newman, is always followed by a process of retrogression and disintegration.

A focus of derivation is created in the diseased gland, which is analogous to what is caused by a profound shock of the muscular system from over-exertion or over-stimulation, and which continues after the cessation of the current; transforming the temporary shock, which the passage of the current has transmitted, to the muscular element of the prostate; and it finally inaugurates a process of retrogression, disintegration, and absorption.

The muscular tissues are relaxed by the powerful stimulating effect of the current; the vessels are relaxed; and the blood-flow is increased by diminishing the capillary resistance; and absorption readily takes place.

Of galvano-chemical absorption, Dr. Davis says: "I understand that it is a chemical decomposition, which borrows its immediate effects from the suppurated albuminous bodies through the constituents of tissue; and not as defined by Newman as ' The process or act of being made passive by the disappearance in some other substance, through molecular or other invisible means, as absorption of light, heat and electricity,' which, though it is Webster's definition of absorption, is only a vague descriptive picture of the disappearance of animal structures."

The author concludes that a favorably-adjusted galvano-chemical current of low intensity will produce a decomposition of the tissues of the body, without resulting in or producing galvano-chemical cauterization of the superficial layers.

Electrolysis, while applicable to all strictures of the urethra, is of permanent benefit in the morbid alteration of the prostate produced by gonorrhœa of the urethra. It has an anæsthetizing influence upon the terminal nerves at the point of application; and by causing muscular exhaustion, it produces early relaxation of spasm, and thus aids in overcoming spasmodic urethral strictures, following the over-stimulation by natural reproductive processes; it excites absorption, and relieves the patient.

Intestinal Obstruction With Linseed.

Dr. Polaillon lately brought to the notice of the Academy of Medicine of Paris a curious effect of linseed, which is frequently prescribed in grain for obstinate constipation. He had under his care a young woman in good health, but habitually constipated, who took daily for three months a tablespoonful of linseed in grain. At the end of this time she showed symptoms of intestinal occlusion, and after complete constipation, lasting for a week, it was found necessary to make an artificial anus, through which an enormous quantity of linseed escaped. Notwithstanding this relief, the patient continued to sink, and died seven days after in a markedly typhoid state. Dr. Polaillon recalled a similar circumstance reported by Professor Verneuil, of obstruction produced by fig-seeds. He thinks that in his own case surgical intervention was too late, and that the woman had succumbed to stercoræmia. Dr. Berger also recalled what takes place in animals which ingest these same products without bruising them, and of which they easily disembarrass themselves. He had seen guinea-pigs fed with Indian corn in grain; their intestines filled like a sack of wheat, and they continued ingesting until the bowel was ruptured. It is probable that these differences between man and animals depend on the nature of the secretions.—*Lancet*, Dec. 15, 1888.

Protection for American Physicians.

Recently actors of the second and third grade have expressed a desire to be protected from the cheaper and perhaps better English article by a non-importation act; for " professional actors " are excluded from the operations of the present law. This actors' movement has struck the average public as absurd, but it is capped by the New York *Medical Record*, which in its issue of December 29 devotes its leading editorial to an earnest plea for protection for American physicians.

It complains that numbers of physicians, so-called, come over from Germany on every steamer. They possess a university diploma of M. D., which entitles them to practice as soon as they get here, though they could not practice in Germany because they have never passed, and are not able to pass, the state examination. Here, however, they have at once the legal status of a physician. They settle down in the German districts, put out a sign and pay visits for twenty-five or fifty cents. England, France and Italy make similar contributions annually to the number of practicing physicians of the United States. On this account, the *Record* says, " there is a growing feeling among physicians in New York City that if the principle of Protection be applied to some class of workers it might with equal justice be applied to the doctor."

It is not disputed that the ranks of physicians in this country are overcrowded. If, however, doctors need to be protected from incompetent Germans they need quite as much to be protected from incompetent Americans, who are turned out of the regular medical colleges by the wholesale and are authorized by their diploma to practice medicine with often an entirely inadequate preparation for their work. One diploma mill, we have in mind, graduates its young men after two terms or a total attendance of six months. Competent doctors may or may not think they require protection from this class of practitioners, but it is certain that the public do. It matters not whether the physician comes from Germany or from Kentucky, the fact that he holds a diploma from some alleged medical college ought not of itself without further proof of fitness to entitle him to practice his probable ignorance upon a suffering and defenseless humanity.

Germany is perfectly right in permitting no one to practice medicine there without passing the state examination. A like provision here would protect the doctors by keeping out thousands of competitors; but its chief recommendation is that it would protect the public in great measure from the quacks and incompetents who, armed with a diploma from some obscure college, now practice unchallenged on whomsoever they can persuade to entrust their health to their keeping.—*Philadelphia Press*, Jan. 3, 1889.

Case of Probable Poisoning with Creolin.

So much has been written lately in praise of creolin as a harmless antiseptic that the following case of probable poisoning with it, which occurred in the wards of Prof. Rosenbach, of Breslau, and is communicated to the *Therapeutische Monatshefte*, merits attention. In a primipara, 27 years old, after evisceration of a dead fœtus the uterus and vagina were washed out with a two per cent. creolin solution, in which procedure about one gallon of the solution was used. As the temperature rose on the next day to 102.4° the uterus was again washed out with one quart of a one per cent. creolin solution. On the following day the temperature was 100.5°, and for this reason and because of a somewhat fetid discharge, the uterus was washed out with about one quart of a one per cent. creolin solution, making the third washing out since the delivery of the woman, without any change in the good health of the patient occurring. In the evening about half-past six the uterus was washed out a fourth time. About nine o'clock the patient became suddenly pale and cold, and vomited violently. The temperature was 99°. The vomiting did not cease, sweating occurred, and at eleven o'clock the patient died in collapse and unconscious, after the temperature had fallen to 96.3°. The brownish-green vomitus smelt of creolin with extraordinary intensity. The distillate treated with bromine water gave a rich precipitate which had the characteristics of tribromphenol. The urine also smelt strongly of creolin.

The result in this case can not be attributed to heart failure, because the patient was pretty well just before death; nor to puerperal sepsis, for the result of the autopsy is opposed to this. Poisoning with creolin is indicated by the similarity of the symptoms to those of carbolic acid poisoning, by the unexpected death in collapse, the negative result of the autopsy, and by the character of the urine and vomitus.—*Wiener med. Presse*, Nov. 11, 1888.

A Threatened Revolt of Medical Students.

The trouble in the Medical Department of the University of the City of New York, to which reference was made in the REPORTER, Dec. 29, is not yet at an end. The students, it may be remembered, objected to the selection of a son of ex-President Woolsey, of Yale College, to be Professor of Anatomy, when they desired a favorite instructor, Dr. Weisse, to receive the appointment. In an address to the students, Jan. 2, Vice Chancellor MacCracken said that Dr. Woolsey had been definitely decided upon as the new Professor, and that Dr. Weisse's resignation had been accepted. Dr. Woolsey gave his first lecture Jan. 3, and the threatened revolt did not come off at that time. A few of the students left the room, but almost all remained, listened to their new lecturer with respect, and applauded him when his lecture was completed.

On Jan. 14, however, 86 dental students presented a paper to the Faculty formally notifying them of their withdrawal from the University. This secession includes all of the dental students in attendance. It is also said that the withdrawal of A. J. Walsh has left the College without anyone who knows the secret way of preserving bodies. The Faculty is therefore obliged to secure fresh bodies for dissection.

Treatment of Acute Coryza.

Dr. F. H. Potter, Lecturer on Laryngology in the Medical Department of Niagara University, makes some timely remarks on the treatment of acute coryza, in the *Buffalo Med. and Surg. Journal*, January, 1889. He considers pernicious the prevalent custom of sleeping with the windows open when the external temperature is below a certain point. At this time the temperature may suddenly fall, or through some restlessness on the part of the sleeper he may expose a part of his body to rapid cooling, and so contract a coryza. A cold bath should be taken in the morning in a warm room. If a bath-room is convenient, the water should be drawn and allowed to stand over night. The bath should be taken rapidly, so that the whole body will glow afterward.

No part of the body should be under-clothed or over-clothed. It is important to keep the feet warmly covered, and to remove outside wraps upon going indoors where the atmosphere is warm. The neck-scarf should be worn according to the temperature of the day, when its use has become necessary to the wearer. Chronic affections of the nose and throat should be treated, for in patients so afflicted acute attacks of coryza may be only symptomatic of the chronic disorder.

If the cold comes on toward evening, the patient should take a hot bath, then 1-100 to 1-60 of a grain of atropine, and go to bed and be well wrapped up. If the atropine should disagree, a full dose of quinine, about ten grains, may be substituted. During the next day the nose and throat should be thoroughly washed with a warm alkaline spray. But a better plan is to employ the post-nasal syringe for irrigation; contract the turgescence of the nasal tissues with cocaine; and, finally, cover the entire surface with a coating of an unirritating oil. For this purpose he has found *oleum petrolinum* (fluid cosmoline) the best. The applications should be made three times a day. If the cold is first noticed in the morning, the process should be reversed—the local treatment given during the day and the general treatment at night.

By this method of treatment he says that colds which generally last from ten days to two weeks can be limited to about two days. When it fails some chronic intra-nasal disease will usually be found, or else some constitutional disorder which makes the attack of extraordinary obstinacy.

Idiosyncrasy as to Antipyrin.

Dr. F. Brandenberg, of Zug, relates a singular instance of idiosyncrasy as to antipyrin. A man who was suffering from acute articular rheumatism, and could not tolerate salicylate of soda, took fifteen grains of antipyrin in powder. About five minutes later there suddenly appeared violent toothache along the whole lower jaw, then headache, an intense "tearing-asunder" pain in the ear and the parts adjoining, with profuse flow of tears and nasal mucus. The symptoms ceased in the reverse order of their appearance, the toothache lasting for three to four hours. To elucidate the matter, Dr. Brandenberg requested the patient, a very intelligent man, to take another dose. The patient consented, but this time took only seven and one-half grains of the drug. In ten minutes, precisely similar symptoms developed, the toothache lasting for about twelve hours. Curiously enough, the articular pain had disappeared almost completely before the appearance of the other symptoms.—*British Med. Journal*, Dec. 15, 1888.

The Anatomical Tubercle.

Dr. William Osler writes as follows in the *Montreal Med. Journal*, Dec., 1888 : There have been of late years several very interesting observations upon the common post-mortem wart, or as it was named by Wilks, who first described it, *verruca necrogenica*. It is now very generally regarded as a local tubercle, the result of inoculation. The presence of bacilli has been demonstrated in several instances. The tubercles consist chiefly of granulation tissue, occasionally with giant cells, and with papillomatous outgrowths of the epidermis, which give the tubercle the wart-like character. They are met with in persons who perform many post-mortems, and in those whose business brings them into close contact with animals and animal products. Their occurrence is by no means infrequent. In Germany it is quite common to see the hands of the demonstrators of pathology (and more especially the attendants in the autopsy rooms) disfigured by these structures.

I have myself eight or ten scars from these warts, which I have had at times on my hands during the past fifteen years. They rarely increase in size beyond a quarter of a dollar piece, are seldom painful, and are only unpleasant on account of the disfigurement. In my case they have lasted variable periods, from four or five weeks to eight or nine months. I have usually found them to disappear spontaneously. Thus, the last one I had was the result of accidental inoculation made from a phthisical subject early in November. I persistently refrained from local treatment in order to watch its development. It gradually spread, and after attaining the size of a ten-cent piece remained quiescent, but did not disappear until June. As is often the case, it had several small colonies in its neighborhood. In the treatment of these structures, I have usually found that the oleate of mercury persistently applied with friction causes rapid disappearance.

In Hutchinson's lectures on Lupus, which appeared in the *British Medical Journal* during the early part of this year, the anatomical tubercle is classed as "lupus necrogenicus," and a very good case is made out in favor of placing it among the lupoid affections. He mentions an interesting instance in which a post-mortem wart has persisted for nearly forty years. Although harmless in the majority of instances, there are cases on record, some of which are quoted by Ruhl and Paltauf in their exhaustive article in vol. xiii of *Vierteljahres-schrift für Dermatologie und Syphilis*, in which systemic inoculation has resulted from the local sore. Verneuil suggests, in this connection, that the phthisis with which Laennec suffered might possibly be associated with the wound which he received many years before at a post-mortem on a phthisical subject. No doubt the reason why systemic infection is not more frequently observed is owing to the unfavorable soil which the skin offers for tubercular processes.

Formula for Producing Local Anæsthesia.

Dr. J. M. Lewis, of Mexia, Texas, gives the following formula for injection before extracting teeth, in *Daniel's Texas Med. Journal*, Oct., 1888 :

R .Cocaini muriat. . . . . . . gr. viii
Chloralis hydrat. . . . . . gr. v
Acidi carbol. . . . . gtt. iii
Aquæ destil. . . . . f ℥ iii
M. Sig. Inject two or three drops into the gum.

Swallowing Sovereigns.

Dr. Siotis reports the case of a patient who had swallowed fifteen sovereigns. He complained of severe pain in the epigastric region. Auscultation revealed the distinct clinking sound of the coins when the patient moved. Purgatives were useless. Pills of opium and belladonna were then administered. The next day three gold pieces were found in the fæces, and a painful cylindrical tumor was detected in the rectum. On the following day four other pieces were expelled, and severe pain was felt in the right iliac fossa. When percussed, this region gave a metallic sound. The remaining gold pieces were shortly afterward expelled, and the patient completely recovered.—*British Med. Journal*, Dec. 22, 1888.

Association of Acting Assistant Surgeons, U. S. Army.

The Annual Meeting of the Association of Acting Assistant Surgeons of the U. S. Army, an announcement of which was published in the REPORTER Nov. 24, will be held in Newport, R. I., Monday, June 24, 1889, at 8 P. M. Members of the Association are cordially invited to read or present papers concerning the history and the welfare of the corps.

Members who intend to be present are requested to notify the Recorder, W. Thornton Parker, M.D., Newport, R. I., at the earliest possible date.

NEWS.

—Dr. Amos Walker, formerly of Philadelphia, died at Doylestown, Pa., January 10, 1889, in the 95th year of his age.

—Several families in Albany, New York, are reported to have been poisoned by eating cheese and pickles. No deaths have occurred.

—Lieutenant Miles, of the United States Steamer Yantic, which recently arrived in New York from Hayti, died of yellow fever January 14.

—Dr. B. F. Kane, Professor of Clinical Medicine and Pathology, Medical Department of the University of California, died Dec. 29, 1888.

—The eleventh public congress of the section in Balneology of the German *Gesellschaft für Heilkunde*, will be held in Berlin in March, 1889.

—Prof. Liebreich announces in the November number of the *Therapeutische Monatshefte* that he has succeeded in producing cocaine by synthesis.

—Dr. Thomas Goodwillie, of Vernon, Vt., died of pneumonia Dec. 22, 1888. He was graduated from the Medical Department of Dartmouth College in 1866.

—Dr. George A. Bodamer has resigned his position as Resident Physician in Chief of the German Hospital, and intends to go abroad for purposes of study and recreation.

—Dr. Nathan Allen, of Lowell, Mass., died Jan. 1, 1889, at the age of 76. He was graduated from Amherst College in 1836, and from the Pennsylvania Medical College in 1841.

—The President of the Board of Health and the Health Officer, of Jacksonville, Florida, have issued bulletins declaring the city of Jacksonville and the county of Duval free from yellow fever and perfectly safe to visit.

—A cable dispatch to the daily papers states that the Royal College of Surgeons of England has passed a vote of censure on Sir Morell Mackenzie for publishing his book on the case of the late Emperor Frederick. The vote was twenty-one to two.

—The number of deaths in Philadelphia last week numbered 360, a decrease of 29 as compared with the same period last year. As usual the number of deaths from diseases of the lungs and bronchi largely predominated, numbering 121 in all. There were 9 deaths from scarlet fever, and 10 from typhoid fever.

—The *New York Med. Journal*, Jan. 12, in its statement of the infectious diseases in New York, gives the following figures for the two weeks ending Jan. 8: Typhoid fever, 29 cases and 11 deaths; scarlet fever, 544 cases and 87 deaths; measles, 809 cases and 35 deaths; diphtheria, 296 cases and 93 deaths.

HUMOR.

A CALL TO ARMS—a wail from a baby at 2 A. M.—*Burlington Free Press.*

EMPEROR WILLIAM has instructed the army physicians not to be afraid of making their treatment Teutonic. — *Pittsburgh Chronicle.*

SURE CURE.—Family Doctor—"Your wife needs outdoor exercise more than anything else." Husband—"But she won't go out. What am I to do?" "Give her plenty of money to shop with."—*New York Weekly.*

MRS. VENEERING—"Really, my dear doctor, you must come to my ball. It is Lucy's coming-out affair, you know, and I shall take no refusal; none at all." Doctor Bygfee—"Well, you see, my dear madam, I am a very busy man. My time is not my own—" Mrs. Veneering—"Say no more. Include the visit in your bill. There, I shall expect you. Good-bye."—*Pittsburg Bulletin.*

SMALL PRACTICE.—Young Doctor—"Yes, I expect that it will go pretty slow when I first open an office until I get started a little." Old Doctor—"Well, you bet it will. Why, when I first hung out my shingle I sat in my office for three months and only had one case." "Whew! That *was* pretty tough, wasn't it? Only *one* case! and what was that a case of?" "A case of instruments."—*Puck.*

OBITUARY.

JOHN J. SINNICKSON, M.D.

Dr. John J. Sinnickson died recently in Salem, N. J. His family is one of the original Swedish families which came to this country in 1638. Dr. Sinnickson was graduated from the University of Pennsylvania, and served in the war with Mexico. He was wounded in battle and remained disabled from his injuries to the end of his life. He was engaged largely in mercantile pursuits.

MEDICAL AND SURGICAL REPORTER

No. 1665.　　　PHILADELPHIA, JANUARY 26, 1889.　　　VOL. LX.—No. 4.

CONTENTS:

COMMUNICATIONS.

TUBERCULOSIS.[1]

BY J. H. MUSSER, M.D.,

PHILADELPHIA.

Stenographically reported by Wm. H. Morrison, M.D.

My object, Mr. President, in presenting this account of tuberculosis—of tuberculosis in its entirety—is not to announce anything original, even if it were possible, in regard to the subject, but rather to present it as I think the present state of our knowledge warrants us in considering it, and, in the course of the statements which I shall make, to illustrate the various phases of the subject and its various anatomical and clinical points by the citation of some cases which have occurred to me during my study of it.

I regret very much that, for want of time, I shall be unable to present a series of speci-

[1] An address delivered before the Philadelphia County Medical Society, December 26, 1888.

mens illustrating the various forms of tuberculosis, not only of pulmonary tuberculosis in which I am more especially interested, but also of the other varieties which I shall mention later. I, however, trust that it will not be long before I shall be able to show both macroscopical specimens and microscopical preparations illustrating the various points which will be brought out in the discussion of this subject. My remarks are based largely on the views of the later workers in tuberculosis, and my support of their statements is based upon the autopsies of some seventy cases carefully recorded, which I have made in the Philadelphia Hospital.

In the first place, in order to be precise, I shall state what I mean by the term tuberculosis. Tuberculosis is a specific infectious disease, the phenomena of which are due to the presence, in one or more organs or universally throughout the body, of the tubercle bacillus. Such is the definition warranted by our present knowledge. Whether or not the phenomena of tuberculosis are due to the tubercle bacillus alone, I am unable to say, but there undoubtedly is present in

97

every lesion tubercular in character, sometime in the course of its development; this micro-organism. Just here let me state the varieties of tuberculosis which we are called upon to see. I do not refer alone to pulmonary tuberculosis in all its phases, but in addition, to the so-called joint tuberculosis, the fungous disease of the joints; to the so-called scrofulous disease of the lymphatic glands, the cheesy glands, lymphatic tuberculosis; and also to tuberculosis of the genito-urinary tract, to tuberculosis of the serous membranes, as tubercular pleurisy, tubercular meningitis, and tubercular peritonitis. Then too, included among the forms of tuberculosis, we have the well-known disease, lupus. From recent observations, I have no doubt that this disease is of tubercular origin. Finally to tuberculosis belongs that most interesting general infectious disease, miliary tuberculosis.

A word in regard to tuberculosis of the lungs. I recognize in pulmonary phthisis only one condition, namely, tubercular phthisis. Such has been my experience. This, however, has its varieties. There is in the first place simple tuberculosis of the lungs—the racemose variety of tubercular infiltration; there is the cheesy variety, caseous phthisis, pneumonic phthisis; there is tubercular catarrhal pneumonia, and fibroid phthisis. These are the forms of tuberculosis found in the pulmonary structure.

By a tubercle I mean a specific inflammatory growth characterized by the presence of round cells, epithelioid and giant cells, and in addition by the presence of the specific irritant, the tubercle bacillus. This organism is present in all forms of tuberculosis. In the tubercle itself, it is universally present. The relation of it to the causation of tubercle depends upon a number of causes which I shall endeavor to detail. The bacillus is the specific element of the inflammatory growth, and the tubercle therefore is nothing more than an inflammatory growth characterized by the presence of this specific element. Round cells, lymphoid cells, epithelioid cells and giant cells are frequently found under other circumstances; but in tuberculosis we never find them without also finding the tubercle bacillus. In the tubercular process a tubercle of the histological characters mentioned need not necessarily be present. These inflammations occur without organized tubercle, as in tubercular catarrhal pneumonia. In this, as in all tubercular processes, whether or not a tubercle is found, the tubercle bacillus is present. On account

therefore of the universal presence of this organism—for it is found not only in pulmonary tuberculosis, but also in the other forms of tuberculosis which I have detailed—on account of the fact that by the methods comparatively recently introduced by Koch, this organism can be isolated by means of cultures—and it is the only organism that is isolated by the culture process from any tubercular lesion whatsoever; and because by the inoculation of the organism tuberculosis is produced, we are warranted in giving to it the highest etiological prominence.

For these reasons we are warranted in emphasizing the unity of tuberculosis, the common element being the bacillus. Moreover, the organism is found in the products of tuberculosis, as for instance in the sputum, in the pus from caseous glands or from diseased bone, or in the fluids that come in contact with infected centers, such as the urine in tuberculosis of the kidney and the stools in intestinal tuberculosis. It is found here not because the urine is pathogenic, but because the bacillus is washed out by the urine. It is found in all the discharges that arise from the irritation of this organism. When I say that it is found in all the discharges, some limitation must be made; for instance you may tap a tubercular pleurisy and fail to find any bacilli; or, more likely still, a caseous gland will be aspirated, and while we should expect to find the tubercle bacillus in the products of suppuration, this is not always the case, and for two reasons: In the first place, and this is the minimum reason, the bacillus is not abundant in the pus from tubercular lymphatic glands. There is not an excess of growth. In the second place, it is well known that the organism, especially in suppuration, may escape and not be detected by our cultures and staining. It is said that it is more particularly apt to escape in the process of suppuration, and while found in the tissues is not found in the degenerated products. There is, however, this point to prove the specificity of the product, namely, that if you take the product, even where you have failed to find the bacillus, and inoculate with it, tuberculosis is invariably produced, so that by inoculation of the bacillus isolated by culture, or by inoculation of the products of inflammation or by the inoculation of the inflammatory growth itself, tuberculosis is induced. The law is absolute that tuberculosis alone produces tuberculosis and that nothing else whatsoever will do it. An explanation of the fact that the inoculation of products of inflammation in which the tubercle bacillus may not be found, causes tuberculosis, is said by careful workers in this subject to be found in the presence not of the fully developed bacillus itself, but of the spores of this bacillus.

While therefore a tubercle is nothing more than an ordinary inflammatory growth, the result of the action of the specific irritant differs very much and does not necessarily cause tubercle alone. Thus in tuberculosis, the further process in the development of the disease, or perhaps in the immediate effect of the irritation, is frequently seen in caseation. This is most marked, and it is almost one of the specific elements of tubercular disease. It is true that caseation takes place under other circumstances. It is found, for example, in carcinoma and gumma, but it is especially characteristic of tuberculosis. There is one form in which caseation or caseous necrosis is so common, that it is known as caseous pneumonia or caseous tuberculosis: the cheesy variety of tuberculosis. I can give no explanation for the presence of the change. Coates has recently stated that caseation is so general, so universal in tuberculosis that it may be considered part and parcel of the tubercular process. Another feature of this specific inflammatory growth is its marked tendency to fibroid change. Anyone who has examined the various forms of tuberculosis, and particularly pulmonary tuberculosis, will have often seen this. There is almost constantly a marked tendency in some areas for the occurrence of an overgrowth of connective tissue. This is conservative, and part of the process which leads to healing, which is much more frequent than we generally admit.

I have said that tuberculosis is an infectious disease. That this is so is well known, particularly from the fact that it can be reproduced by inoculation of the tuberculous inflamed mass or its products as I have already pointed out, as for instance serum or sputum from tubercular lesions. As you well know, Tappeiner, long before the discovery of the tubercle bacillus, found that he could set up tuberculosis in animals by the inoculation of sputum from tubercular subjects. The pus from caseous glands, from a suppurating lung or from a pulmonary cavity will also, by inoculation, produce tuberculosis. I will refer later to a further proof of the infectious nature of tuberculosis, as proved by the fact that eating the flesh of tuberculous animals or drinking the milk from tuberculous cows

has frequently caused the disease. Moreover, one characteristic which belongs to all forms of infectious disease, obtains also in tuberculosis: I refer to incubation. This is definitely and quite positively proved. It is well known that in tuberculosis artificially produced, the disease arises in from fifteen to twenty days after inoculation of the tubercular matter. The experiments on this point are absolute and final, and cannot be gainsaid. This is proved not only by the experiments of Koch and his fellow-laborers, but even by experiments made before the period of the full knowledge that the tubercle bacillus existed. It was well known that in a definite period after the inoculation of certain materials, tuberculosis would develop.

Not only is this period of incubation shown in the production of tuberculosis artificially, but it is also occasionally seen in the human subject. It has been traced in some epidemics and outbreaks of tuberculosis, where in a definite period after the ingestion of flesh or of milk from diseased animals, tuberculosis has developed. It is, however, very difficult to determine this period of incubation in the human subject, and in fact, if we had not the results of experiments on animals, we should not be warranted, for reasons which I shall refer to further on, in stating that a certain number of days was the period of incubation. Attention has been called by Coates and Woodhead to the fact that in cases of old quiescent tuberculosis, there has been after the occurrence of hemorrhage the involvement of the general system in the course of fifteen to twenty days. After such a hemorrhage, tuberculosis sets up and from that time the progress is rapid. At the autopsies the lesions of general tuberculosis are found and also the lesions of the old, quiescent local disease. Just such a case presented itself in my wards of the Philadelphia Hospital, in the person of a healthy-looking, burly negro who had for a long time been the subject of a cough. There were present the physical signs of a circumscribed pulmonary cavity, but that the disease was not making any inroads upon his health, his condition testified; and that the lung was not generally involved, the physical examination showed. A short time after coming under observation, he had a hemorrhage, and about twenty days after the bleeding fever made its appearance with all of the phenomena of tuberculosis, and in five weeks he died of general tuberculosis, infected by the local disease of the lungs.

If the tubercle bacillus is related to the causation of tuberculosis—I have merely affirmed that it is universally present in the tubercular products—its mode of introduction into the system must be accounted for. It can be introduced by inhalation. Experiments have proved this. There is a fair amount of clinical and experimental evidence, if properly weighed and sifted, to show that by the inhalation of the products of tuberculosis, the disease can be set up. Tappeiner many years ago produced tuberculosis by causing animals to inhale the dried sputum from phthisical patients. There is no doubt that this is a common source of the disease, perhaps more common than we are willing to admit. In hospital wards where there are a large number of cases of tuberculosis, there is no doubt that the air is fully infected. The air in the Philadelphia Hospital at one time was examined by processes which all sanitary experts and others who work in this subject well know, and in some of the wards it was found to have the tubercle bacillus floating freely through it.

The tubercle bacillus is also taken into the system by means of the food. There is no doubt about this, and there is no necessity to cavil about it. The eating of the flesh of animals infected with tuberculosis has frequently caused epidemics of this disease. More especially may it be caused by milk from infected animals.

Here comes up an interesting remark made by Woodhead on this very point, that cases of infantile tuberculosis, and of local epidemics of tuberculosis, have been undoubtedly traced to the use of milk from cows in which there has been tuberculosis. The tuberculosis need not be general in the animal, and hence no general symptoms, for in several instances it was limited to the udder, and thus infected the milk. Not only is the tubercle bacillus found in the tissue of the udder, but also in the milk with the other secretions. Animals, as for instance, pigs that were fed with it, died of tuberculosis, and by staining the fluid, as well as by cultures, the organism was found. Heubermaas, more wonderful still, reports eight cases of infants, infected from their mothers, on account of tubercular mammitis.

Another way in which the tubercle bacillus may enter the system is by absorption. There has recently been sufficient evidence produced to show that by the absorption of the tubercle virus through the skin, the disease may be set up. In all probability caseous glands are thus caused. There is skin irritation, exposure to the tubercle bacilli, and as a result secondary disease of the glands. This is not as positively proved as the other modes of introduction of the poison ; but there is strong evidence that it may occur. That we have tuberculosis of the skin is well known, as seen in lupus.

One of the most interesting facts, or series of pathological facts, in regard to tuberculosis, is its method of spreading throughout the system after being introduced. It is of course known that it is locally infective and that it usually extends along the course of the lymphatics, but it is also important to remember, as Coates points out, that tuberculosis is a disease of surfaces and channels, and that the organism, or the products containing this organism are moved about over these surfaces and in that way infection takes place.

If there is tubercular disease anywhere, local infection is very readily seen in the tissues about the lesion. This is particularly seen in phthisis. Around the old lesion—a cavity or caseous mass—a dense area of tubercular infiltration is seen, and then an area of scattered tubercles, more and more separated, and younger and younger, until the healthy zone is reached. Along the course of the lymphatics the disease develops and has often been seen. This is possibly seen more frequently in tabes mesenterica than in any other variety. Even in adults you can often trace from a local area the course of the infection throughout the body. In a case which was under observation some time ago, there was tubercular disease of the lymphatic glands around the bronchi at the root of the lung, the lymphatics coursing toward the pericardium were markedly tuberculous and at the autopsy the disease could thus be readily traced to the pericardium. The pericardium was infected, tubercular pericarditis was set up and the patient died as a result of the enormous pericardial effusion, thus excited. Over and over again this has been seen. Coates, and a number of others, have reported examples in which, from old lesions, which were undoubtedly present, in the mesenteric glands, the tubercular process spread to the remainder of the lymphatic system, to the peritoneum, spreading over the surfaces of the diaphragm, from thence extending to the pleura, and in some instances even to the bronchial lymphatic glands. Subsequently the lung became infected. This is one method of the origin of pulmonary tuberculosis. Koch, Woodhead and others mention such cases, and those who have made many *post-mortems* have seen old lesions of the bronchial, the cervical and axillary or the mesenteric glands with secondary infection of the lungs or the entire system. In one recorded instance the ulceration extended from a caseous gland into a bronchus and thus the lung was rapidly studied. While the patient had been in ill health for some time, yet the occurrence of general tuberculosis was shown by the acute manifestations, and at the autopsy the lesions were found.

I shall not speak in detail of the different channels through which the disease may extend, but shall for a moment refer to a form which anyone can prove for himself. It is well known that after laryngeal tuberculosis begins, general pulmonary tuberculosis takes place sooner or later, and this readily, because the products of the laryngeal disease are aspirated into different areas of the lung, and thus the pulmonary structure is infected. In the same way the disease may extend throughout the lung. There is, for instance, infection of one apex, and fluids from this area are drawn, by aspiration and the position of the patient, into other parts, which are secondarily involved. As long as consolidation alone is present—there is usually no secondary involvement, and, indeed, if caseation and ulceration do not take place, but on the other hand the opposite process, fibrosis, ensue, there will be no secondary involvement. The occurrence of intestinal tuberculosis following pulmonary tuberculosis is due to the fact that the products of the disease in the lungs are swallowed and thus the intestinal canal is infected. And in a manner similar, tuberculosis of the genito-urinary apparatus is evolved, either from the kidneys to the remainder of the apparatus, or more frequently from a tubercular testicle along the lymphatics to the other strictures.

A word in regard to some interesting evidence as to the manner of general infection of the body from local disease as shown in miliary tuberculosis. For a long time we were unable to explain miliary tuberculosis, and how it was that the organism became infected. While even yet there are many cases of which we can not speak positively, yet the researches of Ponfick, Weigert and Coates leave no doubt that if careful search is made it will be found that the organism has been infected through the thoracic duct from an infecting tubercular mass in any portion of the body or from extension of the tuber-culous process to the veins. This latter method is discussed by Weigert. If a careful search is made the origin of the affection can usually be explained. I have seen it once or twice and demonstrated its course once this year and once last year. It is not often that opportunities for studying acute miliary tuberculosis present themselves. Coates explains the occurrence of the disease by involvement of the veins adjacent to or supplying the diseased lymphatic glands and by infection of the system through the blood. We know that tubercle bacilli are found in the blood and in the spleen, as well as in the infected tissues.

There are a few characteristics of the growth and development of the tubercle bacillus which explain very well the clinical course of tuberculosis, and in studying tuberculosis it is most important to consider them. From a knowledge of these features we know why it is difficult to reckon the period of incubation or the date of first infection; why the disease is one of long duration; why it is so frequently cured, and why it is so difficult to determine the contagiousness of the disease and the relation of predisposing causes—such as sex, age, occupation, climate, etc.—to the origin of the disease. In the first place it is well known that it develops slowly. This is seen in culture preparations. It is also seen when inoculation is performed. It is true that local irritation is set up, but the general development is slow; hence the disease is always of long duration. It is particularly on this account that we are unable to tell when the person has been infected. For instance, I may be exposed to the tuberculous poison now, I may have inhaled the tubercle bacilli in large numbers, but my tissues may not be in a condition to afford a place for their rapid development. There is not epithelial abrasion to admit of the introduction of the bacillus, or there is not that low vitality of the cells which must exist before there can be bacillary growth. But the organism is not readily destroyed. It may find a lodgment, but not a soil for growth. It may, however, retain its vitality for a long period of time, a second peculiarity of its life. It will live for a long time under unfavorable circumstances and for a long period of time remain quiescent. It can not, indeed, be definitely estimated how long this may continue. In scrofulous disease of the glands we know how long the duration of the disease is. I have now under my care a colored woman who has been under my observation for two years, in whom a long time ago tubercular disease was shown to be present by the discovery of the tubercle bacillus in a section of a gland taken out. The patient is still in fair health. The disease is progressing, but only slowly. This is also illustrated in the case of a man who recently came under my care, from whom a large number of lymphatic glands were removed by Dr. Pancoast in 1876, at the Jefferson clinic. Only the glands on one side were removed. The glands of the other side continued to grow and from the glands of the neck, the disease extended to the bronchial glands, thence to the mesenteric glands. The relation of the different growths, as regards the point of time, was distinctly shown at the autopsy by the characters of the inflammatory growths of the different parts. It could be seen that the older lesions were in the neck.

We have every reason to think that the primary disease was in these glands, from the clinical course of the disease. After slowly increasing in these glandular structures, acute tubercular catarrhal pneumonia developed and then general tubercular disease, tubercular meningitis being the immediate cause of death. This case shows the slowness of the growth and its power of the bacilli to live under ordinary circumstances of human life without destruction, and this fact explains the long duration of all forms of tuberculosis.

Remember too that the duration, as well as the virulence of the disease is influenced by the number of organisms which have been introduced, as has been shown by many and recently by the experiments of Dr. Trudeau. As you know, he has recently published a report of experiments in which, after the introduction of a certain dose, the disease developed in some up to a certain point and in others lasted for a certain period of time. If a larger dose were given, the course was much more rapid, the general infection more acute and more pronounced. Therefore the slowness of growth, and the number of bacilli introduced are all points explaining the duration of the disease.

As is well known, tuberculosis, including pulmonary tuberculosis and all varieties of the disease, is frequently cured or rather gets well. Under ordinary circumstances, tuberculosis tends to heal. Anyone who has followed the course of a large number of autopsies will have frequently seen instances of arrested tuberculosis, not only in the lymphatic glands but in other structures, as in the bones and in the lungs and even in the intestine. Not long ago, Dr. Osler made an autopsy on a patient in whom there were tubercular lesions in the intestine, some of which were progressing, while others were healed, and cicatrices were found.

In regard to the method of healing I shall not speak for want of time, except to say that it is by an overgrowth of connective tissue surrounding the specific inflammatory growth, the tubercular mass itself.

If, as is stated, one-seventh of all deaths are due to phthisis, the number of cases of tuberculosis must be very great, much greater than is generally admitted. Gardner in speaking from his own experience of tabes mesenterica, and also of other forms, says that they are much more prevalent than was formerly admitted. If one-seventh of all deaths are due to tuberculosis, we would almost be warranted in saying that one-fourteenth of the human race are infected with tuberculosis without evil results. In the autopsies made at the Philadelphia Hospital it is surprising to see the almost universal presence of this disease in a more or less active state, in patients dying from other affections, such as Bright's disease or carcinoma. In a patient recently under my care, for instance, who died of carcinoma of the stomach, there were found tubercular foci and ulceration in the lungs, and this observation could be multiplied. An abundance of examples of healed tuberculosis, as the puckered apices and the encapsulated nodules show, are constantly found.

With regard to contagion. I am inclined to the belief that tuberculosis is contagious, but only feebly contagious. And this is due to the peculiar characteristics of the tubercle bacillus itself. The reason why the disease is not more contagious and more prevalent is because the tissues are not in such a state of vitality as to be receptive to the bacillus, or to form a nidus or a soil for its development, and because there are no pathological processes present through which the tubercle bacillus can enter. Just as it is difficult to determine the period of incubation and the manner of introduction of the bacillus, so it is difficult to determine whether or not the disease is contagious. I may be exposed to the tubercular poison and have inhaled quantities of it at a certain period. This may find a resting-place in my lungs or it may have been taken into the lymphatics; and yet my health and the condition of my bronchioles and alveoli or gland structures may be such that there is nothing whatsoever to encourage the development of the bacillus, and it will remain quiescent. It is difficult to kill the organism. It will remain quiescent for long periods of time under the ordinary conditions of life, and then from one cause or another, as a long period of indigestion, worry, strain, or break-down of any kind, there is lowering of the vitality of the cells sufficient to allow the growth of the micro-organism and then it is that it develops. This period between the reception of the poison and the development of the disease may be so long that we can not positively trace its cause. It may have been forgotten. The predisposing factors just mentioned become operative in this manner.

I shall not enter into a discussion of other phases of this subject. Already sufficient time has been occupied. The prevention of tuberculosis or its treatment will not be spoken of. Practically, however, the treatment consists in prevention or in attending to the wants of the economy so as to prevent cell life of low grade. I have taken up more time than was intended, but the subject is one of such great interest that it is proper to present some conclusions in the manner which I have done. It is true it has been done in a most cursory and rather unscientific manner, and yet I trust I have shown that tuberculosis is an infectious disease of bacillary origin. A strictly scientific method of presentation of the subject has been sacrificed to one that is truthful, and yet at the same time clear, I trust. The evidence has not been presented as forcibly as my convictions are strong on the subject, and yet it seemed advisable to present the truths in a semi-popular manner. If these remarks are sufficiently clear and earnest to interest and arouse you all, I am content.

N. E. corner Locust and Fortieth Streets.

—The *New York Medical Journal*, Dec. 15, says "Away with the cant that anyone can write too well, or draw too well, or speak too well. Boorishness in style is not evidence of intellect, nor slovenly expression the necessary accompaniment of cultivated observation. Such defects are to be deplored. Their meaning goes deep. A university graduate suggests that it should be a point of honor among medical men to write in such form that an educated person can tell what the subject matter is, though not himself an expert in medical lore."

THE IMMEDIATE TREATMENT OF FRACTURES OF THE EXTREMITIES.

BY ERNEST C. HELM, M.D.,

BELOIT, WIS.

All surgical authorities will agree with Wyeth when he says:

"The great end to be achieved in the *treatment* of fractures is a reduction of the displacement to as near the normal as possible, and the absolute retention of the parts as replaced;" and, as Dr. Edmund Andrews of Chicago, Ill., teaches: "Put the parts in correct position and keep them there." The first part of this advice is usually not very difficult of accomplishment, especially if an anæsthetic is used; so assuming that the bones are in correct position, what is the best way to keep them there?

It is probable that no *perfect* dressing will ever be found, and that a plan advocated now will be antiquated in a few years.

The splint that is safest and most comfortable to the patient, and requires the least care or anxiety on the part of the surgeon, will be a blessing to all concerned.

It seems to me that the splint of the future will be a rigid one, and will be applied at once The primary dressings usually advocated in older, and even the most recent, works on surgery are temporary expedients and makeshifts and are to be used only "*until the swelling has subsided,*" and then a rigid apparatus is to be used. This method is all right if the patient lives at a great distance, but in hospital, or where the patient can be seen frequently, for a few days, a splint can safely be used which would absolutely retain the parts as replaced. This fear of swelling is a great bugbear to most young physicians, and therefore with the dread of constriction and mortification before them, temporary dressings are used until swelling has subsided. The patient's sufferings are greatly increased, the provisional callus is much greater, and the cure less rapid and satisfactory than it would be if an immediate fixed splint had been applied.

When the patient has not been seen until the swelling has become great, the surgeon may be forced to use temporary expedients; but if he is seen early, or before there is great swelling, a firmly yet smoothly applied fixed dressing, extending from near the tip of the extremity to well above the seat of fracture would hold the parts as replaced, and moreover, by affording firm and even support of the tissues, would prevent much swelling. The fragments being immovable, there could be very little callus, and repair would be rapid and uninterrupted. Swelling usually results from an uneven or tight dressing, and from not extending splint (or at least a bandage) well down toward the tips of the extremities. Levis's splints, strengthened by gypsum, have proved very satisfactory in my hands. The Levis splints being moulded to the shape of the limb, and being very light and strong, aid greatly in retaining the limb in proper position while the plaster is "setting."

There are two great objections to plaster of Paris alone: First, while the plaster is "setting," the limb has no support except the hands of the assistant, which often cannot keep the parts exactly as placed; second, the hands, and especially the fingers, deeply indent the soft plaster and make corresponding ridges on the inside of the cast, which may become very painful to the patient.

The use of the Levis splint with the gypsum obviates these difficulties. The objections to the perforated tin splints alone are that they are not rigid enough, and are rather short. But as they are strong and light, their conjoined use with plaster of Paris renders the latter lighter than it would be without them, as less plaster is required to obtain the needed firmness. There is nothing new in my mode of application, which is to apply a well-padded Levis splint to the adjusted fracture, securing it there by a few turns of a roller bandage; then to wrap the limb and splint in a thin layer of cotton, and apply plaster-of-Paris bandages until the desired firmness is obtained. The plaster extends from the base of the phalanges to considerably above the fracture—above the next upper joint if possible. In fractures of the femur or the humerus the gypsum may not have to extend so far down, but then a bandage would have to be used from the base of the phalanges to the plaster, otherwise swelling would ensue.

The patient will have to be seen in a few hours, and if there is little pain, and the fingers or toes, as the case may be, are not cold or blue or swollen—in other words if the circulation is good in them—the patient may be left. It is well to see him several times during the first four days, and to instruct the nurse to call you instantly if there is much pain or swelling. After four days the patient will require little care. Should pain or swelling be great the bandage can be loosened by a longitudinal incision, and a roller applied. This in itself is a fine and quite rigid dressing. Usually, however, the circulation continues good and the patient comfortable.

The advantages of immediate fixed dressings are so obvious that I need not refer to them here. Their dangers have been greatly exaggerated, for if carefully and intelligently watched for the first few days, they are probably safer than any other. As there is little if any movement, there is much less provisional callus, and consequently, if the fracture is near or involves a joint, there will be less danger of anchylosis; though in joint injuries the splint should be removed and passive motion practised as soon as it is deemed safe. I could cite many cases in which this mode of treatment has been used, but will mention only four or five very briefly.

On July 4, 1888, my brother, Dr. A. C. Helm, and I treated a case of Pott's fracture in the manner indicated. It was a railroad injury and there was great displacement, yet the recovery was almost painless and both rapid and uninterrupted. A few days later we treated a fracture of both bones of the forearm in the same manner, with very satisfactory results. This was originally a case of green-stick fracture, but both bones were broken in the attempt to straighten them. A fracture of the femur in a child three years old was easily treated by this method of dressing, and so was a fracture of both bones of the leg, just below the middle.

An old man last February broke his arm at the elbow, the fracture extending through the humerus just above both condyles, the splitting between them into the joint. The method of treatment I have described was as satisfactory here as in the other instances. In none of these cases, indeed, did the dressings have to be loosened or changed on account of swelling.

Whether this plan meets the approval of the readers of the MEDICAL AND SURGICAL REPORTER or not, I can only say that in my hands it has not disappointed me once, but has always exceeded my most sanguine expectations. I hope others who may have adopted the same method of treatment will give the result of their experience.

—Typhoid fever is said to be prevalent in Vienna. There were 10 cases in June, 32 in November, and 40 up to the 17th of December. This shows an increase of about 50 per cent. over the total for 1887.

THE TURKISH BATH AND ITS USE AS A THERAPEUTIC AGENT.[1]

BY A. HAMILTON DEEKENS,

UNIVERSITY OF PENNSYLVANIA.

The subject I wish to bring before you this evening is one in regard to which, as future physicians, I think we should be to a certain extent familiar, *viz :* "The Turkish Bath and its use as a Therapeutic Agent." A certain amount of knowledge of this now popular mode of treatment is demanded both in our own and our patients' interests. The attention of the laity has been attracted, during recent years, toward the Turkish bath, as a means of cure for various disordered conditions of both body and mind ; and they naturally turn to the physician for his professional opinion on the subject, and it is but fair to them, that he should study its merits and demerits, according to his best judgment, and give his patient the benefit of any good there may be in this system.

Until quite recently, most people, including the majority of physicians, have had exceedingly erroneous and exaggerated ideas concerning the Turkish bath, and have conjured up the most frightful visions of the barbarities and tortures the poor victim underwent, who dared enter the portals of this relic of heathenism. No doubt many of these ideas originated in the writings of various humorists—of Mark Twain, for instance, who, in his inimitable book "The Innocents Abroad," gives a vivid description of the tortures he underwent in this Purgatorial region, winding up with his being almost flayed alive with the jack-plane, as he facetiously terms the shampooing brush.

It is true, that when first introduced into England and this country, too much physical energy was occasionally expended on the devotee of the bath ; but this, with many other ignorant and unnecessary customs, has almost entirely disappeared, and in modern well-conducted bathing-establishments, everything is carried out according to the most approved anatomical and physiological principles.

The Turkish bath is no new invention. It is as old as the human race. It has been found in all climes and ages, and in every grade of social condition. It is one of the most ancient therapeutic agents of which we have any record. *Heat is its vital*

[1] A paper read before the D. Hayes Agnew Surgical Society of the University of Pennsylvania.

principle. Most nations of the world have recognized this fact. The greater part of Europe used the Turkish bath in one form or other ; even the Indians of America were familiar with its application. The ancient Phœnicians used the bath daily, as did also the Greeks. The Romans received the idea from the Greeks, and thus originated the famous Roman baths. When Constantine founded Constantinople he took with him the system so general in Rome, and constructed baths which were among the most magnificent structures in the world, and thus they came to be called Turkish baths.

Our modern so-called Turkish bath, however, would be more appropriately named the "Anglo-American" bath, as to this country and to England belongs the honor of having first introduced the dry air system. Dr. Barton, of England, was the first to discover that the real value of the bath lay in its heat, and was the first to put this discovery to a practical use. He built the first bath ever constructed on the dry air principle, at St. Anne's on the Hill, near Blarney, in Ireland, in 1856. Mr. Urquahart, who has written a well-known book on the Turkish bath, was the first to introduce this system into England, and we are indebted to Dr. Sheppard, of New York, for its first appearance in America. He erected a bath on Laight St., New York City, in 1862. In Ireland, even at the present time, are to be found "sweat-houses," as they are called, the use of which has not entirely died out, and which stand as heirlooms of an ancient people, who in their simple and practical way knew more of the hygienic conditions of life than most of us, in this scientific age, find it possible to put in practice.

One of the national characteristics of the Finlanders of Northern Europe was their constant use of heat, as a means of health, and their manner of using it. Nearly every peasant had a small private bath-house, for his own immediate use. It consisted of one small chamber, in the innermost part of which was placed a pile of stones, which were heated until they became red hot, then a stream of water was directed on them, and the Finn luxuriated in a true Russian or vapor bath. Their power of endurance of heat was wonderful. They would remain in a moist atmosphere at a temperature of from 130° to 150°, for half an hour or more at a time, at the same time going through a system of rubbing, and lashing every part of their bodies with birch twigs, until they presented a very raw appearance. In the winter season, they would frequently go out of the bath in a perfectly nude state, and roll in the snow, when the thermometer stood at 20° or 30° below zero. These hardy natives claim that their strength is recruited as much by the hot vapor baths as by rest and sleep, and such a thing as gout or rheumatism was unknown among them. I do not think, however, that I should advocate their form of bathing, as it would scarcely be suited to the American constitution.

To give you a general idea as to the proper manner of taking a Turkish bath, I will describe the different stages of the process, as carried out in our better class of bathing-establishments. The bather first registers his name and pays his fee, one dollar is the usual price, with half rates to physicians at most places; the bather's valuables are checked and deposited in a safe and the bather is shown to a private dressing-room, where he disrobes and arrays himself in a sheet, after which he is conducted by an attendant through the vestibule to the *tepidarium.* Here a sheet is spread over a reclining chair and the bather takes his place in it. The temperature of this room usually varies from about 110° to 120° or 125°. The air, although so much above summer heat, is not oppressive to most persons, and, owing to good ventilation, it is delightfully pure and soothing. Here the bather remains for a variable length of time, according to his feelings, stretching out his limbs in comfort and allowing care and anxiety to drift from his mind. After being thoroughly heated here, the bather next enters the *sudatorium.* This is a large, well-lighted and well-ventilated room with a temperature of from 140°— 160°. Here the flow of perspiration, which began in the *tepidarium,* increases and some of the pleasantest features of the bath are experienced. To give you some idea of the effects of this stage of the proceedings I cannot do better than to describe the sensations as told by Prof. Erasmus Wilson, who is an ardent advocate of the bath.

He says: "The air is clear, no vapory mists. It is fresh, for there is a free circulation of air through the room, and how marvellously soothing! All care, all trouble, all anxiety, all memory of the external world and its miserable littleness is chased from our mind; our thoughts are absorbed in rapturous contemplation of the delights of the new world, the Paradise into which we have just been admitted. The tyrant *Pain!* even loses his miscreant power. The *toothache,* where is it gone? The *headache* disappears, the *spasm* no longer abides, the grinding aches of craving appetite, the pang of *neuralgia,* of *rheumatism,* of *gout,* all have fled, for this is the region where the suffering find a soothing relief from all their torments, and over the door, is it not written, *This is the Calidarium, pain* enters not here."

The temperature of this room is sufficient to secure all needed physiological effects, but for certain diseased conditions a still higher temperature is needed, and for this purpose most establishments have a room with a temperature range of from 200°— 250°, this is the so called "*Torridorium,*" and although the heat is not sufficient to kill bacteria, it undoubtedly has a specific action on various morbid diatheses, and it is at this temperature that some of the best results of the bath have been attained.

The next move is to the shampooing-room, where the bather stretches out on a marble slab, and gives himself up into the hands of a manipulator, who effectually rubs and kneads, squeezes and percusses, wrings and manipulates his skin until the effete matter and worn out *débris* which has been brought to the surface by the opening and flooding of the pores forms in rolls upon his surface and is rapidly washed away. The process generally removes from one to three pounds of superfluous matter which had been clogging up the system. Shampooing is not the joint-cracking, neck-snapping and generally painful operation which so many imagine it to be. On the contrary, it is a thoroughly pleasant and enjoyable part of the programme, and a skilfull operator soon learns to graduate his muscular force to the requirements of the patient. After the manipulation is over, the bather is led to a shower bath, and thoroughly rinsed off with water at first warm and gradually made cooler, and then allowed the choice of either taking a plunge in a tank of cold water, large enough to swim in, or of first taking the Russian part of the bath, which consists in staying for awhile in a small room filled with hot steam, and following this with the cold plunge. It is not necessary to take the plunge at all, and the bather may merely cool off his body in order to avoid taking a cold when he goes out. After a brisk rub down the bather proceeds, enveloped in a sheet, to the *Frigidarium* or cooling room, where, resting on an easy couch and sipping a cup of coffee, he gradually dozes off into a refreshing slumber, where, in the words of Bayard Taylor, "mind and body are drowned in delicious rest, and we no longer remember what we are; for gently sleep steals upon our senses; as gently the clouds dissipate, and we are born again into the world, and walk forth instinct with a new life."

The indications for the use of the Turkish bath are numerous, both as a prophylactic and as a means of cure. Physicians of eminence, both in this country and in Europe, have testified repeatedly as to its value in various ailments and diseased habits of body. I cannot give you a better idea of its usefulness in disease than to quote you a few of their public opinions on the subject.

Dr. Austin Flint says that, as a remedy for sleeplessness, it is better than bromides, chloral, or opiates. Dr. Lewis Sayre says that when the medical profession arrives at a thorough knowledge of the value of hot air baths, they will prescribe them more frequently, and medicines less, and be of more service to their patients. Dr. L. W. Thudichum, of London, thinks the Turkish bath, the most powerful and certain, and at the same time the safest and most agreeable therapeutic agent in existence. He says one can remove as much of the poisonous and effete matter from the body in one hour in a Turkish bath as can be removed by other means in twenty-four hours, and that it is a common experience, that persons who have been liable every winter to attacks of catarrh, bronchitis or neuralgia, acquire an almost perfect immunity by the regular use of the bath. Sir Benjamin Brodie, M.D., of London, says it is of great use in dyspeptic and gouty diatheses, and to those who lead inactive or sedentary lives. Professor Erasmus Wilson, says that in the Turkish bath the skin acquires color, freshness, firmness and elasticity; it loses the muddy and faded hues of ill-health, and the parched and wrinkled aspect of infirmity and age; and that it procures for the habitual bather exercise, health and life. Sir John Fife, M.D., of Edinburgh, who was the first to establish a bath in connection with a hospital, at the great Newcastle Infirmary, says that its effects are most remarkable in obviating disorders and palliating diseases of the liver and kidneys, the passage of gall stones and the relief of kidney obstructions often occurring almost immediately after the use of the bath.

I could give you much other testimony of the same character; but these quotations are sufficient to show you that many of the leading physicians of the world are firm believers in the therapeutic value of this agent. As far as my own personal experience and observation go, the indications for the use of the bath, seem to point most strongly to its use as a diaphoretic, a general tonic, and a febrifuge. It is roughly estimated that there are seven million pores opening on the surface of the skin. These are the vent holes, or sluice gates, for over twenty-five miles of drainage. To insure health, it is necessary that the greater part of this system of drainage should be in proper working order. If the sluice gates are blocked up, the waste matter must find an outlet in some other quarter, and naturally it permeates the tissues of the body, enters the blood current and produces diseases of various kinds. The Turkish bath, by opening the pores, by flushing and allowing free egress to this deleterious matter, cleanses the blood from impurities, gives an impetus to the circulation, and invigorates the entire organism. It is one of the best remedies I know of for relieving a "general cold," and it acts well as a mild febrifuge. I have reduced my own temperature a degree and a half when suffering with a slight fever, by a stay of about 20 minutes in the hot room. There are many instances on record, of ladies who on first entering the bath would not sweat below their waists, and who, by continuing its use, have procured a uniform opening and cleansing of the pores, followed by a general improvement of health, and disappearance of nervous and dyspeptic symptoms. In cases of chronic eczema, some most happy results have been reported from the continuous use of the Turkish bath. Unlike many rules the Turkish bath works both ways: it will reduce superfluous tissue, and, by its action in restoring the system to a normal condition, it will also increase the bodily weight. If time permitted, I could give many more instances of the remedial power of this great therapeutic agent, but I hope I have said sufficient to give you an idea of its power for good when rightly used under the directions of a competent medical adviser.

—The *Western Med. Reporter*, Dec., 1888, says that in a recent suit the Supreme Court of Indiana decided that unless damages are collected during the lifetime of the physician, they cannot be collected. No action for damages in a malpractice suit can be maintained after the death of the party sued.

SOCIETY REPORTS.

OBSTETRICAL SOCIETY OF PHILA-DELPHIA.

Stated Meeting, Thursday, January 3, 1889.

The President, THOMAS M. DRYSDALE, M.D., in the chair.

DR. PARVIN presented the ·

Sexual Organs of a Young Girl,

and said that they are among several which he procured in Munich last summer for the purpose of teaching students practically many of the operations upon such organs by the method proposed and pursued by Prof. Winckel. His method is as follows: The organs being properly fastened within and upon Schultze's obstetric phantom, many of the more common operations can be done by the student as upon the living subject. This much was said to explain why he had no history of the subject from which the specimen was taken. In the specimen there is a very perfect annular hymen, one of the rarer forms of this structure, and its borders are quite regularly dentated. The bladder apparently has its walls somewhat thickened, though probably not really; but certainly they seem very thick in comparison with the uterine walls. These latter are so thin that there is in this regard a hypoplasia of the uterus, and thus a uterus membranaceus; but the organ in length and breadth seems fairly developed.

DR. PARVIN also presented

An Obstetrical Manikin.

He had the obstetric phantom made in Munich; it represents a design he had entertained for many years, in fact since the beginning of his obstetric teaching. He wished a complete human form, which could be put in the different positions a woman occupies in labor—natural, manual, and instrumental. The joints are sufficiently mobile to permit the model to be placed on the side or on the back, the limbs put in any position desired. The pelvis is of iron, covered with leather and has a movable coccyx; while the external parts are made of rubber which will dilate so as to admit the passage of a fœtus. The abdominal cavity is ample for the introduction of two fœtuses. One or both may be included in the rubber uterus designed by Prof. Winckel,

and thus placed in that cavity. For the suggestion of a cast-iron pelvis, a model of the best one found in the Museum of the Munich *Frauenklinik*, I am indebted to Dr. J. Clifton Edgar, of N. Y., then a resident obstetrician in the *Klinik*. Dr. Edgar, who remained in Munich several weeks after I left, during his stay superintended the work, and doubtless I· am indebted to his intelligent supervision, suggestion and direction for the successful manner in which the workman carried out the original design. The model will be useful in gynæcological as well as in obstetric teaching, in that the different positions in which the patient is placed in examinations and in operations can be readily and plainly illustrated. The only addition which it seems to me at present might be usefully made is a rubber abdominal wall, similar to that of Budin's well-known obstetric manikin.

DR. J. C. DA COSTA did not think that annular hymen is so very rare. He had seen some cases and among them one that was very marked. The woman had been married some two years, had been pregnant and had aborted at four or five months. Coitus was excessively painful both to the husband and to the wife, and in the wife was frequently followed by attacks resembling epilepsy. The hymen was annular, smooth, unbroken and elastic, grasping the finger when introduced, like a firm rubber ring. Cutting the hymen cured all the trouble, both of husband and wife.

DR. KELLY remarked that the condition of the hymen is a subject of much interest, about which many erroneous views prevail. It was by no means uniformly ruptured by coitus. In other cases coitus alone was as capable as numerous pregnancies of obliterating all traces of the hymen. He had made many observations and careful drawings of a number of cases, which showed a definite relation between a certain condition of the hymen and the severity of a preceding labor; that is, when the vaginal outlet has been broken down, with extensive laceration, the hymen remained *intact* except at the split posteriorly, being saved by the vaginal tear. On the contrary, the surest way of thoroughly destroying the integrity of the hymen is the equable, all-around dilatation of a *normal* labor. In a forceps case, examined some months after labor, the hymen, elsewhere intact, was as cleanly cut into halves as a lacerated cervix. It is unquestionably, as Budin has shown, the pointing terminus of the vaginal canal.

Dr. B. C. Hirst showed a specimen of

Endometritis Gravidarum Polyposa

from the University Museum. There are in the Museum two other examples of the same condition, one recently contributed by Dr. R. Deaver, of Germantown. In the last case the embryo was certainly not over three weeks old ; the ovum corresponded to the third month and had been retained in the uterus some six months after the death of the embryo. They are all very good specimens of a very rare disease.

He also showed a

Pregnant Uterus

removed from a woman with chronic nephritis, who died suddenly from apoplexy within three months of term. She had been blind for three weeks before her admission to the hospital, and was œdematous in face and extremities. As soon as his attention was called to the case, he ordered premature labor to be induced, but before this could be done the woman died. The uterus showed on abdominal palpation an apparent right lateral version. On opening the abdomen this was seen to be due to the attitude of the fœtus—vertex presentation, L. O. A. The uterine body extended equally to both sides of the median line, but had not the pyriform shape supposed to be characteristic of the pregnant organ. It was irregularly triangular in form, the base of the figure being to the right side, the apex to the left. This would give one the impression on abdominal palpation of right lateral version, from the fact that the highest point of the uterine fundus was to the right side ; but this point corresponded to that angle of the uterine cavity on which lay the trunk and extremities of the fœtus.

Dr. Hirst then read the following :

M. M., 39 years old, widow ; has had four children ; youngest six years old. Six weeks ago the patient attempted to lift a heavy weight, and was immediately seized with sharp pains in the left groin. This occurred just at the commencement of a menstrual flow, which was unusually profuse and painful. The bleeding had in fact continued until the present time (Nov. 8). On this day the woman came by a rather long horse-car journey to the Philadelphia Hospital, to visit her daughter, a patient in the wards ; in the hospital she was suddenly seized with great pain and sank to the ground from weakness. She was carried to the medical wards where an examination showed some form of pelvic or abdominal tumor. She was consequently transferred to the gynecological floor. A vaginal examination showed a mass of considerable extent to the left of the uterus, and apparently a cystic tumor in Douglas's pouch. Laparotomy was done the next morning. As soon as the peritoneum was cut through, a large quantity of dark-colored blood welled out of the opening. The incision was enlarged, the intestines turned out and wrapped in warm towels, a pint or more of blood sponged out, and a careful examination made by inspection and touch. The left broad ligament was distended by a tumor, made up, as far as he could tell, of clotted blood ; near the uterus there was a ragged opening into which he could put the tip of his little finger. During the half-hour the abdomen remained open there was no hemorrhage from this spot, and had evidently been none recently, for there was no fresh blood in the abdominal cavity. His diagnosis, naturally enough, was ruptured tubal pregnancy. As the embryo, if one existed, was too small to give future trouble, and would be absorbed, he simply cleaned the abdominal cavity, picked adherent clots off the intestines and closed the wound without drainage. The convalescence was entirely favorable. He has been inclined since to alter the diagnosis. The woman, on close questioning, absolutely denied the possibility of impregnation. This fact, together with the history of great muscular effort at the beginning of a menstrual period, and the subsequent behavior of the patient, would naturally suggest the possibility of a rupture of a blood-vessel in the broad ligament. The acute attack of pain and weakness two days before the operation might be explained by a rupture of the peritoneal covering of the effused blood, with an escape of clots and a fresh hemorrhage into the peritoneal cavity.

The following officers were then elected : *President*, Theophilus Parvin, M.D. ; *Vice Presidents*, W. H. H. Githens, M.D., and J. C. DaCosta, M.D. ; *Secretary*, J. M. Baldy, M.D. ; *Treasurer*, Alfred Whelen, M.D.

———◆●◆———

—A chemist named Halffpap, who practised medicine under cover of a fictitious American diploma, is said by the *Bulletin Medical*, Dec. 30, 1888, to have been sentenced to imprisonment for two years on the charge of homicide. It seems that he prescribed for an infant two months old, suffering with convulsions, one-sixth of a grain of morphine, to be repeated every two hours.

NEW YORK ACADEMY OF MEDICINE.

Meeting of January 3, 1889.

The President, A. JACOBI, M.D., in the Chair.

The annual reports of officers and committees were read, and an oil portrait of the late Dr. Samuel Purdy, was accepted with thanks. Dr. John C. Peters read a memorial of him.

. DR. MALCOLM McLEAN read a paper on

Intra-Uterine Cry after Expulsion of the Waters,

in response to the President's call for the narration of interesting cases. He stated that in August last he was asked to assist Dr. Tracy in delivering a woman at term. Dr. McLean had attended her in four previous normal confinements. On this occasion the occiput was in the posterior position, and while he was trying to rotate the head forward with his hand the nurse drew the patient into a hollow in the bed, whereupon the abdominal organs receded from the pelvis, air rushed into the vagina and uterus, and immediately the child began to cry. The crying continued while he rotated the head, applied the forceps, and extracted, or during about five minutes. It was somewhat remarkable that material was not insufflated, interfering with breathing. The case, he believed, was unique.

The following named members were elected to office: *President,* Dr. A. L. Loomis; *Vice-President,* Dr. D. B. St. John Roosa; *Recording Secretary,* Dr. A. M. Jacobus; *Corresponding Secretary,* Dr. M. A. Starr; *Treasurer,* Dr. O. B. Douglas; *Trustee,* Dr. A. Jacobi; *Treasurer for the Trustees,* Dr. F. A. Castle; *Member of Committee on Admissions,* Dr. Robert Abbe; *Member of Committee on Library,* Dr. E. S. Peck. Five delegates were elected to the State Medical Society.

Stated Meeting, January 17, 1889.

The President, A. JACOBI, M.D., in the Chair.

DR. PAUL GIBIER, of Paris, read a paper entitled: .

Yellow Fever; Experimental Researches on its Etiology,

in which he gave a *résumé* of his researches in Florida, instituted under the direction of the government of the French Republic. These experiments were a continuation of certain investigations into the etiology of yellow fever which he had formerly made and reported, once in a paper and again in a lecture, before the Academy of Medicine, Paris.

When he arrived in Jacksonville, Florida, the severity of the epidemic was diminishing. Yet a few cases which he had an opportunity to study and to make bacteriological observations upon were undoubtedly of yellow fever. In one instance especially the symptoms and the pathological lesions were distinctly those of yellow fever. The disease terminated fatally on the fourth day. The intestines contained a large quantity of black liquid, which was alkaline, while the contents of the stomach were acid. This fact is noticeable inasmuch as the bacterium to which he has ascribed the origin of typhoid fever existed only in the intestinal contents; acid fluids would destroy it. In this case, as in all others, this microbe was absent from the blood, liver, spleen, and kidneys. If this microbe is the cause of yellow fever, its absence from the intestines in some cases may be accounted for by the fact, which is well known, that when a culture medium becomes saturated with it its growth stops, and if then another bacterium is introduced it will displace the former. It is his intention, as soon as opportunity presents, to examine the dejecta in a number of cases from the beginning of the disease; and he would not be surprised, he said, if the microbe were present only during the first days of the disease. The theory which he has supported is that yellow fever is an intestinal disease, due to a microbe, and that it must be treated with disinfectants directed to the intestinal tract— such as bichloride of mercury, naphthalin, and tannic acid. The microbes are the origin of certain poisonous ptomaines which enter the circulation and give rise to certain symptoms.

DR. L. D. BULKLEY read a paper on

Unusual Methods of Acquiring Syphilis, with Reports of Cases.

The subject, he said, is a vast one, and could not be fully covered in one paper. He called attention to a few of the innocent methods by which syphilis is acquired, methods which commonly are wholly unsuspected and unprovided against.

When non-venereal methods of acquiring the disease are generally recognized, its dangers will become more apparent and be better guarded against; syphilis will then also be oftener recognized by the patient and physician when there is no history of venereal exposure, and less stigma will be attached to it. As a result of this, syphilis will be placed where it belongs, among the infectious diseases, and will be placed under the care of health authorities who will aid in stamping out a malady which has caused untold misery both to those guilty and those innocent of sexual transgression.

The relative frequency of the different modes of acquiring the affection is not generally appreciated. Literature contains accounts of dozens of epidemics during which thousands have acquired the disease. There are also reports of cases in which thousands have been infected with the disease in ways hardly suspected before. Fournier has recently declared, from a study of his cases, that in about twenty-five per cent. of all cases of syphilis in females the disease is innocently acquired, and during the discussion of his paper Ricord stated that his experience fully corroborated Fournier's statement.

Dr. Bulkley stated that in looking over the more or less complete records of his cases, numbering something more than 1500, he had found that the larger proportion came under care after the primary sore had disappeared, and in a large number there was no account of the primary lesion or character of the infection. Yet among the 1500 cases notes of extra-genital chancre occurred in 65 instances, or in four and three-tenths per cent. In most of these instances the disease had been acquired in an innocent manner. Thirty-four of the 65 cases were in males and 31 in females. The disease occurred in females in one-third of the whole number of his cases and of these cases it was hereditary in ten per cent. ; in the larger share of the rest of the cases the disease seemed to have been acquired in an innocent and unsuspected manner. It was safe to say that in forty per cent. of his cases seen in private practice syphilis had been acquired innocently and undeservedly.

Of his 65 cases of extra-genital chancre, the location of the chancre was on the lip in 30, on the finger in 7, on the breast in 6, on the tonsil in 5, on the tongue in 5, on the cheek in 3, on the chin in 2, on the eyelid in 2, on the nose, ear, hand, forearm, and sacral region in one each.

The unusual methods of acquiring syphilis, or those other than by venereal contact, he classed under three grand groups, which permitted again of numerous subdivisions.

The first was syphilis economica, in which, in the ordinary economic or domestic relations, the disease was transmitted innocently. Second, syphilis blephatrophica, in which the disease was acquired by or through infants. Third, syphilis technica, in which it came from body service.

He subdivided syphilis economica into three sub-groups : syphilis by domestic, industrial, and personal transmission. Of domestic transmission, that by means of spoons, forks, knives, jugs, tobacco pipes, is familiar. The author recited one case in his own practice of transmission through the tobacco pipe. Other methods are through wearing apparel, such as shirts and pantaloons. He cited an interesting case in which the chancre was contracted in the sacral region by the wearing of a public bathing suit.

Beds, toilet articles, sponges, toothbrushes, etc., have transmitted the disease. In one of his cases it seemed altogether probable that chancre of the tongue had been caused by pins, which the girl was in the habit of putting into one side of the mouth. It is rather remarkable, he said, that he had failed to find a single authenticated instance of syphilis being acquired in public urinals. Under industrial transmission, he stated that numerous cases had been recorded in which the disease was transmitted through common use of a glassblower. Not a case had been found in which the disease was attributed to handling paper money. It is commonly supposed laundresses frequently acquire the disease in washing soiled linen of syphilitics, but this mode of transmission has not been proved.

Personal transmission is common, and next to the venereal act, kissing is probably the most common mode of communicating the disease. Dr. Bulkley cited one case in which a man transmitted the disease by kissing the lady to whom he was engaged, and this was the cause of breaking of the engagement ; the man soon married another girl, and she acquired the disease in the same manner, that is, by kissing. In one instance a lady gave the disease to a lady friend by kissing.

Many cases have been recorded of transmission of syphilis through nursing and attendance on infants. An instance is recorded in which over forty women and children were infected from one syphilitic child. Individual instances are still common. Of his own 65 cases of extra-genital chancre, 6 were on the breast. Children sometimes infect attendants and attendants sometimes infect children.

The third great branch, syphilis technica, includes cases in which the operator is the victim ; cases in which he, not having the disease, is yet the means of conveying the poison to others, and also includes those in which he is the direct medium. The author cites one instance in which the surgeon acquired a chancre on the finger, and then, notwithstanding his precautions, conveyed syphilis to his wife. There are cases in which, during an examination, the surgeon has got the virus upon the uninjured finger, then scratched the eyelid or other portion of the face, and there a chancre has developed. More than one instance has been recorded in which the patient has projected the virus while coughing, and thus infected the medical attendant. There are a number of instances of syphilis being conveyed to the eye by quacks attempting to remove a foreign body from the eye with the tongue. One of Dr. Bulkley's cases came from tattooing. Cases in which the physician has been the medium of infection were seen in syphilis contracted from vaccination, during ritual circumcision, wetcupping, ordinary surgical operations, in dentistry, etc.

The question of prevention of syphilis is one which should receive the best attention of physicians and of the community.

DR. S. W. HUBBARD cited a case in which an infant acquired syphilis from the nurse when the latter had no lesion on the body, and he expressed the belief that the disease was transmitted through the milk.

DR. BULKLEY, being asked if he thought milk could transmit syphilis, expressed himself in the negative.

THE PRESIDENT remarked that milk from the healthy mother is a seeretion, composed mostly of transformed epithelium, while that from one in reduced health is a transudation, composed largely of blood serum and the poisons of the blood which it may carry, and hence it is capable of transmitting syphilis.

—The Empress Augusta has offered, in connection with the German Society of the Red Cross, a prize of $2,500 for the best portable military hospital. The award will be made at an exhibition to be held in Berlin, in June. Prizes will also be given for the best collection of medicines or surgical instruments. All countries are invited to exhibit.

PERISCOPE.

A Few Points in Macewen's Operation for Radical Cure of Hernia.

In a paper on this subject in the *Boston Med. and Surg. Journal,* Dec. 6, 1888, Dr. Herbert L. Burrell says that the indications which have governed him in advising the operation have been the existence of hernia uncontrollable by truss, or rendered painful by truss, or, as in one case, coincident mental depression. In discussing the technique of the operation, he takes it up in sections. He then speaks as follows :

1. The finding of the sac. In performing this operation, the strictest of antiseptic precautions have been attempted, but unfortunately have not always been successfully carried out. The patient having been thoroughly anæsthetized, an incision of two or two and a half inches has been made directly over the external abdominal ring, great care being exercised to bring the incision directly over the middle of the lozenge-shaped opening and running in its direction. Then I have carefully avoided attempting to isolate the different layers which are ordinarily distinguished as covering a hernia. This I have done by having an assistant take a pair of anatomical dissecting forceps, and I have taken another, and then deliberately we have carefully divided every structure for the whole length of the incision that we have met, the assistant carefully grasping the new structure to be divided in the very depth of the incision, and I grasping the tissue directly opposite to him, and then between the two forceps I have divided the elevated layer of tissue. In this way I go on until I meet a rather thick white layer, which on being divided shows that I have entered a cavity, when I know that the sac has been reached. I never attempt to isolate the sac without opening it, for the recognition of the cavity of the sac is its distinguishing point. Therefore the whole attention of the surgeon should be devoted, from the time that he makes the primary incision in the skin, to the finding of the sac. By this means I feel that I have been enabled to save time.

If I cannot readily distinguish the sac, I allow the patient partially to recover from the ether, and very quickly the sac is distended.

2. The isolation of the sac. When I recognize that I am in the sac, from this time on I prepare it for restoration to the abdominal cavity. Should I find it adher-

ent, as so commonly occurs, I fill the sac, through the small opening that I have made in it, with iodoform gauze, distending it, in the same fashion that a mending-ball does the heel of a stocking. Having accomplished this, there is not the slightest difficulty in dissecting out, with the point of a knife or the handle of a scalpel, the distended sac, and separating it from the cord and its accompanying vessels.

When, however, the sac is filled with omentum, implanted directly on and about the testicle, as it was in one of the congenital cases operated upon, one has a difficult, tedious dissection before him to separate it carefully from the testicle and return it to the peritoneal cavity. Occasionally I have had to divide the omentum into various parts and return the carefully secured ends to the peritoneal cavity.

When one has a congenital hernia to deal with, the simplest way, after carefully exposing the sac, is to fill the processus vaginalis with the "iodoform gauze darning-ball," and then to divide the sac into two parts, forming a distinct tunica vaginalis for the testicle, and then sewing up the proximal part of the sac and returning it to the abdominal cavity.

3. The troublesome hemorrhage and the manipulation of the tissues. In the first few cases that I did I had considerable difficulty in identifying the sac, and hence I had once a troublesome hemorrhage from the vessels that accompany the cord. Further, in pulling on the different structures to make them out, I did an amount of damage to their vitality which should be avoided. In two of the cases I feel quite sure that the manipulation of the tissues, especially the dragging of the testicle out of the scrotum, had much to do with the formation of scrotal abscesses. This I believe can be avoided by the "darning-ball of iodoform gauze."

4. The introduction of the sutures. I can only say that I have tried almost all of the different patterns and forms of needles, and have found that I could place the stitches more accurately, and this is really one of the most important points in the whole operation, by a Hagedorn needle in a good needle-holder. I have, after carefully separating the sac the whole length of the inguinal canal and for a half an inch around the intra-abdominal surface of the internal ring, placed a stitch in the very extremity of the sac and transfixed it through and through, and brought it out, after traversing the inguinal canal, through the muscles of the abdomen, pulling up the sac inside the abdomen; the suture pulling up the sac in the same way that a Venetian blind is raised. This suture is not fastened in position until the end of the operation, its protruding extremity being caught in position on the abdominal muscles by a pair of pressure forceps. Then I carefully attempt to restore the valve-like form of the inguinal canal by stitching the conjoined tendon with strong silk or stout catgut to the aponeurotic structures of the transversalis, internal and external oblique. I usually place two, if not three, sutures in position, and as I tie them, have the assistant introduce his finger in the canal, and he can then determine how tightly I bring the parts together, and I run no danger of cutting off the circulation in the cord.

5. Dressing. I always consider that the point where the operation proper is finished and the dressing begins is when I have tied the last suture which closes the inguinal canal. Of course, strictly speaking, this is not the case, but it serves to emphasize the importance of the foregoing procedures.

I have in the last cases closed the opening completely, and have not used any drainage-tube; of course this means that I have had to take a great deal of time in carefully rendering the wound perfectly free from fluids. A thorough and effective flushing at the end of the operation of the whole surface of the wound with 1-1000 corrosive sublimate is, I believe, of the greatest importance. The wound is superficially closed with a continuous catgut suture. The dressing proper is applied as follows: six sterilized gauze pads 6x8x½ are superimposed, covering the wound surface and the scroto-femoral cleft; this is held in place by a carefully applied gauze bandage four inches in width, just enough being used to steady the dressing in place. Over this is laid a piece of Macintosh, with a hole in it large enough for the penis to protrude; then this is covered in by sterilized sheet-wadding.

This is secured in position by a cravat gauze bandage six inches in width and long enough to form a double spica bandage. Over this is placed another piece of Macintosh, with a hole in it for the penis, and this is secured in position by two safety pins placed on either side of the penis and at various other points on the abdomen and thighs as may be found necessary.

6. The question of the necessity of a truss. There can be but little doubt that

the wearing of an ordinary truss after a hernia operation is open to the objection that pressure on cicatricial tissue is usually followed by gradual absorption. I have never felt quite safe in recommending the entire neglect of a truss in the after treatment of this operation, and have therefore been led to use a worsted truss in much the same way that is recommended by Pye. This does not exert any undue pressure on the cicatricial tissue.

These are a few of the points that I have found of interest in performing the operation, and I can only say that they have been derived not alone from my own experience, but from that of my colleagues.

Relation of Acetonuria to Diabetic Coma.

Before the Royal Medical and Chirurgical Society of London, Nov. 27, 1888, Dr. Samuel West read a paper on acetonuria and its relation to diabetic coma, of which the following is an abstract. The relation of acetonuria to diabetic coma had been investigated by experiment and by clinical observation, and this paper was a contribution to the clinical side of the problem. The results of experiment were briefly referred to, and the conclusion to which they led. Clinical observation was for a long time difficult from the want of trustworthy tests. A short account of the chief ones was given: 1. Lieben's iodoform test. 2. Gunning's and Le Nobel's modification of it. 3. Reynolds' test. 4. Legal's test with nitro-prusside of potassium. 5. Le Nobel's modification of it. 6. Penzold's test. Legal's test was found to be the most convenient for use in the urine direct, and Lieben's in the distillate, but this reaction was also obtained if alcohol was present. But if the urine gave Legal's, and the distillate both Legal's and Lieben's tests, the presence of acetone might be accepted. As control experiments two series of convalescent cases were examined. In the first thirty cases, a doubtful Legal's reaction was obtained in three. In the only urine which was distilled neither test was obtained in the distillate. In the second series of about the same number no evidence of acetone was obtained in any. Of non-diabetic patients actually suffering from illnesses at the time of examination, acetone was found in fifteen cases. Acetonuria is therefore very rare in healthy or convalescent persons, but common in various forms of acute and chronic disease. Of diabetic patients fourteen were examined, four being at the time

comatose. In some of these cases the examination was continued for many days. The following conclusions were arrived at: 1. Acetonuria is common in diabetics without coma. 2. It is not constantly present in cases of diabetic coma. 3. It varies greatly in the same case from time to time without definite cause. 4. It varies independently of variations in the amount of sugar, specific gravity, etc. 5. It may even disappear when coma develops. The iron reaction shows also no relation either to coma or to acetone. Experiment and clinical observation therefore lead to the same conclusion, viz., that acetone can not be the cause of diabetic coma. Clinical observation, however, seems to show that acetonuria has a clinical value as indicating that the patient is in a more critical condition than when it is absent. The symptoms of diabetic coma depend, in all probability, upon acute intoxication by some substance rapidly generated within the body, but at present unknown. It may be that in the perverted chemical processes which develop it, acetone and the allied body giving the iron reaction are produced, so that the presence of these bodies in the urine may serve as "danger signals."

Dr. Maguire said that acetone is evidently not the poison which produces diabetic coma; nevertheless, the condition is undoubtedly due to the presence of a poison. The liver either may split it up or the kidneys eliminate it, so that, although it may be found in the blood, serious symptoms may not develop. He looks upon the presence of albuminuria as a valuable danger signal when occurring in the course of diabetic coma, its presence being probably due to renal irritation. In every case he has examined, the kidneys have presented extreme parenchymatous inflammation, and such a condition can be brought about by the injection of diacetic ether or acetone into the blood. He thinks that, if albumin is found after acetone has been ascertained to be present, the case is graver than if acetone is found alone.

Dr. Angel Money has on two occasions found hyaline necrosis in the kidneys from cases of diabetic coma. The iron reaction is a sign of danger, and he has never failed to find it when the knee jerk is absent. Albumin is generally present in fatal cases.

Dr. West replied that albumin, like acetone, is by no means a constant phenomenon in fatal cases, and therefore may or may not be a "danger signal."—*Lancet*, Dec. 1, 1888.

The Removal of Hook-Shaped Foreign Bodies.

One of the most acute of American physicians, Dr. Morrill Wyman, of Cambridge, Massachusetts, is reputed to have once relieved a small boy of a fish-hook that he had swallowed by the clever device of slipping a perforated bullet over the line, which fortunately was hanging from the boy's mouth, causing him to swallow the bullet, and then drawing upon the line, the bullet guarding the tissues against injury from the hook during the process of extraction. But the small boy, owing doubtless to the special Providence that watches over him, rarely feeds on fish-hooks, so that Dr. Wyman's expedient, ingenious as it was, is more likely to be handed down in anecdote than to serve as a precedent in actual practice. Most of us are not in pressing need of a device for removing fish-hooks from the stomach—not so much, indeed, as of a trick for enticing hairpins from the urethra —but it happens now and then to almost every practitioner to find himself face to face with the task of disengaging some hook-shaped body that has become imbedded in the tissues. In such a case M. Le Fort, of the Necker Hospital, Paris, lately made use of a procedure which we find detailed in a clinical lecture published in the *Union Médicale* for October 18. The manipulation, however complicated it may seem at first thought when described as *par version*, *bascule et propulsion* was really very simple. Undoubtedly it has been resorted to by many practitioners, for it would suggest itself at once to a man of ordinary ingenuity; but, as we do not remember to have seen it described in print, we think it may prove of interest to our readers.

The patient was a lad who, nine months before his admission into the hospital, had been struck upon the cheek by a person who held a button-hook in the hand with which the blow was given. The pain of the blow was very great, and the lad at once perceived that the person who had struck him now held only the handle of the button-hook. There was a punctured wound of the cheek, from which a free flow of blood took place, situated in front of the masseter muscle and at the level of the lower teeth. An hour afterward there was considerable swelling of the cheek, and on the following morning, the swelling being persistent and accompanied with rather sharp pain, a pharmacist was consulted, who, as the patient said, "corked up the hole in his cheek." At the end of two or three days the wound had healed and the swelling had subsided, but there was some induration perceptible to the patient, who, however, felt no further pain and no embarrassment of the movements of the jaw. This quiescent state of things continued until about a month before the lad's admission into the hospital, when an inflammatory redness appeared at the site of the wound, and an opening formed from which a little shaft of iron protruded to the extent of about a third of an inch. The hooked extremity was directed backward, and was so engaged in the masseter muscle as not to admit of removal by direct traction without great risk of serious injury. Having enlarged the opening by a slight cut, M. Le Fort depressed the presenting end of the piece of iron and gradually worked it backward until he had reversed its original position. The hooked end now lay forward, and was easily made to emerge from the wound. Reference was made also to a somewhat similar case in which, some years before, M. Le Fort had extracted from a lady's hand a hook-shaped English implement for drawing corks.—*N. Y. Medical Journal*, Dec. 22, 1888.

Abscess of both Testicles Consequent on Urethral and Prostatic Irritation.

Mr. J. Newton Burns reports a case of abscess of both testicles consequent on urethral and prostatic irritation, in the *British Med. Journal*, Nov. 3, 1888. As abscess of the testicle, except in connection with tubercular or scrofulous disease, seems to be rare, he thinks the following notes of abscess of both testicles may be of interest.

Until a week before Mr. Burns saw him, the patient, a hale man 72 years old, had not suffered from any disorder of the genitourinary apparatus. During that week he had frequency of micturition, and was found by Mr. Burns with bladder distended above the umbilicus. Examination *per rectum* revealed an enlarged and tender prostate. A prostatic catheter was passed with difficulty, and the bladder emptied of over two quarts of smoky urine, mixed toward the end with bright blood and mucus. Catheterization was continued for several days. When the prostatic region became less tender and swollen, and it became possible to pass the ordinary rubber catheter, this was regularly used night and morning by the patient himself. All vesical irritation ceased after washings out with antiseptics, and the patient soon regained health and strength, though he still continued the use of the rubber catheter.

About a month after Mr. Burns's first visit he received an urgent call, and found the patient in great agony, with his left testicle very much swollen, hot, and tender in the region of the epididymis. At first the enlarged testicle could be distinctly felt at the bottom of the scrotum, but it gradually became indistinguishable from the surrounding infiltrated tissues. The exudation into the skin and tissues overlying the testicle rapidly increased, and in about twenty-four hours the testicle measured twenty inches in circumference.

The usual treatment soon alleviated his distress, and in a few days the measurement was reduced to sixteen and then to twelve inches. Signs of abscess having developed, a free incision was made, and about four drachms of pus and black blood were evacuated. The cavity was then irrigated with water containing a few drops of liniment of iodine, and healed in about ten days. Six weeks later Mr. Burns treated by the same means a similar affection of his right testicle, which, as in the former instance, got well. Both testicles returned to their normal size.

Hill-Climbing for Heart-Disease.

At the seventh Congress for Internal Medicine, held this year at Wiesbaden, an animated discussion took place on Oertel's treatment of chronic diseases of the heart by diet and exercise. Briefly stated, Oertel's aim is to strengthen the heart-muscle by a course of heart-athletics—*e. g.*, hill-climbing, the steepness of the paths being carefully graduated to suit the condition of the patients. In addition, he endeavors to lighten the work of the heart by limiting the amount of fluids supplied to the system and promoting their elimination. He puts great stress on the amelioration of the watery condition of the blood as being an important item in the treatment. In compensatory hypertrophy and dilatation, in acute diseases of the heart-muscle following on sclerosis of the coronary arteries or hæmorrhagic infarct, in myomalacia, and in cases of aneurysm of the heart, the "dietetic-mechanic" method is contra-indicated. In conclusion, Oertel gives the result of three years of his method at Meran, Ischl, Reichenhall, Liebenstein, Abbazia, Baden-Baden, Kreuth, and Wildbad. These results are necessarily valuable, independently of all theories, and are as follows: 1. In cases of fatty heart in elderly people, where there is no perceptible sclerosis of the coronary arteries, and where there is serous plethora, turgid veins, and frequently œdema, the results have been decidedly favorable. 2. Re-establishment of lost compensation and compensatory hypertrophy in valvular lesions, and in impediments of the pulmonary circulation due to diseases of the spinal column. 3. Recovery of the heart-muscle from extensive dilatation (in so far as non-compensatory) following weakness of the heart-muscle, and when caused by heightened intra-cardial blood-pressure due to valve lesions. 4. The best possible balance restored between the arterial and venous systems, decrease of the cyanosis, of the plethora of serum, and of the watery and even œdematous condition of the tissues. 5. Abatement and complete disappearance of the respiratory disturbances.—*Medical Chronicle*, Sept., 1888.

Fœtal Blood at Birth.

Dr. Scherenziss, of Dorpat, has published some interesting observations on the condition of the blood at birth. The specific gravity is, he finds, markedly lower than that of the blood in the adult. The hæmoglobin is also much less than in adult blood, the proportion being 76.8 to 100. The amount of fibrin is only about two-sevenths of that in the blood of the mother. Fœtal blood cannot be analyzed quantitatively by washing with saline solutions, a large part of the constituents of the corpuscles which appear to be in a very loose state of combination, especially the hæmoglobin, going over in the filtrate. Fœtal blood is richer in saline matters than the blood of adults, especially in insoluble salts. The sodium salts are somewhat greater in amount than in the blood of adults, but the potassium salts decidedly less. The sex and the weight of the child appear to have no influence on the quantitative constitution of the blood at birth.—*Lancet*, Nov. 24, 1888.

Frequency of Cancer of the Larynx.

B. Grimme (Inaugural Dissertation, Munich, 1888) states that he has found 15 cases of cancer of the larynx in a total of 13,517 autopsies, a percentage of .11; or, deducting two doubtful cases, .09 per cent. Seven of these fifteen cases were primary, seven secondary, and one doubtful. Epithelial cancer preponderated. The male sex was most frequently affected, in the ages from 40 to 49 and 60 to 69.—*Schmidt's Jahrbücher*, Nov. 15, 1888.

THE
MEDICAL AND SURGICAL
REPORTER.

ISSUED EVERY SATURDAY.

CHARLES W. DULLES, M.D.,
EDITOR AND PUBLISHER.

The Terms of Subscription to the serial publications of this office are as follows, payable in advance:

Med. and Surg. Reporter (weekly), a year, **$5.00**
Quarterly Compendium of Med. Science, - 2.50
Reporter and Compendium, - - - - 6.00
Physician's Daily Pocket Record, - - - 1.00
Reporter and Pocket Record. - - - 6.00
Reporter, Compendium, and Pocket Record, 7.00

All checks and postal orders should be drawn to order of

CHARLES W. DULLES,
N. E. Cor. 13th and Walnut Streets,
P. O. Box 843.   Philadelphia, Pa.

☛SUGGESTIONS TO SUBSCRIBERS:
See that your address-label gives the date to which your subscription is paid.
In requesting a change of address, give the old address as well as the new one.
If your REPORTER does not reach you promptly and regularly, notify the publisher *at once*, so that the cause may be discovered and corrected.

☛SUGGESTIONS TO CONTRIBUTORS AND CORRESPONDENTS:
Write in ink.
Write on one side of paper only.
Write on paper of the size usually used for letters.
Make as few paragraphs as possible. Punctuate carefully. Do not abbreviate, or omit words like "the," and "a," or "an."
Make communications as short as possible.
NEVER ROLL A MANUSCRIPT! Try to get an envelope or wrapper which will fit it.
When it is desired to call our attention to something in a newspaper, mark the passage boldly with a colored pencil, and write on the wrapper "Marked copy." Unless this is done, newspapers are not looked at.
The Editor will be glad to get medical news, but it is important that brevity and actual interest shall characterize communications intended for publication.

STATE BOARD OF MEDICAL EXAMINERS.

Probably no single movement of medical progress in our country, within the last decade, has been so marked as the steps taken by several of our States in regard to the requisitions for practising medicine within their boundaries. It is somewhat remarkable that this reform should have commenced, not where one would most naturally have looked for it—in Pennsylvania, New York, or Massachusetts, the old centres of medical instruction—but in some of the more youthful and vigorous members of the Union—Illinois, Ohio, Minnesota, California, and others. These States have set a good example in the legislative enactments which they have made to regulate the practice of the healing art.

For years we have been impressed with the importance of a change in the general methods of licensing practitioners of medicine in this country, simply upon the guarantee afforded by the possession of a *diploma.* Along with many others, we have realized the utter inadequacy of such a certificate. To put the matter in its most favorable light, suppose the diploma to be issued from one of the first-class schools in the land, one where scrupulous care is exercised in the admission of matriculates, where a three years' graded course is required, and where the branches taught even exceed the traditional "seven," is it not a matter of common observation that a student may manage to pass his final examination, and obtain his diploma without any real, practical understanding of his professional duties? If this is true of our best schools, how much worse is the case in those which do not deserve this designation?

As already intimated, we have long been in favor of having a State Board of Examiners to determine the proficiency of the students of the different medical schools of the State, before conferring on them the right to practise medicine. In other words, transferring the licensing power from the professors or instructors in medical schools to an entirely independent Board of qualified and experienced practitioners of medicine.

An obstacle to this plan, often cited, is the difficulty of an amicable arrangement between the various schools of medicine, both as to the manner of appointing the Board of Examiners, and as to the examination of candidates. This difficulty is a very real one and requires wisdom and discretion in dealing with it. Just here, there are certain established principles not to be lost sight of. The law places all medical systems as on a perfect equality, and it cannot be expected to make any distinction between the graduates of a regular college and those of the homœopathic medical schools. To attempt to exclude candidates from any of the latter from the privileges of examination for a license to practise when their schools are recognized by the very State which creates the Board of Examiners would be unreasonable. The only feasible plan would be to open the examination freely to all who may wish to apply, with the understanding that the subjects for examination would include those taught in the most advanced regular schools.

This is essentially the plan pursued by the Army and Navy Boards. The point to be ascertained is whether the candidates can satisfactorily answer the questions propounded to them by the Board.

A Bill on this subject is now before the Legislature of Pennsylvania. As may be supposed, it has its warm advocates and its strong opponents. But from the powerful testimony brought from those States that have adopted the plan of State Examining Boards as to the uniform good results produced by their operation, both in diminishing the number of incompetent practitioners in the State and in elevating the standard of medicine, we have little doubt of the feasibility of the Act contemplated for our own State, and we hope for its speedy adoption.

TREATMENT OF DIPHTHERIA.

The treatment of diphtheria presents one of the most serious problems which confront the medical man. For years the methods in vogue have been of the most heroic sort ; forcible removal of the membrane, active cauterization, and the administration of drugs often most repugnant to the palate and sometimes dangerous to life. Of late there has been a growing tendency to adopt the teaching of Oertel that violent local treatment is useless and dangerous, and less confidence is placed in the virtues of chlorate of potash. Mild local applications like that of lime water or solutions of papayotin have to a great extent taken the place of nitrate of silver and mineral acids, which were once regarded as almost indispensable.

We have already, at different times, called attention in the REPORTER to methods of treating diphtheria which were free from the objections to which some of the older methods are open, and which have already proved of value under our own observation, or that of other practitioners. We now call attention to another which is exceedingly simple, and has proved useful elsewhere.

This method is strongly recommended by Dr. C. Lorey, of Frankfort-on-the-Main, in the *Deutsche med. Wochenschrift*, Nov. 15, 1888, and has been referred to at some length in the letter of our Berlin correspondent, in the REPORTER, Dec. 22, 1888. It consists in insufflation of finely powdered sugar. It is carried out with a tube preferably of glass—charged with pulverized sugar, and armed with a rubber ball, compression of which propels the sugar against the fauces.

Dr. Lorey has used this method in eighty cases, in patients both old and young, and in all forms and grades of the disease. In his hands it has brought about a notable shortening of the duration and limitation of the extent of the disease process, diminution of the foul odor, and loosening and removal of the membrane.

If such results can be obtained with an agent which is absolutely harmless, and by no means unpleasant, the fact deserves careful attention from medical men everywhere, and, in considering it, it is proper to note that Dr. Leroy advises accompanying the local treatment with the administration of a mixture containing from three-quarters of a grain to a grain and a half of apomorphia in three and a half fluid ounces of menstruum, of which a teaspoonful would contain about one-twentieth of a grain. When the acute stage is passed he gives tincture of the chloride of iron with glycerine.

ALEXANDER'S OPERATION.

Shortening the round ligaments, is one of the various methods of treating retroversion, retroflexion, and prolapse of the uterus. It was first done on the living subject by Alexander, and appears to the student both logical and based on correct anatomical principles. Its claim to validity, however, has been more vigorously assailed perhaps than that of any other operative procedure. Both those who deny the importance of versions and flexions, and those who maintain the importance of these displacements, alike contend that by the use of pessaries all needful aid can be rendered, and therefore they condemn the operation as unnecessary. Those who oppose operative procedures in general condemn this operation on account of its supposed dangers, and also, with considerable justice, because operators have sometimes failed to find and draw out the round ligaments. Others have opposed the method on the ground that the principles upon which it is based are wrong; that retroversion, retroflexion, and prolapse of the uterus depend primarily on relaxation of the utero-sacral ligaments, or on relaxation or laceration of the supporting segment of the pelvic floor, or on both; and therefore, since shortening the round ligaments cannot remedy any of these conditions, they assert that a permanent cure cannot be produced by Alexander's operation.

In a conservative and valuable paper read before the Medical Society of the County of New York, Oct. 22, 1888, and abstracted in the REPORTER, Nov. 10, Dr. Mundé discusses the status, indications, limitations, and technique of this operation, and reports his experience with it. He considers that the round ligaments can always be found and drawn out, and the uterus thereby anteverted and elevated, whenever the fundus uteri is not bound down by adhesions, and the ligaments possess their normal play in the inguinal canal.

The principal field for Alexander's operation is in the cure of long-standing cases of retroversion or retroflexion of the uterus, especially when the displacement is associated with descensus, or actual prolapse, of that organ and more or less protrusion of the vaginal walls, together with the bladder and rectum; in other words, when the pelvic floor is either injured or relaxed beyond non-operative restoration. It is taken for granted that treatment by pessaries has been tried and has failed. Alexander's operation is not indicated in cases of backward displacement, or descensus of the womb of moderate degree, as these are comfortably managed by vaginal supporters; adhesions of the uterus absolutely contraindicate the operation. The free, even excessive, mobility of the uterus is considered the one condition justifying it.

If the pelvic floor is intact and the displacement is merely a retroversion or retroflexion with but slight descensus, Dr. Mundé says his experience entitles him to state that the operation of shortening the round ligaments is sufficient to bring about a cure. If the operation is a success, the suspension of the uterus is permanent. When, however, the perineum is destroyed, or the pelvic floor injured or so relaxed as to give no support to the vaginal walls—which in consequence prolapse and drag down the uterus —or when there is complete prolapse of the uterus and vagina, it is necessary to supplement Alexander's operation by an operation to narrow the vagina, and restore the perineum. Under these conditions it seems like trifling with the operation to employ it alone.

Dr. Mundé reports twenty-three operations, of which nineteen were successful; in two, the ligaments were not found, and in two they were both torn off. The nineteen cases remained under observation for periods varying from three months to three and one-half years, and in all but one of these cases the uterus was retained absolutely in the position it occupied at the conclusion of the operation. In one case the fundus dropped slightly backward, but the elevation of the whole organ was maintained, and the operation was a success. The danger of Alexander's operation is regarded by Dr. Mundé as practically *nil*, if proper antisepsis is maintained.

This paper of Dr. Mundé's is a timely one, pointing out as it does the true field of usefulness for Alexander's operation, a field which is occupied neither by vaginal pessaries, by plastic operations on the vagina and perineum, nor by the newer operation of hysterorrhaphy, or ventro-fixation of the uterus.

PHTHISIS AS A NEUROSIS.

It is somewhat remarkable to find an earnest and industrious student of phthisis, at the present day advocating a theory in regard to its nature which almost entirely—if not quite—ignores the bacillus tuberculosis. We say "almost entirely" because, as we understand Dr. Mays's lectures on Pulmonary Consumption considered as a Neurosis, which were published in the *Therapeutic Gazette*, November 15 and December 15, 1888, he discusses more especially that form of phthisis which begins with a catarrhal inflammation in the alveoli of the lungs, and describes lesions which some students of the subject would say were not really tubercular. We say "if not quite," because we believe he has little faith in the etiological *rôle* very generally attributed by pathologists to the tubercle bacillus, and because his lectures make no distinction between the kind of phthisis to which he refers and any kind in which this bacillus is found.

The substance of his argument is that certain unquestionable neuroses are found associated with phthisis, or alternating with its exacerbations. He describes a number of cases, the histories of which he has collated, which seem to support his view, and claims that it is supported by a study of the nervous element to be found in the fatigue, the aphonia, the dyspnœa, the sweating, the anorexia, the diarrhœa, the hæmoptysis, the œdema and the thoracic pain of phthisis. His conclusion is that a proper interpretation of all the facts shows that pulmonary consumption is a peripheral disease, connected with a depreciation of the whole nervous system caused by a central lesion. He thinks that it is possible for a neurosis of the pneumogastric nerve to give rise to all the lesions generally found in phthisical lungs, although this may not be demonstrable by experiment.

The nearest analogue to the *rationale* of phthisis which he presents, is found, he says, in herpes zoster, in which a neurosis is accompanied by manifestations on the surface, which are characterized by an inflammatory process and destructive lesions.

This theory of phthisis is too startling to be accepted at once; and yet there may be more in it than appears at first sight. It is certainly ingenious, and deserves careful consideration. To our mind the argument of Dr. Mays, while interesting, is by no means conclusive. There can be no question that the nervous system suffers very seriously in phthisis, and that some of its phenomena—such as sweating—are plainly of a neurotic character; but to attribute all of its phenomena to a central nervous disturbance seems to us a step by no means warranted by the evidence adduced.

It is to be hoped that others, who have made consumption the subject of special study, will take up the theory proposed by Dr. Mays, and test it by their own observations; so that, if correct, it may receive the stamp of their approval; and, if incorrect, it may be clearly disproved.

A BILL TO INCREASE the salary of the Surgeon General of the Marine-Hospital service from $4,000 to $5,500 has been introduced into Congress by Senator Cullom. This increase would make the salary equal to that received by the Surgeon General of the army. As the present incumbent of the office of Surgeon General of the Marine-Hospital Service has just entered upon the office of editor of the *Journal of the Amer. Med. Association*, which has heretofore carried with it a salary of $6,000, the bill referred to, if it should become a law, will make his income a very good one.

THE CASE OF DRS. McCOY AND WILDMAN.—Drs. McCoy and Wildman, who are practising medicine in Philadelphia and advertising extensively in the daily papers, were formerly located in Chicago, where their certificates were revoked for alleged unprofessional conduct by the Illinois State Board of Health. It seems that Dr. McCoy appealed to the Supreme Court against the decision of the Board, and swore that he had never been served with a notice to appear before the Board, and that, therefore, the revocation of his certificate was illegal. The Court, in the absence of sufficient evidence of service, decided in favor of McCoy. As Wildman's certificate was revoked because of his association with McCoy, the Governor under the circumstances was obliged to reverse the decision of the Board. The Chicago *Medical Standard*, Jan., 1889, says that in the case now pending before the Supreme Court there is reason to believe that a real and not a pseudo-McCoy has been served, and that the glowing miraculous "cures" reported by hypochondriacs will disappear from the advertising pages of the great dailies.

—D. M. Burgess, Sanitary Inspector Marine-Hospital Service, reports to Surgeon-General Hamilton, under date of Jan. 2, that there were 571 deaths in Havana, Cuba, during the month of December. Twenty-six of the deaths are reported to have been caused by yellow fever, 26 by pernicious fever, 1 by paludal fever, 7 by typhoid fever, 2 by small-pox, 1 by diphtheria, 2 by croup, and 3 by glanders. Twenty-six dying of pernicious fever, while during the same time only one died of any other form of paludal fever, leads to the suspicion that pernicious symptoms due to yellow fever may have been confounded with those produced by malarial poison.

BOOK REVIEWS.

[Any book reviewed in these columns may be obtained upon receipt of price, from the office of the REPORTER.]

BASHORE'S IMPROVED CLINICAL CHART OF TEMPERATURE, PULSE AND RESPIRATION, DESIGNED FOR DAILY RECORDING OF CASES IN HOSPITAL AND PRIVATE PRACTICE. BY HARVEY B. BASHORE, M.D. 50 charts, in tablet form. Size, 8 by 12 inches. Price, 50 cents net. Sold by F. A. Davis, Philadelphia.

These charts are arranged so that the variations in the Temperature, the Pulse, and the Respiration are recorded in spaces provided as in most "temperature sheets." The specimens sent us are not in tablet form; but are detached sheets. Each sheet contains spaces for three weeks' time. They are fairly well printed, but would be more desirable if better paper were used.

QUESTIONS AND ANSWERS ON THE ESSENTIALS OF ANATOMY. BY CHARLES B. NANCREDE, M.D., Senior Surgeon to Episcopal Hospital, etc. With 117 illustrations. Small 8vo, pp. 352. Philadelphia: W. B. Saunders, 1888. Price, $1.00.

This volume of "Saunders' Question Compends" is the largest of the series, and one of the most important. Its bulk is partly due to the space occupied by the questions; but principally to the fullness with which the author has treated his subject. It is quite a complete treatise on anatomy, and its descriptions are clear and distinct. Its illustrations are chiefly made from plates used in the first edition of Leidy's Anatomy, and show the marks of use. The printing and binding are good, and the book, as a whole, is creditable to both author and publisher.

QUESTIONS AND ANSWERS ON THE ESSENTIALS OF OBSTETRICS. PREPARED ESPECIALLY FOR STUDENTS OF MEDICINE. BY WILLIAM EASTERLY ASHTON, M.D., Demonstrator of Clinical Obstetrics in the Jefferson Medical College, etc. 8vo, pp. xi, 220, with Illustrations. Philadelphia: W. B. Saunders, 1888. Price, $1.00.

The "Essentials of Obstetrics" is the fifth in the series of question compends issued by the same publisher. These compends are intended to be an aid to the student in preparing for examination. Dr. Ashton has written a book which is well adapted to this end; the subject matter is given in clear concise English, and is unusually free from errors of statement, and typographical errors. He has undoubted authority for the principles and practice advocated, but he has not selected his "authority" wisely in all instances. The chief fault of books of this kind is that they give an incomplete representation of the subject. Although Dr. Ashton has not entirely escaped errors of omission, he has done unusually well. As examples of incomplete statement, we note the subjects of the perineum, and Hegar's sign of pregnancy. No one could gain a proper conception of the anatomy and functions of the perineum, or of the technique of Hegar's sign from this book. Also under the head of puerperal septicæmia no mention is made of fevers caused by the absorption of the products of putrefaction within the birth-canal—a large and important class. With some slight exceptions there is only good to be said of this compend as an aid to students preparing for examination.

PAMPHLET NOTICES.

[Any reader of the REPORTER who desires a copy of a pamphlet noticed in these columns will doubtless secure it by addressing the author with a request stating where the notice was seen and *enclosing a postage-stamp*.]

189. THE TREATMENT OF THE FINAL STAGE OF PHTHISIS. BY J. H. MUSSER, M.D., Philadelphia. From the *Medical News*, Oct. 15, 1887. 8 pages.

190. TWO CASES OF MALIGNANT ENDOCARDITIS. BY J. H. MUSSER, M.D., Philadelphia. From the *Transactions of the College of Physicians of Philadelphia*, Third Series, vol. ix. 12 pages.

191. REMARKS ON VOMITING, PHYSIOLOGICAL AND CLINICAL. BY J. H. MUSSER, M.D., Philadelphia. From the *Transactions of the Medical Society of the State of Pennsylvania* for 1887. 8 pages.

192. IS THE AVERAGE DENTIST OF TO-DAY A SPECIALIST IN MEDICINE? BY B. H. CATCHING, Louisville, Ky. 7 pages.

193. THE GREAT VALUE OF A 0.25D. CYLINDER IN THE RELIEF OF HEADACHE AND EYE PAINS. BY JULIAN J. CHISOLM, M.D., Baltimore, Md. From the *Journal of the Amer. Med. Association*, Oct. 27, 1888. 12 pages.

194. CATARACT EXTRACTIONS, WITH ONLY THE EYE OPERATED UPON CLOSED BY ADHESIVE STRIPS. BY JULIAN J. CHISOLM, M.D., Baltimore, Md. From the *Journal of the Amer. Med. Association*, Nov. 3, 1888. 11 pages.

195. THE PREFERABLE CLIMATE FOR PHTHISIS. BY CHARLES DENISON, M.D., Denver, Colorado. From the *Transactions of the Ninth International Medical Congress*, vol. v. 15 pages.

196. PHILOSOPHICAL PRINCIPLES OF EDUCATION AND THEIR SCIENTIFIC APPLICATION TO THE DEVELOPMENT AND PERFECTION OF MEDICAL SCIENCE. BY JOSEPH JONES, M.D., New Orleans, La. 114 pages.

197. THREE SUCCESSFUL CASES OF CEREBRAL SURGERY. BY W. W. KEEN, M.D., Philadelphia. From the *American Journal of the Medical Sciences*, Oct. and Nov., 1888. 43 pages.

189. This is an admirable paper giving instructions in regard to the management of patients in the last stages of phthisis, when the hope of a cure has been abandoned. The subject is one which has received little attention in the books, but it is one of the greatest importance. The details mentioned by Dr. Musser are calculated to be of great service at a very trying time.

190. This pamphlet gives the histories of two cases of malignant endocarditis : ·one somewhat incomplete, derived from notes of the author's father and conversations with him ; and the other very full, from observations of the author himself. They are of value as a contribution to the literature of a subject which has only recently received the attention which it deserves.

191. Dr. Musser's paper on vomiting contains an interesting study of the *rationale* of this symptom, illustrated by brief descriptions of a variety of cases in which its cause was traced to obscure conditions, which might easily be overlooked. These descriptions and the comments on the cases are of the most instructive sort, and furnish an admirable example of the habit of careful observation, and intelligent association of the phenomena presented in the practice of medicine.

192. The question which forms the title of Dr. Catching's presidential address before the joint meeting of the American and Southern Dental Associations, in 1888, must be answered in the negative; but he makes a strong plea for a different state of things, and holds that every dentist should be a Doctor of Medicine in order to reach the proper level of scientific attainment, and the greatest measure of success in practice.

193. The contents of this paper have been laid before the readers of the REPORTER more than six months ago. Dr. Chisolm has found the use of a weak cylindrical glass of the greatest service in the treatment of the nervous strain and pain caused by low degrees of astigmatism, and urges ophthalmologists to look carefully for the condition for which such glasses are suitable and to apply the remedy which has proved so useful in his experience.

194. The ideas contained in Dr. Chisolm's pamphlet were laid before the readers of the REPORTER in an Editorial, in the issue of June 2, 1888. They are sufficiently indicated by the title of his paper, and are now no longer strange to ophthalmologists. Dr. Chisolm has had most excellent results by the method he advocates, and he is naturally a warm defender of it.

195. Dr. Denison is well known as an advocate of the suitability of the climate and other conditions found in Colorado to the treatment of pulmonary consumption. In the present pamphlet he goes very thoroughly over the evidence in favor of his belief, and gives a very interesting statement illustrated by two colored maps of the relative humidity and cloudiness of different parts of the United States. He also discusses briefly a very important phase of the climatic treatment of phthisis, namely, the condition of the patient, which may make removal to a high, dry and cool region wise in one case and very unwise in another.

As a whole, his paper may be commended to the attention of our readers ; for serious mistakes are sometimes made in sending phthisical patients away from home, when no possible good can come of the change.

196. Dr. Jones's elaborate and interesting essay on the principles of medical education goes over a great deal of ground, including the nature of the human body and mind, and of the vital principle, as well as the general principles of reasoning and logic. It covers a large extent of time, from that of the earliest Hindoo writers to the present year. Its wide scope can only be indicated here, and it is remarkable how much the author has found to say on the subject.

197. Dr. Keen's paper, which was read at the last meeting of the American Surgical Association, contains a full account of three difficult and successful operations upon the brain. It is written in the clear and attractive style for which the author is well known, and illustrated by admirable wood-cuts. It is much more than a report of the cases described : for the author's account of his operations would serve as an excellent guide to other surgeons even if he had not concluded his paper with a summary of the technique of cerebral surgery.

The paper contained in this pamphlet was regarded as one of the most important scientific features of the recent Congress of American Physicians and Surgeons, and would well repay the careful perusal of all of our readers.

CORRESPONDENCE.

Identity of Scarlatina and Diphtheria.—A Reply.

To THE EDITOR.

Sir: The article by Dr. Trent, in the REPORTER Jan. 12, on the Identity of Scarlatina and Diphtheria is an interesting and striking contribution to the history of a well-known fact—the frequent coincidence, or close association, precedent or subsequent, of epidemics of scarlatina and of diphtheria. All of us have noticed this close association, and all of us have doubtless seen different members of the same household affected simultaneously, one set with one disease, one with the other; all of us have seen convalescents from one disease contract the other; and some of us have had occasion to question whether the throat affection in a child suffering from scarlatina was simply that of the exanthem, or part of a superimposed diphtheria. The clinical courses of the two diseases differ essentially. But diphtheria does not protect either against scarlet fever or diphtheria, while scarlet fever does protect against scarlet fever, though not against diphtheria; this fact is sufficient in our present state of knowledge to necessitate the maintenance of the distinction between the two diseases. Though their identity has frequently been asserted, this and other considerations have prevented the acceptance of the view.

All that we are justified in asserting from observed facts, is that similar climatic and other conditions, general and local, favor the development of both diseases, and hence they are frequently associated. That some other association underlies this, as well as the association between tonsillitis and rheumatism, and between both of these and scarlatina and diphtheria, is highly probable; but just what it is the bacteriologists or the ptomainologists must be left to discover.   Yours truly,   S. S. C.

—The *Canadian Practitioner,* Jan., 1888, says that Miss Florence Nightingale has never recovered from the severe strain to which she was subjected in her noble work of nursing during the Crimean war. She is now an invalid from spinal disease, in her seventieth year, and is an inmate of St. Thomas's Hospital, where she will probably end her days, tenderly cared for by the nurses who in that excellent training school are reaping such benefit from the Nightingale fund of $250,000, which was raised in 1858.

NOTES AND COMMENTS.

Clinical Report on Sulphonal.

Dr. William H. Flint, attending physician at the Presbyterian Hospital, New York, in a communication to the *N. Y. Med. Journal,* Dec. 15, 1888, gives the results obtained in the employment of sulphonal in 33 cases. The clinical features upon which special stress was laid in the investigation are: The primary disease of the patient suffering from insomnia; his previous history; the dose of sulphonal administered; the time elapsing after the exhibition of the drug before sleep ensued; the duration of the sleep, its quality, and the after-effects of the remedy.

While he admits that the cases reported above are too few to justify any generalizations regarding the exact indications and effects of sulphonal, they yet offer some interesting corroborative testimony regarding its great hypnotic value already established by earlier observations. The general conclusion which may be drawn from these observations is that sulphonal, even in single doses of 20 or 30 grains, is a safe and, in the main, reliable hypnotic, free from unpleasant concomitant effects, and usually from all undesirable sequelæ. The single objectionable after-effect witnessed by Dr. Flint was moderate somnolence on the morning following the administration of the remedy. In none of the cases was there the slightest derangement of appetite or digestion, and the circulation and respiration have not been appreciably affected at the time of awaking. The cutaneous and renal secretions have neither been increased nor diminished; nausea, vomiting, and constipation have not followed the use of the drug. Several of the cases seem to show that an increase of the original dose is often not required, and that, after a certain time, natural sleep being restored, the sulphonal may be discontinued. This, he says, is the only light thrown by his cases upon the important question as to the possibility of engendering a sulphonal habit or of prejudicially affecting the organism by the continued use of sulphonal. The doctrines that sulphonal is of exceptional value in insomnia occasioned by debility, neurasthenia, and mental perturbation, and that it has no appreciable anodyne properties, receive support from the history of several of these cases. Thus, in one case, the happiest results followed the use of the drug in a destitute, homeless, neurasthenic, and exhausted patient. The same was true in two cases of hysteria. In six cases the pain of acute rheumatism, of pelvic peritonitis, of chronic·rheumatism, of sciatica, and of dysentery was not sufficiently controlled by the remedy to permit of quiet sleep. On the other hand, the pain of splenitis, of cerebral gumma, of pharyngitis, and of alcoholic gastritis, was not of sufficient violence to prevent the patients from sleeping under the influence of sulphonal. The effect of sulphonal was especially fortunate in the cases of those patients who had previously been addicted to the use of opium and of other hypnotic drugs, or were suffering from insomnia due to the withdrawal of these remedies. In four cases of insomnia due to the dyspnœa of cardiac and Bright's disease, sulphonal was powerless to produce sleep, and morphine was alone perfectly adequate to meet the indications. In a case of cardiac dyspnœa, the hydrate of amylene proved fairly successful. In two cases insomnia was occasioned by the harassing cough of pulmonary tuberculosis, but, under the influence of sulphonal, the patients slept better than usual, and although the cough continued during sleep, they were not awakened by it. Sulphonal also rendered excellent services in the insomnia of typhoid fever, as was shown in three cases.

The average length of time at which sleep ensued after the administration of the sulphonal was about an hour. The average duration of sleep was a little over six hours, and success attended the use of the sulphonal in about 82 per cent. of all the trials, and this high average of successes occurred in a series of unselected cases, many of which were plainly unsuitable for experiment with a pure hypnotic.

Danger of White Phosphorus.

At a recent meeting of the Academy of Medicine of Paris, M. Brouardel spoke on the danger of allowing white phosphorus to be employed in the manufacture of matches, and proposed that the Academy should insist that the Government prohibit it absolutely. He considered that all the prophylactic precautions advised would be without effect, inasmuch as the workmen would not follow them, preferring rather to run the risk of getting disease of the jaw than be compelled to adopt an irksome *régime*. He advises the use of red phosphorus, which has proved inoffensive in the different factories in which it has been used. Several members spoke in the same strain, and the proposition of M. Brouardel was unanimously approved.

Primary Sarcoma of the Heart.

At the meeting of the *Aerztlicher Verein zu Hamburg,* July 10, 1888, Dr. Mennig reported a case of primary sarcoma of the heart. The patient was a strong girl, 18 years old, without hereditary taint, and was well up to February 7, 1888. Her health became slowly impaired, and she became affected with loss of appetite, vomiting, dyspnœa, and finally cough with bloody expectoration.

On March 1, great dyspnœa and cyanosis, and a small, irregular and undulating pulse led to the diagnosis of an infarct in the lower lobe of the right lung, and an enormous pericardial exudate. The pericardium was tapped with a fine trocar in the fifth interspace one-finger's breadth from the left border of the sternum, and 9½ ounces of a bloody serous exudate removed. There was at once considerable improvement, which lasted eight days. The temperature during the whole disease continued normal. The pulse, in spite of the use of digitalis, did not fall below 120 after the puncture. On March 4 the presence of an infarct was no longer recognizable. On March 9 there was again great dyspnœa, cyanosis, and a thready pulse. The pericardium was punctured a second time, and within three-quarters of an hour 30 ounces of fluid removed. The pulse then improved, sleep returned, and profuse diuresis set in, and for some days the patient felt comfortable, in spite of the great frequency of the pulse—120 to 140. On March 20, the patient was punctured for the third time, and 24 ounces of fluid removed; on the 25th, the fourth puncture became necessary, and 22½ ounces were removed. Nevertheless dyspnœa and cyanosis did not disappear, œdema occurred, obstinate vomiting set in, and on the 29th of March the patient died in profound exhaustion.

The autopsy disclosed an enormous dilatation of the pericardium, which filled the whole left thorax and had compressed the left lobe of the lung from above downward into a thin leathery mass. The pericardium contained about three pints of a serous fluid, which in its upper layers was clear and yellow, in its lower thick and bloody. The pericardium itself showed no significant changes. The heart was small and flabby. In the anterior wall of the right auricle was a tumor the size of a walnut, which further investigation proved to be a spindle-celled sarcoma. There was nothing abnormal in the right lung and in the abdomen.— *Deutsche med. Wochenschrift,* Dec. 27, 1888.

Salol in Dysentery.

Dr. R. B. McCall writes to the *Medical Brief*, Nov., 1888, that in treating a case of dysentery in a child five years old he tried the methods of treatment which an experience of fifteen years had made familiar; but, as the boy continued to grow worse, he resolved to try salol, which he administered in two-grain doses every three hours. In speaking of the marked and rapid improvement which followed, he says: "In all my experience I never saw the efficiency of a medicine so unmistakably portrayed by characteristic results—the effects following close in the wake of the cause. Dose for first two days was two grains every three hours, increased to three grains, and continued at that as the maximum for three days longer; after which it was given for five days longer in diminishing quantities until left off.

"In about ten days nearly 200 grains were taken, by a child five years old, and that without the least sign of oppression, disturbance of any kind, of stomach, heart or kidneys, or of brain or mind. I believe salol is perfectly safe to be used in suitable doses at any age, and am persuaded from the above case and from a little experience in summer diarrhœas, wherein its influence was unquestionably kindly and effective, that it is destined to be a valuable agent."

Preparations of Sozoiodol in Diseases of the Nose, Throat and Larynx.

Dr. Seifert communicates to the *Münchener med. Wochenschrift*, No. 47, his experience with preparations of sozoiodol in fifty cases. Sozoiodol with talc in the strength of one part to two, or equal parts, is best for application to the mucous membrane of the nose, throat and larnyx. It is preferable in those forms of chronic rhinitis which are accompanied with abnormally profuse secretion. Sozoiodol with sodium in one-half strength was employed, only in the form of insufflations, in tuberculous ulcers of the larynx, with very satisfactory results. The powder adheres firmly to the ulcers and has, on account of its ready solubility, an intense antiseptic effect. But he used most frequently the zinc salt, in those forms of chronic rhinitis which are marked by abnormally small secretion—as isolated forms of hyperplastic rhinitis, and the different forms of atrophic rhinitis. In the first form the secretion was not only made more profuse, but also the mucous membrane of the muscles diminished in bulk in a very striking manner after one or two weeks' treatment, consisting of an insufflation once or twice a day. In atrophic rhinitis the secretion was greatly increased and the fetor obviated. The dry pharyngitis which in most cases coexisted was also considerably improved. In the majority of the patients the strength was one part in ten; in many cases, however, in which this mixture caused disagreeable symptoms, such as violent burning in the nose, headache, and dizziness, the proportion was changed to one part in twelve. The strength must not be greater than one part to seven and one-half. The mercury salt cannot be employed because of its strong corrosive action on mucous membranes.—*Wiener med. Presse,* Dec. 16, 1888.

American Medical Students in Vienna.

Dr. G. C. Simmons, in a letter from Vienna to the *Occidental Medical Times*, Jan., 1889, says that at present among foreigners studying in Vienna, Americans take the lead, outnumbering the English by 100 to 50. The English-speaking students can always be found in company with each other. They go to the same cafés and restaurants, and in general establish the customs of their country. Their patronage is evidently desired, for the cafés subscribe liberally for English and American periodicals. The restaurants announce American dinners, and further, even in the hospital, courses in English are announced. As a consequence of this seeming partiality, an envious feeling has arisen in the minds of Austrian students, and perhaps rightfully. The foreigners crowd the best courses, pay liberally for them, and the poor Austrian student finds them too expensive. This results in the native being often compelled to receive his instruction from inferior teachers and with poor opportunities for clinical study. On the other hand, this liberal feeling for the best courses is becoming a drawback with foreigners, each year the teachers demanding higher honorariums. Such a policy will prove harmful to the success of the Vienna school, for even at this time, it is customary for the American students to stay but a few months, spending the remaining time, and money, in a centre perhaps less famous, but certainly more reasonable in its financial demands. With this single exception, there is no cause for complaint.

Removal of Nasal Polypi During Hypnotism.

The Vienna correspondent of the *Occidental Medical Times*, Jan., 1889, says: Regarding the extirpation of nasal polypi under hypnosis, Professor Schnitzler gives the following details of a case in which the patient had suffered from deafness and disturbances of respiration, owing to obstruction of the nasal passages with polypi. Hypnosis in this case was also produced by an intense light. Several large polypi, and some small ones, were extracted from both nares with the wire snare, and the pedicles touched with the galvano-cautery. The operation lasted about ten minutes, the patient remaining in a deep sleep, similar to that of chloroform narcosis. Upon regaining consciousness she had no recollection of anything that had occurred. She complained of headache for about half an hour. Later on, she was again hypnotized and the mucous membrane of the lower and middle fossæ of the nose was thoroughly cauterized with a platinum point without the patient's experiencing any sensation whatever.

Prevention of Food Adulteration.

A bill for the Prevention of Adulteration of Food has been introduced in the House of Representatives of Pennsylvania.

The bill provides for the establishment of a chemical laboratory in all boroughs and cities having Boards of Health. The laboratory is to be conducted under rules formulated by the State Board of Health, and the borough and city boards are to appoint for the enforcement of the act such chemists, inspectors and clerks as are recommended, as necessary by the State Board. It is provided that the boroughs and cities shall pay the expenses. No person is to manufacture or sell, or offer for sale, any article of food or drugs adulterated within the meaning of the act. The penalty is to be a fine or imprisonment or both. The bill does not apply to cases in which any ingredient not injurious to health is added to the food or drug because of the necessity of such addition in preparing articles of commerce, and not fraudulently to increase the bulk, weight or measure, or to conceal inferior quality.

It is also provided that no person, with the intent of selling in the altered state, without notice, shall abstract from an article of food or drug any part of it, so as to affect fraudulently or injuriously its quality, substance or nature ; nor shall any article so altered be fraudulently sold. Under the penalty mentioned, no person shall fraudulently sell any compound article of food or drugs not composed of the ingredients demanded by the purchaser. The inspectors are required to inspect all breweries, distilleries, bakeries, factories, dairies, stores and markets where food or medicine is prepared or offered for sale, and secure, by purchase, if necessary, daily, excepting legal holidays, samples of articles likely to be adulterated. These samples shall be submitted to the chemists for examination and analysis. Violations of the act are to be reported by the Health Boards to the proper prosecuting officers. The Health Boards are directed to act in like manner, upon ascertaining that the complaint of any citizen about food or drugs is well founded. All fines and penalties are to go into the respective city and borough treasuries.

Poisoning with Antipyrin.

Dr. Rapin communicates to the *Revue méd. de la Suisse romande*, No. 11, an account of a case of antipyrin poisoning. A young woman 28 years old, suffering with sciatica, had obtained great relief several times from fifteen and one-half grains of antipyrin, without untoward attendant symptoms. The patient was dismissed from medical treatment with the advice to take fifteen and one-half grains of antipyrin immediately if the pain should return. This the patient did five days later. Immediately after taking the drug she was seized with violent burning pain in the epigastrium, vomiting and collapse, bluish-black cyanosis of the lips and cheeks, and an itching exanthem over the whole body. The patient recovered the following day. On the other hand, two patients with arterio-sclerosis died soon after taking the same quantity of antipyrin.

Dr. E. Haffter states in the *Correspondenz-Blatt für Schweizer Aerzte*, No. 23, that he has seen fatal collapse occur in the case of a man 63 years old, suffering with severe pneumonia, one hour after he had received fifteen and one-half grains of antipyrin. The question will be asked whether the symptoms were *post hoc* or *propter hoc*. At all events, however, the steadily increasing reports of threatening symptoms after the use of antipyrin demand greater precaution in its use.—*Wiener med. Presse*, Dec. 16, 1889.

The Inoculability of Leprosy.

Dr. Charles W. Allen, in a letter to the *N. Y. Med. Journal*, Jan. 5, 1889, says that Dr. Berger, of Tampa, Fla., who has made extensive personal investigations of leprosy in Key West, Cuba, and Nassau, as well as in this country, writes to him that he is convinced that there are over a hundred cases of leprosy in Key West alone, and that he has personally inspected thirty advanced cases in that island.

Dr. Augustin A. Crane, who has recently gone to the Hawaiian Islands from New Haven and become a government resident physician in the midst of lepers, wrote Dr. Allen under date of October 29, in which he says: "Father Damien is now dying, having had a rather short course of the disease. He gives as his theory of the contagion that he was performing the last rites in an extremely foul case; that the flies were very annoying during the sacrament, and that he thinks he was inoculated upon an abrasion on the scalp by the flies." Dr. Crane describes the sufferer as being in a horrible condition. He further says: "The convict you speak of is now distinctly leprous. These two points are slight in themselves, but, as far as they go, they seem to throw whatever weight they may have on the side of inoculation as against contagion."

Treatment and Prophylaxis of Cholera.

The Paris correspondent of the *Wiener med. Presse*, Dec. 2, 1888, states that at a recent meeting of the Academy of Sciences, Dr. A. Ivert made a very practical and interesting communication upon the treatment and prophylaxis of cholera. During the expedition to Tonking, Ivert had an opportunity to observe a frightful epidemic of cholera, without being able to influence the disease with remedies. In April, 1887, he assumed the direction of the Nam-Dink hospital, and decided, from the bacillary nature of the disease, to try the effect of corrosive sublimate. He began with small doses, and observed an immediate improvement in the local condition. When the dose was increased, the diarrhœa diminished and the stools became semi-solid. In no case did vomiting occur. This is in such contrast with the symptoms produced by corrosive sublimate in healthy persons, that Ivert assumes that the drug has in cholera a specific action upon the bacilli, or upon the poison developed by them. The result of his experiment was so encouraging that Ivert placed upon this treatment all the patients with cholera who came under his observation from May 1 to June 30. The cases, he says, may be divided into three groups: 1. Pronounced cases of cholera, which present all the classical symptoms of the disease, that is to say, cases in which the disease occurs suddenly, and is announced by vomiting, violent colicky pains, numerous rice water-like evacuations, violent cramps, cyanosis, an algid state, and anuria, to which symptoms asphyxia is sometimes added—cases which tend to death. 2. Cases in which the same symptoms as those noted in the first group are present, but the course is not so rapid—cholera sicca. 3. Cases in the first stage of the disease.

The number of cases treated by Ivert was 45. Of those belonging to the first group, 3 Europeans recovered and one died; and 8 Anamites recovered and 7 died. In the second group, 6 Europeans recovered and 1 died. In the third group, 3 Europeans recovered and none died; 16 Anamites recovered and none died. Total for the three groups, 36 recoveries and 9 deaths.

Ivert employed also symptomatic treatment—hot bottles, injections of ether when there was great adynamia, inunctions of camphor or turpentine for the cramps, tea, coffee, etc.

Prophylactic treatment was instituted in all affections which predispose to cholera. In no instance did a case of cholera develop in the hospital.

As a prophylactic Ivert prescribes:

Liquoris Van Swieten . . . . ℞ cl to ccv
Rum . . . . f ℥ i to f ℥ i f ʒ ii
Opii pur. . . . . gtt. xx
Aq. dest. . . . . f ℥ ii
M. Tablespoonful a day.

Liquor Van Swieten has the following formula:

Hydrarg. bichlor. . . . . gr. xvss
Aq. destill. . . . . f ℥ xxvi
Alcoholis (80 per cent.) . . ● . . f ℥ iii

Treatment of Scrofulous Ophthalmia.

Dr. Augagneur says that the true cause of phlyctenular kerato-conjunctivitis is a rhinitis due to microbes, some of which ascend to the eye through the lachrymal duct. Unless the rhinitis is treated, relapses are incessant. He advises insufflation into the nasal fossæ of the following powder:

Powdered camphor,
Boric acid,
Sub-nitrate of bismuth, equal parts.

He thinks the microbes are conveyed to the nostrils upon the fingers.—*Gazette Hebdomadaire*, Dec. 21, 1888.

NEWS.

—A sanitary expert has been engaged to make an examination of the sewage system of Jacksonville, Fla.

—Those who intend to go abroad will be interested in learning that small-pox is reported to be prevalent throughout Italy.

—It is reported that Dr. R. S. Huidekoper intends to resign from the Veterinary Department of the University of Pennsylvania.

—Dr. B. L. Batterbury, in a communication to the *British Med. Journal*, Oct. 27, 1888, recommends coffee as a vehicle for antipyrin.

—The Governor of Indiana advocated, in his inaugural address, a local option law, and recommended severe penalties against adulteration of food.

—Dr. J. D. Mercur, of Philadelphia, was recently so fortunate as to capture a burglar just after he had broken open the front door and was going upstairs.

—In a communication to the *Medical Age*, Jan. 10, Dr. F. T. Paine reiterates his previous assertions as to the anaphrodisiac properties of salix nigra.

—The daily papers state that a colored boy three years old is exciting much interest in New York City through his exhibition of marvelous feats of memory.

—Dr. F. A. Neely has retired from the editorial staff of the *Memphis Medical Monthly*, because the work interferes with his practice and his teaching.

—Dr. Tanner has proposed a fasting contest in which he is to drink only water, while the other participants are to have all the alcoholic beverages they desire.

—A sophomore in Cornell University has developed small-pox. An order has been issued by the President of the college requiring every student to be vaccinated.

—The *N. Y. Med. Abstract*, Nov., 1888, says that M. Gariel, a professor in the Nantes Medical School, proposes a combination of two important therapeutic measures in his method of "general hydropathic electrization." This consists simply of a shower bath to which wires are attached in such a way as to pass electric currents through the water at the time of using it. Patients who have been unable to take the ordinary cold douche appear to have used this modification of it with advantage, on account of the quick reaction which follows its employment.

HUMOR.

MOTHER—I want to get a real sweet, smooth name for my baby daughter.

Gouty Uncle (who is thinking of a salad) —Well, why don't you call her Olive Oil? —*Boston Gazette.*

DOUBTFUL COMPLIMENT. — Hostess—"I hope you are enjoying your dinner, Mr. Fowler." Guest—"Yes, indeed. This country air has given me such an appetite that I can eat most anything."—*Boston Beacon.*

AT THE CONCERT.—"Why are these boys called 'child wonders'?" "First because they are so dexterous with their fingers; second, because they continue to be twelve years old for four or five years." —*Fliegende Blätter.*

TRUTH FROM TRUTHFUL JAMES.—"Do you swear to your circulation?" asked the advertising agent of the truthful country editor.

"No," said the truthful country editor, truthfully, "I swear at it."—*Somerville Journal.*

THE ONLY SAFE PLAN.—Oculist—"When did your eye first become inflamed?"

Patient—"Yesterday. I went up to a lady to speak to her and the peak of her bonnet—"

"I see. We have many such cases. Use this lotion and be careful while the present fashion lasts to do your talking to ladies by telephone."—*Record.*

MRS. DOLLIVER—"Oh, Henry, I have dropped the water pitcher out of the window, and I saw it light on an elderly man." Mr. Dolliver (turning pale)—"Great Scott, Jane! You don't know what damage you may have caused!" Mrs. Dolliver (in tears) —"Yes I do. It's pure china and can't be replaced for less than $20. Oh, what shall I do?"—*Harper's Drawer.*

TOO GOOD FOR LIFE.—Little Edith was required by her mother to assist in the household labor, and it fell to her lot to dust the stairs. When dusting day came around, Edith would moan "Oh, how unhappy I am!" but after she had completed her task, she would change her tune and say "How happy I am!" On the last recurrence of the dreaded day, Edith went about her work without being told. When she had finished, however, she came into the sitting-room with a sad, troubled face. "Mamma," she said, "I'se 'fraid I'se going to die. I've got so good that I love to dust."—*Boston Transcript.*

MEDICAL AND SURGICAL
REPORTER

No. 1666.   PHILADELPHIA, FEBRUARY 2, 1889.   VOL. LX.—No. 5.

CONTENTS:

CLINICAL LECTURE.[1]

A CASE OF SYPHILITIC INFECTION COMPLICATED BY EPILEPTIFORM CONVULSIONS, KERATITIS, ETC.

BY HENRY M. LYMAN, M D.,

CHICAGO, ILL.

PROFESSOR OF PHYSIOLOGY AND DISEASES OF THE NERVOUS SYSTEM, RUSH MEDICAL COLLEGE; PROFESSOR OF THEORY AND PRACTICE OF MEDICINE, WOMAN'S MEDICAL COLLEGE.

(Reported by William Whitford.)

Gentlemen: Here is an interesting case. It is an illustration of the ravages of syphilis. The mother of the patient was infected by her husband, and the first child that was born was also a victim of the disease. This is the second child. The mother has had five miscarriages, and now after that experience the child born since the last miscarriage is healthy—an example of the subsidence of the disease. The second child shows well-marked evidences of infection; and the most prominent symptoms are connected with the eye.

In addition to the symptoms and changes which you observe in the eyes, there have been pain and headache, and at one time the child suffered from pain in the legs, a periosteal inflammation involving the tibia. But the most remarkable thing, and what brings her here, is the fact that about a year ago she began to have convulsions. The child would be taken several times during the day with a fit; she would then run to her mother for shelter, as children are apt to do, and would remain on her lap until the paroxysm was over. After a few minutes the child gradually recovered consciousness. She had eight or ten of these paroxysms during the day. Under treatment they have become less frequent and less severe, until now, after the expiration of one year, she does not have completely developed convulsions.

This case is interesting as showing how

[1] Delivered at Rush Medical College, October 25, 1888.

convulsions may occur as a consequence of disease of the brain, which resembles epilepsy, and yet is not to be considered as true epilepsy. We employ for such cases the term "epileptiform convulsions." Eclampsia is a name that is sometimes used, but the word epileptiform is a good one, because it indicates the resemblance between the phenomena that occur in these cases and the phenomena of epilepsy. True epilepsy is a disease of the brain, which perhaps is as extensive as the brain itself, and is generally incurable. It is characterized by recurrent convulsions, which are repeated, in spite of treatment.

Professor Lyman then introduced to the class Dr. Alfred Hinde, ophthalmologist to the clinic, to explain the condition of the eye. Dr. Hinde spoke as follows:

The affection of the eye in this patient is the one so frequently present in children affected with hereditary syphilis. It shows itself usually after the fourth year, being preceded by a period of latency of the constitutional affection. The affection referred to is known as diffuse parenchymatous, or interstitial keratitis, and is seen most frequently in children and young adults. It usually affects both eyes, though it may be in varying degree. It appears first as a slight opacity covering the surface of the cornea; later the process extends more deeply, and varies in its increasing density in different portions of the same cornea, until the vision of the patient may be greatly reduced, owing to the entire thickness of the cornea becoming opaque.

There is, however, another disease of the eye so frequently present in syphilitic subjects that we must be ever on the alert for it. It often coexists with keratitis, and is known by the name of iritis. Now, on carefully examining the right eye of the patient, and selecting the most transparent portion of the cornea, the iris may be seen to be swollen, muddy-looking, and its pupillary margin irregularly thickened and attached to the anterior capsule of the lens—the latter condition being known as a posterior synechia. Hence we must call the condition present in the right eye kerato-iritis. As the rosy zone of the sub-conjunctival vessels is absent, and there is also a lack of vascularization of the cornea itself, the stage of the disease is subacute or chronic.

Jonathan Hutchinson, of London, many years ago observed that, coexisting with this disease, there is also frequently present in the young subjects of hereditary syphilis a peculiar coloring and conforma-

tion of the teeth, more especially of the two upper permanent central incisors. The peculiarity consists in a dirty brownish coloration, together with a dwarfing, or narrowing and shortening of these teeth, with a gouged-out condition of the central portion of the cutting end, so that a pegged appearance of the two teeth results. At one time he thought that, in a well-marked case, such teeth alone were sufficient to prove the patient to be syphilitic. The observation was a praiseworthy one, but the conclusion is too sweeping. In many cases there would seem to be a strange coincidence to say the least, of the three conditions—syphilis, diffuse parenchymatous keratitis, and Hutchinson's teeth. Yet in our little patient the pegged teeth are not present. About the seventh year the permanent incisors appear, but this child is in her eleventh year, and the upper central incisors are not yet fully grown. Their color is white, the teeth are broad, and their cutting edges are serrated instead of pegged—none of which conditions is characteristic of Hutchinson's teeth; and yet we have a positive history of hereditary syphilis.

The late appearance of the teeth may be attributed to general malnutrition, and the latter is certainly due to the specific disease.

The treatment for the eye is the same as that for the general condition; the time required for cure will necessarily be long; the result will largely depend upon the character of the pathological changes in the corneæ and uveal tracts of the two eyes. The fibrinous exudate and cellular proliferation will, be largely absorbed under appropriate and long-continued treatment. The new connective tissue formation in the corneal layers will, however, remain. Where the iris, ciliary body, and choroid have been involved, these parts will be only partly repaired.

Again, the retina has probably not escaped injury. Unlike other forms of keratitis this variety shows little tendency to ulceration and abscess, hence irritants, judiciously used, are admissible in its local treatment. Therefore, to aid the absorption of the opacity of the cornea a mild vascularization of the latter must be produced and kept up. This condition may be brought about by warm fomentations, frequently repeated, and long-continued; and, as soon as the corneæ begin to clear up, by daily insufflations of pure calomel, or by the daily use of an ointment of the yellow oxide of mercury, together with massage of the eyes. Too much irritation must be avoided, as well as too little, otherwise an increased exudation will result on the one hand, or, on the other, a stationary condition of the eyes will continue. Each case must be treated on its own merits, and strictly routine directions, suitable for all cases, cannot be given.

Again, in those patients in whom the uveal tract is involved, instillations of solutions of atropine are resorted to, and the effect of irritants and astringents must be most carefully watched, lest the iritis be aggravated and an extension of the inflammation to the choroid be brought about. If the latter accident happen, an irido-choroiditis results, which would cause a shrinking and atrophy of the eyeball and result in blindness.

Improvement in nutrition and good hygiene are the main indications in the treatment of these cases. Easily digestible and nutritious food, together with cod liver oil and syrup of the iodide of iron, are the agents most suitable for their cure. Where the greatest improvement in nutrition has been attained, and where evidences of struma are absent, minute doses of the bichloride, long continued, will be found to be beneficial, especially so if combined with the tincture of the chloride of iron.

Professor Lyman, continuing, said : The interesting thing to consider in this connection is the relation between the disease and the convulsions. How does it happen that the patient has been having convulsions—convulsions that did not appear until a year ago ? Why did they not occur during the early years of life when the nervous system was exceedingly sensitive ? How does it happen that the patient passed through the early period of life without convulsions, but developed them at the age of ten years ? I think it is due to peripheral irritation. Where is it situated ? At the periphery of the brain. The convulsive centers, as we may call them, are located at the base of the brain ; they are connected with the pons, the medulla oblongata, with the anterior and lateral columns of the cord, and with the gray matter in the cord. These, then, are the structures principally concerned in the matter of convulsions. It is due to irritation of these centers at the base of the brain that convulsions are usually produced. In many cases of true epilepsy we can trace the connection between the irritation at the surface of the brain and the convulsion that originates apparently in the convulsive centers at the base of the brain.

A patient has, for example, an injury or a blow upon the head, partial fracture of the bone, a depression of the internal table ; subsequent inflammation takes place. There is a localized inflammation of the meninges of the brain. This produces local irritation of the surface of the brain, and, as you will remember, the lateral portion of the cortex of the brain is excitable. Irritation of an electrical character applied to the surface of the lateral portion of the brain adjacent to the fissure of Rolando will produce movements in the muscles that are connected with the spinal cord below. In the event of a disease, or an inflammation produced by an injury in that region, the irritation of the meninges will be communicated in many instances to the cortical structures adjacent to the fissure of Rolando, and may be propagated over the fibres that connect these parts with the ganglia at the base of the brain and in the spinal cord. If these irritations are sufficient in intensity, convulsions will occur. This form of epilepsy is known as traumatic.

Now, syphilis is a disease which very frequently produces inflammations of the covering of the bones of the body, the periosteum. This patient complained of pain in the leg at one time, a pain that was referable to the bone undoubtedly ; it was an inflammation of the periosteum covering the tibia. Similar inflammations attack the bones of the skull, that is, an inflammation of the periosteum lining the cavity of the cranium may take place. This inflammation will run its usual course. It reaches its height, then subsides, disappears, and the patient may recover. This is true of certain cases. In others the severity of the disease is so great that the bones may become ulcerated, excavated, honeycombed here and there by the processes of intense inflammation, destroying the bone, and producing necrosis of its substance. It may go so far as to cause an exfoliation of the bone itself, the dead portions separating from the cranium just as they would be separated from the tibia or from any other part in which necrosis takes place. There is no limit to the ravages which may be produced by the syphilitic process ; when it attacks the structures of the cranium the process is not always so severe as that which I have mentioned ; but a syphilitic inflammatory condition involving the internal lining of the cranium, producing what is called pachymeningitis, would encroach inevitably upon the thinner membranes of the brain, the pia mater and the arachnoid, and produce an inflammatory action which might excite the adjacent cortical structures. It is in this way that we may explain the occurrence of convulsions in certain cases of syphilitic disease of the cranial structures.

An additional support to this view is derived from the effects of treatment. The child, as soon as the disease was recognized, was placed upon anti-syphilitic treatment, which produced an amelioration of the symptoms. The convulsions are not now so frequent as they were formerly. Probably they will disappear as the exciting cause vanishes under the influence of treatment.

The affection in the present instance, then, is different from what is called idiopathic epilepsy, in which the disease comes on as a consequence of interstitial changes in the substance of the brain itself. It is a difficult thing to manage : it is almost uncontrollable with medicines. But where we have mere peripheral irritation, the removal of the irritant is the principal thing needed.

This is an admirable case in which to prescribe mixed treatment. The remark made by Dr. Hinde in the matter of treatment is an important one for you to remember. He says he would recommend the administration of syrup of iodide of iron and cod liver oil, and that is a matter of great importance in the treatment of not only this case, but the majority of cases of epilepsy. Patients of this kind—you may say all epileptic patients—are suffering from a deterioration of the nervous system. There is, even in cases which appear to be quite healthy, less than the normal quality of resistance and nervous energy, so that while you administer medicines which are intended to control the convulsions, such as bromide of potassium, and medicines for the treatment of the syphilis, such as mercury, it is necessary also to administer remedies which build up the nervous system.

It was frequently remarked by Dr. Willard Parker, of New York, that mercury in a case of syphilis should not be given until the patient was ready for it. In the treatment of such cases we often have to treat an anæmic, exhausted patient. The anæmia may be due to insufficient food, bad air, unfavorable surroundings, etc. ; but the effort should first be made to remove the anæmia, for if this cannot be done, there will be failure to secure the desired benefit from the specific treatment. It is sometimes desirable then, as Dr. Parker has said, to forget the fact that the patient has syphilis or epilepsy and address treatment to the condition of general cachexia, endeavoring to stimulate the function of the blood-making organs. It is important to determine if there is actual deficiency of hemoglobin in the blood. This fact can be ascertained in a few minutes, as I showed you the other day. If it is absent, administer iron to the patient. Here the syrup of iodide of iron becomes useful ; it is beneficial in a large proportion of these cases. Give your patient iron and good food ; let him secure an abundance of pure air ; then presently, when the general condition improves, it will be proper to administer the specific drugs that are required for the perfect cure of the patient.

The treatment of epilepsy also requires much attention in the matter of diet. If we neglect the diet of the patient we shall fail to get good results, because the character of the diet determines in a great measure the proclivities of the individual. It is desirable to reduce the excitability of the nervous system, to get the patient into a condition as much as possible like that of the slow moving, torpid class of animals.

If a patient manifests a convulsive tendency, endeavor to get him into the slow, tranquil, quiescent condition of a herbivorous animal ; the only way to do this is through attention to the matter of diet. Patients afflicted with epilepsy are subject to nervous excitability, neuralgia, headache, and various nervous disturbances. Eating of meat, then, should be forbidden in such cases ; the patient should be fed with fruits, bread, vegetables, and substances which tend to limit the consumption of albuminous matter ; thus the whole character of the patient will become modified in a favorable way. Evidence of this fact is seen in the case of children who are not really sickly, but who are brought up on a meat diet. They are excitable, passionate, quarrelsome, ill-tempered, and hard to get along with ; whereas, if they are put on a vegetable diet for a number of months, they will become more tractable and far easier to manage. The same holds true with regard to the different races of the world. Where there is a great deal of meat consumed by any race, that same quarrelsome, active, vigorous, energetic character is manifested.

In the treatment of these cases, forbid animal food ; keep the patients on a vegetable diet, and the severity of the nervous disorder will be considerably diminished. This, then, is a point well worthy of consideration when taken in connection with the diet that Dr. Hinde has already recommended. Cod liver oil, which he has advised, is an article of diet not to be considered objectionable, though it is derived from an animal. In its effects it is bland and un-irritating. It does not introduce into the nervous system those chemical elements which give the nervous system its excitable character. Therefore, cod liver oil is one of the best remedial agents, both as medicine and as food, that you can administer to patients of this description.

Another reason for the old maxim in the treatment of epilepsy holds good, I think, in this connection. It was Hippocrates, who said that patients afflicted with epilepsy should dig in the dirt and live as much as possible near the soil. Now, the reason for that is to be found in the fact that people who live out of doors, and who use their muscles in digging, work off a great deal of surplus energy in that way; and, furthermore, by laboring out of doors, occupying themselves with agricultural pursuits, they are placed under favorable circumstances, other things being equal, for healthful nutrition. Of course, this would not hold good in a malarious climate, or in a place where there were other unfavorable environments. But, as a general rule, the conditions of the agricultural laborer are far more favorable to health in epilepsy than are those of the mechanic in a large city. The mechanic lives in an unwholesome atmosphere during a large portion of the time; his brain is over-taxed in many instances; his associations and surroundings are connected with more or less excitement and turmoil. On the contrary, the agricultural laborer does not over-tax his intellectual faculties; his appetite improves; his digestion is confirmed, and his whole life tends to the production of a tranquil state of the nervous system, which is a great aid toward the prevention of a recurrence of epileptic paroxysms.

—As an instance of how small-pox may be spread, the following story taken from the *Lancet*, Jan. 5, 1889, is not without interest. A supper was held in a certain public-house at Ormsby, near Middlesborough, England, and, in order to provide sufficient accommodation in a long room, a partition was taken down, and what had served as a bed-chamber was added. In this chamber a servant girl had been recently lying ill with small-pox. A few days after the supper, no less than nine cases of small-pox, believed to have originated in this place, occurred.

COMMUNICATIONS.

INCOMPLETE SPONTANEOUS VERSION AFTER A HAND WAS EXTRUDED FROM THE VULVA.

BY C. S. SHEPARD, M.D.,

LA PORTE CITY, IOWA.

On August 21, 1888, Mrs. S., a German woman, 38 years old, of medium build and pelvic capacity, gave birth to twins. She was already the mother of five healthy children. When first seen her labor was well under way, the os dilated to the size of a silver half-dollar, and the membranes intact. A normal vertex presentation was made out. The pains were feeble and irregular, making labor extremely slow. The product of conception had made the abdominal tumor of unusual size, and consisted, as I suspected and predicted, of twins, together with a large volume of amniotic fluid.

The parturient canal seeming to be of ample dimensions, the patient was given ten grains of quinine and fifteen drops of fluid extract of ergot. The effect of the medicines was marked in a short time. The futile, capricious pains became converted into efficient expulsive contractions, which soon caused the extrusion of a fine girl weighing six and a half pounds. The interval of rest that usually occurs between plural births was wanting in this case; for, before the cord could be treated, extremely severe uterine contractions came on, accompanied by a gush of fluid. Upon examining for the presenting part, a hand and forearm were found occupying the vagina. The pains were now expulsive, vigorous, and recurrent at short intervals. In a very few moments the hand and forearm emerged from the vulva, and the shoulder began to press closely the pelvic brim. The position was dorso-anterior, the head lying in the right iliac fossa; hence the left shoulder presented.

In the brief intervals between the contractions I passed my hand into the uterus, grasped and tried to bring down a foot. The waters had nearly or quite all escaped. I was unable to make the desired version, whether because the womb too closely grasped the child or from lack of skill on my part, I do not know. It may be that both were factors in the case, but, after persevering in the effort to what seemed the verge of temerity, I withdrew my hand, leaving matters, as the lawyers would say, *in statu quo.*

The husband was taken aside and informed of the serious aspect of the case and that an operative measure might be required to terminate the labor with safety to the mother. On returning to the patient, having been absent perhaps fifteen minutes, I found her having exceedingly severe pains, and a careful examination disclosed the fact that the prolapsed hand was slowly receding into the uterus, while the shoulder was beyond reach. The head and upper part of the trunk now ascended steadily toward the fundus of the uterus, and the side, back, and finally the breech, of the child presented at the mouth of the womb. The child was born a few minutes later, dead. The cord failed to pulsate, the mouth and lungs contained fluid. The passage of the head through the pelvis was too expeditious, it seems to me, to have resulted fatally. The placenta was single and was readily removed. The mother had no untoward symptoms and the first-born child was hearty and vigorous. The still-born child weighed seven pounds, and was perfectly formed. The mother plainly felt the movements of this child for a short time after the first was born. Both children were females.

Lusk defines spontaneous version as "the process by which either a transverse presentation is transformed through Nature's unaided efforts into a longitudinal one"— or by which a normal position is either partially or completely reversed. This form of version, though often occurring during pregnancy, is seldom met with as a feature of labor. Playfair speaks of it as one of the "possible terminations" of shoulder presentations, and strongly urges that such termination cannot be relied on in practice. Lusk says: "According to the statistics of Housemann, cases of spontaneous version after rupture of the membranes are nearly five times as frequent as those occurring before their rupture. The same author states that the head presented in eighty per cent. of the cases occurring before rupture of the membranes, and the breech in seventy-five per cent. of those taking place after the occurrence of that event." He also states that: "An undilated cervix, powerful contractions of the uterine fibers, and a fully developed child are essential conditions for the occurrence of spontaneous version after rupture of the membranes."

In the case in hand two of these conditions obtained—the powerful contractions and the fully developed child; for, though one of twins, the size of the child was nearly equal to the average size of children singly born. But the other condition—the undilated cervix—was lacking. A number of cases recorded by different observers show that a widely distended os does not necessarily preclude spontaneous version. Playfair says: "A few authenticated cases are recorded in which the same fortunate issue (*i. e.*, spontaneous version) took place after the shoulder had been engaged in the pelvic brim for a considerable time, or even after prolapse of the arm, but its probability is necessarily much lessened under such circumstances." Playfair further states that: "The mechanism of spontaneous version, or the favoring circumstances, are not sufficiently understood to justify any positive statement with regard to it."

Lusk, however, explains the mechanism thus, holding, as will be seen, an undilated os as an essential condition: "The os is only partially dilated. The pains force the presenting part into close contact with the os internum. Owing to the absence of an equally distending bag of waters, the os does not dilate, and soon assumes a condition of tetanic spasm, during which it can be felt as an unyielding, cartilaginous ring. The contractions of the fundus of the uterus having now become more forcible, the fetal head or breech, as the case may be, is subjected to violent pressure. Inasmuch, however, as the unyielding os prevents any progress downward, the presenting part is displaced laterally, and that part of the fœtus which previously occupied the fundus is forced into the pelvic entrance." "Cazeaux believed that it is produced by partial or irregular contractions of the uterus, one side contracting energetically, while the other remains inert, or only contracts to a slight degree. To illustrate how this may effect spontaneous version, let us suppose that the child is lying with the head in the left iliac fossa. Then if the left side of the uterus should contract more forcibly than the right, it would clearly tend to push the head and shoulder to the right side, until the head came to present instead of the shoulder.

"A very interesting case is related by Geneuil, in which he was present during spontaneous version, in the course of which the breech was substituted for the left shoulder more than four hours after the rupture of the membranes. In this case the uterus was so tightly contracted that version was impossible. He observed the side of the uterus opposite the head contracting energetically, the other remaining flaccid, and eventually the case ended without assistance, the breech presenting. The natural moulding action of the uterus, and the greater tendency of the long axis of the child to lie in that of the uterus, no doubt assist the transformation, and much must depend on the mobility of the fœtus in any individual case.''

AMPUTATIONS OF THIGH AND LEG.[1]

BY MORDECAI PRICE, M.D.,
PHILADELPHIA.

The subject I wish to bring before the Society to-night is one of deep interest—to me at least, and to all others who are alike unfortunate in having lost a limb. In performing amputation on the leg, the chief object of the surgeon of the day seems to be to remove the limb and save life—the future comfort and usefulness of the patient being minor considerations. The comfort and usefulness of patients who are subjected to amputation of the leg have received my personal attention through the entire period of my professional life. This has been my latest thought at night, my first consideration in the morning ; and I have been painfully reminded many times during the day of the importance of changes in the present surgical practice. I see no reason why in this department we should narrow our surgery to a strict following of the *dictum* of a school of surgeons a century old : why we should not, in step with other departments of surgery and medicine, adopt those new truths which our advanced art and science and wider experience approve.

I ask your critical consideration of the few changes I propose to suggest. As a student I often marveled at the numerous amputations done near the ankle and through the knee, for the reason then given: to save all the limb possible, apparently without due consideration of the discomfort and suffering to follow, and of the usefulness of the limb. I have waited for years hoping that some of our eminent surgeons, members of this Society, would bring the subject before us, when I expected to be able to say something upon the subject. Like many other departments of medicine and surgery, however, this seems to have been looked upon as one of the subjects forever settled. For as far back as the works of surgery of the

[1] Read before the Philadelphia County Medical Society, Jan. 23, 1889.

18th century I find the same old plates, the same old positions for removal of the limb —where it is a matter of selection with the surgeon—as I find in use to-day. Sometimes the accident comes to the patient's rescue and removes sufficient of the limb to compel the surgeon to give the patient a good stump. In an amputation to-day in the foremost hospital of the world—the Pennsylvania—if the location of the injury left a choice as to where the limb should be removed, it would be done through the ankle or at the lower third of the leg. I suppose you ask "Why not?" I would answer that question by asking : Why do we amputate at all ? The answer would be : first, to save life ; and, second, to make a useful limb. Now, we can save life as easily by one method as by the other. Why not then operate solely for the best interest of the patient? In an amputation of the leg all that is left below the middle of the middle third of the leg is useless and in the way, and gives that much more room for ulceration and friction-sores. Let me tell you, gentlemen, these are weighty considerations in an amputation, for they compel the wearer of an artificial limb either to endure great suffering or to leave the artificial limb off, as I can abundantly testify from personal experience. Nearly three-quarters of a century ago, Gibson used the following language: "As much as possible of the thigh should in all cases be saved. But the rule does not always hold good in amputations of the leg. If, for example, the leg be amputated just above the ankle, the bone, from the deficiency of surrounding muscle, cannot be well covered and is therefore not calculated to bear the pressure of an artificial leg. On this account the patient is obliged to have an instrument of the kind adapted to the knee, and the leg therefore is carried out behind at right angles with the thigh and by its weight greatly incommodes the patient, so much so, indeed, that I have known two or three to submit to a second operation, for no other reason than to get rid of the incumbrance." This Dr. Gibson gives as his professional experience. I personally know of a number of reamputations for no other reason than the suffering, discomfort, or absolute impossibility of wearing an artificial limb upon a long stump. After the application of an artificial limb there is a constant diminution of the size of the stump. Its nutrition being continually interfered with, and the parts being of low vitality, consequently, when we have ulceration or friction-sores, or injuries of any kind, it is with great difficulty that they are induced to heal.

There is another element to be taken into consideration. As soon as the artificial limb is left off, and the patient assumes an upright position, the stump is greatly enlarged by a species of œdema which takes place almost immediately, leaving the parts in no condition to heal. The stump has the feeling of being cold and almost lifeless, and if exposed to cold it would be the first to freeze. It is almost impossible to keep it warm, when the artificial limb is left off.

Amputations through the knee joint give in many cases a very bad surface to bear the weight of the body, and a leg is rarely worn with comfort. Such an amputation absolutely prevents the application of a limb of full length, as the knee joint would have to be lowered some three inches for want of room, making at best a useless appliance. Amputate therefore—if it is a matter of selection —through the lower third of the thigh. An amputation below the middle of the leg is objectionable on account of the length of the stump, which presents occasion for ulceration and is difficult to dress properly so that the limb may be worn with comfort. Every inch of stump over five or six inches below the knee involves that many hundreds of hours of suffering and distress to the patient. The additional chance of life does not add one feather's weight in favor of the long amputation. Amputation at the lower third does not give sufficient room for a strong ankle joint, and therefore adds greatly to the wear and tear of the limb, thus adding largely to the expense. Amputations through the ankle may give the patient something to walk on, but this is oftentimes accompanied with great pain. It often gives him a poor excuse for a limb, and completely prevents any mechanical appliance from aiding him in the least, and forever prevents him from hiding his terrible deformity. If ever there was an appliance to which the term "slip-shod" could be appropriately applied, it is to those intended to imitate nature in these cases. The usefulness of an artificial limb is in proportion to the simplicity and completeness of its mechanical construction. The nearer it resembles the human limb in all its parts, the more perfectly it fills its office. There is one fact associated with these cases to which but few of you, perhaps, have given a thought; that is, the ever present and painful consciousness of physical deformity which the patient has, and the fact that his maimed condition closes

to him many avenues of honorable, useful and lucrative employment. This applies especially to the case of civilians; to the soldier it is different; to him the loss of part of a limb is unchallenged testimony of gallant and heroic sacrifice.

ANTISEPSIS AND THE COUNTRY PHYSICIAN.

BY G. WALTER BARR, M.D.,
BRIDGEPORT, ILL.

The warning by Dr. J. M. Taylor, in the REPORTER of December 8, 1888, regarding antiseptics incites me to contribute briefly my experience on the same subject. I practise in the country, over the worst roads in the nation, and when I leave home have no idea whether I will have a case of placenta prævia, fractured femur, typhoid fever, or hypermetropic headache before I return. Under such circumstances the practitioner must be physician, surgeon and inventor combined. Our city cousins have no idea of our trials and emergencies, but I verily believe that the situation has advantages, as a discipline, over the conveniences of town practice. With experience as a student in several medical colleges, the best training I ever received was the teaching of Professors Gross and Brinton at the Jefferson College, where we saw little intricate mechanism or perfected instruments, but heard much about improvised helps and "trunkmaker's board."

Having used the best possible judgment in discriminating between new remedies and fads, the country practitioner is liable to be shy of furors like Bergeon's treatment, but to take up and hold fast that which is good. The greatest God-send we have received for many a day is antisepsis. No one has a more correct idea of the word than the country doctor. He cannot carry the apparatus of a hospital and must somehow create the condition extemporaneously with all kinds of means. Consequently he can not follow a formula, but must know exactly the end to be obtained and the principles to be followed in attaining it. The most convenient antiseptic for our class is bichloride of mercury, because of its very small bulk in ratio to its efficacy. Ammonium chloride is always carried for cough-mixtures, and this dissolves the bichloride in rainwater. Enough gauze for one dressing has a small bulk, and so has a suitable quantity of iodoform. With these in his case, the country doctor takes whatever is at hand and operates antiseptically. When he insists on having a dish instead of a tin cup for his solution, his learning is wondered at; when he amputates some fingers and tells the patient not to touch the dressings until he returns in a week or so, the old nurses think he is daft; and when he takes off the dressings and shows a healed scar he is regarded as either an angel or a wizard. But aside from the carnal benefits to his purse, antisepsis saves him a world of trouble. I dress an operation-wound antiseptically and tell the nurse to notify me in case the secretions wet through the bandage, or any fever or unpleasant odor is noticed. Then I return when I am next in the neighborhood to remove the dressings. This is somewhat better than riding half the night in the rain. Of course some cases cannot be so treated; but still antisepsis is a great boon. I will not discuss the question of the value of antisepsis *per se*. The country doctors have waited until the matter is past the experimental stage; if they will learn the fundamental principles of the art and use it after their usual customs, they will never discard it.

A PIN IN THE BLADDER.

BY HONORA A. ROBBINS, M.D.,
BLOOMSBURG, PA.

The following case has some points which I have no doubt will prove of interest to the readers of the REPORTER.

A single woman, thirty-nine years old, first came under my care in October, 1887, for chronic metritis. Two months afterward, the following May, I was called to see her, and found her suffering with acute cystitis. For six days there was retention of urine. Several times during the introduction of the catheter, she exclaimed, "There is something sticking me."

At the patient's request, an examination was made, and the point of a pin was felt penetrating the anterior wall of the vagina, and, with some difficulty, an old-fashioned ordinary toilet-pin, an inch and a quarter in length, bent at an obtuse angle, covered with rust, was extracted.

The woman said she had swallowed two pins in 1864. She was in the habit of having pins in her mouth, and, while reading, she thoughtlessly swallowed two. One passed directly into the œsophagus, and the other pin could be felt, by a physician, in the pharynx. During his efforts to extract it, it too passed into the œsophagus.

For seventeen years she was subject to spasms. During the last seven years she has suffered with severe attacks of intestinal colic.

Two years ago a straight tarnished pin was removed from the rectum. It lay transversely just within the sphincter ani.

After I had removed the pin described above, the symptoms of acute cystitis at once subsided, and the woman made a rapid recovery.

PERISCOPE.

Hysterical Traumatic Arthralgia.

M. Charcot (*Progrès Médical*, January 28, 1888) again draws attention to a form of joint affection which may have a traumatism for its origin, but yet rest on a purely neurotic basis. A case of this kind formed the subject of a clinical lecture recently delivered by him. The patient, a young girl, had fallen on her left knee seven months before. Since that time the knee had been swollen, and the patient had kept to her bed. A cursory examination would leave the impression that the patient was the subject of a grave joint affection. The joint was considerably swollen, and its outlines were gone. Movement and manipulations caused considerable pain. The skin over the joint was red and shiny, the local temperature was somewhat higher than that of the opposite side. The limb was in a position of semiflexion, and the muscles were markedly atrophied. Analyzing the case, it was found, however, that there had been no fever, and there was no emaciation such as would attend a serious disease of the joint. The redness of the skin was due to all kinds of topical agents that had been employed by various physicians whom the patient had consulted. On further examination, it was found that the patient had left hemianæsthesia and ovarian pain on the left side. There was anæsthesia of the pharynx, and there was considerable diminution of the field of vision of the left eye. There was hyperæsthesia over the third, fourth, fifth, and sixth dorsal vertebræ. Under chloroform it was found that the joint was quite movable and that there was no crepitation to be felt.

The treatment of these cases must be chiefly moral. Hypnotism and suggestion may be tried. The various means employed in hysteria are here called into requisition. —*N. Y. Med. Journal,* Jan. 19, 1889.

Mode of Action of Antipyrin in Typhoid Fever.

Dr. N. S. Davis, Jr., in a paper read before the Chicago Medical Society, and published in the *Med. Record*, Jan. 19, 1889, says that he concludes from his own study of the action of antipyrin in typhoid fever, that it is certainly not a specific for the disease, and that it is of little or no use because of the antipyresis which it produces, and is of very limited use because of any of its other modes of action. It certainly, he says, cannot replace hydropathic treatment, with which it is so often contrasted. It must be remembered, however, that the chief benefit of the latter is not in its antipyretic effect, but in its stimulating influence upon the nervous system, upon nutrition, upon the circulation, and often upon the excretion of urine.

Suggestion of a New Use for Nitro-Glycerine.

Dr. W. C. Kloman writes to the *Maryland Med. Journal*, Dec. 15, that he has recently had occasion to prescribe nitro-glycerine and to observe its physiological action. He has come to the conclusion that the statement that it abolishes the inhibitory function of the pneumogastric nerve is correct; at the same time he observed that the capillaries, and possibly also the smaller arteries, were conveying far more blood than they had done before its administration. This was evidenced by the flushing of the face and the increased warmth of the extremities, while the radial pulse beat fuller, freer and more rapidly.

Dr. Kloman ordered the drug in a case of cardiac asthma, in a man 82 years old. There was no evidence of cardiac disease *per se*, but simply a weakness of the heart's action, with a want of coördination of the action of the right and left side of the heart, due to senile degeneration. Strophanthus had been given, but it failed to be prompt enough to avert the attacks of asthma. He was obliged to give three drops of a one per cent. solution of nitro-glycerine to obtain any sensible effect in this case. On Nov. 29, 1888, Thanksgiving day, the patient spent the afternoon and evening away from home, and returned thoroughly chilled, feeling also the commencing shortness of breath. His wife administered to him a three-drop dose of the solution of nitro-glycerine, and the patient assured Dr. Kloman the next morning that the effect was almost instantaneous: he soon became warm and was relieved.

Dr. Kloman concludes as follows: "Now, reasoning from its physiological and its therapeutic action in this case, it seems to me that it would act highly beneficially in cases of threatened gangrene of the extremities. So far as I know, this idea is original with me, and I should be glad to hear of the results of a trial in a case of this kind."

•Beta-Naphthol in Typhoid Fever.

J. Mitchell Bruce communicates a paper on β-naphthol in enteric fever, to the *Practitioner*, December, 1888. He gave the naphthol suspended in milk, and a small quantity of pure milk was taken after the dose. It must be given frequently, he says, in order to keep up a constant effect, and small doses have also the advantage of not causing the pungent after-taste in the throat which is liable to be produced. To adults it may be administered in gelatin capsules, or by the following formula, which seems the most satisfactory after several trials:

β-naphthol . . . . gr. xx
Tr. aurantii . . . . f ʒ ii
Syr. limonis . . . . f ʒ ss
Mucil. tragacanth . . . . . . f ʒ iii
Aquam . . . . ad f ʒ vi
M. Sig. Dose, one ounce.

In four cases, two of which were in boys 12 years old, the naphthol was taken in doses of three and a quarter grains every two hours during the whole course of the disease, until the temperature remained normal for five or six days.

The number of cases would seem to be too few to furnish trustworthy conclusions. Nevertheless, Mr. Bruce concludes:

"1. That the production of intestinal antisepsis is a rational mode of treatment of enteric fever, and that β-naphthol is a safe and tolerably efficient agent for this end.

"2. That by its use in the above cases the duration of the disease was shortened, and the intensity of the symptoms directly arising from profound disturbance in the alimentary canal was lessened.

"3. That the tendency to the occurrence of splenic enlargement, albuminuria, and of secondary complications such as boils, abscesses, etc., of purulent infective origin, is diminished.

"4. That complete convalescence is more speedily and satisfactorily attained; and that there is less risk of a propagation of the disease to others.

"Finally, we must bear in mind that in some patients naphthol may excite so much gastric disturbance as to prevent its use."

Treatment of Tubercular Diarrhœa with Lactic Acid and Iodoform.

The effect of lactic acid on the diarrhœa of nursing infants is well known, while its efficacy in the tubercular ulcerations of the tongue and laryngeal disease is generally admitted. It would seem to be indicated on double grounds in the treatment of the rebellious diarrhœa of tubercular cases. Henri Huchard states in the *Revue Générale de Clinique et de Thérapeutique*, November 22, 1888, that he has for the last six months employed lactic acid in doses of from thirty to sixty grains daily in cases of tubercular diarrhœa, but that his results have been almost negative. In such cases he adds that he has frequently arrested the diarrhœa by the use of iodoform in small doses. MM. Sezary and Anne appear, however, to have been more fortunate with the use of the lactic acid, which they have administered in doses of from thirty even up to one hundred and twenty grains daily. It would seem that Huchard's failures are, therefore, attributable to the insufficient quantity administered, for these authors assert that in all cases marked improvement was noticed on the second day, and by the fourth or fifth day the stools had become perfectly normal. They cite in support of this statement nine cases, all of which were cured by this method, and with only one exception did the symptoms return after the cessation of the treatment. It is doubtful if such favorable results can always be obtained; the diarrhœa is so rebellious, and the means of combating it so restricted, that any addition to our means of controlling this affection must be gladly accepted.—*Therapeutic Gazette*, Jan., 1889.

Acute Chorea with Insanity.

At the meeting of the Nottingham Medico-Chirurgical Society, Dec. 7, 1888, Mr. Evan Powell related two fatal cases of acute chorea with insanity. The first was that of a lad, 19 years old, whose father died of phthisis, and whose mother had had acute rheumatism when young. The patient had suffered from some rheumatic symptoms, and had been subject to mental anxiety. The choreic movements began in the left arm, then spread to the left side of the face, and in three days attacked the right side; and on the chorea becoming general he became maniacal, and developed delusions of taste, sight, and hearing. On admission, the spasmodic movements were so strong that he was unable to stand. The heart's action was very rapid, 170 to the minute, and there was a loud systolic apex *bruit*. Temperature normal; urine : specific gravity 1,030, acid, with a trace of albumin. During the first three or four days he continued acutely maniacal, and his chorea only slightly abated; some rest, however, was each night procured by chloral. The movements entirely ceased during sleep. For the next ten days he made rapid progress toward recovery, his mind becoming calm and his movements almost disappearing, whilst he put on flesh at a very rapid rate, gaining one pound and a quarter daily for twelve days. At the end of this period he relapsed, all his symptoms returning in an acute form, and he died from exhaustion five days later. During his lucid interval he remembered all that had taken place throughout his attack. On *post-mortem* examination the brain was found in a state of general hyperæmia, with some effusion of lymph in the arachnoid over the motor areas. There were numerous vegetations on the mitral valve, the edges of which were thickened. The lungs were collapsed; the spinal cord normal to the naked eye.

The second case was that of a single woman, 20 years old. The patient had a good family history, there being no taint of rheumatism, heart disease, or nervous affection. She had never suffered any illness herself until about six weeks before admission, when the catamenia did not appear at the proper time, and she became much distressed about this; she placed herself under treatment, and in about three weeks later she had a sort of hysterical fit; four days afterward choreic movements began in her limbs and face, which gradually became more violent, and a fortnight after this symptoms of insanity showed themselves; she became maniacal, and had hallucinations of sight and hearing. On admission the patient was in a state of acute chorea, but her mania had somewhat abated; she was much exhausted. The spasmodic movements were general. There was no abnormal cardiac sign, except that the beat was very rapid—140 per minute; temperature 102.5°; she was menstruating. The choreoid movements gradually left her limb and trunk muscles, but continued in those of the tongue and pharynx, so much so that swallowing and speech were rendered very difficult; her mind also became calm and apparently clear. She gradually sank, however, from exhaustion, five days after her admission. On *post-mortem* examination the brain was found intensely hyperæmic, but no other diseased condition was visible to the naked eye. The spinal cord was apparently normal. The heart showed slight thickening of one of the cusps of the mitral valve; no vegetations. The other organs were healthy. The uterus showed signs of recent menstruation. These cases show how important a part mental anxiety may play in the causation of chorea. Mr. Evan Powell believes the disease to be due to a condition of the blood, allied to, but not necessarily associated with, rheumatism and endocarditis.

Dr. Handford, before describing the microscopic appearances found in the two cases related by Mr. Evan Powell, gave a tabular statement of 154 cases which had been in the General Hospital within the last 14 years. From these, and from the very large number seen as out-patients, he expressed the opinion that chorea is unusually abundant in the Nottingham district. The table showed two deaths, and also that in the age and sex distribution the males were to the females as 1 to 2.4 before the age of puberty, and as 1 to 4.5 after that age. Thus the liability of the female sex, already unduly great, nearly doubled after the age of puberty. Dr. Handford further expressed the opinion that the endocarditis of chorea, when not rheumatic, is chiefly, if not entirely, of mechanical origin. The endocarditis, which was found almost, but not quite, invariably in fatal cases was of a special character. The numerous small vegetations, chiefly limited to the margins of the valves, with little, if any, general thickening, suggests that the invariable, abrupt, tumultuous, cardiac action in a generally anæmic subject caused a bruising of the valve margins where they came into contact, and thus started the endocarditis. He looked upon the endocarditis as a comparatively trivial complication, so far as its immediate effects were concerned. The microscopic appearances in Mr. Powell's cases were illustrated by numerous drawings, showing small hemorrhages, chiefly in the cord and pons, but also in the motor cortex; thromboses of vessels with hemorrhage into the lymph sheath; rupture of vessels in the commissure of the cord; and one vessel in which there was what appeared to be an incomplete embolus. No change was found in the nervous elements of the cord or brain. Dr. Handford expressed the opinion that all the symptoms of chorea are explicable on the hypothesis of a hyperæmia of the nervous centres, and he thought that this view is amply borne out by the camera lucida drawings he had shown. Chorea appears to be due in mild cases to a hyperæmia of the cord, and perhaps the basal ganglia, the lowest and middle evolutionary levels; and where the mind is affected and insanity ensues, the cerebrum, the highest level, has become involved.—*British Med. Journal,* Jan. 5, 1889.

One Thousand Consecutive Cases of Abdominal Section.

In the *Medical Record,* Nov. 10, 1888, Mr. Lawson Tait reports a general summary of conclusions drawn from a second series of 1000 consecutive cases of abdominal section. This series of operations has been done in the last four years, with a mortality of 5.3 per cent.; the mortality of his first series of 1000 cases was 9.2 per cent. This diminished mortality is attributed by Mr. Tait partly to the fact that he has freed himself from the shackles imposed by the traditions of the elders, partly to increased skill, and partly to the fact that the general profession is beginning to forsake the old, and to follow the new light; hence cases come to the specialist in better condition now than formerly. Two rules are insisted on: first, that the principles which govern our actions in general surgery must apply in abdominal surgery; and, second, that no doubt or difficulty of diagnosis should stand in the way of adopting that means by which the diagnosis is at once made clear, and successful treatment rendered possible by means of abdominal section.

He attacks the doctrine, attributed to Sir Spencer Wells, that an ovarian tumor should not be removed so long as the patient can go about; and maintains that an ovarian tumor should be removed as soon after it is discovered as possible.

In support of the claim to validity of exploratory abdominal section, the histories of two cases are given. The first case was one in which the attending physician diagnosticated simply "a lump in the pelvis," and for which lump he treated the woman "medically" three months, in which time she was brought to the edge of the grave. She was then sent to Mr. Tait for diagnosis and treatment. A large putrid sac of a ruptured tubal pregnancy was removed. The woman had not vitality enough left to recover, and died a few hours after the operation—a victim of an incomplete diagnosis. In the report of the second case the Drs. Keith, father and son, are attacked, more especially because of their opposition to the principle of exploratory abdominal section, and the "restless spirit of abdominal surgery which has lately been let loose." Dr. Skene Keith had diagnosticated the disease as probably sarcomatous, and had recommended a stomach mixture, apparently for the patient's encouragement. When Mr. Tait was consulted, the patient had been twice tapped, and a large ascitic effusion was present. He considered the ascites due to an ovarian tumor jammed into the pelvis, and perhaps fixed by papillomata. An exploration was made, a small papillomatous cystic tumor of the right ovary found, and also secondary papillomata infecting the abdominal viscera. From the history of the case Mr. Tait concludes that papillomatous infection had not occurred when the woman consulted Dr. Keith—the inference being that had a correct diagnosis been made by exploratory section and the cyst removed, the woman would have been saved.

Fifty-three exploratory abdominal sections were made in this series, as compared with 94 in the first series. Exploratory incision is still preferred to first tapping, because a complete diagnosis is thereby possible, and the incision serves the purpose of a complete tapping; and also because, as the patients almost uniformly recover, the incisions do no harm. The smaller number of exploratory incisions is explained by the fact that the patients come to the operator earlier than formerly. Thus results are arrived at exactly the opposite of the disaster narrated in Dr. Skene Keith's case. At least 30 cases in this series, in which tumors have been removed successfully, would have resulted as did the case referred to had removal been delayed; an argument for early operations and for exploratory incisions which is perfectly unanswerable. Of these 53 patients, 2 died, but the operation neither hastened nor delayed this event.

Occasionally the exploration is followed by drainage, and in some of these cases the most marvellous results have followed—the ascitic effusion has not appeared again, and tumors of the spleen, liver, and other organs, the nature of which was not ascertained, have disappeared, and the patients have been permanently cured. No explanation is offered of this extraordinary fact, but its truth is undoubted.

The next group consists of 263 operations for chronic inflammation of the uterine appendages, with a mortality of 3.4 per cent., as against a mortality of 5 per cent., in the first series—a diminution which is attributed to increased experience. All the operations were completed. These opera-

tions are considered more difficult than the removal of tumors of any kind, and the deaths are almost entirely confined to the broken-down condition of the women—the "too late" cases of Mr. Bryant. Mr. Tait congratulates himself upon the fact that the profession and public have accepted his teachings concerning this class of disease. As evidence of this he has 263 cases to report in this thousand as compared with 201 in his first series.

The use of electricity in the treatment of inflammation of the uterine appendages is next considered. Those who claim to be able to cure gonorrhœal inflammation of the appendages are invited to cure gonorrhœal inflammation of the elbow and knee joints, and the promise is made that when the elbows and knees have been restored to their pristine state, more credence will be given to the assertions of cures of appendages infected with gonorrhœa.

Mr. Tait states that he has always maintained that the great majority of cases of inflammatory disease of the uterine appendages get well without operation, though getting well does not necessarily mean that they are cured. He contends, however, that the residuum should not be condemned to live on, hopelessly suffering, while there is a *dernier ressort* at command. When that should be invoked is a matter for determination in each particular case, and depends upon conditions which cannot be formulated into laws, varying as they do in importance, even to the social position of the patient. Electricity may yet prove the means of still further diminishing the number of cases to be submitted to the surgical method.

The treatment of uterine myoma by electricity is considered unsatisfactory and even dangerous. The treatment of myomata by removal of the uterine appendages is believed to be far safer and more satisfactory. The uterine appendages have been removed in 148 women suffering from myoma, with 3 deaths, giving a mortality of 2.03 per cent.; whereas there were 99 cases in the former series, with a mortality of 7 per cent. The two series include 247 cases with ten deaths. Three women subsequently died with cancer, 3 had hysterectomy performed owing to the subsequent growth of the tumor, but no other failures are known.

Eighty hysterectomies are reported with a mortality of 11.3 per cent.; a striking contrast to the previous series of 54 cases with a mortality of 35.7 per cent. This diminished mortality is attributed to the adoption of Keith's method of operating. This method was not known to Mr. Tait until recently, because Keith would not allow him to witness the method of operating. The point is a simple one and consists in tying the broad ligaments separately, and stripping them off the uterus. This prevents occlusion of the rectum by taking off the strain. The fact that there have been 31 consecutive recoveries from hysterectomy shows that the mortality may be made to approximate that of ovariotomy.

Nothing is added to the method already published concerning the operations of cholecystotomy, nephrectomy, nephrotomy, opening and draining pelvic abscesses, and operations for tubal pregnancy.

Twenty-six cases of acute and chronic suppurating peritonitis were treated by abdominal section, washing out, and drainage, with only 4 deaths—a mortality of 15.3 per cent. ; whereas there were nine cases in the first series with a mortality of 22.2 per cent. It is urged that these cases should be treated by early and efficient drainage, just as in purulent pleuritis.

Four cases of puerperal peritonitis have been operated upon, with 3 deaths. The operation is considered as on trial, but it must have a fair trial—must not be left as the closing scene. Mr. Tait believes that in many cases of puerperal peritonitis the chief trouble is in the womb, and that removal of this organ may be necessary to effect a cure.

The article concludes with a presentation of the claims of a modified Porro-operation, for which see the REPORTER, Jan. 5 and 12, 1889.

An Eruption from the Use of Sulphonal.

The employment of sulphonal as a hypnotic has been followed by an eruption in one case occurring in the practice of Dr. Engelmann (*Wiener medizinische Blätter*, November 1, 1888). The patient was a woman, 40 years of age, suffering from chronic metritis with violent dysmenorrhœic pains, in whom sulphonal was given to relieve the insomnia, after chloral had failed. Thirty grains of sulphonal were given at bedtime ; no hypnotic effect was noted, but on the following morning a diffuse scarlet-red eruption appeared, accompanied by itching under both breasts. The red coloration of the skin was sharply separated from the normal skin and rapidly extended, so that on the evening of the same day it had covered the internal sides of both arms in a perfectly symmetrical manner, and reached to the sternum ; on the morning of the following day it had extended to the abdomen, and the eruption, which had been distinct on the two sides of the body, was now confluent. On the third day the eruption, which was now the seat of violent itching, gradually disappeared. It has been noted by Lesser that in the majority of cases the production of eruptions from the use of drugs is to be explained as attributable to vaso-motor disturbances, a theory which in this case appears to be sustained by the perfectly symmetrical character of the eruption.—*Therapeutic Gazette*, Jan., 1889.

Dislocation of the Eyeball.

A singular case of dislocation of the eyeball is related by Dr. Van Dooremaal in the *Donders Fest Bundel*. A butcher's assistant, in passing out of the shop, caught his upper eyelid on one of the hooks. He begged his fellow-shopman to extricate it for him, but the latter performed his task so awkwardly, that the hook pushed the eye forward, and allowed both upper and under eyelid to disappear completely behind it ; even the eyelashes were invisible. The man was brought to Dr. Van Dooremaal. The eye was pushed frightfully forward. The man shrieked incessantly, "Oh, how strong the light is"; and on being asked whether he was in pain, replied, "Yes, but oh, that light, that light!" while he clasped his hands convulsively over his eyes. Dr. Van Dooremaal decided to enlarge the external angle of the eyelids by means of blunt-pointed scissors, which were introduced between the protruding eyeball and the outer angle. After the cut had been made, a strabismus hook was introduced along the under edge of the upper eyelid. As soon as the hook had been pushed somewhat inward under the upper eyelid, a curette was inserted, and then pressed outwardly without exerting pressure on the eyeball, so as to bring the upper lid out. This was accomplished without difficulty, and then the under lid was gently drawn back to its place by the thumb. The wound was sewed up as usual, and the eyes bandaged. The wound healed quickly ; the reaction was extremely small, but the patient complained of excess of light on the removal of the bandage. The discomfort, however, soon disappeared, and the sight was normal.—*British Med. Journal*, Jan. 5, 1888.

Case of Subacute General Anterior Spinal Paralysis.

MM. Pitres and Vaillard report in the *Progrès Médical,* Sept. 1, 1888, a typical case of the affection described by Duchenne under this title. The patient, a robust man 43 years old, took a violent chill, which was followed by shivering fits, a feeling of general malaise, colic, and tenesmus, with slight diarrhœa. A month later, another attack of the same kind came on, with extreme feebleness; and six weeks after the onset of the illness, he came under observation, complaining of general weakness. The muscular feebleness was very marked. Two days after admission, paralysis, without affection of sensation, came on in the right shoulder, and shortly afterward in the left. About a week later, the paralysis had extended to the arms, and to the muscles on the posterior aspect of the forearms. The patient now complained of great weakness in the legs; was barely able to stand, and could not walk at all. Seven weeks after admission, all motor power in the four limbs was completely lost. The muscles now began to waste, and to lose their excitability to the Faradic current in the order in which they had been involved in the paralysis. There was no affection of sensation of the sphincters, nor of the organs of special sense, and no fever. A month later, there was œdema of hands and of the lower extremities, but no albuminuria. Slight signs of bulbar paralysis now showed themselves, with nocturnal delirium. Two months afterward, the patient was in the same condition, except that he was beginning to gain power in the right arm: at this time he died of an attack of lobar pneumonia.

At the autopsy the brain and spinal cord were normal; the only abnormality found, on microscopic examination of the spinal cord, was a slight degree of thickening of the neuroglia in the lateral columns and in the columns of Goll. The peripheral nerves, both in the large nerve-trunks and in their finest ramifications, showed considerable morbid changes of the form described as "degenerative neuritis," differing in degree only, and not in the nature of the pathological alterations, in different regions. Briefly, the changes consisted in breaking up or segmentation of the myelin sheaths (early stage), followed by complete atrophy, leaving empty nerve-sheaths mixed with finely varicose fibrils. The proportion of healthy nerve-fibres mixed with the atrophied fibrils in the nerve-trunks was exceedingly small. These lesions affected without exception the nerve-trunks and their branches in the four limbs. The anterior roots of the spinal nerves were much less altered. Individual nerve-fibres were found to be affected in the same way as the foregoing; but there were few diseased nerve-fibres, and these occurred individually, scattered amongst the very much larger proportion of healthy fibres, whilst here the morbid process never destroyed whole bundles of nerve-tubes as it did in the case of the peripheral nerves.

The symptoms of this affection resemble those of Landry's paralysis; but differ in the slowness of onset and progress. Duchenne thought that the seat of the lesion would be found in the motor cells of the anterior cornua of the spinal cord. The case is interesting, since it shows that in this undoubted instance of the affection in question, the peripheral nerves were affected almost alone, the slight change found in the spinal cord being unimportant. It also shows that profound alterations in the mixed nerves may cause only general motor paralysis without any affection of sensation. The authors give a brief account of the few cases of this rare affection that have been published hitherto. — *Bristol Medico-Chirurgical Journal,* Dec., 1888.

On the Effects of Acids on the Functions of the Stomach, and Their Therapeutic Application.

W. Jaworski (*Ctrlblatt für klin. Med.,* 1888, No. 10) draws the following conclusions, after extensive experiments with acids on the gastric function:

1. The acids throw down a considerable precipitate of mucus.

2. They (especially hydrochloric acid) increase the cellular elements of the gastric contents.

3. Their introduction is followed by intense butyric reaction, most marked after hydrochloric acid.

4. Larger quantities of the acids produce a considerable effusion of bile into the stomach.

5. They stimulate, very actively, the secretion of pepsin, but have no more influence upon the secretion of hydrochloric acid than so much distilled water would have.

6. Their long-continued administration is followed by marked diminution of the secretion of hydrochloric acid.

7. Even in large quantities hydrochloric

acid produces no gastric disturbances. On the contrary, a continued administration of the acid is attended with a feeling of well-being.

8. The difference in the effect between acids and the alkaline salts on the gastric functions consists in the fact that the alkaline salts dissolve the mucus and decrease the secretion of pepsin, while the acids precipitate the mucus and increase the secretion of pepsin. The disappearance of the alkaline salts from the stomach is followed by a decided increase of the hydrochloric-acid secretion. This does not occur, or only to a slight degree, in the case of acids. Both the acids and salts, in large quantities in continued use, have the same effect in lowering the activity, and finally in destroying the function. of the glands secreting hydrochloric acid.

Experiments with the introduction of carbonic acid into the stomach, either in gaseous form or dissolved in water, show that this acid has the property of stimulating the peptic and acid functions of the stomach, and in that way increases its digestive power. — *N. Y. Med. Journal,* Jan. 19, 1889.

Cellulitis of the Neck, with Partial Paralysis of the Right Arm, following Acute Traumatic Otitis Media.

Dr. Christopher Lewis, Assistant Surgeon of the Ear and Throat Hospital, Birmingham, reported a case of this kind to the Section on Otology of the British Med. Association, at its meeting in Glasgow, August, 1888. He was called in consultation to see a strumous, delicate boy, 13 years old, with the following history: some fourteen days before his visit the lad had received a box on the ear at school—a fact not brought before the attendant's notice. The patient complained of sore throat and occasional earache; in a few days these slight symptoms rapidly developed into a more serious condition, for the temperature ran up to 102°, delirium came on at night, obstinate vomiting and pain in the head were present. These symptoms became more pronounced, especially the delirium; deafness became marked, and the temperature ranged between 102° and 104°.

About the ninth or tenth day the 'true nature of the disease showed itself by a swelling and redness over the apex of the mastoid, and the cerebral symptoms, which had been gradually improving for a few days, almost disappeared. The mastoid

puffiness subsided, only to be followed by a deep-seated inflammation of the neck, which rapidly assumed an alarming size. There was a slight muco-purulent exudation in the external meatus of the right side, which was generally congested and tender to touch, but no inflammatory thickening. The tympanic membrane had a boggy appearance, its lustre had gone, and the pyramid of light was obliterated; there was, however, no perforation.

The whole inflammatory mischief was now centred in the neck, where an enormous swelling had developed, as hard as a board. This induration extended to some distance beyond the edge of the sterno-mastoid posteriorly, anteriorly to the median line of the neck, inferiorly on a level with the clavicle, and superiorly in a line with the floor of the meatus. There was some difficulty in swallowing, and the breathing was slightly labored. Singularly enough, Dr. Lewis remarks, there was no history of rigors, nor was there the least tendency to pointing; the pain, however, was so great and the constitutional disturbance so grave that it was a matter for serious consideration whether or not some attempt should be made at once to relieve the pressure. It was decided, however, to wait a day or so. On his next visit, as the symptoms did not appear to subside, it was decided to make an incision, although no fluctuation could be detected. A point was chosen a few inches above the clavicle, and, dividing the skin and superficial fascia, a grooved probe was moved about until a caseous mass was at last struck upon. The wound was then enlarged, and after the caseous substance had reached the surface there was some discharge of pus. As the hemorrhage was rather profuse the wound had to be plugged firmly with strips of lint. The pus welled up freely during the night, and the following morning there was a decided improvement in the patient's condition, and from this time virtually the whole symptoms began rapidly to subside. Dr. MacMunn made a counter opening later on. It was at this stage that some difficulty of movement was noticed in the right arm, owing, of course, to the injury received by the cervical plexus. This in itself, Dr. Lewis thinks, is sufficient to show how deep-seated and extensive the inflammation was.

Owing to some trophic changes, the patient lost the nails from three fingers. He gradually lost his deafness, and his hearing is to all tests and appearances normal. The recovery is said to have been in every way complete, although his convalescence was both prolonged and tedious.

In his remarks on the case Dr. Lewis says that the escape of pus through the mastoid in all probability saved the patient's life and prevented involvement of the brain, for, instead of bursting the membrane, the fluid forced its way into the mastoid cavity, and then through its apex, for it was at this point that the redness and swelling presented itself, and thus the products of inflammation were brought into contact with the deep cervical fascia, accounting for the formation of cellulitis.

Bezold was, he thinks, the first to point out that when the inflammation of the mastoid process is confined to the inner aspect of the apex of the mastoid, extension to the neck takes place, for a very thin osseous layer here protects the air-cells, so that, if any pus is formed, it easily forces its way through it at its inner aspect, and thus readily extends beneath the sterno-cleido-mastoid muscle, and so the pus escapes into the deep tissue. The time from the appearance of mastoid puffiness to the development of the enormous swelling in the neck could be counted by hours rather than by days. Deep-seated abscess not infrequently forms in the muscle of the neck near the affected mastoid cavity, but it rarely spreads so deeply as in the present case. Again, phlebitis of the emissory veins of the mastoid may occur in the course of an inflammation of the ear, but the induration is peculiar; and, although a cellulitis may develop, Dr. Lewis is not inclined to the belief that the case could be classified among those due to such a cause.

Death from the Presence of a Caseous Gland in the Trachea.

A healthy-looking boy, five years old, was admitted at 7 A. M. on Nov. 29, 1888, into St. Thomas's Hospital, under the care of Dr. Ord, suffering from great dyspnœa, lividity, and cough of four days' duration. According to the parents, he had coughed up a thick piece of phlegm the preceding night. Rhonchi were heard over both lungs. An emetic was given, and at 10 A. M. the child seemed fairly well. He continued well until Dec. 9, when he was discharged. During his stay in the hospital his temperature rose, once to 104° and at other times to 102°, for no apparent reason. On Dec. 18 he was readmitted to the hospital, suffering from still greater dyspnœa, especially well marked on expiration. Rhonchi were heard over both lungs, and the child was in very great distress. Stimulants and expectorants were administered, but he died at 2 A. M. on the 19th. At the post-mortem examination, held the next day, both lungs were collapsed, and there was a little inflammation of the bronchi. But in the trachea, just above its bifurcation, springing from the right side, was a caseating gland which had ulcerated through its walls and almost completely blocked it. A few more caseating glands were found round the trachea and bronchi, but none elsewhere. This is a very rare condition, inasmuch as the gland which caused the fatal result was found lying loose in the trachea, having been "shelled out" from the suppurating cavity. A similar case was recorded by Dr. Goodhart in 1879, and another by Dr. Percy Kidd in 1885. It is more common to find caseating abscess cavities communicating with the large air tubes.—*Lancet*, Jan. 5, 1889.

Cancer of the Womb in a Girl Eight Years Old.

F. Gaughofner reports a case of this kind in the *Zeitschrift für Heilkunde*, S. 337, 1888. He first refers to three cases of carcinoma of the uterus occurring in patients under twenty years of age, which have been reported by Schauta, Rosenstein and Eckart, and then gives an account of a case observed by himself. The patient was a girl eight years old, who for two or three years suffered with irregular hemorrhage from the vagina. On examination a large number of soft nodules were found extending apparently from the anterior vaginal wall. The patient was anæsthetized, and a speculum introduced. A tumor was found the size of a hazel-nut, which bled when lightly touched. The tumor was pronounced a sarcoma of the vagina. On Dec. 14, 1887, the sphincter of the vagina was cut posteriorly, a large speculum introduced, the tumor excised with scissors, and its base destroyed with the thermo-cautery. On Dec. 15, fever set in; on the 16th the iodoform bandages were changed, when it was demonstrated that the excised tumor arose exclusively from the portio vaginalis. On Dec. 17 variola developed, and the patient succumbed Dec. 25.

At the autopsy no more tumors were discovered. Microscopic examination of the tumor proved it to be a medullary glandular carcinoma of the portio vaginalis.—*Centralblatt f. d. med. Wissenschaften*, Dec. 15, 1888.

Recent Observations Relating to Intubation.

Dr. Francis Huber, chief of the Clinic for Diseases of Children, College of Physicians and Surgeons, New York, read a paper on Recent Observations relating to Intubation of the Larynx, before the N. Y. Academy of Medicine, Oct. 24, 1888. This paper is supplementary to one read before the Academy June 2, 1887, and is published in the *Archives of Pediatrics*, Jan., 1889. He states that of 94 cases there have been 37 recoveries; about 40 per cent. Patients over three years of age numbered 45; of these 20 recovered—about 44½ per cent. ; while of the 49 under three years of age, 17 recovered—about 35 per cent. This he very properly regards as a favorable showing, especially when it is borne in mind that the larger proportion of the cases occurred in thickly-populated districts under the poor hygienic and sanitary conditions existing in tenements. The cases were not selected. Intubation was resorted to no matter what complication existed, when the stenosis became sufficiently grave to warrant operative interference. He states also that they were late cases.

As regards the time for performing intubation, Dr. Huber says he does not favor early operation, because he has seen a comparatively large number of patients recover under the faithful employment of the bichloride of mercury and steam.

The difficulty in feeding, the strongest and most valid objection to the method, may be overcome in great measure by the employment of a trained nurse, personal supervision on the part of the physician (the idiosyncrasies of each patient as regards the ability to swallow liquids being carefully studied), the use of solid and semi-solid nourishment, rectal or forced feeding through the stomach-tube by the mouth or nares, and intermittent intubation.

If the symptoms in a case lead to the belief that the trouble is localized in the larynx and trachea, a full-sized tube should be inserted. A smaller tube may be inserted (with a view to being coughed out after a variable period of time) when membrane is suspected in the bronchi, or to relieve the recurring dyspnœa occurring in some cases upon the removal of the larger tube at the fourth, fifth, or sixth day.

Intermittent intubation, he says, offers the following advantages: Food, medicines, and stimulants may be administered in the interval. If membrane exists or is loose below the tube, there is less danger of occlusion, for the tube is readily coughed out, and with it the membrane. The time of wearing the tube is materially shortened. The spasm which sometimes occurs when the larger tube is removed on the fourth to the sixth day is relieved by the insertion of a smaller tube, and when the latter is coughed out, usually in from six to twenty hours, the patient will be found to breathe without difficulty.

He asserts that his deductions are not theoretical or imaginary, but are based upon numerous and careful observations, verified in a number of cases. He admits that intermittent intubation has been advocated before, but the plan proposed differs from the one he uses, in that the tubes (full sized) were removed at intervals and reinserted after the child had been fed. Dr. O'Dwyer, in detailing his second series of cases, incidentally refers to the advantages afforded by employing smaller tubes in certain cases. Dr. Huber's investigations in this respect were conducted without a knowledge of what had been accomplished by Dr. O'Dwyer.

Nasal Bougies.

Dr. H. C. Wood states in the *Therapeutic Gazette*, Jan. 15, 1889, that having had a severe case of hay-fever in his own household he was led to make experiments upon nasal bougies. He tried gelatin without success. When fresh, bougies made of it have not sufficient stiffness to be inserted into a partly occluded passage, but in a few days they become so hard as to be distinctly irritating. Cocoa-butter seems to be free from objection, though some skill is required to make bougies of it when it is used alone. The employment of wax is altogether objectionable.

If the patient is lying down, the bougie should be pushed forcibly upward, so as to jam itself between the two sides of the upper nostrils, closed by the swelling of the erectile tissue ; it will then be held firmly in place, and in a few minutes will melt. After the insertion of the bougie, the patient should continue to lie down, with a pledget of absorbent cotton wet with cocaine pushed up the nostril, so as to prevent the cocoa-butter as it melts from running over the lip.

The only medicine that Dr. Wood has found of service in hay-fever is cocaine, which, he says, seems to act better when added to a little atropine. Each bougie should be made to contain one grain of hydrochlorate of cocaine and one-twentieth grain of atropine.

THE
MEDICAL AND SURGICAL
REPORTER.

ISSUED EVERY SATURDAY.

CHARLES W. DULLES, M.D.,
EDITOR AND PUBLISHER.

The Terms of Subscription to the serial publications of this office are as follows, payable in advance:

Med. and Surg. Reporter (weekly), a year, **$5.00**
Quarterly Compendium of Med. Science, - **2.50**
Reporter and Compendium, - - - - **6.00**
Physician's Daily Pocket Record, - - **1.00**
Reporter and Pocket Record, - - - **6.00**
Reporter, Compendium, and Pocket Record, **7.00**

All checks and postal orders should be drawn to order of

CHARLES W. DULLES,

N. E. Cor. 13th and Walnut Streets,
P. O. Box 843.   Philadelphia, Pa.

☞SUGGESTIONS TO SUBSCRIBERS:
See that your address-label gives the date to which your subscription is paid.
In requesting a change of address, give the old address as well as the new one.
If your REPORTER does not reach you promptly and regularly, notify the publisher *at once*, so that the cause may be discovered and corrected.

☞SUGGESTIONS TO CONTRIBUTORS AND CORRESPONDENTS:
Write in ink.
Write on one side of paper only.
Write on paper of the size usually used for letters.
Make as few paragraphs as possible. Punctuate carefully. Do not abbreviate, or omit words like "the," and "a," or "an."
Make communications as short as possible.
NEVER ROLL A MANUSCRIPT! Try to get an envelope or wrapper which will fit it.
When it is desired to call our attention to something in a newspaper, mark the passage boldly with a colored pencil, and write on the wrapper "Marked copy." Unless this is done, newspapers are not looked at.
The Editor will be glad to get medical news, but it is important that brevity and actual interest shall characterize communications intended for publication.

A CONFIDENTIAL WORD TO OUR READERS.

It is with much pleasure that we acknowledge the gratifying response of our subscribers to the effort of the publisher of the REPORTER to get the mail-list in first class shape. There is a great difference between the cleanness of the mail-list to-day and the state in which it was nearly two years ago. There were on it then names of men who had not paid up for some time, and who apparently never meant to. These have been asked to pay, then asked more firmly, then drawn on, and then—if they did not settle—they have been cut off. There were on it also the names of men who had asked to have it stopped. These it took some time to discover. But the work of straightening things out has gone on steadily, and now the mail-list is one which can be regarded with great satisfaction by all the real friends of the REPORTER. It is larger than ever within our knowledge, and the subscribers seem to share the opinion of the publisher that good business principles are the best all the time.

It may surprise some of our readers to know that it has been necessary to part with a certain number of subscribers who had been getting the REPORTER at a reduced rate, for no other reason than that they were not willing to pay the usual price. This unjust discrimination is no longer made; and those who regard the REPORTER as a first-class publication, and treat it as such, will be pleased—we trust—to know that the publisher endeavors to treat all who have business dealings with it exactly alike. This applies to advertisers and subscribers both ; and we can heartily recommend each of these classes of our patrons to the other ; in the full belief, from our own relations with them, that both are honorable and upright, and that it is to the advantage of both to be brought into such relations as a medical journal may properly secure. In saying this, we desire to thank all those—both subscribers and advertisers—who have seconded our efforts to make the REPORTER a good medical journal, and promise—so far as our judgment shall extend—to keep it honest, impartial and fearless. We shall take kindly any friendly corrections which may be offered, and hope for continued support in every endeavor to do what is right.

AN ARTIFICIAL BLADDER.

Among the recognized operations of surgery total extirpation of the urinary bladder is one of the most formidable, and most rare ; but it is performed often enough to make it desirable to have some way of providing a receptacle for the urine which will measurably, at least, obviate the inconveniences of a continuous discharge from the

ureters.· ·Up to a very recent date the best
method consisted in turning the ends of the
ureters into the rectum, and imitating the
mechanism found in birds.　The most successful experiments in this direction with
which we are acquainted are those of
Novaro, of Siena, in Italy, who carried the
operation out in two sittings.　More recently
Tizzoni and Foggi, of Bologna, have on
June 22, 1888, tried a new way of replacing
the bladder, which consisted in isolating a
portion of the small intestine, by dividing
it at intervals of about two and a half
inches, leaving its mesenteric attachment
undisturbed, suturing its two ends so as to
make a closed cavity, and joining the two
ends of the intestine itself, so as to restore
its continuity.　At a subsequent sitting,
about a month later, the ureters were
separated from the bladder, and the latter
was excised.　The ureters were then inserted
into two incisions in the now somewhat
contracted cavity of the section of intestine and were stitched in place, while the
lower end of the new receptacle was incised
transversely and the edges of the incision
were carefully stitched to the stump at the
neck of the bladder.

The result of the operation, which is
fully described in the *Centralblatt für
Chirurgie*, Dec. 15, 1888, was entirely satisfactory.　After a short period of relative
incontinence, the new bladder began to
perform its office in a very excellent manner,
and the dog was able to hold its water for
an hour or more and to pass it naturally.

This interesting experiment indicates that
it is possible to obtain in animals an organ
lined with mucous membrane and surrounded with a muscular wall, as a substitute for the urinary bladder in cases in
which this has to be removed or in which it
cannot perform its usual functions.　It may
be that the experiment would not prove so
successful if performed on a human being;
but the result obtained on a lower animal
encourages the hope that it may be possible
to extend its benefits to mankind as well.

THE PHILADELPHIA HOSPITAL.

There are few persons, not officially connected with the Philadelphia Hospital, who
are aware of its value as a place of refuge
for the sick and injured, and as a teaching
institution.　The service of the staff of this
hospital will compare favorably with that
of any hospital in this city, and the results
obtained are as good as is usual in hospitals,
and wonderfully good in view of the character and physical condition of many of the
patients, and the arrangement of the buildings.

These facts, added to the fact that in the
Philadelphia Hospital almost all of the
students of medicine in this city receive a
considerable part of their clinical education, are sufficient to attract to it the
attention of the profession as well as of
the citizens at large.

Just at present this attention is especially
keen because an effort is being made by
those who are interested in the Hospital to
increase its dignity and improve its opportunities for usefulness by freeing it from an
element which has always been a source of
prejudice against it on the part of those who
might enjoy its hospitality, and an obstacle
to securing the best results of the work of
its staff of physicians and nurses.　This element is the presence of thousands of paupers in the vicinity of the hospital wards.
The hospital was originally but an adjunct
of the Philadelphia Alms-House—its Infirmary, in fact; but it has grown now to be a
large municipal Hospital and its importance
as a Hospital and as a teaching institution
requires that it shall now be treated as a
distinct establishment, and freed from the
embarrassments caused by its attachment
to the parent institution.

All of the friends of the Hospital—and,
we may say, of medical education in Philadelphia will be pleased to know that there
is a good prospect that the authorities of
the City will soon take steps to remove the
Alms-House to some place better suited to
the requirements of its inmates, and make

the alterations needed to complete the organization of the Hospital on an entirely independent basis.

It is to be hoped that all of our fellow citizens will share the unanimous opinion of the members of the medical profession that this step is a most desirable one, and aid those who are trying to have it carried out, by their personal influence and co-operation.

STATE ASYLUMS OR ALMS-HOUSES FOR THE INSANE.

The care of the insane has been the subject of a number of Communications and Editorials in the REPORTER during the past two years, and it is one to which attention will be called as often as occasion seems to demand.

Just now it seems proper to say a few words in regard to it, because the Governor of Pennsylvania in his last message to the Legislature has recommended a step which is directly opposed to principles which we have advocated in the REPORTER for April 14, and May 12, 1888. The Governor recommends relieving the crowded condition of certain of the State Hospitals for the Insane by sending part of their inmates to the County alms-houses. This is a suggestion which is opposed to the opinion of all who have made the care of the insane a matter of special study, and its adoption would be a step backward toward the customs of fifty years ago. Last April we cited the evidence on this subject presented to a Committee of the Senate of New York and especially that given by members of the New York Charities' Aid Society, showing that the pauper insane are not as well cared for under the jurisdiction of county authorities as they are in establishments under the management of the State. In May we cited the opinion of the State Lunacy Commission of Pennsylvania that State hospitals are much preferable to alms-houses for the care of the insane.

The recent recommendation of the Governor of Pennsylvania is the subject of an extended article in the *Pittsburgh Commercial Gazette*, January 7, 1889, part of which gives the opinion of Dr. C. C. Wiley, of Pittsburgh, and all of which we can endorse as reflecting the humane and scientific views in regard to the care of the insane which prevail among medical men at the present day.

We invite the attention of the readers of the REPORTER all over the United States to this matter, because it concerns them all. In Pennsylvania it merits immediate notice, because an unwise step might be taken at any time, unless its true character is made clear to the Governor and the Legislature, which is now in session. But it deserves notice everywhere, because a similar step may be next proposed when it is least expected. A year ago the Legislature of New York considered and refused to pass a bill to transfer the care of the insane to the State hospitals, and we spoke in support of that measure little thinking that before a year had passed we should be called on to protest against a proposition to degrade Pennsylvania to a level from which good and true men were then trying to elevate New York.

So our readers may bear in mind that the question which is of such immediate urgency in the State just now may at any moment confront them, and they may as well prepare to meet it when it comes, and lend their assistance to those who are facing it now.

PHILADELPHIA POLYCLINIC.—Among the interesting signs of enlargement of the scope of the Philadelphia Polyclinic we note the fact that its Trustees have founded a chair of Diseases of the Mind and Nervous System, and have elected Dr. S. Weir Mitchell to the Professorship. The prosperous condition of the institution is further indicated by the announcement of the purchase, for twenty-five thousand dollars, of a large property on Lombard Street above Eighteenth.

BOOK REVIEWS.

[Any book reviewed in these columns may be obtained upon receipt of price, from the office of the REPORTER.]

LECTURES ON ECTOPIC PREGNANCY AND PELVIC HÆMATOCELE. By LAWSON TAIT, F.R.C.S., Edin. and Eng., LL.D., Professor of Gynecology in Queen's College, Birmingham, Surgeon to the Birmingham and Midland Hospital for Women, etc. Octavo, pp. 107. Birmingham: The "Journal" Printing Works, 1888.

At this time when the subject of ectopic pregnancy occupies the attention of the profession to a considerable degree, any contribution to the subject is very welcome. This is especially true when the contributor has had the large and exceptional experience of the author. In these lectures Mr. Tait gives his views concerning the nature and natural history of ectopic pregnancy, and his experience in the management of these cases, together with a cursory review of some of the literature of the subject in an entertaining but rather rambling manner. The allied subject of hæmatocele is also discussed. Bernutz and Goupil are quoted as having made the first important contribution to the literature of pelvic hæmatocele. This is striking. Bernutz was perfectly familiar with the true nature of pelvic inflammation and abscess, but it remained for Mr. Tait to discover the method of cure. And now the same is true of hæmatocele—more especially hæmatocele caused by the rupture of a tubal pregnancy. While all may not agree *in toto* with Mr. Tait, his extensive and successful experience in the management of ectopic pregnancy demands and will ensure a wide circulation of these "Lectures" among all students in this field.

QUESTIONS AND ANSWERS ON THE ESSENTIALS OF SURGERY: TOGETHER WITH A FULL DESCRIPTION OF THE HANDKERCHIEF AND ROLLER BANDAGES. By EDWARD MARTIN, A.M., M.D., Instructor of (sic) Operative Surgery, University of Pennsylvania, etc. With ninety illustrations. Small 8vo, pp. 314. Philadelphia: W. B. Saunders, 1888. Price, $1.00.

Dr. Martin's book contains a very good summary of what may with propriety be termed the essentials of surgery. It is—as the title indicates—arranged in the form familiar to all who have enjoyed the benefits of a "quiz"; and the questions and answers are clear and concise. In most respects it is thoroughly reliable. In some it is open to improvement. In the examination which we have been able to make of it, we have been struck with the inadequate consideration of fractures at the elbow-joint, and the omission of certain points in the treatment of impacted fractures of the neck of the femur which we regard as of great importance. It would be too much, perhaps, to expect a book like this to mention properitoneal hernia; but it would be an advantage if it did. The description of suprapubic lithotomy is also open to criticism.

We have made these comments not to disparage the book before us, but rather to suggest improvements in subsequent editions. As a whole we can heartily recommend it; for it contains, in a comparatively small space, a great deal of valuable surgical teaching. Its style is interesting, and its illustrations are admirable. On its general appearance, we can congratulate its publisher as well as its author.

PAMPHLET NOTICES.

[Any reader of the REPORTER who desires a copy of a pamphlet noticed in these columns will doubtless secure it by addressing the author with a request stating where the notice was seen and *enclosing a postage-stamp.*]

198. THE YELLOW FEVER PANIC. BY J. C. LE HARDY, M.D., Savannah, Ga. 14 pages.

199. CONSEQUENCES OF ACUTE SUPPURATION OF THE MIDDLE EAR, WITH SPECIAL REFERENCE TO OPENING THE MASTOID. BY A. R. BAKER, M.D., Cleveland, Ohio. From the *Transactions of the Ohio State Medical Society*, 1888. 20 pages.

200. HEART WITH THREE CAVITIES. PARTIAL TRANSPOSITION OF ABDOMINAL VISCERA. BY M. HOWARD FUSSELL, M.D., Manayunk, Philadelphia. From the *Medical News*, Nov. 3, 1888. 11 pages.

201. THE HOMING INSTINCT. AN EXPLANATION SUGGESTED. BY GEORGE M. GOULD, M.D., Philadelphia. From *Progress*, October, 1888. 24 pages.

202. SOLUTION OF THE PHILADELPHIA WATER QUESTION. BY EMILE GEYELIN, Philadelphia. 7 pages.

203. A CONTRIBUTION TO THE STUDY OF BONE REPAIR. BY JOHN S. MILLER, M.D., Philadelphia. From the *Transactions of the Philadelphia County Med. Society*, June 27, 1888. 7 pages.

204. THE TREATMENT OF PERITONITIS BY ABDOMINAL SECTION. BY L. S. McMURTRY, M.D., Danville, Ky. From the *Annals of Gynecology*, September, 1888. 16 pages.

205. A CASE OF TYPHLITIS, WITH DOUBLE PERFORATION OF THE CÆCUM, AND PERITONITIS, IN WHICH LAPAROTOMY AND SUTURE OF THE GUT WERE FOLLOWED BY RECOVERY. BY L. S. McMURTRY, M.D., Danville, Ky. From the *Journal of the Amer. Med. Association*, July 7, 1888. 8 pages.

198. In an Editorial in the REPORTER, Jan. 5, we have already cited some of the views expressed by Dr. Le Hardy in his pamphlet on the yellow fever panic of 1888; but our readers will find it to their profit, we believe, to make themselves acquainted with the whole of it. There is much instructive reading here, and much which, if taken to heart, would tend to prevent the repetition of follies committed during 1888, which were of the most damaging character. Dr. Le Hardy has had opportunities of studying yellow fever such as few men can enjoy, and what he writes has the impress of great sense and judgment.

199. Dr. Baker's pamphlet is one which might well be studied by every medical practitioner. He dwells upon the importance of early recognition of suppurative disease of the mastoid and early and vigorous treatment of it. This he does with an earnestness which is fully justified by the fact that many lives are lost every year because the principles which he inculcates are not appreciated as they should be. He describes clearly the best method of operating upon the mastoid process, and gives accounts of a number of cases in which he himself has performed the operation.

200. Dr. Fussell describes the appearances in a case of malformation of the heart, in a child that died when nearly two years old, in which there was practically but one ventricle and one auricle, the other

corresponding parts being very imperfectly developed. The description of the specimen is preceded by an account of the history of the case from the birth to the death of the little patient, which forms a very interesting part of the paper and one of great practical value considered in connection with the findings of the autopsy. Cases of this kind are exceedingly rare, and such a carefully observed and described one is of unusual interest and instructiveness.

201. Dr. Gould's little pamphlet contains a number of interesting stories about the return of various animals to places from which they had been removed, and the suggestion in regard to the homing instinct is that it depends upon some unconscious relation between the animal and the magnetic currents of the earth. The author recognizes the purely speculative character of his suggestion, and invites experiments to test it which he has not yet been able to make himself.

202. Mr. Geyelin has for years been an interested student of the condition of the water-supply of Philadelphia, and has come to the conclusion that, for this city—as for all cities—it is important that sewage shall not be poured into the rivers from which the drinking water is obtained, and that the latter should be filtered to free it from solid matters held in suspension in it.

203. Dr. Miller describes two cases of bone repair occurring in his practice, in one of which the cavity of an involucrum of the tibia seemed to become filled with bony tissue, while in the other a button taken by trephining from the lower jaw bone, after removal of the periosteum, became consolidated when restored to its former position, although rotated through an arc of ninety degrees.

204. Dr. McMurtry describes a case in which opening the abdomen and washing out the peritoneal cavity led to great and long continued amelioration in the condition of a woman whose peritoneum was found to be studded with tubercles, and another in which he removed the ovaries and an offensive blood clot. Both patients are examples of the advantages of laparotomy in the treatment of peritonitis, when done according to the methods now approved by the best surgeons.

205. Dr. McMurtry reports the case of a physician upon whom he performed a laparotomy, and found two gangrenous perforations of the cæcum. These he treated by trimming their edges and suturing them. The patient made a good and uninterrupted recovery. The history of this case is well described, and is of exceptional interest, because the case is the first on record of such an operation for the relief of non-traumatic perforation of the cæcum.

LITERARY NOTES.

—A new German medical journal has just been started in New York, with the title *Medicinische Monatsschrift.* The first number is dated January, 1889, and contains 56 octavo pages of reading matter. It is edited by Dr. A. Teibert, and published by the Medical Monthly Publishing Company. The January number contains a good deal of interesting reading. The Editorial entitled "Unsere Berechtigung" has a boastful tone which we hope to see modified; but the magazine as a whole has a strong and incisive character, and is both interesting and instructive.

CORRESPONDENCE.

"Good Form" in Doctors' Cards.

To the Editor.

Sir: Will you kindly say what is good form for the cards of physicians, both for office and social use? Should either contain "M.D.," and if the doctor is "F.R.C.S." may the letters follow his name? If "M.D." may be used, may "(Jefferson)," "(Univ. Penna.)" or "(Harv.)" follow? May the visiting card contain the office hours? I do not wish to start a discussion, but to know the usage of the *élite* in the profession.

Yours truly,
Country Doctor.

[The visiting cards of physicians are usually engraved with the full name preceded by the letters *Dr.* and with the street address in the lower right hand corner. Business cards are rarely used by physicians in the city; but when used they ought to bear the address and office hours.

It is not usual to have a visiting card contain any titles except as stated above. Business cards may contain the letters referred to, or others of like character, or the abbreviation for the place of graduation in medicine.—Ed. Reporter.]

Advertisement of a Physician.

To the Editor.

Sir: Herewith I send you an exact copy, *verbatim et literatim* (except name) of a card which is being circulated *in extenso* by a young would-be disciple of Æsculapius, and his agents, at various places in the neighborhood, more especially at church.

Dr., What Is Your Bill?
Visits . . . . 75 cents
Plus 15 cents per mile and first cost of medicine.
Obstetrics : $5.00, and two extra visits.
Consultation . , ... $5.00
One dollar extra is charged for the night.
——, M.D.

This is certainly as unique as it is indefinite, and a good specimen for your "curiosity box," as showing one of the means of advertising which may be resorted to by the unscrupulous, in an extremity. It is perhaps proper to state, in justice to the character of the Greene County Medical Society of Pa., that the author of the card is not a member, although a resident of said county.

Yours truly,
Regular.

Greene Co., Pa.,
Jan. 19, 1889.

Typhoid Fever, its Care and Treatment.

To the Editor.

Sir: The communication of Dr. B. M. Smith, of Parsons, W. Va., in the Reporter, Dec. 17, 1888, regarding his experience with typhoid fever leads me to make the following remarks as to the proper management of cases of this disorder. The first step should be a free and thorough disinfection of every house where there is a case of the fever, while especially care is taken to render the dejecta innocuous. The general treatment of the patient should consist in sponging, once in twenty-four hours with a weak solution of permanganate of potash—about a violet color; of course tepid water is desirable, as it is more agreeable to the patient. The medical treatment is not of much importance, and is simple in application. First, of the patient. To reduce the temperature, the administration of three or four doses of eight or twelve grains of antipyrin usually has the desired effect. Then the following has proved very satisfactory in my hands.

R   Tr. Iodi . . . . f℥iii
    Ac. carbolic . . . . f℥ii
· Sig. Three drops in a tablespoonful of water every two hours.

If there is any malarial complication, I frequently combine, in pill form, the following :

R   Quininæ sulph. . . . . gr. xxiv
    Acidi arseniosi . . . . gr. i
    Ferri carb. . . . . · . . gr. xxiv
M. Div. in pil. No. xvi.
Sig. One every three or four hours.

The employment of the latter prescription is seldom required, the carbolic acid and iodine, when employed with plenty of cold water to drink and judicious feeding, is probably all the treatment that a typhoid patient will require. Dr. Da Costa lays much stress on the early morning food; he advocates plenty of milk, broths, beef-tea, etc., and says they must be given *early* in the *morning*, say at two or three o'clock A.M. I have found this early morning feeding to be of incalculable benefit. In the later stages, during the third or at the beginning of the fourth week, the heart will be found weak and crippled from excessive work. So lame will this organ become sometimes that it will intermit in its systolic effort, dropping one beat in three, thus claiming eight hours of rest in the twenty-four. The pulse may be found very weak and intermitting, probably imperceptible at the wrist. The heart flutters and apparently is about to stop. In this condition no time should be wasted, lest the patient die. This heart must have a crutch to hobble on, and that crutch is alcohol; and whiskey is probably the best form in which to administer it. The quantity must be regulated by the effect. Thus, with the temperature under control, plenty and suitable liquid food at the proper time, and the heart sustained with alcohol, there need not be much fear regarding the prognosis.

Yours truly,
J. C. Ellis, M.D.
Philadelphia,
January 18, 1889.

Heroic Method of Removing Gunpowder from the Face.

To the Editor.

Sir: On the evening of November 10, 1888, a boy, 12 years old, came into my office with his face looking hideous by having a few moments before had gunpowder blown into it. Having always failed with the ordinary means, recommended and used in such cases, to obtain pleasing results, I decided to do nothing until festering had taken place, and then vigorously to rub it out with a very coarse towel wet with warm water. This, at the expiration of twenty-four hours, I satisfactorily accomplished in about ten minutes, and to-day there is hardly a vestige or mark of powder to be seen on the boy's face. I report this method of treatment because I have never read or heard of its being used before.

Yours truly,
John Gray, M.D.
Mystic River, Conn.

—The *Ledger*, January 15, 1889, says that an opinion has been rendered in the case of Frank H. Dent, plaintiff in error, against the State of West Virginia. Dent was convicted of unlawfully engaging in the practice of medicine without a diploma, in violation of a statute of the State. Dent appealed to the State Court of Appeals, asserting that the act was unconstitutional, inasmuch as it deprives him of liberty and property without due process of law, contrary to the Fourteenth Amendment to the Constitution. The Court of Appeals gave judgment against Dent and the Supreme Court has affirmed that decision.

NOTES AND COMMENTS.

Hemorrhagic Variola.

In a communication in the *Archives générales de Médecine*, Dec., 1888, F. de Grandmaison gives an interesting account of hemorrhagic variola as observed in Paris in 1887. After remarking that the cases of hemorrhagic variola were furnished by the most infected quarters of the city, he states that there are two forms of this variety of smallpox, differing both in their symptoms and in their terminations. One is relatively benign; this he designates as cutaneous hemorrhagic variola. The hemorrhages take place only into the pustules; the general symptoms are not grave and improve in a few days; the eruption is discrete, the suppuration is slight, and the termination rarely in death.

The other form is grave, almost fatal. It is characterized by multiple, profuse, repeated hemorrhages; by marked general symptoms, which grow progressively worse; by very characteristic visceral complications; by a rapid course and generally fatal ending. This is true hemorrhagic smallpox. The physician should always have in mind these two forms of hemorrhagic variola, so as to be guarded in his prognosis, and not be exposed to unfortunate surprises.

Antipyrin in the Pains of Labor.

Auvard and Lefebvre have been unable to convince themselves of the far-famed action of antipyrin in the pains of labor. They tried it in ten cases in the maternity of the Paris Charité. Only three patients showed the effect of antipyrin; of these a marked relief was produced in one, and a slight relief in two cases; in seven the effect was *nil*. The solution used by them is as follows:

Antipyrin . . . . gr. cviii
Muriate of cocaine . . . . . gr. iss
Distilled water . . . . . . f℥ v

A syringeful, containing four and one-half grains of antipyrin, was injected three or four times.

In reviewing this experience, a writer in the *Wiener med. Presse*, Nov. 11, 1888, remarks that in a case of his own fifteen and one-half grains of antipyrin internally and the same amount hypodermically had not the slightest influence upon the intensity of the labor pains.

Care of the Insane in Pennsylvania.

That portion of Gov. Beaver's message which condemns the policy of sending the indigent insane from county almshouses to State asylums is being severely criticized, especially in this Western part of the State. The remedy he recommends—that of returning this class of insane to the county institutions and suggesting that the Board of Charities be empowered to insist on the proper maintenance of them, does not meet with the general approbation of persons interested in that branch of charity.

A remedy for the overcrowded condition of Dixmont, the State asylum in this portion of the State, has been suggested and is embodied in a bill which is being drafted under the supervision of Chief Elliott, of the Department of Charities. This bill which will be introduced into the Legislature at an early day will provide for the erection of a hospital for the insane, to be located in this county, and to be for the use of the contiguous counties of Beaver, Lawrence, Washington and Butler. The idea is to accommodate the indigent insane in this institution, and thus relieve Dixmont, which at present is overcrowded and cannot admit any more patients. This bill is gotten up for the relief of the poor insane whose friends are not able to support them in private asylums, and for whom there is no room in State institutions. It is a humanitarian move, as the fact can not be disputed that cases of this class can not be properly treated in a county or township home. The facilities of treatment in almshouses are very limited, and justice cannot be done the patients.

This bill will be supplemented by another now in course of preparation, or it may be that the two will be merged into one. The last bill recommends the erection of a hospital in the western part of the State for the maintenance of acute, or curable, cases of insanity. The object is to remove all cases of this class from the present State institutions and leave the latter solely for the accommodation of chronic cases. By so doing, and with proper arrangements, which will be specified in detail in the bill, the acute cases can receive immediate and positive attention from experts, and every facility offered that would tend to their rapid restoration to reason. Both these bills are intended as a remedy for the present state of affairs which is lamented by the Governor, and for which he proposes the relief mentioned above.—*Pittsburgh Commercial Advertiser*, Jan. 7, 1889.

Solidified Petroleum Fuel.

According to the *Revue Scientifique*, the problem of reducing petroleum to a solid state, available for practical purposes, has been solved by Dr. Kauffman, who has followed up the experiments made in the United States with the admixing of soap. He heated the liquid, to which from one to three per cent. of common soap had been added, half an hour, until the soap was completely dissolved, when the mixture acquired the consistency of tallow. The article thus obtained may be cut into pieces of suitable size for feeding to furnaces. Solidified petroleum, although it does not kindle readily, burns slowly and steadily and without smoke. The residual ash amounts to only two per cent. The combustion is only one third as rapid as that of an equivalent of anthracite coal, while the amount of heat evolved is more intense.—*Sanitarian*, Oct., 1888.

Absolute Signs of Death.

At the meeting of the Medical Society of London, December 10, 1888, Dr. B. W. Richardson read a paper on the absolute signs of death, which he took up in the following order: 1. Respiratory failure, including absence of visible movements of the chest, absence of respiratory murmur, and absence of watery vapor from the breath; this test is, he said, a fallacious one, for apparent movement and murmur might be absent, and the mirror test is useless. 2. Cardiac failure, including absence of arterial pulsation, of cardiac motion, of cardiac sounds, and absence of turgescence, or filling up of the veins on making pressure between them and the heart. The pulse as a sign is of more value than the cardiac motion or sounds, and yet even it may be undetectable, although the body may be alive and capable of recovery. He had written a paper some time ago on the maintenance of life when the circulatory apparatus was working at low pressure. An animal under chloroform may pass into this condition, the heart being only partially filled and emptied at each beat, and yet this partial action is sufficient to keep the animal alive, though scarcely any of the signs of life may be manifest. This cataleptic, syncopal, or hibernating condition is seen in animals while in a state of suspended animation. The proof by pressure on the veins was one not likely to deceive. A band should be bound round the wrist, a cardboard being arranged in front so as to relieve the arteries from pressure.

If life were not extinct, turgescence of the dorsal veins of the hand would soon be apparent. 3. Reduction of the temperature of the body below the natural standard. A diminution of a few degrees does not signify death, as recovery has taken place even after a falling of the temperature to as much as 7° F. below normal. A fallen temperature as a proof of death should always be considered only in combination with others. If the temperature within the mouth were found lower than that of the surrounding atmosphere, it would be a strong presumptive sign of death. 4. Presence of rigor mortis and muscular collapse. Rigor mortis may be imitated by rigidity from cold or by tetanus, but the history will distinguish, and tetanic spasm produces distortion of the limbs. 5. Coagulation of blood in the veins. This, when present with rigor mortis, is an absolute sign of death, but both may be absent for even a long period. 6. Presence of putrefactive decomposition. Its presence in the eyeball indicates certain dissolution; but it is not in all animals an invariable sign of death, for frogs have been kept by amyl in a state of suspended animation until the web of the foot had commenced to decompose, and yet the animal has recovered. 7. Absence of red color in semi-transparent parts under the influence of a powerful light, such as that from a magnesian lamp. 8. Absence of muscular contraction under the stimulus of an electric or galvanic current. The handiest apparatus for this test is a small Faradic battery, and needles should be thrust into the muscles of the forearm. 9. Absence of a red blotch under the skin after the subcutaneous injection of ammonia. This test the author looked on as especially valuable. 10. Absence of signs of rust—oxidation—of a bright steel needle after plunging it deep into the tissues. This test is only of value for a short time after death, as later rust will follow from oxidation of the needle by the acid products of decomposition.

In the last part of his paper Dr. Richardson indicated the precise mode in which the practice named should be directly applied, taking up the steps of the necessary examinations one by one, pointing out the relative values of each, and giving, so to speak, in a condensed form, the diagnostic formula for an absolute proof of death in every doubtful case, without any operative procedure that was itself inimical to life. He recommended the practical application of tests in the following order :

1. Apply the fillet to the wrist and examine the veins at the back of the hand. 2. Open a vein at the bend of the elbow and seek for stringy coagula; open, if necessary, two or more veins. 3. Apply the electric test. 4. Inject ammonia hypodermically. 5. Examine by strong light for absence of red color from the transparent tissues. 6. If any doubt still remained, and rigor mortis had not developed, let the body be kept in a damp room at 84° F.; this would speedily bring about decomposition if the body were dead, and would favor recomposition or restoration if life were not extinct. This last test had the great recommendation that it could be carried out in those cases where it was forbidden to touch the body.

Dr. C. H. F. Routh said he had observed in persons dying from pneumonia, especially if the disease were double, a remarkable preservation of natural color. He referred to a case under his care in which, after death following ovariotomy, the temperature went up to 111°, two degrees higher than it was immediately before death. Speaking of post-mortem movements, he referred to the custom at Vienna of placing a bell-rope in the hand of the corpse; the bell had only been rung once, and that was after death from Asiatic cholera. In catalepsy some amount of respiration went on, and the limb, if put in an extraordinary position, remained so; he found that a blow upon the spine brought these patients round. In deaths from lightning, he was under the impression that the electric fluid usually made a mark of entrance and of exit, and that the blood remained fluid. —*Lancet*, Dec. 15, 1888.

Infanticide in China.

The *Sei-I-Kwai Medical Journal*, of Tokyo, Japan, publishes in its September issue the following account of infanticide in China, which shows a lamentable prevalence of the crime: In a series of papers on infanticide in China, read at a meeting of the North China Branch of the Royal Asiatic Society in Shanghai on May 14, 1885, Dr. Edkins and Mr. Balfour both allude to a bullock cart which perambulates the city, collecting the corpses of infants for burial. It is extremely difficult to obtain accurate information upon any subject in China, and the particulars given concerning the details of this charity vary with each informant, but the following may be taken as a fairly correct account of the matter: Except in the more respectable families with some money to spare, it is considered useless extravagance to bury with any formalities a child under ten years of age, and going lower in the scale we find that infants of the poor are often simply thrown out into the fields or canals, where they are at the mercy of dogs, instead of being properly interred. To meet this distressing state of things, at any rate inside Peking, there are two carts in connection with the Imperial Foundling Hospital, which make daily rounds to collect the little corpses for burial in ground set aside for that purpose. Each cart has its district, one for the East city and one for the West, which it visits daily. Here it may be well to mention that some informants state that there is only one cart actually, which visits different parts of the city in turn. The carts are each drawn by a bullock and driven by an old man—the object being that they should move slowly and reverently. They always take the right of way as being Imperial equipages, and everyone, even high officials, must yield the road to them—which most people are only too glad to do, especially in hot weather. They are the ordinary travelling carts with the cover, which in their case is black, and are known as "compassionate dry land ferry," being an allusion to the ferry "in which Kwan-yin carries souls to rest." Outside each gate are established stopping-places, generally in connection with a temple, where the bodies are brought by women to await the cart, which carries its pitiful freight to cemeteries outside the Southeast and Southwest corners of the city. These burial grounds are either Imperial property or the gift of the charitable. The person bringing a corpse to the Niu ch'e Fang pays 400 cash. The bodies are sewn up neatly in matting, or very occasionally enclosed in a rude coffin. They are not buried separately, but in a common grave. It occasionally happens that a cry reveals the fact that a little one is not dead, in which case it is taken to the Foundling Hospital, where its life hangs on a very slender thread, unless it is speedily adopted. The most significant fact in connection with the institution is that *no examination is made of the bodies*, a startling proof that whether infanticide does or does not exist to any great extent, the Government does not regard it as a matter of the slightest consequence. As for the quantities buried no statistics are obtainable, but the cart has been seen crammed full of these abortive attempts at increasing the population, even the rest at the back being piled high with the little packages.

Pseudo-scientific Humbuggery.

In a letter to *Science*, December 7, 1888; Charles F. Cox, of New York, says:

The more mysterious a thing is, the more do ignorant people think they know about it. The learned man alone recognizes the limitations of his knowledge. On our maps the thoroughly explored regions have strict boundaries: only the *terræ incognitæ* shade off into infinity.

Now, of all the uncertain subjects at present passing under scientific scrutiny, the etiology of infectious and contagious diseases is probably the most occult; but, for this very reason, it offers irresistible attraction to all sorts of rash theorizers. At the same time, the excitement occasioned by the visit of an awful plague, like yellow fever, discloses a ready soil of credulity for the reception of every wild dogma, and starts into life the germs of superstition everywhere lying dormant in men's mental substratum. If you care to see how charlatans take advantage of such a concatenation of circumstances, you have only to walk through upper Broadway, and drop in at the headquarters of a certain "microbe-killer," which you will have no difficulty in finding. Even if the proprietor's explanation of his wonderful invention does not strike you as being altogether lucid and ingenuous, you will surely be impressed with his apparent knowledge of and faith in human nature, as shown in the certainty with which he reckons upon a paying market for his extraordinary nostrum. This is evinced also by the fact of his occupying a conspicuous place of business, for which I suppose he has paid a good rent, and, perhaps even more indisputably, by his having risked the expense of a two-column advertisement in one of the daily papers a few weeks ago. The astonishing effrontery of that advertisement is manifested, not only in the ingenious nonsense put forth as a history of the alleged discovery, but also in the impressive pictures with which the highly imaginative article is adorned. These profess to be likenesses of the "deadly microbes" for which the infallible "killer" has been providentially provided. Of course, there is not a microbe among them. They are, however, with one exception, rude reproductions of photographs of diatom valves. The exception is a representation of a part of the tracheal system of a butterfly or moth. . . .

It is the greatest shame of these impositions under the guise of science that professional men of some reputation at times lend them their countenance and aid. And, even when the thing recommended is not itself fraudulent, the mode of indorsing it often becomes so. An example of this came under my notice not long ago, when, in looking over a newspaper, my eye was caught by the word "microscopical" occurring in a rather prominent advertisement of a certain soap, and upon examination I found that a gentleman of scientific claims had undertaken to give a certificate to the merits of the article advertised. Now, soap seems to be a thing about which comparatively little can be said from a sanitary point of view, except that a free use of it is desirable. But in the testimonial of which I am speaking there was manifested a wide-awake disposition to make the most of the passing public interest in infection and contagion. With remarkably lame logic, the scientific attorney of the manufacturer declared, in substance, that, having submitted the soap to microscopical examination, and having found it free from disease-germs, he was prepared to recommend it for its detergent qualities.

While we do not wonder to see a Wiggins rush forward, upon the very slightest excuse, as he did but lately, with a sixteenth-century astrological theory of yellow fever, we cannot but feel both astonishment and mortification when a good chemist publicly dispenses bad microscopy, or an eminent physicist plunges headlong into hygiene and therapeutics, as one did the other day. A man may have almost superhuman insight as to the laws of electricity and yet be as ignorant as the rest of us about the how and why of a bacillus or a spirillum. It was not very strange that a gentleman hitherto absorbed in physics and mechanics should prove to be uninformed as to the unsuccessful endeavors that had been made to isolate and identify the microbe of yellow fever, for he had come across-lots into a scientific region of which the literature and even the language was unfamiliar to him. For the same reason, how was he to know that what would kill an ant would not necessarily kill a bacterium or a vibrio?

The trouble is, that a large part of the people who are most ready to discuss the new phase of biological science have not the faintest idea of what a microbe is. Most of them seem to fancy that merely a new name has been invented for what used to be called a spore or a germ; and of course everyone knows what a germ is, for he has only to look at the seed of any well-known plant! This seems to be the difficulty with a famous military commander who has recently taken up the weapon more powerful than the sword, and, by means of it, given to the world, through one of our magazines, his *a priori* exposition of the mode of origin and spread of epidemic diseases. He may fairly claim experience in keeping yellow fever out of a community, but, after reading his article, we may well doubt whether he really has much information as to how it gets in.

In short, pseudo-scientific humbuggery is very prevalent just now; but I suppose we may console ourselves by regarding it as a popular tribute to the worth of true science, since we are told that "hypocrisy is a sort of homage that vice pays to virtue."

Medical Missions in the East.

In an interesting article in the *Sunday School Times*, Jan. 12, 1889, Dr. George E. Post, of Beirût, Syria, says:

A few years ago the illustrious Abd-el-Kadir, the Algerine hero who saved thousands of Christian lives in Damascus at the time of the massacres, was taken ill. I was sent for to attend him, and succeeded, by a surgical operation, in relieving his sufferings and prolonging his life. Since that time his eldest son has been under my care, and thus an influence secured in one of the most powerful families of the East. I shall never forget the evening when the success of the operation gave relief to the obstruction under which he was sinking. His large harem was assembled under the windows of his suburban home near Damascus. It was an early evening hour, and, by the faint moonlight, their sheeted forms could be seen, like ghosts, among the trees of the garden. When the news of the relief experienced by the aged prince was sent down to them, they set up a shout of triumph and thanksgiving which echoed far away among the chalk cliffs of the Abana valley, and then crowded around the door to catch up and transmit each item of encouragement, while the noble sufferer threw his arms around my neck, and kissed both cheeks, in token of his gratitude.

It would be easy to prolong this list by adding the names of governors and mayors, and military commandants, and even the ecclesiastical dignitaries of the Christian and Jewish and Mohammedan and Druze and Mutawâli sects; kadis, muftis, zaptiehs, sheiks, pachas, rabbis, bishops, patriarchs. To name them all would possibly seem like egotism, and would only confirm the fact insisted on at the outset, that the medical man has access to those whom no other can reach.

Let it not, however, for a moment be supposed that the writer, or any missionary, attaches too much importance to the high station of some of his patients. Even as the result of medical evangelism, "not many wise, not many noble, not many mighty," are called. It is from the weak ones, the lowly classes, that God constructs his kingdom. But here the same principle obtains. The medical man can enter *by invitation* doors that would be slammed in the face of any other missionary. Nay, the candidates for healing come from all parts. I have just discharged a patient from the hospital, who walked from Mosul to receive treatment. Forty days' journey on foot did not discourage him from seeking and finding relief. They come from Tartary and the Sahara, from Arabia and Asia Minor, from Palmyra and Bagdad. On any clinic day the dispensary ministers to people of a dozen nationalities and creeds; and at the hospital service these patients hear the gospel, which no other influence could bring to bear on them. The power which the medical man has over the great ones of the earth gives him influence over the feeble. His reputation as the counselor of princes, the guest of Pharisees, the healer of kings, the friend of priests and bishops, is the substratum on which he builds his influence with the outcasts and the oppressed. Picturesque as is medical work among the lordly in their castles, the power of the healing art is in the cabins of the poor, in the halls of the dispensaries, and the wards of the hospitals. A commodore of the United States Navy, who did not believe in missions, once told the writer that there was one sight which impressed him as the most Christ-like he had ever witnessed. It was a medical missionary, in his dispensary in Singapore, toiling all the morning long with those wretched outcasts, in the stifling air of a pest-stricken city, and all for the love of Christ. Against such an exhibition of unselfish benevolence no cavil can be brought. And the same effect is produced on the native mind. Such a service, so above all that their religions can match, so without precedent or basis in their own experience, is from another world. They are accustomed to see Europeans and Americans as conquerors, as seekers after commercial gain, as travelers searching for knowledge or pleasure, but here are persons who offer them a living demonstration of the Golden Rule, and although using science and art, yet using them under the inspiration of a purpose from on high.

Phenacetin.

Pesce has communicated to the Royal Academy of Turin some clinical observations upon phenacetin. It effects pronounced and lasting fall of temperature and has a favorable influence upon the general condition of the patient. This fall and the subsequent rise of temperature occur nearly always slowly and gradually. Seven and a half grains usually produces a fall of two or three degrees C. ; this dose should be given once. The fall of temperature usually occasions no disagreeable. or dangerous symptoms, apart from perspiration, which is never copious.

Phenacetin also possesses a powerful antirheumatic action; it suppresses the fever and the pains in the joints, lessens the feeling of oppression, and makes the movements of the joints freer. It also exerts a favorable influence upon apyretic rheumatism, but upon the disease process itself it has no effect. It is of service as an analgesic in neuralgia, headache, migraine, and conditions of irritation of the sensory nerves. As a rule, seven and a half grains are sufficient to cause disappearance of the pain ; where it is necessary this dose can be repeated after two or three hours. In disturbances arising from compression or from anatomical or functional lesions of the nerves, such as neuritis, fifteen and a half grains must be employed, and repeated if necessary.—*Deutsche med. Wochenschrift,* Dec. 6, 1888.

Is Instrumental Delivery a Cause of Idiocy?

Drs. Winkler and Bollaan have written a paper in a Dutch medical journal on "The Forceps as a Cause of Idiocy." They mention a case of bilateral, almost symmetrical, damage to the cortex of the brain, found in an idiot. The boy had been born with the aid of forceps. Only part of the vertex could be examined. There were no marks of the forceps, yet there were strong reasons for belief that the injury was caused by them. In another case there was still more ground for the opinion that injury had been caused by forceps. In this child, who was an idiot from birth, there were marks of the forceps on both sides of the skull corresponding almost exactly to the damage done to the brain. This coincidence was too remarkable to be accidental. Drs. Winkler and Bollaan performed necropsies on ten idiots, and examined twenty-five living idiots, of whom six had bilateral depressions in the skull. Another case was that of a woman born with the aid of forceps, an inmate of the Utrecht Asylum for four years. She was very short, being only 1.27 metres high, and small in proportion. She could make all movements, isolated movements being difficult to her. There were but two words which she could say, and she never gave any sign of understanding what was said to her. She died at the age of sixty, and at the necropsy the brain was found to be very small, weighing only 742 grammes (31½ oz.). All the organs at the base of the brain, the optic nerves, olfactory nerves, etc., were found to be very small. Deep depressions were found on either side of the sagittal suture, the right side being the more indented. The depth of the depression was two millimetres, and its greatest breadth twelve millimetres. The brain was much atrophied. The authors believe that depressions of the skull caused by instrumental delivery, even when no fracture occurs, tend to damage the cortical substance of the brain, and that this leads to general atrophy of the hemispheres, thus producing idiocy. They are disposed to think that the use of forceps is much more frequently the origin of idiocy than is generally supposed.—*Lancet,* Jan. 5, 1889.

A Doctor's Perilous Experience.

On the night of Wednesday, January 9, 1889, the suspension bridge just below the Falls of Niagara was blown away in a terrific windstorm. It is not known that any one was upon it at the time ; but the last man to cross it before its fall was a physician. Dr. J. M. Hodge, of Niagara Falls, N. Y., started across the bridge about midnight on his return from visiting a patient on the Canadian side. Believing the bridge to be perfectly safe, he started without any fear. When but a short distance from the Canadian side he realized that something was wrong. As he neared the centre he was obliged to get down on his hands and knees and creep along. At times he did not dare to move. The bridge, he says, rocked like a boat in a heavy sea, and at times it seemed to tip up almost on its very edge. Not for an instant did the Doctor dare let go the iron railing, but he found several places where it was bent so that he was obliged to feel his way around.

There was no light on the bridge, the night was very dark, and, to add still further to his discomfiture, great volumes of spray from the Falls swept over the bridge, drenching him to the skin. The wind actually tore open the struggling physician's overcoat. At that hour evidently the shore guys were broken, for the Doctor could hear them flapping, and the bridge must have first begun to give way about that time.

___

Electricity for Executions.

The correspondent of the Philadelphia *Ledger* writes from New York, under date of Jan. 6, that it is not unlikely that, at the present session of the Legislature, the law which went into effect the first day of the year, providing for the execution of murderers by electricity, will be repealed, or the time extended for its going into effect. It is not altogether sure, he says, that executions by electricity can be made without pain or mutilation. Electricians are divided on the subject, and the majority seem to be opposed to the law. It is noticeable that every electrical journal opposes the electrical method of execution as inexpedient and inhuman, and in a recent address Professor Brackett, of Princeton College, spoke of execution by electricity as an outrageous thing and the degrading of a noble agent to an ignoble use.

___

"The American College of Health and Vitapathic Institute."

The great need of effective State Licensing Boards is made apparent to everyone on reading such items as the following, which is taken from the Philadelphia *Ledger*, Jan. 25, 1889: "A man recently applied for registration as a practising physician to the Secretary of the Board of Health in Baltimore, exhibiting a document purporting to be a diploma issued by 'The American College of Health and Vitapathic Institute' of Cincinnati, J. B. Campbell, President (which, it is said, turns out doctors in five weeks). The caller was refused registration on his diploma, but he afterward showed a letter from J. B. Campbell, which said: 'Vitapathic Minister Physicians need not register; Health Boards have nothing to do with us, as we never let our patients die, but if they do, or will die, call in an M.D. in time.' The Secretary informed him that the laws of Maryland in regard to the practice of medicine are so loose, that almost any one can practice, but in the event of a patient dying the coroner would order an autopsy, and should any malpractice be revealed, the practitioner would be summoned before the Grand Jury."

A Three Thousand Dollar Prize Offered.

A committee of the Caspian Sea (Russia) fishing firms offers a prize of 5,000 roubles (nearly $3000 nominal) for the best pamphlet in English, French, German, Russian, or Latin on the subject of the nature of the poison which is formed in raw salted fish. The pamphlet should explain the physical and chemical nature of the poison; its effect (as demonstrated by experiments on animals) on the heart, the circulation of the blood, the digestive organs, and the nervous system; the time required for the absorption of the poison into the digestive organs; the methods by which contaminated fish may be distinguished from sound; the indication of means by which the development of the toxic elements can be arrested; and the indication of the antidotes and medical assistance required in cases of poisoning. Information may be had and answers should be addressed to the "Imperial Ministry of Domains, St. Petersburg."—*Chemist and Druggist*, Jan. 5, 1889.

___

The Hunt Memorial Hospital.

Dr. J. H. Hunt, of Port Jervis, N. Y., has erected a hospital in that town, in memory of his father, the late Dr. Isaac S. Hunt. The building, which is a three-story brick structure, contains a ward in which are ten beds, eight rooms for private patients, three offices, an operating room, a hall, a dining-room, and a kitchen. The hospital is intended for the reception of injured employés of the Erie Railroad and for the personal patients of Dr. Hunt. The sanitary arrangements and equipments of the building are all that could be desired for the comfort of patients.—*N. Y. Med. Journal*, Jan. 19, 1889.

___

The Philadelphia Hospital.

A bill has been introduced into the City Councils of Philadelphia providing for the setting aside of a certain portion of the House of Correction property for the erection of buildings to be occupied by the indigent poor of Philadelphia. This bill, if passed, will result in the very desirable separation of the Philadelphia Hospital and the Blockley Almshouse, the former of which is much over-crowded and should, moreover, be relieved from the stigma which intimate association with an almshouse imposes upon it.

NEWS.

—Small-pox is said to be epidemic at Azalia, Dundee and Milan, Michigan.

—It is reported that there are twenty-one cases of small-pox in Oberlin, Kansas.

—Scarlet fever and diphtheria are reported to be prevalent at College Point, New York.

—Eighteen cases of small-pox are reported from Milan township, Monroe county, Michigan.

—The Lehigh Valley Medical Association held a Winter Conversational Meeting at the Hotel Allen, Allentown, January 31, 1889.

—Dr. William Osler gave the first of three lectures on Cerebral Localization at the Orthopædic Hospital in Philadelphia, Jan. 19, and the second, Jan. 23.

—Dr. E. B. Brant, a well-known physician of Mechanicsburg, died Jan. 19, at the age of 60 years. He was graduated from Jefferson Medical College in 1855.

—The proprietors of the *Lancet* have set apart $1,500 to be used for the pecuniary assistance of medical men, and of their widows, orphans, or dependent relatives.

—Prof. L. B. How will deliver the next course of lectures on Anatomy at the Medical School of Maine, in place of Prof. Gerrish, who is in California recruiting his health.

—The clinical service at Vienna is said to be seriously embarrassed by the great number of students, native and foreign, and by the enormous increase of patients for consultation.

—At the festival *de Noël* Mme. Carnot sent to the Director of Public Assistance, of Paris, one thousand francs for the children of the hospital Trousseau, and the hospital for Sick Children.

—The hospital collections in New York, up to Jan. 16, amounted to $38,000. The Childs' Nursery and Hospital is said by the *Med. Record*, Jan. 19, to have realized $19,000 from the Charity Ball.

—Passed Assistant Surgeon W. G. G. Willson was found dead on the U. S. Receiving Ship St. Louis, at League Island, Philadelphia, Jan. 23. He is supposed to have died from the effects of a dose of chloral, which he had taken for insomnia.

—The *Lancet*, Jan. 19, announces that an International Congress of Physiology will be held at Basle, Sept. 10, 1889. The Congress will also embrace the subjects of anatomy, histology, physics, chemistry, experimental pathology and pharmacology.

HUMOR.

FEELING HIS OATS.—George—"I say, Gus, what's happened? You strut along the street as if you owned the whole city. Fallen heir to a fortune?" Gus—"No, but I've been dodging my tailor for eighteen months, and to-day I've got the money in my pocket to pay him."

THE EDITOR OF A RELIGIOUS PAPER in Michigan solemnly promised his subscribers that he would sample all the patent medicines offered to him by advertisers before he would insert the notices. This was four years ago. He is now an inmate of an inebriate asylum.—*Burlington Free Press.*

MORE PROTECTION WANTED.—(The effect of an editorial in a contemporary)—Workingman—"See here, I want protection." Great Statesman—"Certainly, certainly; you shall have it. What's the matter?" "Well, sir, some of these 'ere foreign doctors know so much that they keep folks alive too long. I want foreign doctors kept out o' this country. I'm a grave digger."—*Philadelphia Record (Dem.).*

BETTER THAN NOTHING.—Mr. Dickinson Compton says: A very handsome man, of large form, fell off the railway platform at Camp Hill, falling under the train, and had one thigh and the leg of the other below the knee completely smashed. He was brought to the General Hospital and both limbs were at once amputated. The patient gave me much anxiety; but he continued to live, the wounds healing well. I found he was engaged to be married to a very nice, respectable young woman, whom I found one evening sitting by his side. I said I thought she should think very seriously about her engagement, hinting that I thought it had better be broken off; but she most naïvely said: "Oh! sir, I am quite content to take the rest of him."—*Guy's Hospital Reports.*

OBITUARY.

JOHN M. JUNKIN, M.D.

Dr. John M. Junkin, of Easton, Pa., died of apoplexy Jan. 18, while in the office of the Adams Express Company. He was 67 years old and was well known throughout Eastern Pennsylvania. He was graduated from Jefferson Medical College in 1845. His father was President Junkin, formerly of Lafayette College. Dr. Junkin served during the war as surgeon in the Ninth, and later in the Fourth, Pennsylvania Cavalry. He recently returned to Easton, his former home, from Bucks county.

MEDICAL AND SURGICAL REPORTER

No. 1667.   PHILADELPHIA, FEBRUARY 9, 1889.   VOL. LX.—No. 6.

CONTENTS:

CLINICAL LECTURE.[1]

CASE I: CEREBRAL SYPHILIS; CASE II: ASTHMA CAUSED BY A FOREIGN BODY.

BY J. M. DA COSTA, M.D., LL.D.,

PROFESSOR OF THEORY AND PRACTICE OF MEDICINE IN JEFFERSON MEDICAL COLLEGE, PHILADELPHIA.

Cerebral Syphilis.

Gentlemen: The patient now before you (a man, about 40 years of age) you saw at our last meeting, when I read you his clinical history. Briefly, it was this: He had had frequently recurring attacks of convulsions, limited to the left arm, occasionally the right arm also would participate in the spasmodic movements, though not to the same degree. He never had general convulsions, and the lower extremities were never involved. These attacks were attended by vertigo and confusion of ideas. He had

[1] Delivered at the Pennsylvania Hospital, December 1, 1888.

constant tinnitus aurium, and in addition to the ordinary sounds of escaping steam and chiming bells, he heard sounds resembling a band of music and even human voices; all these being increased during and after the attacks, which came on several times a day before his admission. We ascertained that he had no paralysis of the extremities, and sensation is well preserved. He does not suffer with headache. He does not lose consciousness during the attack, and does not vomit. There is marked diminution of the power of hearing in both ears, but he is more deaf on the left side than on the right. His eyes were examined, and, beyond some error of refraction, nothing abnormal was found. There is no heart-lesion; and no albumin was detected in the urine.

In seeking an explanation of these symptoms, which I have briefly detailed to you, two possibilities are presented: in the first place, is this a tumor of the brain? In favor of this view, we have the convulsions limited to the muscles of the left arm. Limited convulsive movements point to an irritative cortical lesion, such as a tumor would

161

cause. The vertigo aggravated during the attacks, but occurred also at other times, is one of the symptoms of brain tumor. Then the deafness, unconnected with ear disease, and therefore central, might be caused by pressure of a new growth upon the auditory nerve. Why do we have the ear-affection upon the same side as that of the arm affected by convulsions? Because the law is that while a destructive lesion will cause paralysis upon the opposite side of the body, an irritative cortical lesion causes spasm upon the same side as that upon which it exists. But why does the right arm participate at times? I can only conclude that its movements are reflex. Brown-Séquard would have no difficulty in thus explaining it, because he believes that most of the phenomena of brain disease are due to the reflex action of one part of the brain upon another.

In spite of the reasons given for assuming that the symptoms are due to a cerebral tumor, I must decide against this view for several reasons. In the first place, the symptoms just mentioned are not sufficiently persistent. The symptoms of brain tumor are progressive, and constant. Moreover, one very prominent feature of cases of brain-tumor is entirely absent; he has no headache. He has no vomiting. Finally, the ophthalmoscopic examination does not show the choked disc which is so generally found in cerebral tumor. The report is that the eye-ground is quite normal, his ametropia being simply an ordinary fault of refraction which can be remedied by appropriate glasses.

The case not being one of tumor, my diagnosis would be disease of the brain or of its vessels, due to syphilitic infection: cerebral syphilis. His marked improvement since his admission a fortnight ago, while he has been taking a drachm of potassium iodide daily, would favor this view of the case. He has also had some bromide at night. He is doing well and has no vertigo at present, although he still has ringing in his ears. Standing or walking with his eyes closed, he gives no evidence of incoördination. He has not had a convulsive seizure since he was before you last; the treatment will be continued for the present.

[Feb. 1. The patient is still in the Hospital, but has very greatly improved.]

Asthma Caused by a Foreign Body.

The next case is peculiar and possibly unique in character. It is also one of convulsions, and therefore very properly discussed in connection with the preceding case, although it presents special features which are of more interest than the brain symptoms.

This boy, white, sixteen years of age, was admitted November 26, having been brought to the Hospital by the Police Patrol, who found him lying on the street in a fit, which was clearly epileptic in character. We learned that this boy received an injury by being struck with a brick on the left side of his head, about six years ago. He tells us that about two years after he was struck upon his head, convulsions came on. In spite of treatment, the convulsions persisted, and they became so frequent that he had to seek surgical advice. Two years ago, at the Hospital of the University of Pennsylvania, Dr. John Ashhurst trephined his skull at a point which can be still recognized; it is above and on a line with the left ear, at about the centre of the parietal bone, where a depression can still be felt. He says that, at first, no relief was obtained from the operation, but that lately there has been improvement; the convulsions now occur about once in three weeks; he had them sometimes twice a day before the operation. It is a fair inference that he was benefited by the operation, although he says that for about eighteen months there was no benefit, yet since that time he has markedly improved.

The special point to which I wish to ask your attention is this: On the 26th of November, the day he was brought into the Hospital, he had a fit or attack of convulsions upon the street, and became senseless. As he was recovering from the attack, he experienced great difficulty in breathing. When he came to the Hospital he was conscious, but was suffering intensely with difficulty in breathing. His respiration was labored and noisy, like that of asthma, and the expression of his face showed that he was laboring under great respiratory distress. He was seen by one of my colleagues, who happened to be present when he was admitted, and who kindly went into the ward and prescribed for the patient. Partly from his account and partly from that of the Resident Physician—for I did not see the patient until half an hour later, when he was somewhat relieved—we learn that the breathing was noisy, the inspiration weak, and the expiratory sound was prolonged. It was especially upon the left side that the expiratory sound was asthmatic; in fact, he presented the symptoms usually seen in a case of asthma. He was distressed and struggling for air; respiration labored, expiration very distinct and noisy. The heart rate was accelerated, but presented no signs of organic disease. He was ordered tincture of belladonna in ten drop doses with a little ammonia and subsequently ergot; and his chest was dry cupped. The prescriptions, all of which had for their line of thought the relief of spasm, were followed by great benefit. The breathing became better and easier, and he went to sleep. It looked as if all these antispasmodics had accomplished their work, and that the attack had passed away, when, about twelve hours after admission, during the night, he had a severe attack of dyspnœa with coughing, lasting about fifteen minutes, and, while the physician had gone for the laryngoscope, up came the piece of apple which I now show you. It is a little shrunken from the action of the alcohol in which it was placed for preservation, but it is still a piece of considerable size, longer than broad and irregular in shape. (It was about ⅞ of an inch in greatest length and about ½ by ⅝ in cross section.)

We then got this strange history that when the epileptic fit seized him he was eating an apple. During the convulsion this piece slipped from his mouth into his. windpipe, and owing to the insensibility during the attack it was drawn into the trachea and lodged below the bifurcation, obstructing the left bronchus rather more than the right, and thus explaining the difficulty in breathing. He subsequently had a severe attack of dyspnœa in the middle of the night, in which he nearly died, and which was terminated by the expulsion of the foreign body. He has since had no signs of asthma; but was allowed to continue taking bromides, simply with the view of preventing the recurrence of the epileptic fits.

There are several points of clinical interest in this case. One of these is the way in which the symptoms of spasmodic asthma were closely simulated by the presence of this foreign body in the trachea lying at its bifurcation into the bronchi, which caused intense distress and labored respiration. But what was curious, he had also the physical signs of asthma; intense dyspnœa, noisy breathing, prolonged expiration, and weak inspiration; the percussion note was clear. There were no rales in the finer tubes; but, with this exception, he had all the symptoms which we would expect to find in a case of asthma.

. Now what were these signs due to? A condition of spasm in the bronchial tubes.

Therefore, if I say that it is like a case of spasmodic asthma, I may go further and state that this foreign body provoked an attack of asthma. There is almost identity of pathological condition.

Again, as bearing upon this view of the case, look at the results of treatment! They were most remarkable, and I might say most decisive. If it had not been for our getting the piece of apple, it would never have been supposed that a foreign body in the air-passages had caused the symptoms.

From the free use of belladonna and free cupping, there was most evident relief; the spasm, which had been evoked by this foreign body, yielded, and the patient breathed more easily and even went to sleep. Therefore the means employed largely removed the irritation, notwithstanding the cause remained.

Lastly, I may call your attention to this fact, that this foreign body had passed beyond the trachea, because if it had lodged in the wind-pipe, it would have given rise to much greater difficulty in breathing, and would have impaired his voice. As you heard in his history, his voice was distinct, but was feeble on account of his respiratory distress. So that in the violent convulsion which came on while he was eating the apple, this piece was inspired into the larynx, which, owing to the insensibility produced by the convulsive attack, allowed it to pass into the trachea, and into the left bronchus just at the bifurcation, where it caused irritation and set up spasmodic asthma, due to a foreign body.

At present his breathing is easy and natural. Upon auscultation, the inspiratory sounds are well marked on both the right and left side; nor is the expiration either prolonged or abnormal in character. The same condition is found posteriorly as anteriorly. The breath-sounds are not quite so strong at the lower part of the left lung anteriorly as at the corresponding part of the right lung. The percussion note is clear. The heart, which was feeble, has regained its tone. There is nothing abnormal.

His temperature is rather low. On admission it was 98.6° (F.), and it has since declined. This morning it is 96.4°; his usual evening temperature is 97.8°. Possibly the morning temperature may be lower on account of being taken after his ablutions, but the evening temperature is also low; since admission it has not exceeded 98°.

He has been taking twenty grains of

potassium bromide three times a day; but considering that he has this tendency to coldness, we will give him aromatic spirits of ammonia, half a drachm (f℥ss) three or four times daily. He shall also take exercise in the open air, and he shall have a nourishing but not too stimulating diet.

---•••---

COMMUNICATIONS.

THREE REMARKABLE CASES OF REFLEX NEUROSES DUE TO EYE-STRAIN.

BY GEORGE M. GOULD, M.D.,
PHILADELPHIA.

There are some physicians who are at once seized with an acute attack of mental strabismus when they are told stories of peripheral irritation inducing functional disturbances, such as the following cases. The *superior oblique*, not the *internal rectus*, is the muscle affected. They distrust the Greeks even when bearing therapeutic gifts, and smile incredulously. For this reason I have hesitated to publish the notes of the following cases; but since the facts are well-known to several reputable physicians and may be substantiated at any time, and since, moreover, I believe all these cases range themselves under a common law that explains their apparent illogicality and makes them intelligible, I conclude it best to make them known to others.

Case I.—Chorea of Several Years' Duration Relieved at once by Correction of Ametropia.—Susie H., aged 14 years, came to me, Nov. 7, 1888, with the following history and complaints: Twitching of the right hand was first noticed two or three years ago, coming on without noticeable cause. Since then up to this date she has been treated for chorea at one of our best Hospitals for Nervous Diseases. She gets somewhat better during summer, but when school again begins, she gets worse. Latterly and just previous to coming to me, she had been having frontal headaches every day with attacks of giddiness or dizziness. Her mother and sister complain of her violent outbursts of temper. Sometimes, even in street-cars, and upon the slightest provocation she will burst out crying, or jump up and down and scream. The chorea, however, was the chief cause of complaint, and this seems to have continued during sleep, her sister being frequently disturbed or awakened by the jerking. The right shoe was worn out much

sooner than the left, and as the child sat before me the motions of the hand and foot were continuous and painful to see. Menstruation began three months ago, but certainly had not made the chorea any better. In the history of the case I particularly noted that there had never been any blepharospasm or tic of the face. The child was physically a robust, well-built young woman, otherwise in excellent health, without a sign of hysteria, and whose parents were likewise of non-neurotic healthy temperament. When she came to me she was taking twelve drops of Fowler's solution three times a day, which had been ordered by the physicians of the hospital. The arsenic had no evident effect upon the disease and the order was to increase the dose until certain well-known symptoms were noted, or until she became sick from the effects. Under a mydriatic I ascertained her refractive error to be alike in both eyes, and corrected it by the following combination of lenses: Sph. + 1.00 D. = Cyl. + 0.75 D. Ax. 90°. Spectacles were prescribed and the arsenic treatment wholly and suddenly suspended. Instead of the choreic symptoms being thereby increased, her sister a week later told me that she was no longer troubled by the child's movements at night. In fact the involuntary movements of both foot and hand slowly disappeared, so that in three weeks after the application of glasses none were noticeable. The headaches, etc., have disappeared and the disposition changed for the better. So far as the chorea is concerned, it does not exist to-day.

Case II.—Flatulent Dyspepsia of 20 Years' Standing Cured by the Application of Spectacles.—On Nov. 11, 1888, Mrs. E. G., aged 44, was kindly recommended to me by her physician, Dr. O. P. Rex, who had after oft-repeated advice, finally got her to consult an oculist. Her complaint was of certain ocular and cerebral troubles, asthenopia, difficulty in near work, etc. She had had headaches for most of her life. She did not complain to me of her gastric troubles, naturally thinking these had no connection with an oculist's work. But inquiry soon elicited the information that her flatulent dyspepsia ("wind-colic," as she called it) was her greatest trouble, and that her life for at least 20 years had thereby been rendered most wretched. At once upon entering I noticed the constant eructations which were very unpleasant and continuous. The knowledge of the fact of the disgust excited in others, together with the disease itself had rendered her very despondent and subject to melancholia. There were evident lassitude, prostration, a look of 'suffering in the countenance. She complained of a constant "load upon her stomach," and of loss of appetite, which .last had been a great cause of weakness and debility. In the past 20 years she had had the services of several excellent physicians and had taken a great deal of many different medicines, all without relief. The least conversation with the woman showed the complete absence of any hysterical element. She had healthy parents, and had been a plucky, hard-working woman all her life, enduring and fighting her affliction with a heroism that few would under like circumstances have shown.

I was put upon the track of my diagnosis by the following fact: When I put her in position to examine her eyes with the ophthalmoscope, the unpleasant eructations were as usual constantly taking place; but, upon throwing the light from the mirror full into the eye, such an instantaneous and frightful paroxysmal attack took place that I hastily ran for a vessel, convinced that violent emesis was taking place. But it was only flatus. A repetition of the attempt had the same result, and I had to give it up; but the thought at once came to me that I now had to do with a reflex neurosis. To be brief: I found her refractive error indicated by the following combination: For Distance:— R., Sph. — 0.25 D., = Cyl. + 0.75 D. Ax. 110°; L., Sph. — 0.25 D., = Cyl. + 1.00 D. Ax. 70°. The presbyopic correction was Sph. + 1.50 D. added to the above. It was highly interesting to notice that the application of the distant glasses, in the trial-frame, as effectually quieted the gastric volcano as the ophthalmoscopic mirror had previously aroused it. So long as the lenses were in place, no eructations took place; the effect was so pleasant she was unwilling to have them removed, but when this finally became necessary the eructations instantly recommenced. On November 24, having procured and worn the prescribed glasses *ad interim*, my patient returned, saying she had had none of her old symptoms during the time she had worn the glasses. I remarked a look of zest and happiness in her face in marked contrast to that of her first visit. Her appetite had greatly improved, the "load" had disappeared from her stomach; she had had no "belching"; the headache and the lassitude had disappeared; she had been heard to sing at her work, and all her friends remarked the change in her appearance. She said she could not leave the glasses off a minute without trouble. Without apprising her, I fixed her gaze upon small distant letters, so to put the accommodation to a tension, and, while thus looking, I suddenly raised the glasses away from her face, and like a flash the eructations broke forth. I dropped the glasses, and they disappeared. Here was evidently as pure an example of neurotic reflex as one could wish. The improvement in health and the complete absence of gastric, cerebral, and psychological symptoms continues up to the present time.

Case III. — Cardiac Palpitation, etc., relieved by Correction of Astigmatism.—I am indebted for the following notes to the courtesy of Dr. A. P. Brubaker, of Philadelphia, and Dr. Lewis H. Taylor, of Wilkesbarre, Pa. The patient was referred to me by Dr. Brubaker, but could not stop in Philadelphia sufficiently long to undergo examination and treatment of the eyes, which were carried out by Dr. Taylor.

Mrs. J. N., aged 24, married, without children, had 'enjoyed good health until during the summer of 1887, when, following a great deal of reading at night, she was troubled with severe pain and burning sensations in the eyes. Shortly after this, she began noticing how rapidly her heart was beating, and this symptom increased until the heart's action numbered as high as 130 strokes a minute. Then began a decline in health, with loss of appetite, feeble digestion and nervousness. She soon lost something over 20 pounds in body-weight. When seen by Dr. Brubaker in the spring of 1888, the rapidity of the cardiac action was still as great as ever, and slight cardiac enlargement was noted. She was placed upon the tincture of aconite for several weeks, without deriving any benefit from it. I should have added that treatment by other physicians prior to consulting Dr. Brubaker had also proved ineffectual in relief of the palpitation. On June 12, 13, and 14 Dr. Taylor tested the refraction, etc., of her eyes under atropia, and prescribed, for constant use, the following glasses: R. Cyl.— 0.75 D. Ax. 180°, ◯ Cyl. + 0.25 D. Ax. 90°; L. Cyl. — 0.75 D. Ax. 180°. Upon wearing the spectacles the rapid action of the heart began at once to subside, and within two or three months all the symptoms, ocular, cerebral and cardiac, had passed away, the heart's action had become entirely normal, the body had regained its entire loss of flesh, health, etc.

REMARKS.—To understand these cases and bring them under a common law we may be helped by likening the nervous system to the switch-board of a great telegraph-office. With every plug properly in place, every wire ends so that its messages are shunted to the proper table and operator and the out-going answers correspond to the call made. This corresponds to the physiological condition of the body when response is rightly co-ordinated to stimulus; when an outflow of saliva follows the placing of a sapid substance upon the tongue, when the capillaries expand by friction, when motion, secretion, etc., are the correspondent consequences of stimulus. If a careless or ignorant hand misplace a key of the telegraph switch-board there is chaos in the office, the messages do not reach the proper instruments, and replies are sent to the wrong far-away stations. Reflex neuroses are precisely such results in the body: the return messages do not reach the point of irritation, but some non-irritated organ which must then vicariously suffer for the sins of another.

Those who reluctantly admit the possibility of reflex neuroses, say that they cannot take place unless intermediated by centers in topographical proximity. They would say, for example, that an irritational strain of the oculo-motor could not result in choreic discharges from the phrenic or pneumogastric or cardiac centers, because of the distance of the "jump" or transfer. But may it not be that distance has little or nothing to do with the matter? This is not a saltation of the electric spark across a blank or insulated space. The number of associate fibers between centers is of course proportional to the functional relations of their peripherally located co-related mechanisms: but no center is wholly disconnected from any other, though the fact may not be anatomically demonstrated. The brain is certainly an organic unity and this is only possible by the means of myriads of commissural fibers proceeding almost everywhither and binding all ganglia together directly or indirectly. It is well established that chorea of the extremities may be caused by phimosis or other genital derangement, by a carious or impacted tooth, etc., etc., and yet the Rolandic centers are far-removed from those of the other organs. In place of topographical proximity, may there not be another law having a much more dominant power, that is, the law, or a corollary of the law, of the conservation of energy? Every irritational stimulus that from a peripheral organ proceeds inward may be viewed primarily in its dynamic aspect: it is force, and its function is to bring about another discharge of force whose nature and outgoing should correspond to the want indicated by the stimulus. If it is so correspondent, it is physiological; if it is not so, it is pathological, it is a reflex neurosis. But again this derouted discharge is also subject to the law that it must follow along the line of least resistance, and in accordance with this, its outlet will lead to those muscles and functions most easily moved. In irritational choreas the hand or foot or other small muscles are the most frequently set in motion. May it not be that sometimes when these channels become too small to drain off the overflow, other and greater centers are inundated, and that chorea thereby may even pass over into epilepsy? When slight irritational stimuli do not find such outlets, a general irritability and motility give vent and relief: a man with the toothache will walk the floor, a boy with "acute indigestion" will writhe and dance, a girl with eye-strain is restless and inattentive, etc. This overflow of unutilizable stimulus may according to peculiarities or habits become a tic, a strange habit of gesture, a chorea of the extremities, or, as it seems may have been true in my cases, what might analogically be called a chorea of the diaphragm, or a chorea of the cardiac muscle. But, whatever the explanation, such cases overlooked every day are doubtless more frequent than we suspect. This must be true when we think of the growing complexity of strain and nervous disease consequent upon our high-pressure civilization. Such deroutation and irregularity of outflow cannot help constituting in the future a prolific source of pathologic facts,—but a no less fertile source of brilliant therapeutics for the intuition and art sufficiently subtle and far-seeing to track out the hidden and distant *fons et origo mali.*

There can be no doubt that eye-strain is far above all others the one preponderant source of irritational neuroses. The incredulous smile at the hobby-riding specialist must give way to facts and the logic of facts. Here is a mechanism the most delicate, and moved by the slightest forces, of any in the organism; it is the most complexly constructed of all, its function most important of all and the most used of all; its nuclear associations are the most wide, intimate and direct with all other centers, and every process of thought or emotion is inextricably bound up with its functions and memories; language and intellect may be justly considered its products. And yet with all this, it must be remembered that within one or two centuries this wonderful mechanism is put to a strain for which it was never planned and to which in its evolution or history it has never been subjected. I allude, of course, to the persistent exercise at near range that is the necessary outcome of the art of printing, of schools, of commercialism, of urban life—in a word, of nineteenth century civilization. The natural eye is hyperopic and nature so forms it now. Ocular disease is growing as fast or faster than civilization. The sudden strain does not give time for the adaptation, even if one of these adaptations, myopia, be not a disease itself. If the naturally hyperopic eye, with nature's customary obstinacy persist in its hyperopia, and if in addition, corneal asymmetry (astigmatism) be superadded, even muscular insufficiency—then there can be but one result of the forced work at short range to which every servant of civilization is subjected. Unless every ametropic child have its ametropia corrected, either ocular disease, cerebral disease or reflex neurosis must ensue. This seems a certain result of the law of the conservation and equivalence of force. Pathology is but disordered, unregulated physics and physiology. In fact, the ophthalmic surgeon has not ridden his hobby half hard enough. He has been frightened by a sneer. If held "well in hand," his horse will not soon be winded. My own limited experience has convinced me that many general physicians are strangely obstinate in ignoring ocular strain, for years drugging their patients with bromides, iron and tonics, for cerebral or gastric derangements that disappear as if by magic when the eye-strain is relieved. Cases of tragic suffering due to such mistaken diagnoses are constantly turning up.

The cases I have described are all examples. Even where eye-strain is acknowledged to cause such neuroses, it is thought that several dioptres are necessary to set up the trouble. On the contrary, I have had cases where one-half and even one-fourth of one diopter is quite sufficient. Neither can such quantities be diagnosticated by the ophthalmoscope. To me the report from a hasty ophthalmoscopic examination that no eye-strain exists, is *per se* an evidence either of ignorance, or carelessness, or worse.

I have intimated that in my view the three cases described are essentially alike in cause and method of production: the chorea proper, the flatulent dyspepsia and the cardiac neurosis were all due to a peripheral irritation, eye-strain, that, derouted in its reflex course, returned somehow, directly or indirectly to other organs than to those concerned in the irritational stimulus. For other illustrations of this proceeding, see the excellent article of Professor Brubaker, *The Reflex Neuroses of Dental Pathology* in Lea's American System of Dentistry. There is no logical reason for limiting the term chorea to certain muscles, and a chorea of the diaphragm or of the heart muscle may prove as scientifically justified as one of the hand or foot.

As regards the details of the cases cited there is little to be objected to in the first case. It was a typical case of chorea, wholly uninfluenced by arsenic, and yielding quickly and completely when the irritational strain was removed. It may be said of the second case that too much is proved, because the 20 years of functional derangement must inevitably have set up organic changes that would not disappear in a day. I can only answer that the most brutal fact is worth more than the most beautiful theory; that the case is accurately reported; that a study of the symptoms, etc., seemed to show me that the gastric derangement was not due to imperfect secretion, was not chemical or organic, but was due to a spasmodic action of the diaphragm or of the muscular walls of the stomach. The fact, however, may bear other explanations, which I leave to others to give. As to the third case it may be true that the cardiac acceleration was due to a stoppage of the normal inhibition of its rhythm, and not to a positive increase of its innervation. In this case the force of the derouted reflex would find its own force neutralized in overcoming the cerebral inhibition.

—The *Ledger* says that Dr. Weisbach has been making careful measurements of the skulls of Beethoven and Schubert for the Vienna Anthropological Society. In his report he says that Schubert's skull, compared with measurements taken of 30 German-Austrian skulls, is slightly larger, longer and broader, but also somewhat flatter, than the average. Compared with Schubert's, Beethoven's face was altogether smaller, and much narrower between the cheek-bones, and especially about the lower jaw.

TECHNIQUE OF ABDOMINAL PALPATION.[1]

BY CHARLES P. NOBLE, M.D.,

PHILADELPHIA.

The following paper has been prepared as an addition to that on the "Value of External Examination in Obstetric Practice," which was presented to the Association September 26th, 1888, and published in the REPORTER, Oct. 20, p. 488. The request of some of the members is my excuse for bringing before you a brief and incomplete account of the technique of abdominal palpation—a subject which has been so ably presented to the profession by others, notably by Pinard. The subject of abdominal palpation as applied to the diagnosis of the presentation and position of the fœtus *in utero* only, will be considered.

Before proceeding to discuss the subject proper it will be well to recall certain physiological and mechanical facts which serve to render the results of palpation more exact, and at the same time more easy to attain.

It is now certainly known that while the head, breech or lateral plane of the fœtus may *offer* at the superior strait prior to labor, the vertex alone *engages*. The pains of labor are necessary to cause the engagement of the other presentations. The reason why only the vertex engages prior to labor is that the diameters of the vertex alone bear such a relation to the diameters of the pelvis as to make engagement possible, without the moulding effect of labor. It is also known that the head engages in a state of flexion—in obedience to the same law of accommodation which governs the attitude of the fœtus during pregnancy, and the imparted movements of the presenting part during labor. The knowledge of these two facts—that prior to labor, of the various possible presentations only the vertex engages, and that it engages in a state of flexion—is of immense importance in practising palpation. When the pelvic excavation is found full, that is, when the presenting part has engaged, we are at once assured that the vertex is presenting.

Since the vertex engages in a state of flexion, the occiput descends more deeply into the pelvis than the brow, and hence the brow is more accessible to the hand palpating from the abdomen; or, in other

words, when the two hands palpate the abdomen above the occiput and the brow, if both hands are depressed, the hand corresponding to the occiput will sink more deeply into the pelvis, before it is arrested by the resisting occiput, than will the one corresponding to the brow. A further point to aid in the differentiation is that the brow feels harder to the touch than the occiput does. This may be owing to the relative thinness of that part of the scalp which covers the brow, when contrasted with that which covers the occiput, or it may be due to the more advanced degree of ossification of the frontal bosses as compared with those of the occiput ; or, again, it may be that the greater accessibility of the brow makes it feel harder to the examining finger. I am inclined to believe that all three factors unite to create the difference in sensation imparted by touch. By thus discriminating between the brow and occiput, the position is determined.

It is important to know that the difference in the character of the articulations between the head and neck and the breech and trunk assists in differentiating between breech and head presentations in some cases. This differentiation is based on the wide range of mobility of the head, and the limited range of mobility of the breech. The head can be moved widely without disturbing the trunk, but it is not possible to move the breech independently of the trunk. Owing to these anatomical peculiarities the head can be ballotted, but the breech cannot. This cephalic *ballottement* can be obtained in head presentations (prior to engagement), in breech, and also in trunk presentations.

The thorough appreciation of these facts is of the greatest assistance in palpation. The practice, then, is based upon scientific data, and the method is rendered systematic and very uniform in its results.

The dress and position of the woman to be examined by abdominal palpation, are by no means matters of indifference. The less clothing worn, the better. Hence it is best to examine the patient in bed, and to see that she is clad only in her night-dress. When the skirts are simply pushed down below the nates, and the upper garments drawn up, to expose the abdomen, especially if corsets are worn, so much discomfort is caused that respiration is more or less disturbed, resulting in quickened respiration, which embarrasses the examiner.

The woman should occupy the dorsal decubitus, with the arms along the sides,

[1] Read before the Northern Medical Association, Dec. 14, 1888.

the thighs and legs extended, and the legs slightly separated. This allows the examiner to explore the false pelvis with ease, and the pelvic inlet with considerable facility. This position, which is that insisted on by Pinard, alone enables the examiner to explore the pelvic cavity. When the thighs are flexed upon the abdomen, and the legs on the thighs, the hypogastric region is so encroached upon by the thighs as seriously to embarrass the examiner in his manipulations, and even to prevent absolutely a satisfactory exploration of the pelvic cavity. The decubitus should be as nearly horizontal as possible—only a low pillow should be placed under the head. Occupying the horizontal decubitus, the woman has little temptation to contract the abdominal muscles, because no *point d'appui* is provided.

The bowels, and especially the bladder, should be emptied before beginning palpation. When the bladder is full the presenting part is inaccessible, and the sensations perceived are indefinite and untrustworthy.

The temperature of the room in which the examination is made should be such as not to chill the patient, who must lie with her bared abdomen exposed for some minutes.

The examiner's hands should be warm. It is well to wash the hands in warm water not only to secure the necessary warmth, but also to render the tactile perception more acute. Should palpation be attempted with cold hands, disappointment will surely result. The reflex contraction of the abdominal muscles from cold is prompt, and sometimes the shock causes the uterus to contract also—painless contraction of pregnancy.

Palpation can be practised only in the intervals between the contractions of the uterus; hence, when a contraction occurs during the examination, exploration must cease until this passes off. In practice this time can be usefully employed in listening to the fœtal heart-sounds, the location of which is of value in diagnosis, and the recognition of which establishes the fact that the fœtus is living.

While not strictly *apropos*, it is not unimportant to observe that the frequent recognition by the practitioner of these painless uterine contractions of pregnancy, during the routine examination of pregnant women, will effectually prevent such glaring errors in diagnosis as have occurred in the past, and are occurring even now. Were obstetric palpation generally practised, the pregnant womb would never be mistaken for a neoplasm, and unpremeditated Cæsarean sections would cease to occur.

With the foregoing principles in mind, and the conditions insisted on having been complied with, the examiner stands indifferently to the right or left of the woman, who is placed on a hard mattress sufficiently near the edge of the bed to be within easy reach. It is well to stand about opposite the umbilicus. Palpation is begun by estimating the thickness of the abdominal wall. This is done by picking up a fold between the thumb and fingers. The diagnosis of pregnancy having been established, it remains to determine the presentation and position of the fœtus. I have found it best to follow the teaching of Pinard, who examines after a uniform method, taking the bony pelvis of the woman as a fixed land mark. The horizontal rami of the pubes are sought for, and the hands, separated four or five inches, are placed upon the abdomen, the finger tips resting upon the upper margin of the pubic rami. This is easy under ordinary conditions, but when the abdomen is pendulous it is necessary first to raise up the sagging abdomen with the palms, before proceeding as indicated. The abdominal wall is then depressed from above downward and from before backward, the finger tips just grazing the pubic rami. The inlet of the true pelvis is thus explored and one of two conditions is found—that the cavity is *full* or that it is *empty*.

When palpation is practised in the last six weeks or two months of pregnancy, in the immense majority of cases the pelvic cavity is found full, the presenting part has engaged. Thus the diagnosis of vertex presentation is usually readily made. The presenting part is felt to be round, regular, and resisting. The head may be deeply engaged—and usually is in primiparæ—and immovable; slightly engaged and movable in the pelvic inlet; or it may simply rest at the pelvic inlet. When the head is found well engaged not only is the diagnosis of the presentation determined, but also that a proper relation exists between the diameters of the pelvic inlet and those of the fœtal skull. This condition is of prognostic as well as of diagnostic importance. Moreover, it is known that the presentation is fixed and definite—the uterine, fœtal, and pelvic axes coincide, accommodation is complete, and change of presentation impossible; only change of position can occur.

The diagnosis of the position is made by finding upon which side the cephalic tumor is more accessible. This is determined by depressing the abdominal wall by the two hands, in the manner already described, until the palpating hands are resisted by the cephalic tumor. The hand upon one side will descend more or less deeply into the pelvic cavity, while that upon the other side will be arrested at a higher point. That portion of the head which is more prominent and accessible is the brow. These points are most easily determined in primiparæ, because in primiparæ engagement is more complete than in multiparæ—the vertex sinks into the pelvis, carrying the inferior segment of the uterus before it, at times almost to the pelvic floor; in which case flexion is very marked, and the different level occupied by the brow and occiput is easily determined.

When engagement is not so marked, as in the occipito-posterior positions, flexion is not so great, and the differentiation is correspondingly difficult to make. In my experience it has been at times impossible to say that the cephalic tumor was more accessible upon one side than upon the other, and I have been obliged to rely on other signs for the diagnosis of the position.

To sum up, then, when the pelvic cavity is full, the vertex is presenting. If the cephalic tumor is more accessible to the right, the position is left, and *vice versâ*.

Having explored the region of the superior strait and recognized the depending fœtal head, it remains to examine for the trunk, breech and extremities of the fœtus. Pinard recommends that the breech be searched for in the region of the fundus uteri, but I have usually proceeded to examine the uterine contents systematically, from below upward. In many cases it is possible distinctly to define the groove between the head and shoulders. Passing upward, palpating gently with the finger tips, upon one side at a time, a resisting plane, more or less broad, can be made out; this corresponds to one lateral half of the uterus. The fingers meet with little resistance in the other lateral half of the uterus. The abdominal and uterine walls can be more or less deeply depressed. Usually in making these manipulations the fœtal small parts can be felt. If the resisting plane is broad, it is the fœtal dorsal region; if not so broad, it is the lateral plane of the fœtus. In the one case the occiput is anterior, in the other it is posterior. Again, if the small parts are very accessible, that is, if they are anterior, the position is posterior; while if the small parts are accessible with difficulty, that is

if they lie posterior in the uterus, the position is anterior. Should the fœtal dorsal region or lateral plane be separated from the uterine wall by liquor amnii, and not be easily reached by palpation, the manœuvre of Budin, which consists in depressing the breech—that is, increasing the natural anterior curvature of the fœtus—is useful. By this means the fœtal dorsal or lateral region is brought in contact with the uterine wall, and is then easily examined by palpation.

In head presentations the breech is found in the fundus uteri, in one or other hypochondriac region. The breech is best found by following upward the resisting plane of the fœtus (dorsal region, or lateral plane), which begins at the shoulder below and ends at the breech above. The breech gives the sensation of a voluminous, irregular body, less resisting than the head. The fœtal small parts are often felt in close proximity. The breech has not such a characteristic "feel" as the head.

Palpation after the method described usually gives positive results. When the sensations felt are typical, a diagnosis can be made of single pregnancy, of the presentation and position of the fœtus, and that pregnancy is not complicated by large intra-uterine or extra-uterine tumors. Cases of the class just considered form the immense majority of those seen in practice.

Instead of finding the pelvic cavity full, however, the palpating hands may find it empty. In this case, the lower end of the fœtal ovoid is usually found in one of the iliac fossæ, or it may be found resting on the pelvic brim, or above the plane of the superior strait. Almost never do the two extremities of the fœtal ovoid occupy the opposite flanks. Since one extremity of the fœtal ovoid is always in relation with the false pelvis, this region should be explored first. Whether the head or breech occupies the inferior uterine segment can be determined usually by recognizing the proper characters of these parts; and by finding the opposite extremity of the fœtal ovoid and the back, the exact location of the fœtus can be determined. If it is not possible to differentiate between the head and breech by recognizing the characters proper to each part, nor to locate the furrow between the head and shoulders, the head can be distinguished from the breech by a resort to *ballottement*. The head can be ballotted, but the breech cannot. As already pointed out, this fact is due largely to the different character of the connection between the head and trunk and the breech and lumbar region. It is due partly to the fact that the head is spheroidal in shape, and hence touches the uterine parietes at one point only, while the breech is in contact with the wall of the uterus by an extended surface.

It seems to me that it will be sufficient to give the diagnostic signs of the first and third positions of presentation of the vertex, and to refer briefly to the other presentations and positions.

Presentation of the Vertex: First Position.—The patient having been placed in the proper position for palpation, and the conditions which promote success having been complied with, the examiner begins to palpate. The thickness of the abdominal wall is estimated by picking up a fold between the thumb and fingers. The horizontal rami of the pubes are then found, and the hands, separated four or five inches, are placed upon the abdomen, the finger tips resting on the rami of the pubes. The abdominal wall is depressed from before backward and from above downward, which allows the inlet of the pelvis to be explored by the finger tips. Usually the cavity of the pelvis is found full—occupied by a round, regular, resisting body, which can be nothing but the engaged head. This being determined, the hands are placed at a slightly higher level (nearer the umbilicus) and depressed as before, to discover which side of the cephalic tumor is more accessible. This side corresponds to the brow, the other to the occiput. In the first position of the vertex presentation, the brow is found to the right. The diagnosis of this presentation and position is made usually in this way very readily. The diagnosis is confirmed by further palpation, or, should the diagnosis of the position be doubtful at this point, it can be made by finding the location of the back, small parts and fœtal heart sounds.

The examination is continued by palpating the abdominal contents systematically, from below upward, making light pressure with the finger tips, first on one side, then on the other. A broad resisting plane will be found, in the first position, in the left half of the uterine cavity; while the fingers will sink deeply on the right side, depressing the abdominal and uterine walls. The plane which resists the fingers is the fœtal dorsal region. Resistance is not felt on the right side because the liquor amnii, which occupies the space between the curled-up body of the fœtus and the uterine wall, is readily dis-placeable. The breech is found continuous with the "resisting plane." In primiparæ, and in multiparæ with tense abdominal muscles, the breech is found usually in the left hypochondriac region, while in women with lax abdominal and uterine walls it is more likely to be found in the epigastric or right hypochondriac regions. Owing to the anterior position of the dorsum, the small parts are posterior and relatively inaccessible. (In practice, the diagnosis is confirmed by finding that the fœtal heart-sounds can be heard plainest to the left of the median line at a point about halfway between the umbilicus and the middle of Poupart's ligament.) Thus it is seen that the diagnosis does not depend upon the recognition of any one point, but upon the determination of the location of the various anatomical regions of the fœtus; and for this reason the diagnosis is very reliable.

In case the vertex has not engaged it is of little importance to determine the position of the fœtus, since under these circumstances the position is very unstable. It can be done, if desired, by locating the back, and fœtal small parts.

Second Position.—This position is very seldom encountered. The description of the diagnosis of the first position is applicable to that of the second position if the words "right" and "left" are transposed.

Third Position.—Owing to the less degree of flexion of the head in posterior positions the relative accessibility of the brow is not so marked as in anterior positions; hence the results gained are not so definite. Usually, however, it can be determined that the position is right by finding the brow to the left. This is confirmed by finding a resisting plane in the right side of the uterus, and by the absence of a resisting plane on the opposite side. The resisting plane, felt to the right is narrow—it is the lateral wall of the fœtus. The small parts are anterior and can be readily felt in the left side of the uterus The breech will be found in the right hypochondriac, epigastric, or left hypochondriac regions, according as the abdominal and uterine walls are tense or lax. (The fœtal heart is heard plainest far to the right of the median line.)

Fourth Position.—The description of the diagnosis of the third position is applicable to the fourth position, the words "left" and "right" being transposed.

Presentation of the Breech.—The pelvic cavity is found empty. The breech is found in relation with the false pelvis. If it be impossible to recognize the breech by its proper characters the diagnosis can be made by finding the head at the fundus uteri. (The fœtal heart is heard at or above a horizontal line dividing the uterus into two equal parts.) The position is made out by locating the dorsum and fœtal small parts.

Presentation of the Trunk.—The pelvis is found empty. The long axis of the uterus is oblique and not parallel with the long axis of the body. One extremity of the fœtal ovoid is found in one iliac fossa and the other in the opposite flank. The dorsum or fœtal small parts are felt in relation with the anterior wall of the uterus. Pinard found the head in one flank and the breech in the other only twice in the 100,000 women examined by him.

Presentation of the Face.—It is practically certain that presentation of the face never occurs prior to labor. Those who have examined women per vaginam only, admit that primitive face presentations are exceedingly rare. Naturally these examinations have seldom been made until the advent of labor. The fact that Pinard has never met with a face presentation prior to labor is strong evidence that this presentation is produced after labor has set in.

The description of presentations of the vertex already given was restricted to women with normal proportions. Pinard states that in women having pendulous bellies (ante-version of the pregnant uterus) a special accommodation is found. The occiput is in relation with the middle of the iliac bone, and not with either the acetabulum or the sacro-iliac synchondrosis. The breech is found near the ilium opposite to the occiput, and the feet are felt very near the brow. That is, the fœtus is very much curved on itself, and a considerable part of the dorsum runs transversely across the uterus, instead of approximately parallel with its vertical diameter. A resisting plane is felt on each side of the uterus, and the elasticity of the liquor amnii is perceived as easily above as below. Unless this peculiar accommodation of the fœtus is known, a mistake in diagnosis is easy.

When the vertex presents in women whose pelves are deformed by rachitis (rickety flat pelvis) the head is found at the level of the superior strait or slightly engaged—depending on the degree of contraction. As is well known in this variety of contracted pelvis, the long, *antero-posterior*, diameter of the head is parallel with the long, *transverse*, diameter of the pelvis. Flexion is slight. The brow can sometimes be felt at a higher level than the occiput, and at times can be recognized by its marked hardness. The dorsum is felt in relation with one lateral wall of the uterus, the narrow lateral plane of the fœtus being directed anterior. The breech is found in the fundus when the uterus is not anteverted. The small parts are felt in the lateral half of the uterus opposite the dorsum.

In the other varieties of contracted pelvis, when the degree of contraction is at all great, the head rests at the level of the superior strait, and is freely movable by the palpating hands. It is impossible to force the head down into the cavity of the pelvis, *i. e.*, to make it engage, by making pressure from above. The same is true in cases in which the disproportion between the head and pelvis is due to abnormally large size of the head, as from hydrocephalus, being especially marked when the disproportion is great.

ERYSIPELAS OF THE PHARYNX AND FACE.

BY EDWARD P. DAVIS, A.M., M.D.,

OBSTETRICIAN TO THE PHILADELPHIA HOSPITAL; PHYSICIAN TO THE FOULKE AND LONG ORPHANAGE FOR GIRLS, AND TO THE CLINTON ST. BOARDING HOME FOR WOMEN, ETC.

The following case, while not rare, furnishes a clinical study of practical interest:

R. F., 17½ years old, a robust girl of full development, had formerly had diphtheria and scarlatina. Examination of the pharynx, when in ordinary health, revealed slightly enlarged tonsils with chronic catarrh of moderate severity of the pharynx and posterior nares. She had, at intervals of 6 or 8 months, several attacks of tonsillitis from which she recovered under the use of sodium salicylate, and a gargle of boracic acid, potassium chlorate and glycerine. On Dec. 14, 1888, the writer's attention was directed to the patient who was said to be suffering from "a cold," contracted 48 hours previous. The face was flushed, the pharynx uniformly reddened and swollen, the tonsils enlarged: moderate constitutional disturbance was present. As the symptoms were those of previous attacks of tonsillitis treatment for that condition was ordered.

Twenty-four hours later the nature of the infection from which the patient suffered was apparent. The face exhibited the diffuse lymphangitis present in facial erysipelas ; the pharynx was intensely reddened, uniformly swollen, without membrane ; the tonsils swollen, but not greatly in excess of the swelling of the surrounding parts. The lymphatic glands of the neck were enlarged and tender. A marked febrile disturbance .... with severe frontal headache, back-

purulent fluid, which left the surface of the mucous membrane a bright pink. The stools were voided with pain and difficulty, and were streaked with mucous and grumous coffee-ground material. A slight urethral and vaginal discharge was also present. Convalescence was established at the end of three weeks.

The treatment consisted in the regular and persistent administration by a competent nurse, of whiskey and milk, the amount of alcohol given varying with the pulse and temperature, as indicating the severity of the septic intoxication. High temperature was treated by sponging with alcohol and water; no antipyretics were given. Suppositories of glycerine were used to relieve constipation, and soap and water enemata were occasionally employed. Boracic acid was used as a local antiseptic; the conjunctivæ were douched with a saturated solution diluted one third; the pharynx was treated with a saturated solution in glycerine,

employed as a gargle; the nares were thoroughly douched with a glycerine and water solution. An ointment:

Acid. boracic. pulv. . . . . ℥ i
Lanolin . . . . ℥ i
Vaseline . . . . q. s.

was thoroughly employed in anointing the lips, nostrils and abraded surfaces on the face.[1]

Alcohol was the only constitutional antiseptic and cerebral sedative given; the quantity administered varied with the indications and effect desired. As the fever declined a mercurial purge was given, followed by salines. The urine was rich in urates and phosphates, with a trace of albumin. Easily digested food was allowed in abundance as soon as the condition of the intestines warranted its administration. The case was considered infectious and contagious, and was isolated: the apartments occupied were thoroughly fumigated and disinfected after the patient's convalescence: the patient received an antiseptic (carbolic acid) bath, and especial attention was given to cleansing and disinfecting the scalp and hair.

The point of practical interest to which attention is directed is the centre for septic infection afforded by an enlarged tonsil. In the case in question no caries of the teeth or jaw and no ozæna existed in which the infection could have originated.

It has been shown by numerous observers that "catching cold" is not an adequate cause of erysipelas of the face; while exposure to cold may cause congestion, predisposing to inflammation, yet the specific germ of septic infection is needed to produce erysipelas. Tissues in which necrosis of the cellular elements has occurred furnish a peculiarly favorable culture field for such infective micrococci. This has been especially well shown by Kaposi,[2] who considers the most frequent sources of facial erysipelas to be a carious tooth; a patch of facial eczema; lupus; scrofula or syphilis of the nose, or retro-pharyngeal abscess. Strümpell[3] regards nasal catarrh, acute or chronic, as a common predisposing cause of facial erysipelas. Koch and Fehleisen have shown

[1] Some samples of lanolin are too stiff for a convenient ointment, and can be mixed to advantage with vaseline or cosmoline.

[2] Pathologie und Therapie der Hautkrankheiten Erste Hälfte. 1886. § 406.

[3] Lehrbuch der Specieller Pathologie und Therapie der innerer Krankheiten. Erster Band, 1886. § 95.

the possibility of direct infection and contagion when the infective germ finds a favorable culture-field. It is for this reason that persons whose nasal and pharyngeal mucous membrane and cutaneous surfaces are intact may come in contact with erysipelas with impunity, while another who possesses a focus of former suppuration is readily infected. As the patient was in an institution in which other inmates were living who had formerly had tonsillitis or other inflammatory affections of the pharynx, jaws or nares, her isolation was necessary.

Regarding the treatment of such a septic infection, the value of alcohol is especially noteworthy, when combined with easily digested food. No other antiseptic can be introduced into the blood in efficient quantities without danger to the patient. The use of antipyretics which act by depressing the nervous system is contra-indicated in septic fever; in the present state of knowledge of pathology it is not known that fever is not a conservative process by which the spores of septic cocci are destroyed as soon as formed.[1] An antiseptic which can circulate in the blood, destroying septic germs, and in proportion to the dose exciting or exercising a sedative influence upon the cerebro-spinal centres, is needed in the treatment of septic fever. Among other objections to the depressing antipyretics is the fact that secretion and excretion are impaired by their use in large doses. In this connection Runge's method of treating puerperal septicæmia by alcoholics, baths and packs and forced feeding is instructive; his cases now number 20, with 15 recoveries.[2]

The local treatment of facial erysipelas is important, as Kaposi has shown. The mouth, pharynx, nares, and ears should be thoroughly cleansed and disinfected by an innocuous antiseptic, iodoform, thymol or boric acid.

A vaseline or lanolin ointment containing one of these antiseptics may be employed to advantage in carefully healing fissures or abrasions on mucous membranes or skin.

Erysipelas, or infection of the mucous surfaces of the body by Fehleisen's micrococcus, is sufficiently common to afford abundant opportunity for its clinical study, and with other septic infections offers some of the most interesting problems in modern pathology.

[1] Welch; Pathology of Fever; *Medical News*, May 26, 1888, p. 568.

[2] *Archiv für Gynäkologie*, Band 33, Heft 1.

A FORMULA FOR CROUP.

BY J. B. JOHNSON, M.D.,
WASHINGTON, D. C.

—The *Boston Med. and Surg. Journal*, Jan. 17, 1889, says that the German societies of Brooklyn, N. Y., interested in the establishment of a German hospital, have appropriated about $10,000 from the regular society fund to the purchase of a hospital site in the 18th ward, near the routes of the Brooklyn Elevated and other city railroads. The twenty-seven parcels of land bought aggregate 50,000 feet or more.

—The *Western Druggist*, Jan., 1889, says that quinine, under a recent decision of the Illinois Supreme Court, is not a "domestic remedy" and cannot be sold except by a registered pharmacist. An Illiopolis barkeeper has been recently fined for selling it. In view of the late crusade of saloon-keepers against alleged dramselling-druggists, the compliment should be returned by prosecuting quinine-selling liquor dealers. Absinthe is also a drug, and an attempt might be made to suppress its sale also.

SOCIETY REPORTS.

MEDICAL SOCIETY OF THE COUNTY OF NEW YORK.

Stated Meeting, January 28, 1889.

The President, A. S. HUNTER, M.D., in the Chair.

DR. H. D. CHAPIN read a paper on

Septic Poisoning in Early Life.

Cases of septic poisoning in early life, he said, are conveniently divided into those which occur in the newly born and those which occur in older infants. In the newly born the seat of entrance of the poison is usually the umbilicus, and may, according to J. Lewis Smith, be by way of the vein or by way of the lymphatics. The abrasion giving entrance to the poison may be caused by the forceps; after birth and after healing of the cord, the genitals are likely to be the vulnerable point. The infection often starts as an erysipelatous inflammation upon the surface, and some poison enters the system, giving rise to inflammation of the peritoneum and other serous membranes, etc. In older children the upper part of the body, especially the scalp, mouth, etc., become the vulnerable parts. Pediculi, which cause the child to scratch and thus introduce matter from ulcers into the system, are not infrequently the cause. The germs when introduced in small quantity may be entirely or largely disposed of by the inherent vitality of the lymphatics, and cause only local symptoms; but if introduced in larger numbers constitutional symptoms develop. Dr. Chapin thinks aphthous mouth with small ulcers may be the source of septic poisoning, as also may otitis media purulenta, etc. In closely crowded apartments with imperfect ventilation, sewer-gas and foul air, the germs are constantly brought in contact with the air passages, and doubtless often give rise to mild forms of septic poisoning, which are commonly attributed to malaria.

The treatment should be prophylactic; but when septic poisoning has occurred, the seat of entrance of the poison should be sought for, cleansed, and healed, and, in addition, general measures are indicated.

DR. J. LEWIS SMITH thought the severest cases of septic poisoning in infants took place at the umbilicus. He suggested filling the umbilical fossa with iodoform in the newly born. He believes scarlet fever and diphtheria often prove severe or fatal on account of septic material finding entrance at the seat of lesions occurring in those diseases. Strict cleanliness and antisepsis should be observed. Vapor of carbolic acid, turpentine, and eucalyptus (the latter to mask disagreeable odor) should fill the room; and a spray of bichloride of mercury, in quantity sufficient for an internal dose, should be used in diphtheria, allowing it to pass on down the throat.

DR. A. H. SMITH urged the importance of stripping gelatinous material from the cord and thus hastening mummification.

DR. SIMON BARUCH read a paper on

The Value of Water in Therapeutics,

in which he sought to give an impartial review of its value as established by clinical evidence, and not simply to praise the water-cure system. During his service as army surgeon in the late war it was the custom to use water freely in dressing wounds, and the mortality from suppuration and gangrene was greater than has attended the more recent dry dressing. In laparotomy boiled water has been demonstrated to be of value. It is the author's belief that the antiseptics of the surgery of the future will be largely cleanliness, obtained by boiled water, and not so much by antiseptic drugs. The value of hot water as a styptic has been established; it is especially serviceable in *post-partum* hemorrhage. The marked value of vaginal douches in certain inflammatory conditions has been established by Dr. Emmet. Water is of benefit also in certain skin affections, but is contraindicated in eczema. The treatment of otitis media purulenta by irrigation has been abandoned for the dry treatment, and with great advantage. The custom of employing vaginal irrigation in normal labors has been shown to be bad.

Speaking of the internal use of water, the author passed by its diuretic and diaphoretic effects, and first considered the advantages of washing out the stomach in dyspepsia and indigestion. In recent cases a few washings with some care in diet often cure; but in chronic gastritis the treatment has to be continued for some time. The sipping of hot water at intervals before breakfast is of benefit in indigestion, but it should not be taken just before the meal. Of recent date also is the introduction of the treatment of gastric disturbance in infants by washing out the stomach. In summer diarrhœa no treatment is more beneficial than irrigation of the large gut. It is also of value in catarrhal jaundice.

Cold water to the surface of the body acts chiefly through mechanical and thermal influence, and has a wide field of usefulness. The reaction which follows the application of cold water to the surface has a remedial effect in many affections, among which are certain neurasthenias in robust patients; it takes the place frequently of so-called tonic medicines. Dr. Baruch reviewed the use of cold or tepid water in the reduction of the temperature of the body in fevers, and the mortality statistics of typhoid fever, according as the disease had been treated by the usual method or by the employment of the bath. The usual mortality, he said, has been from 21 to 26 per cent., or higher, whereas Brandt and others show a mortality rate under the treatment by water of only 7 per cent. or less. He concluded his paper by strongly recommending Brandt's method of treating typhoid fever. The bath employed by him has been of a temperature of 65° F., but he suggested that it it may be better to employ a higher temperature, gradually lowering it by adding colder water, which, of course, would necessitate leaving the patient in the water a longer time.

Dr. J. Harvie Dew read a paper on the same subject, viewing it rather from the standpoint of physiology. At the beginning, he said, it is necessary to recognize the following facts: 1. The chief component part of human bodies in fair condition is water. Its relative proportion to all the solid constituents has been estimated at from two-thirds to three-fourths the entire weight. 2. Water constitutes almost the total volume of each of the circulatory fluids, including those of digestion. 3. It is the essential medium by which digestion is accomplished, absorption is made possible, and the transportation of the elements of nutrition to the various tissues of the body is made easy. 4. As water enters so largely into the composition of the tissues, it becomes of corresponding importance to every process of assimilation. 5. Water is not only the medium of transportation of nutritive elements introduced by absorption, but it is also the medium by which all waste matters are held in solution and are conducted to their several points of exit. 6. Observation and experiment have shown that from three to four pints of liquid food are required to maintain the normal functions and weight of an individual weighing from 140 to 150 pounds. 7. It is a clinical fact that wherever we find persons thin in flesh it can be noted that by habit or for other reasons they are taking very small quantities of liquid food; while, on the other hand, all well preserved or fleshy persons will be found to be copious drinkers of fluids in one form or another. 8. It is also a clinical fact that in every morbid or diseased condition of the system, whether organic or functional, primary or secondary, the functions of digestion, absorption, assimilation, secretion, and excretion, embracing elimination, become in one way or another disturbed—sometimes one or more of these functions, at other times all of them to a more or less degree in the same patient. 9. It is not only important to note these disturbances as they are exhibited in well defined diseases, but it is equally important to recognize the fact that a very large proportion of the diseases and troubles to which the human body is liable have their origin primarily and absolutely in some improper performance of these functions.

From these facts one would recognize at once the necessity for a plentiful supply and use of fluids, both in the maintenance of health and in the restoration thereto from disease.

The discussion of these two papers was made the special order of the next meeting.

FOREIGN CORRESPONDENCE.

LETTER FROM AUSTRALIA.

The Theories and Treatment of Snake-Bite in the Australian Colonies.

In an interview with Dr. Creed, of Sydney, I gained the following opinions on the treatment of snake-bite. Dr. Creed said:

From the experience which I have had of cases of snake-bite in New South Wales, and from inquiries I have made as to the particulars of others which have occurred in the practice of my friends who have kindly given me an account of them, I have been obliged to arrive at the conclusion that, with the exception of the species of *Hoplocephalus*, especially the "large-scaled snake," or, as it is called in Tasmania, the Diamond snake (*Hoplocephalus superbus*), and the brown banded or tiger snake (*Hoplocephalus curtus*), the death adder (*Acanthophisantaretica*), the brown snake (*Diemenia superciliosa*), and a large and vigorous specimen of the black snake (*Pseudechis porphyriacus*), the danger of death from the effects of the bite of the numerous venomous snakes common to the colony is very much exaggerated, and that in the majority of cases showing serious symptoms, these symptoms are really the effect of intense fear and not of snake poison.

The doctor says that the essential object to be attained in the treatment of every bite from a venomous snake is the prevention of the absorption of the poison, and this can be done only by the stopping of the circulation as quickly as possible between the bite and the heart, and the prompt and efficient excision of the punctured part to such a depth as shall insure either the absolute removal of the injected poison, or at all events, its exposure to such an extent that it can easily be removed by washing with the nearest attainable fluid, preferably water. He strongly insists on the advantages of the excision of, instead of incision into and about, the puncture caused by the teeth of venomous snakes, for the following reasons: As the longest poison-fang of the largest Australian snake is less than one-fourth of an inch in length, excision of the very lowest point of the puncture is easily practicable by any intelligent person, without danger of causing more serious hemorrhage than can easily be controlled by the application of a pad. If done in this way the whole of the poison will be removed. On the other hand, incision made into and about the wound may or may not remove the venom, which might easily be retained at the original spot into which it was injected by the bite, if the cut made did not actually enter into and freely expose it. In addition, the danger from hemorrhage would be very much greater from the wound made by the incision, as the point of the knife would probably enter to a greater depth than the wound made in excision. In fact, unless the operator has a fair knowledge of anatomy, he might easily in many places wound an artery lying comparatively superficially, and cause death by hemorrhage in a few minutes.

With regard to sucking the wound, the entire removal of the poison by its means is problematical, and such treatment is not without danger to the person sucking. Unless made by a person with some knowledge of anatomy, he thinks the excision should be made by pinching up the parts to be cut away, and then removing them with the middle of the blade, and not by inserting the point of the knife and cutting round the bite. The wound should be well washed and moderate bleeding encouraged. It would be well to wash it with a weak solution of permanganate of potash, or it might have an application of strong nitric or carbolic acid, or the actual cautery. The permanganate is probably an antidote if brought in direct contact with the poison, but when thrown into the general circulation it can be only of little if any use, for it will attack not only the snake poison but will oxidize all organic matter with which it comes in contact. After the ligature is removed the patient should be carefully watched and symptoms treated, the best stimulant being ether under the skin. Compulsory exertion or walking the patient about is forbidden. This notion of keeping the patient awake is carried even to a ludicrous extent. In a case in New South Wales the local brass band was hired to play their most fierce tunes to keep the patient from sleeping ; the patient made a recovery from the bite as well as from the infliction of the music. Dr. Creed uses alcohol for the treatment of the symptoms of exhaustion but not as a special treatment of the poison.

By experiments made by Mr. Krefft, in Sydney, it has been demonstrated that no effect follows the infliction of a bite by one of the most venomous snakes either on itself or on another venomous snake of the same or a somewhat similar class. From this Dr. Creed argues that if a physiological antidote is to be discovered, it must be sought in this peculiar property inherent in the snake, which can hardly be merely consequent on structure, but may be the result of some substance diffused in the snake itself, which diligent research may demonstrate to be capable of isolation, and, if so, of use in the treatment of snake-bite. Dr. Creed is of the opinion that in order to prevent fear from acting harmfully on the patient he would when needed use ether as an anæsthetic. He would keep the patient barely unconscious for an hour or two, then allow him to recover enough to judge of his condition, watching pulse and respiration all the time carefully. If necessary he would bring the patient again and again under the influence of the ether, so long as might be required.

He feels there is a germ of useful treatment in this suggestion. I am told that the treatment of snake-bite by ether has been tried by Dr. Bancroft, of Brisbane, with most encouraging results. Dr. Creed feels that there has not been up to the present time a physiological antidote found for this terrible poison of snakes. This is not the opinion of other members of the profession, and I now ask your attention to views held by a prominent physician of Victoria.

An interesting article on snake-bite and its treatment was read recently by Dr. Augustus Mueller before the Victorian Medical Society. The doctor stated that his experience and observations have made him acquainted with the poison of the black, the brown, and the tiger snakes only, and he did not extend his views to the poison of any other varieties of Australian snakes, nor for those of America and India. Inferences might be drawn that the antidote he suggested would be useful in all ; but inferences were not proofs.

To be brief, I will state that the doctor's theory is that the poison of the snake does not act as a special blood poison ; all the symptoms are due to deficient nerve action. The insidious venom travels quickly to the nerve centers, affecting in rapid succession the anterior columns of the cord, the vaso-motor centers of the brain, and causing paresis and paralysis of the muscles of the lower extremities, accompanied by rapidly diminished force of heart action and blood pressure, and in a very short time by sleep, which in severe cases deepens into coma ; the latter sometimes remains till death, but more frequently passes off again, even in fatal cases. The usual method of death is by syncope. Dr. Mueller then made some interesting comparisons between the effects of the poison of the Australian and the Indian snakes. Both are without doubt nerve poisons. The Australian snake-poison seems more diffusible and develops its effects more quickly, and is distributed uniformly over the whole motor system. It is on this account, and also on account of the smaller quantity of poison at the disposal of Australian snakes that their bite is less frequently fatal than those of the Indian snakes of the East Indies.

The poison of the latter snakes, especially of the cobra, seems less diffusible, and takes a longer time as a rule to develop its effects ; but once fully developed the course is much more quickly fatal, owing to the fact that the poison concentrates its action on special nerve centers, instead of being equally distributed over all. Dr. Mueller has had thirty years' practice in a district in which snakes abound, and he has unusual opportunities of studying the effects of snake-bite, both on men and the lower animals. He tells how he came to have his attention called to the use of the antidote that he now so strongly recommends, viz., strychnia.

Strange to say it was in a case of spider-bite in a child two years old. He asserts that effect of spider-bite differs only in degree from that of snake-bite. Incidentally it may be mentioned here that there are a number of fatal cases of spider-bite on record in the Colonies ; in Queensland they are not at all of very rare occurrence. In commenting on this case the doctor says he was at once struck by the close resemblance, if not identity, of symptoms here present with those of snake-bite—loss of power in the legs, extreme pallor, coldness of skin, feeble heart action, with pulse scarcely perceptible at the wrist, dilated pupils insensible to light, and inability to move either arms or legs.

Treatment was begun with the usual orthodox remedies—eliminative, stimulating, alkaline, etc., etc., but all failed. The collapse increased rapidly, respiration became difficult, eyes glassy, heart's action barely perceptible, pulse gone at the wrist. In short, the patient would die in a few moments to all appearances. Now came to me a happy thought, says the doctor ; like a flash it passed through my mind that the child's inability to walk soon after being bitten might have been caused by the subtle poison exerting a specific depressing effect on the motor cells in the anterior columns, gradually extending over the rest of the motor and also the vaso-motor centers. All the ominous symptoms thus found a ready explanation, and strychnia suggested itself as the remedy for this condition of things. To use his own words, " I hastily procured some strychnia, and injected ten minims of the official solution into the arm. In a half hour's time my little patient was sitting up, snatched, I have reason to believe, from the very jaws of death." He then relates a case in which he used this remedy in a venomous snake-bite, with equally good success. In another case he produced, through the agency of the strychnia, a marvellous change in a desperate case in less than an hour, watched the patient for a number of hours and then gave his sanction to his going home. The lad felt strong and entirely well, mounted his horse and rode off ; but he died next morning before the doctor could reach him. " I did not know then, as I do now, that even strychnia is more quickly decomposed and thrown out of the system than the snake-bite poison and that the latter will lurk about in the holes and corners of the system and resume its work of destruction as soon as the antagonist is removed that kept it in check. I had injected into the system of a mere boy, within half an hour not less than one-third of a grain of strychnia; but even this comparatively large quantity was evidently only just enough to counteract for a time, and as long as it lasted, the deadly venom. If I had only dared to push the use of the drug a little further, until it produced the usual symptoms in a moderate degree; if I had only directed it to be taken internally, from time to time in ordinary doses as I do now, after the painful lesson this case gave me, I have not the remotest doubt, from what I have seen of its action since, that the life of this lad would have been saved.''

Notwithstanding the fatal termination of this case, however, his faith in the antidote was confirmed rather than shaken, for he felt convinced that its failure was wholly and solely due to the mistake he made in not continuing in it small doses, until it produced slight muscular spasms. Though the lad had received within a half hour four times the quantity we are allowed to give in ordinary practice in one dose, it was evidently not sufficient to counteract completely and effectually the deadly venom with which his body was saturated, but only checked it for a time.

Dr. Mueller feels quite confident that snake-bite and strychnia react on each other in the human organism with the unerring certainty of two chemical tests. The dose of the antidote must be in proportion to the severity of the symptoms, but even a little more than is required can do no harm, for its effects pass away very quickly in snake-bite. A few muscular twitches, a little stiffness about the neck or about the mouth, are nothing compared with the horrid sensations which the deadly snake-poison produces.

Dr. Mueller then produced some collateral evidence in regard to this treatment. In China and India where the terrible raja commits its destruction of human life each year, a famous antidote with the natives is a pill which is called in China Nooang. On examination this is proved to belong to the strychnos family; that is, the pill is made from a plant of this family. Another famous antidote is the nuts of the Simaba Cedron, among the natives of Central and South America. Its active principle resembles strychnine; it probably resembles more closely quassine, yet this leads us to the point that it is among the bitter tonic alkaloids that we are to look for the antidote for snake-poison. The doctor concludes with his opinion of alcohol: "Stimulants are,

no doubt, of use in stimulating the heart; but their action is transitory, because they do not attack the enemy in his stronghold; they do not permanently raise and alter, as the strychnine does, the depressed and partly suspended function of the motor centres, which lies at the root of all the mischief, and is, beyond doubt, the cause of death in snake-bite.''

C. C. VANDERBECK.

PERISCOPE.

Hereditary Syphilis.

The Vienna correspondent of the *British Med. Journal*, Jan. 12, 1889, states that at a recent meeting of the Imperial Royal Society of Physicians of Vienna, Professor Neumann read a paper on hereditary syphilis. The questions with which the lecturer dealt were the following:—1. What is the condition of the offspring when the father and mother were healthy at the time of conception, and the mother became infected at a later date (pure post-conceptional syphilis)? 2. What is the effect of post-conceptional syphilis with reference to the offspring when the father was already syphilitic at the time of procreation? 3. What is the effect of post-conceptional syphilis with reference to the offspring when the condition of the father's health at the time of procreation is unknown, and the mother was healthy at the time of conception, and became infected at a later date? 4. What is the condition of the offspring when the infection and the conception took place at the same time? And, 5, when the infection of the parents occurred before conception?

Professor Neumann's paper was based on cases most of which he had observed during eight years in his clinic. Of these only 102 were available for the purpose he had in view, as accurate data concerning the offspring could not be obtained in the rest. The physicians of the three obstetric clinics of the General Hospital and those of the Vienna Foundling Hospital also took an active part in the investigation. With regard to pure post-conceptional syphilis, Professor Neumann had observed 11 cases; of these 5 patients were healthy, and the rest, in part, presented the appearances of syphilis, and, in part, miscarriage occurred. As regards post-conceptional syphilis, where the father was syphilitic, 5 children were found to be healthy, 2 children were affected with syphilis, and in 5 cases miscarriage had occurred. In the cases of post-conceptional syphilis, where the father was unknown, there were 10 healthy, 1 syphilitic, and 7 dead children; 2 children were still under treatment. In the cases in which conception and infection took place at the same time, 15 children were healthy, 1 died of peritonitis, 4 were syphilitic; the fate of these cases could not be ascertained, and in 21 instances still-birth occurred. Among 25 cases of syphilitic infection before conception, there were 10 healthy children, 8 cases of miscarriage, and 4 of maceration; 3 were still under treatment.

Professor Neumann arrived at the following conclusions: 1. A syphilitic mother may convey the disease to her offspring at any stage of her affection, whether the infection has taken place before or after the conception. 2. A mother who has contracted the disease after conception sometimes transmits it to the fœtus. In the case of pure post-conceptional syphilis the transmission of the affection to the child is extremely rare, especially when the mother has become infected in the last months of pregnancy. 3. When the infection of the mother has taken place after conception, and the father was syphilitic at the time of procreation, the effect on the offspring is greatly intensified; the children in these cases die *in utero*, or are born with signs of syphilis. 4. In the case of post-conceptional syphilis, where the infector is unknown, the proportion is the same as in pure post-conceptional syphilis; syphilis acquired in the last months of pregnancy is usually transmitted to the offspring. 5. When infection and conception occur at the same time, the children die in one half of the cases. It is nevertheless remarkable that a great part of the offspring remain free of syphilis, in spite of the fact that the disease was in an active state in both the parents at the time of conception. This disproves the assertion that a healthy child can never be born when both parents are syphilitic at the time of conception. On the other hand, the assertion that healthy children are born only when the syphilis of the parents is seven years old, is also negatived. 6. In the case of infection before conception, the period at which conception occurred has to be taken into account; the longer the interval between infection and conception, the more favorable is the prognosis for the offspring. 7. The offspring has the best chance when the mother only contracts syphilis in the last months of pregnancy, while the father was healthy at the time of procreation; the same is also true of the offspring of parents suffering from tertiary syphilis. The offspring has the least chance when infection and conception have occurred simultaneously, or when the father was suffering from recent syphilis at the time of procreation. 8. This last observation also elucidates the question as to paternal syphilis. It is especially the cases in which the father was syphilitic at the time of procreation, and the mother became infected only after conception, and the child was soon after the infection born in a macerated condition, which prove the extremely injurious nature of paternal syphilis. This is opposed to the observations of Boeck and Dewere, who state that the child of a syphilitic father is always healthy.

These data, concludes Professor Neumann, show the sad fate of the children of syphilitic parents, as, out of 109 cases, only 44 were born healthy; and, according to inquiries made by Dr. Friedinger, director of the Vienna Foundling Hospital, only the minority of them live. Hereditary syphilis must, therefore, be considered one of the most terrible plagues of infant life.

Two Cases of Thyrotomy for the Removal of Malignant Disease of the Larynx.

At the meeting of the Clinical Society of London, Jan. 11, 1889, Mr. Butlin read notes of these cases. In pursuance of an opinion expressed by him in a previous paper, that it is not necessary to remove the cartilaginous or bony framework of the larynx in certain cases of intrinsic carcinoma of the larynx which are suitable for operation, two cases were reported. The first was a case of squamous-celled carcinoma (epithelioma) of the larynx in a woman 27 years old. The thyroid cartilage was divided in November, 1887, and the disease was cut and scraped out. She made a good recovery, and was well a year later, and free from every sign of cancer. The second was a case of the same disease in a man 51 years old. A similar operation was performed in 1888. The man recovered without hindrance, and was well in September. The author pointedly drew attention to the comparatively trivial nature of the operation in cases of malignant disease of the larynx of limited extent. In another instance in which he performed an exploratory thyrotomy in a man advanced in years, and found the disease too extensive for removal, he closed the wound, and the man recovered and left the hospital wearing a tracheotomy tube.—*British Med. Journal*, Jan. 19, 1889.

THE

MEDICAL AND SURGICAL
REPORTER.

ISSUED EVERY SATURDAY.

CHARLES W. DULLES, M.D.,
EDITOR AND PUBLISHER.

The Terms of Subscription to the serial publications of this office are as follows, payable in advance:

Med. and Surg. Reporter (weekly), a year, **$5.00**
Quarterly Compendium of Med. Science, -   2.50
Reporter and Compendium,   -   -   -   - 6.00
Physician's Daily Pocket Record,   -   -   1.00
Reporter and Pocket Record, -   -   -   - 6.00
Reporter, Compendium, and Pocket Record, 7.00

All checks and postal orders should be drawn to order of

CHARLES W. DULLES,

N. E. Cor. 13th and Walnut Streets,
P. O. Box 843.   Philadelphia, Pa.

☞ SUGGESTIONS TO SUBSCRIBERS:
See that your address-label gives the date to which your subscription is paid.
In requesting a change of address, give the old address as well as the new one.
If your REPORTER does not reach you promptly and regularly, notify the publisher *at once*, so that the cause may be discovered and corrected.

☞ SUGGESTIONS TO CONTRIBUTORS AND CORRESPONDENTS:
Write in ink.
Write on one side of paper only.
Write on paper of the size usually used for letters.
Make as few paragraphs as possible. Punctuate carefully. Do not abbreviate, or omit words like "the," and "a," or "an."
Make communications as short as possible.
NEVER ROLL A MANUSCRIPT! Try to get an envelope or wrapper which will fit it.
When it is desired to call our attention to something in a newspaper, mark the passage boldly with a colored pencil, and write on the wrapper "Marked copy." Unless this is done, newspapers are not looked at.
The Editor will be glad to get medical news, but it is important that brevity and actual interest shall characterize communications intended for publication.

THE DANGER OF CALOMEL INJECTIONS.

The recent studies in connection with the use of calomel injections in the treatment of syphilis have led to a revival of interest in this subject on this side of the Atlantic. But there are two reasons why those who are not yet committed to it may hesitate about adopting this method. One of them depends upon the fact that so eminent a syphilographer as Neumann, of Vienna, has recently pronounced against the general utility of calomel injections, and the other is that these injections may be dangerous to health or life.

Attention has recently been directed to this point by an article by Prof. J. W. Runeberg, of Helsingfors, in the *Deutsche med. Wochenschrift*, January 3, 1889, who refers to a few cases of mercurial poisoning caused by the medicinal administration of salts of this metal, and describes in full a case coming under his notice in which death was attributed, with much show of reason, to the absorption of mercury from points at which calomel had been injected.

The form of disease caused by accidental and chronic mercurial poisoning is usually that of an acute dysentery, and this was seen in Runeberg's case, while the autopsy disclosed the presence of a cavity containing unhealthy pus and a considerable quantity of mercury.

The case referred to indicates that one of the chief merits of the hypodermic use of calomel has associated with it a feature of danger. It is an advantage to have a method by which mercury can be administered by the physician with the expectation that it will be gradually absorbed; but the disadvantage is that the rate of absorption is not determinable, and some injections may be carried into the system promptly, while others may be taken up slowly and produce, with later ones, a culminating effect. And if such an effect makes its appearance, it is no longer possible to limit it by discontinuing the administration of the medicament. The quantity already in the body cannot be withdrawn, and it may continue poisoning the system long after it was first deposited.

These dangers deserve consideration, although in practice they have not proved to be very imminent. The cases of mercurial poisoning caused by calomel injections are very few and most of them have occurred in persons in an anæmic condition, predisposed to general disturbances. Still in one case, reported by Kraus, the patient was in good condition, and it must be remembered that syphilitics are not rarely in this very state and that always when they are so, and generally when they are not, some other way of administering mercury may well be chosen for them.

TETANUS NEONATORUM.

There was a time when tetanus of the new-born was so frequent that it was more or less an object of fear to physicians and parents. But in these days it has become so rare that it is hardly ever taken into consideration in estimating the perils of the first period of life. When it occurred, in former times, it was generally attributed to traumatism, and charged to improper management of the stump of the divided umbilical cord. Nowadays the germ theory of disease has come in to suggest a totally different conception of the nature and mode of origin of tetanus, and on the one hand we are asked to make our views in regard to it conform to the possibilities of infection with the germ found in earth by Nicolaier, and on the other hand we are confronted with the claims of Verneuil that tetanus is of equine origin and can always be traced to some direct or indirect infection from horses.

The arguments in support of both of these theories have much that is plausible about them, but nothing which to a keenly critical mind can be said to be conclusive. Both earth and horses are widely enough distributed to make it possible to invoke either of them to explain what takes place in almost any land; and certain experiments have been performed which indicate that tetanus may be produced in some of the lower animals with matters derived from the soil or found where horses are kept. But, none the less, the subject is still involved in much obscurity, and cases of tetanus in human beings occur which are as inexplicable to-day as were those which were observed many years ago.

An illustration of this fact is found in a recent study of trismus neonatorum, as it is seen in Iceland and in the Faroe Islands and the Hebrides, by Dr. H. Labonne, the results of which are published in the *Gazette Hebdomadaire*, January 11, 1889. Dr. Labonne makes the mortality from tetanus neonatorum in these islands range from thirty to sixty-seven per cent. In studying the causes of this frightful mortality he finds nothing to support the theory that the tetanus neonatorum found here is due to infection with a microbe, although he hazards a guess that the birds which furnish so much of the food of the natives, and so much of their bedding, may also supply them with some bacterium of tetanus. On the other hand, certain practical experiments which he cites indicate that the almost exclusive use of the flesh and oil of birds as food by nursing women brings about states of the milk which directly or indirectly induce tetanus in their nurslings.

The report of the investigations of Dr. Labonne is interesting, although it is not conclusive. It would be more valuable if it gave an account of the management of labor in the lands he visited, and the entire care of infants during the first days of their life. Both of these matters are of great importance in estimating the probable cause of any disease like trismus neonatorum; and without a knowledge in regard to them it would be impossible to form a rational theory of the etiology of the disease.

TREATMENT OF PUERPERAL SEPSIS.

Grave septic intoxication during the lying-in period is one of the most formidable conditions which confront the medical man, and one which sometimes puts his resources to the sharpest proof. For this reason it is desirable to give the widest circulation to any method for the treatment of puerperal sepsis which seems, on its face, to be rational and to have stood the test of experience in a sufficient number of cases.

Such a method has been in use for some time by Prof. Max Runge, of Göttingen, and is described in full in the *Deutsche med. Wochenschrift*, Jan. 3, 1889. In brief, the method consists in the employment of the customary local treatment, with the addition of lukewarm baths and the administration of large doses of alcoholic liquors and full nourishment. Runge calls attention to the improvement in the prospects of women with puerperal sepsis which came with the introduction of an intelligent method of local treatment, and the comparative powerlessness of general medication. Of all the medicaments used in this condition, he thinks alcohol to be the only one of real value. Antipyretics he unqualifiedly condemns, as generally useless and often dangerous. This for two reasons: One, that the fever in puerperal sepsis is not usually of a high grade, and that mere elevation of temperature is a symptom which does not demand active interference; and, two, that antipyretics almost invariably ruin both appetite and digestion.

On the other hand, he finds that the administration of large quantities of wine and brandy, and the use of one or more lukewarm baths (22° — 24° Reaumur, or 82° — 86° Fahr.), improved the appetite of his patients so that it was not difficult to get them to take large quantities of nutritious and satisfying food.

The quantity of alcohol which may be given to a patient with puerperal sepsis may be gathered from the fact that one of Runge's patients took within a week over ten bottles of port and Madeira and about two quarts of Cognac. It is noticeable that even such large quantities of alcohol do not produce symptoms of intoxication, and that intolerance of large quantities is usually a sign of beginning convalescence.

As to the baths, Runge used them—not to reduce temperature, but to improve the general condition of his patients and to increase their disposition to take food. The idea of placing a lying-in woman in a full bath may seem startling to others; but Runge has never seen it do any harm, and has always seen it do good. The operation to be successful must be conducted by a skilled nurse or a physician, the temperature of the water and of the room must be right. The bath may last from three to eight minutes, and it is to be used according to the indications. The most that Runge ever administered was four in a day; usually he found one or two sufficient. The highest number he used in any one case was nineteen, in the majority of his cases from five to seven baths were sufficient, and in some of his cases only two or three were used.

The treatment outlined above is presented to his professional brethren by Prof. Runge in a manner which cannot fail to impress any one who reads his paper. In it there is no attempt to overrate the value of the method, and the whole argument bears the impress of careful thought, close observation and wise deduction. In theory his method commends itself to one's judgment, and in practice he has found it successful. We believe our readers will find it to their interest and helpful to their patients if they will give the method a trial, remembering that it can be expected to succeed only when combined with judicious local measures.

REGULATING THE SALE OF MILK.

We call attention to the suggestions—which are published in this number of the REPORTER—made by a Committee of the Board of Health of Philadelphia in regard to a law to regulate the sale of milk in this city. The fact that more than two hundred and fifty thousand quarts of milk are used in Philadelphia every day indicates the importance of some such legal regulation of its sale as is here proposed. Our only comment on the plan of the Committee is that it might well be incorporated in and assimilated with a more general law, securing a systematic inspection of all articles of food and drink. If such a measure could be adopted soon, it would be better than a law for only one article. But if the former is not attainable at present, we hope a carefully prepared law in regard to regulating the sale of milk may speedily be passed.

AN ABRUPT ENDING.—We have information from a trustworthy source that the official connection of Dr. John B. Hamilton with the *Journal of the American Medical Association* terminates this day, February 9. This sudden relinquishment of an office which he entered upon so recently will be a cause of surprise to those who have followed his vigorous editorial policy for the past six weeks. The reason for the step has not reached us when this note is written, but it may be public by the time it is printed.

THE MIDDLETON GOLDSMITH LECTURE for 1889 will be delivered by Dr. Reginald H. Fitz, Shattuck Professor of Pathology in the Harvard Medical School, in the hall of the New York Academy of Medicine, on Saturday, February 16, at 8½ o'clock P. M. The subject will be: "Acute Pancreatitis, with an especial consideration of Pancreatic Hemorrhage, Hemorrhagic Pancreatitis, and Subperitoneal Fat Necrosis."

BRITISH STUPIDITY.—The *British Medical Journal*, Jan. 12, contains a letter from a correspondent in Paris, in which the prizes awarded by the French Academy of Sciences are mentioned. In this letter the following statement occurs: "The Prix Cuvier in Geology was awarded to Mr. Joseph Leidy, of Harvard University." This statement is no reflection upon the fame of Dr. Leidy, but is rather an illustration of editorial ignorance or carelessness.

THE DOCTOR'S BADGE.—The *Medicinische Monatsschrift*, January, 1889, turns its attention to the question of a distinguishing mark for physicians, which has been seriously discussed during the past year by some of the medical journals. It quotes the *Medical World* as asking those who have courage enough to make themselves heard on this subject, and adds: "We accept this invitation, but would prefer to substitute for the olive green coat proposed by the *World*, a gray one. Instead of the letters M. D. on the collar, we would regard as more practical large ear trumpets of the same material, as a distinguishing mark of the bearer which would be visible from a great distance, and because they would serve as collectors of sound vibrations and facilitate the approach of the call of suffering fellow men to the membrana tympani of the wearer."

ELECTION AT THE UNIVERSITY OF PENNSYLVANIA.—At their meeting on Tuesday, February 5, Dr. J. William White was elected Clinical Professor of Surgery, and Dr. John Guitéras was elected Professor of Pathology and Morbid Anatomy.

Dr. John Guitéras is a native of Cuba, where he received his preliminary education, graduating from the Medical School of the University in 1873. In 1879 he was appointed by the President of the United States a member of the Havana Yellow Fever Commission, and took charge of the investigations in morbid anatomy. In 1880 he was appointed in the Marine Hospital Service, serving in St. Louis, New Orleans, Key West and Charleston. He was ordered by the Government to investigate epidemics of yellow fever in Vera Cruz, 1883; Key West, 1887; Florida, 1888. Dr. Guitéras has lectured in various medical colleges, and has made valuable contributions to medical science. In order to accept the Chair of Pathology he will resign his commission as Passed Assistant Surgeon U. S. Marine Hospital Service.

Dr. J. Wm. White, the new Professor of Clinical Surgery, is a Philadelphian, and was graduated at the University in 1871. Since then he has been surgeon to several hospitals in Philadelphia.

Besides these changes, a Clinical Chair of Orthopædic Surgery in the University Hospital was created, and a Chair of Histology and Embryology in the Medical Department. The former position will be occupied by Dr. De Forest Willard, and the latter by Dr. George A. Piersol.

BOOK REVIEWS.

[Any book reviewed in these columns may be obtained upon receipt of price, from the office of the REPORTER.]

A COMPEND OF THE DISEASES OF THE EYE; INCLUDING REFRACTION AND SURGICAL OPERATIONS. By L. WEBSTER Fox, M.D., Ophthalmic Surgeon to the Germantown Hospital, etc., and GEO. M. GOULD, M.D. Second edition revised and enlarged, with 71 Illustrations. Philadelphia: P. Blakiston, Son & Co., 1888. Small 8vo, pp. 164. Price $1.00.

That this little book has grown in usefulness there can be no doubt. Nearly all of the chapters have undergone revision, and many have gained by rearrangement. Treatment has been brought to date, and puzzling technicalities have been carefully replaced by either proper terms in full or by common expressive equivalents. Of the newly added cuts, however, all but one are taken from Meyer, without any indication that they have been borrowed.

Taken as a whole, the book is a good and trustworthy guide for its intended readers—undergraduates and busy general practitioners—but to them it is only fair to say: to cultivate a habit of close and accurate observation of the eye. The successful ophthalmologist often suspects or bases diagnoses upon a perception of subtle and delicate differences in the external appearance of an eye that he would have difficulty in explaining to another "—as this is the only way by which they may hope to arrive at correct diagnosis, proper prognosis, and judicious treatment in cases of ophthalmic disease.

ELEMENTS OF PRACTICAL MEDICINE. By ALFRED H. CARTER, M.D., Lond., Physician to the Queen's Hospital, Benningham, etc. Fifth edition. Small 8vo, pp. xvi, 472. London: H. K. Lewis, 1888.

The purpose of this book is stated by the author to be: to provide students with a simple introduction to the study of systematic medicine, and to bring the essentials of the subject clearly and tersely within the grasp of those unable to master larger treatises. It is high praise to say that Dr. Carter has attained his object. His book is both terse and clear; and its terseness is not secured by sacrificing anything essential to such a work. His descriptions of diseases and morbid states are simple and yet full enough to be very useful, and his recommendations in regard to treatment are judicious and easy to remember. He avoids excess of detail in the former, and in the latter he lays down general principles and has not burdened his book with prescriptions.

As a whole his work is excellent, and would prove of value to students if its reading were made to accompany their attendance on didactic and clinical lectures. Equally is it calculated to be a help to busy practitioners—especially those who have not the time or inclination to consult elaborate treatises.

—Messrs. J. B. Lippincott Company announce to the profession the publication of a Cyclopædia of the Diseases of Children, medical and surgical, by American, British, and Canadian authors, edited by John M. Keating, M.D., in four imperial octavo volumes; to be sold by subscription only. The first volume will be issued early in April, and the subsequent volumes at short intervals. This is the only work of the kind that has been published in English.

PAMPHLET NOTICES.

[Any reader of the REPORTER who desires a copy of a pamphlet noticed in these columns will doubtless secure it by addressing the author with a request stating where the notice was seen and *enclosing a postage-stamp.*]

206. SOME ACCOUNT OF THE MEDICAL PROFESSION IN NEW HAVEN. By FRANCIS BACON, M.D., New Haven, Conn. 44 pages.

207. TWO SUCCESSFUL CASES OF BRAIN SURGERY. By CHARLES B. NANCREDE, M.D., Philadelphia. From the *Medical News*, November 24, 1888. 14 pages

208. IS THE ELECTRIC LIGHT INJURIOUS TO THE EYES? By GEORGE M. GOULD, M.D., Philadelphia. From the *Medical News*, Dec. 8, 1888. 23 pages.

209. EXPLORATORY TREPHINING AND PUNCTURE OF THE BRAIN ALMOST TO THE LATERAL VENTRICLE. By W. W. KEEN, M.D., Philadelphia. From the *Medical News*, Dec. 1, 1888.

210. PRELIMINARY REPORT OF AN OPERATION FOR THE FORMATION OF AN ARTIFICIAL PUPIL THROUGH THE SCLEROTIC COAT OF THE EYEBALL. By GEORGE STRAWBRIDGE, M.D., Philadelphia. From the *Medical News*, Dec. 15, 1888. 12 pages.

211. CONDITIONS RENDERING DIAGNOSIS DIFFICULT IN PELVIC AND ABDOMINAL DISEASES. By T. B. HARVEY, M.D., Indianapolis, Ind. 14 pages.

212. EL PASO, TEXAS, AS A WINTER HEALTH RESORT. By W. M. YANDELL, M.D., El Paso, Texas. 10 pages.

206. The history of the medical profession in any part of the United States, if well written, could not fail to be of interest; but that of the older sections of the country has a peculiar charm, because it takes the student back to the time in which our forefathers were laying the foundation for the superstructure which in our day extends so far and towers so high. In the pamphlet before us Dr. Bacon has brought together, in most attractive and entertaining shape, reminiscences of the early practice of medicine in and near New Haven, which have a much more than local interest. The work is done with a grace of style and a shrewdness of commentary which are characteristic of the family to which the author belongs.

207. In one of the cases which Dr. Nancrede reports he trephined the skull to find a bullet, the course of which he traced to the base of the skull but could not follow further; in the other he excised the thumb-centre for Jacksonian epilepsy. Both patients recovered. The description of these operations is both interesting and instructive, and the paper which contains it is a valuable contribution to the literature of surgery of the brain.

208. Dr. Gould, after a careful review of the evidence in regard to the effect of the electric light upon the eyes, answers the question of the title of his paper in the negative. More than this, he shows that the cases in which the electric light has proved injurious to the eyes are to be attributed to its improper use, and he urges the general adoption of electric lighting for all public halls. His pamphlet contains a valuable bibliography of the subject.

209. The literature of brain surgery bids fair soon to rival that of abdominal surgery; and Dr. Keen's contributions to it are always of great interest and

value. In the pamphlet before us he describes, with excellent illustrations, the history of a case of abnormal intracranial pressure, in which he trephined the skull, and punctured the brain, in the hope of giving vent to the fluid which caused the trouble. Unfortunately he failed to reach the fluid, although he came very near to it. His patient died, and the autopsy showed that Dr. Keen's exploratory puncture had come within a quarter of an inch of the fluid, which was contained in a distended left ventricle.

The experience of this case, added to the operator's general experience, leads him to propose tapping the ventricles of the brain as a definite surgical operation, and he describes the method by which he thinks this operation may be most safely performed. Such a proposal challenges the thoughtful attention of all surgeons and students of injuries and diseases of the brain, and Dr. Keen's pamphlet cannot fail to attract very wide spread notice.

210. Dr. Strawbridge makes an exceedingly ingenious suggestion for the treatment of incurable leucoma, and one which is likely to attract as much attention as Von Hippel's method of trephining the cornea. At the time of publishing his article he had made a number of successful experiments by his method upon the eyes of rabbits, and he had done two operations upon human eyes. Sufficient time had not elapsed in the latter cases to demonstrate what the ultimate result of the operations would be; and this result will be looked for with the deepest interest.

211. Dr. Harvey calls attention to the necessity for examining patients carefully in order to avoid the error of overlooking unconspicuous, but important disorders. The special field which he considers is that of the abdominal and pelvic viscera of women; but what he says has a still wider range of applicability.

212. Dr. Yandell has taken up the teaching of Dr. Denison, of Denver, and applied it to the case of El Paso, in such a way as to indicate that the latter is a very desirable place for the residence of persons affected or threatened with consumption. He claims that El Paso has, in common with southern New Mexico and southern Arizona the best Winter climate in the United States for consumptives and asthmatics, as well as persons suffering with other chronic pulmonary affections.

LITERARY NOTES.

—The *Independent Practitioner,* a dental journal published in New York and Philadelphia, has changed its title to *The International Dental Journal.*

—The *Journal of the Respiratory Organs* is the name of a new magazine, edited by J. Mount Bleyer, M.D., and published by Napoléon Thompson, of New York. The first number is dated January, 1889, and contains 13 octavo pages of reading matter. It is to be issued on the fifteenth of each month; subscription price $1.00 a year.

—The American Biographical Publishing Co., Philadelphia, announces that a work on American Resorts, with notes upon their climate, by Bushrod W. James, A.M., M.D., with a translation from the German by Mr. S. Kauffman of those chapters of "Die Klimate der Erde," written by Dr. A. Woeikof, of St. Petersburg, Russia, that relate to North and South America and the islands and oceans contiguous thereto, is in press and will shortly appear.

CORRESPONDENCE.

A Defense of Homœopathy.

To THE EDITOR:

Sir: A few days ago, I was shown an editorial in the REPORTER, Oct. 6, 1888, entitled "The Homœopathic State Medical Society of Pennsylvania." I am sorry it had not come to my notice earlier, as I should have had a reply in your hands long ere this.

Your reference to the fact that the Homœopathic State Medical Society of Pennsylvania had just concluded an interesting meeting in Philadelphia, and had displayed a fitness for the discussion of important medical questions which would hardly be expected by those who are not familiar with the advances made of late by those who bear this designation," is perfectly correct; but. you err when you say that "the proceedings at this meeting were so like those of any 'regular' medical society that it is hard to discover any homœopathy in them at all."

You err, however, when you state that "the tenets of Hahnemann have come to occupy but a minor and subordinate position in their (*i. e.* the Homœopaths') thoughts and practice." I doubt if there was one in all the large gathering of members of our school at the session of the society who subordinated the Homœopathic principle in his thoughts or practice. Never have the laws of Hahnemann been so well understood, or so freed from the things that unfortunately since his day have somewhat hampered the growth and development of his system. The law of *similia similibus curantur* is upheld by our school no less vigorously to-day than formerly. But time and the progress of things have taught us wherein we were weak and needful of strength. The transactions of our societies are therefore more liberal. We are striving to give the principle of the *similars* its proper value, and to that end we investigate and court investigation. If our law of cure is universal in its application, our effort is to prove it; if it is not, still we aim to seek the truth and in the finding give it proper place. The old school is in need of an intelligent understanding of what we are really doing and of what we are really accomplishing. The time will surely come when the old school will believe as fully as we do, that the Homœopathic law is at least one of the laws of cure.

Is there not some mistake in the following

taken from your article: "The time will "yet come when . . . such men as made "the last meeting of the Pennsylvania State "Homœopathic Medical Society almost "undistinguishable from a similar meeting "of 'regular' physicians will not debar "themselves from association with all other "scientific medical men by holding fast to "a name which misrepresents them, and dis- "credits them in the opinion of men who "have no desire to be unjust or uncharita- "ble"?

Can you in all earnestness believe that such a time is near or ever likely to come? Is there a place in the old school of this city for the physician who has the courage of his convictions that Hahnemann demonstrated a principle in the laws of the similars? It is essential to the believers in Homœopathy that they class themselves together under the name which Hahnemann adopted ; and this is true even for those who deny the *universality* of the Homœopathic law. What opportunity is afforded in the "regular" school for the study of the "similars"? Do you throw open to us your hospitals and your journals? Are we given fair-handed opportunity to demonstrate what we can do? When you allow us the freedom of action for which for years we have been pleading, then, and only then, can the two schools hope to commingle, and our title of "Homœopath" give place to that of plain "Doctor of Medicine."

I am glad that your article shows in some respects a spirit of fairness on your part. It is only by an unimpassioned, unprejudiced inquiry into the relative merits of the claims of the two rival schools that there can be entertained any hope of an ultimate solution of the problems of the hour.

Yours truly,
G. MAXWELL CHRISTINE, M.D.
2043 N. Twelfth St., Philadelphia.

[This letter is given place in the REPORTER because the writer has desired to have it published as a sort of justification of those who, he thinks, have been misrepresented in our columns. But, in doing so, attention is called to several points in it.

1. The writer cannot be aware of the belief and practice of many of his fellows in this city, or he would not venture the assertion that he doubts if there was one in the gathering spoken of who subordinated the homœopathic principle in his thoughts or practice.

2. He cannot be a careful reader of the journals of his own school if he believes that the law of similars is upheld as vigorously by his school to-day as formerly.

3. In reference to the appeal for a chance to work out homœopathic theories in regular hospitals: this is a most impracticable idea. There may be something more than coincidence in the fact that certain drugs produce in health symptoms similar to those of disease in which they may be administered with advantage ; and this is a proper subject for unprejudiced investigation ; but the claim that homœopathy, or any other "pathy" furnishes a universal law of treatment is condemned by all unbiassed scientific men. This condemnation is usually spoken of as if it applied only to homœopathy ; but it applies equally to every exclusive dogma, whether it be homœopathy, or hydropathy, or electropathy, or vitapathy.

As asserted in our editorial, we believe the time will come when the rational men who bear the name of homœopath will drop this inappropriate and deceptive designation, and leave the title to those to whom it properly belongs—to the advantage of all concerned. It is not possible for assimilation to take place between such miscalled homœopaths, and those whose scientific methods they approve and imitate, until the former refuse to be called by a name which is practically false, and announce their adherence to those principles of reason which alone deserve the name of scientific. We know that this fact is appreciated by some who still permit themselves to be denominated homœopaths, and we hope that they will yet find occasion to declare publicly that what they believe of homœopathy is but a part of what experience teaches, and not what the real homœopath thinks it—an exclusive and universal law.]

Nasal Bougies.—A Correction.

TO THE EDITOR.

Sir: May I make a correction in the article on Nasal Bougies (REPORTER, Feb. 2, p. 146), which you did me the honor to republish?

The strength of the nasal bougie is given as one-twentieth of a grain of atropine; it should be one-one hundred and twentieth of a grain of atropine.

Yours truly,
H. C. WOOD, M.D.
Philadelphia, Feb. 4, 1889.

—Dr. Oliver Wendell Holmes has presented his medical library to the Boston Medical Library Association.

NOTES AND COMMENTS.

Regulation of the Sale of Milk in Philadelphia.

The Sanitary Committee of the Board of Health of Philadelphia at its meeting, January 29, 1889, presented a petition to be submitted to the State Legislature with reference to a regulation applying to the sale of milk in Philadelphia. The petition is rather voluminous, and states that the Board of Health, recognizing the necessity. of a strict supervision over the milk supply of the city, whereby the purity of a most important article of food shall be secured, petitions the Legislature to adopt such legislation as will best effect this object.

It suggested that in order to protect the public health a law be enacted which shall embrace a number of provisions contained in the petition. Among these suggestions are: That if any person or persons shall sell or exchange, or offer for sale or exchange, or have in his, her, or their premises, with intent to sell or exchange, milk to which water, ice, coloring matter, or any other foreign substance shall have been added, or milk from which the cream, or any part thereof, shall have been removed, or milk taken from a cow fed upon distillery-waste or any other substance tending to make her milk unwholesome, or milk taken from a sick or diseased cow, or milk exposed to infection or unhealthy exhalations, or not of standard quality, shall be guilty of a misdemeanor, and upon conviction shall be sentenced to pay a fine not exceeding $100 or be imprisoned not over six months, or both or either, at the discretion of the Court.

Evaporated or condensed milk shall contain 25 per centum or more of fat, and milk containing 12 per centum of milk solids shall be deemed of standard quality, and all other milk shall be deemed not of standard quality. This does not apply to buttermilk.

In cities of the first class the Director of Public Safety is directed to appoint an Inspector of Milk, with assistants, clerks, analysts, and collectors of samples. The latter are directed to take a fair sample of any milk offered for sale, and for such purpose may enter all places where milk is stored or kept for sale, and have access to all wagons, carts, or other vehicles used for the conveyance of milk and open any vessel or package containing milk for sale or exchange. Whenever an Inspector or Col-

lector takes a sample of milk he is required to divide it into two parts and put each into a separate can or vessel and seal (it) in the presence of the owner or owners or their agents or employes from whom the sample was obtained. One part shall be offered to the owner or owners, agents or employes, and the other shall be retained and analyzed or tested. Unless the provisions of this section are complied with the result of the test shall not be received in evidence in any. prosecution brought under the Act. If any person or persons shall hinder, obstruct, or interfere with any Inspector, or Collector of samples in his collections, or if any person or persons use or have any imitation of the Collector's seal, they shall be guilty of a misdemeanor, the punishment, on conviction, being the same as referred to above.

It shall be unlawful in any city after an Inspector has been appointed for any person to sell or exchange milk without a license. All applications for a license are required to be made in writing to the Inspector of the Milk for the city for which the license shall be desired, which application shall contain the location of the place or places and the number of vehicles for which licenses are desired. It also provides that, unless City Councils make other provisions, the sum of $10 shall be tendered for each place, $5 for each vehicle, for which a license is desired. After application has been made, the Inspector shall issue a certificate to the applicant showing whether the license is for a place or vehicle. These licenses shall expire on the 1st of May of each year, and the Inspector is required to keep a record of all the licenses granted. Cities of the first class are empowered to substitute for the license charges named any sum deemed expedient. In cases of removal of location a fee of 25 cents is to be charged for changing the certificate and records.

Licenses may be transferred upon personal application to the Inspector and the payment of the fee of 25 cents for the changes made on the records. In all cases the certificates of licenses must be displayed conspicuously. If any person not licensed shall sell or exchange milk, or if any person make a false statement in application for a license or transfer, or if the certificate be not conspicuously displayed, or if milk be sold from a vehicle not properly marked, such person or persons so offending shall be guilty of a misdemeanor. It will be the duty of the Inspectors to cause the arrest of any person against whom they have sufficient evidence.

All moneys received from licenses, charges, and fees are to be paid into the City Treasury and shall constitute a separate fund to be appropriated by Councils.—*Telegraph*, Jan. 29, 1889.

New Method of Illuminating Internal Organs.

The Vienna correspondent of the *Lancet*, Jan. 5, 1888, says that the well-known experiment for showing total reflection of light in a jet of water or in a glass rod has been made use of in Vienna by Dr. Roth and Professor Reuss in devising a new method of illuminating from outside some cavities of the body, such as the larynx and nose. The instrument used for this purpose is a well-polished (not blackened) glass rod, to one end of which a small electric incandescent glow lamp, like those used for electric breast pins, is attached. The light of the lamp is reflected equally through the whole glass rod to its other end, which is placed on the skin of the throat in the case of a laryngoscopical examination being required; then the interior of the larynx becomes illuminated sufficiently for laryngoscopy. If this luminous glass rod is applied to the sclerotic, the interior of the eyeball can be examined in the same way as by using an ophthalmoscope, the structure of the posterior parts of the vitreous body being very well seen and studied. As the glass rod remains cold, it can be employed in operative surgery to light the natural and artificial cavities.

Evil Effects Following the Administration of Sulphonal.

Dr. Schotten, of Cassel, reports a case of this kind in the *Therapeutische Monatshefte*, Dec., 1888. A woman 45 years old, a hemiplegic since her twentieth year as the result of chronic myelitis, was a victim of wakefulness. Schotten gave the patient sulphonal, three days in succession, in doses of fifteen and 45 grains. Under its influence she was affected with extreme prostration, headache, anorexia, and a bitter taste in the mouth. Four days later her body was covered with an eruption resembling measles; at the same time the other symptoms attributed to the sulphonal disappeared. The eruption was accompanied with a sensation as of burning and of heat in the skin, and lasted fifteen days.

A sister of the patient had presented a similar eruption following the use of antipyrin.—*Gazette Médicale de Paris*, Dec. 29, 1888.

Therapeutics of Iodol.

Prof. Dante Cervesato, of Padua, has communicated to *Lo Sperimentale*, September, 1888, his experiences with the therapeutic use of iodol in internal diseases. It was first tried in scrofulosis, in all forms of which it acted well. It was most active in the torpid form, especially in torpid, swollen lymph glands which had not yet suppurated—and not only in the peripheral glands but also in the bronchial and mesenteric. It was less favorable in its action upon scrofulosis of the mucous membranes, especially of the nose and ear. It has very little influence upon scrofulous dermatoses. It was employed internally in doses of seven and a half, fifteen, and twenty-two and a half grains in older children, and the treatment could be kept up without harm for two or three months uninterruptedly. Iodoform ointment (one part to fifteen of vaseline) and insufflations of iodoform were useful adjuncts. The iodol was well borne; not only did no digestive disturbances occur, but the digestion even improved. In diseases of the respiratory organs iodol was given in doses of fifteen to forty-five grains a day, in addition to inhalations with the following solution: one part of iodol is dissolved in five parts of warm absolute alcohol; to the filtered solution ten parts of glycerine (at 60°—70°) are added. Before the solution cools, ten parts of water are added with constant stirring. The iodol remains proportionately suspended for a long time. Four drachms of the emulsion are used for each inhalation, which is given two or three times a day. He has observed marked improvement in primary tuberculosis of the larynx. In acute and chronic catarrhal laryngitis, and in different forms of bronchitis, the results were brilliant. In tertiary syphilis it was employed with very favorable results. Two patients with extensive ulcers on the palate and pharynx recovered after the internal and local use of iodol for two months. Internally iodol was given in doses of fifteen to forty-five grains; the following solution was used locally:

Iodol	gr. xv
Alcohol	f ʒ iv
Glycerine	f ʒ viii

M.

In a case of tertiary syphilis with lesions of the liver and of the larynx, the internal use of iodol achieved wonders. No iodism nor any other disagreeable accompanying symptoms whatsoever occurred in any of the cases.—*Wiener med. Presse*, Dec. 2, 1888.

The Doctor as a Civilizer.

The large part played by medical travelers and missionaries in the most remote and uncivilized parts of the world in attracting the affection of savage populations, and leading them in the path of civilization, is not the least glorious page of medical history, and would afford material for an interesting research. Mr. George Curzon, in his account this month of a *Visit to Bokhara the Noble*, gives a highly interesting sketch of Dr. Heyfelder, who was chief of the medical staff in Skobeleff's Turcoman campaign. "It would be hard to exaggerate the part which his manners and generosity have played in the pacification of this whilom haunt of fanaticism. As early as six in the morning people crowd into the Embassy to see him. Very often so childish is their faith that they do not ask for a prescription, but simply implore his touch. . . . A fat old Bey, he told me, came to him one day and said : 'Can you make me better ? I suffer from eating four dinners a day.' 'Certainly,' said the doctor, 'eat three.' Thereupon the old gentleman became very angry, and retorted, 'How can I eat less when I am called upon to entertain venerable foreigners ?' I asked the doctor whether it was out of benevolence that he continued to reside in Bokhara. 'Yes,' he replied, 'and as a pioneer of civilization.'"—*British Med. Journal*, Jan. 12, 1889.

Statistics of Operations on the Gall Bladder.

Dr. A. Depage, in the course of a paper upon Surgical Intervention in Biliary Lithiasis (*Journ. de Méd. Brux.*, 1888, No. 24), says that up to the present there have been 78 cholecystotomies performed. Of these operations, 6 were done according to the method of Spencer Wells, 72 with suture of the gall bladder to the abdominal wall. Of the first-named series, 3 patients died from acute peritonitis, in 1 cured case there was recurrence, and 2 patients were completely cured. Of the second series there were 11 deaths, 5 from hemorrhage and collapse, 2 from biliary retention, 2 from effusion of bile into the peritoneum, and 2 from undetermined cause ; there were also 4 deaths from secondary complications. Amongst the "cures" are 24 cases of biliary fistula, some permanent. The number of cholecystectomies has been 22, with 2 deaths from obstruction of the bile duct, and 1 after recovery from the operation from a cause independent of biliary lithiasis.

Thus in cholecystotomy with suture of the gall bladder, and its return free into the abdominal cavity, a mortality of 50 per cent. resulted ; in cholecystotomy with suture of the bladder to the parietes, 15.27 per cent.; and in cholecystectomy, 9.99 per cent.; and as the last-named figure comprises the two cases of permanent occlusion of the common bile duct, the result, if they be excluded, is to enhance greatly the position of cholecystectomy as an operation to be preferred to cholecystotomy.—*Lancet*, Jan. 12, 1889.

Frequency of Diseases of the Nose and Throat.

Dr. W. Franklin Chappell, Attending Physician to the Chest and Throat Department, Presbyterian Hospital, New York, has undertaken to ascertain the frequency of diseases of the throat and nose. In his paper, published in the *American Journal of Med. Sciences*, Feb., 1889, he gives some interesting details of his examination of the noses and throats of two thousand children. Nine hundred and fifty-five of these were from the New York Juvenile Asylum, six hundred and forty-five from the Grammar School No. 49, and two hundred from the Half Orphan Asylum in East 10th Street, and the remaining number from various sources.

In the entire number the following abnormal conditions were found : Adenoid growths, 60 ; enlarged tonsils, 270 ; deviated septa, 330 ; spurs on septa, 150 ; hypertrophy of inferior turbinated bodies, 260 ; hypertrophy of middle turbinated bodies, 161. This shows that 1231 were suffering from some anatomical abnormality, and usually with its accompanying symptoms of respiratory obstruction and catarrh.

After an analysis of these statistics, he expresses the opinion that enlarged tonsils and adenoid growths are the only anatomical abnormalities that can be classed as belonging to very early life. The other abnormal conditions are acquired usually after the age of six years, increasing rapidly with each succeeding year until puberty. All social classes are liable to them in about equal proportions, and at the same age. Males, he says, suffer more frequently than females, probably owing to greater exposure to the causes which produce catarrhal congestion and inflammation. In glandular organs it is but a step from congestion to hyperplasia, and an increased afflux of blood being once established, a slight irritation will serve to keep it up, and hypertrophy is the necessary result.

Hospitals for Contagious Diseases in Tennessee.

In his report to the State Board of Health of Tennessee, Jan. 8, 1889, the Secretary, Dr. J. B. Lindsley, spoke as follows:

"As to yellow fever we must not conceal the fact that the outlook is ominous. All sanitarians in the Southern States familiar with the past are very uneasy about the coming summer. There is but one way open to us, namely, to look the possibilities fairly in the face and be ready for any emergency.

"In this connection a local matter of great importance should not be overlooked. The four cities—Memphis, Nashville, Chattanooga, and Knoxville—each centres of great travel and traffic, visited by thousands annually, not only from Tennessee, but from States near and far, with large floating populations, should, without delay, provide suitable accommodations for the care and treatment of persons suffering from communicable diseases—ordinarily termed contagious or infectious. Such hospitals should be isolated, but not at too inconvenient a distance. They need not be large, but should be always equipped and ready for use, and competent physicians and nurses constantly retained for service. No one can tell when such hospitals will be wanted. These four cities are already noted and populous, rapidly growing also, and are without excuse for not making such provision for the stranger within their gates or their own people, many in number, who cannot be well cared for at home."—*Tennessee State Board of Health Bulletin,* Jan. 15, 1889.

What are we to Know?

Canon Isaac Taylor, in an address on "Literature and Culture," published in the *Church Worker,* has given some advice which, with some obvious modifications, doctors and medical students would do well to lay to heart. He said : "It is impossible for any one man to know everything—*omne scibile.* Two hundred years ago it was possible; but now the domain of knowledge has been so vastly extended that it is impossible. In these days, to be distinguished, a man must be a specialist—he must devote himself to some department of knowledge. It is impossible, for instance, that the same man can be at once a great historian and a great chemist. It was said of Whewell, that while science was his forte, omniscience was his foible. Because he knew so much, he thought he could know everything; and so, if you strive after universal knowledge, what you will attain will not be science, but sciolism. Strive after universal knowledge, and you will become a universal smatterer. On the other hand, the mere specialist tends to become a narrow pedant. How shall we avoid these opposite dangers—sciolism and pedantry? I think the best rule for a young man to set before him in his studies is, to resolve to know something of everything, and everything of something. To know everything of something is to choose some one branch of science for your specialty, and to learn everything that can be learned about it ; this will give you accuracy and precision. To become 'an authority,' as it is called, on some one subject, however small—on butterflies, birds' eggs, or even on postage stamps—is better than nothing. Still better is it to take some department of history, or of geology, or of philology, and master it thoroughly. But this is not enough. You will thus learn to be accurate, exhaustive ; but you will be narrow. You must not only know everything of something ; but, to gain breadth of mind, you should also resolve to know something of everything. Strive to take a general interest in every department of human knowledge. Strive to know enough of every science to enable you to listen intelligently to any great specialist you may chance to meet, and to read with profit any great epoch-making book that may appear. Such knowledge cannot be deep; but such an imperfect knowledge adds immensely to the intellectual pleasures within your reach, and will constantly throw light on that one branch of knowledge which you have specially made your own."— *Bristol Medico-Chirurgical Journal,* Dec., 1888.

Naval Board of Medical Examiners.

The Board of medical officers is now convened at Philadelphia for the examination of applicants for appointment as assistant surgeons in the navy, and will remain until March 31 ; it has been ordered to meet at the Naval Hospital, Brooklyn, April 1, and to remain there until the following October. The change is made to enable students at the New York and Brooklyn hospitals to be examined by the Board without the expense of leaving their homes. There are fourteen vacancies in the grade of Assistant Surgeon. Further information may be obtained by addressing the President of the Examining Board.

NEWS.

—Small-pox of a malignant type is reported to be increasing in Nanticoke, Pa.

—Dr. Heinrich A. Pagenstecher, the eminent zoologist, has recently died at Hamburg.

—Dr. John A. Fisher died in New Orleans Jan. 15. He was a native of Lebanon, Pa.

—Dr. W. R. D. Blackwood was elected President of the Anti-Vivisection Society at its recent meeting Jan. 28, 1889.

—Dr. Charles Bliss died in New York City Jan. 23. He was graduated from the Berkshire Medical College in 1865.

—Prof. Ziegler of Tübingen has been invited to take to Professorship of Pathological Anatomy in the University of Freiburg.

—Dr. E. A. Neely, who has just withdrawn from the editorial staff of the *Memphis Medical Monthly*, was married at Memphis Jan. 23.

—Dr. John Underhill died in Cincinnati, Ohio, Jan. 28, from the effects of cocaine, to which he is said to have become habituated through experimentation.

—Typhoid fever is epidemic at Lake View, Cook county, Illinois. The *Journal of the Amer. Med. Association*, Feb. 2, says that there are now nearly fifty cases of the disease.

—The Eighth German Congress for Internal Medicine will be held in Wiesbaden from April 15 to April 18, 1889, under the presidency of Prof. von Liebermeister, of Tübingen.

—Dr. William A. Edwards has established a private Hospital at San Diego, Southern California. The nursing will be conducted by graduates of the Philadelphia Hospital Training School.

—A disease presenting some peculiar symptoms has made its appearance in Webster county, Kentucky. It seems to be traceable to impure water and poisoned atmosphere, and is said to be rapidly fatal.

—Another doctor has been beaten by White Caps who have committed some outrages at North Manchester, Indiana. Dr. W. H. Clair was assaulted on the principal street of the place and ordered to leave town. He was beaten over the head and shoulders with clubs, and then shot at, one of the bullets inflicting a painful wound.

HUMOR.

A FOND MOTHER of a smart boy was making a lot of nice preserves one day, and as she sealed them up she labelled them thus: "Gooseberry jam put up by Mrs. Mason." Johnnie soon discovered the shelf on which they were deposited, and fell to work. Having emptied one of the jars, he took his school pencil and wrote underneath the label: "Put down by Johnnie Mason."—*Am. Druggist.*

"MAY I LOOK through your wastebasket?" inquired a young man, entering timidly. "Certainly," said the editor. "What do you want to find?" "A little poem on 'Mortality' that I sent in yesterday." "My dear sir, that poem was accepted and will appear to-morrow. I will draw you a check for $25, and I assure you—" But he spoke to lifeless ears. The young man had fallen to the floor. The shock had killed him.

A DERMATOLOGIST, being seated by a lady unknown to him, at dinner, when conversation lagged, remarked interestedly, "Have you noticed the spots on that man's face across the table?" To which she indignantly replied, "Excuse me, sir; that is my husband!" The skin man, being a Briton, and so never to be crushed by circumstances, most enthusiastically said: "Ah! that *is* fortunate; then *you* can tell me whether he is spotted like that all over, *cawn't* you?"

OBITUARY.

MARTIN L. WEAVER, M.D.

Dr. Martin L. Weaver died at his residence in Germantown, Feb. 1. He was born in Germantown about eighty-four years ago. His grandfather, Martin Webber, came to America about 1714.

Dr. Weaver was graduated from the University of Pennsylvania in 1829, receiving his preliminary education at Princeton College. At one time he contemplated entering the ministry of the Presbyterian Church, and took a theological course at Carlisle. He never took a regular charge, but employed the greater portion of his time as co-executor of his father's estate.

Dr. Weaver came into prominence in the newspapers several years ago through the trouble between his daughter and his second wife. Efforts were made to have him adjudged insane and his marriage set aside, but the Courts decided in his favor.

MEDICAL AND SURGICAL
REPORTER

No. 1668.   PHILADELPHIA, FEBRUARY 16, 1889.   VOL. LX.—No. 7.

CONTENTS:

CLINICAL LECTURE.

RHEUMATISM WITH ARTICULAR, CEREBRAL AND VISCERAL SYMPTOMS.[1]

BY PROFESSOR M. PETER,

PARIS, FRANCE.

(Reported specially for the MEDICAL AND SURGICAL REPORTER.)

Gentlemen: We saw for the first time, this morning, a patient in the Laennec ward, who struck me as furnishing a good lesson for you. In examining him I was first of all taken aback with the lamentable aspect of his face and the deplorable state of his pulse, which is irregular and almost imperceptible. The disease is what I call *"mad rheumatism."* The patient is pale, his nose is pinched, and his aspect is not that of a person with a febrile malady, but rather that of one profoundly depressed. The tongue is dry, the abdomen swollen,

[1] Delivered at the Hospital Necker, Paris.

and there was an involuntary stool this morning; so that those who noticed these symptoms will say, "It's a typhoid fever case;" but it is not. I will explain why. The patient is lying in the dorsal decubitis, it is true, but when an attempt is made to move his arm he has an intense pain in the scapulo-humeral articulation. The disease is rheumatism. But, you will say, a singular rheumatism to be accompanied with swollen abdomen, involuntary stools and irregular heart action. Talk to him, however, and you will find out that he is a market porter, and that he has been in the habit of "drinking without counting." You know the habits of these men—always a drink after each basket they carry, so that they take as much as four or five quarts of wine a day. The patient is then an alcoholic; he says it is part of his profession. It will always be found that disease in an alcoholic patient will differ from the usual type. The patient says that some seven or eight years ago he had articular rheumatism, for which he was treated in this same hospital with salicylate of soda, and that he recovered. It does

193

not appear that he had endocarditis afterward, with a mitral insufficiency. I say this because we cannot tell, in organs that have been drenched with alcohol for eight years, whether there was a lesion of that kind or not. As to his present trouble, he says that fifteen or twenty days ago he was taken with pulmonary congestion, for which leeches were applied over the right lower thoracic region. The redness still persists there, which shows the bad state of his skin, which consists in a tendency to lymphangitis of a sub-inflammatory order; it also shows that his tissues are just as weak as his other organs. It seems that he was cured of his pulmonary congestion when he commenced to have delirium, and his doctor said: "I don't understand this; he is delirious and yet better of the pulmonary trouble." And now fever lights up again, and he has pains in all his joints. In a word, he had rheumatism in the first place, and it is probable that his congestion was rheumatic. He is a rheumatic subject, as these visceral localizations indicate.

When asked to show his tongue, he simply turns it as he would a ball, with the greatest difficulty, and puts out the tip, which is dry and of a typhoid look. The patient says he cannot put it out further. If the finger is pressed below the temporo-maxillary articulation, it will be noticed that he says nothing; but if it is pressed on the articulation itself, he screams with pain, so that he has a bi-lateral temporo-maxillary arthritis. This is rare in rheumatism; but as I led you to expect, all is unusual in such cases. Has he then acute articular rheumatism? No; he has what I call "*fievre rhumatismale typhoidique*," called also rheumatic fever. It cannot be doubted that he had visceral rheumatism. From the start his congestion was rheumatism, his delirium was cerebral rheumatism. But this rheumatism shows itself not only in the brain, but also in the heart symptoms; there is no rhythm in the heart beat, and we never find that endocarditis produces arhythmia. It determines mitral insufficiency, by default of tension or by alteration of the valvular surfaces; it can only produce trouble in the circulation by a reflux of the blood—a physical fact that shows a physical lesion. But a rhythmic disorder of the pulse such as this, is only seen when the heart-muscle itself is altered. There is present in this case an alteration of the innervation of the heart, analogous to the trouble in his intelligence, which came from a like disorder of the brain. The patient has, therefore, a rheumatism of the heart, not endo- but myocardial, and perhaps also neuritis by fluxion on the nerves of the cardiac plexus.

Is this all he has? No; because the swollen abdomen and the involuntary stools show that there is also an intestinal, visceral rheumatism. The digestive tube is in somewhat the same state that it is in typhoid fever; that is to say, there is a paralysis of the muscular tunic of the intestines, which causes a swelling of the abdomen, and a fluxion of the glands, giving rise to the diarrhœa; but there are no lesions of Peyer's patches.

I must try now to give you an idea as to what ordinary rheumatism is, and what cerebral rheumatism is like. More than half a century ago, Bouillaud wrote a treatise on "Acute Articular Rheumatism," and he made it out a prototype of inflammation; but notice that he called it acute articular rheumatism, and not rheumatic fever. He thought it was an inflammatory malady of the articulations, and he called valular endocarditits an arthritis, as though the valves were articulations and the trouble was the same; so that for Bouillaud it was an inflammation that was pathologically localized in articulations for the body, and on the valves when the heart was affected; but all this is an absolute error, for in an autopsy of a case of acute articular rheumatism as given by Bouillaud, it will be noticed that he tries to prove that the troubled aspect of the heart, or rather of the pericardium, is owing to inflammation; but both the endocardium and the articular surfaces are intact; there are not even any signs of vascularity of the tissues. In fact, there are none of the lesions found in arthritis, and we are obliged to say it is not an inflammation of the articulations. It is a fluxion which had already left the articulation; and just because it is a simple fluxion, there is produced in these cases a wandering of its manifestations; during several days it will appear at many different points, but a real arthritis never does this. It is, therefore, a malady with a flux from the natural tissues, which appears at different articulations, and may also appear on the endocardium, the brain and the intestines, as it has done in this case. Remember this fundamental fact: acute rheumatism is a general malady with fever. It is a fever; so we shall say, acute rheumatism with fever. It is articular as a rule; but it may not be so, and in our case there was delirium, which the doctor did not understand. Do you know what is found at the autopsy of a person who dies of cerebral rheumatism? Why, nothing; no more than is found in the articulations in acute rheumatism; because, as I said before, it is not a cerebritis but a simple fluxion, which goes away after death. A little cerebro-spinal liquid has been found in a few cases, owing to an intense flux of the meninges. But it is a very serious affair to have a flux in the brain, much more so than to have one in the articulations; the last gives great pain, but is rarely mortal; while the first is often fatal, especially after delirium.

I say that rheumatism is a malady which strikes wildly at different organs; but why was the brain attacked in our patient's case? Simply because he, like many others who get this trouble, was a weakened man. We most often see attacks of cerebral rheumatism in private hospitals, because they are the homes of patients who have met with bad fortune, or who have wasted their health and abused life in many ways, and end by going to such places for care. Many of these people suffer from cerebral rheumatism. Or it may be that the patient at such places is a ruined banker, or perhaps a writer, or a poet; and in such persons the brain is the part of less resistance. I won't say such patients have poor brains, although I may think it as regards poets; but they are all persons who have used up what brain power they had, so that the brain is in a state of hyperemia, and in a condition predisposing to cerebral rheumatism. Vigla, who wrote a work on this subject, was influenced by the reigning ideas of the time, and thought the affection was an inflammation; but in searching for the lesions Vigla, with scientific sincerity, was compelled to say that he could not see any; he was therefore reduced to making only a clinical description of the disease. But to return to our patient. The large quantity of alcohol that this man put into his brain easily accounts for his having cerebral rheumatism. The brain was a weak point with him, and he had so badly treated the whole of his organism that the rheumatism quickly became grave, and attacked the brain, the myocardium, and the intestines. It is a serious matter to have these organs attacked in such a manner.

Here I am obliged to take up a question of doctrine. A form of rheumatism has been described called infectious; which is distinguished from acute general rheumatism, and in particular from visceral rheumatism. This form is born of the microbe doctrine and is supposed to be engendered by a micro-organism, and to differ from another form called suppurative, which is engendered by a special micro-organism called after Heront. So that in these modern days, we have the frank acute form of rheumatism, or articular, which is the prototype of rheumatic fever; then we have a visceral rheumatism, which strikes at certain viscera; and cerebral rheumatism, although this is the same as the last; we have also the so-called suppurative form; next typhoid rheumatism, as in our patient, and lastly, infectious rheumatism. Is this last infectious on account of some micro-organism? No. I do not think so. It is infectious because of the bad state of the organism through some of the causes I have given, which produce the suppuration in an articulation, or the typhoid state. In the case of our patient, it was simply the hard work and harder drinking which depressed his organization so that he was left open to these maladies. I saw him for the first time this morning a little while before this lesson which I improvised for you at once, as his case teaches us an important practical matter in therapeutics. Besides, he may die and you will see my statements borne out by the autopsy, and you will know what to think of visceral rheumatism, as well as of the so-called infectious form.

What shall we do for him? Do *not* give him salicylate of soda. That would only make him go into a delirium again; perhaps the flux would be displaced and rush to one spot. His temperature was 102.2° F. yesterday, and this morning it is 100.4°, so that fever exists. Be careful in such a case not to give salicylates, as they may provoke cerebral symptoms which cannot be controlled, and the patient may die of cerebral trouble. What then shall be done? Give him Todd's potion (which is only one and a half fluid ounces of Cognac in four fluid ounces of water or other vehicle); then give thirty grains of watery extract of cinchona, just as though he was a patient with typhoid fever. Keep up his strength with good food, let him have soup and milk, and do not keep wine from him. Drunkards must never be deprived of wine, but it must be given with care. Then give sulphate of quinine, which does not act as the salicylates do, as it sustains nervous force, as coffee does. I should be disposed to give him also a hypodermic injection of caffeine. I should give only seven and a half grains a day of the quinine, enough to keep up nerve strength, and yet not cause congestion of the brain. You see I act with care in this case. Then to night, if he is as weak as he appears this mòrning, I should give a hypodermic injection of one-sixth grain of caffeine; and this is all I would do. But if he become delirious, then I should not hesitate to put six wet cups on the cervical region, or two leeches behind each mastoid process, to attempt to take away the congestion; because his life would be in danger.

We are far from theory here; we do not give this man who has rheumatism salicylate of soda, the remedy that is best adapted to that trouble, because he is menaced with a cerebral affection. This is how you should learn pathology; not as you do your catechism, but by seeing the patients. You will then find out that your books on therapeutics do not contain all the truths necessary to practise medicine.

COMMUNICATIONS.

ABLATION OF TONSILS WHEN SMALLER THAN NATURAL.

BY GEORGE TROUP MAXWELL, M.D.,
JACKSONVILLE, FLORIDA.

Excision of the tonsils, when by increased size they cause danger or discomfort, is a common operation; but the removal of them, when from disease they become smaller than is natural, is an operation which, according to my information, has neither been performed nor advised by others. Nor, so far as my knowledge extends, has attention been directed to the pathological action which causes the reduction in the volume of the tonsils.

Although enlargement of a tonsil may be properly regarded as a hypertrophy, the result of excessive nutrition, it cannot be said with exactness that diminution of size is in all cases, if in any, due to the opposite condition, known as atrophy. Indeed, decrease in the dimensions of a tonsil is not usually due to failure of nutrition, but to destructive, suppurative inflammation.

The tonsils, it will be remembered, are not single glands, but are congeries of minute glands or follicles, bound into almond-shaped masses by connective tissue. With this anatomical fact borne in mind, it may be readily understood that the condition found in the single, isolated follicles of the pharynx, especially those of its posterior wall, in chronic follicular pharyngitis, may possibly exist in few or many of the follicles constituting the tonsils. This is, indeed, what frequently happens. A very common, if not an invariable, concomitant of that inflamed condition of the isolated pharyngeal follicles, which has given its name to the disease, is a slow but progressive destructive inflammation of the tonsils—one or both. Indeed, during the last thirty years I have found chronic suppurative inflammation of the tonsils, with loss of substance, associated with follicular pharyngitis so often, as to induce the belief that it is probably a very important factor in the etiology of that disease. I believe that chronic suppurative inflammation of the tonsil is the *causa causans* of follicular pharyngitis.

All are familiar with the phenomena of acute tonsillitis. The great distress caused by swelling and pain compels attention. But few if any have given thought and care to the organs when undergoing slow destructive inflammation. This is due to the almost complete freedom from pain located in the tonsils, to their decrease in size, which causes them to be overlooked upon inspection, and to the extension of inflammation to more conspicuous adjacent parts. The diffused redness, swelling and marked inflammatory action in the neighboring isolated follicles attract attention upon even a casual inspection, whilst the delinquent, painless, shrunken tonsil, partly hidden by the anterior pillar of the fauces, escapes notice. Not unfrequently the patient not having experienced pain or discomfort in the tonsil, is slow to credit the assertion that that organ is probably chiefly responsible for his "sore throat." In some cases nothing short of a demonstration, easily made, will convince patients that the charge against the tonsil is founded in fact. The explanation of the painlessness of the diseased tonsil, upon which the incredulity of patients is based, is that pus escapes with every act of deglutition, especially of solid food, through natural and abnormal openings; and there is consequently no distension of the tissues. Thus nature and disease provide ways of ready egress for pus from organs poorly supplied with nerves of sensation.

In examining patients suffering with follicular pharyngitis it is my habit gently to press the tonsils with a forefinger. If there is pus, which is more likely to be present several hours after meals, it will be seen escaping from minute orifices, and may be caught upon the end of the finger. I have often demonstrated in this way, for the satisfaction of patients, the real seat of trouble. This done, there is rarely opposition to operative procedure.

Applications to the mucous membrane covering the tonsils, in the condition described, are absolutely profitless. They are, on the contrary, often hurtful. They do no good, because they do not reach the diseased tissues. They sometimes do harm, because by their irritating properties they cause swelling of the mucous membrane, and consequent temporary occlusion of the vents. Pus is thereby retained, and pain from distension results.

My method of operating is first to anesthetize the parts with cocaine, seize the mucous membrane covering the tonsil with a double tenaculum (Green's), and, with Green's probe-pointed long-handled bistoury, remove the membrane. Then the pyogenic tissues are exposed to the direct application of a strong solution of the crystals of nitrate of silver, four grains to one fluid ounce. When the wound thus made and treated heals, healthy tonsils remain; and usually the follicular pharyngitis is cured.

The principle of this operation is the same as that recommended by Solis-Cohen in the treatment of intractable, inflamed, isolated follicles, by splitting them with a knife before making application of nitrate of silver.

Thirty years ago I performed the operation I have described upon a man who had follicular pharyngitis, who, every winter, for ten successive years, suffered with one or more attacks of acute tonsillitis. He is still living, and has ever since enjoyed uninterrupted exemption from follicular pharyngitis, or acute tonsilitis. I could report hundreds of similar results were it necessary.

———

—Dr. Kruss, a chemist of Munich, Germany, is said to have succeeded in decomposing cobalt and nickel, both of which have hitherto been supposed to be elementary substances.

—The Sanitary Superintendent of New York City, says the *N. Y. Med. Journal,* Feb. 2, has reported to the Health Board that water contaminated with sewage is being used in some instances in the manufacture of carbonated waters. Physicians should bear in mind the possibility of such contamination when prescribing artificial carbonated waters.

RETAINED PLACENTA DUE TO SPASMODIC CONTRACTION OF THE UTERUS.

BY J. B. CARRELL, M.D.,
HATBORO, PA.

———

At 6 P.M., August 4, I was called by a neighboring physician, a man of much skill and experience in obstetrics, to assist in the removal of an adherent placenta.

The patient was a primipara of fine physique, and had given birth to her child at 9 A.M. of the same day. There was nothing unusual about the case, except the violence of the expulsive pains; the last pain forcing the child unaided entirely from the mother.

Unfortunately, in this case a dose of ergot was given and the delivery of the placenta not at once effected. Pain not coming on, the doctor attempted to deliver, and, not succeeding, concluded to wait. After an hour, he was unable to introduce his hand, on account of the powerful contraction of the uterus. There being no hemorrhage, he waited until 5 P.M., and then, finding no relaxation, sent for me to assist him. In my practice I had, by the free use of chloroform and perseverance, overcome several cases in which the womb was strongly contracted, and fully expected to overcome this one. However, I was much surprised after chloroforming the patient to the surgical degree, to find I could not introduce even the index finger through the strongly contracted os. Our efforts being unavailing, we concluded to wait until the next morning. Meeting again, we found the same condition as on the previous evening, and again decided to wait until 6 P M. The os was well smeared with belladonna ointment and free doses of Hoffman's anodyne and opium given. At 6 P.M., we found the patient under a high state of excitement, temperature 104°, pulse 120, and a fetid discharge from the vagina. The uterus was still firmly contracted. After thoroughly anæsthetizing the patient, my friend attempted to pass his hand, while I steadied the uterus with both of mine. His hand becoming tired out, he took my place and I his. After ten or more minutes of persistent effort, I succeeded in passing my index finger, then the second, and finally the entire hand. Passing it up along the left surface of the womb, I found the placenta firmly adherent at the fundus, and with much effort peeled it off. Immediately, the womb contracted and forced both hand and placenta from the cavity. The vagina was cleansed with an antiseptic solution, and from then on no difficulty was experienced.

This was certainly a remarkable case, and I have not read of or met its like. In cases in which the placenta is retained, it is usual for the uterus to relax in the course of a few hours, or, under the influence of an anæsthetic, it is possible by perseverance to succeed in passing the hand into the uterus. Although each of us was strong and determined, it was absolutely impossible for either to pass a hand. The uterus remained firmly contracted for thirty-three hours after delivery of the child, and then only by the most determined effort was it possible to succeed in passing the hand.

REPLACEMENT OF THE BUTTON OF BONE AFTER TREPHINING: WITH A SUCCESSFUL CASE.[1]

BY WILLIAM R. BALLOU, M.D.,

NEW YORK,

LATE HOUSE SURGEON, BELLEVUE HOSPITAL; ATTENDING SURGEON OUT-PATIENT DEP'T, BELLEVUE HOSPITAL.

In these days of exact and antiseptic surgery, recoveries after the operation of trephining for compound depressed fractures of the skull are sufficiently common not to warrant one's taking much time or space in their discussion. There is, however, one feature in the case I present this evening, somewhat out of the usual course, and for this reason I invite your attention to it.

The patient, a groom by occupation, while harnessing a horse, August 9, 1888, was kicked in the head by the animal. He was brought to the Hospital, and on admission was semi-unconscious and rambling and delirious in his speech.

A scalp-wound was found over the upper central portion of the right parietal bone, which led down to a depressed fracture of the skull.

Trephining and removal of the depressed portions was done under the most thorough antisepsis, the details of which I need not describe. The button of bone removed by the trephine was found to be healthy, and not contused, and it was immediately placed in a warm solution of mercuric bichloride (1-2000) until elevation of the depressed bone—which involved an area of one and one-half inches by three-fourths inch—was effected.

The button was then replaced, the peri-

[1] A paper read at the meeting of the Alumni of Bellevue Hospital, New York, Feb. 6, 1889.

osteum carefully sewed over it, deep and superficial drainage-tubes were introduced, and the incisions in the skin were closed. The patient rallied well from the anæsthetic and had absolutely no unfavorable symptoms after the operation. On the fourth day, the drainage-tubes were removed, and the wound was found healthy. On the seventh day, there was a slight elevation of temperature; the edges of the incision, being raised at one point, were opened, and a small amount of purulent serum was evacuated.

The wound healed rapidly, and, on the eighteenth day, the patient was discharged. He has since reported regularly at my office. The wound has entirely healed, and the button has united to the rest of the bone. The man is in perfect health, and has pursued his vocation as groom for several months.

The points of interest in this case briefly summed up are: (1) that healthy bone may be replaced if the pericranium be sewed over it and the fragment be kept in a perfectly aseptic condition from the moment of its removal; and (2) that meningitis will not occur if all sharp spicules are removed and thorough antisepsis be carried out.

I would not recommend replacement of the button of bone in all cases, though Macewen, of Glasgow, and Barker, of the University Hospital, in London, have gone so far as to divide the bone into small fragments, which were placed on the dura, covered with the periosteum, and left as centres for ossification.

I have reports of six cases in which this procedure was resorted to, with two successes and four failures.

In one of the failures, meningitis is said to have developed.

In two cases, the buttons underwent necrosis and were removed within a few weeks. In one of these cases, the trephining was done for epilepsy, resulting from an old fracture of the skull; in the other, for a depressed pistol-shot fracture.

In both these cases, the bone was undoubtedly of low vitality. In such cases, replacement should not be attempted. In two of the three remaining cases, the operation was performed for old head injuries. In one case, the attempted replantation of the bone was successful; in the other it was not.

The sixth case is the one you have seen this evening.

The case I have just described occurred during the service of Dr. W. F. Fluhrer, with whose kind permission I report it.

No. 236 East Thirty-first Street.

BEDFORD SPRINGS AS A HEALTH RESORT.

BY H. B. RUNNALLS, M.R.C.S., L.S.A. ENG.,
BEDFORD SPRINGS, PA.

So much has already been written regarding mineral waters and climatology, that it is with some amount of diffidence that I add one more article to this, as yet, little understood subject. I doubt whether I should have done so now, but being acquainted with the various Spas in England, and on the European Continent, I was so struck with the many advantages of, and the general superiority of the Bedford Springs, although a much less known health resort, that I felt it would be more or less a boon to the profession, if I laid before them a few facts respecting this place.

In these days of mental strain and struggle for existence, the relationship between mind and body is only too often witnessed by the city physician, and how futile our attempts are to bring about a healthy equilibrium in such cases by the aid of medicine alone is too well known to all of us. The morbid conditions resulting from an unbalanced nervous system are indefinite, and we are only acquainted with the grosser symptoms accruing from a disordered state of the digestive system, which in our larger centres of population displays itself as gout, diabetes and the various kinds of kidney trouble; and in older countries, where the struggle for existence is more keen, pessimism and a distaste for life generally may be added. Shakespeare recognized the relationship between mind and body when he asks, " Can'st thou minister to a mind diseased?''; and we all know the difficulty of solving that problem. Perhaps no class of men more thoroughly appreciate and derive more benefit from a change of air and scene than physicians. To be hastened away from the worries and troubles of a seething mass of humanity, to the country town or hill-side village, where the air is pure and laden only with life supporting properties, makes life once more a joy, so that one does not ask himself now whether life is worth living.

Having had personally a considerable amount of experience in hospital surgery in London and also in the country I have been struck with the vast difference in the process of repair. The ruddy cheeks and sturdy limbs of the country-raised child, and the leaden complexion and emaciated condition of those born and bred in cities and large towns prove conclusively that pure air and good water are very important factors in the healthy growth of the human body, and valuable adjuncts or rather absolutely necessary aids when it is wished to repair a constitution broken down from disease or mental strain.

To appreciate thoroughly the advantages of pure air and pure water one should have lived in England during the last ten or fifteen years, during which time a revolution has taken place in the sanitary condition of houses and towns. When every house had its cess-pit and well of drinking water, with badly ventilated rooms, typhoid, typhus, diphtheria and many other of the diseases resulting from such causes, were rampant and numbered their victims by thousands every year; but now with uncontaminated water supply and the abolition of the cess-pool, these diseases have almost disappeared, and are considered preventable diseases, and sanitary authorities are liable to be sued for damages if these diseases arise within their precincts. One need but go to those countries where cholera and yellow fever produce their ravages, to understand the reason why these disease germs show such a decided predilection for those countries. The same causes though in a less degree are present in all large centres of population, and especially in low-lying lands, or where towns are encompassed by hills, thus preventing a free circulation of air, and the substitution of healthy atmosphere, for that impregnated with the exhalations of thousands of people with the odor arising from decaying animal and vegetable matter and with the fine particles of dust and soot arising from so many fires.

These causes to a great extent are responsible for the puny and ill-developed children; for the languor, lassitude, loss of appetite, sleeplessness, nervous irritability and other symptoms showing only too plainly the deficient supply of oxygen. All these cases defy medicinal treatment, but it is surprising to see how quickly these symptoms disappear after a short sojourn in an unvitiated atmosphere. To the poor these valuable aids toward recovery as a rule are not obtainable, and it is useless for the physician to advise change of air; but to the man of means it is a want that can be supplied, and the question arises as to the choice of place. There are many Spas, but few really good ones; and to decide upon any one in particular, where natural conditions are accompanied with the comforts of home life, becomes a difficult matter.

All these requirements can be obtained at the Bedford Springs. They are situated in the Allegheny mountains, 256 miles west from Philadelphia *via* Penna. R. R.; and 160 miles from Pittsburgh. Here for centuries nature has been pouring forth with her usual lavishness, one of her remedial agents for dyspeptic troubles. The action of this water upon the system might be termed a magnesia purgative, but the purgative action is very pleasant and gentle. Sulphate of magnesia is the principal ingredient, from which the purgative action results. And this effect is much improved by the lime and iron it contains, as it builds up the system at the same time it is helping to remove the waste material. The accompanying accurate and complete analysis of the water by Prof. Leffmann, of Philadelphia, will speak for itself:

BEDFORD MAGNESIA WATER.—*Results of Analysis of Water from Springs known as Magnesia Springs, Bedford, Pa.*

	Grains to O. S. G.
Calcium carbonate	7.55
Ferrous carbonate	0.06
Calcium sulphate	103.61
Magnesium sulphate	41.34
Potassium sulphate	0.09
Sodium sulphate	0.34
Sodium chloride	0.45
Silica	0.42
Calcium phosphate	0.01
Lithium	Traces
Strontium	Traces
Nitrates	None
Nitrites	None
Fixed organic matter	None
Total solids	153.87

The water of the magnesia spring is noticeable from its large proportion of active mineral ingredients, especially the magnesium sulphate (Epsom Salts) which confers upon it a mild aperient quality. The high degree of organic purity is also to be noted. The absence of organic matter, nitrates and nitrites, together with the very low figure for sodium chloride, indicate that this water arises from sources deep in the earth, and free from any of the polluting influences to which surface waters and superficial springs are liable. As drawn from the spring the water is perfectly clear, and retains its qualities unchanged for a long period, the active ingredients being held in solution by their own properties, and not by any accidental association.

This shows that the chief remedial agent present is the magnesia sulphate, slightly combined with the iron. How valuable these products are combined, in the treatment of the many diseases resulting from an abnormal condition of the digestive system, is well known to all of us, and particularly so to the hospital physician.

I remember when I was connected with the London hospitals, that the most favorite medicine called the "white medicine" was a combination of magnesia carbonate and sulphate. How quickly does the anæmic woman who comes complaining of irregular menstruation, fainting attacks, constant headache, costiveness and general depression, regain her strength when she takes the magnesia sulphate and iron combined. Here we have a natural combination and it is surprising to note the rapid strides toward health that the invalid makes after he has been taking the water for only a short time.

To the gouty dyspeptic the water is a most valuable aid toward complete restoration of health. I have always been forcibly impressed with the fact that the action of mineral waters generally is considerably enhanced when they are taken when the brain and nervous system are resting; and the greater the change of scene that is provided for the over-taxed nerve centres, the greater is that rest. The natural surroundings of the Spring cannot be equalled; mountain and valley are intermingled in that artless manner so characteristic of the designing hand. The eyes are enchanted with the majestic growth of forest trees, the luxuriance of the vegetation, the gorgeous colors of the flowers and insect life, and the ears are lulled with the rippling music of the mountain streams as they rush over their pebbly beds. Any taste for natural pursuits can be cultivated. The shooting and fishing are extremely good. Here the visitor finds he can wander for miles where he likes with rod or gun, and need not fear to be disturbed by the game keeper, as would be his fate in the neighborhood of the English or European Spa.

Added to this there is a hotel fitted up with the latest improvements and requirements of the nineteenth century. It is situated about one mile from the town of Bedford, and lies pleasantly situated amongst the trees in a pretty vale. The drives and walks are numerous, most of them meandering for miles through forest vegetation, teeming with objects of interest. With such surroundings the invalid or holiday seeker cannot help being restored to health; and when he returns to the busier tasks of every day life, he has a brain stored with the reminiscences which are always so pleasant to recall.

NEW YORK CORRESPONDENCE.

Clinics by Drs. Polk, Bulkley, Loomis, and Peabody: Views of Prof. Polk on Alexander's Operation.

PROF. W. M. POLK, at the clinic at Bellevue Hospital showed a patient, a domestic, 23 years old, who was sent to the hospital Jan. 17, by a reputable physician, as a case of simple chronic gastritis. Her history revealed that in the third week of last October she menstruated for three days and then ceased until December 1, after which she flowed profusely, at intervals. On January 1, a small grape-like mass came away with much blood. Nausea and vomiting began early in December, and became so severe that the patient could eat nothing and became very weak. On her admission to the hospital her temperature was 100°, her pulse 112 and very weak, her mouth and tongue brown and dry, and her breath offensive. Physical examination showed a tumor in the pelvis extending up to the umbilicus, of the size and shape of a uterus in the fifth or sixth month, and slightly tender on pressure. The os was not soft, but was dilated enough to admit the end of the index finger. January 19 and 20 more of the grape-like gelatinous masses with a decided odor of decomposition, came away, and the tumor declined in size. Dr. Polk made the diagnosis of hydatiform degeneration of the chorion, differentiating it, chiefly by the length of the history, the appearance of the masses, and by exclusion, from endometritis, polypus, fibroma, and mole. The os being sufficiently dilated, he emptied the uterus with a double curette, washed it out thoroughly with hot water and packed it with weak iodoform gauze, which was renewed after twenty-four hours. The patient had no fever and is now on the high road to recovery.

This treatment of curetting, washing out with hot water, or 1 to 5000 solution of bichloride of mercury, and then packing with weak iodoform gauze is one constantly used by Prof. Polk in chronic endometritis of the hemorrhagic or fungosum type, in septicæmia from retention of membranes, and similar conditions. With him and in Bellevue Hospital it has yielded brilliant results.

The REPORTER, January 26, contained an editorial on Alexander's operation of shortening the round ligaments, its indications value, etc. This is an operation introduced into the United States and advanced to its present high standing by Prof. Polk, and as his views differ somewhat from those advanced in the REPORTER, they are herewith presented.

The effect of shortening the round ligaments is to draw the uterus upward and forward, so that the fundus can be placed directly behind the symphysis pubis. Consequently the operation is indicated in procidentia. This is the joint result of rupture of the perineal structure and stretching of the uterine ligamentous supports, chiefly utero-sacral, and the basic lines of the broad ligaments. The principal perineal support is the pubo-coccygeal division of the levator ani muscle. Prolapse is usually accompanied by backward displacement and hence Alexander's operation corrects both conditions, and then, when supplemented by restoration of the pelvic floor, it is both rational and satisfying. Among other indications are retroflexions and retroversions of the uterus, in which the organ can be placed in the normal position by the sound, and yet a pessary cannot be comfortably worn. So long as the uterus cannot be replaced easily, it is outside the domain of the operation, and the only alternative is abdominal section, tearing up the adhesions and removing the tubes if necessary. Another indication is prolapse of the ovary, provided it is reducible and not large enough nor diseased enough to require removal. The objections raised, that sometimes the ligaments cannot be found, and that they are not strong enough to hold the uterus, are unfounded. Dr. Polk, in more than half a hundred operations, has never had the slightest trouble in finding them, and experiment has proved that they are capable of supporting four to five pounds or more. So far as he has had opportunity to observe, the shortening does not interfere with pregnancy. One of his cases went to term and another is now pregnant and soon to be confined. As to danger, he thinks that, with thorough cleanliness and antisepsis and a knowledge of the anatomy of the parts, there is practically none. Up to Jan. 1, 1889, he had operated on fifty-five cases—more than any other man in America has performed. His results have been uniformly good, and only in one known case has the malposition recurred.

DR. L. D. BULKLEY, at his clinic on diseases of the skin, in New York Hospital, Jan. 28, had a typical case of lupus erythematosus, for which he recommended, internally, Thompson's tincture of phosphorus, ♏xv, t.i.d.; and locally:

℞ Potass. sulph.,
   Zinci sulph. . . . . āā ℨ j
   Glycerini . . . . f ℥ j
   Aquæ rosæ . . . . f ℥ iv

M. Sig. Apply freely.

PROF. A. L. LOOMIS, in a lecture on the treatment of acute lobar pneumonia last week, recommended the following: Counteract the shock of the first few days with opium (morphine hypodermically); keep the temperature down with quinine; when the heart begins to fail, *and not before*, use your stimulants, giving brandy at first. If this fails, sustain the heart and carry it past the crisis with citrate of caffein, in five grain doses every five or six hours. It acts on the nervous system rather than on the heart muscle itself, and is not diuretic. Digitalis he thought contraindicated in an uncomplicated case, and convallaria and strophanthus too unreliable for use. If pulmonary œdema comes on, relieve it with dry cups. Calomel, to unload the portal system, is dangerous because of its depressing effects. Counter-irritants are also bad, and he uses instead the flannel and oil-silk jacket or a hot mush or flax-seed poultice that completely encircles the thorax. This should be applied as hot as can be borne every two hours, and will give much better satisfaction than a poultice over only a portion of the lung. Expectorants are of no service unless the mucus is very tenacious, when small doses of the muriate of ammonia can be given. Large doses are contraindicated, as they upset the stomach, while as a heart stimulant the drug is inferior to champagne. The use of cold is likely to do harm. To this treatment he adds absolute rest, a diet of milk, eggs, broth, etc., and uses the ordinary remedies for cough and other symptoms that may arise.

DR. G. L. PEABODY, on Jan. 31, held the last clinic of his spring course in New York Hospital. It consisted mainly of an array of old cases. Among them were several convalescing cases of typhoid fever which had been treated with resorcin. The results seemed very satisfactory, though the Professor was unprepared to give an opinion of its comparative utility. A case of chronic gastritis which had been treated with daily washings of the stomach, with steady improvement, showed a relapse, having great pain, vomiting, temperature 102°, aching bones, etc. The patient—a young woman—is taking extract of malt and a fluid diet, and her secretions are being regulated with aloes and myrrh. It was

decided to withhold the washings for a few days.

A case of peripheral neuritis of alcoholic origin showed marked benefit from a long course of strychnine. His insomnia was best treated with paraldehyde in doses of f ℨ j–ij, though urethan, in doses of gr. 100, did very well.

A painter with wrist-drop from lead-poisoning was regaining the power of extension under iodides. His face presented a well-marked iodide eruption, being covered with pustules. He was a man who had suffered with rheumatism and gout, and during his present illness a joint affection came on at the knee. To be sure to strike the disease, the doctor prescribed (successfully) medicines to meet both conditions, viz: iodide of sodium and wine of colchicum. This brings to mind a similar double-barrelled prescription, it being the rheumatic mixture of Bellevue Hospital. It is:

℞ Sodii salicylat. . . . . . gr. x
   Vini colchici . . . . . . ♏ v
   Pot. iodidi . . . . . . gr. x
   Aq. cinnamomi . . . . ad f ℨ j

M. Sig. One dose.

Perhaps the most interesting case presented was one which has baffled Prof. Peabody and the entire staff. It is that of a servant-girl, aged 17, single, and coming from Denmark. Last summer, the patient entered the hospital with a high temperature. There was no apparent cause for it, but up it stayed, reaching normal about twice every three weeks or so. Pain was developed in the right iliac fossa, the diagnosis perityphlitis made, and laparotomy performed. The appendix was found in a healthy condition, and no pathological state could be found in the neighborhood. The patient left last September and was gone three months, returning in November in the same condition. Since then, her temperature has ranged constantly from 102° to 105° and even higher. Quinine seems to act best in controlling it. Besides the temperature, until January 30, she had no other symptoms; none in the chest, abdomen, nor kidneys—though sometimes her pulse and respirations became very rapid. She eats well, suffers no pain, and loses little or no weight. January 30, she had a chill, and her fever went up to 108 ⁶⁄₁₀°. Next day, she had a similar experience, and then under phenacetin the temperature was kept down to 103°. What the affection is, the Doctor does not know. All that can be done is to combat the fever.

FOREIGN CORRESPONDENCE.

LETTER FROM BERLIN.

An Ideal Laxative Suppository—An Interesting Demonstration of Hypnotism—Vile Abuses of Hypnotism—Singular Results of Arsenical Poisoning—Thiol and Ichthyol —The Wachsmuth Treatment of Diphtheria—The Bee-sting in Rheumatism— Medical Candidates in Germany.

BERLIN, Jan. 25, 1889.

The history of the at present fashionable employment of glycerine as a laxative is rather interesting. Dr. Oidtmann, a physician of Maastricht, Holland, who cared less for the Dutch code of ethics than for the almighty dollar, did for years a flourishing business by advertising his infallible and instantaneously acting purgative. As he did not appear to get rich fast enough the German government came to his assistance by forbidding its sale as a secret remedy, and publishing at the same time an analysis of it. The natural result of this proceeding was a tremendous demand for Dr. Oidtmann's purgative on the part of all who were troubled with constipation. The analysis having proved that its essential constituent was simply glycerine, the profession itself soon took hold of this drug in the treatment of constipation. The fact is that glycerine applied to the rectum, in slight cases of constipation, acts really as a prompt, though scarcely as an energetic laxative. The question why glycerine exerts a laxative influence has been answered variously, though it cannot be said that its *modus operandi* has as yet been definitely established. Some regard its action as a reflex phenomenon due to the local irritation of the drug ; others believe that glycerine acts like an alcohol, causing (like ethylic alcohol, for example) a rapid abstraction of water from the part, which in turn causes increased peristaltic movements of the bowels. It has been suggested that a similar process—on a grand scale—takes place in cholera, where the rapid desiccation of the mucous membrane of the bowels leads to muscular cramps.

The application of glycerine by the mouth and by the rectum by means of a syringe was soon superseded by suppositories prepared from glycerine and oil of cacao, which again were replaced by hollow suppositories, filled with glycerine. But the greatest improvement was reached by the introduction of glycerine toilet-soap as the most perfect and most convenient laxative suppository. The soap, being very plastic, the patient can make suppositories from it at any time without any preparation whatever. The action of the glycerine-soap suppository is very prompt, a few minutes sufficing to produce a gentle movement of the bowels. It must be admitted that for ease and convenience of application, for economy and prompt action, this new form of glycerine suppository is an ideal laxative which, especially for women and children, cannot fail to become popular soon.

Hypnotism, in spite of its highly interesting features, many physicians are loth to approach, partly because they regard their established prejudice and skepticism as invincible, and partly because they do not care to enter a new domain of science, in which there is demonstration but no explanation. It seems that the German physicians, who thus far have left the exploration of this interesting field to their French colleagues, have of late taken more interest in the matter. Prof. Mendel, the eminent neurologist of the Berlin University, recently gave a highly interesting representation of hypnotism before a small and select group of medical men. The patient was a young man, 25 years old, who, on account of weakness in the lower extremities, could only limp in walking. Prof. Mendel told the patient to close the eyes ; this he did and immediately fell asleep. He remained in a sound sleep even after having opened his eyes again at the word of the Professor. Then the patient at once showed no more traces of his former disability, but could walk as easily and uniformly as a sound man, could mount a chair and perform other movements regarded previously as absolutely impossible. To increase the surprise of the gathering the patient, who previously stammered to such an extent that he was unable to enunciate two consecutive words, began now with considerable oratoric skill to recite *"Des Sänger's Fluch"* (the minstrel's curse), by Uhland. When told that an organ was close at hand, he directed the hymn "Jesus, Lover of My Soul " to be sung, and he intoned it at once. Another interesting feature of the *séance* was the following performance: The patient was given five blank postal cards with the " suggestion " that on one of them the letter A—the beginning of the patient's name—was written. This card was then marked by a dot on the other side, and five cards, after having been thoroughly mixed, were handed to the patient, who without hesitation selected the marked card. Prof. Mendel regretted his inability to give a satisfactory explanation of the remarkable facts witnessed. Regarding the card feat, he thought that the hypnotic state possibly sharpened the optic faculties of the medium.

This hypnotic performance recalls to your correspondent two cases of vile abuse of hypnotism, which some time ago came before the French law courts and created a profound sensation. A crippled beggar, 25 years old, went to a farm-house occupied by an intelligent and wealthy family, and asked for alms. He represented himself as being a deaf-mute and in need of something to eat. During the meal he made some strange gestures, for instance the sign of the cross over his face and over everything he ate or drank. Asking for a piece of paper he wrote down the following: "I am the Son of God; I come from heaven and my name is 'Our Lord'; you see my small miracles, later you will see grander ones; do not be afraid, for I am sent by God."

These words made a deep impression upon all present, especially on the daughter, a young lady of beauty and accomplishment. The beggar spent the night in a barn and next morning went to the house again, where he found the young lady alone. He conversed again with her by gestures and made the sign of the cross repeatedly with his fingers on her back and forehead. During the meal he stared at her so intently that she suddenly sank from the chair in utter exhaustion, whereupon he disgraced her. Though she knew what was going on she could offer no resistance nor utter a cry; she was restrained by some strange, powerful force and evidently in a state of lethargy. At his suggestion the lady left her home, went along with him, stopped with him at night in a neighboring barn, and was a powerless tool for the vilest of his designs. If at any time she was about to return to consciousness regarding her situation, a mere touching of her hips (hypnotogenic zone) sufficed to put her again into somnambulism and bondage. Witnesses testified that she executed automatically all movements suggested by him, laughed convulsively, glided on her knees about the room, mounted a ladder, caressed him with erotic fervor, etc.

Before the court he acknowledged having seduced the lady through hypnotism and suggestion, and that he had previously ruined several girls by the same method. He boasted before the jury that he could overpower the strongest and most unwilling girl and declared himself ready to prove it in court. He also volunteered to hypnotize the president of the court by the mere power of his eyes; but the latter avoided this predicament by turning his back to the defendant. The latter was sentenced to the penitentiary for twenty-one years.

The second case is that of a dentist, who hypnotized a lady patient in his operating chair, and disgraced her. This villain was also sentenced to the pentitentiary.

That an intoxication with such a poisonous drug as arsenic may have highly beneficial results must certainly be regarded as exceptional. A child two and a half years old, affected with obstinate enuresis and incontinence of the bowels, took by mistake some rat-poison and developed severe arsenical poisoning. Both conditions mentioned above were found to have disappeared after the child had recovered from the effects of the poison. But still more remarkable was the change noticed in the mental condition of the child. Before the accident it could say only the single word "mamma," and was exceedingly peevish; while after recovery it learned to talk rapidly, played alone for hours, and turned out to be a bright and good child. It is clear that the gratifying changes mentioned are to be ascribed to the alterative effects of the arsenic. Possibly two doses a day of Fowler's solution may be indicated not only for the disorders of the bladder and bowels, which existed in this case, but also for children with a retarded mental development.

"What's in a name?" In medicine, at least, we should think nothing; as long as the action of a drug is a desirable one, its name should neither favor nor check its popularity. Still it seems that even in legitimate therapeutics, especially among the lately discovered remedies, those with a soft-sounding and harmonious name have been victorious over those with less happy designations. There is, besides, an evident tendency to apply to newly discovered remedies names closely allied to successful predecessors. This is noticeable in the names of antipyrin and antifebrin; salicylic acid and salol; iodoform and iodol; ichthyol and thiol. Thiol, the latest claimant to professional favor, was discovered by Jacobsohn, who prepared it by distillation from brown coal-tar by the addition of flowers of sulphur. The mass is heated in an oil-bath up to $215°$ C. ($419°$ F.); the sulphurated hydrates of carbon are first converted into sulpho-acids by the aid of sulphuric acid, and then by treatment with ammonium or sodium hydrate into thiol salts. Thiol, or German ichthyol, closely resembles ichthyol, and is easily soluble in water or in a mixture of alcohol and ether. Its reducing power is shown by its conversion of ferric chloride into ferrous chloride and by instantly decolorizing permanganate of potash. Dr. Reeps, assistant of Prof. Schweninger, has subjected thiol to clinical trials and has pronounced it as the medicinal equivalent of ichthyol. The thiosulphate of sodium contains twelve per cent. of sulphur and is asserted to have anti-rheumatic virtues. A great advantage which thiol possesses over ichthyol is its cheapness. If Dr. Reep's statement should be confirmed, thiol has every chance of becoming a popular remedy. The value of ichthyol in rheumatism and skin affections is at present well established.

The vexed question of the most successful treatment of diphtheria is certain never to disappear from the professional forum. Recommendations and alleged miraculous successes have in this direction been so plentiful of late that the average practitioner has long ago ceased to be credulous. Still it is our duty at least to take notice of all novel suggestions of treatment. The so-called Wachsmuth treatment of diphtheria is at present, in Germany at least, attracting considerable attention. It is always applicable in children under five years of age, in adults, however, in graver cases only. The child is stripped, wrapped up in wet linen sheets, so as to leave only the head uncovered, and then covered with warm blankets or a feather-bed. The first application is best made by the physician himself, and the others can be made at intervals of several hours by a member of the family. Wachsmuth himself recommends to make an application lasting three hours and then to pause for two hours, and to prolong the period if improvement sets in. Gargles with a greatly diluted solution of corrosive sublimate, or better with a two to three per cent. solution of acetic acid, should be used also. Careful ventilation of the sick-chamber and a change of room for the nights, if possible, are likewise recommended. The results obtained with this treatment are said to be highly satisfactory; the fever being lowered in height and duration, the membranes being expelled rather easily, and the period of convalescence also shortened.

So-called household remedies and methods of treatment have been adopted by the regular profession not infrequently. A singular illustration of this is the employment of the bee-sting in gout and rheumatism, as originally advocated by Dr. Tere, of Marburg. This practitioner has used this old-fashioned and empirical treatment on 173 patients, on whom he produced altogether 39,000 stings. As the sting is manipulated by the practitioner, the latter, of course, has to avoid being stung himself. Light and acute cases are said to improve, or to be cured after a few stings, while in chronic cases hundreds of stings are required to produce a curative effect. In acute articular cases the bee-sting is said to have no advantage over antipyrin and salicylic acid, and is therefore here only applicable when the other remedies have failed. In chronic and complicated rheumatic processes especially, the bee-sting deserves to be tried. The application is also said to act with remarkable promptness in rheumatic pains of the heart when endocarditis and myositis are threatening. On account of its cheapness the bee-sting cure might be tried in the treatment of the poor.

It may be of interest to the readers of the REPORTER to learn of the number of medical candidates from States within the German Empire who failed last year in their final examination. The percentage of those who failed is 28 ; in Berlin and Breslau this percentage rose to 42 per cent., in Halle to 34 per cent. These figures are a fair criterion of the almost fatal severity of German medical examinations. It would really be a highly desirable improvement if the requisites of graduation in American medical schools were raised. There is no use denying the deplorable fact that with only a few exceptions the requisites of graduation in America are far below the European standard. Before attempting, however, any improvement in the direction indicated it is necessary that the course of medical training should have the compulsory length of four years, and above all that the preliminary examinations should be rendered more rigid. Unfortunately a uniform governmental supervision and regulation of medical education, which is found all over Europe, cannot well be introduced into America.

—The State Board of Health of New York notified the health boards in all parts of that State on Jan. 30, that small-pox has become threatening in the Onondaga county poorhouse, the penitentiary at Syracuse, and at Lyons and other places in Central New York. The Board urges all persons to be vaccinated, and a special lockout for tramps.

PERISCOPE.

Albuminuria of Pregnancy and Puerperal Eclampsia.

Dr. Lantos, of Buda Pesth, has recently made a series of observations on albuminuria of pregnancy in the wards of Professor von Kézmársky. His paper will be found in the *Archiv für Gynäkologie*, vol. xxxii, part 3. In over 18 per cent. of 70 pregnant women he found albumin in the urine, whilst in nearly 60 per cent. of 600 newly delivered women the urine was albuminous. Albuminuria was detected in over 70 per cent. of 268 primiparæ, and over 50 per cent. of 332 multiparæ. The percentage was distinctly lower in premature labor, and 50 per cent. lower in abortion cases. Out of 10 cases in which albumin was abundant so that Dr. Lantos used the microscope, he found pus in 3 and casts in 5, but no foreign elements in the remainder. He examined the kidney in 39 cases in which the patients had neither died from eclampsia nor from nephritis. In 15 of these cases the kidneys were very anæmic, in 21 pale, and only in 3 full of blood. Amongst the local changes in other cases he found acute parenchymatous nephritis in 2 cases, acute hæmorrhagic nephritis in one case, parenchymatous degeneration in 9 cases, and in 4 albuminous degeneration.

Dr. Lantos therefore concludes that, putting aside all evident and probable cases of nephritis in pregnant women, albuminuria is not rare in pregnancy, and very common after parturition. He refers the phenomenon to reflex irritation of the vasomotor nerves of the renal vessels; it has, he says, no pathological significance, and, in conjunction with other symptoms, is a valuable diagnostic sign of pregnancy. Out of 14,815 labors observed in the course of fifteen years, he noted 53 cases (0.36 per cent.) of puerperal eclampsia, a ratio of 278 to 1. Over 78 per cent. out of 42 eclamptic cases occurred in primiparæ, over 21 per cent. in multiparæ; 15 out of the entire 53 died.

Dr. Lantos thinks that the rate of mortality is increased when instruments are used, and as the convulsions often do not cease after delivery, he thinks that the forceps should not be used unless there are strong indications. Convalescence is much prolonged after eclampsia. In 23 of the eclampsia cases the urine was examined; in 21 it was albuminous, casts being found in 4.

At the necropsies of fatal cases of convulsion, Dr. Lantos found constant changes in the brain, but only once acute, though frequently chronic, renal changes. Like Osthoff, he traces puerperal eclampsia to violent reflex vasomotor disturbance, and classes it as acute peripheral epilepsy.— *British Med. Journal,* Jan. 12, 1889.

Button-hook in the Intestines.

Mr. A. B. Kelly communicates the following account of this interesting case to the *Lancet,* Jan. 5, 1889.

On Oct. 31, 1888, I was summoned to see Mrs. D——, who, I was informed, had swallowed a steel bow-handled button-hook, three inches and a half in length. On arriving at the patient's house about a quarter of an hour after the occurrence, I found her seated in a chair, apparently more frightened than hurt. She stated that she had been picking her back teeth with the point of the hook, and the article slipped out of her hand during an act of inspiration and went down her throat. Evidently it had not lodged in the œsophagus, but had descended to the stomach. I requested the patient to assume the recumbent posture; and directed an attendant to administer some bread-and-milk as quickly as possible, and an ounce of castor oil about an hour afterward. On visiting the patient later on, I learned that there had been a copious motion, but nothing particular to note. I saw the patient daily afterward for about a week, she remaining in bed for a few days. There was a daily evacuation, but no sign of the hook. I recommended food consisting of pudding of doughy material, and a moderate allowance of meat, hoping to form a coating round the hook. Further, I gave directions for castor oil every other day, and a mixture of linseed decoction to be administered three or four times daily. I asked the patient to send for me should any urgent symptoms arise; but I heard no more of the case until Nov. 23, or just three weeks after the hook was swallowed. The defecations had been passed daily into a night-stool and watched, when, to the patient's great relief, on the day just mentioned, she found the hook had passed from her bowels, but without any coating of food. There was, however, a brownish-black discoloration over its entire surface.

Pins, coins, etc., have repeatedly been swallowed, but I have seen no case recorded in which such an article as a button-hook has been swallowed.

A Good Bread for Diabetics.

In a communication published in the *Boston Med. and Surg. Journal*, Jan. 24, 1889, John A. Jeffries spoke of a good bread for diabetics. All are now doubtless aware, he said, that the so-called gluten flours are not what they should be, and will agree that the first thing in the treatment of diabetic patients is the avoidance of starches and sugars. It is therefore very desirable to get a bread, or more accurately a substitute for bread, which will satisfy the cravings of the patient for bread and yet fill the therapeutic indications. Experience seems to show that the craving is not for starch but for the form and taste of the bread; that is, for the sensations produced by such food in the mouth and nose by the senses of touch, taste, and smell, not for starch in the stomach and intestines. Were this not the case, he said, it would be impossible to satisfy the patient's wants.

He showed samples of bread which he thought much more nearly fulfilled the requisites of the case than any now in use. He has succeeded in preparing two kinds, one simply an improvement on those now in use but easily procured and inexpensive; the other a great improvement, but at present difficult to procure and expensive.

The first is made by using equal parts of bran and graham flour, or, put in accurate form: One cup of graham flour; one cup of best bran previously scalded with one cup of boiling water; two eggs; German yeast or baking powder; salt to taste; one cup of milk or water. To be mixed with a *spoon.* Such a bread contains 17.72 per cent. of starch, the equivalent of 19.68 per cent. sugar.

The second is made from the gluten of the starch factories ground to a fine flour. In the ordinary method of manufacture, he said, the gluten is fermented out and lost, but lately efforts have been made to separate it out by machinery for sizing. The bread is made as follows: One cup gluten flour; one cup best bran previously scalded; one teaspoonful of baking powder; salt to taste; two eggs; one cup of milk or water.

To be mixed with a *spoon.* If the hands are used the result will be even more disastrous than in the making of ordinary bread. This bread is wholesome, palatable, nutritious, and contains but 4.57 per cent. of starch, equal to 5.08 per cent. of sugar. The analyses were made by Dr. Charles Harrington.

Dr. Jeffries thinks this bread is practically the same as that described by Waltering in the *Allgem. med. Central-Zeitung*, August 4, 1888.

In answer to the question by Dr. A. N. Blodgett, why Dr. Jeffries thought it is so essential that this bread should be made with a spoon, Dr. Jeffries said that all bread, even ordinary bread such as everybody has, is much better when not touched with the hand, and this is especially true of this gluten bread. Some of the gluten he exhibited is separated out for manufacture and used as shoemakers' wax in Germany. If it is worked with the hand it is apt to be soggy and not rise at all; if worked with the spoon it will rise nicely.

Lactic Acid in Chronic Suppurative Otitis Media.

Isidor Herrmann, according to the *Therapeutische Monatshefte*, Dec., 1888, has obtained the best results in chronic suppurative otitis media from the use of lactic acid, and this in cases which defied other treatment. He instils daily into the middle ear a few drops of the diluted acid, which is allowed to remain there about twenty minutes. Usually the bad odor, due to the purulent excretion, disappeared after three or four applications of the acid. The discharge itself ceased after about six weeks' treatment. Moderate ulcerations in the drum healed, after topical treatment with the mitigated stick of nitrate of silver, within a few weeks after the discharge had entirely ceased.

Before the acid is applied, both the external meatus and the outer surface of the drum-membrane should be protected with vaselin, oil, or some such agent, in order to avoid direct contact of the acid with parts which are so prone to inflammation. A twenty per cent. solution of lactic acid is first used, and gradually increased in strength up to forty per cent., if the patient bears the weaker solution well. After the application of the acid finely pulverized boric acid is blown into the ear, under the employment of which small perforations in the drum-membrane heal. If moderate ulcerations in the drum-membrane show no tendency to heal, then the employment of an artificial drum-membrane is indicated, which the patients for the most part bear. If they do not, then a relatively large quantity of boric acid is blown into the middle ear, to give adequate protection to it. Usually the boric acid melts with the secretion of the ear and forms a moderately resisting circular wall with only a small opening in the centre; in this way an artificial drum-membrane is formed and the hearing decidedly improved.—*Wiener med. Presse*, Dec. 30, 1888.

Treatment of Typhoid Fever.

Ziemssen (*Centralblatt für klin. Med.*, No. 6, 1888) attributes the lowered mortality of typhoid fever within the past few years to improved therapeutics. Only a few of the more important features of his very extensive and scientific paper can be given. The patient's room should be capacious, quiet, and well ventilated. Water-pillows should be used, and, when possible, a second bed. The author is in favor of easily digested albuminates during the fever. Beef-juice extracted from fresh beef is the most suitable, and of this the patient should have 150 to 200 grammes (5 to 6½ oz.) in twenty-four hours. Regarding other forms of nutriment, the author follows the prevailing methods. Gelatin is often given in form of calves'-foot jelly with wine. The author gives but few medicines, and these only when specially indicated. Calomel, he thinks, has a decidedly beneficial effect when given at the right time—that is, within the first five days of the illness. He gives seven and a half grains three times within two hours. Strong emphasis is laid upon his method, which is so well known, of reducing the temperature by graduated cold baths. He speaks warmly of antipyrin as an antipyretic, of which he administers 5 grammes (grs. lxxv), in three divided, hourly doses, beginning the administration after 6 P.M. Thallin and acetanilid receive praise from him, but he condemns quinine, because it is attended with untoward effects—such as noises in the ears and an indescribable sensation all over the body. Kairin and salicylate of sodium as antipyretics he considers antiquated. In slight cerebral symptoms an ice-bag should be applied to the head, but not continuously; in severe cerebral symptoms, graduated baths, with cold affusions, are indispensable. Insomnia and restlessness are best combated by an injection of morphine. A tendency to cardiac weakness is best met by excitants, the best of which are camphor and wine, champagne and brandy. Severe diarrhœa is best treated with starch and opium enemata. Intestinal hemorrhages call for ice-bags on the abdomen, and subsequently for ice-water enemata, which act reflexly. The intestinal hemorrhages which occur between the fourth and sixth weeks offer a much worse prognosis than those that occur during the second and third weeks. Bed-sores can be avoided by care, cleanliness, cold-water treatment, and a water-pillow.

During convalescence great care must be exercised regarding the diet. For five days, at least, after the non-febrile period has set in, the diet should continue to be of a liquid nature. After this it may be given in a semi-solid form for a few days, and then solid food may be cautiously given. The patient should keep in his bed for fourteen days, even after a mild attack, and for three or four weeks after a severe one.—*N. Y. Med. Journal*, Jan. 19, 1889.

Tumor of the Brain and Accidental Injury.

The following case, observed by Dr. Kaufmann (*Vierteljahresschrift für gerichtliche Medicin*), is interesting chiefly from a medico-legal point of view. A house-painter was thrown from a ladder, striking in his fall the corner of a piece of furniture. From this time on, violent headaches and pains in the back were frequent. Immediately after the fall he remained for several hours unconscious. After slight and transitory improvement, during which he returned to his work, the head pains returned, mental weakness, slowing of pulse, narrowing of the field of vision, and loss of appetite came on. Transitory mania was also observed during the cephalalgic attacks; finally almost total blindness and paralysis of the left arm supervened. Death took place six months after the accident. Post-mortem examination showed death to have resulted from a sarcoma. The tumor was of comparatively recent growth; the oldest pathological cerebral lesion was evidently an apoplectic cyst which was surrounded by a cheesy tumor. This cyst was pronounced by the pathologist to correspond to an effusion of blood of such amount that it could not have taken place without visible symptoms. It was extremely probable that the hemorrhage was the result of the fall, and that the loss of consciousness noted was dependent on it. The hemorrhage was the direct cause of the development of the tumor, as injuries, falls, and the like were undoubted and recognized causes of cerebral tumors and their most frequent explanation, especially in the case of sarcomata. All other explanations were only hypotheses. The histological examination of the tumor explained its rapid development in so short a time. The conclusion was that the fall led directly to the development of the tumor, and through this to death.—*Med. Record*, Jan. 26, 1889.

The Place of Saccharin in Pharmacy.

Under this title, Professor Attfield, F.R.S., one of the editors of the *British Pharmacopœia*, gives some very practical information as to the formula and uses of saccharin, in a pamphlet just issued from the press. By way of introduction, he observes that saccharin will be of good service in pharmacy in four ways. First, it will give patients an opportunity of taking certain medicines in comparatively small bulk. Many medicinal confections, powders, and lozenges have hitherto necessarily contained large proportions of sugar. A mere trace of saccharin put in place of sugar, while rendering the medicament as sweet as before, will give such a reduction in bulk that, for example, a bismuth lozenge will become a mere pellet, and compound liquorice powder, or confection of senna, be reduced to half their old volume. Second, the intensity of the sweetness of saccharin will enable it to mask the nauseous taste of certain medicines, the flavor of cod-liver oil, for example, being well disguised. Third, patients who are obliged to avoid sugar will no longer be deprived of its property of sweetness, for not only tea, coffee, cocoa, etc., but many medicines also, containing saccharin in place of sugar, will once more become palatable—sweet, but not harmfully sweet. Fourth, saccharin not being liable to ferment, while sugar is specially prone to ferment, its use will afford permanent preparations where those made with sugar will frequently spoil. The exhibition of saccharin will present no difficulties. In prescriptions for fluids, such as gargles, mixtures, and emulsions, where physicians would have ordered a given quantity of solution of sugar (syrupus) they will prescribe an equal volume of simple solution of saccharin (sol. sacc. simp.). In prescriptions for a powder, or a confection-like mass, saccharin itself might be prescribed. And most of the large number of galenical preparations, as commonly ordered by physicians, and now made with sugar, would be prepared with saccharin, and would be set forth in prescriptions under distinctive names—mist. cretæ sacc.; pulv. glycyr. co. sacc. concent.; conf. sennæ sacc. concent., etc. Concerning incompatibles, saccharin is a tolerably indifferent substance. It is unaffected by the fluids of the body, acid or other, for it has been proved to pass through the system unchanged. Fusion with caustic alkali gives a salicylate, hence prolonged contact with strong alkalies is probably undesirable ; and, obviously, acids would precipitate saccharin itself from a strong, though not from a weak, solution of a soluble saccharinate, that is, "soluble saccharin"; but saccharin is quite anaffected by the ordinary materials used in medicine. Professor Attfield regrets the name saccharin, and suggests "neo-saccharin," or an equivalent. He furnishes a considerable number of interesting formulæ.—*British Med. Journal*, Jan. 26, 1889.

Communication of Tuberculosis.

An instructive case of communicated tuberculosis is related by Dr. E. von Duhring, who states in the *Monatshefte für prakt. Dermatologie*, No. 22, 1888, that a girl 14 years old sprung from a family uncontaminated with phthisis, was in friendly relations with a young girl who died of consumption. At the time when this girl died the patient, E. Z., was in good health. Shortly after the death of the friend she removed the earrings which the other wore from the ears and fastened them in her own. The mother stated that the girl who had died had no wound in her ear, but E. Z. herself, on the contrary, states that her friend had frequently blood and matter on her ear. The patient E. Z. herself had up to that time never worn earrings, although the ears had been bored for the purpose. Shortly after she began to wear earrings the hole through which they were fastened began to secrete freely, notwithstanding which she continued to wear them, and she had continued to wear them up to the time when Dr. von Duhring saw her. It was on account of the condition of her ears that she was brought to him. He found her pale, somewhat thin, but well built and well developed for her age. Where the left ear had been pierced there was a shallow ulcer with undermined borders, and on the left side of the neck there was a slightly enlarged gland adherent to the skin, which was ulcerated on the surface and covered with a dirty scab. On removing the scab a somewhat abundant thin secretion escaped. The borders of this ulcer were irregularly dentated. On examining the lungs, there was dulness detected in the left apex. Granulations removed with a sharp spoon from the wound in the ear showed the presence of tubercle bacilli. The further progress of the case was rapid, and at the time Dr. von Duhring wrote his paper the patient was rapidly sinking from phthisis.—*British Med. Journal*, Jan. 19, 1889.

Action of Ergot on the Uterus.

Dr. Lombe Atthill, in a communication published in the *Dublin Journal of Medical Science*, Dec. 1, 1888, says of ergot that it is most uncertain in its action and in its effects. In some cases it causes pain, and when it does it always, he thinks, lessens hemorrhage from the uterus, the pain being evidently due to clonic contraction of the muscular fibres. But sometimes the same dose of the same preparation which caused pain previously, does not do so on another occasion, though apparently no change has taken place in the patient's condition. Dr. Atthill thinks that ergot will not induce clonic contraction of the uterine fibres unless something acting as a foreign body is present in it. The mere presence of a foreign body is not sufficient; it must be acting. Pedunculated polypi, he says, are commonly enough met with in the uterus, but their expulsion by painful uterine action is quite rare, and it is most likely that the seat of the tumor is the main element of its tendency to excite uterine action. The portion of the uterus between the entrance of the Fallopian tubes is the sensitive portion of the organ, and, in his opinion, it is necessary for a tumor to be situated there for it to act as a foreign body.

He regards it as very doubtful if ergot ever originates clonic contractions of the uterus during pregnancy, unless the organ is prepared by some pre-existing cause to expel its contents. When engaged formerly in midwifery practice he was in the habit of frequently prescribing ergot as a preventive to *post-partum* hemorrhage, commencing its administration a week or ten days before the expected advent of labor, and he says he has never once had reason to suppose that it hastened that event ; on the contrary, in several instances the period of utero-gestation seemed to be lengthened. In like manner, in cases of a threatened abortion, he has seen the hemorrhage checked, and pregnancy proceed normally under the administration of ergot ; it seemed, indeed, to act as a uterine tonic, if such an expression be admissible. In others, and perhaps the majority, it seemed to produce no effect at all ; in a few it induced clonic spasms, but in these there was always reason to think that the ovum was already blighted. In cases of uterine fibroids, he says, ergot will, in general, be found to act most beneficially in lessening hemorrhage when the tumor is embedded in the muscular tissue, and as thinning of the wall takes place, and as the tumor consequently comes in closer contact with the uterine mucous membrane, the result of its administration will be less satisfactory ; but in all cases much will depend on the preparation used and upon its freshness.

Rickets, Rheumatism, Chorea, Cancer, and Urinary Calculus in the British Islands.

The *British Med. Journal*, Jan. 19, contains the report of the Collective Investigation Committee of the British Medical Association regarding the geographical distribution of rickets, acute and subacute rheumatism, chorea, cancer, and urinary calculus in the British Islands. The following is a summary of the report:

1. That there is no district in the British Isles in which acute and subacute rheumatism and malignant disease are not common in the sense defined in the inquiry paper. Of varying degrees of prevalence above that point this inquiry was not designed to furnish a criterion.

2. That rickets, though not unknown in rural districts, is mainly a disease of towns and industrial regions, and especially of large industrial towns ; that it is rare in the rural districts of Scotland, the North of England, North Wales, and Ireland, Ulster excepted ; that it is more common in the rural districts of Ulster and of the rest of England, and exceptionally prevalent in Cornwall, Kent, and North Essex.

3. That chorea, like rickets, is mainly a disease of towns and industrial regions, though by no means unknown in rural districts ; that it is fairly evenly distributed in the rural districts of the four countries ; that it is rare in seaside watering-places ; and that it is, by exception, somewhat rare in the south as well as the west of London, and not, generally speaking, common in Glasgow, even in the poorer quarters.

4. That the distribution of chorea is further affected by that of acute and subacute rheumatism, its prevalence diminishing as the latter disease becomes rare.

5. That urinary calculus exhibits a decided tendency to affect the eastern sides of the two islands; that its chief seat in South Britain is the county of Norfolk, from which it radiates into the neighboring counties, and in North Britain the angle of land above Aberdeen, from which it extends down the east coast to the Forth ; that it shows a less decided tendency to appear in the coalfields, being especially prevalent in the Black Country ; and that its prevalence does not otherwise seem due to geological conditions.

THE
MEDICAL AND SURGICAL
REPORTER.

ISSUED EVERY SATURDAY.

CHARLES W. DULLES, M.D.,
EDITOR AND PUBLISHER.

The Terms of Subscription to the serial publications of this office are as follows, payable in advance:

Med. and Surg. Reporter (weekly), a year, **$5.00**
Quarterly Compendium of Med. Science, - 2.50
Reporter and Compendium, - - - 6.00
Physician's Daily Pocket Record, - - - 1.00
Reporter and Pocket Record, - - - - 6.00
Reporter, Compendium, and Pocket Record, 7.00

All checks and postal orders should be drawn to order of

CHARLES W. DULLES,
N. E. Cor. 13th and Walnut Streets,
P. O. Box 843.   Philadelphia, Pa.

☞SUGGESTIONS TO SUBSCRIBERS:
See that your address-label gives the date to which your subscription is paid.
In requesting a change of address, give the old address as well as the new one.
If your REPORTER does not reach you promptly and regularly, notify the publisher *at once*, so that the cause may be discovered and corrected.

☞SUGGESTIONS TO CONTRIBUTORS AND CORRESPONDENTS:
Write in ink.
Write on one side of paper only.
Write on paper of the size usually used for letters.
Make as few paragraphs as possible. Punctuate carefully. Do not abbreviate, or omit words like "the," and "a," or "an."
Make communications as short as possible.
NEVER ROLL A MANUSCRIPT! Try to get an envelope or wrapper which will fit it.
When it is desired to call our attention to something in a newspaper, mark the passage boldly with a colored pencil, and write on the Wrapper "Marked copy." Unless this is done, newspapers are not looked at.
The Editor will be glad to get medical news, but it is important that brevity and actual interest shall characterize communications intended for publication.

DECEPTION OF A MEDICAL WITNESS.

The daily papers report from Chicago that at the trial of a woman for murder, Dr. Kiernan, while testifying as a medical expert, was made the victim of a shameful trick by one of the attorneys for the defense. The latter held in his hand a volume of Ray's Jurisprudence and read an account of a case, pretending it was printed in the book. It was, however, written on pieces of paper which he had concealed between the leaves, and when Dr. Kiernan—as the story goes—said he was familiar with the case, the lawyer took the paper out and said he had concocted the account himself.

According to the published reports, this *dénouement* filled Dr. Kiernan with mortification, and the prisoner and her counsel with delight. This might well be; but there is another way of looking at the matter. As to Dr. Kiernan's part in it: it is not strange that he was caught in the trap set for him; because—as he stated—the account read was similar to many published in the books, and he might think he recognized it, and believe it was in almost any book on jurisprudence. In a similar case hereafter, he will no doubt ask to see anything read to him by an attorney at a trial; and this would be a good rule for all witnesses.

The lawyer's part in the occurrence merits the severest condemnation. Such dishonorable tricks are not indulged in by men of high character; and we know, from personal inquiry, that they are indignantly repudiated by the best members of the legal profession. To physicians the matter is one of more than general interest; because they are unfortunately often called to the witness-stand, and usually have an uncomfortable enough time there when attorneys keep within civil and considerate bounds. But the case will be far worse if physicians have added to the ordinary perplexities of examination and cross-examination the fear that they may be exposed to attempts to entrap them by what is virtually lying.

It is to be hoped that the occurrence which has prompted these comments will lead to some expression of opinion in regard to it on the part of representatives of the legal profession; for while a physician has been mortified and hurt by it, a lawyer has been disgraced.

There is no good reason why lawyers and doctors should not be the best friends in the world—many of them are; and we trust that the principles of professional comity will prevent a repetition of such an unfortunate occurrence as is described above.

ARTIFICIAL STIMULATION OF THE GROWTH OF BONE.

One of the well recognized curiosities of medical experience is the observation that the bones may sometimes rapidly increase in size under the stimulus afforded by disease or accident—or perhaps rather of the recoil from depressing influences. Similarly the bones of pregnant women increase in size under the influence of the heightened physiological activity of the state.

The occurrence of what may be called—somewhat inaptly—the pathological increase in size of bones was the subject of a careful study by Bergmann some years ago, who published the results of his investigations in the *St. Petersburger Zeitschrift*, Bd. xlv., and Ollier and Langenbeck have made valuable contributions to the literature of the subject.

In a very recent article in the *Berliner klinische Wochenschrift*, Prof. Max Schüller, of Berlin, presents an interesting, though brief, review of the hitherto recorded observations in connection with the, so-to-speak, spasmodic growth of bone, and an able study of the application of the teachings of these observations to attempts at producing such growth by artificial means.

From his own investigations and experiments, as well as those of others, it seems clear that this form of growth can be looked for only during the usual period of development of the skeleton, and that it depends upon some stimulus acting upon the cartilage between the diaphysis and epiphysis of long bones. A few cases are on record in which the bones have suddenly increased in length after the apparent end of the growing period, and these seem to make it probable that an interstitial growth may take place after the connecting cartilage has ossified. But such observations are very rare; and it is difficult to understand how a bone can increase in length, except at its extremities.

Among the conditions which have given rise to lengthening of the bones are aneu-rism, and angiectasis, and universal development of the blood-vessels; but ulcers, fractures, inflammations of the joints, and even infantile paralysis have been followed by a similar result.

Ollier experimented on animals, with various irritations of the periosteum and medulla of the long bones, and found they provoked an increase in length of the bones. Schüller has had a similar experience, and finds that the growth is caused by communication of the stimulus to the connecting cartilage.

A number of surgeons have attempted to make practical use of the suggestions afforded by observation and experiment, and Schüller has followed up the idea of producing an artificial congestion in the bones with the object of increasing their length. This congestion he produces by means of a constricting rubber tube applied some distance above the point to be influenced so as to compress the veins, but not the arteries, of the parts. The application is made at first for only an hour or two, then for gradually lengthened periods, until it is continuous during the day and night. The application must be graduated so as to produce no pain, and so as to accustom the patient to it.

Schüller does not depend on this measure alone to provoke growth in the bones, but adds massage, exercise and careful nourishment of the patient, including the administration of food containing salts of lime. He has practised his method in two cases, with quite satisfactory results, and recommends it for further testing.

This interesting subject is worthy of careful study in this country, and it would be useful to have it taken up by those who have cases suited to experimentation with Schüller's method. In the many hospitals and homes for the crippled in America there must be many patients who might with advantage furnish an opportunity for confirming or correcting Schüller's opinions; and we commend them to the attention of the surgeons in charge of these institutions, in the hope that they may prove to be correct, and be applied for the benefit of those who are deformed or injured.

HYSTERORRHAPHY.

Among the most trying and intractable cases which the gynecologist is called upon to treat are those of retroflexion of the uterus with fixation in the malposition. These cases are trying not only because it is difficult to treat them successfully, but also because it is often difficult or impossible to make out the extent of the diseased conditions present, and hence to decide upon the line of treatment indicated. Inflammation and prolapse of the ovaries, and disease of the tubes of varying degree, quite frequently complicate the retroflexion. Under these circumstances the practitioner, in order to effect a cure, has need of all his energies, and his best efforts will sometimes be without avail. It is especially in this class of cases that the comparatively new operation of abdominal section, separation of adhesions, and fixation of the body of the uterus to the abdominal wall above the pubes promises to do much good. Treatment by pessaries can seldom be employed in these cases ; vaginal packing often fails to effect even a symptomatic cure ; the operations of Alexander and Schücking are contra-indicated by the adhesions present ; often the uterine appendages are healthy or but slightly diseased, and exsection of these structures is not indicated. Nothing remains to be done except the application of Brandt's system of massage, or hysterorrhaphy.

The name hysterorrhaphy, was given to the operation by Dr. Howard Kelly, of Philadelphia, one of the earliest, and an original worker in this field. It is evident that the nature of the operation is different, when on the one hand the abdomen is opened for the sole purpose of suturing the fundus to the abdominal wall—separating adhesions when necessary ; and when on the other hand the abdomen is opened in the performance of some operation, such as removal of the uterine appendages, or ovariotomy, and the ventro-fixation of the uterus is simply supplemental to the procedure first undertaken. As more distinctly setting forth the nature of the operation done, Dr. C. C. Lee, of New York, speaks of primary and secondary—supplemental—hysterorrhaphy. While this classification is evidently of practical importance, it is plain that it can not be applied to all cases. The operator may purpose to do a primary, formal hysterorrhaphy, but after opening the abdomen, he may find greater disease of the uterine appendages than he had suspected, or some other condition requiring operative treatment, and thus the suturing of the uterus may become supplemental or secondary. As thus defined, secondary hysterorrhaphy has been performed for some years, Kœberlé having operated as long ago as 1869, and Tait and Thomas within the present decade. There seems to be no question as to the propriety of fixing the fundus uteri to the abdominal wall, whenever in the course of an intra-abdominal operation it is found retro-flexed and fixed, or markedly prolapsed.

Primary hysterorrhaphy was first done by Olshausen. According to Lee, it is indicated in cases of malposition of the womb with fixation from adhesions, which resist milder methods of treatment. Kelly and Sänger extend the indication to cases of intractable prolapsus, and retroflexion without fixation, thus bringing this operation in competition with that of Alexander.

While to many it may appear that already enough operations have been invented to be practised upon women, and that in the future progress should be made in prophylaxis, and in perfecting the technique of methods of treatment already in use, still we believe that there is a field of usefulness for this new operation in the cure of stubborn cases of retroflexion of the uterus with adhesions, and in exceptional cases of prolapsus.

IODOFORM AND CADAVERIN.

It is interesting to note that an explanation of the antiseptic properties of iodoform is offered by Behring, in the *Deutsche med. Wochenschrift*, Aug. 9, 1888, which calls in a chemical reaction between iodoform and cadaverin. Behring says that unadulterated cadaverin causes pus formation, but that when mixed with iodoform it has no such effect. In regard to its constitutional effect, Brieger has asserted that cadaverin was not a toxic alkaloid; but Behring says that it is, and that it gives rise in mice to a definite and regular set of symptoms. None of these symptoms, however, arise when mice are treated with cadaverin mixed with iodoform.

These assertions are laid before our readers as medical news. It will be seen that, in order to complete the Behring's theory in regard to the antiseptic properties of iodoform, it is very convenient to dissent from Brieger in regard to the action of cadaverin on the general system. Whether Brieger or Behring is right in this connection we cannot say; but iodoform will probably be used as an antiseptic for some time to come, no matter how its action may be explained by laboratory investigators.

ARTHRECTOMY AT THE ANKLE-JOINT.

The usual line of approach to the ankle-joint, for the purpose of removing from it tuberculous or fungous deposits, is behind the external malleolus. In this line the access to the joint is relatively easy, and the incision here does not implicate any important structures. But Dr. Meinhard Schmidt, of Cúxhaven, proposes a new method as specially adapted to the removal of the products of tuberculosis in the talo-crural, or ankle-joint. His method, as described in the *Centralblatt für Chirurgie*, Jan. 12, 1889, consists in making a vertical incision alongside of and parallel to the outer border of the tendo Achillis, the middle of which crosses the line of the joint, going through the deep fascia, and opening the capsule of the joint. After clearing out the posterior part of the joint through this incision, the anterior part is approached through a vertical incision carried over the front of the joint in a line passing between the tibia and fibula.

In this way Schmidt found that he could explore and operate upon the ankle-joint better than in any other; and he calls attention to the fact that the arrangement of the ligaments of the ankle-joint is such that effusions or growths within it protrude from it in front and behind, and so, as it were, approach the surgeon.

This is not the first time that it has been suggested to employ an anterior incision in approaching the ankle-joint; but it is, so far as we know, the first recommendation to combine an anterior and a posterior vertical incision for this purpose. The proposition seems entirely rational, and has been carried into execution by Dr. Schmidt with ease; so that it deserves the consideration of other surgeons.

THE PHILADELPHIA POLYCLINIC.

A few years ago the meaning of the word "Polyclinic" was almost unknown in this country, except to those few fortunates who had enjoyed the advantages of study in one of the teaching establishments called by this name in Germany or Austria. Now, however, the term is well understood, and polyclinics have been established in several cities in the United States. One of the first of this class was the Philadelphia Polyclinic, which was organized in 1883 by Drs. Levis, Morton, and others, and which has continued its work ever since. At present—as our columns have from time to time indicated—it is enlarging its facilities for clinical instruction of graduates in medicine, and making an appeal to the Legislature for a grant of money to aid it in erecting a building better suited to its needs, and to those of its students, than the one now in use.

We sincerely hope that this grant will be

made; and we call the attention of our readers in this State to the Philadelphia Polyclinic, because we believe it deserves their hearty support. It is, in the first place, the only institution of the kind in Pennsylvania, and for this reason has a peculiar claim for sympathy and support—if it deserves them. In the second place, it is an excellent institution, managed by competent and honorable physicians and surgeons, and calculated to be of great service to medical men, who have recently graduated and need closer clinical opportunities than teaching in medical schools or general hospitals affords, as well as to active practitioners, who can spare a few weeks at a time to revive their knowledge or to improve themselves in special branches or phases of medical science or art.

In this connection, we note that there seems to be a disposition, on the part of the two most important medical schools in this city, to encourage the development of the Polyclinic, which is in agreeable contrast to the attitude at one time assumed toward it. This is as it should be. The medical schools cannot successfully combine the teaching of under-graduates and post-graduates, and they do well to encourage those who can relieve them of part of the work. We therefore regard with pleasure the evidences of sympathy with the Polyclinic shown by the University of Pennsylvania and the Jefferson Medical College; for we believe that its success will not only prove an advantage to the whole profession in Pennsylvania, but also add to the reputation of Philadelphia as a medical centre.

BRITISH AND AMERICAN CONTINENTAL MEDICAL SOCIETY.—Our correspondent in Paris writes that it is proposed to form a Society under the above, or some similar, title, with a view to promote social Intercourse and maintain good fellowship between British and American physicians who practise on the Continent. The membership is to be limited to British and American subjects who are actually engaged in the practice of medicine abroad.

It is suggested that the Paris exhibition will attract many medical men to that city during 1889. The French medical Societies will hold meetings, and much of interest to doctors will be seen, so that it would be a favorable time to hold a first meeting there, which might take the form of a dinner (after a preliminary sitting) when it could be decided what form the present idea should take.

A letter has been issued to a number of American and British medical men practising in Europe; and on receipt of answers, a local committee of ten or twelve English and American physicians will combine to make the temporary arrangements so as to suit the wishes of the largest number as to time of meeting.

THE PRESBYTERIAN HOSPITAL.—At the annual meeting of the Trustees of the Presbyterian Hospital, Jan. 22, a very encouraging report was read of the work accomplished during the past year. It is a pleasure to note that this admirable institution, which stands so high in the estimation of patients and of the community, is to be still better equipped for the coming year. The want of a suitable administration building has been a great hindrance to the work of the hospital, but such a building is now to be supplied through the liberality of one of the members of the Board of Trustees, who has authorized the announcement that he will submit to the Board for consideration plans for the building, and assume the entire cost of its erection, should it be the pleasure of the Board to accept his offer. The Ladies' Aid Society of the Hospital is also pledged to raise thirty thousand dollars for a new surgical ward. With certain changes and additions the hospital will then be able to accommodate about two hundred patients, provided the increase in its endowment and in the annual contributions from churches will be adequate to meet the running expenses.

BOOK REVIEWS.

[Any book reviewed in these columns may be obtained upon receipt of price, from the office of the REPORTER.]

THE FUNCTIONS AND DISORDERS OF THE REPRODUCTIVE ORGANS, ETC. BY WILLIAM ACTON, M.R.C.S., ETC. Seventh edition. 8vo, pp. xii, 263. Philadelphia: P. Blakiston, Son & Co., 1888. Price, $2.00.

Dr. Acton's work on the reproductive organs is too well known to need extended notice now. It contains a full and scholarly discussion of the normal phenomena connected with the function of the reproductive organs of both sexes, and of the disorders and abnormal exercise of these organs. It is a book full of wise counsels, and written in the spirit of a true moralist. It contains much that is interesting, and treats of a delicate subject in the most prudent manner. No attempt is apparent in it to attract readers by dwelling too long or too curiously on matters which are proper subjects for scientific investigation, but which cannot be dallied with without offending against chastity; and everywhere its tone is pure and its language carefully guarded.

There is no book which can well be compared with this one in the English language; and it is likely long to hold its position as a classic on the subject of which it treats.

The present edition is poorly printed—apparently from old stereotype plates, and has unfortunately no index.

FAVORITE PRESCRIPTIONS OF DISTINGUISHED PRACTITIONERS, WITH NOTES ON TREATMENT. COMPILED, ETC., BY B. W. PALMER, A.M., M.D. 8vo, pp. 256. New York: E. B. Treat, 1888. Price, $2.15.

It is rather the fashion with reviewers to abuse books of this sort; and, we confess, it was with no predisposition in favor of the class to which it belongs that we took it up. But justice requires the admission that a list of the prescriptions of men who have been successful in the practice of medicine may be very useful to men whose general notions in regard to treatment need to be put into definite shape before they can make good use of them. Such books as this have a legitimate field, and in their proper field they are not to be sneered at.

The volume before us has some merit. It would never do to follow its implied directions too blindly; but a judicious culling from its formulæ would probably help many a man in a strait.

In commenting upon it, it is hard to keep a just balance between commendation and warning; but the reader of it will have to exercise great caution lest what may be useful, if used wisely, prove a snare to his unwary feet.

DISEASES AND THEIR COMMENCEMENT. LECTURES TO TRAINED NURSES DELIVERED AT THE WEST LONDON HOSPITAL. BY DONALD W. CHARLES HOOD, M.D., Cantab., Physician to the Hospital, etc. 8vo, pp. vii, 138. London: J. & A. Churchill, 1886. Price, two shillings sixpence.

This book consists of a series of five lectures on some points in pathology, symptomatology and therapeutics, delivered to nurses. All who have lectured to nurses upon elementary facts in medicine appreciate the difficulty of presenting these facts to them so that they will be of value in their practical work. The danger is that such necessarily incomplete information will spoil good nurses by giving them an exalted opinion of their knowledge of medicine. Dr. Hood has succeeded well, and nurses will be less likely to make this error after than before reading his book. The nature of the subject makes the lectures rather rambling, but they will prove interesting and instructive to nurses and the laity, and in some respects physicians.

PAMPHLET NOTICES.

[Any reader of the REPORTER who desires a copy of a pamphlet noticed in these columns will doubtless secure it by addressing the author with a request stating where the notice was seen and *enclosing a postage-stamp*.]

213. THE TREATMENT OF EMPYEMA: THE PROCESS OF REPAIR, ETC. BY G. J. ROBERTSON, M.B., Oldham, England. From the *Medical Chronicle*, March, May, June and July, 1888. 60 pages.

214. THE ANOMALIES OF THE OCULAR MUSCLES. BY GEORGE T. STEVENS, M.D., New York. First Paper. From the *Archives of Ophthalmology*, 1887. 28 pages.

215. THE ANOMALIES OF THE OCULAR MUSCLES. SECOND PAPER. BY GEO. T. STEVENS, M.D., New York. From the *Archives of Ophthalmology*, 1888. 33 pages.

216. HOT WATER IN THE MANAGEMENT OF EYE DISEASES. BY LEARTUS CONNER, M.D., Detroit, Mich. 16 pages.

213. Mr. Robertson's pamphlet contains a complete and scholarly study of the conditions of empyema, and of the process of repair which takes place when different forms of treatment are carried out. It also contains a well described and well illustrated account of a method of subcutaneous drainage and irrigation which he has used with the best results in a number of cases. The pamphlet is of the most interesting and instructive character, and a careful study of it could not fail to be of advantage to all medical men.

214. Dr. Stevens, as is well known to the readers of the REPORTER, attaches great importance to what some medical men have considered slight defects in the action of the muscles of the eyeball, and in the pamphlet before us he discusses the effects of such abnormal action—especially hyperphoria, and their treatment. In regard to the latter, he favors tenotomy, when this is practicable, and the use of prisms when an operation is not possible or desirable. He describes the method he follows, and the instruments he uses, the latter being illustrated with a wood-cut.

215. This pamphlet continues the discussion begun in pamphlet No. 214, in regard to the symptoms and treatment of certain abnormal conditions of the muscles of the eyeball. The symptoms are described with technical precision, and the treatment suited to different conditions is clearly stated.

216. Dr. Conner has prepared a very instructive paper on the use of hot water in diseases of the eye, such as blepharitis, corneitis and conjunctivitis, as well iritis and ophthalmia. The method of using hot water is fully and admirably described. This paper is not written so as to interest specialists alone, but all practitioners of medicine; and any physician who masters its contents will have gained information which will prove of service many a time in his experience.

CORRESPONDENCE.

Superfluous Hairs.

To the Editor.

Sir: Could you inform me of any safe and sure means of removing superfluous hairs from the face of a lady?

Yours truly,

H. J. Stubbs, M.D.

Wilmington, Del.,

Feb. 3, 1889.

[There is one way only of removing superfluous hairs, and that is by destruction of the papilla. Several methods for accomplishing this have been suggested from time to time. The most successful, and that at present employed by dermatologists, is by means of electrolysis. The operation requires a galvanic battery of ten to twenty cells, a needle-holder, and a fine needle. When done by a skillful and practised operator, the results are satisfactory, not more than ten per cent. returning. The operation is, however, tedious, and requires keen sight. The various details of this method may be found in all recent American works on dermatology.—Editor Reporter.]

Result of a Herniotomy.

To the Editor:

Sir: In the Reporter May 26, 1888, I reported an operation for radical cure of hernia. About that time the patient became entirely paralyzed on the left side, and he died yesterday morning. Ten hours after death, at the *post mortem*, I made a careful dissection of the site of operation. No person would have thought of there having been a hernia, except for the cicatrix left by the incision in the integuments. The opening through the conjoined tendon was entirely obliterated, being filled by dense connective tissue, which was strongly adherent to Pouparts ligament, the pubic bone and all the surrounding tissues, making that side much stronger and thicker than the opposite one. The spermatic cord and vessels were found in their proper canal. The internal abdominal ring had never been disturbed. Looking at the site of the hernia from the inside there was no depression, and nothing indicating a pathological condition, except adhesion of the peritoneum where the hernia formerly protruded. Those who saw it considered the result of operation perfect.

Yours truly,

A. Ady, M.D.

Muscatine, Iowa,

Jan. 22, 1889.

Father Damien.

To the Editor.

Sir: The statement made in your issue of Jan. 26, as to the condition of Father Damien dying of leprosy, has led me to think that possibly some of your readers may not know the history of this noble man in his self-sacrificing work. I therefore take the liberty of quoting the following utterance of Sir Risdon Bennett, M.D., made some two years since: "We cannot refrain from making reference to the case of the heroic Father Damien, which has excited so much painful sympathy. This young Belgian Roman Catholic priest, after his ordination in 1873, volunteered his services in the leper settlement at Malakoi, one of the Sandwich Islands. When he arrived there the lepers numbered 800, of whom between 400 and 500 were Romanists, and were dying from 8 to 12 per week. After ministering to these for 13 *years* (!), in every possible capacity, spiritual and temporal, as doctor, cook, carpenter, and even grave-digger, he has himself fallen a victim to the disease, and has resigned himself with the most touching Christian submission to all its well-known consequences, saying daily to God, '*Fiat voluntas tua.*'"

Yours truly, * *

A Question of Etiquette.

To the Editor.

Sir: Suppose Dr. A. upon request of Mrs. B. attends her family in sickness during the year. Mrs. B. is the widow of a Doctor who died years ago, and whom Dr. A. never had any acquaintance with or even any knowledge of. Mrs. B. is a lady of affluence. Is there anything in medical etiquette which would make it improper for Dr. A. to make out a bill against the widow?

Medicus.

[If the widow in affluence were a person of proper feeling, it would not be necessary for our correspondent to ask this question. If she is not, there would probably be some risk of being abused if a bill were sent. But, as a matter of morals and of etiquette, it would be perfectly right to send a bill in such a case as is described.—Editor of the Reporter.]

—Diphtheria is reported to be epidemic in Hancock county, Ohio. The schools in Big Lick, Blanchard and Marion townships have been closed, and others will have to be unless the progress of the disease abates. It is fortunately not of a malignant type, and deaths are few.

NOTES AND COMMENTS.

The New Hypnotic, Sulphonal.

Constantin Paul spoke of sulphonal before the Therapeutic Society of Paris, Jan. 9, 1889 (*Bulletin Médical*, Jan. 13, 1889). After referring to the observations of Kast, which have been noted already in the REPORTER, he said that when fifteen grains are given to a patient in the evening, he generally falls asleep in a half-hour, but sometimes only in an hour or two. The sleep is light and without either dreams or night-mare, and is followed by a feeling of comfort without gastric uneasiness on awaking.

Sulphonal is especially indicated, he says, in nervous insomnia, in doses of fifteen or thirty grains. M. Paul has employed it with variable success in toothache, in a case of cellulitis of the face complicated with neuralgia, after a fracture, in alcoholic delirium, delirium tremens, in mania, in hypochondria, and in acute diseases, fevers, etc. Sulphonal, he says, may be substituted for morphine; thirty grains produce sleep in morphinomaniacs. In a case of hypertrophy of the heart no intolerance was produced; the cardiac distress was not increased, respiration remained quiet. He regards sulphonal as an adjuvant in rheumatism when the pain has been previously allayed with salicylate of soda; so also in acute or subacute bronchitis. In the latter he first allays sensibility with codeine and then obtains restful sleep with sulphonal, which he says is well borne even by children.

M. Huchard was more guarded in his statements. He gave a brief account of fourteen cases in which he had employed it; in five of them it was unsuccessful. He stated that sulphonal has no anæsthetic power. Its greatest action is produced in nervous insomnia and is prolonged for four or eight hours, rarely longer, although Kiffer has observed a patient in whom sleep lasted thirty-six hours. Because of its slow action it is necessary to give at the outset a large dose. It sometimes occasions slight diuresis. Its principal inconvenience is its being followed by a painful awaking, with a feeling of hesitation in walking, resembling cerebellar tottering rather than ataxia. Some eruptions and hallucinations of hearing have also been noted. If sulphonal is a substitute for chloral, he says, it is not superior to it, its only advantage being its prolonged action.

Treatment of Baldness.

Dr. Lassar has a communication on the treatment of the hair in the *Therapeutische Monatshefte*, Dec., 1888. He regards alopecia as a parasitic disease, and he recommends an antiparasitic treatment which has commended itself in more than one thousand cases. The scalp should be soaped by an expert hand for ten minutes daily for the first six or eight weeks, later less frequently. For this purpose a strong tar soap is best. After the scalp is well lathered the soap is carefully washed off with tepid followed by cool water, contained in an irrigator or watering-pot. The washing with cool water hardens the scalp in a happy manner against the colds to which patients with alopecia are usually disposed. The scalp is then dried gently and rubbed with:

Sol. hydrarg. bichlor. . . . gr. viiss to f ℥ iv¼
Glycerini,
Spir. Cologn. . . . . . aa f ℥ iss

It is then dried and rubbed with absolute alcohol, to which one-half per cent. naphthol has been added; and then as much of the following as possible is rubbed into the scalp, which is now quite free of fat:

Acidi salicylici . . . . gr. xxx
Tinct. benzoini . . . . ℳ xlv
Olei pedum tauri (neat's foot
oil) . . . . ad f ℥ iii

The soaping removes all adherent substances, the sublimate solution is readily absorbed by the mouths of the hair follicles, the alcohol dries the scalp, removes the fat and disinfects it, and finally the mixture of salicylic acid and oil is taken up by all the pores and exerts its action in the interior of the glands.

A daily use of this treatment will bring about a favorable result in the majority of the cases. This is especially true in the cases of young women and girls. The brittle, lustreless hair becomes flexible and elastic. Hundreds of new, vigorous hairs shoot up. —*Wiener med. Presse*, Dec. 23, 1888.

Regeneration of the Hair.

In the *Semaine Médicale*, Nov. 28, 1888, Besnier recommends the following treatment for alopecia: The neighborhood of the bald spot is shaved, or the hairs which come out easily are removed, and an application is made of a mixture composed of equal parts of chloroform and glacial acetic acid. This mixture has caustic properties, and must be applied lightly with a camel's hair brush each evening; and if the bare spot be large only part of it can be treated at a time, or too much pain will be caused.

The Transmission of Leprosy.

Amongst instances which have lately been published which tend to show that leprosy is communicated by contagion, none are more striking than those which have been related by Dr. Zuriaga in the *Annales de Derm.*, vol. ix, No. 6. In 1849 leprosy did not exist in the village of Parcent, in the province of Alicante. In 1850 a leper, from the neighboring town of Sagra, in the province of Alicante, district of Pego, came to reside in Parcent with one of his intimate friends, Vincent Poquet Andres. The two friends ate from the same plates, with the same spoons, drank from the same glasses, and slept together. The effects of these close relations were not slow in making themselves evident. In the first year Poquet had acquired the leprosy which infected his friend. A nephew of Poquet, called Ramont Poquet Perez, who frequented the house of his uncle, was not long in becoming affected. Ramont had three married brothers, Baptiste, Joseph and Rosa. Fearing contagion, Baptiste and Rosa ceased to have any relations with Ramont. Less careful, Joseph and his children continued to have communication with him. Soon afterward leprosy became apparent in the house of Joseph. He had seven children; five of them were attacked. The two others were so impressed by this fact that they left their father's house, established themselves elsewhere, and ceased to have any relations with their family. They have remained free from leprosy. Joseph Perez died of disease of the heart. His wife still lives and is free from leprosy. The five sons who were leprous are still alive, and have reached the period of exhaustion. Joseph Mora lived close to the first leper in Parcent, being an intimate friend of Vincent Poquet. Soon afterward he developed leprosy. Joachim Guier, a friend of Mora, also became a leper, and some years later his two brothers were also attacked. They lived in the same house. Without following Dr. Zuriaga's paper further in detail, suffice it to say that two sisters appear to have been infected by Guier, and that shortly afterward their five brothers were in their turn attacked. Of five young soldiers more or less associated with Ramont Perez, three avoided him, and two were careless as regards contagion. The three remained healthy, the other two became lepers. Soon afterward other inhabitants of the village became lepers. Without there being apparent cause of contagion of late years, a considerable part of the population has become lepers. Since 1850, in this small village, there have been about sixty cases of leprosy; forty-five of these lepers have died. According to the statement of the Mayor of Parcent, by whom these facts have been communicated, fifteen are still alive.—*British Med. Journal*, Jan. 12, 1889.

Treatment of Typhoid Fever with Naphthalin.

Dr. Gennaro Petteruti communicates his experiences with naphthalin in the treatment of typhoid fever to the *Giornale internaz. delle scienze mediche*, No. 10. Naphthalin is borne by the organism in doses up to sixty grains daily without noteworthy disturbance. The only disturbances caused by it when introduced into the stomach are a brownish coloration of the urine and more or less severe pains on micturition. The brown color of the urine begins five hours after administration of the drug and lasts during the whole course of the treatment; it is due to resorption of small quantities of naphthalin by the bowel and their excretion in the urine. The pain on micturition is also produced by the presence of naphthalin in the urine. Diarrhœa was observed rarely.

Naphthalin, he says, exerts not only an antipyretic action analogous to that of antipyrin, thallin, and the usual antipyretics, but it also has a direct healing influence upon the typhoid fever. In Petteruti's cases the fever ceased upon the administration of the naphthalin and did not return, even when the drug was no longer given. The fall in temperature, which begins after two or three days' treatment, proceeds until the fever completely disappears. The healing, or better, the abortive action, of naphthalin is explained by its direct influence upon the chief seat of the disease. It is to be preferred to other antiseptics because it is well borne by the mucous membrane of the bowel, is absorbed only in very small quantity from the intestine, and therefore remains longer in contact with the diseased part upon which it exerts its action.

In children under four years of age, Petteruti began with fifteen grains, and never exceeded thirty grains a day. Adults received on the first day seven and one-half grains four times daily, given at intervals of an hour, and increased on the following days up to seven or eight hourly doses of seven and one-half grains.—*Wiener med. Presse*, Jan. 6, 1889.

Antipyrin in Obstetric Practice.

Dr. Talbot Jones, of St. Paul, Minn., communicates an interesting article on antipyrin in obstetric practice to the *North-western Lancet*, January, 1889. He has employed antipyrin in seven cases of confinement with the very happy effect in six cases of subduing the labor pains without checking the contractions of the uterus. He injects from twenty to thirty grains into the rectum, and repeats the injection if it is necessary. This treatment has also been used in two cases of inevitable abortion, one probably due to syphilitic degeneration of the villi, the other to causes unknown. In both cases, the ovum was thrown off without suffering by either patient, after one or two rectal injections of antipyrin.

In concluding his paper, he remarks that its anodyne effect is probably due to the quieting action exerted upon the spinal nerves supplying the uterus. That it lowers reflex irritability, and markedly dulls, where it does not wholly abolish sensibility, must be patent to everyone who has prescribed it in other conditions, as, for example, hemicrania, neuralgia, migraine, the darting pains of locomotor ataxia, *crises gastriques* with shooting pains in the legs, and in that large and varied class of nervous disorders in which sensibility is affected.

Clinical Experiences with Sulphonal.

Mr. Conolly Norman, Medical Superintendent of the Richmond Asylum, contributes an interesting paper on sulphonal to the *Dublin Journal of Medical Science*, January, 1889. He has employed it in twenty-two cases, and summarizes his experiences as follows: 1. Out of the twenty-two persons observed, in only two were any bad results noticed. These were specially unfavorable cases, and cases in which other sedatives had failed. 2. In no case was gastric or intestinal trouble observed. 3. In eight cases refusal of food, or a tendency thereto, existed. This was overcome, and the appetite seemed to improve under the use of sulphonal. 4. In six cases masturbation and tendency to sexual trouble existed. The drug appeared to lessen the tendency to self-abuse and erotic excitement. 5. In some recurrent cases it appeared to check or shorten the attack. 6. Out of the limited number of cases treated the majority happened to be melancholiacs, but the drug seems to exercise a hypnotic and sedative effect in various forms of insanity. 7. No patient complained of the drug, or refused it for other reasons than delusional ones. 8. Sleep produced appeared to be natural, refreshing, and undisturbed by dreams.

In comparing sulphonal with other medicines having similar effects, it is needless to refer to the products of opium, or to chloral. Of the more modern drugs paraldehyde is, perhaps, the most used. Its great disadvantage is that it requires constant increase in the dose. As far as Mr. Norman is able to judge, this does not apply to sulphonal. Paraldehyde long continued is also stated by Fröhner to cause destructive changes in the blood corpuscles, while Krafft-Ebing points out that it occasionally produces symptoms resembling alcoholism. Urethan, to which Mr. Norman has given a pretty extensive trial, he declares to be uncertain, and of no great strength. Amylene hydrate is uncertain and dangerous, as Schlöss's cases prove (*Jahrbuch der Psych.*, VIII., 1 and 2). Methylal is liable to the same reproaches. Hypnone, he says, is undoubtedly of some value; he once thought highly of it, but has found it uncertain, and it appears indisputable that patients soon become habituated to its use. All the three last-named drugs, he says, are so abominable in taste and smell that it is almost impossible to get patients to swallow them, and, as might be expected from this, they all upset the stomach.

The advantages of sulphonal he states to be: 1. It is absolutely free from smell. 2. Otto states that it leaves on the mouth a faint bitter after-taste. This Mr. Norman noticed, but it is very slight, and patients always say it is tasteless. 3. It produced, in his cases, no gastric derangement, and no troublesome head symptoms; it does not affect the appetite. 4. The sleep which it produces is relatively "natural."

Its disadvantages are: (1) that it is bulky and practically insoluble, therefore difficult to administer; and that, perhaps owing to its insolubility (2), it is slow in action. A further practical disadvantage hitherto has been its very high price.

Mr. Norman quotes Otto to the effect that in a few of the sixteen cases in which he used sulphonal solely as a hypnotic—*i. e.*, giving a single dose at night—a slight degree of giddiness and unsteadiness, with a sense of weariness, was experienced next morning. The same phenomena occurred in some of Rosin's and Schwalbe's cases. Otto gave the drug with excellent effect as a calmative, in small and repeated doses during the day, in nineteen cases. He observed not only the head sensations referred to, but the occurrence of transient digestive disturbances—vomiting and slight diarrhœa—in less than half his cases. These troubles soon passed off, though the drug was continued; and he notes that in most cases the appetite was good. Schwalbe observed in some cases similar digestive troubles, but attributed no consequence to them. Funaioli and Raimondi, who appear to place sulphonal at the head of the list of hypnotics, have observed no unpleasant after-consequences. Cramer, writing in June, 1888, as the result of Rabbas's and his own experiments, conducted on forty-nine patients, could record no unpleasant consequences save an occasional slight drowsiness on the morning after a dose.

Mr. Norman has no doubt that unpleasant and even injurious results will be found to occur from the injudicious or continual use of sulphonal, and that it will be found to have its peculiar dangers, like every other potent drug. The use of any drug to procure sleep or rest must at best be regarded as a deplorable necessity, and dangers should be apprehended from what must always be, to some extent, a blind interference with natural laws. It would seem, however, that we are justified in saying that in sulphonal we possess a powerful and not disagreeable hypnotic, free from any immediate danger, and followed by very trifling, if any, unpleasant after-effects.

Treatment of Thrush.

Dr. F. Forscheimer takes up the symptomatology and treatment of stomatitis mycosa, or thrush, in the *Archives of Pediatrics*, Feb., 1889. Prophylaxis, he says, is as important as the treatment proper. All slight abrasions may become infected with the parasitic cause of the disease, the saccharomyces albicans. The mother or nurse should be taught how to keep the nipples clean, and how to cleanse the mouth of the infant. The best disinfectant for the feeding utensils is exposure to the temperature of boiling water for a little while. Every part of the apparatus should be so arranged that the boiling water can gain access to it, and that any deposit can be removed mechanically. When this is rigidly carried out, infection becomes impossible even in hospitals.

The treatment proper consists of two parts: the mechanical removal of the fungus, and its destruction. To accomplish the first, the attendants must be told to wash out the mouth at stated times—for instance, between the times of nursing and immediately after nursing. For this purpose, a solution of one drachm of bicarbonate of soda to a tumbler of water is very serviceable. The remedies used must be applied four or five times daily, with a brush. He avoids syrups. In his own experience, he has rarely found it necessary to use anything except sodium bicarbonate. Occasionally, when ulcers are produced, it becomes necessary to touch them with nitrate of silver; but in uncomplicated cases this is exceedingly rare. There are some cases, he says, which will resist any or all methods of treatment.

Calomel in small doses or corrosive sublimate very much diluted almost always acts as a specific in intestinal troubles which are due to thrush. But the relation between intestinal troubles and thrush must always be kept in mind, and the indiscriminate use of cathartic alkalies or other laxatives must be prevented as doing the patient more harm than good, reducing his strength and being absolutely harmful and needless. Baginsky, he says, claims good results from resorcin, and warns against the use of too large a dose (from one-half to one per cent. solution—never more than one teaspoonful every two hours). But Dr. Forscheimer does not see how this, or any other remedy, can produce an effect upon an œsophagus stopped up completely with plugs of parasitic growth. When a conjectural diagnosis of œsophageal thrush has been made, he regards it as most expedient to introduce the soft catheter into the œsophagus. In one case, he succeeded in gradually working his way into the stomach with a catheter; some of the masses were pushed into the stomach and were then removed by vomiting. The patient, however, died a few days afterward, and postmortem examination showed that the œsophagus had been again filled up.

"Semelincident" Diseases.

The *Pittsburgh Med. Review*, Jan., 1889, says that no medical word at present expresses the fact that certain diseases occur only once in the individual—disorders, such as small-pox, in which one attack usually confers immunity from subsequent infection. Prof. R. E. Williams, of Allegheny, has suggested a new term descriptive of this class of maladies. It is "semelincident," from the Latin *semel*, once only, and *incido*, to happen or occur. The word appears to be a useful one; it has the added merit of being properly formed and is worthy of adoption.

Treatment of Syphilitic Disease of the Eye-lids.

P. Silex states in the *Deutsche med. Wochenschrift*, No. 43, 1888, that the best method of treatment of syphilitic disease of the eye-lids is a sweat "cure" combined with inunctions and followed by the use of about two hundred grains of iodide of potash. Injections of corrosive sublimate and of calomel do not give correspondingly good results. Fourteen patients who had been treated with injections of corrosive sublimate acquired specific disease of the eye in one and one-half years at latest; while of fifty others who had neglected their syphilis up to the outbreak of the eye disease, but then underwent the treatment first mentioned, twenty-five remained free from any symptoms whatsoever for at least one and one-half years; the remaining twenty-six in part had slight relapses and in part had withdrawn themselves from control. In the interstitial keratitis that is frequently associated with hereditary syphilis, the best results were obtained with iodide of potash. To avoid errors in estimating the results effected by a drug, Silex cautions against assuming that every eye affection occurring in a syphilitic is in causal connection with syphilis.—*Centralblatt f. d. med. Wissenschaften*, Jan. 5, 1889.

A European View of the "Pneumatic Cabinet."

Dr. Moeller, of Brussels, who has, according to the preface of his little pamphlet, "Un Mot sur L'Aérothérapie," had considerable experience in the use of compressed and rarefied air, says concerning the "Pneumatic Cabinet" practically the same thing that Solis-Cohen, Platt and others in this country have consistently maintained. "The procedure of Dr. Williams," says Moeller, "possesses no novelty except the name, which appears to be indeed very happy. How does it in fact work? The patient is placed in a partial vacuum, but he continues to breathe air at the ordinary pressure, impregnated with some medicament. In other words, the air of bronchi and lungs is in communication with an atmosphere *relatively compressed* and charged with antiseptic vapors. . . . The procedure of Dr. Williams produces the same result as the portable apparatus of Waldenburg and others with this sole difference—which however is not to the advantage of the new procedure—that Dr. Williams obliges the patient not only to inspire air relatively compressed, but also to make expiration into the same air, while with the portable apparatus, expiration is made into the free atmosphere. It is indeed true that Waldenburg at first essayed equally to make this twofold use of compressed air, but in view of its disadvantages he was not slow to abandon the practice." . . . "What is the advantage of medicating the air? The practice has been long since thoroughly tested and abandoned as well at Berlin by Waldenburg as at Brussels by Tamin-Despalles and his successors. We ourselves have repeated the same efforts both with pneumatic chambers and portable apparatus. We have at last fully recognized the perfect inutility of the combination of the two methods (inhalations of compressed air and of medicinal substances) and are convinced that it is far preferable to submit the patient to aërotherapy alone, and if indications for medicamentous inhalations are presented to administer them separately by means of vaporizers, or atomizers, or respirators constructed for that special purpose."

"The method of Dr. Williams, then, offers nothing new from the double point of view (aërotherapy and inhalation), and experience has demonstrated that it is of no advantage to employ simultaneously the two therapeutic procedures."

Purpura from Iodide of Potassium.

M. Besnier has recently had an old syphilitic as a patient, who showed a remarkable intolerance to iodide of potash, which produced a purpuric eruption upon the lower limbs each time he took it. M. Besnier had made him take five drops of tincture of iodine. The patient was seized with symptoms of idism—dyspnœa, anxiety, acceleration of pulse—to such a degree that the iodine had to be stopped; but he had no purpura. It seems, therefore, that iodic purpura is not produced after the employment of iodine, but only in patients who take iodide of potassium. — *Gazette Hebdomadaire*, Jan. 18, 1889.

Remedy for Erysipelas.

Dr. W. L. Schadkewitsch records in the *Medozinskoie Obosreny*, No. 12, 1888, that he has found a mixture of equal parts of ammonium-sulphoichthyolicum and lard an admirable application in erysipelas. The effect of its use was to shorten the duration of the disease, and to dissipate remarkably soon the burning pain.

Cirrhosis of the Liver in Cats.

Professor Greenfield reports in the *Journal of Comp. Pathology*, Dec., 1888, the results of his examination of two well-marked examples of hepatic cirrhosis in cats. In the one specimen the organ was much enlarged and smooth, resembling to the naked eye a leucocythæmic liver. Microscopically, however, the lobules were found to be separated by wide bands of connective tissue, within which were dense plexuses of young bile ducts and bile capillaries, the formation of which appeared partly to be by fission of the liver cells. In the other case, a successful injection of the bile ducts revealed a large number of such plexuses, and a comparison with a healthy liver proved that in the cirrhotic the plexuses were of new formation. Each animal had ascites, and the cirrhosis was monolobular. Professor Greenfield points to the similarity in anatomical character between the conditions here found and those met with in hypertrophic or " biliary " cirrhosis, the difference being that in these cats there was no evidence of obstruction of the duct, or any jaundice, whereas there was marked ascites. In man hypertrophic cirrhosis is characterized by pronounced jaundice, and ascites is usually absent or is slight.—*Lancet*, Jan. 12, 1889.

Athletic Sports and Scholarship.

The Phila. *Ledger*, Feb. 1, says that Prof. Richards, of Yale College, has made a study of the records of 2425 students in order to determine, if possible, the relations of athletics, in Yale, to scholarship. The general result is that the athletes fall slightly behind the non-athletes in scholarship, but not so much as to demand a suppression of such exercises. In some branches of athletic exercises the students who engage in the sports are above the average of the non-athletes in scholarship. For the slight difference noted between the two great classes, there may be greater strength and endurance or physical development compensating for the loss of scholarship. This does not appear from the report, but a healthy, energetic man with fair scholarship is a better product of college education than a debilitated student with higher average in book studies. So far as statistics go, however, the most that can be claimed for Prof. Richards's report is that it is negative in its results, and shows that athletic games do not seriously interfere with the scholarship of students.

Saccharin.

A commission appointed by the Belgian Academy of Medicine has come to the conclusion that saccharin cannot be considered a substitue for sugar in foods ; but that, although differently borne by different persons, it is not poisonous. They are of opinion also that it is not wholly excreted by the kidneys, but is liable to find its way into the milk and saliva. Consequently the commission has reported that in its judgment all persons selling wholesale or retail articles sweetened with saccharin should be compelled to indicate the fact in a conspicuous manner.—*Medical Press and Circular*, Jan. 9, 1889.

Prophylaxis in Cerebro-Spinal Meningitis.

The Berlin police intend to issue the following regulations to prevent the spread of cerebro-spinal meningitis : 1. Every physician shall at once report to the police any case that comes to his knowledge. 2. Patients are to be isolated. 3. The children of families in which there are cases are to be kept from school. 4. The sick rooms, expectorated matter, linen, handkerchiefs, clothes, and other belongings of the patient used during the illness are to be cleaned and disinfected.—*Lancet*, Jan. 5, 1889.

A Gallant Act.

It is our pleasant duty, says the *British Med. Journal*, Jan. 5, 1889, to record another of those acts of heroism on the part of Army Medical officers, which are so often displayed under circumstances of peculiar difficulty and danger. The facts, as given in the *Civil and Military Gazette*, of Lahore, show that on November 4, during the Black Mountain Expedition, when our troops were retreating, one man was severely wounded and placed on the shoulder of a comrade, who, however, was soon exhausted ; Surgeon Heuston then took the man on his own back and conveyed him, under a heavy fire of shot and rock from the enemy, to a place where the troops were forming, and where a stretcher could be procured.

—For the week ending Feb. 2, the Sanitary Bureau of the Health Department of New York City reports the following numbers of cases of contagious diseases and deaths : Typhoid fever, 6 cases and 2 deaths ; measles, 324 cases and 21 deaths ; diphtheria, 178 cases and 39 deaths.

NEWS.

—Dr. N. F. Bosley died in New York City, Feb 10. He was a surgeon in the navy during the late war.

—A man in Mt. Vernon, New York, on Feb. 4, took strychnine supposing it to be quinine, and died in a short time.

—A despatch from New Brunswick to the daily papers states that cerebro-spinal meningitis prevails in that region, and is said to be spreading.

—The *North Carolina Med. Journal,* Jan., 1889, states that a call has been sent out for a Sanitary Convention to be held in Raleigh, N. C., Feb. 6, 1889.

—It is stated by the *Lancet,* Jan. 5, 1889, that the professors at the University of Tomsk have given up the whole of their first half-year's fees for the benefit of the students, nearly all of whom are poor.

—Emin Bey has been commonly spoken of as Dr. Schnitzler, an Austrian; but a gentleman living in New York, and who claims to be a first cousin of Emin, says his name is Dr. Edward Schnitzer, and that he was born in Prussian Silesia.

—Press despatches state that at the fire in the hospital at Madrid, on Feb. 7, the helpless sick were carried out by doctors and nurses, the Governor himself removing several who were suffering from contagious diseases, and not a life was lost.

—The *British Med. Journal,* Jan. 26, says: Dr. W. R. Gowers, F.R.S., has resigned the appointment of Physician to University College Hospital. We believe that the motive which has prompted Dr. Gowers to take this step, which will be felt to involve a serious loss to the teaching power of University College, is that he finds himself unable to meet, with impunity, the increasing claims of consulting practice, and at the same time to perform the duties of Professor of Clinical Medicine and of Physician with the regularity which is desirable at an important medical school. While relinquishing the more arduous post, however, he retains his appointment as Physician to the National Hospital for the Paralyzed and Epileptic, Queen Square. Dr. Gowers possesses qualities as a clinical teacher in nervous disease which could ill be spared, and his retention of the last-named office will enable him to continue the "clinical afternoons" at Queen Square, which have become so well known to medical visitors and senior students in London.

HUMOR.

THE DRUGGIST charges the soda fountain and makes the customer pay cash.—*Providence Journal.*

RELATIONS between a milkman and a millionaire are naturally strained. — *New Orleans Picayune.*

A HORSE in Dakota has eight feet. He must be the "Lost Cord" we heard sung about so much.—*Lowell Courier.*

MRS. PALLID—"Don't you find that the noise of the boiler foundry across the street affects your nerves, Mrs. Youngwife?"
Mrs. Youngwife—"I seldom hear it."
"How strange!"
"Well, you see, baby is teething now."—*Drake's Magazine.*

DR. BUSHY, whose figure was beneath the common size, was one day accosted in a public coffee room by an Irish baronet of gigantic size, with "May I pass to my seat, O giant?" The doctor, politely making way, answered, "Pass, O pigmy." "Ah, sir," replied the Baronet, somewhat nettled, "my expression alluded to the size of your intelligence!" "And my expression," said the doctor, "to the size of yours."—*Lancet.*

OBITUARY.

JOSEPH S. LUSK, M.D.

Dr. Joseph S. Lusk, of Butler, Pa., died Feb. 2 of heart disease. He had been seriously ill for several months and his death was not unexpected. Dr. Lusk was the oldest son of Dr. Loring Lusk, who was one of the earliest settlers in Harmony, Butler county, and died a few years ago at a great age. The son chose his father's profession and studied medicine at the Western Reserve College, Cleveland, O., in 1850, and soon after began practising in Harmony. In 1886 he went to Butler, where he soon came into a very extensive practice, and was beloved for his talent, learning and unaffected ways. During his life of 63 years Dr. Lusk, besides pursuing a successful professional career, found time for extended reading, study and other pursuits. He was a member of the State Legislature for three terms and held various local offices. He was at the time of his death a member of the Pension Board for the Butler district, and had held numerous offices in medical societies. He was an enthusiastic geologist and mineralogist and had many rare and curious specimens.

MEDICAL AND SURGICAL REPORTER

No. 1669.   PHILADELPHIA, FEBRUARY 23, 1889.   VOL. LX.—No. 8.

CONTENTS:

COMMUNICATIONS.

STOMATITIS GANGRENOSA; A NEW TREATMENT.

BY LLEWELLYN ELIOT, M.D.,

WASHINGTON, D. C.

In selecting "Stomatitis Gangrenosa; A New Treatment," as my subject, I do so in the hope that my success in the treatment of my cases, will encourage others to give the plan a trial. At the outset I shall state my position and belief in a few words, and then endeavor to sustain them.

Stomatitis gangrenosa is dependent for its existence upon a germ, a parasite, a fungoid growth; the corrosive chloride of mercury has the power, when employed in sufficiently strong solutions, of destroying germs and parasites, therefore the application of this germicide is the correct treatment of this disease.

A few observations upon this affection will not be amiss. Dr. Battus, a Dutch physician, gave the first correct description of this disease, as far back as 1620, in his "Manual of Surgery." Since then various writers, Swedish, French, English, American and German have described it as water kanker, noma, gangrene of the mouth, gangrenous scorbutus of the gums, necrosis infantilis. In America, the best articles on this subject are by Gerhard, Coates, Meigs and Pepper, and Cohen. This is not a disease of private practice nor is it frequently seen in hospital or asylums. It attacks children between their first and the sixth years, as a rule, and those older as the exception. Only those children who are constitutionally run down by long and severe illness, by improper feeding, by unsanitary surroundings or the various concomitants of the poorer classes, are affected by it. Although not considered a contagious affection, I believe that one case of gangrenous stomatitis, admitted into an asylum for foundlings and not subjected to restriction, such as isolation and the use of special towels, cloths, clothing and bedding, will prove the starting point for an epidemic of this disease. I write this from firm conviction and, I think, from the point of view of experience.

The disease sets in without special symptoms and may so escape detection, although there is a gangrenous odor to the breath. The mucous membrane ulcerates and the cheek or lips become tumefied, shining, pale and hard, and the disease may either spread externally or follow the mucous membrane of the mouth, perforating the cheek or laying bare the alveolar processes, or even an entire section of the maxilla, superior or inferior, with subsequent necrosis. The patient's strength does not fail, unless the previous condition of debility increases. Death supervenes in the second week, either from entero-colitis, pneumonia, pulmonary gangrene, or collapse. When recovery follows it is only with loss of much tissue and with more or less deformity. The diagnosis is easy, for the odor of the breath and the appearance of the eschars are sufficient to set aside all doubts as to the nature of the affection. The death rate is stated at from seventy-five to eighty-five per centum, but is less in private practice than in hospital or asylum practice, and as a matter of course depends somewhat upon the simple or complicated condition of the case.

As to the treatment, I believe that the internal administration of chlorate of potash with the tincture of the chloride of iron, sulphate of quinine, stimulants, and the local application of caustics, is the only treatment worthy of mention. As to caustic applications to the diseased parts, hydrochloric acid is preferred, although nitric acid, the actual cautery, acid solution of nitrate of mercury, and undiluted carbolic acid are employed. Gerhard employed undiluted tincture of the chloride of iron, Maguire uses the subnitrate of bismuth. Condie used sulphate of copper, thirty grains to the ounce of water. As an application, my preference is decidedly in favor of the corrosive chloride of mercury in strong solution, and my prescription is:

R Hydrargyri chloridi corrosivi . . gr. j
Aquæ destillatæ . . . . f ℥ j

M. Sig. Apply with a cotton probang twice a day if necessary to remove the eschars.

These applications are to be made twice a day if necessary; if the eschar is removed and no further extension of the disease takes place, then there is no further need for such a strong solution. I then make a solution of 1 to 2000 and continue its use as a wash until the suspicious appearance of the ulcer has left, when a solution of tincture of myrrh is employed. To be effective any application must be thorough and be repeated as long as there is any evidence of the continuation of the disease. Internally, I order:

R Potassii chloratis . . . . ℥ iss
Tincturæ ferri chloridi . . . . . . f ℥ j
Aquæ destillatæ . . . . f ℥ ij

M. Sig. Teaspoonful every three (3) hours.

In reviewing the experience of the past fifteen years, I find that I have treated five cases of stomatitis gangrenosa, two of which rapidly went to a fatal termination, the other three recovering after a long convalescence. In treating these cases the approved methods of procedure were faithfully and religiously followed in two cases. The nitric acid applications were made without fear, chloride of iron and chlorate of potash were administered to the point of tolerance, quinine and alcoholics were not spared, but both the patients died in spite of the care and treatment they received. The three remaining patients were treated with free applications of the corrosive chloride of mercury in strong solution, with the iron, the potash, the quinine, the stimulation and the full diet of the other two, and they recovered from the disease. The eschars separated much sooner than when the acid was employed. In each of these cases there was a relaxed condition of the bowels, which was controlled with paregoric.

I am not a believer in the antiseptic treatment and methods of the day, for I do not think they are applied in sufficient strength, and I do not believe that a douching, an irrigation, a washing, a spraying—call it what you will—with a quart, a gallon, yes, a barrel, if needs be, of a solution of the corrosive chloride of mercury, of a strength of 1 to 3000 or 1 to 4000, will do as much good as the same douching, irrigation, washing, or spraying with clean water. With this belief, different as it is from that of the majority of my professional brethren, I employ the very antiseptic I decry. Compare the difference in strength, and then see "the faith that is in him." Not for one moment do I doubt the records of experimenters in this line of study, nor the favorable reports following the use of such weak solutions; but I still assert, that to get the germicide effects of the corrosive chloride of mercury, it must be employed in very strong solutions.

THE CLIMATIC TREATMENT OF PULMONARY CONSUMPTION IN THE DRY ELEVATED REGIONS OF THE ROCKY MOUNTAINS.

BY L. HUBER, M.D.,

ROCKY FORD, COLORADO.

Each year develops fresh discussions of the climatic treatment of pulmonary consumption. In these discussions there is much difference of opinion and teaching as to what part altitude takes in the treatment of the disease; some advocate its beneficial effects, others deny them. Another matter of contention is as to the aseptic qualities of the atmosphere in many parts of the region specified. This condition is little understood by physicians outside the limits in question, and hence is overlooked in the discussions of the present question. That an old and thickly settled region, into the atmosphere of which the smoke, dust, and effluvia of long years have ascended, should differ in the amount of "atmospheric dust" and in its quality from that of a comparatively recently settled country, is quite reasonable. In truth, the fact has been demonstrated by scientists and observers. What relation this condition of the atmospheric air should have to the climatic treatment of consumption will subsequently receive due consideration, it being sufficient now to mention simply the fact of such a difference of air, and to note that in the present inquiry it is often disregarded.

Another source of disagreement among physicians on this subject is the misleading views and erroneous notions entertained as to the bodily temperature changes in pulmonary consumption. Let us briefly discuss this subject and remove its obscurities. Dr. Williams, in his masterly work on "Pulmonary Consumption," by innumerable clinical observations, substantially concludes as follows: The active deposit of tubercle (tubercularization) produces an irritative condition of the system and increases the heat-producing functions. But tubercularization, in taking hold of the system, produces a tendency to collapse. Now, the changes of bodily temperature, wherever present, are the resultant, as it were, of these two opposite conditions. To quote the exact words of the author: "To understand the temperature chart of phthisis, we must bear in mind that it is due to two principal agencies:

"1. Excessive action of the processes by which the heat of the body is maintained, the processes of oxidation and disintegration, combined with a weakening of the inhibitory action of the nervous system in these phenomena, such as is present in all inflammations and fevers.

"2. A collapse of the constitutional powers, which characterizes the natural course of consumption. These two influences act on the patient, and according as one or the other predominates, is shaped the course of the temperature. When they are equally balanced, a chart hardly differing from the normal, results. When collapse prevails, subnormal temperatures appear, and, when inflammatory processes are in the ascendent, pyrexia shows itself."

This teaching is essentially different from that propagated in many text-books on practice, and that entertained generally by medical men. It contradicts the erroneous notion that the temperature rise in phthisis is commensurate with the extent of tubercularization.

Having a proper conception of the temperature changes attending the active deposit of tubercle in the lungs, or coincident with the primary changes in phthisis, let us examine whether these have the same cause as the febrile phenomena attending softening and extrusion of tubercular masses, during the later stages of the disease. That the latter depend upon other conditions, is beyond dispute. There is now some absorption of septic matter and consequent irritative or hectic fever. Dr. Williams supports this view with observations upon many cases, but our common text-books fail to make this distinction.

We are now prepared to analyze to advantage the relation of pulmonary consumption to the climatology of the Rocky Mountain regions. If the climate of this region, with the effects of elevation, tends to make the system more tolerant of tubercularization and to limit this process by any counter virtues it may possess, then, surely, improvement is to be hoped when patients seek this resort in the *early* stages of the disease. What do experience and observation teach? They tell us of almost invariable improvement and recovery at this time. Altitude contributes largely to this end. It is on these elevated plains and mountain slopes that a rarefied atmosphere and a diminished atmospheric pressure effect important changes in the breathing capacity of the lungs, which expand especially at the apices. This removes the susceptibility to apical consolidation and impairment and effects a change sought to be attained by proper gymnastics, when altitude is unavailable. Add to this effect of altitude the benefit of a dry soil and a sunny climate, which will admit of out-door life during nearly the whole year, and a combination of circumstances exists highly favorable to the arrest of phthisis in its early stages. Usually these conditions lead to a vigorous appetite, a desire for increased exercise, and ultimately to permanent recovery.

When hemorrhages or local congestions are imminent in this stage, then great care is needed as to the elevation sought. Too much altitude will lead to undue expansion of the lungs and increase these susceptibilities. Hence judgment is required in sending patients into the regions in question. This cannot be too strongly enforced. Some patients need an elevation of only two thousand feet, while others will do well at five thousand or six thousand. Any attending heart lesion must be duly regarded, as a damaged heart is often taxed in its functions as the elevation increases. It is best always in cases of phthisis complicated with heart disease, to proceed cautiously into elevated districts, directing the patient to low or medium altitudes at first. He may be able to ascend as improvement follows.

Before leaving this subject of altitude, it may be well to quote some observations and conclusions from Dr. Williams's treatise heretofore cited, relative to the effects of rarefied air and elevation upon phthisical patients. These are thus summarized in different parts of the work: " Hypertrophy, or more development of the healthy lung tissue, shown by the physical signs and increased respiratory power.

" In consequence of the above changes, there is expansion of the thorax, which increases in circumference at various levels from one to three inches, such increase being independent of any augmentation of fat or muscle, as it takes place in patients who are losing weight, and occasionally in bed-ridden ones.

" The above thoracic expansion is always accompanied by diminution in the number of respirations, which become deeper, and by a slowing of the pulse.

" Absorption of atmospheric oxygen by the blood takes place more readily, while at the same time the carbonic acid formed within the body passes outward through the pulmonary tissue into the air, which is breathed with a greater degree of facility than at lower altitudes (Marcet).''

These observations are not by · one observer only, nor are they confined to any special mountain region. They are summations from the best authorities and confirm the general tone of this paper.

Lastly, the aseptic quality of the atmosphere in much of the region designated is another important factor in the treatment of consumption by climate. It has been stated that in the stage of softening and extrusion of tubercular masses from the lungs the accompanying fever is due largely to blood poisoning. But sepsis is set up only in the presence of germs that float in the surrounding air. Where these germs do not exist, septic processes should be absent. This is, indeed, the case in the Rocky Mountain districts, as many observations show. There are many localities in which meats will not putrefy for many days even during mid-summer, and when they do undergo changes, they are those of mummification rather than of putrefaction. Wounds rarely take on an unhealthy condition. During the year, the writer treated a number of gun-shot injuries, without meeting with a single instance in which there were any signs of sepsis whatever. Often persons far removed from a physician, in filthy camps or in other extremely unhygienic surroundings, will go days and weeks with severe injuries to the tissues, without developing blood poisoning. This .insusceptibility to putrid and septic changes must be due to the aseptic quality of the air. And what direct bearing has this fact upon the consumptive? Evidently in such an atmosphere he should be in little danger of hectic fever in the later stages of his disease. And this is a confirmed fact. It is true the physician may be misled with cases sent here in a very late stage, as in these, as a rule, when there are cavities and solidified areas, softening sets in so rapidly and tissue changes go on so extensively that there is complete overwhelming of the system. While touching upon this point, it cannot be made too emphatic that it is very injudicious for consumptives to resort to most mountain climates late in the progress of the disease, as the final catastrophe is generally precipitated.

Whether bacteria are absent from the air in these regions, or only exist under conditions inimical to their development and activity, are questions which as yet, so far as the writer's knowledge goes, have not been decided. Bacilli are found in the sputa of consumptives here as elsewhere. Where many phthisical patients have long resorted, as in some of the older and larger cities, an honest expression of the profession would no doubt favor the idea that the *climate has lost its virtues.* This may be due to impregnation of the soil, houses, and the atmosphere with germs, or to the fact that the comforts and confinement of city life are unfavorable to the disease. Much of the Rocky Mountain region being new or almost uninhabitated, new health resorts with accommodations for invalids continually springing into existence, the physician is left to exercise his judgment and preference where to send his patient.

During the writer's residence here he has met and had under treatment a large number of phthisical patients who had already tried the Pacific coast for relief. The change from the moist atmosphere to this dry climate was almost invariably attended with great relief to the attending catarrhal and bronchial disease, which in these subjects is quite noticeable and common. Even retirement from the coast to elevated districts failed in a number of cases to relieve the sufferer to the same extent he improved here. Hence it may be inferred that the slight humidity incident to many sections of this country can be always made available in the treatment of phthisis. A dry soil is usually associated with a dry atmosphere. By many authorities the former is held to be just as important as the latter.

The chief disadvantage to patients resorting to these elevated districts is that, after a period of residence, however great their improvement, they incur great risk of new and extensive outbreaks of the disease, in case they return to places nearly on the sea-level, or to a climate having a damp cold winter. The proper way to get the chief and lasting benefit of this climate is permanently to reside in it, if improvement follow one's advent. This fact has come to be pretty generally appreciated, and not a small percentage of the yearly immigration to Colorado, at least, is due to it.

The most common-sense deductions to be drawn from what has been said so far are these :

1. There is something to be gained by the climatic treatment of pulmonary consumption.

2. The time to begin it is at the first outbreak or manifestation of the disease. In those families in which the disease is hereditary, resort to this region should be made even earlier.

3. After the disease has made considerable inroad upon the system and medical measures have been exhausted, do not then advise the patient to seek a new climate with the hope of speedy improvement and ultimate recovery.

4. Physicians should always consider well the prognosis of the phthisis, when it is complicated with intercurrent trouble. A bad valvular lesion might of itself make the forecast of the disease unfavorable. So also certain organic affections of the liver and kidneys. It is not an unusual experience to meet with patients sent here for the benefit of their lungs, whom some intercurrent disease is sure to carry off.

In this shape we dismiss the present subject, hoping that what has been said will contribute something to the better selection of patients to be sent hither, and to the comprehension of the treatment of a disease which makes such fearful ravages upon the human family.

REMOVAL OF TWO-THIRDS OF A RIB.

BY J. A. MINICH, M.D ,
WORTHINGTON, IND.

John Hixon came to me in June, 1888, to consult me in regard to a tumor on his left side, which I found to contain pus. I lanced the abscess and it discharged about eight or ten ounces. This gave him some relief, but he returned again complaining of his side. I found crepitation in the rib at about its middle portion some distance from where I had lanced it, and with the probe I discovered the bone was diseased, but how extensively I did not know. He grew gradually worse and finally a troublesome cough also set in, and he could get no sleep or rest, and he became very much emaciated. I finally decided to remove as much of the rib as was diseased, which I did on January 7, 1889. I removed all of the sixth rib on the left side except about four inches next to the spine. It was so much diseased that it broke very easily in several places on removing. At one place beneath the rib there was about a teaspoonful of thick cheesy substance imbedded ; this seemed to have no connection with the opening which had been discharging all summer and fall. Fortunately there was no opening through into the cavity of the pleura, and I succeeded in removing the rib without injury to the membrane.

The patient told me he had the best night's rest that night he had had for a year. And now, January 26, his cough has left him, the wound has healed, and he is free from all pain and is happy.

THE CONJUGAL STATE.

BY J. B. JOHNSON, M.D.,
WASHINGTON, D. C.

The experience of the world has long since declared that the union of one man and one woman in the association known as marriage, is the best possible relation for the sexes to assume or maintain in order to attain the most happiness, as well as the greatest degree of welfare and comfort, that the natural relations of the sexes demand. That such does not always lead to success, and prove a blessing, by bringing as a reward, happiness, prosperity and congeniality, is a fact beyond contradiction ; and the question, why it does not always lead to the fruition of the object of its institution, is answered by the fact, that the preliminary courtship which leads to it, is not conducted with the same caution, judgment and frankness, which are brought to bear upon other important transactions of life. Courtship, instead of being conducted in a frank, honest and sincere manner, is marked by a system of concealment, disingenuousness and deception which endeavors to hide the multitude of faults that marriage generally discloses.

Those who associate with each other for the purpose of marriage, should be sincere, and endeavor to ascertain each others likes and dislikes, habits, mode of life, thoughts and sentiments ; for it is important for each of the parties to it to learn the opinions of the other upon every subject in common between them, in order to insure harmonious action when brought into such intimate relations as exist between man and wife. It is the studied concealment of the true character of each from the other, during courtship, that gives rise to injury to the marital state. After marriage, those traits of character which were so studiously concealed before the nuptial relations were established, are recklessly and unreservedly manifested ; and thus often results in a want of congeniality and harmony of feeling, thoughts and sentiment. The husband does not find the recent sweetheart in the new wife, nor does the wife find 'her lover in the husband ; and often before a month has passed, their want of congeniality, and their unfitness for a life-time association with each other, is brought home to them in a most unhappy and disastrous manner.

If, after marriage, a want of harmony exists between man and wife, patience must take the place of affection, and forbearance with each other's faults becomes a duty ; then discrimination and tact will make life not only bearable, but pleasant, and other ties may be formed which will bind the husband and wife in a firm, strong bond, such as they would at one time have deemed impracticable. Should husband or wife, or both, not possess this capacity, or disposition to make the most of an unpropitious marriage, a worse condition of affairs is usually excited. The husband becomes cold and careless in his attentions, while the wife grows indifferent, and shuns, rather than invites, his caresses. This growing indifference toward each other soon degenerates into estrangement, and as soon as this occurs, there often arises in the hearts of the self-deceived husband and wife a feeling of absolute disgust toward the other ; and they find, alas ! when it is too late, that there exists neither love nor congeniality between them. When this condition is fully realized by both, the disappointed husband, or it may be, the disappointed wife, sometimes looks abroad for that kindness and love which he or she expected from the other ; and then the door is open for the temptation to conjugal infidelity. If the case goes on to extremities the husband seeks his affinity in another woman, while the wife gives her ear and smiles to some man who is polite and kind to her ; and these associations soon produce a total and permanent disruption and abandonment of all their marital ties. Their marriage bed has no attractions for either, and each becomes cold toward the other.

The negligence of the beau and sweetheart in failing to ascertain before marriage the habits and sentiments of each other, preparatory to the establishment of matrimonial relations, is the cause, not only of many unhappy marriages, but also of many divorces. A husband who loves his wife, will make any sacrifice for her, and the wife who loves her husband is willing to risk her life in the duty of trying to please him. Like a true woman, every effort of her mind and body is dedicated to his pleasure and welfare ; and every act she performs toward him is but the offering of an unselfish love ; and when she feels the product of conception, the offspring of a holy marriage-bed, fluttering within her womb, her love toward her husband grows stronger, and no wicked thought of destroying it ever enters her mind. Under the influence of such love, the pains and suffering of maternity, and the duty of taking care of the babe of her bosom become a pleasure. A wife who does not feel this is a selfish woman, and is true neither to herself, to her husband, nor to her offspring. Her selfish conduct may drive her husband to sexual depravity, and force him to those necessities of evil which vice always imposes upon the transgressor. Every effort a married woman makes to prevent conception is sinful, and in direct violation of God's command : "*Be fruitful and multiply;*" and a conscientious physician cannot afford to compromise his manhood by lending his professional advice to an interruption of a normal operation of the laws of nature, in order to gratify immoral motives, or the caprice or the temporary inconvenience of the effects of procreation.

STRANGE EFFECT OF NERVOUS SHOCK.

BY J. C. MILNER, M.D.,
COMANCHE, TEXAS.

Allow me through your valuable journal to report the following case :

J. W., five years old, was burned when six months old on the right side of his face, the burn destroying the orbicularis palpebrarum. Cicatricial eversion of upper and lower lids followed, exposing the eye ball and a large area of epithelial tissue. The sight of the eye up to the time I now speak of remained good.

Some time in November last, the child, with his mother, was on a visit in the country, and in playing became fastened under the floor of an out-building. When discovered by his mother he was so impacted that it was necessary to dig him out. The mother reports the observance of nothing unusual except that the child cried, and finally sobbed himself to sleep. On the following day the child refused food. He did not appear to be sick, but had lost his usual energy and refused food altogether. The next day the mother, fearing he would be sick, returned home with him. Under the expectation of going home, he was induced to eat a small piece of bread, with sugar upon it.

About ten days after the fright, I was called in to see the boy. The father said that "Jimie had lost ten pounds in the last ten days." I found the patient greatly emaciated, without fever, refusing to lie in bed, his bowels and kidneys acting, but he rejecting food totally, having eaten not as much as one ounce since his fright.

I diagnosticated the case to be one of inanition, caused by nervous shock. I could not bring the electric current to bear; hence it was not used. The line of management consisted in sponge baths with warm water, in which were put soda and mustard, with nerve tonics, peptonized food, fruit, etc.—all of which had to be forced upon him. This continued for ten or twelve days, during which time I was satisfied the system was consuming by absorption and thus producing a state of blood poison, which I expected to end in death. The first indication of blood poison (if my theory be correct) manifested itself ten days after I first saw the case, and twenty-one or twenty-two after the fright, in a nervous rigor, lasting about one hour, followed by rise in temperature to 103° or 104° and loss of muscular power, with mental disturbance and prostration upon the bed. This condition was met with antipyretics and antiseptics. The patient now resisted swallowing everything offered either in the shape of liquids, food, or medicine. A wretched and aggravating cough now set up. We met that as best we could with a flannel jacket saturated with mutton tallow over which was sprinkled powdered capsicum mixed with sulphate of quinine, and adjusted closely to the surface of the chest. Cod liver oil was freely rubbed on the remaining part of the body. For three more weeks the little fellow continued in this condition, refusing all manner of food and drink except as it was forced upon him. When food was swallowed, it was only to undergo fermentation in the stomach, and to be passed off with the odor of sulphuretted hydrogen. During this time a corneal ulcer formed in the eye which had been burned, completely destroying the sight. Abscesses formed also over different parts of the body.

After about five weeks from the time of the fright, though every day for the last two of the five I expected death to end the scene, the system again rallied and small teaspoonful doses of some kind of nourishment could be taken. No medicine was given except a few drops of a hypnotic as required, to procure sleep ; but gradually the desire for food returned, and the powers of digestion were restored, until now, eight weeks after the child received the fright, he is beginning to walk a little over the floor, holding on to articles of furniture. Am I correct in my diagnosis ? Was I correct in assuming a blood poison by absorption ? If so, how was the system sustained, and what were the eliminating forces that freed the system from the poison ? A correct solution would be appreciated.

SOCIETY REPORTS.

PHILADELPHIA COUNTY MEDICAL SOCIETY.

Stated Meeting, January 23, 1889.

The President, W. W. KEEN, M.D., in the chair.

DR. MORDECAI PRICE read a paper on

Amputations of Thigh and Leg.[1]

DR. L. K. BALDWIN, in opening the discussion, said : I have been much interested in the remarks of Dr. Price, partly because a gentleman called at my office this afternoon and asked me to look at an abrasion on the stump of an amputated limb. The amputation had been performed at the junction of the middle and lower third. It was just such a stump as I thought that he ought not to have had. The operation was performed ten or twelve years ago, and although he has worn a number of legs, the stump is always getting rubbed. The remarks of Dr. Price in regard to amputations near the joint are very good. There is no one more capable of speaking upon this subject than Dr. Price himself, for there is nothing like practical experience. His remarks are worthy of all consideration, and it would be well if they were followed out.

DR. JAMES COLLINS : I have listened with a great deal of earnestness to the remarks of Dr. Price on this question. He comes rich in that experience of suffering that makes men wise. I therefore attach great weight to his words. I could, however, but think that while the doctor is entirely right in his opinions, he may have forgotten the lectures given at the time he graduated. I have heard the professor of surgery say, and have seen him demonstrate, that the point of election for amputation of the leg was three fingers' space below the tubercle of the tibia. I think it well to mention this, and while I admit the great advances which have been made in surgery, yet, I think, that we should not cut entirely loose from all that has been done in the past. With reference to what has been said in regard to long stumps, I think that the surgeons of twenty years ago were deluded by the promises of the artificial-limb makers. The artificial-limb makers made demonstrations before classes in surgery, and led the surgeons to believe that if they had a certain form of stump they could apply the

[1] See REPORTER, Feb. 2, p. 135.

limbs better. They described their wonderful limbs that could almost walk without a man attached to them, and thus to a certain extent deceived the surgeon.

DR. O. H. ALLIS : I would ask Dr. Price if in a case of injury to the foot, he would take off the limb say at the tarso-metatarsal joint, or go to the point of election below the knee ?

DR. M. PRICE : I should prefer to operate at the point of election. I think that even in an injury which would require amputation of the great toe, the patient would be more comfortable and walk better if the limb were taken off below the knee, although I do not say that I should do it.

DR. H. R. WHARTON : I agree very thoroughly with Dr. Price as to the necessity of securing a good stump, and as to the point of election in amputations through the leg. I have for some time made it a rule not to make any amputation near the ankle-joint, preferring to go some distance above, if I have to go above the ankle.

I, however, disagree with him in regard to the discomfort which a patient suffers with a Syme or a Pirogoff amputation. I have seen such patients get along very well, and walk with comfort. I also disagree with Dr. Price in regard to knee-joint amputations. I, of course, refer to amputation through the joint, the condyles being saved and the patella being left. I have seen these patients apparently walk with comfort and have a good stump. Where the amputation is one at the knee-joint, a portion of the condyles being sawed off and the patella removed, a square stump is secured which can be well covered. I have seen a number of cases of this operation, and in these the patients had good stumps.

I think that the main element of a good stump is a movable covering, the skin being perfectly movable over the bone. If the skin is bound down and is subjected to pressure, the patient will suffer from constant irritation, and will be apt to exhibit some of the forms of mechanical ulceration seen in stumps.

I agree in regard to the uselessness of trying to save too much time in amputations.

DR. JOHN B. DEAVER : In the large number of amputations I do in the hospitals of Philadelphia, I never do a Syme, but I do a Pirogoff and a Chopart. We often have to be governed by the wishes of the patient. I have had cases where I advised an amputation of the leg in order to render the use of an artificial limb easier, but where the patient has insisted that as much as possible of the limb should be saved. A Pirogoff does well. It answers better for a working man than for one under better circumstances. Osteoplastic resection of the foot gives the patient an almost useless limb. Yet it is a very nice and a very difficult operation. It has been performed only twice in this city, once by Dr. Hopkins, and once by Dr. F. H. Gross, at the German Hospital. The patient of Dr. Gross is still in the hospital. He is able to get around, but I do not think that he will be able to do hard work.

In amputations through the knee-joint I think that it is important to leave the patella, which serves partly to carry out the theory of Dr. Price of leaving a plane surface. When the patella is removed there are left two irregularities caused by the condyles. We must here be careful not to divide the ligamentum patellæ. If that is divided the action of the quadriceps causes retraction of the patella. I have, however, seen retraction in cases where attention was paid to this point. In such cases it would be better to do the amputation at the knee. This, of course, opens up the medulla, and exposes the patient to the dangers of septicæmia, but with antiseptic surgery I think that the risk would not be increased.

DR. J. PRICE: Attention has been called to the locomotion of persons wearing artificial limbs. Dr. Price has not said very much about his own locomotion. He is very fond of using the gun, and I have often hunted with him from morning until evening, and can speak of the tolerance of a good stump and a good artificial limb. In his own case he has wonderful tolerance for prolonged walking and climbing.

I have watched many cases of amputation where the operation was performed years ago. One case, operated on by Dr. John Mitchell, I see sometimes with one crutch and sometimes with a crutch and a cane. In none of these cases is the locomotion good. The amputations were made at the points criticized this evening.

DR. A. HEWSON, Jr.: The only point which I have to offer is in regard to Pirogoff amputations. It has been suggested that no artificial appliance could be employed in these cases that would look well. In several of these operations, done by my father, I have seen a shoe so well applied to the stump that it was almost impossible to tell that the man had an artificial foot. The difficulty was overcome by a large spring being put in the place occupied by the ball of the foot, i. e., extending from the heel toward the toe, so that when the heel was put to the ground there was not that sagging in of the shoe as occurs when simply a filled shoe is worn.

DR. O. H. ALLIS: My own feeling is that where amputation is very low down near the ankle-joint, the limb is used almost as a crutch, whereas if the amputation is a little below the knee, the instrument maker can make so good an ankle-joint that the wearer can walk on any declivity almost as well as with the natural limb. When you try to piece out an ankle, the part cannot be used as a foot, but is more like a crutch.

DR. FRANK WOODBURY: I should like to say a word in regard to a class of cases to which reference has not yet been made, that is, to amputation for disease, and particularly tuberculous disease of the joints. I would refer to a series of observations made by Ogille, in which it is stated that the prognosis of tuberculosis of the lungs is improved by an amputation, and that the larger the portion of the body removed, the better chance there is for the entire recovery of the patient. It seems that in certain cases of phthisis the nutritive powers are not sufficient to maintain the nutrition of the entire body, so if we can remove say one-eighth, or a larger portion of the body, the digestive function and the blood-making function are more than sufficient for the remainder of the body, and the nutrition is therefore improved.

This is directly to the point of operating in cases of joint tuberculosis, and also in the direction of the paper, that we should not endeavor to save all the tissue that is available.

DR. M. PRICE: I agree with the statement of Dr. Allis that such appliances are just like crutches. A man with a well-made foot can readily go up stairs giving a little spring with the sound foot. I was able to play base-ball, foot-ball, and the like, and was at school for a long time before it was known that I had an artificial limb to any one with the exception of my room-mate.

In regard to Dr. Collins's statement as to the teaching when I was a student, Dr. Smith, who was at that time professor of surgery, was one of the most conservative of men. His statement was that we have to consider what we are doing in amputating, and consider the influence upon the man himself. As many of these patients are led into bad habits of dissipation by being invited to drink by every one they meet, it might, in these cases, be better to amputate around the throat. I am not surprised that Dr. Collins·has called attention to the fact that Dr. Smith amputated three finger's breadth below the tubercle of the tibia. Dr. Smith had been in the war, and had seen much to show him the usefulness of a proper-length stump.

If I were going to amputate near the knee, I would operate below the joint, giving the patient a knee-bearing leg, with the patella and all its attachments in place. As soon as you amputate the leg, retraction takes place. It·is one· of the secrets of treating, a man with amputation to keep the stump straight. If the limb is left lying loosely on a pillow, there will be retraction of the muscles. Now and then I have to wear a peg, and it is then two or three days before I can straighten the leg. I would not suggest an amputation that opens the knee-joint. Where the operation suggested cannot be done, I would amputate at the junc-tion of the lower and middle third· of the thigh, and thus the knee-joint could be brought in the proper position.

In the case of workingmen who have passed that period in life when there is no chance of advancement, I have no objection to a Chopart,·or any other amputation that will give the ·man a limb that he can walk upon. I·am speaking of amputations that will give the man the same appearance that he originally had. I think we err in dis-cussing the question of what ought or ought not to be done with the patient. We are there as his adviser, and it is our business to do the best for the patient. I say to·him, such and such should be done. If he says that he will not have it, I decline to treat him.

—Dr. John Marshall, whose address· is Chemical· Laboratory of the Medical Depart-ment of the University of Pennsylvania, is engaged in examining the matters vomited or obtained by lavage in cases of supposed cancer of the stomach, and also of the blood in cases of sarcoma· and carcinoma. Any physicians who have such cases, are requested to send the specimens of the vomit and of the blood (the last· especially from an operation) to Dr. Marshall, at the above address, as soon as possible after obtaining them. A small quantity of ordinary ether should be added· to the specimens before sending them to Dr. Marshall, so as· to pre-vent ·decomposition. A ·statement of the nature of the case, and the results of any microscopical examination, together with the name and address, should accompany the specimen.

REPORTS OF CLINICS.

PHILADELPHIA HOSPITAL, JAN. 23.

CLINIC UPON DISEASES OF CHILDREN AND
　　　OBSTETRICS—DR. PARVIN.

Facial Paralysis of the New-Born.

I present to you an infant delivered six days ago. You observe that one side of the face is·paralyzed, this paralysis manifesting itself if the child cries or sucks. An injury was done the right facial nerve by the blade of the forceps upon that side· on which the palsy is now found, for in consequence of narrowing of the pelvic outlet—the pelvis was. kyphotic—it was necessary to end the labor instrumentally. This accident is by no means a rare one following the use of the forceps. Yet it may occur, but very seldom, though the delivery is spontaneous. Still more, there may be the same paralysis in consequence of an intra-cranial lesion, but when this exists other parts are paralyzed also, and not merely the external parts ; thus you will then find, for example, that the loss of power involves the veil of the palate.

In the variety of what is called obstetric paralysis here presented, the prognosis is favorable, while in that just referred to, it is the opposite. Almost all cases, scarcely an exception is ever seen, of facial paralysis from the forceps, recover, and usually within a few days. Therefore there is no indication for any treatment. But if by exception the paralysis should continue for a month or six weeks, the use of electricity would be indicated.

Cephalohæmatoma.

I showed you a week since this child suf-fering with a hæmatoma situated upon the right parietal bone, and then called your attention to the means by which you dis-tinguished such a tumor from the caput succedaneum, or sero-sanguineous effusion occupying·the presenting part of the child, which is so common a condition observed in the new-born that it may almost be regarded as physiological. But this is a rarer condition, occurring not oftener prob-ably than once in 200 cases. Let me direct your attention to the bony margin lifted up, and so distinctly felt around the base of the tumor: this is one of the distinguishing marks of a cephalohæmatoma. It is possi-ble such a tumor might for a moment be confounded with a cerebral hernia; but such hernia would increase when the child cries, it might be partially reduced, pressure on it would cause nervous accidents, and possibly the opening in the skull through which the hernia escaped could be felt.

The rule is that such a tumor disappears in a few weeks whether anything or nothing is done, and therefore no active treatment is indicated. Very rarely suppuration occurs, and then of course the abscess must be opened, proper antiseptic precautions being used.

Jaundice in the New-Born.

I present you three infants with jaundice, that which is sometimes called physiological jaundice to distinguish it from a graver form usually associated with septic infection. This generally manifests itself three or four days after birth, and spontaneously disappears in a week or ten days. The most important points in the care of an infant affected by physiological jaundice are to see that the child has its daily bath, and that regular evacuations from the bowels are secured, calcined magnesia, for example, being given, if any medicine is necessary.

Changes in the Areola and in the Nipple caused by Pregnancy. Care of the Nipples in Pregnant Women.

You are all familiar with the fact that important, and in some cases distinctly characteristic, changes occur in the areola surrounding the nipple as a consequence of pregnancy, such as the swollen or puffed condition of this part, its becoming notably darker, and the greatly increased size of the glands opening upon its surface, glands which notwithstanding the differing statements of observers are most probably miniature mammary glands, and are commonly known by the name of Montgomery, a distinguished Dublin obstetrician many years dead, who very carefully observed and described the changes in them consequent upon pregnancy: my belief, however, is that they were first called after Morgagni. Now, one of the women before you is in the 8th month of pregnancy, and you see there is not the slightest darkening of the areola, and no enlargement of the glands opening upon its surface. You usually get no information in regard to pregnancy worth having if you examine the mammary areola in a blonde, or in a woman with red hair, or, finding it so free from changes, may hastily conclude that pregnancy is improbable, and thus be led astray.

The other women are presented that you may see in one the normal form and size of the nipple, and in the other a small and retracted nipple. And this leads me to say a word in regard to the care of the nipples in pregnancy, especially important if the woman be a primigravida. It is all-important if the mother is to suckle her child, that the nipple shall have a suitable form and size; a bad nipple may foretell fissures, abrasions, and ulceration, and consequent mammary inflammation and abscess. Now I believe very much may be done to educate, or educe a retracted nipple. Teach the woman by the use of the index finger and thumb to draw out the nipple, spending a few minutes two or three times a day in this process of education, for education it is in the etymological sense of the word. Let the woman too, wear a nipple shield of firm material that will not only prevent compression of the organ, but also secure for it ample room to grow outward. This treatment ought to be begun at least two months before the end of pregnancy.

Several years ago I lost faith in the prophylaxis of "sore nipples" commonly employed then, and commonly employed to-day, that is, by the application to them of alcoholic and astringent preparations. Nature meant the skin of the nipple to be pliable, and she also has protected it from the injurious effects of the fluids, contact with which it is normally subjected to, by an almost infinite number of fat glands. But the treatment mentioned hardens the skin, dissolves away the protective glandular secretion, and lessens the activity of the glands. Therefore I believe it to be utterly irrational, and I have seen no satisfactory results from its employment. It is wiser, I think, to keep the nipples clean by the occasional use of a little warm water, possibly soap sometimes employed with the water, and then only apply a little cocoa butter to them at night. Of course this treatment is not required until the latter part of pregnancy.

CLINIC ON NERVOUS DISEASES—DR. F. X. DERCUM.

Gentlemen: I shall bring before you to-day a number of cases of spinal disease, not so much because they are interesting in themselves as because they illustrate, in addition to gross disease of the spinal column, focal disease of the cord. It is by the study of just such cases that we can best prepare ourselves for recognizing focal lesions of the cord, when no evidence of the same is afforded by an examination of the spinal column.

Pott's Disease.

Let us take, for instance, the case of the woman before us. It is a simple case of Pott's disease. The body of the first lumbar vertebra and to a lesser extent the bodies of its immediate neighbors are badly necrosed, so much so, indeed, that the spinal column has, as you see, a sharp bend in this region. The angle formed is so small that it is impossible for the patient to lie upon the back, but she is forced to rest upon either side. You can readily see what must happen to the contents of the spinal canal at the point of flexion. The calibre of the spinal canal is so much diminished that the cord is compressed, and we have very much the same set of symptoms as those derived from a transverse section of the cord in an animal or in a man whose spinal cord has been compressed by a tumor, or which has been cut across, it may be, by a bullet. Of course, there are certain differences, but they are matters of detail, and do not affect the general principles.

In the first place, we have, as you see, a paralysis of motion below the point of disease. I ask her to move her legs, and you see that she is powerless to do so. I next prick her limbs with a pin, and you observe that she gives no sign of pain. Repeating the test in various ways, you observe that she has lost all power of recognizing either touch or pain in the legs. Thus far we have established paralysis both of motion and sensation. In addition, we have, in this case, the added symptom of pain near the site of the disease. This pain is described by her as sharp and shooting, and radiates in a belt-like manner around her body. It is intense in character, and for a time was so severe that the patient was kept more or less under the influence of morphia. We must look for an explanation of its presence in the extreme distortion of the bodies of the vertebræ and the consequent compression of the nerves as they make their exit through the intervertebral foramina. Regarding the question of pain in focal diseases of the cord generally, for instance in tumors, I may say in passing that it may be absent or but slightly pronounced in growths having their origin in the substance of the cord, and is especially marked where the lesion involves the membranes or the posterior nerve-roots.

It is almost invariably a prominent symptom and radiates along nerve-trunks having their origin at or below the level of the lesion.

In studying our patient more closely, we become aware that the paralysis of sensation and motion does not begin at the level of the flexion of the spinal column, but some distance below it. This is to be explained by the oblique and descending course of the nerves in this region. Take, for instance, the ilio-hypogastric nerve. You will remember that it takes its origin from the first lumbar nerve, its fibres therefore gaining an exit from the spinal canal between the first and second lumbar vertebræ. You will remember further that it is ultimately distributed to the skin of the hypogastric region and the buttocks. In testing our patient carefully, we find that as we proceed downward from the region of the diseased vertebræ, the patient continues to recognize the touch of the finger or the pin-point until the buttocks are reached. Here her responses become uncertain, and finally cease altogether.

You see at once then that to make a successful diagnosis of the level of a given lesion you must be thoroughly familiar with the origin and course of the various nerve trunks, while you should also bear in mind that the point of spinal exit of a nerve by no means corresponds to its level of origin in the cord. In fact the latter is usually much above the former, the difference in level being more pronounced as we go from above downward. In the present instance, the actual level of origin of the first lumbar nerve, of which the ilio-inguinal is a branch, is just beneath the lamellæ of the *eleventh dorsal* vertebra ; so that a lesion in the cord causing paralysis of this nerve would have to be sought for at this level instead of at the first lumbar vertebra.

Our patient presents in addition other symptoms which I prefer merely to mention, my object being rather to indicate general principles. You observe that her legs are in a condition of spastic contraction, and further that the muscles are much atrophied. These conditions are the result of degenerative changes in the segment end nerves below the seat of compression, as I may have further opportunity to point out. Both sphincters are also, as you would naturally expect in so complete a lesion of the cord, paralyzed.

But one more point of interest remains, to which I shall call attention. If you will observe her very closely while I again test her for sensation you will notice that the latter is not as absolutely lost as is motion; and this is probably to be explained by the fact that the spinal cord, being compressed from in front, the motor tracts suffer *first* and suffer *most* while the posterior tracts are compressed later and less effectually. The posterior tracts indeed suffer in such a case by transmitted pressure from in *front*. The surgical indication in such a case would therefore be—extension having been tried and proving useless—to remove the lamellæ and spines of the diseased vertebræ. In the patient before us, however, the pronounced character of the disease and the extensive secondary changes that have ensued would discountenance any such procedure.

Crossed Spinal Paralysis.

In the next case we have before us a middle aged man who, while in a condition of good health, was struck on the shoulders by a heavy bale of rags, the bale falling from the height of a third floor. The man was walking at the time. The blow caused him to sit down forcibly on the pavement while his thorax was forcibly flexed upon his abdomen. Strange to say, after recovering from a momentary shock, he got up and walked home, and for a number of months thereafter attended to his occupation, that of carpenter. It was not indeed until seven months after the accident that he began to have difficulty in walking. His condition at present is extremely interesting. On asking him to move his legs as he sits in his rolling chair you observe that he moves his left leg quite readily while the right leg fails utterly to respond to the will. Testing him now for sensation you notice at once that he responds instantly when the paralyzed leg is touched and fails to recognize any impression on the leg in which motion is still preserved. In other words we have paralysis of motion on one side with paralysis of sensation upon the opposite side. We have here then exactly the same condition as we would find in an animal in which a hemi-section of the cord had been made. A tumor compressing one-half the cord would of course produce a similar set of symptoms. The seat of the growth would then be determined by the level of the anæsthesia plus the point of origin in the cord of the nerve fibres supplying the area above and below this level. Pains radiating around and down one side would probably, as in the present case, be an additional symptom.

It is hardly necessary to relate to you the explanation of crossed spinal paralysis. You remember, doubtless, that the motor fibres decussate in the anterior pyramids of the medulla, while the sensory fibres decussate along the entire length of the cord. Let us see how they were interfered with in the present case. On carefully examining the patient we find that the spines of the twelfth dorsal and first lumbar vertebræ are markedly deflected to the right, and it therefore appears that the bodies of these vertebræ underwent gradual softening after the accident, and that a *lateral* displacement finally resulted.

If I have succeeded merely in impressing you with the general method of examination for localized diseases of the cord, and in that term I include also the membranes, my object has been accomplished. One very important group of symptoms, however, I have not even touched upon, as a full discussion is not permitted by the time at our command. I refer of course to the tendon phenomena and reflexes. However, the following rule with regard to them holds good: You all know that if the cord of an animal be cut, just as soon as the shock of the operation passes away, the tendon phenomena, *e. g.*, the knee jerks, are increased. This of course also holds good in man. A division of the lateral tract by a bullet or by a tumor results in an increased knee jerk— *i. e.*, other things equal. Long continuance of the lesion may result in the contracture and wasting and so, as in the case of the woman you saw, the reflexes may be abolished. You should also remember, that if the lesion be lower down in the cord, *e. g.*, in the lumbar portion and termination, the end of the cord being destroyed the paralysis in the legs cannot be accompanied by reflex action, as there are no centres below the seat of lesion.

SURGICAL CLINIC—DR. M'CLELLAN.

Case of Dog-Bite.

Gentlemen: The first patient whom I shall show you this morning is a woman who received a few days since a very ugly bite from a dog, the injury involving the ala of the nose and the lower lip. There was no reason in this case to suppose that the animal was rabid: but I have known very troublesome results from similar injuries which were much less severe than those in the present case. It is well always to cleanse thoroughly a wound of this nature when it is first seen, and then to cauterize it. Punctured wounds are bad things to deal with, owing to there always being a probability of inflammatory products being imprisoned; and when they occur from the teeth of animals they should, when it is feasible, be carefully sucked out before a caustic is applied. It is well also to administer a cathartic, to put the patient on light diet, and, when it is applicable, the wound should be treated antiseptically. In this case, as you see, such a course has been well rewarded.

Two Cases of Punctured Wound of the Scalp.

, Here are several cases of punctured wounds of the scalp, from an examination of which you may gain some practical hints. The first was inflicted by a stick falling on the man's head; caries of the frontal bone resulted, and subsequently the dura mater became involved, and the operation of trephining had to be done to relieve distressing symptoms. The other man fell a week ago, striking his head against some sharp object. The wound healed quickly, but there is evidently fluctuation beneath the scalp tissues. I think, as a general rule, punctured wounds of the scalp should be converted into incised wounds, so that they may be cleansed of all foreign matter and washed out.

In both of these cases the damage done involved the entire scalp, and owing to the loose connection of the latter to the pericranium, if inflammation occurs and results in suppuration, pus will often burrow away from the site of the injury to some dependent position.

Case of Felon.

The next patient has had a felon. This is a most painful affection. It is not always easy to determine the cause, but most frequently felons occur from bruises in persons whose vocation subjects the fingers to much use in hot or cold water. There is very apt to be more or less injury to the deeper parts, and if the periosteum becomes involved the bone is often destroyed. The great pain is due to the blood-pressure on the nerves at the ends of the fingers. It is less severe if only the soft parts are concerned, as the swelling then becomes diffused; but when the trouble is with the tendon or periosteum the theca confines the pus to a very limited area, and the peculiar, intolerable, throbbing pain occurs. The treatment of felon consists in preventing suppuration, or if that is unavoidable, in hastening it. If it is tried early, the inflam-

mation may often be aborted by painting the finger with strong iodine liniment, or with nitrate of silver, followed by strapping. This will cause a few moments' suffering, which will speedily diminish and disappear. If, however, suppuration has begun it should be encouraged by hot dressings, and when fully established the felon should be freely incised in the middle line over the tendon down to the bone. If you apply poultices, do so warily, and for a few hours, for they are a remedy almost as bad as the disease, if improperly used. I am sure I have seen numbers of fingers lost through over-poulticing by ignorant persons. From their excessive use the soft parts become macerated and boggy, and the pus finds easy inducement to travel toward the hand. After incision, a soothing mild dressing may be used, and, if you prefer it, one which is antiseptic.

General Lipomata.

Here is a man about forty years old, who is afflicted with a number of growths upon his back, neck, throat, arm, groin, and thigh, which upon examination feel doughy and lobulated. They are insensible to pressure and are evidently fatty tumors, or lipomata. They occur generally in parts exposed to friction and pressure, but it is rare to meet with a patient presenting so many of these tumors at the same time.

Epithelioma.

Here are two cases of epithelial cancer. The one on the lower lip has possibly been caused by smoking a clay pipe. Its removal before greater involvement of tissue occurs would certainly lessen suffering, and perhaps not be followed by a return of the growth. The other case, in which the epithelioma is on the anterior part of the neck, involves many great blood vessels and nerves on both sides, and is not amenable to operation. Fortunately the man is not now suffering.

———◆◆◆———

—The number of cases of infectious diseases in New York City shows some diminution over that of a few weeks ago. For the two weeks ending Feb. 12, the following statement is furnished by the Sanitary Bureau of the Health Department: Typhoid fever, 14 cases and 2 deaths; scarlet fever, 666 cases and 96 deaths; cerebro-spinal meningitis, 5 cases and 2 deaths; measles, 595 cases and 40 deaths; diphtheria, 388 cases and 103 deaths; small-pox, no new cases, one death.

PERISCOPE.

Recurrent Pneumothorax.

Dr. Samuel West, Assistant-Physician to St. Bartholomew's Hospital, refers to a most important and interesting case, published by Mr. Gabb, in which there had occurred three attacks of pneumothorax, with complete recovery. He says he had a similar case under his care at the beginning of this year at the Chest Hospital, Victoria Park. The history of the case is as follows:

W. H. D., 22 years old, was admitted on January 3, 1888, into the Chest Hospital, Victoria Park, complaining of shortness of breath. The attack came on, he stated, without any apparent cause, on the morning of December 23, on getting out of bed. The breathing was so short that he found it necessary to remain at home, though he did not lie in bed; and, as after some days it still continued short, he applied for admission into the hospital. He had not felt ill or suffered in any way except with the shortness of breath.

The patient was a healthy-looking young man, slightly built, but well-developed and muscular. There was no dyspnœa evident. The shape and movements of the chest were symmetrical, but the percussion note was tympanitic over the whole right side from the apex to the base, back and front. The tympanitic resonance extended to the left edge of the sternum right down to the xyphoid cartilage, and the liver dulness did not rise above the seventh rib. The heart was displaced to the left, the apex beating under the léft nipple. The vocal vibrations could be feebly felt and heard over the whole side, but the respiratory murmur was absent except at the base behind, where weak and distant amphoric breathing was audible. There was no bell sound or succussion. The lower edge of the liver could not be made out. The opposite lung was completely healthy, and the other organs seemed normal. The case was clearly one of pneumothorax without effusion, and in the process of resolution.

The subsequent history of the case is simple. The shortness of breath quickly disappeared. The patient looked and felt well, and gained flesh. The abnormal physical signs gradually vanished, and on February 6 the following note was taken: "The shape of the chest is symmetrical, the movements free, but, on deep inspiration, there seems to be a little more expansion on the left side, especially in the axilla. The liver dulness begins at the sixth rib in the nipple line. The cardiac dulness is of its normal size, and the apex in the proper place. The percussion note is still a little more resonant on the right side; the breath sounds are distinctly audible and vesicular in character over the whole side down to the base. In the mid-axillary region a little fine crepitation is heard, probably pleuritic, for it is in this place that the patient has complained of pain for the last few days."

The patient's previous history was good. He had had no serious illness except scarlet fever and measles, but he had been regarded as a rather delicate child, having been subject to a cough on catching cold ever since an attack of bronchitis at the age of 3 years, but he lost his cough as he grew older. His father was living and well, but his mother died after a confinement. He had a brother and a sister, both strong; and he considered himself strong and active, and enjoyed athletic exercises.

Now comes the interesting part of his history. Last August, while walking quietly, he was suddenly seized with pain above the right clavicle, and felt a bubbling sensation in the right side. The breath at the same time became very short, and he had a rather violent cough—as he called it a " churchyard cough"—which he had not suffered from before the breath became short. He was able to keep at his work, however, but had to avoid all hurry and exertion for about a fortnight, when he appeared to get quite well. In the beginning of November, the morning after a game of football in which he was several times charged violently, he became again short of breath. The breathing continued short for about a month, but at the end of that time he found himself quite well again, and continued well until the present attack three weeks later. The two previous attacks were, he stated, all similar to the present one.

In the absence of direct evidence, there is a very strong probability that the previous attacks were, like the present, due to pneumothorax. The last attack was without doubt pneumothorax, but he came under observation rather by accident than of necessity, for it was not until he had had the dyspnœa for ten days that he presented himself at the hospital, and even then the dyspnœa was so slight that he grumbled at being kept in bed.

There are two facts about pneumothorax,

Dr. West remarks, which, though well established, are not generally known: that it is of not uncommon occurrence in the apparently healthy; and that it may develop in the latent insidious way it did in this case, and without the violent symptoms which frequently accompany it. The interest of this case and of that published by Mr. Gabb does not lie in their illustrating these points, but in the fact, which they establish, that a patient may have more than one attack of pneumothorax and recover completely. Dr. West says he does not see any reason why this should not be so, but he does not recollect any recorded case of the kind, so that Mr. Gabb's case is a very important contribution to the literature of the subject.—*British Med. Journal*, Jan. 12, 1889.

Biology of the Pancreas.

Dr. Polïkarp D. Küvshinsky, of St. Petersburg, has published recently (*St. Petersburg Inaugural Dissertation*, 1888, pp. 56) a valuable contribution to the biology of the pancreas, based on a number of laborious and careful experiments on dogs with a permanent pancreatic fistula. The scientific chapter in question attracting as yet relatively little attention, the following short summary may be placed before the readers of the REPORTER. 1. The pancreatic secretion never ceases altogether, not even in sleeping or fasting animals. 2. It manifests, however, considerable variations in regard to its hourly and daily amount, as well as to its physical and chemical properties; and that not only in individual animals, but even in one and the same dog examined on various days, all other conditions being equal. 3 Given a healthy dog under normal conditions, some of the variations prove to be distinctly determined by taking food; some by mental, some by physical, state. 4. As to the influence of food, a daily course of the secretion is, generally speaking, this: As a rule, shortly after the meal the secretion increases until it reaches its primary maximum during the second half-hour, less frequently during the first half-hour; after a more or less short interval, it decreases fairly markedly to rise and sink slightly again and again, the secondary maxima being reached at about four-hour intervals after the meal. 5 An average daily quantity of the juice in a non-fasting animal, weighing about nineteen kilogrammes, amounts to 335 cubic centimetres (eleven fluid ounces). 6. The pro-

portion of solid constituents in a normal pancreatic juice varies between 1.6 and 7.7 per cent., gradually rising to its highest point about seven hours after taking food. 7. The "secretory pressure" in a dog's pancreas amounts to 280 milligrammes of an aqueous column, or to 21.4 of a mercurial one. In a rabbit's gland it is equal to from 219 to 225 (Heidenhain). It is probable that in man, too, the pancreatic tension is nearly as low. Since a catarrhal condition of the duodenum in dogs and rabbits seriously interferes with the escape of the juice into the bowel, we may safely assume that duodenal catarrh in human beings must similarly give rise to a more or less complete cessation of the juice's flow. 8. The secretion is most distinctly influenced by psychical agents. In a dog, kept fasting for twenty-four hours and then excited by having food placed before it, a considerable increase in the secretion takes place, fairly rapidly. The juice secreted contains a relatively low proportion of solids (3.5 per cent.), but still possesses a normally energetic digestive action. 9. Hence, we are justified in assuming that in man, too, appetite plays an important part as a stimulant for the secretion and, consequently, as a powerful promoter of digestion and assimilation. 10. During sleep the secretion gradually sinks to a fairly low level, the fall going on synchronously with deepening sleep; while on awakening the secretion gradually increases. 11. Alcohol in a diluted form and in moderate doses, is a powerful stimulant to the pancreas, since it rapidly causes a very considerable and fairly prolonged increase in the amount of the juice, which acts energetically. This increase lasts twenty-four hours. 12. Hence, the internal administration of spirits before and during meals can be actually beneficial in anæmic and weakened persons, convalescents, etc. 13. Morphine, however used—hypodermically or internally—is a powerful pancreatic depressor, since it in two minutes inhibits, and subsequently, in thirty to twenty minutes, completely arrests the secretion for from one to three hours, the effects being very pronounced even after small doses (*e. g.*, one-tenth of a grain to a dog of 21.5 kilogrammes in weight. The effect corresponds generally to the size of the dose. 14. Cocaine similarly manifests an inhibitory action on the pancreas, which, however, on the whole, is less powerful and by far less prolonged as compared with morphine.

Spasmodic Urethral Stricture from Anal Fissure.

In the *Med. Record*, Jan. 26, 1889, Dr. L. Bolton Bangs communicates an account of a case in which he believes a more or less permanent stricture of the urethra was due to reflex action of the spinal cord from an irritation at the anus.

The patient was forty-one years old, a painter by trade. Twenty years ago he had syphilis, followed by secondary symptoms, but for many years subsequently he had no evidence of it whatever. For several years he had been subject to attacks of painter's colic, and at such times the associated constipation was very obstinate. About six years ago he began to have indescribable sensations in the region of his bladder, and pain during urination, but he had never had any urethritis or disease of the urethra or bladder to which these sensations could be attributed. About two years ago. he acquired a specific urethritis which lasted acutely some weeks; then became chronic, and finally terminated at the end of six months. About eighteen months ago he had an attack of painter's colic, accompanied with constipation, and then experienced intense pain in the rectum, which was most marked after defecation. This pain became constant, gradually increased to extreme intensity, and he suffered from it, both after and before a stool. With this pain in the rectum, he had a gradually increasing difficulty of urination, the urine passing in a small stream, and at times only in drops, accompanied with pain in the penis and in the pelvis generally.

At length the difficulty of expelling the urine became such that his physician was compelled to resort to the use of the catheter, in order to relieve the bladder of a certain amount of urine which was retained. For the two months preceding his coming under Dr. Bangs's observation his troubles, both as regards the pain in the rectum and the dysuria, increased so greatly that the use of the catheter was continuous, and the latter finally set up a mild form of urethritis, which aggravated his symptoms. The pain referred to the rectum and to the bladder became so severe that he was obliged to resort to hypodermic injections of morphia. When Dr. Bangs first saw him, the man was anæmic, weak, and in constant pain, unable to empty his bladder without the use of the catheter, and under the necessity of being constantly under the influence of morphia. He was unable to discriminate between the pain in his bladder and that in his rectum.

He was tormented with frequent desire to urinate, and although he could expel some urine with great straining, the feeling that his bladder was not emptied was so intense that he could hardly be restrained from passing his catheter, which he always carried in his pocket for the purpose. His meatus urinarius admitted a 32 French *bougie à boule*. At four and three-fourths inches was a stricture of 26 French. A solid sound of the latter size (26 French), after being obstructed for a few seconds at the membranous urethra, slipped into the bladder. On withdrawing, it was strongly held by the urethra, which alternately relaxed and contracted upon the instrument until the latter was free in the penile portion. There was evidently a spasmodic condition of which there could be no doubt. It is true, Dr. Bangs remarks, that such a condition in the deep urethra might be due to a stricture of large calibre in the penile portion, and if it had been nearer to the meatus he would have paid more attention to it; but inasmuch as the patient complained so greatly of the pain in the rectum, he thought that perhaps the secret of the trouble might be found in or about the latter. On exposing the anus it was found to be violently contracted. The anal region was very sensitive and it was only with great difficulty that the patient could be induced to relax the sphincters sufficiently to enable Dr. Bangs to find that he had three bluish-red exceedingly painful fissures of the anus. This seemed a good opportunity to test the question of cause and effect by observing the result of treating the anus alone. Accordingly the patient was etherized, and the sphincter-muscles were paralyzed digitally. Nothing whatever was done to the urethra, and the catheter was taken away. This was on June 7. On the 9th it was recorded: "The patient passed urine and fæces spontaneously, and with much less pain, being but slight during urination and not nearly as great after defecation."

From this time on improvement was progressive. There was none of the spasmodic straining to empty the bladder, there was no retention of urine, and the urethritis gradually subsided. Ten days later, a sound as large as could be insinuated through the stricture at four and three-quarters inches, namely, 30 French, was easily passed into the bladder, without any resistance and without any spasmodic contraction about the instrument upon its withdrawal.

On June 26 the patient was discharged from the hospital cured. Dr. Bangs states that for the past six months he has been intermittently under observation. He has been treated for "painter's colic," and has had none of the obstinate constipation, no pain in his rectum, and no trouble whatever with his urethra or bladder.

Intubation with an Ordinary Rubber Tube.

Dr. Geo. O. Williams says, in the *Med. Record*, Jan. 26, 1889, that quite a number of patients die of diphtheria in consequence of the obstruction to respiration caused by the closure of the fauces from tumefaction of the tonsils and uvula, the larynx at the same time being intact. The majority of those who die within the first forty-eight hours die in this way. He then refers to a case of this character. The disease had existed forty hours. The child was eleven years old. The fauces and soft palate were covered with exudation. The throat was closed. Respiration very labored. Constant restlessness had been present for thirty-six hours. All the indications of slow suffocation were present. The child was informed of what it was desired to accomplish, and his promise to assist as much as possible was secured.

A soft rubber tube was then passed beyond the obstruction, and its extremity left just at the larynx. The boy nodded his head to indicate that it gave him relief and was in proper position. Within three minutes he dropped into a motionless slumber of absolute rest. The distressing breathing was instantly relieved. The sleep continued an hour. At the end of that time a little mucus obstructed the tube, and he awoke and pulled the tube from its place. It was immediately replaced. The tube extended six inches from the mouth. An attendant constantly supported this extremity. An ink mark on it, on a line with the teeth, designated the proper distance for introduction. After a few hours the care of the tube was intrusted to the friends. It was maintained in use for seventy hours. It was removed for cleansing, and for nutrition and medication at proper intervals. At the end of that time the subsidence of the tumefaction permitted its discontinuance. The tube measured seven-eighths of an inch, outside measure. No complication occurred in the case and a good recovery followed. He says he does not recall any published account of such a procedure in diphtheritic cases, but thinks it likely, from its simplicity and efficiency, that it must have been in use by others.

Inoculation with Tuberculosis by way of the Skin.

Von Lesser states in the *Deutsche med. Wochenschrift*, No. 29, 1888, that a woman 48 years old, who had been previously always healthy, had frequently washed the clothing of her husband who died of general miliary tuberculosis. In this patient a tumor the size of a cherry was found on the lowermost part of the volar surface of the right arm. The tumor proved on extirpation to consist of an alveolar structure with giant cells and central caseation; ascending from it caseous infiltrated streaks of tissue could be traced upward on the skin. Microscopically the skin appeared unchanged; only in the deep layers around the bases of the sweat glands there was great infiltration of cells. On the eighth day after extirpation of the tumor a tuberculous paronychia developed on the left ring-finger, which healed after being scraped.

Von Lesser regards it as probable that in this case the tumor developed through penetration of the virus by way of the sweat glands. The skin was intact as far as could be discovered by microscopic examination, and for the virus to cling to it under such circumstances seems to the author to require, next to hereditary taint, long maceration of the skin in a fluid containing the tuberculous poison.—*Centralblatt f. d. med. Wissenschaften*, Dec. 15, 1888.

Naphthalin Rash.

In the Moscow bi-weekly *Meditzinskoïé Obozreniïé*, No. 16, 1888, p. 316, Dr. S. Prëobrajensky communicates an interesting case which tends to upset the common opinion that naphthalin, when administered internally, produces no accessory symptoms, since it is not absorbed by the gastro-intestinal mucous membrane. A boy, 16 years old, suffering with obstinate diarrhœa, took sixty grains of the drug in the course of forty-eight hours. By the end of this time diarrhœa ceased, but the patient's whole body, except the face and neck, became covered with a slightly itching, profuse rash, in the shape of fairly regular, circular, slightly prominent, brown-red patches one-half centimetre in diameter. After other two ten-grain doses, the face and neck became similarly studded. When naphthalin was discontinued the rash gradually disappeared, to be followed about the fifth day by a free desquamation. The temperature remained normal throughout.

Slight Aortic Insufficiency.

Some instructive experiments on artificially induced aortic murmurs were published some months ago by Dr. Timofejew (*Berlin klin. Wochenschrift*, Nos. 24 and 25, 1888), in which he showed that a very slight aortic insufficiency may exist without producing a diastolic murmur, but that in such cases a distinct accentuation of the second sound can then be heard ; he also found that with greater but still slight insufficiency, though a murmur is produced, this can be made to cease by diminution of the blood pressure, either by venesection or by section of the spinal cord. These experimental observations are in full accord with the well-known clinical fact that an aortic bruit is sometimes temporarily much less pronounced than usual, and may even occasionally disappear. An interesting paper has just been published by Professor Carl Dehio, of Dorpat (*St. Petersburg med. Wochenschrift*, No. 50, 1888), in which he gives the details of a case which illustrates this variability of some aortic bruits very well. The patient was a student who had suffered from syphilis. At times he experienced severe pain in the region of the heart, accompanied by dyspnœa, headache, giddiness, and faintness. He had consulted several physicians, some of whom had detected a murmur, while others had declared there was none. Professor Dehio found at first, while the patient was sitting, merely some accentuation of the second sound, but as soon as he stood up, a blowing murmur was audible over the whole of the body of the sternum synchronous with the second sound, and prolonged to the end of the diastole. After a time, this became less and less perceptible, and finally vanished, but, on the patient moving or working his arms about, it reappeared. Tracings taken with a Dudgeon's sphygmograph showed that while the patient was in a recumbent posture, there being no murmur, the pulse, which was beating 80 per minute, was of a normal but weak character, with a slight distension wave and a low blood pressure, the secondary waves being only just perceptible. On standing up, the beats increased to 88 per minute, the bruit becoming then audible, the tracing assumed the character frequently observed in cases of neurotic cardiac palpitation, the pulse wave being higher, but falling rapidly, and the secondary and tertiary waves being well marked. After considerable exertion, when the bruit was louder still, the beats being, however, only 76 per minute, the distension wave was three times as high as when the patient was lying down, and it fell very quickly, being in fact the typical *pulsus celer*. It is seen that the bruit was dependent on the initial blood pressure due to the force of the contraction of the left ventricle, rather than on the mean intra-arterial pressure, which was probably not increased, since, according to the researches of Riegél and of Wetzel, there is no increase in the mean pressure, where the secondary waves become more pronounced. It is evident from the tracings that whenever the primary wave increased, the secondary waves increased also ; and thus that, while when the patient was in a recumbent posture, there was but a gentle backward stream through the defective valves, yet, upon a slight amount of exertion, the velocity of this stream was greatly increased, and thus became capable of producing a murmur. This difference between a gentle and a rapid stream can be easily illustrated by compressing an india-rubber tube through which water from a cistern is flowing, when the murmur, which can both be heard and felt, is readily found to depend on the velocity of the water. Dr. Dehio remarks that he cannot well have mistaken a murmur of hæmic origin for a slight aortic insufficiency in this case, for the whole history, the dilatation of the heart, the occasional whistling character of the murmur, and the serious subjective sensations of pain and palpitation all point to organic mischief. Again, the insufficiency must, he thinks, be of slight extent, as the dilatation of the left ventricle was but very moderate, and as Duroziez's double bruit was not audible in the femoral arteries. —*Lancet*, Jan. 19, 1889.

Case of Sebaceous Cyst of the Groin.

At a meeting of the Brooklyn Surgical Society, March 15, 1888, Dr. Rockwell presented a photograph of a case taken at the moment of operation, with the following history :

A woman had been brought to his office by a physician, who supposed her to be suffering from inguinal hernia, but was not quite satisfied with the diagnosis. On examination, a tumor, which had been slowly developing for two years, was found in the left inguinal fold, where it lay parallel to Poupart's ligament, which it directly covered. It was about nine inches long and two or three inches in diameter, looking like a large sausage. It had never been reducible, nor had it given any pain. Impulse on coughing and resonance on percussion were wanting. The finger could readily be passed under the tumor and into the inguinal canal, outside of the tumor's wall. It was flat on percussion, and gave the impression of containing fluid or colloid material. A diagnosis of cyst was made, and, on opening the tumor at the time of operation, it was found to contain about half a pint of fluid rendered semi-solid by the presence of enormous quantities of cholesterin crystals, though little if any true sebaceous matter was found. It was probably a sebaceous cyst modified by location and pressure to its peculiar shape. The sac was dissected out, and the patient rapidly recovered. The case was of interest from a diagnostic point of view, as it might easily have been mistaken for one of femoral hernia pushing up over Poupart's ligament, or hydrocele of the round ligament, both of which it resembled in many of its clinical features. —*Brooklyn Medical Journal*, Jan., 1889.

Origin of Human Diphtheria from a Similar Disease in Birds.

At the time when Nicati published some statements tending to demonstrate the identity of the contagious element of diphtheria in children and in chickens, Mágnin, as the result of numerous observations and microscopical investigations, also published statements denying such identity. This was in 1879. Since that time, thanks to the development of bacteriology, Loeffler, and Cornil, and Babés have shown the almost complete identity of the bacilli found in the false membranes of children and birds. More recently this statement has been confirmed by the investigations of Menziés, Delthil, Pamard, Bouchard, and Leissier. Menziés has endeavored to show that diphtheria was caused by the dejections of birds, through the medium of water which has percolated through the deposits of dove-houses or poultry-yards into wells. In the epidemic, which was reported by the author, the atmosphere seems to have been the medium of propagation. He believed that the disease was carried to the island in which the epidemic occurred, and in which nothing of the kind had previously been known, by diseased turkeys. In the course of five months, 125 of a population of 4,000 were attacked with diphtheria, and 36 of them died. This island was in the northern part of the Greek Archipelago, Skiatoes by name, and the epidemic continued during five months of the year 1884. The diseased turkeys showed false membranes of a gray color upon the velum of the palate and upon the pharynx. In one of them, the process extended to the larynx; the membranes were not very closely adherent, and could be readily removed. The underlying mucous membrane bled but little, and the glands of the neck were not very much swollen. In one of those which recovered, there was paralysis of the feet, and the animal was unable to walk. The conclusions which were drawn from this epidemic are:

1. There is in turkeys a kind of diphtheria which resembles that which occurs in human beings in its symptoms, its evolutions, and its gravity.

2. Its virus may be transmitted by the atmosphere to man, communicating the disease to him, and then developing into an epidemic.—*Glasgow Medical Journal*, Jan., 1889.

Hereditary Chorea.

The Lyons correspondent of the *Bulletin Médical*, Jan. 6, 1889, says that G. Lenoir has devoted an interesting thesis to hereditary chorea. He concludes that there exists a special form of chorea deserving the name hereditary, and that it should be placed in the group of arhythmic choreas. It is a disease of adult life and of maturity. As regards etiology, only one essential and so to speak necessary influence is found, namely, heredity. In symptomatology it is characterized by an insidious appearance and by the slowly progressive march of the choreic symptoms, which, at first sight, do not differ from those of the common chorea of Sydenham. A more attentive examination, however, shows as an essential difference that the patient is able to stop the movements by an effort of the will. Disturbances of intelligence and of memory are very frequent. The diagnosis is easy enough. Convulsive tic is perhaps the only affection with which hereditary chorea may be confounded. A number of cases described under the names chorea of adults and of the old should in future be studied with more care with reference to heredity. It is very probable, indeed, that a large number of these cases should be classed as hereditary chorea. The progress of disease is slowly progressive, and it ends in loss of mind and in death. While the prognosis is fatal for the disease it should be reserved for the children and the descendants up to the age of fifty years at least. But it is very interesting to note that hereditary chorea never skips a generation. If a child of a choreic escapes the disease his own children will be free. No treatment up to the present time has given satisfactory results.

THE
MEDICAL AND SURGICAL
REPORTER.

ISSUED EVERY SATURDAY.

CHARLES W. DULLES, M.D.,
EDITOR AND PUBLISHER.

The Terms of Subscription to the serial publications of this office are as follows, payable in advance:

Med. and Surg. Reporter (weekly), a year,   **$5.00**
Quarterly Compendium of Med. Science, -   2.50
Reporter and Compendium, -   -   -   6.00
Physician's Daily Pocket Record, -   -   -   1.00
Reporter and Pocket Record, -   -   -   - 6.00
Reporter, Compendium, and Pocket Record, 7.00

All checks and postal orders should be drawn to order of

CHARLES W. DULLES,
N. E. Cor. 13th and Walnut Streets,
P. O. Box 843.   Philadelphia, Pa.

☞ SUGGESTIONS TO SUBSCRIBERS:

See that your address-label gives the date to which your subscription is paid.
   In requesting a change of address, give the old address as well as the new one.
   If your REPORTER does not reach you promptly and regularly, notify the publisher *at once*, so that the cause may be discovered and corrected.

☞ SUGGESTIONS TO CONTRIBUTORS AND CORRESPONDENTS:

Write in ink.
Write on one side of paper only.
Write on paper of the size usually used for letters.
Make as few paragraphs as possible. Punctuate carefully. Do not abbreviate, or omit words like "the," and "a," or "an."
Make communications as short as possible.
NEVER ROLL A MANUSCRIPT! Try to get an envelope or wrapper which will fit it.
   When it is desired to call our attention to something in a newspaper, mark the passage boldly with a colored pencil, and write on the wrapper "Marked copy." Unless this is done, newspapers are not looked at.
   The Editor will be glad to get medical news, but it is important that brevity and actual interest shall characterize communications intended for publication.

THE STATE BOARD 'OF MEDICAL EXAMINERS.

As the fate of the bill to establish a State Board of Medical Examiners in Pennsylvania has not yet been settled by the Legislature, we would add a few words to what has · already been said in the REPORTER about it.

Just at present the opposition to the passage of this bill is being pushed with great vigor and, while nothing new is said against it, the old objections are brushed up and brought out in a way to mislead those who are not familiar with them and their history.

The opponents of the bill may, we believe, be divided into the following classes: First, and most influential, a large part of the homœopaths, who fear that a board containing—as it ought to—a majority of men of the "regular" school would have a prejudicial influence upon the maintenance of their separate existence. This opposition is natural; but we are happy to believe that the most intelligent and honest so-called homœopaths are not afraid to rely upon the justice and fairness of such a board as is proposed, and that they see the need for examining boards unconnected with medical schools as clearly as any medical men do.

Second, there are among the opponents of the bill certain men who pose as the most orthodox of the "regular" school, who go about talking of the "Code of Ethics" and trying to work up a scare about homœopathy, which is in ludicrous contrast to the fear of some of the homœopaths just spoken of. These men do not represent the mass of the regular profession, either in their abject fear of homœopathy or in their intemperate assaults upon the character of homœopaths in general.

A third class of opponents is found in the teachers and *attachés* of certain medical schools which make a pretense of maintaining a high standard of medical education, but whose graduates have hitherto found it harder to pass the examinations of State Boards than it was to get their diplomas. This kind of opposition is easy to understand, if its motive is known; and when its motive is known it will no doubt meet with the contempt which it deserves.

The last class of objectors to which we wish to allude is made up of those who are the open supporters of fraudulent and ignorant methods—or no-methods, as Carlyle would say—of treating the sick. This is a motley crew of vitapaths, electropaths, eclectics, Christian scientists, pow-wow doctors, and who can tell how many more. These are not very conspicuous in their opposition to a State Board of Medical

Examiners—although they are deeply concerned—because their cause is being maintained much better than they could maintain it, by the homœopaths who are afraid of the "regulars" and the "regulars" who are afraid of the homœopaths. We believe we voice the best and fairest professional sentiment in Pennsylvania, when we say that the most upright and intelligent members of the medical profession want what the general community wants, viz: that a license to practise in this State shall be given to those only who can pass an examination before a Board chosen by the State, and subject to the scrutiny of all of its citizens, and that the possession of a degree shall not carry with it the right to practise after a mere registration. We believe that all who oppose a law of this kind are consciously or unconsciously working to keep the practice of medicine open to the ignorant and unprincipled, and we trust that nothing will prevent the adoption by the Legislature of the Bill now before it.

TREATMENT OF LOCOMOTOR ATAXIA BY SUSPENSION.

In a recent lecture at the Salpêtrière, in Paris, Professor Charcot has called attention to a very interesting suggestion in regard to the treatment of locomotor ataxia, or tabes, which was first made by Motchoukowsky, of Odessa, in Russia, and which Charcot has adopted with very striking results. In introducing this method to his hearers, as reported in the *Gazette Hebdomadaire*, January 25, 1889, Charcot took pains to make it clear that he had used every care to avoid the error of being carried away by the fascinations of a new method, or of attributing to it what might more properly be credited to other factors in the case. He also stated that the cases in which he had treated it were actual cases of ataxia— a statement which is hardly needed from so eminent and experienced a clinician.

The method of Motchoukowsky is simply suspension, as usually practised when a plaster jacket is applied for disease or deformity of the spinal column. The discovery of the method was purely accidental. Motchoukowsky was treating a patient with tabes, who had also a scoliosis. To remedy the latter, he suspended his patient and applied a plaster-of-Paris jacket. In a very short time the patient found himself very much relieved of the fulgurating pains with which he had suffered; and careful testing assured Motchoukowsky that this relief was caused not by the jacket, as he at first supposed, but by the suspension. After this he used suspension upon a large number of ataxia patients, with marked advantage to almost all of them.

This interesting result has now been confirmed by Charcot, who, since last October, has treated fifteen patients by suspension, with remarkable success. The method has been used two or three times a week, for a minute or two for the first few times and for two or three minutes at the succeeding ones.

The relief experienced by the patients consists in a marked diminution of the characteristic pains of locomotor ataxia, and of the inco-ordination. One of the most striking results of the method of treatment is the restoration of the sexual functions; and an investigation disclosed the fact that suspension was actually employed in establishments which exist in Paris for the cure of impotence!

It will prove of value to those who take an interest in this subject if they can go over the details given by Charcot of the effect of suspension in four or five of his cases; but without this, our readers may well believe that a method endorsed by so famous a teacher must have something of actual value in it. Its extreme simplicity, the ease with which it can be carried out, and the results attributed to it entitle it to the serious consideration of all medical men. If—as is to be sincerely hoped—the experience of Motchoukowsky and of Charcot are repeated in other lands than Russia and France, it will revolutionize the treatment of locomotor ataxia, and perhaps influence the treatment of other organic or functional diseases of the spinal cord.

If any of our readers have under their care patients with locomotor ataxia, we would be glad to have them apply this method and report its results for the benefit of their fellows, and as a contribution to medical science.

INFECTIOUS ULCERS OF THE CORNEA.

At the meeting of the Société d'Ophtalmologie of Paris, January 8, 1889, M. Abadie called attention to the conditions essential to the production of serious infectious ulcers of the cornea. These are: Erosion of the epithelium; inoculation with a pathogenetic microbe; and sufficiently prolonged contact of the organism and the denuded corneal tissue. The last condition might be considered to be included necessarily in the second; but M. Abadie points out that time is an important element, and that this accounts for the fact that serious ulcers of the cornea are perhaps never met with except in patients who are careless in their habits, and not strict in regard to cleanliness.

The treatment of these ulcers is indicated by their etiology. In the earliest stages they may be combated—and sometimes cured—with repeated washings with an antiseptic solution, and the insufflation of finely powdered iodoform. At a later period they require section, according to the method of Sæmisch, or cauterization with the galvano-cautery, with opening of the anterior chamber. In some cases a cure cannot be effected without thorough disinfection of the nasal cavity; for which purpose M. Abadie has used, with excellent results, a solution of mercuric chloride, one part to two thousand of water.

This last suggestion, in regard to the treatment of grave ulcers of the cornea, is one which may well be borne in mind; for it is easy to carry out, and as rational as it has proved to be useful in M. Abadie's hands.

CLASSIFICATION OF ABSCESSES.

As a result of his interest in bacteriological studies, Prof. Verneuil has recently proposed to classify abscesses according as their pus contains only the micrococci constantly found in pus, or also other microbes not characteristic of pus. This is in our opinion a somewhat premature suggestion. It might be interesting and instructive to have a collection of carefully observed data in regard to the distribution of the various microbes according to the character of the abscesses in which they are found; but far too little is known now about the relation of microbes to pus formation to justify any attempt to classify abscesses in the way Verneuil suggests.

More than this, an attempt of this sort leaves out of sight the fact that the mere presence of an abscess or its peculiar character often signifies less from a practical standpoint than the state or condition of the patient or the situation of the abscess. These are at present the things to be regarded in estimating the significance of abscesses; although it would undoubtedly enlarge our knowledge if it could be shown that abscesses of certain sorts are caused or always accompanied by certain microbes, and that the absence of such microbes is evidence that pus is of a more—or less, as the case may be—malignant character. With some definite information of this sort, the treatment and prognosis of abscesses might perhaps be modified, and certainly would be more accurate than they are at present.

Unfortunately, however, there is nothing of this sort known now. The bacteriological theories in regard to the formation of pus are still in a very immature state, and by no means ready to pass from the laboratory to the clinic.

REMOVAL OF FOREIGN BODIES FROM THE NOSE.

In a letter to the *Lancet*, Nov. 3, 1888, Dr. Charles W. Dodd describes an ingenious method of removing certain foreign bodies from the nose, which is worthy of extensive notice. He introduces a tube into the free nostril and blows suddenly into it so as to cause a strong pressure of air, passing back of the septum, behind the foreign body. He recommends, if this does not succeed at once, that the opposite nostril be closed by the surgeon while he blows, and the closure suddenly removed when the pressure is strong enough.

For the carrying out of this method Dr. Dodd uses a soft rubber tube provided with a hard rubber end made to fit the nostril; but almost any tube could be made to do the work if the surgeon is possessed of a little dexterity.

TREATMENT OF TONSILLITIS.

The treatment of tonsillitis is unfortunately by no means established upon a firm and uniform basis; and, so long as this is the case, it is worth while to call attention to methods which are said to have proved useful at the hands of intelligent medical men. For this reason, it is interesting to note that Dr. A. Hillaby, in the *Therapeutische Monatshefte*, December, 1888, speaks very highly of the results obtained by administering at the outset a simple carthartic, such as the infusion of senna, and following this up with doses of nine or twelve grains of salicylate of soda, several times a day. Under this treatment, he says, the fever and the local inflammation subside rapidly; the activity of the skin is re-established and the formation of abscesses in the tonsils is prevented. He recommends diminishing the dose of salicylate of soda when the inflammatory process is subsiding, but to continue it in small quantities until a cure seems assured.

—Small-pox prevails among the Indians at Fort Buford, Dakota.

BOOK REVIEWS.

[Any book reviewed in these columns may be obtained upon receipt of price, from the office of the REPORTER.]

DOSE AND PRICE LABELS OF ALL THE DRUGS AND PREPARATIONS OF THE UNITED STATES PHARMACOPŒIA OF 1880, ETC. BY C. L. LOCHMAN, Translator of the first and second editions of the German Pharmacopœia, etc. Third edition, revised and enlarged. 9 x 4¼ inches, pp. xvi, 201.

We have already noted with approval a former edition of this excellent book. It is primarily intended for the use of pharmacists; but is of such a character as to be very useful to medical men. It gives, in alphabetical order, the Latin and English names of all the drugs and compounds contained in the last U. S. Pharmacopœia, with a brief statement of their derivation, dose, and medical properties, with blanks for writing in the price of different quantities. It contains also an appendix, in which a number of common mixtures are described and a short account is given of many new drugs which have not yet been placed in the Pharmacopœia. A full index adds to the value of the book.

TEXT-BOOK OF MEDICAL JURISPRUDENCE AND TOXICOLOGY. BY JOHN J. REESE, M.D., Professor of Medical Jurisprudence and Toxicology in the University of Pennsylvania, etc. Second edition. Revised and enlarged. 8vo, pp. xvi, 646. Philadelphia: P. Blakiston, Son & Co., 1889. Price, $3.00.

Those who have had the pleasure of attending upon the lectures of Prof. Reese at the University will look upon the appearance of this second edition of his excellent manual as the return of an old friend. In it are found the same charms of a clear and graceful style, and the same merit of thorough and accurate teaching. The book covers the whole range of subjects coming under the general term medical jurisprudence and toxicology, and gives in admirable shape what physicians and lawyers ought to know about the medico-legal relations of deaths from suspected violence and poisoning, about feigned diseases, pregnancy, abortion, feticide, infanticide, legitimacy and inheritance, rape, insanity, medical malpractice and life insurance.

The author discusses all these subjects with due consideration of the medical and legal sides of each, and with a judgment and discrimination which are the result of years of practice as a teacher and as an expert witness in the Courts.

It is a pleasure to be able to speak in such unqualified terms of approval of any book; and we feel sure that those who turn to it on our recommendation will not be disappointed in it. It is a work which does great credit to its author, and its paper, printing and binding are equally creditable to its publishers.

LITERARY NOTES.

—*The North American Practitioner* is the name of a new medical magazine to be published monthly by Charles Truax and Company, Chicago. It will be edited by Drs. Bayard Holmes and Junius C. Hoag in the interests of the Post-Graduate Medical School of Chicago. The first number presents a good appearance and makes a favorable impression.

CORRESPONDENCE.

The Medical Examining Board.

To the Editor:

Sir: I see the fight on the Medical Examining Bill has begun, and the warring factions may think it senseless. It might be better for us to yield a point to the other fellows than to have the whole thing "dished." For instance, give them a show on "theory and practice," for an examination their own way. I am no lover of the homœopathic system; but we must recognize that there are just as true gentlemen, loyal citizens, and Christians practising in the other schools as in our own, and legally we are compelled to recognize them, if not professionally. So we may as well yield to the "legal," and be done with it. I have therefore suggested to Representative Randall to amend the "Walk bill" by making the number of the Board twelve, instead of nine: six to be chosen from the Regular, three from the Homœopathic, and three from the Eclectic school, to be chosen from the registered lists of practitioners of over ten years' practice, regardless of political faith. This is only simple justice; there are many excellent doctors who are not members of any medical society, and it is not right to debar these men from positions on that account. Cases of gross injustice in medical societies are not uncommon, nor is professional courtesy or ability confined to them alone. Besides this, in a work of this kind the support of every good practitioner and man is wanted, and no society should put itself as the arbiter of his fate or promotion. Also, that eight members be a quorum; this keeps the representation even. That the Secretary and President be not of the same school. That the examinations on anatomy, physiology, chemistry, toxicology, pathology, hygiene, surgery, and obstetrics be before the whole board (or quorum); that no applicant be obliged to state his or her school of practice, or exhibit any certificate or diploma until after this examination. On the branches of "Theory and Practice of Medicine" and "Materia Medica," the examination to be before the examiners of the Board belonging to the school to which the applicant belongs. That the exclusive use of Latin names in answering questions shall not be required; and that all practitioners of medicine now registered according to law have issued to them a license to practice, and all be obliged to post the same in their office.

On such a bill all fair-minded doctors could agree; the gentlemen of the different schools could surely repress their prejudices while examining on the branches that all concede to be essential and in which there is no difference of opinion.

The above is merely suggestive, but I hope it will be of some help to the brethren who are trying to improve the quality, if not the quantity, of the profession.

Yours truly,
Marienville, Pa.,   S. S. Towler, M.D.
Feb. 7, 1889.

Removal of Gun-Powder From the Face.

To the Editor.

Sir: In the Reporter, Feb. 2, p. 152, Dr. John Gray reports his method of removing gun-powder from the face. I cannot quite agree with him in his method, although he was successful. In allowing supuration to take place scarring is more likely to occur. This I always try to avoid, but it cannot always be done when the entire structure of the skin is burnt through. If only the outer layer is destroyed the supurating method can be used without much danger of destroying the deeper structures by subsequent inflammatory action. I will report a case which I saw with another physician, and give you my method of treatment.

W. J., about 21 years old, was standing over a blast in a slate quarry when it was discharged unexpectedly; his face was filled with powder, and so deeply that in many places the powder penetrated through the skin; his eyes were filled with powder, the cornea of one was deeply burnt, and powder lodged in its structures. The patient was almost insensible to any manipulations about the face. We removed every particle of powder or colored tissue from the face with scalpels, simply scraping the face clean; iced water was used to wash off the detached particles. This was a slow process, but it was a success. The same method was used to remove the powder and burnt tissues in the eyes, using finer instruments, however. Instead of washing the eyes with lint, they were freely syringed out with ice-cold water. The powder and burnt structures of the cornea were completely removed by the scraping and syringing. The only dressing used was lint, repeatedly changed to keep the face cool. The young man made a complete recovery. The cornea was restored entire. There was no scarring of the face, nor did any specks of powder remain. The face was kept covered with moistened lint as long as the structures remained unhealed. There was no suppuration, and consequently no scars. After the necessary cold water dressings to the eyes, small powders of calomel were dropped into them two or three times a day; whether the latter were of benefit or not I cannot say.

Yours truly,
JOHN M. CURRIER, M.D.
Newport, Vermont,
Feb. 6, 1889.

A Plea for Skimmed Milk.

TO THE EDITOR.

Sir: I want to call your attention to one matter in the milk bill now before the legislature. I think it should be altered so as to permit of the sale of pure unadulterated and undiluted *skimmed* milk. The only way to encourage temperance amongst the laboring classes is to give them a substitute for alcohol, which they will otherwise drink. *Unless food is made cheap high license or prohibition will be valueless in saving the laboring class.* As medical men we all know that to the laborer a pint of *skimmed* milk, otherwise pure and undiluted, represents a value as a force-producer and muscle-maker which the addition of the ordinary percentage of cream by no means increases in equal ratio to the additional expense. For the one he will probably pay five cents a quart, for the other ten cents a quart. I am heartily in favor of the heaviest penalty for milk, and indeed all food adulteration and dilution, but I am much opposed to the restriction of the sale of pure unadulterated skimmed milk, which is nutritious, healthful and within the means of the poorest laborer. Let him have it and plenty of it, in fact, let all his food be cheap and pure—milk, meat, bread and water, and in that way there will be a marked difference in the health and sobriety of these classes.

Yours truly,
JOHN M. KEATING, M.D.
Philadelphia,
Feb. 9, 1889.

—The Philadelphia *Ledger*, Feb. 16, says that physicians in Lowell, Mass., have formed an association "to guard themselves from imposition by transient people who have been in the habit of evading payment, going from one physician to another after having exhausted their credit."

NOTES AND COMMENTS.

The Welfare of Pharmacy.

The *Pharmaceutical Era*, Feb., 1889, says: The welfare of pharmacy depends upon the emphatic maintenance of special skill as a condition of its practice. As a mere division of commerce, without special learning, it is evident that the business of pharmacy must go under. The man who is to supply medicines, duly apportioned not to prove poisons, cannot take all his risks and pay all his expenses if he undertakes to trade wholly upon the business plane of the grocer, the clothier, the hardware dealer. A few weeks ago, a country grocer sold what he supposed to be "salts." It was sulphate of zinc. The wife of the purchaser took three teaspoonfuls. He is a man of grim determination. The grocer has made a hurried inquiry into the differences between kinds of salts, but one thing he is now sure of, it will not pay him to deal in any kind of salts for medicine. It is true all the way up, it does not pay any man to deal in chemicals unless he knows what they are. If the pharmacist reaches out of his proper pursuit and deals in certain common wares to eke out the scantiness of cheapened reward, let him all the more hold fast to his anchor of special skill in his proper calling, unless indeed he is ready to give up altogether. The welfare of every pharmacist stands with his professional training, and the good of the body of pharmacists stands or falls with the general basis of learning in pharmacy.

Cocaine in Cancer of the Breast.

J. F. Somerville states in a letter to the *Lancet*, Jan. 26, 1889, that a patient was operated on about two years ago for cancer, the entire left breast being removed. Twelve months after the operation the disease reappeared and developed so considerably that the same surgeon was again consulted, and he pronounced the case hopeless. Three months later the usual intense pain which accompanies such cases set in, and it became simply a question of alleviating suffering. After the usual remedies for relieving pain had proved ineffectual, Mr. Somerville tried a cocaine ointment (one part in twenty). It had, he says, a marvelous effect; the pain was subdued almost immediately, and remained continually subdued by its use. He states that it was used for two months, there being no occasion during that time even to increase the strength. The patient died Dec. 24, without the least suffering.

Oil of Turpentine in Diphtheria.

In the *Omaha Clinic*, Jan. 1889, Dr. J. H. Peabody has a communication on the treatment of diphtheria with oil of turpentine. He refers to a former communication by him published in the REPORTER Sept. 9, 1876, at a time when the use of the oil of turpentine for this purpose was not mentioned in most if any of the current textbooks.

Dr. Peabody says: "I have carefully selected from 613 cases of throat disease, occurring in my practice during the last fifteen years, 175 cases of diphtheria. I say carefully, for I do not wish you to think that any case of follicular tonsillitis has been included in the 175 cases. If any error has been made it is in placing some mild cases of diphtheria among my 438 cases of tonsillitis, as I treat them at the onset with exactly the same remedies used in diphtheria; and I am confident I have jugulated many a case of this fell disease and prevented its spread in schools and homes where I have used turpentine."

During the past four or five years he says he has employed the following:

R Ol. terebinthinæ . . . . . . f℥ ii
Sacch. albi . . . . ℥ ii
Pulv. acaciæ . . . . ℥ ii
Aquæ . . . . f℥ iv

Misce. Sig. Shake up and give a dessertspoonful every three hours to an adult or to a child twelve years old. Alternate with two grain doses of quinine given in coffee.

In sthenic cases in the adult he allows a dessertspoonful of liquor ammoniæ acetatis with five drops of the tincture of aconite root, every three hours until there is some abatement in fever. If the patient is not decidedly better by the second or third day, tincture of the chloride of iron is given in large doses, and the patient is sustained with brandy in proper doses. By this means, a child 12 years old gets about twelve drops of the oil of turpentine every three hours. He also has a vapor diffused through the room by pouring turpentine and water on a hot brick, or by a water-bath. Strangury has in several instances occurred to a slight extent in his practice with the dose mentioned.

He says he has been called in consultation in a number of cases after violent septic poisoning has occurred, and has derived no benefit from turpentine in the heroic dose of a teaspoonful. Tincture of iron and chinoline with brandy in large doses are then indicated; but under any and all treatment the mortality is fearful.

A Characteristic Reaction of Bismuth.

A solution of iodide of bismuth in iodide of potassium is sometimes used, under the name of iodobismuthate of potash, for the research of the alkaloids. It gives insoluble, orange-yellow compounds with many natural inorganic bases, but gives no indication of the nature of the alkaloid found. I have thought, writes M. E. Léger, in the *Journal de Phar. et de Chim.*, Dec. 15, 1888, that this would be otherwise should we use such a reagent in finding bismuth. I used a reagent composed of cinchonine, 1 part; iodide of potassium, 2 parts; distilled water, 100 parts. The cinchonine is dissolved in water with the aid of a few drops of nitric acid; the liquid is heated and the iodide added. This solution, added to one of nitrate of bismuth, gives an orange-yellow precipitate. It should be used in excess, avoiding solutions containing hydrochloric or sulphuric acid; it must not contain too much nitric acid. This reagent may be used for metals precipitable by sulphuretted hydrogen, whose sulphides are insoluble in sulphhydrate of ammonium. It gives, with minimum solutions of mercury, a greenish-yellow precipitate, turning black with excess; maximum solutions give yellowish-white; cadmium, white or yellowish; silver, the iodide if the argentic salt is in excess, yellow if the reagent is in excess; copper (minimum), precipitate of cupric iodide; maximum, brown maroon, containing iodine, copper, and cinchonine; lead, sulphur-yellow precipitate, soluble in an excess of nitrate of lead, and containing iodine, lead, and cinchonine.—*Amer. Jour. Pharmacy*, Feb., 1889.

Lanolin in Suppositories.

According to M. L. Broutin, *Bull. Com.*, Nov., 1888, lanolin greatly facilitates the introduction into suppositories of extracts or other substances soluble in water. He thinks that when the choice of an excipient is left to the pharmacist, the latter may properly replace a small quantity of the cacao butter with lanolin. The following formula is cited as having given excellent results: Dry extract of hamamelis, gr. xii; lanolin, gr. cxl; cacao butter, ℥ vii; for 25 suppositories. The extract is heated with a sufficient quantity of water, to which the melted butter is added by degrees. The mass should be run off as soon as it commences to thicken. The suppositories are entirely homogeneous.—*Amer. Jour. Pharmacy*, Feb., 1889.

Incubation of Scarlet Fever.

At the meeting of the Nottingham Medico-Chirurgical Society, Jan. 4, 1889, Dr. Whitelegge read a paper on the duration of the incubation period in scarlet fever. Dealing first with experimental evidence, he took exception to Trousseau's view that inoculation is the only means of determining the latent period of a disease, pointing out that the period is not always constant even in inoculated diseases, and that the latency of an inoculated disease is usually shorter than that of the same disease when acquired without inoculation. The latent period of inoculated small-pox, for example, cannot be accepted as even approximately true of ordinary small-pox. A similar consideration applies to cases of infection by milk, and to surgical scarlet fever. For practical purposes, reliance has to be placed mainly on the result of observation of individual cases, and the evidence of this kind is divisible into four classes: (1), cases following a single exposure; (2), cases in which a maximum limit can be fixed; (3), cases in which a minimum limit can be fixed; and (4), indirect evidence derived from massed observations of a certain kind. The first and third are open to error, since infection may be carried for a time before infecting the system; the value of the second and third is mainly confirmatory or corrective. The estimate given by earlier authorities is much too long. In many instances the range adopted is so wide as to be useless for guidance in practice, and it becomes necessary to ask if there is not some well-marked usual period which would hold true of the great majority of cases. Murchison and Squire have shown that the usual latency is short, not exceeding three or four days at most.

Many cases were cited in support of this view, including fifteen which had come under Dr. Whitelegge's own observation; and stress was laid upon the constancy of the three days' incubation in the cases of definite limited exposure in infected ambulances recorded by Dr. Tonge Smith and others. Among the confirmatory indirect evidence, he said, is the comparative rarity of appearance of rash on Wednesdays, possibly accounted for by exceptional conditions on Sunday; and also the sudden reduction in the average number of second attacks in infected households about three days after the average date of cessation of acute symptoms in the respective first cases, followed by an increase about three or four days after the average date of commence-ment of desquamation in the first cases. It has been found that, of the new cases occurring in a house after removal of a patient to hospital, three-quarters presented a rash within five days of the removal. Instances of protracted incubation are to be regarded with suspicion, partly for the reasons already stated, but also on account of the difficulty or impossibility of excluding more recent sources of infection. The majority of ordinary cases are infected from unknown sources, and, if they happened to be exposed to known infection a week or two previously, they might rank as examples of prolonged latency. After reviewing the evidence, Dr. Whitelegge expressed the opinion that the usual period of incubation is three days, or, at all events, between two and four days; and that it is rarely less than one day, and very rarely, if ever, more than seven days.—*British Med. Journal*, Jan. 26, 1889.

Case of Acute Cirrhosis of the Liver.

Körner communicates an account of this case to the *Deutsches Archiv für klin. Medicin*, xlii, S. 615. A woman 20 years old was received into the hospital after she had been sick some days with headache, lassitude, nausea, and, more frequently, vomiting. On her admission the patient had no fever, the thoracic viscera were healthy, the liver and spleen not enlarged, the uterine adnexa free. The belly was a little swollen, and somewhat tender on pressure in the neighborhood of the pylorus and cæcum. The breath was fetid. The urine contained no albumin. The bowels were moved first on the day following admission, after the administration of castor oil.

In a few days there was slight rise of temperature in the evening and slight jaundice. On the fourth day after admission the lower border of the liver was felt in the mamillary line one centimetre (.39 inch) below the edge of the ribs; the liver itself was very tender. The patient was very restless. Two days later jaundice was very marked. The liver now projected five centimetres (about two inches) below the ribs, and extended into the left hypochondrium. The urine contained much bile pigment, and was only secreted in small quantities. There were hemorrhages from the nose and gums. Some days later there was a subsidence of the swelling of the liver. Numerous crystals of leucin and tyrosin were present in the urine. On the tenth day after her admission the patient died with symptoms of acute œdema of the lung. At the autopsy numerous hemorrhages were found in the skin, and in the mucous and serous membranes. The liver was nearly normal in size, ochre-yellow in color, its capsule opaque in places and thickened. A microscopic examination of the tissue demonstrated the disease to be an acute cirrhosis of the liver.—*Centralblatt f. d. med. Wissenschaften*, Jan. 5, 1889.

Nikiforow's Carmine.

Dr. Nikiforow (*Zeitschrift für Wiss. mik.*) recommends a formula for a carmine stain which acts intensely on the nucleus, and can be used with advantage for staining specimens in toto, and which does not require after treatment with the strong acids which act harmfully on the tissues. It is prepared as follows: Take three parts of carmine, 5 parts of borax and 100 parts of water, and boil in a porcelain dish until a small portion of the carmine has dissolved. Add sufficient ammonia to dissolve the remaining carmine, and the liquid takes on a deep cherry-red color. The mixture is now evaporated by boiling to somewhat more than one-half its volume. Carefully neutralize with dilute acetic acid, when the cherry-red color gives place to one of a carmine tint. The secret is not to get too much acid (Grenacher's carmine), for such a preparation will require after treatment with an acid (? alkali). The safest way is to add the acid slowly and experiment from time to time. When the solution is prepared, a few drops of carbolic acid may be added, and it will keep indefinitely. Tissues which have been preserved in alcohol are stained by it in about fifteen minutes, though no overstaining takes place after twenty-four hours.—*Microscope*, Jan., 1889.

A Beautiful and Durable Cement for Ringing Balsam Mounts.

Mr. J. D. Beck sends the following to the *Microscope*, Jan., 1889: To a thick solution of gum arabic add a little glycerine to prevent cracking. Ring balsam mounts with this first, then finish with the same cement colored with magenta, or fuchsine, or the "Diamond" black dye dissolved in water. Ornament with gold paint, etc., and finish with "Winsor & Newton's" mastic picture varnish. Try cement on a blank slide; if brittle when hard, add a little more glycerine, so that it will harden in twenty-four hours without brittleness.

Surgical Treatment of Chronic Cervical Adenitis.

The Lyons correspondent of the *Bulletin Médical*, Jan. 23, 1889, says that M. Poncet has made a communication to the Academy of Medicine on the surgical treatment of chronic adenitis. He distinguishes two kinds. In the first the glands are superficial, although sub-aponeurotic, and extirpation can often be accomplished with the knife or the scissors. In the second the deep carotid or subclavian glands are affected, and the difficulties of extirpation are increased.

Surgical intervention may be divided into several steps. In the first the glands are exposed by incising the skin and soft parts. The incisions should be long, even measuring at times fifteen centimetres (nearly six inches). The second step comprises the extirpation or the destruction of the diseased glands. The use of the knife is simple and easy for superficial glands, but becomes dangerous in deep glands on account of the risk of wounding the vessels and nerves. The diseased gland must first be fixed with the left index finger and then punctured with the point of the knife. Through this opening a small curette is introduced and part of the diseased tissue removed; a larger curette is then inserted and the sub-capsular enucleation of the gland completed in a few seconds. The same operation is repeated for each gland, and in this way as many as ten or fifteen may be removed at one sitting.

The third step consists in covering the whole wound with a layer of iodoform, inserting a drainage tube through the whole length of the wound, letting it just come out of the inferior angle, and in taking a number of stitches to insure immediate union. He states that recovery is very rapid, occurring in from fifteen to twenty days, and that it is permanent, several patients having been seen completely cured two years after operation.

Combination of Syphilis and Cancer.

Lang states in the *Wiener med. Blätter*, No. 10, 1888, that he had previously observed three cases in which cancer had arisen from syphilitic ulcers; in one case the ulcer was upon the face (rodent ulcer), in another under the tongue, and in the third upon the lower lip. He then presented a fourth case in which a carcinoma had developed upon the anterior edge of a syphilitic ulcer of the palate. The diagnosis was established by microscopic examination in all cases.—*Centralblatt für Chirurgie*, Dec. 15, 1888.

Benefits of Vaccination.

In Paris, where the law requiring vaccination is feebly enforced, the mortality from small-pox ranges from 136 to 10.1 to the 100,000 inhabitants, while in the principal German cities, where the vaccination laws are rigidly enforced, the death-rate is but 1.44 to the 100,000 inhabitants. London, under compulsory vaccination, has a death-rate from small-pox of but .6 to the 100,000 inhabitants. On the other hand, in the Canton of Zurich, in Switzerland, since the compulsory vaccination law was repealed in 1883, the death-rate from small-pox has risen steadily from 8 to 85 to the 100,000 inhabitants.

A report lately published by Mr. Ritchie, President of the British Local Government Board, with reference to the recent epidemic of small-pox in Sheffield, shows that of the children under ten years of age, 95,000 were vaccinated and 5000 were not. Among the vaccinated there were 189 cases of small-pox with 2 deaths; among the unvaccinated there were 172 cases and 70 deaths. Keeping these proportions, if all the children in Sheffield had been vaccinated, there would have been 200 cases of small-pox among them and a fraction more than 2 deaths; if none of the children had been vaccinated, there would have been 3337 cases and 1330 deaths, 600 times the mortality with universal vaccination.—*Sanitarian*, Jan., 1889.

Alcoholic Solution of Hæmatoxylin.

Dr. G. Cucatti (*Centralblatt für Bakteriologie und Parasitenk.*) gives the following formula for making a hæmatoxylin solution which possesses the advantages of never turning bad and of staining only the chromatic part of the nuclei, the color being fixed most deeply in the karyokinetic figures.

Dissolve 25 grm. (6½ drachms) of pure potassium iodide in 25 ccm. (6¾ fluid drachms) of distilled water, and pour the mixture into a glass-stoppered bottle containing 75 ccm. (2⅓ fluid ounces) absolute alcohol, shaking the whole repeatedly. Then grind together in a mortar 75 c.grm. (12½ grains) of hæmatoxylin crystals and 6 grm. (1½ drachms) of alum. When these are intimately mixed, add 3 ccm. (50 minims) of the iodide solution. Keeping the mixture well stirred, add little by little the rest of the solution, and then pour into a well-stoppered bottle, and leave for ten to fifteen days. At the end of this period,

shake up well again and in an hour or two afterward filter, and preserve the filtrate very carefully to prevent evaporation and deposit of iodide crystals. This solution only stains up to a certain point, consequently the sections may be left in it almost indefinitely.—*Microscope*, Jan., 1889.

Toxic Effect of Cocaine.

Dr. Moizard reports in the *Journal de Médecine*, Dec., 1888, that a child 4 years old took by accident four grains of cocaine. There was no immediate effect; the child went quietly to sleep. One hour afterward he awoke in frightful agony. The face was pale, the respiration difficult; there were nausea, pains in the upper portion of the chest, formication, cramps of the limbs, and great muscular agitation. The child could get no rest, and was a prey to terrifying hallucinations. An enema containing eight grains of chloral, followed two hours later by one containing five grains, was given. The child began to get quiet. During the night it slept, but was frequently awakened by convulsive movements. On the following day it was perfectly well.—*Amer. Jour. Pharmacy*, Feb., 1889.

Relative Age in Procreation.

At a recent meeting of the Hungarian Academy of Sciences, Prof. Korösi read a paper on the influence of parents' ages on the vitality of children. The point is one which has hitherto received but scant attention at the hands of ethnological statisticians, but M. Korösi has collectd some 30,000 data, from which he deduces the following conclusions: Mothers under the age of twenty, and fathers under twenty-four, procreate children endowed with a less aggregate vitality than the offspring of parents of maturer ages. These children are especially liable to lung diseases. The healthiest children are those whose fathers are from 25 to 40 years of age, and whose mothers are between 20 and 30. He affirms that the best results are obtained from the union of a man the senior of the wife, but a woman between 30 and 35 will fare best with a somewhat younger husband. The wife of a man between 30 and 40 should not exceed 30 years of age, and whenever the mother's age exceeds that of the father by more than five years the health and vitality of the offspring are likely to suffer.—*Medical Press and Circular*, Jan. 23, 1889.

The Nature of Milk.

The results of a study of this subject were lately submitted by M. A. Béchamp to the Paris Society of Pharmacy. The author's conclusions are (*Union Phar.*, Dec., 1888): Milk is not an emulsion. The milky globules are not simply fat globules, but true adipose vesicles in a freed condition. Cow's milk contains, beside casein, albuminoid substances which are not free, being dissolved in combination with alkalis. Human milk is not, strictly speaking, a casein milk; it contains a ferment which is peculiar to it. (See *Comptes rendus*, xcvi, p. 1508). Milk coagulates spontaneously, *i.e.*, without the aid of vibriones.—*Amer. Jour. Pharmacy*, Feb., 1889.

Food for Shipwrecked Seamen.

The Prince of Monaco lately read a paper before the French Academy of Sciences, in which he said that shipwrecked seamen who have to take to the boats without provisions on the high seas can obtain food from the ocean itself by trailing a drag net made of any light stuff along the surface during the night. The net will, in the morning, be found to contain some small shell fish available for food. In the sea to the west of the Azores, the Prince added, the vegetable matter on the surface teems with animal life and fish which are capable of affording substantial nutriment.—Phila. *Ledger*, Feb. 11, 1889.

Eczema of the Anus and Genitalia.

In the *Deutsche med. Wochenschrift*, Jan. 17, 1889, the following method of treating eczema of the anus and genitalia is given: Hot sitz-baths, and washing with soapy water, followed by inunction twice a day of

℞ Cocain. oleat.	4–10 parts
Ol. olivæ	20 "
Lanolin	100 "

—Dr. C. Meymott Tidy has been awarded the Swiney prize, consisting of a silver cup and 100 guineas. It is given by the Society of Arts and the Royal College of Physicians of London conjointly, for work in jurisprudence.

—The hospital of the Johns Hopkins University will be formally opened May 1. Its organization has been entrusted to President Gilman, who, it is said, will reside in the hospital and exercise a close personal supervision over its executive management.

NEWS.

—Dr. J. W. Cox, of Pine Bluff, Arkansas, was shot in that place, Feb. 12.

—Dr. J. B. Taylor died while attending a patient in East Cambridge, Mass., Feb. 15.

—Dr. Herman von Meyer, Professor of Anatomy in Zurich, has just died, at the age of seventy-four years.

—Boston physicians have been ordered to make a monthly return of the number of births attended by them.

—Dr. Henry F. Formad has withdrawn his resignation as Demonstrator of Pathology in the University of Pennsylvania.

—A disease described as resembling membranous croup is reported to be raging among the children at Wabash, Indiana.

—The William F. Jenks Prize for the best essay on the "Diagnosis and Treatment of Extra-uterine Pregnancy" has been awarded to Dr. John Strahan, of Belfast, Ireland.

—Dr. D. W. Cheever has given $5,000 to the Medical Department of Harvard University to establish a scholarship to be known as the "David Williams Cheever Scholarship."

—Dr. Francis B. Kane, Professor of Clinical Medicine in the Medical Department of the University of California, died recently in San Francisco of pneumonia, after a very short illness.

—Dr. F. G. Mitten reports a case to the Cincinnati *Lancet Clinic*, Feb. 16, in which he suggests that a certain deformity, which is present in a child five months old, is due to a supernumerary clavicle.

—Dr. Carl Zoller, of Philadelphia, has been bound over by United States Commissioner Bell to answer the charge of sending obscene postal cards to the Medico-Jurisprudence Board of Pennsylvania.

—The New York Postgraduate Medical School and Hospital has obtained a lease for ten years of the property adjoining its present location, and will use the addition for increasing the babies' wards of the Hospital.

—The *Chemist and Druggist*, Jan. 26, says that a pharmacist in Warsaw was recently making up a prescription consisting of 32 parts of chlorate of potassium and 4 parts of tannic acid, and on adding a few drops of oil of peppermint to flavor it, the mixture exploded with great force, doing considerable damage. A St. Petersburg pharmacist has dispensed the prescription with the same result.

HUMOR.

"GEORGE, dear, what kind of fruit is borne by an electric-light plant?" "Electric currents, of course."—*Terre Haute Express.*

WHAT "FAMILY PHYSICIAN" MEANS.— "Who is General Bickett's family physician?" was asked of a doctor. "I guess I am," was the reply; "at least, he owes me three hundred dollars."—*Puck.*

A NEW WAY OF DIAGNOSTICATING SHOULDER PRESENTATION.—Quiz Master— How do you diagnosticate a shoulder presentation? Student—By feeling for the hair in the axilla.—*Medical Record.*

MINISTERIAL RISK —"I'm very glad to have been of any comfort to your poor husband, my good woman. But what made you send for me, instead of your own minister?" "Well, sir, it's 'typhus' my poor husband's got, and we dinna think it just reet for our ain minister to run the risk!"— *Punch.*

PRECAUTIONARY.—Quilpin—"And now, sweetest, what kind of an engagement ring will you have? Shall it be a diamond?" Sweetest (hesitatingly)—"O, Algernon, pardon me, but—but—" Quilpin—"But what love?" Sweetest—"You newspaper men have so much to do with paste, you know, that—suppose you let me go with you when you select it?"—*Burlington Free Press.*

HISTORIC JOKES.—Napier's famous despatch from India announced his victory in one word, "Peccavi"—which is, by interpretation, "I have Scinde." Very much of the same kind was Gen. de Bourmont's message to the French War Minister in 1830, when the Dey of Algiers escaped him after being taken. "Perdidi Diem"—"I have lost a Dey." It is said that Drake, when the ships of the Armada turned their sails, sent to Elizabeth the word "Cantharides"—that is, "The Spanish fly." This last is probably a fable.—*Temple Bar.*

"WHAT a QUICK-TEMPERED FELLOW Gapeleigh is!"

"Why, what has he been doing now?"

"We were at dinner the other day, and Gapeleigh—who never has any use for a fork, you know—was quite in earnest in what he was pleased to call the unreasoning prejudice against the knife at table. He contended, with much warmth, that the knife was the proper thing to eat with. It was the most convenient, every way—at least, he found it so."

"Well, and what then?"

"Oh, I simply remarked that all persons were not gifted with a mouth like the mouth of a river; and, if you'll believe it, Gapeleigh took it as a personal affront, and he hasn't spoken to me since. But then he's so quick-tempered it's hard to get along with him, any way."—*Boston Transcript.*

OBITUARY.

MARY H. STINSON, M.D.

Dr. Mary H. Stinson died at Norristown, Pa., Feb. 11, of erysipelas. She was born on November 14, 1819, and was therefore in the 70th year of her age. After studying at the female seminary in Charlestown, Mass., she studied medicine and was graduated in the class of 1869, from the Woman's Medical College of Pennsylvania, the Faculty of which College recommended her for the position of assistant physician in the department for women at the Massachusetts State Lunatic Hospital at Worcester, a position to which she was elected by the Trustees in July, 1869. This was the first appointment of a woman to such a position. In 1875 Dr. Stinson resigned, and the next year visited Europe to make a study of the manner of conducting the hospitals for the insane and the sick, and the medical departments of the universities. When the Hospital for the Insane for the Eastern District of Pennsylvania was organized at Norristown, she was offered the position of resident physician of the Women's Department, but declined it.

JOHN C. DALTON, M.D.

Prof. John C. Dalton, of New York, died Feb. 12. Dr. Dalton was born 64 years ago in Massachusetts, and was graduated from Harvard University in 1847. He served successively as Professor in the Medical Departments of the Universities of Buffalo and Vermont, and of the Long Island Hospital College, and in 1855 began his long service with the College of Physicians and Surgeons of New York, a service broken only by his term in the army, where he became brigade surgeon. He was the author of the well-known text-book on physiology. He was the first in this country to teach physiology with illustrations by vivisection. In the International Medical Congress, held in Philadelphia in 1876, Dr. Dalton was a delegate from the American Medical Association, and was chosen President of the section on Biology.

MEDICAL AND SURGICAL
REPORTER

No. 1670.   PHILADELPHIA, MARCH 2, 1889.   VOL. LX.—No. 9.

CONTENTS:

LECTURE.

FAILURE OF VISION IN OLD AGE.[1]

BY EDWARD JACKSON, A.M., M.D.,
PROFESSOR OF DISEASES OF THE EYE IN THE PHILA-
DELPHIA POLYCLINIC.

It is a general law that the more highly differentiated or developed an organism or an organ, the more liable it is to injury by violence from without, or defect of nutrition from within. From this liability the delicate and complex visual apparatus is not exempt. It is universally understood that some sort of loss of visual power is a necessary condition of old age; but few appreciate how often remediable conditions are taken as part of the inevitable, and submitted to without any attempt to get relief.

The conditions causing impairment of vision coming on with age might be grouped under two heads: physiological, those arising in what must be regarded as a strictly normal course from development to dissolution; and pathological, or those diseases to which age renders the eye especially liable. But between the two groups no hard and fast line can be drawn. There are conditions, such as senile nerve-atrophy and cataract, which, though commonly classed with diseases, are so closely allied to the normal senile degenerations, that the placing of them in the one group or the other would seem to depend mainly on the age at which they occur, or the relative advancement of other processes of bodily decay.

Failure of Accommodation.

Among physiological conditions, most important is failure of accommodation, beginning in infancy and almost complete at the period when other senile changes are fairly begun. Primarily the loss of power to focus the eye for near objects depends on increased rigidity of the crystalline lens. The lens, jelly-like and extremely elastic in infancy, becomes progressively harder and

[1] One of the Tuesday Evening Lectures, delivered at the Philadelphia Polyclinic.

257

less elastic year by year. So that while during adolescence the ciliary muscle actually increases in strength, its power of changing the shape of the crystalline lens and rendering it more convex steadily diminishes. As the process continues the near point of perfect focussing, and distinct vision, recedes; until between 40 and 50 years, in the normal course of the change, ordinary close work, such as reading, writing, sewing, etc., is interfered with, and *presbyopia* is said to begin. Yet even when this occurs there may still be no diminution in the muscular power brought to bear on the crystalline lens, but simply an increased resistance to any change of shape. Later when the power of accommodation has been still farther diminished, so that what remains is of but little practical importance to its possessor, and he comes to rely on glasses for any change of focus, the ciliary muscle often undergoes atrophy, caused or accelerated by disuse; and the remnant of accommodative power is entirely lost. After this failure, which for all emmetropic and hyperopic eyes has necessitated the wearing and frequent strengthening of glasses, is complete, there can be no farther loss of sight from this source. It is popularly regarded as remarkable that a person of eighty or ninety should be able to read with the same glasses as he wore twenty or thirty years before; but really the failure that glasses were sought to make good, is commonly complete at sixty, and unless the eye is changed in some other respect, no other glasses could be so satisfactory.

Senile Ametropia.

The loss of the power of accommodation does more than simply interfere with the seeing of near objects. While emmetropia is the standard aimed at in the development of the eye, few eyes accurately attain it. In nearly all there is present a perceptible amount of ametropia, usually in the direction of hyperopia; which the power of accommodation enables one to correct. This power being gone the ametropia becomes absolute, and distant vision also becomes imperfect. Hence the large majority of persons, through changes strictly physiological, suffer some failure of vision with age. But this failure can in a manner be compensated by the use of glasses.

The same compensation is available in the case of ametropia not formerly present and unmasked by loss of accommodative power, but arising from senile changes in the form or refractive power of the cornea or lens. Such ametropia generally takes the form of hyperopia, the so-called "H. acquisita"; but in quite an important class of cases there is an increase in the refractive power of the lens leading to myopia. These latter are the cases of "second sight." After having been compelled for years to wear convex glasses for near vision, they discover that they can again read with weaker lenses, or without any such aid at all. But this does not come through any recovery of power to change the focus of the eye, but through a gradual shifting of the point for which the eye is adjusted, from a distance to somewhere about the point at which objects are commonly held for near vision. The adaptation for near-seeing is gained by loss of distinctness in far-seeing. These same senile changes of the crystalline lens occasionally give rise to considerable degrees of regular astigmatism; and very generally in their more advanced stage cause irregular astigmatism. These same changes, carried but a little farther, result in opacity of the crystalline lens, or cataract.

Cataract.

This condition is of importance, not only because it is common and often causes the loss of all useful vision, but especially because its management often requires the reversal of the rule which applies to all other conditions likely to cause blindness. In other conditions treatment does most good, or only does good, when commenced at the earliest possible moment. In cataract radical treatment can be resorted to only after a longer or shorter period of delay. If, as happens not rarely, a diagnosis of cataract is made when the failure of vision is really due to something else, the patient is likely to be advised to enter upon a course of waiting which never can do any good, and that may consume the precious time, during which alone therapeutic measures could have been resorted to with any chance of benefit. On this account, I hold that every one offering himself to the people as a general practitioner of medicine or surgery, and undertaking to give any opinion as to a failure of sight, should be able to recognize with certainty whether, in any given case, cataract be, or be not, present to such extent as probably to cause the given impairment of vision.

Among methods that may be employed for the recognition of cataract, that of simple inspection, or inspection under the most favorable conditions, called *oblique illumination*, may be mentioned, only to state that no reliance whatever should be placed upon it. The experienced ophthalmic surgeon knows that while in some cases he can recognize cataract in this way, that any senile eye with a dark enough choroid, and large enough pupil, will present a striking appearance of opacity of the lens, although the lens may be absolutely normal and transparent. So that the largest experience will not enable him to judge whether it really is a case of cataract or not. Again, there are some cataracts, so-called black cataracts, in which the appearance of the pupil is quite normal. And even in ordinary forms of cataract, if the pupil be small and the opacity not immediately beneath the pupil it may not, in this way, be possible to recognize its presence.

The diagnosis of cataract is generally to be made with the *ophthalmoscope*. But by ophthalmoscope I do not mean any elaborate or high-priced instrument. The cheapest, the common "Liebreich" form, which cannot be spoken of as *good* for any thing else, answers this purpose as well as the most costly. The perforated concave mirror commonly used for illuminating the ear, nose, or throat, answers admirably; or, lacking all these, any piece of looking-glass with a little opening scratched in the silvering will be found quite satisfactory. Throwing the light into an eye with the ophthalmoscope, held ten or twelve inches distant, and placing his own eye at the aperature in the mirror, the observer sees the pupil of a normal eye occupied by a uniform red glare, paler in persons having a light choroid, or when the optic disc comes opposite to the observer, and more dusky as the choroid is darker. When however cataract is present, this red glare from the fundus of the eye is interrupted. If the cataract be advanced toward maturity, no red light from the fundus is perceived by the observer; but if even the smallest speck of lens substance has become opaque, it will appear as a black spot very noticeable against its brilliant red back-ground. Specks of opacity in the cornea, or upon the lens capsule, may cause the same appearance; but if the observer will move his position up and down, or from side to side, specks in the lens will seem to move across the pupil in the same direction as he moves, those in the cornea will seem to move in an opposite direction, and those on the lens capsule will appear to remain stationary. In the very few cases in which the ophthalmoscope does not entirely settle the diagnosis as to cataract, the *catoptric test* may be resorted to. In it we look for the little and rather faint inverted image, formed by the posterior surface of the normal lens, of a candle-flame held before the eye. We recognize this inverted image in this way. The cornea always gives us a bright erect image of the flame; and the inverted image we seek is situated on the opposite side of the pupil, and on moving the candle, while the corneal image moves with it, the image in question moves in exactly the opposite direction. Of course any opacity of the lens or its capsule prevents the formation of any such image.

You must not regard the certain recognition of the presence of lens opacity as completing the diagnosis of cataract. It only begins it. Many old people have some opacity of the crystalline lens, whose impairment of vision is due, perhaps entirely, to other causes. For cases occur in which, with very marked opacity of one portion of the lens, other portions are so little affected that the vision remains normal, or very nearly normal. But on the other hand, when the lens by its opacity gives evidence of damage by imperfect nutrition, it does not generally suffer alone. As a rule other parts of the visual apparatus suffer with it; and to their impaired function the lowering of vision may be due, quite as much as to cataract. So, while it may be quite unjustifiable to make a diagnosis of cataract when there is no cataract, it may be almost as bad for the patient to rest on the diagnosis of cataract, even though it be present, if along with it some other unrecognized lesion exists, which is equally or to a greater extent the cause of the impairment of vision. One other point about cataract is to be remembered, namely, its extreme frequency. After a certain age a majority of eyes present some lens opacity; and in extreme old age it is quite general; but the majority of persons die before the opacity has involved enough of the lens to deprive them of useful vision.

Glaucoma.

An affection frequently confounded with cataract, and always with most disastrous results, is glaucoma. In it the pupil is commonly rather large, and the lens looks gray, or greenish and partially opaque, to simple inspection, even though it is perfectly clear. The essential fact of the disease is increased tension or hardness of the globe. It occurs after middle age; and this has been ascribed to the increased size of the lens, which continues to grow throughout adult life. It is supposed that the lens pressing on the periphery of the iris hinders the out-flow of fluid from the eye, and thus causes the increased tension. The course of the malady is invariably, unless checked by treatment, toward absolute blindness, usually with great pain in and about the affected eye. But its progress is often very insidious and deceptive. Exacerbations occur during which the sight grows suddenly worse, followed by partial recoveries during which some of the visual power is gradually regained. The patient is inclined to hope that each "relapse" may be the last, and may be followed by more complete recovery; and fails to realize that each is a positive advance of the morbid process covering ground never to be regained, and with an ever increasing tendency toward accelerated movement. These exacerbations are commonly attended with pain and hyperemia of the globe, which ought to distinguish the affection absolutely from cataract, but which are too often ascribed to "neuralgia" and a "simple inflammation" of the eye-ball. Glaucoma is not a very common affection; but its strongly malignant tendency gives it a great claim on the attention of the general practitioner.

Passing over certain other pathological conditions which might claim notice here, such as albuminuric retinitis, and a form of chorio-retinitis that might well be designated as senile, as of comparatively less importance, let me call your attention especially to

Senile Amblyopia and Atrophy of the Optic Nerve.

Of course, I use the term amblyopia in its modern sense, to designate imperfect vision, which cannot be accounted for by any fault of refraction, or pathological process making itself manifest in any other way. The impairment of function must in such a case involve some portion of the nervous apparatus concerned in the act of seeing. Amblyopia occurring in old people is often to be regarded as strictly physiological, as merely a part of the general diminution of capacity of the organism to respond to external stimuli, which constitutes a true decline of life. Often the amblyopia is accompanied by or depends on a lessened blood-supply of the parts, which is shown by a pallor of the optic disc; and in many cases this local anemia is but part of a lessening of the general blood-supply, another kind of vital decline. But marked amblyopia may exist without perceptible local anemia, and a very noticeable pallor of the disc is not incompatible with perfect acuteness of vision. When both pallor of the disc and impairment of vision

are especially well-marked, the case may be regarded as one of optic atrophy. In cases of atrophy, however, there is also contraction of the field of vision. In senile atrophy, this contraction is concentric and most regular, and is especially great for color vision, red and green being distinguished only in the immediate vicinity of the fixation point.

A point which I wish in this connection especially to impress upon you is that you should not conclude that any given case is one of merely senile, or irremediable amblyopia, or nerve atrophy, until all other possible explanations of it are proved unsatisfactory. My experience indicates that in old people with inferior blood-supply, with diminished power of resistance, with lessened capacity for repair, the nervous portion of the visual apparatus is especially susceptible to the actions of certain substances that influence it injuriously, such as tobacco, lead, quinine, large doses of the bromides, etc.; and that these agents may produce amblyopia or atrophy, even though they are taken only in amounts that have previously produced no injurious effect whatever. For instance, I have now under observation a man, 60 years old, who had used tobacco very moderately, and only a little alcohol occasionally, ever since he was a boy, and who is using less now than in earlier years. His sight had been failing for six months, and was less than half the normal. Stopping the tobacco and alcohol, and taking full doses of strychnia gave him full vision within a month. Had I rested in a diagnosis of senile change, probably neither my patient nor I would have been the better off for our coming together.

━━━━━◆●◆━━━━━

—The *Medical Press and Circular*, Feb. 6, says: Fears have been expressed lest the Paris schools should be overrun with foreign students, and it would even seem that endeavors have been made to impose certain onerous restrictions on their attendance. A recent number of the *Revue Scientifique* contains a very eloquent protest against so unworthy a sentiment, especially on the eve of an international exhibition. The prestige of the ancient Faculty of Paris would suffer sadly were foreign visitors to be driven away, and its influence as an intellectual centre diminished. University teaching in France is practically free to all comers, and it is one of its most noble attributes. It is satisfactory to find that the *Chauvinists* are not likely to have it all their own way.

COMMUNICATIONS.

PRACTICAL ASEPTIC SURGERY.[1]

BY J. W. LONG, M.D.,

RANDLEMAN, N. C.

Mr. President and Gentlemen: On this occasion I hope to speak not so much *to* you as *through* you to the great body of patient toilers throughout the South. Southern doctors are beset by many trying difficulties. In the first place, most of them are dependent upon their practice for a living, while many have large families to support; besides, those of us who do not live where we are accessible to a drug-store are compelled to furnish our own medicines and surgical supplies. Add to these difficulties broken-down health—which is often the case—from overwork and exposure, and, I am sorry to say, sometimes from dissipation, and is it any wonder that the average Southern doctor buys so few new books and periodicals and so seldom reads them when he does get them? The subject which I shall endeavor to present to you to-day has invited so much speculation and given rise to so many varying methods, each claiming to be the right one, that our minds have become confused and we overlook the principles involved by considering the hypotheses and paraphernalia incident to the subject. If I can even to a small extent strip this great question of some of its extravagances and impracticabilities and present it to you in a practical everyday form, then I shall count myself most happy.

We all know that in these latter days the *technique* or management of accidental and surgical wounds is entirely different from what it was one or two decades ago. Formerly the operator expected suppuration; now he is disappointed if it occurs. Then surgical fever followed almost every operation as a matter of course; now its presence indicates some defect in the management of the wound. Aseptic surgery has come to be the order of the day, and it simply means surgical cleanliness as applied to the treatment of wounds. Aseptic surgery has made dangerous operations safe, and legitimized many heretofore unjustifiable procedures. It is the outcome of common observation that devitalized animal tissues when brought under favorable conditions putrefy. These favoring conditions are warmth, moisture,

[1] An address delivered before the Southern Surgical and Gynæcological Association, Dec. 4, 1888.

and certain micro-organisms. The absence of any one of these conditions will prevent the fermentive changes which in the living animal result in suppuration and septicæmia. Now I am not here to champion asepsis, nor to dispute with any one the validity of its principles, for I consider that these have already been established upon an immutable basis; and he who does not believe in aseptic surgery must necessarily believe in septic surgery. Notice, please, that I did not say *anti*septic but *a*septic; for antiseptics are only methods, while asepsis is a science involving great and unvarying principles: the one may change, the other never. Carbolic acid and corrosive sublimate may be forgotten, iodoform may be relegated to the realms of obscurity, but surgical cleanliness will ever be counted the greatest safeguard to life and health that man has yet devised.

The object of this paper is purely practical, and the hope is earnestly entertained that aseptic surgery may be set forth in such a light, stripped of all technicalities as well as of all unnecessary expense, that any regular doctor possessed of a fair knowledge of anatomy may at comparatively small cost fit himself to do in an aseptic manner all the operations which occur in every-day practice. After having once tried aseptic surgery and mastered its principles, I am sure no conscientious man will ever go back to the old ways of long finger-nails and rusty instruments.

To this end I have devised two bags, the smaller of which is my daily companion, the larger being used only in the more important operations. Prof. Gerster presented to the New York County Medical Society a bag to be used in "surgical emergencies," and while it is a capital thing, it is not adapted to the everyday work of the average practitioner. My larger bag is somewhat like his. I have been led to the construction of these bags by the repeated annoyance which arises from not being prepared to do the operations, great and small, that constantly come up in my practice. Not only has this been true of myself, but I know numbers of good men who believe in asepsis and antiseptics, and would like to do their operations aseptically, but they are not prepared to meet the emergencies as they arise, and they go along in the old slip-shod way. Furthermore, they are deterred from trying to get ready by the controversies and mystery which surround the subject and the supposed great expense of the necessary appliances. As a matter of fact, I do not know of one man in fifty who is prepared at any moment to amputate even a finger, or do a herniotomy, or any other operation in an aseptic manner.

The rules and formulæ of aseptic surgery are simple but comprehensive, and may be briefly stated as follows:

The proper cleansing of the surgeon's hands and arms and the parts to be operated on deserves the first consideration. The surgeon's coat should be removed, his sleeves rolled above the elbows, the finger-nails carefully pared and all dirt removed from under them by means of a sharp-pointed pen-knife. The hands and arms should then be scrubbed and soaked in hot water and soap. Lye soap is preferable because of its solvent properties. The hands ought to be kept in the water for at least five minutes, that the hard places and crevices may become thoroughly softened and cleansed. A stiff nail-brush is indispensable in cleansing the hands. After this the hands and arms should be placed for one minute in a solution of corrosive sublimate, 1 to 1000. During the operation a basin containing a similar solution is placed convenient to the operator, who dips his hands into it whenever he chances to touch anything that has not been sterilized, as a chair, his nose, a sponge picked up from the floor, etc. This same care of the hands is required of all the assistants. Surgical cleanliness means more than some people imagine. I remember seeing a doctor, who does a large amount of surgery and who professes to believe in and practice antisepsis, apply an ointment to the lids in a case of syphilitic conjunctivitis, then examine and make application to a case of hemorrhoids, catheterize a patient, and finally operate for double pterygium— all without washing his hands either before, during, or after treating these several cases. As Gerster says, "the new surgery of cleanliness does not tolerate pretense and imposition."

If possible, always have the patient bathe and change his clothing before an operation. When on the table the parts to be operated on must be carefully cleansed with hot water and soap, shaved, and finally washed with sublimate solution, 1 to 1000. Towels wrung out of a warm sublimate solution should be arranged around the field of operation.

It is impossible to do work aseptically with instruments that can not be rendered aseptic. The ingenuity and workmanship displayed in complicating instruments is simply wonderful—double joints, screws, rough handles, and every other device imaginable to make an instrument difficult or impossible to be cleaned. I am glad to note that modern surgery is demanding instruments more simple in construction, the revolution exhibiting itself in open joints and hard-rubber handles. An instrument should have as few joints as possible; most jointed instruments can be made with one joint, and this must be an open joint, either like the American bullet forceps, which have the French joint, or the Jones joint. Very few instruments indeed can not be made to come apart easily. Toothed instruments should have coarse teeth, with the angle between the teeth obtuse and rounding, so that all particles of matter may be readily dislodged by a stiff nail-brush. Those instruments not having solid metal handles should have baked-rubber handles. Such handles will withstand the effects of boiling water, which is the best medium for cleaning instruments. Wooden handles or rough handles are entirely unsuitable and should be discarded. Even the name of the manufacturer should not be stamped on an instrument. The Sims' dull curette is a beautiful example of an aseptic instrument, while the sharp curette is a typical example of a non-aseptic instrument. Horn handles like this scalpel are objectionable, as hot water causes the sides to spring away from the metal shank, leaving crevices in which particles of matter may lodge; we can never be sure they are clean. The Volkmann scoop is also perfectly aseptic, while the periosteal elevator is "a thing of beauty and a joy forever." These instruments were selected at random, and presented simply to show the difference between the perfect and faulty. I have been thus careful to particularize concerning the make-up of instruments for the reasons given above, and the additional fact that there is not a single pocket or operating case on the market, so far as I know, which meets the requirements of modern aseptic surgery. Every surgeon should select each individual instrument— don't buy anybody's "case," and see to it that in every respect each one is genuinely aseptic.

The care of instruments is an important item and has given me much concern. Half an hour before an operation they should be placed in a five per cent. solution of carbolic acid. For small operations a shorter time and a three per cent. solution will do. Knife blades remain in the solution only a few minutes, as the acid dulls the edge. Immediately after an operation place the instruments in a pan and pour very hot, even boiling, water over them. They should then be scrubbed thoroughly with soap and a brush, and dropped back into the carbolic solution, from which they are taken and dried with a soft cloth. It is very necessary that all toothed instruments be carefully brushed with a stiff nail brush in order to remove particles of blood and *débris* which invariably lodge between the teeth. For transportation instruments should be wrapped in a clean towel, or placed in canvas case, as either can be washed, but a leather case can not be washed and causes instruments to rust. No rust speck should be tolerated. The rust must be removed or the instrument laid aside. For permanent keeping a dust-proof drawer or case in a dry room is the best place to prevent instruments from rusting.

I am constrained to specify the care of catheters, because of the imperfect manner in which they are usually cared for. Before using, the cleansed catheter should be placed in three per cent. carbolic solution; a 1 to 1000 sublimate solution may be employed for rubber catheters. In either case, transfer the instrument to a solution of common salt 6 to 1000 (heaping teaspoonful to the quart of water, previously boiled), after which anoint them with iodoform ointment (gr. viii to ʒi). After being used in a septic case soft rubber and woven instruments should be destroyed. To cleanse rubber catheters, wash them in hot water and soap, and flush by means of a small syringe; then wash and flush in a five per cent. carbolic solution. Metal catheters can be properly cleaned only by prolonged boiling (an hour), or by passing through an alcohol flame until all smoke and steam cease to issue from them. An observance of these precautions will greatly lessen the number of cases of urethral fever and catarrh of the bladder.

If we could always have our hands, instruments, the parts to be operated on, the atmosphere, etc., in the ideal aseptic condition, there would be no need of germicides; but, unfortunately, we can not be sure of this happy condition. Therefore we resort to the chemical antiseptics, by means of which we keep a wound aseptic, or render it so by sterilization.

Antiseptics.—For irrigation, disinfecting hands, preparing sponges and gauze corrosive sublimate is the best and most convenient germ-killer. For the hands, arms, and the parts to be operated on, solutions of the strength of 1 to 1000 are necessary; while for irrigating ordinary wounds solutions of from 1 to 2000 to 1 to 5000 are strong enough. Irrigation of the greater cavities require the solutions to be of only 1 to 8000 to 1 to 20000 strength. The following formula will answer every purpose:

℞ Corrosive sublimate . . . . . . ʒi
    Water . . . . f ℥ ii

M. S. Teaspoonful to one pint of water = 1 to 2000.

Some add twenty grains of common salt to the above formula, which prevents the mercury from decomposing so soon. Tablets of corrosive sublimate containing the proper amount to be added to a pint of water may be purchased from any manufacturing chemist or large dealer. They are more convenient, but more costly than the salt prepared as above. In all solutions boiled water is preferable, but not indispensable, in the majority of instances.

For disinfecting instruments and keeping sponges aseptic, carbolic acid excels any known agent. A five per cent. solution is made by thoroughly mixing one ounce of the acid with one and one quarter pints of water; a three per cent. by adding one ounce of acid to two pints of water.

The Thiersch solution consists of boracic acid ʒi; salicylic acid gr. xv; water Oi. This solution may be used with impunity in the abdominal cavity or elsewhere, as it will cause no irritation.

No surgeon can afford to be without iodoform. Its desiccating properties render it invaluable in the treatment of the vast majority of wounds, both accidental and surgical.

I have given but a few of the well known germicides, for the reason that if we thoroughly understand the use of a few they may be made applicable to every case, and such knowledge is preferable to having an imperfect knowledge of many. Besides, it relieves the mind of the tedium and strain incident to frequent changes; for when one habituates himself to the use of any particular thing, its application becomes a matter-of-course and requires little thought.

Sutures.—Silver wire may be kept wrapped in protective or in a metal cylinder. The cylinder is costly and not indispensable. Silk may also be kept wrapped in the protective. Both silver and silk are rendered aseptic by placing them in a three to five per cent. carbolic solution for half an hour, or by boiling for an hour. Cat-gut is made aseptic by soaking in the so-called oil of juniper berries[1] for twenty-four hours, then transferred to ninety-five per cent. alcohol; or it may be kept in the oil indefinitely. The bottle contains spools holding gut of several sizes, the ends passing through a perforated stopper, and any desired amount may be drawn from the bottle without removing the spools.

The best drainage tubes are of soft black rubber, with a lumen of one-sixteenth to one-half inch. These may be kept in a tightly corked glass jar dry, or in a five per cent. carbolic solution. Bone drains are useful in permanent dressings and are kept immersed in oil of juniper berries.

Dressings.—To prepare sublimate gauze, divide say twenty-four yards of cheese cloth into four pieces. Double each piece several times, and tie a string around it. Place these pieces in water with two pounds of bicarbonate of soda and boil for an hour or more. Then rinse the cloth through clear water and place it in a solution of corrosive sublimate, 1 to 1000. After twenty-four hours it may be wrung out and hung up in a dustless place to dry. For permanent keeping, either a stout jar, tight drawer, or a can with the lid held down by adhesive plaster will do. Excellent prepared gauze may be bought at about fifteen cents a yard; but it can be made by any one disposed to try at a cost of only about four or five cents a yard.

Iodoform gauze is made by sprinkling gauze freshly wrung from a 1 to 3000 sublimate solution with iodoform from a pepper box; Gerster's, or an ordinary tin box with perforated top, will answer.

Absorbent cotton can be purchased at small cost, or can be prepared in an emergency by dipping cotton batting in a fifteen per cent. boric acid solution (boracic acid ℥v, water Oii).

Protective is thin rubber tissue and costs about fifty cents a yard.

Bandages, both cotton and flannel, should be made from cloth previously treated as described for gauze. As a matter of economy a cigar-box will make an excellent bandage roller. Near one end pass a stiff wire through from side to side, and shape one end of the wire into a crank. Toward the other end of the box arrange three or four wires or rods so that the cloth will pass over and under them in succession.

[1] In a private note from Dr. Squibb he says: "The best oil of juniper berries in the market is obtained by distilling the fresh twigs of a different Variety of juniper from that which bears the berries."

Every operating case should have one or two rubber bandages.

Sponges.—Florida sponges are cheap and are better than the fine silk ones. They are beaten well and washed to remove all grit; soaked for fifteen minutes in dilute muriatic acid; thoroughly kneaded in hot water and soft soap; rinsed through clear water till they loose the soapy feel; finally transferred to a five per cent. carbolic solution, where they may be kept indefinitely. After use in an aseptic case sponges are cleansed by repeated washings in warm—not hot—water, and immersion for one hour in 1 to 500 corrosive sublimate solution. Never use a sponge that has been used in a suspicious case, nor to dress a wound with; pellets of cotton are infinitely better and can be destroyed when once used. I have seen one little sponge do service in every case occurring in the practice of a distinguished (?) surgeon.

The irrigator is indispensable, the ordinary fountain syringe being one of the best for a surgical bag. On a pinch, the irrigating fluid may be poured from a pitcher.

In considering the types of dressings we will notice just three with their modifications; and these keep the wound in an aseptic state by desiccation, sterilization, or hermetical sealing of the surfaces, or by two or more of these principles combined.

Desiccation.—Small wounds, especially about the face and neck, may be kept aseptic by freely dusting them with iodoform, or equal parts of iodoform and subnitrate of bismuth. These drugs, especially the former, have the peculiar property of drying a wound by checking the secretions, while the secretions that do escape are rapidly desiccated to a pasty crust, which protects the wound from contamination by infectious substances and in turn is rendered aseptic by the antiseptic properties of the powders. When there is much oozing the parts should be dusted every half-hour until a crust has formed.

Sterilization.—By this is meant the moist dressing. The wound is gently packed with gauze squeezed from a fresh sublimate solution, 1 to 1000 to 1 to 2000. The field of operation and contiguous parts are lavishly padded with gauze and cotton previously treated as above, the whole being covered by a piece of protective, held in place by a roller bandage. This dressing will absorb discharges more readily than the dry dressing, and is applicable in cases in which we may expect profuse oozing or fear the drainage tubes will become clogged. When no impervious outer dressing can be had, the gauze may be kept moist by pouring a drachm or two of an antiseptic solution into it every half hour.

Desiccation and Sterilization.—These two types of dressing are happily confined and modified in the *dry dressing*, in which the wound and parts around are thickly covered with gauze and cotton, previously sterilized by chemicals. A few strips of iodoform gauze are laid directly over the line of incision to facilitate the drying of the deepest portions of the dressing. No protective is applied to the outside, as the free access of dustless air is necessary to hasten the drying process.

Schede's modification of the dry dressing.—The prime object in this dressing is organization of the blood-clot. Asepsis must be perfect. A piece of protective just a little larger than the wound is laid directly on the parts, and iodoform gauze thickly applied above this. No protective is used on the outside of the dressing.

Hermetical sealing of the wound.—I do not think any paper relating to the modern treatment of wounds complete that does not give credence to the hot water method, so ably promulgated by the late Dr. Varick. This is specially indicated in amputation wounds, and consists in applying water only a little below the boiling point to the freshly-cut surfaces until they are thoroughly glazed with a coat of albumin. This effectually occludes the mouths of all lymphatics and small vessels, including the capillaries, so that contamination is impossible. The parts are next brought together, and little dressing is applied. The success of this method is truly wonderful. Small wounds may be hermetically sealed by touching them with acetic acid.

(*To be continued.*)

A CASE OF MENINGOCELE.

BY CHARLES BAUM, M.D.,
PHILADELPHIA.

On September 18, 1888, I was summoned to attend Mrs. N——, æt. 37, American, of large frame, very fat figure, and nervous temperament, being in labor with her eighth babe.

Two abortions had occurred in her early married life. No history or evidence of syphilis could be elicited. At a preliminary visit she stated that in her former labors she had acted like a crazy person, screaming, pulling out her hair, striking her head and attempting to bite her attendants.

When I entered the room she was highly excited, walking the floor, wringing her hands and declaring she would "die this time." Her former children had been very large and forceps had been applied on one occasion to hasten delivery for the relief of nervous agitation.

Dilating pains had continued six hours. As the woman was in the act of placing herself in position for a digital examination, the amniotic fluid escaped with a gush. Upon examination, her pelvic diameters were found to be larger than normal, the os uteri was fully dilated and the finger came in contact with an elastic tumor, covered with the hairy scalp. Owing to obliteration of the usual fontanelles and sutures a right occipito-anterior position was determined by the relation of the ears to the swelling and the neck. The woman was at times entirely uncontrollable, but the labor pains were active and in two and a half hours the delivery was accomplished, manual assistance being demanded to liberate the shoulders and hips. Before the hips were delivered the child cried loudly. In deference to a superstitious notion of the mother, the extremely large male babe was not weighed, but was thought by the nurse to be about fifteen pounds; it surely weighed twelve pounds.

On the right side of its head was found an elastic, prominent tumor, which arose from the posterior fontanelle and extended along the sagittal and a portion of the lambdoidal suture. This entire region was bulging, while the edges of the occipital and parietal bones were everted about half-inch. Longitudinally over the prominence the measurement was $5\frac{1}{4}$ inches, transversely, $4\frac{3}{4}$ inches. Light was readily transmitted through the swelling. As the child grew, it was noticed that pressure upon the tumor caused drowsiness. In addition to this defect there was right sided scrotal hernia; otherwise, the child seemed healthy and natural in appearance.

To satisfy the demands of the parents, as well as to try the experiment, one gramme of potassium iodide dissolved in compound syrup of sarsaparilla and water was administered internally three times each day, and this was continued until the swelling was absorbed; locally, an application of ammonium chloride gr. xv, alcohol f ℥ j, was ordered to be made every six hours, but as was learned later, the parents made it every three hours.

By degrees the swelling disappeared, and on November 27, 1888, the bones were united along the suture lines, there being, however, a general prominence, which has remained unchanged, over the region involved. Excepting slight constipation during the second week the child has remained perfectly well, never having displayed any nervous symptoms. At present it is teething easily, and was vaccinated January 24, 1889. He is large, fat, solid, bright, laughing and playful.

630 N. Broad St.

CASE OF SUB-SPINOUS LUXATION OF THE HEAD OF THE HUMERUS.

BY T. Y. SCOTT, M.D.,
BENTLEYVILLE, PA.

The reading of the report of Dr. Cate's case of sub-spinous luxation of the humerus, in the REPORTER of January 19, 1889, brings to my mind a similar case that occurred in my own practice, being the only case of sub-spinous luxation that I have met with in eighteen dislocations of the head of this bone. By referring to my note-book, I find the following particulars of the case, under date of Jan. 16, 1884:

Mr. J. C., æt. 70 years, a small man and very spare, apparently devoid of any adipose tissue, was thrown down while feeding his hogs by a large hog running against him from in front, tripping up his feet and pitching him forward, he alighting, with extended arms, upon his palms, while his feet were elevated in the air upon the back of the hog. I saw him within four hours after the happening of the accident. I found him sitting in a chair with the right arm resting upon pillows, and extending forward, slightly downward, and very slightly outward, the forearm flexed at a right angle with the arm. He was suffering much pain in the right shoulder. Examination of the shoulder showed no contusion or swelling, other than a hard rounded prominence on the posterior surface of the scapula, below the spinous process; absence of the head of the bone from the axilla, and a depression beneath the anterior portion of the acromial process. The sub-spinous tumor was firm, rounded and resisting, and its movements, in obedience to rotation and other movements of the humerus, were, owing to the marked scarcity of adipose tissue, very perceptible both to the eye and the finger.

In this particular case the prominence of the coracoid process was very marked.

Repeated attempts at reduction, both by manipulation and extension and counter-extension with the heel in the axilla, failed, but it was very readily accomplished by an assistant making extension forward, slightly downward and outward, while counter-extension was secured by means of a sheet carried over and down in front of the shoulder and brought back under the arm, traction being made with the two ends of the sheet widely separated, so as not to make pressure upward into the axilla, while I made pressure upon the head of the bone from behind forward toward the glenoid cavity.

Securing the arm to the side, with the forearm in a sling for two or three days, and the use of an evaporating lotion to the shoulder constituted the after treatment. The pain ceased with the reduction, and all the functions and strength of the joint were fully re-established in four weeks.

ACETIZED COTTON.

BY THOMAS W. HARVEY, M.D.,
ORANGE, N. J.

The value of acetic acid as a styptic is often forgotten. In its common form as vinegar, it is familiar to most every general practitioner as a ready means of controlling parenchymatous hemorrhages generally. The nose, gums, and uterus are the situations in which it has been frequently used.

I have recently had prepared by the lint-makers an absorbent cotton, impregnated with acetic acid, of three grades—5 per cent., twelve and one-half per cent., and twenty per cent. Cotton so prepared should be kept moist and be preserved in air-tight bottles. The advantages of the acetized cotton are that, while styptic, it is not corrosive and does not form sloughs; its taste is not unpleasant, and while the 20 per cent. cotton causes smarting when laid npon a denuded surface, yet it is not very irritating, and is antiseptic.

The conditions in which it will be found useful as a styptic are numerous. Some of these conditions are as follows: Epistaxis; hemorrhage from the gums after tooth extraction; in menorrhagia, as a tampon to be placed immediately at or within the os uteri; in cancer of the uterus—indeed in ulcerating cancer wherever located. It is also useful in prolonged flowing from a subinvoluted uterus, or from lacerations of the cervix or vagina after labor. It will control hemorrhage from organs such as the liver, when wounded by the separation of adhesions in operations in the abdominal cavity—continued pressure for a few moments with the prepared cotton will stop persistent oozing that has resisted hot water and other measures, and which would require otherwise the use of the cautery and result in the formation of a slough.

I have not had sufficient opportunity to determine the relative values of the different cottons, but the stronger will act pretty sharply when there is an abraded surface on the skin. The twenty per cent. cotton may be used about the cervix uteri without pain, and also in many cancerous ulcerations.

The chief advantage of the acetized cotton is that it avoids the disadvantages of the iron styptic cotton now found in the shops.

SOCIETY REPORTS.

PHILADELPHIA COUNTY MEDICAL SOCIETY.

Stated Meeting, January 23, 1889.

The President, W. W. KEEN, M.D., in the chair.

DR. EUGENE P. BERNARDY read a paper on

Biniodide of Mercury—Its Antiseptic Use.

He first referred to his second paper " On the Value of Biniodide of Mercury as an Antiseptic in Obstetrics," read before the Philadelphia Obstetrical Society (April 1, 1886), and said that he had fully intended leaving the results of his investigations to the medical profession, and letting them, by further trial, confirm the correctness of his conclusions. As regards the solubility of the salt he said that in several papers on antiseptics, the biniodide of mercury is declared insoluble, and therefore difficult to use; in one paper, the cost is the objection, it being stated to be more costly than the mercuric chloride. It is to be sincerely hoped that pecuniary considerations will never interfere in the use of any medicine that will assist in saving a human life. The biniodide is rendered a soluble salt by the addition of iodide of potassium. After mentioning a number of references to the use of the biniodide in current medical literature, he reported several obstetrical cases :

Case I.—Mrs. L., aged nineteen, first pregnancy; was called to attend her (January 24, 1886) in a premature labor; she was pregnant about six and a half months; when I arrived, I found she had been delivered of a dead male child; the placenta came away in two hours; the patient did well up to the evening of January 27th, when she was taken with a chill, which was repeated in three hours; when I saw her on the morning of the 28th, her skin was hot and dry, face flushed, pulse 112, temperature 102°; tongue thickly furred, abdomen slightly swollen and very sensitive; lochia offensive. Ordered quinæ sulphatis, gr. xx.; morphiæ sulphatis, gr. ¼, night and morning; poultice over abdomen, and hot vaginal injections of 1 to 4,000 solution of the biniodide of mercury every four hours; at the second injection the discharges became free from any odor. January 29th, pulse 100, temperature normal. This treatment was kept up, with the exception of the large doses of quinine, to October 5th, when the injections were reduced to one a day for about four days, when the patient was discharged cured.

I have confined this patient since of a full-term, living child; the biniodide injections were used at once; she had a good lying-in; discharged on the ninth day, well. (The above case really belongs to my second series, but the manuscript was mislaid at the time, and found too late to be incorporated in my second paper.)

Case II.—Mrs. M., age thirty-five; fifth confinement; during her pregnancy she had worked very hard, doing almost the work of a man. Was called to attend her in labor, March 18, 1886; when I arrived at her bedside I found she had been in labor since the previous day; she appeared completely worn out, having hardly any strength to bear down; the family refused positively instrumental interference. I gave two doses of the fluid extract of ergot, teaspoonful, repeated in half an hour; under its influence the child was born; the placenta soon followed.

The patient did well up to March 24th, when, in the evening, she had a severe chill, which again occurred the following morning (March 25th). I saw the patient on the following day; she seemed to have aged fully ten years; her face was drawn, and of a deep yellow color, eyes bright and sparkling with delirium; pulse 140, temperature 105°; the abdomen was immensely swollen, and could not bear to be touched, more especially on the right side. Diagnosticated metro-peritonitis. Lochia arrested. Ordered quiniæ sulphatis, gr. xx., night and morning; morphiæ sulphatis, gr. ¼, whenever pain was severe; hot poultice over the abdomen, hot vaginal injections of 1 to 4,000 solution of biniodide of mercury. March 28th, pulse 120, temperature 101°; lochia returning, abdomen not so sensitive. This treatment was continued up to March 31st; the abdomen now allowed of closer examination; in the right inguinal region could be detected a large mass; vaginal examination showed the uterus bound down and completely surrounded by lymph. Dr. W. Goodell, being called in consultation, verified the diagnosis. The biniodide injections to be continued; internally, quinine sulph., gr. iij., three times a day, besides an alterative tonic. The patient gradually recovered her health, without any additional treatment.

In this case the injections of the biniodide were constantly used for a space of three weeks, first every four hours, then three times a day, then once a day, without the slightest systemic action of the drug occurring.

Case III.—On July 11, 1886, I was asked to see Mrs. W., in consultation with her family physician; on entering the house a most sickening odor struck my nostrils; it reminded me of uterine cancer in its last stage; the more I advanced, the worse the odor became; at last, I reached the room and bedside of the patient; of all odors, I never want to smell the like again; as the nurse remarked, it was worse than decayed carrion; how the patient lived through such a condition was simply miraculous.

I found she had aborted about two weeks previously, and had declined any interference in regard to extracting the placenta, saying "it will come away." On examination, I found the vagina full of sticky, horribly-smelling, broken-down placental tissue, the mouth of the uterus opened, the uterus full of the same kind of material as found in the vagina; the patient declined the use of any instruments, so I broke down and pulled out all that came within reach of my finger; I then washed out the uterus with hot 1 to 4000 solution of the biniodide of mercury; not yet satisfied, I washed out the parts with another quart of the solution (1 to 4000), until the water came back clear.

I did not see the patient again, and, in answer to a letter to the attendant physician, I received the following:

"PHILADELPHIA, May 20, 1887.

"MY DEAR DOCTOR: I am glad to inform you that Mrs. W. did very well. The iodide of mercury pellets acted like a charm.

There was no unpleasant odor attached to the discharges after we began their employment. . . . I have been an ardent advocate of potassium permanganate, but I am now a convert to the biniodide as an antiseptic."

Case IV.—Mrs. H., primipara, aged thirty, fell in labor November 18, 1886. On my arrival at her bedside, I found she had been in labor for some time, the mouth of the uterus wide open, bag of waters unruptured, vertex presentation. On making abdominal palpation, detected at once a twin pregnancy; after a somewhat lingering labor, the first child (boy) was born; on examination, I found the second child (girl) presenting with vertex left posterior; the head came down very slowly, and, on the solicitations of the patient and family, the labor was terminated with forceps. The patient did well up to the evening of the second day, when, about midnight, she was taken with severe frontal headache and chills. I saw the patient in the chill; half an hour after, her temperature was 104°, pulse 140; delirious; ordered quinine sulphat., gr. xx, at once, and repeat next morning. Next day (November 21), temperature and pulse the same, completely out of her mind; lochia almost ceased flowing, and what was present was offensive; abdomen extremely sensitive to the touch. Ordered the quinine to be continued, gtt. x. tr. digitalis four times a day; hot flaxseed-meal poultices over abdomen, hot injections in the vagina of 1 to 4000 biniodide of mercury every four hours. The following day, the lochia returned normal. The condition of things remained about the same up to November 25, when the symptoms were improved; the patient was discharged well, December 4, 1886.

(The following case was the first patient on whom I used the biniodide of mercury injections, and whose history is given in my first paper, June 4, 1885.)

Case V.—Mrs. D., third confinement (being compelled to leave the city, she fell into the hands of another physician), fell in labor September 6, 1886. After a lingering labor, she was delivered of a still-born child; on the second day, as far as I can learn, all the symptoms of an attack of puerperal fever set in; she remained very sick for several days. No vaginal injections of any kind were used. When I saw the patient, on September 19, 1886, she was suffering with an extremely tender abdomen, more especially on the right side, on which side could be detected a small lump. Vaginal examination disclosed the uterus partially surrounded by lymph. Discharges from the vagina very offensive. Pulse 100, temperature 101°-102°. Nothing could be retained on the stomach; as a drink, frozen champagne was ordered. Quinine sulphate, gr. x, once a day; equal parts of ungt. hydrarg. and belladonna to be rubbed over the abdomen once a day, followed by hot poultices, hot injections of the 1 to 4000 biniodide three times a day. My following visit found my patient improved, and in a week she was discharged, but it was some time before she regained her usual strength.

On November 1, 1887, I delivered the above patient, after an easy labor, of a large, female child; immediately after the placenta came away, I washed the uterus out with a 1 to 4000 injection of the biniodide; the injections were ordered to be used three times a day throughout the lying-in, which was perfectly normal, and the patient discharged, well and strong, on the ninth day.

Case VI.—Mrs. C., aged nineteen, first pregnancy; was called to attend her on the morning of August 19, 1888. After an easy labor, she was delivered in the afternoon of a large male child; the placenta came away in about twenty minutes. The following day the patient was doing well, but had not been washed, and the odor in the room was very disagreeable. On my following visit I found the patient in a high fever, temperature 103°, pulse 130, full and quick; tongue dry and chippy; the skin from the posterior part of the vulva back to beyond the anus was raw and covered with minute bloody points; abdomen very tender; lochia, what there was, was extremely offensive.

On close inquiry, I found that the mother of the patient, who was supposed to be nurse, had gone on a drunken debauch since the birth of the child, no doubt celebrating her " grandmotherhood "; the patient was placed at once in charge of a competent nurse; hot poultices were ordered over the abdomen; quinine sulph., gr. v, morphia sulph.. gr. ¼, every four hours; hot injections in the vagina of 1 to 4000 biniodide of mercury every three or four hours, equal parts of zinc ointment and Goulard's cerate were applied over the raw surface.

August 24th, pulse 110, temperature 101°; lochia coming freely and without odor. August 26th, pulse 100, temperature 99°; 4 P. M., pulse 100, temperature 101°. Condition better, treatment continued; patient discharged, entirely cured, September 1, 1888.

With the three cases reported in my first paper, eight in my second, and the six cases just detailed, in all, seventeen (obstetrical) cases in which the biniodide of mercury had been employed, gives us, certainly, sufficient data to draw positive conclusions.

Abdominal Abscess Intercurrent with Typhoid Fever.—On April 20, 1887, I was requested to see Mary B., aged five years. The little patient had been ailing for the past week, suffering from constant frontal headache; she was very feverish, had lost appetite, and had a diarrhœa. I found her in bed, with a temperature of 103°, very quick, compressible pulse, tongue dry, and a number of rose-colored spots over the abdomen and chest. The case was running the ordinary course of typhoid fever, when, on May 5th, the child was taken with a sudden, sharp pain in the right iliac region; my visit found the child suffering agonizing pain in the abdomen, which was tense and swollen; in the right iliac region could be felt a lump the size of an egg; under appropriate treatment the acute pain somewhat subsided. On May 8th, my attention was called to the navel, which had become red, inflamed, and pouting; on touch, a feeling of fluctuation was imparted to the finger. May 10th, the child passed from the bowels a large quantity of pus; the angry appearance of the navel disappeared, all acute symptoms seemed abated. On my visit of May 12th I found the navel again inflamed, with positive indications of pus underneath; the following day it broke, discharging about a cupful of pus. I now suggested a consultation in regard to the advisability of an operation. It was declined. Same condition continued up to the first of June; the child by this time had become greatly emaciated, constant discharge of pus from the navel, and symptoms of septic poison were commencing to show themselves. At last, on June 12th, consent was given to an operation. June 13th, Drs. Allis, F. Elder, and C. Reed were present. The patient was etherized by Dr. Reed; after a close examination, and taking the weakened condition of the child into consideration, and also that the abscess cavity having made an opening at the navel, it was decided that, instead of opening the abdominal cavity, a counter-opening in the left iliac region be made, and a drainage-tube, extending from the navel to it, be introduced, and the abscess cavity washed out. I washed out the abscess cavity through the tube with a two-quart solution of 1 to 4000 biniodide of mercury; the abdomen was then covered first with biniodide gauze, over which was laid a layer of the biniodide wool, all held in position by a bandage that had been washed in a 1 to 4000 solution of the biniodide of mercury. The abscess cavity was ordered to be washed out morning and night with a 1 to 8000 solution of the biniodide; the child rallied well from the effects of the ether. While washing out the cavity, on May 17th, a piece of straw came through the drainage-tube. May 22d, discharge of feces through the lower end of the tube, which occurred two days in succession; for the following ten days, when the child partook of food, more especially if this was an egg, within a half hour some of it partially digested would appear at the end of the upper part of the tube; if the discharge occurred later than a half hour, it would appear at the lower end of the tube: this clearly demonstrated a fecal fistula in connection with the abscess cavity. Gradually all discharges ceased, and the tube was taken out July 23, 1887; a week later both openings were closed, but it was several months before the child could resume her ordinary diet; apples would invariably bring on severe colic.

None of us at the time of the operation went further than to "hope" that the little patient would get well. The case demonstrates well the antiseptic properties of the biniodide. It was an extremely warm month, and, with the exception of the two or three days on which the feces passed down through the tube, the odor of the discharges was held in abeyance.

Double Laceration of the Cervix.—Mrs. F. had a large, double laceration of the cervix following a natural labor. I first saw the case in May, 1885, and advised operation. Operated October 5, 1885. Extensive denudation had to be made; fourteen silver stitches were necessary; hot water was used to cleanse the parts during the operation. On the second day a very offensive bloody discharge occurred. The vagina was washed out with a hot 1 to 4000 solution of biniodide of mercury three times a day; at the first injection all odor disappeared, and did not return throughout the rest of the treatment; the stitches were taken out on the tenth day, with perfect union.

Abscess of Right Foot.—In February, 1887, I was called to see Master McG. About a week previous a heavy box fell on his foot; painful at the time, but not painful enough for him to give up his work, he continued to work up to February 10, 1887; on the previous evening his foot became swollen and painful; under poultices the inflamma-

tion centred, and on February 20th the abscess broke. The opening was stubborn to heal; offensive pus was discharged; every day I injected the cavity with a 1 to 2000 solution of the bichloride of mercury and packed; this treatment was kept up for ten days without any change; the bichloride was then changed to a 1 to 4000 solution of the biniodide of mercury, the discharges were made pure, and in the course of another ten days the opening closed, but the foot remained tender for several weeks.

Abscess Extending from the Right Axilla.—W. S., aged thirty, barber, of scrofulous habit, somewhat dissipated, having a wart on the right middle finger, picked it with his finger-nails; the result was an acute inflammation of the entire arm. I saw the case July 16, 1888; under cooling applications, the inflammation soon abated. About July 21, 1888, the right side, extending from the axilla down to midway between the last rib and the crest of the ilium became intensely inflamed; the pain was excruciating, and large doses of sulphate of morphia gave only momentary relief; large flaxseed poultices liberally sprinkled with laudanum were applied. On the 24th I detected fluctuation at the lower border, made an exploratory incision, and obtained half a cupful of fetid pus and broken down blood; this gave slight relief. On the 26th the pain returned tenfold; the same evening, the patient having been etherized by Dr. S. Solis-Cohen, I enlarged the previously made incision to three inches, and about half a pint of extremely fetid pus was discharged; the finger was then introduced, and two encysted pus sacs, situated at the edge of the scapula, were ruptured, and another half pint of pus was discharged; the cavity was then washed out with a 1 to 4000 solution of the biniodide of mercury, a drainage tube introduced, flaxseed poultice applied, and over all a layer of biniodide wool.

Next day I found the patient had had a good night's rest; I removed the poultice; cavity to be washed out three times a day with the biniodide; drainage tube taken out on the fourth day, and within a week the patient was discharged well. It is hardly necessary to state that good nourishment, iron, and quinine were ordered. After using the biniodide no odor was perceptible in the discharges.

Three Cases of Carbuncle.—April 23, 1887, I was asked to see Mrs. P., aged seventy-two, and found her suffering with a carbuncle on the back of the neck, six inches long and four inches wide. It was riddled with a number of suppurating points; on the previous day the patient had been given up by her medical attendant as incurable. On Sunday, April 24, 1887, after the patient had been etherized, the wound, instruments, and sponges were made antiseptic by being washed with a 1 to 4000 solution of the biniodide, after which a crucial incision was made and all the hardened tissue dissected out, down to healthy tissue, thoroughly washed out with the biniodide, and a flaxseed meal and charcoal poultice applied; the sore to be well washed three times a day with the biniodide, when a fresh poultice was applied. Internal treatment, iron, quinine, and full diet. In twenty days the patient was discharged well. The disagreeable odor in this case was not entirely dissipated, but was held under control.

Case II.—Mr. B., coal merchant, aged forty. Carbuncle in right shoulder, size of an egg, hard, indurated, extremely painful to the touch, and a point of suppuration at the centre; the case was seen April 7, 1888. The next day, after the patient had been etherized, I made a deep crucial incision, and dissected out all the hard indurated tissue; the same treatment was used as in Case I. No odor connected with the discharges. Patient discharged, cured, in two weeks.

On October 20, 1888, I was again asked to see the above patient. I found him suffering from an attack of herpes of the back of the neck, which was, in a few days, followed by a number of abscesses, two of them resembling small carbuncles. A charcoal poultice was applied, and in three days all the abscesses were opened, but during the following week there seemed to be no change for the better. I then ordered a piece of linen to be saturated with a 1 to 4000 solution of the biniodide and applied to the surface, and over this a flaxseed-charcoal poultice; within forty-eight hours, the angry appearance of the abscesses and skin abated, and in four to five days more, all inflammation had disappeared, when the patient was discharged.

Case III.—J. E., aged sixty-nine, was taken sick about three weeks previous to my seeing him. It first commenced with a painful tumor on the neck. When I saw the patient (July 19, 1888), the entire surface from the superior curved line of the occipital bone down to the seventh cervical vertebra and from ear to ear was one immense suppurating surface, covered with a thick yellowish green membrane. The discharges were highly offensive. Pulse quick and compressible; slightly delirious; tongue covered with a thick, black, highly offensive membrane. Ordered a piece of linen to be saturated with a 1 to 4000 solution of the biniodide and applied over the surface, and over this a charcoal-flaxseed poultice every three hours. The odor was held in abeyance. This treatment was continued for about ten days, when the surface became clear of all adventitious membrane. Poultice was continued; carbolic acid was ordered in place of the biniodide. Patient discharged, cured, September 20, 1888.

Dr. S. Solis-Cohen saw the case for me in August, and we concurred in one prognosis, which was death; but we were more than agreeably surprised.

Biniodide of Mercury Wool as an Application over the Chest in Pulmonary Troubles. —When, in the winter of 1886, I first ordered the chest of a child suffering with catarrhal pneumonia to be enveloped in a layer of the biniodide of mercury wool, it was simply to overcome the disagreeable matting of the cotton. The child, previously to its use was very restless, and seemed to suffer pain. On the following visit I found that the little patient had had its first quiet sleep since the commencement of its sickness; since then I have almost entirely discarded the use of cotton. The results in a number of cases lead me to believe that there must be something more than the warmth of the wool. Can it be that the heat of the body disengages the biniodide, and as the consequent result, the patient is constantly surrounded by an antiseptic atmosphere?

In a case operated on for cancerous constriction of the bowel, by Dr. Charles B. Penrose, the patient, about the fourth week, was seized with a sharp pain in the right side below the nipple; counter-irritants did not relieve her; on auscultation, crepitant rales were easily detected in the lower right portion of the lung, under the point where the pain was complained of; the side was enveloped in the biniodide wool, and within twelve hours the pain had entirely disappeared. In the neuralgic pains always present in a case of phthisis, I have found the wool invariably to diminish, if not entirely dissipate the pains, and the expectoration seems easier and in smaller quantities.

My attention was called to the following by my office-pupil, J. N. England: "Biniodide of Mercury Pulverization for Tuberculosis" (*American Journal of Pharmacy*, October, 1888). Miquel and Rueff's formula is given by the *Arch. de Phar.*, September 5, 1888, as follows : Biniodide of mercury and iodide of potassium, of each 1 gramme ; distilled water, 1000 grammes. The solution is stable. At the beginning 10 c.cm. are sprayed once daily ; to be increased to 25 c.cm. twice daily. The larger portion of the liquid should be inspired. It reaches the lungs, says the author, but salivation does not follow, even after months of treatment. The sputa changes in character and diminishes in quantity ; the number of microbes is lessened, but these organisms rarely disappear completely. The cough increases at first, and afterward subsides.

If my theory of the disengagement, by heat, of the biniodide from the wool be correct, its action will readily be explained by the above experiments of Miquel and Rueff.

Disinfectant of Typhoid Fever Stools.— For the past two years I have used the pellets of the biniodide dissolved in the alvine discharges of typhoid fever, and the results have always been satisfactory.

In the spring of 1886 I treated an extremely bad case of typhoid fever ; the patient was broken down from dissipation, having had, about two weeks prior to his illness, an attack of delirium tremens ; the alvine discharges numbered from twenty to thirty a day, and were highly offensive ; chloride of lime, and different forms of chloride and sulphate of iron were used without any diminution of the sickening odor. I then ordered two (1 to 4000) pellets of the biniodide of mercury to be dissolved in a half pint of water and placed in the bed-pan, to be renewed every time the pan had been used by the patient ; the odor was completely dissipated, and kept so.

In another case the bichloride of mercury pellets were used without success ; the biniodide pellets gave the desired result. In a case of labor which, at the end of the lying-in, terminated in an attack of typhoid fever, the nurse used the biniodide pellets on her own account in the bed-pan, there was no disagreeable odor throughout the course of the disease.

The description of the action of new medicinal preparations or new properties to an old medicine necessitates tedious histories of cases ; this must be my excuse for dragging through such dry details.

It is not my intention to present to you the biniodide of mercury as the one and only infallible antiseptic ; I simply present my results, and have tried to give impartial histories, without exaggeration, simply as they have occurred. But the action and results of the biniodide of mercury fully strengthen my belief in its stronger antiseptic value and non-irritating properties over the bichloride.

After some remarks by Dr. Woodbury, Dr. Bernardy closed the discussion. He said : From the start I objected to the shape of the pellets, thinking that they looked too much like candy, and I think that there will soon be a change, so that this danger will be avoided. The pellets of bichloride look very much like chlorate of potassium lozenges, with the exception that the word " poison " is stamped on them.

In regard to this being a double salt. This was the first thing that struck my attention. When I first used this preparation, in 1884, I dissolved the biniodide in alcohol. This was found to be inconvenient, and through the kindness of Mr. Hayes, who allowed me the use of his laboratory, his assistant and I worked up this subject. We added iodide of potassium, and then found that the slightest moisture imparted to one pellet was enough to destroy the entire bottleful. We then decided to add the muriate of ammonium, which prevents this chemical reaction until the pellet is thrown into water. The pellet goes in as the biniodide of mercury, and the iodide dissolves it, but before the change takes place it has been used upon the patient.

In regard to my use of this preparation. I have studied it faithfully, and have tried to look upon the cases in an unbiassed way, and to give a fair history of them. I have sometimes first used the bichloride, and it has not fulfilled the indications as the biniodide has done.

◆◆◆

—The *Medical Press and Circular*, Feb. 6, states that an action was recently brought against M. Poncet, Surgeon to the Val de Grâce Military Hospital, for $10,000 damages for having performed the operation of breaking down the adhesions in an anchylosed knee, the result of which did not fulfil the expectations of the patient. The Tribunal declined to enter into the technical question of the propriety of the operation, and restricted their consideration to proofs of negligence or manifest incapacity. A verdict was arrived at exonerating the defendant on the ground that although unsuccessful, the operation had been performed after due deliberation and with every necessary attention.

REPORTS OF CLINICS.

BELLEVUE HOSPITAL, NEW YORK.

MEDICAL CLINIC—PROF. A. A. SMITH.

Broncho-Pneumonia.

Prof. Smith presented a patient to illustrate an important fact which he had just previously laid stress upon in his lectures; namely, the great significance of the combination of the three physical signs— broncho-vesicular breathing, increased vocal resonance, and slight dulness. The patient, a man 36 years old, had been an inmate of the Hospital for many years, on and off, and always had a simple bronchitis. Dr. Smith himself had examined him many times before. A short time ago he was again admitted with the same trouble, the physical examination of his chest showing nothing but a general bronchitis. Three days ago, however, he suddenly had a chill, his temperature went up to 105° F., and his cough and dyspnœa increased. He complained of no pain. His fever continued, controlled to some extent with five-grain doses of antifebrin, and to-day is 102° F. The examination of his urine is negative.

The question arises, is his present condition the result of his bronchitis alone, or of something else? Physical examination of his lungs shows the presence of dry and moist rales all over, and posteriorly at the right apex a very localized spot presenting dulness, broncho-vesicular breathing, and increased vocal fremitus. This small area of consolidation did not exist before the occurrence of the chill three days ago, and it is so limited in extent that the most careful examination is necessary to determine it. It is a broncho-pneumonia; and what is its significance? There is no heart disease, and examination of the abdomen is negative. It is probable, therefore, that the inflammation is tubercular. The sputum has not yet been searched for the tubercle bacillus: but even if it is not found the diagnosis is not rendered clearer. A good prognostic sign and one against a tubercular process is the non-involvement of the pleura. And it is not altogether unlikely that the pneumonia may clear up and the patient recover. But if this does not occur in two weeks time we may quite positively diagnosticate phthisis.

These cases often occur in practice and are sometimes not so clearly defined as this one. With the bronchitis there may be no increase of cough or fever, and only the most careful examination will reveal the presence of consolidation. Moreover, the physical signs of this condition may not be very pronounced.

Lobar Pneumonia; Pericarditis.

The second patient was a man, 25 years old. Six days ago he was attacked with chill, fever, pain in the left side, cough, etc., and on admission to the Hospital he presented all the signs of lobar pneumonia. During the night he had mild, muttering delirium. After three days, his delirium suddenly became violent; he jumped from bed and rushed to the window and would have thrown himself out if he had not been promptly restrained and by force carried back to his bed. His temperature increased, and cyanosis developed. With this history pericarditis was at once suspected to have developed, and examination revealed a marked pericardial friction sound, which had not previously existed.

This sudden delirium in pneumonia very often signifies the access of pericarditis. To be sure the delirium may be due to other causes, as alcoholism or renal disease, or occur independent of any complication; but the frequency of its connection with pericarditis is more than a coincidence.

The patient has been taking half an ounce of brandy every half hour, day and night. His delirium is much improved and his cyanosis diminished. His pulse is now 140, compressible, but not very feeble. The rules laid down in a previous lecture relative to the use of alcohol are: consideration whether the illness be of long or short duration; the presence of a dry brown tongue; a feeble pulse of 120 or over, and increased first sound of the heart; and cyanosis. In this case we cannot be guided by the pulse altogether, and by the heart not at all. We notice the tongue to be dry and brown and fissured (what is called semi-typhoid), and we have the cyanosis—sufficient indications for stimulants. It is now the sixth day of the disease, and in twenty-four hours there will be, probably, a fall of temperature, for Dr. Smith believes the prognosis to be good.

In these cases of pneumonia the diagnosis is easy. There is almost always a chill (in 59 cases recently observed there was no chill in 14); and it is usually well marked, as in this case, lasting one-half hour. The pain in the side, the cough and finally the physical signs, are usually prominent and characteristic.

With reference to treatment: if there be much cough, dyspnœa or nervous symptoms, give opium and control the nerves. If complications arise, give more opium and add alcohol. Dr. Smith believes opium the most valuable drug in pneumonia. It does not treat the pneumonia, but the patient. Give sufficient to relieve the pain and just moisten the skin. It certainly renders the patient comfortable.

Phthisis.

The third patient was a woman, 37 years old, the mother of eleven children. Six years ago the patient had pneumonia of the right lung, and at that time was in bed six weeks. She has had no sickness since. For some weeks previous to three weeks ago she had had slight cough but no fever and no physical signs of consolidation of the lung, so we are told. Three weeks ago she began to expectorate blood and complain of moderate pain in the right side, high up.

To-day, physical examination shows, at the right apex, retraction and diminished movement, dulness, to three or four inches below the clavicle, bronchial breathing, and rude voice. The patient has laryngitis, and her voice and vocal fremitus are not therefore reliable. The patient has had several slight hæmoptyses since the first attack; sometimes the blood is bright and frothy, sometimes it is dark and clotted. It is probable that this condition of the lungs has existed longer than three weeks.

Hæmoptysis does not make the prognosis in this case more favorable or more unfavorable. The late Dr. Flint has said that life is longer in those patients who had this symptom.

Dr. Smith would prefer, were he the subject of phthisis, to have a moderate hæmoptysis occasionally, and would then consider his chances better; for this symptom seems to occur in the long-continued cases. There are to-day, among many such examples, several practising physicians in New York, old men, who had hæmoptysis thirty and forty years ago.

The treatment in this case should be toward improving the general health. Astringents do no good.

Typhoid Fever.

The fourth patient was a man 20 years old, a machinist. He had been nine months in the United States. He is not intemperate. He was well up to five days ago; he then complained of chilly sensations, cough, headache, and feeling "light and dizzy." There has been no nose-bleed and no pain. The bowels move once a day; are free, but not watery, and are of natural appearance.

The temperature is 103°; pulse; 110. The patient is pale and dull of apprehension. There are slight diffuse bronchitis; enlarged and tender spleen and liver; gurgling and tenderness in both illiac fossæ.

The diagnosis rests between malarial and typhoid fevers, and quinine, in sufficient doses, should be administered to settle this point. If after three days, the temperature is not controlled, the case is probably one of typhoid fever.

NEW YORK CORRESPONDENCE.

Treatment of Club-foot at the University Medical College.—A good caustic for Cancer.—Clinics of Drs. Bull, Thomson, and Winters.

NEW YORK, Feb. 16, 1889.

Two years ago Dr. N. M. Schaffer was succeeded as lecturer in orthopædic surgery in the University Medical College by Dr. A. M. Phelps. A more radical change would be hard to conceive. Prof. Schaffer is a disciple of braces and similar instrumental appliances, rather than of the knife; while Prof. Phelps is directly the opposite. The latter has now operated on nearly one hundred cases of club-foot without a failure and without a death, his highest temperature being 103°. He says he has never seen the case that operation will not cure. His good results are explained by his perfect knowledge of the subject, his skill and fearlessness in operating, and by the strictness of his antisepsis. He lays down the following rules of treatment: If a foot can be reduced by a reasonable amount of force in a reasonable time, do not operate; if not, the foot should be treated first by subcutaneous tenotomy; if this fails make a large open incision and cut everything; should this fail because of deformity of the bone, perform linear osteotomy of the neck of the astragulus; if the deformity is still unreducible, cut out a V shaped piece of bone; and lastly, if it remains then unreducible, cut off the foot. He considers it better to have a shoe stuffed with cotton and going naturally forward than one filled with a deformed foot and going backward like a crab. Prof. Phelps is also lecturer on orthopædic surgery in the Postgraduate School.

In cancers unamenable to treatment by the knife, Prof. Stephen Smith uses the following caustic: Heat sulphate of zinc till the water of crystalization is driven off and the sulphate falls into a powder. Add pure sulphuric acid to any desired consistency, that of mortar being preferable. This paste when applied produces a granulating surface that heals with surprising rapidity.

At the clinic of Prof. W. T. Bull, in New York Hospital recently, ovariotomy was performed for pyosalpinx. The tubes and ovaries were found bound down behind the uterus. They were torn loose without rupture and without great bleeding, and then, after the usual ligatures had been applied, they were removed. The Doctor feared hemorrhage and left in the wound a large glass tube, to which the nurse was instructed to apply suction with a syringe at intervals. Bleeding would thus be detected and free drainage at the same time obtained. He next operated on a case of ventral hernia. The patient was forty years of age and a janitress by occupation, compelled to do a great deal of walking up and down stairs. The hernia when tense was as large as a hen's egg, and gave considerable pain. Though the hernia was of long standing, no truss had ever been worn for it. It was easily reduced. Dr. Bull said he had not had a large experience in this variety of hernia but he believed that the results of operation were not brilliant, especially when the walls of the abdomen were weak and flabby. In this case they were strong and muscular and by excision of the sac and careful approximation of the edges of the muscle he hoped for a good result. A number of large vessels were found in the sac, but no serious trouble resulted.

At the clinic of Prof. W. H. Thomson, a policeman presented himself who apparently was the picture of health. His pulse, however, was irregular. He complained of headache and disordered secretions, sometimes diarrhœa at other times constipation. His worst symptom, however, and the one for which he came for relief, was insomnia. He could find nothing that helped him. Dr. Thomson said it was due to disordered circulation and fermentation in the intestine. He ordered:

R Tr. strophanthi . . . . gtt iv
    Spir. ammoniæ aromat. . . . . . f ʒ j

M. Sig. Take on retiring. To be repeated in four hours if the first dose does not put him to sleep.

After two weeks ten to fifteen grains of chloral hydrate with gentian, whiskey and iron may be substituted. If strophanthus fails to regulate the heart, digitalis may be tried. For the intestinal fermentation salicylate of soda and salol were given. The Doctor said insomnia may be the result of habit, in which case it should be treated with chloral hydrate until the habit is broken. Another cause is worry or mental strain. This variety is most dangerous and may lead to epilepsy or insanity. In this case give:

R Dilute hydrocyanic acid . . . gtt xvj
    Majendies sol. morphine . . . f ʒ j
    Chloral . . . . ʒ jss
    Syrup of ginger . . . . . f ʒ j
    Camphor water . . . . . ad f ʒ vj

M. Sig. Dose, for ordinary case, tablespoonful; for severe case, two tablespoonfuls.

This prescription is also good for the sleeplessness of fatigue.

Prof. J. E. Winters, in a course of clinics and lectures on diphtheria in children, at the University Medical College, has laid down the following rules for its treatment. It is the treatment followed in his private practice and in the University and De Milt Dispensaries, and he vouches for its results. Exhaustion and laryngeal complications are the chief causes of death, and are the things to combat. To prevent the former put the patient in bed and keep him there, no matter how mild the case may be. The latter cause of death is always brought on by exposure, and hence the bed should be placed out of reach of all draughts and the patient's neck should be kept warm. If flaxseed poultices are used they must be kept hot and changed every hour at least. A good method is to apply fat pork or bacon well sprinkled with pepper, both to the neck and up the sides of the face. Use heat by the inhalation of steam. As it is exhausting do not use it constantly but for ten or fifteen minutes, several times daily. Sulphurous acid, obtained easily by burning a piece of sulphur in the room, aids in the exfoliation of the membrane, reduces congestion and promotes the health of the sore. Local treatment: When the diphtheritic inflammation is under direct observation, as on the tonsils, local treatment is of little avail, and, as it causes struggling and consequent exhaustion, is contraindicated. In nasal diphtheria, however, the local treatment is most important and can be had without exhaustion. Place the patient on the edge of the bed and use a Davidson syringe until a passage is obtained through the nostrils. The saturated solution of boracic acid is the best application and, if there is putrefaction, alcohol can be added (f3ss to Oj). General treatment: Begin with calomel (gr. ij into ten powders, one every hour) as it stimulates all the secretions. Iron in full doses is indicated. Ten drops of the tincture of the chloride can be given and, if borne, doubled after twenty-four hours. If there is sepsis even (f3j) doses can be given. If quinine does not irritate, it should be given in tonic doses (to a child two or three years old, gr. j t. i. d.). Give alcohol only when the pulse indicates its necessity, beginning with gtt. x. If the disease is extending downward, in addition to the above burn tar in the room. Its *modus operandi* is unknown, but it relieves the symptoms and also spoils all clothing with which it comes in contact. Carry the nutrition of the patient to the highest pitch with milk and beef tea.

PERISCOPE.

On Gas-Cysts of the Vagina.

Professor Obrzut (pronounced "Objüt"— a Polish name), of Prag, Bohemia, says (*Wiadomosci Lekarskie,* Aug., No. 2, 1888) that Dr. Jacobs, of Bruxelles, working under his guidance, has succeeded in elucidating the pathogenesis of a rare and curious affection of the vagina. This consists in the development of multiple small-sized cysts with gaseous contents, described by Professors Chiari and Breisky under the name of "emphysematous vaginitis." While both of the authors just named, as well as Dr. Piering, believe that the disease represents primarily a lesion of the vaginal lymphatic apparatus, Drs. Obrzut's and Jacobs's researches have shown that the cysts originate solely in the vaginal blood-vessels, the lymphatics remaining wholly intact. According to the latter authors, the first stage of the pathological process seems to consist in œdematous swelling affecting fairly circumscribed isolated areas over the vascular wall; the second stage is a progressive, correspondingly limited or localized obliteration of the vascular lumen; while a third stage consists in a more or less considerable gradual dilatation of the vessel above its stenosed portion. Those dilated departments of the vascular tube in the course of time are transformed into cystiform structures, while their bloody contents undergo disintegration which, amongst other products, yields odorless and colorless gases.

As to the microbes described by Eisenholz, they could not be discovered in the cysts by any method of examination.

Friedreich's Disease.

At the meeting of the Medical Society of London, Jan. 28, Dr. Harrington Sainsbury brought forward two cases of Friedreich's disease. The first occurred in a compositor, twenty-three years old, single, who was treated at the age of fourteen for St. Vitus' dance. The ataxia, the patient says, developed a year or two later. He had an attack of abdominal symptoms of obstructive character at the age of nineteen, and since then the ataxia had increased. The incöordination presented the characters usual in locomotor ataxia, affecting the arms and legs, but being most marked in the latter. There appeared to be some muscular weakness, the head was occasionally unsteady, the speech was thick, and the eyes showed slight lateral movements when looking upward. The pupils were equal, contracting to light and accommodation; the discs were normal. Sensations as of "pins and needles" were felt occasionally in the hands and feet, and cramps sometimes in the legs; the patient felt the ground under him. On testing the sensation, it was found slightly dulled in the feet and legs; there was no delay in perception. Muscular sense for posture and estimation of weight was fairly precise; the superficial reflexes and knee-jerks were absent, and there had been no urinary trouble. The facial expression was blank.

The second patient was a brother of the first, two years younger, presenting a similar condition, but the thickness of speech and blankness of expression were more marked. There was a third brother in the family affected in a like manner. The lesion was identical in position with that of tabes, but there was absence of pain and of cramps.

Dr. Ormerod quoted several cases which had at first, and often for considerable periods, been mistaken for St. Vitus' dance. Looking at the constant unsteady movement in these cases, it was very hard to say that chorea was altogether absent. Dr. Sainsbury's case became worse after an acute abdominal attack; he had noticed a similar tendency to development of the affection after acute diseases—*e. g.*, scarlet and typhoid fevers.

Dr. Sainsbury, replying to a question from Dr. Beevor, said that the father was a drunkard, but there was no family history of neurosis.—*Lancet,* Feb. 2, 1889.

Bacteriology and Antisepsis of the Conjunctival Sac.

In the St. Petersburg weekly *Vratch*, Nos. 43 and 45, 1888, p. 879, Dr. Joseph S. Felser, of Kazan, describes his instructive bacterioscopical researches, undertaken for the purpose of studying mycotic life within the human conjunctival sac, as well as with the view to discover the best method of aseptic and antiseptic management of the conjunctiva in cases of ophthalmic disease and operations. The main outcome may be condensed thus : 1. The conjunctival sac in man always, both in health and disease, contains large numbers of microbes of different species. 2. This mycotic "store" is incessantly kept supplemented and refreshed by a free supply from enormous masses of microörganisms invariably present in the surrounding air. 3. The numerical strength of the conjunctival microbes is directly proportionate to that of the air bacteria. 4. Of pathogenic microbes, the predominating species are the *staphylococcus albus, citreus, aureus*, and *diplococcus*, the first two forms prevailing also under absolutely healthy conditions. 5. In conjunctival catarrh, the *staphylococcus pyogenes aureus* occurs most constantly and in greatest numbers. 6. In inflammation of the lachrymal sac the diplococcus is invariably present, and that usually in a "pure culture." 7. Panophthalmitis developing after extractions of cataract is caused by the *staphylococcus pyogenes aureus* present in the conjunctival sac. 8. Of antiseptic ophthalmic means in vogue, corrosive sublimate (in the form of irrigations with a solution of 1 to 6,000) is exceedingly weak and untrustworthy in its action, while boracic acid (in the form of irrigations with a three per cent. solution) and iodoform (in powder) are ineffective altogether—they are powerless to destroy the vitality of the microbes or even to arrest their proliferation. 9. The best aseptic and antiseptic means yet known for use in eye practice, is, undoubtedly, trichloride of iodine (ICl_3) recently introduced into surgical practice by Drs. O. Riedel and C. Langenbuch. 10. While being wholly innocuous and void of any irritant properties, the trichloride is most effective in the destruction of microörganisms of any species. 11. In suppurative affections of the conjunctiva, the irrigation with a weak solution (1 to 6,000), repeated three, four, or five times a day, never fails to bring about rapid and striking amelioration. Even after the first three or four sittings, the purulent discharge becomes trifling or often ceases altogether, congestion lessens, and all unpleasant subjective sensations disappear without leaving any trace.

A New Deodorant.

Bromine has for a long time been recognized as being valuable in the treatment of gangrene and foul-smelling ulcers, but until recently its merits as an effectual and cheap deodorant have not been appreciated. It was brought into prominence a few months ago by Mr. Martin, the chemist of the Health Department of New York City, who suggested its use upon the earth thrown up in laying the electric subways. As it is a by-product obtained in the manufacture of salt and is not used extensively in the arts, it is sold at a very reasonable price—about seventy cents per pound. It has the property of precipitating the hydrocarbons of illuminating gas, and thus can be used to deodorize the earth exposed in excavations in the vicinity of gas-mains. More valuable than this is its effect upon decomposing organic bodies, which it renders completely inoffensive. This property renders it especially valuable for use in stables, privy-vaults, urinals, cess-pools, or in any place which may contain foul-smelling organic matters. It is soluble in about thirty-three parts of water, but a solution of this strength is not advisable, as there is a constant escape from it of the vapor of bromine, which is very irritating to the eyes and air-passages, and which may even attack wood and metals. For ordinary purposes it is used in solutions containing one part by weight to about eight hundred of water. In this strength it may be used freely without its affecting anything which it may touch. A few gallons used daily will remove all ammoniacal odors from stables, or a few quarts will thoroughly deodorize the entire plumbing system of an ordinary house. It also might be used with advantage upon ordinary house garbage, which usually becomes offensive so speedily in warm weather. There would appear to be scarcely any limit to its usefulness in this branch of sanitary science, and it will, as soon as its merits are better known, undoubtedly be adopted universally as a substitute for the deodorants now in use, which usually act by substituting one unpleasant odor for another. The only drawback in its use lies in the fact that the undiluted bromine is strongly corrosive, and, if it touches the skin, causes a painful burn. Where it is used in large quantities this can be obviated by opening the bottle or, what is simpler, breaking it under water. As its use becomes more extended it will undoubtedly be put up in pearls or tubes containing only as much as would be needed at one time in the average household.— *N. Y. Med. Journal,* Feb. 2, 1889.

Compound Gonorrhœal Infection.

Bumm, in prosecuting his studies upon the gonococcus, has discovered that infection by two distinct varieties of microorganisms can take place, the first preparing the way for the entry and development of the second.

Thus pyogenic microbes may enter one of Cowper's glands after the gonococcus has destroyed its glandular tissue and caused cystic degeneration, and produce suppuration. The mucous membrane of the bladder or urethral follicles may be affected by the staphylococcus in like manner, and the pelvic connective tissue may be invaded. Tubercular disease of the epididymis and tuberculosis of the Fallopian tubes have been known to follow closely upon a gonorrhœa, and are explained in the same way. In gonorrhœal rheumatism the micrococci found in the fluid of the joints are pyogenic, but why they should make their way to the articulations, and the gonococci not do so, is a question still unexplained.

Another source of error is the nodular lymphangitis of blennorrhagia. Small olive-formed tumors are produced along the course of the lymphatics as large as a cherrystone or a small nut, and are firm, hard, and resistant. They arise insidiously upon the prepuce, but their seat of predilection is the glando-preputial groove, and when hidden by a phimosis they are especially liable to cause an erroneous diagnosis. The diagnosis can, however, be made with almost certainty by the adenopathy, when multiple indolent and long-lasting ganglionic enlargements are present.

These lymphatic nodules are essentially prone to resolution, but when they ulcerate, as they sometimes do, typical indurations characteristic of chancre are presented. Here the only element of diagnosis is found in the evolution of the disease. The indurated chancre never begins as a nodular lesion which opens like an abscess. The diagnosis of chancre should never be made from the objective signs alone. The ecthyma of scabies may easily lead into error, resembling, when covered with a crust, the *chancre croûteux;* or when excori-ated, red, and ulcerating, the ordinary chancre. The glands are often implicated in scabies, and the error of overlooking a chancre in a patient with lesions of scabies upon the genitals must be borne in mind. Treatment directed against the itch will soon make the diagnosis clear.—*Journal of Cutaneous and Genito-Urinary Diseases,* Feb., 1889.

Absorption of the Tissues of the Mouth from Pressure.

The absorption which occasionally takes place from constant pressure upon the tissues of the mouth was well exemplified by two cases brought forward at the Odontological Society of London recently by Mr. Hern and Mr. E. Lloyd Williams respectively. In the first case, the patient had been wearing a set of artificial teeth, the upper and lower of which were attached by means of springs. She had not removed these teeth from her mouth for several years, and, as a result, the lower had become buried in the floor of the mouth; it was also so twisted round as nearly to sever the anterior pillar of the fauces. There was found to be complete anæsthesia of the right half of the tongue and corresponding portion of the floor of the mouth, also complete loss of the sense of taste on that side. There was no pressure on the inferior dental nerve, as sensibility was present in the skin over the chin. The plate was removed with considerable difficulty, and caused much hemorrhage. Some weeks later Mr. Hern observed a whitish cord passing across the gap in the anterior pillar of the fauces; this proved to be the gustatory nerve, and on pinching it with tweezers a tingling sensation was felt in the tip of the tongue. Nine months later sensation had partly returned in the tongue.

Mr. Lloyd Williams showed a man who had extracted two loose molars for himself, the sockets of which probably communicated with the antrum. The patient, being annoyed by the cavity, plugged it with gutta percha, gradually increasing the size until a plug was used measuring more than an inch in diameter. The hole, however, was much larger than this, as the patient was in the habit of encircling the gutta percha with a piece of lettuce leaf. The walls of the antrum presented in places foul ulcerated spots, which, however, speedily disappeared when an obturator was placed in the mouth and antiseptic injections were used.—*Lancet,* Jan. 19, 1889.

THE

MEDICAL AND SURGICAL REPORTER.

ISSUED EVERY SATURDAY.

CHARLES W. DULLES, M.D.,
EDITOR AND PUBLISHER.

The Terms of Subscription to the serial publications of this office are as follows, payable in advance:

Med. and Surg. Reporter (weekly), a year, **$5.00**
Quarterly Compendium of Med. Science, -   2.50
Reporter and Compendium, - - - - 6.00
Physician's Daily Pocket Record, - - 1.00
Reporter and Pocket Record, - - - 6.00
Reporter, Compendium, and Pocket Record, 7.00

All checks and postal orders should be drawn to order of

CHARLES W. DULLES,

N. E. Cor. 13th and Walnut Streets,

P. O. Box 843.   Philadelphia, Pa.

☞ SUGGESTIONS TO SUBSCRIBERS:

See that your address-label gives the date to which your subscription is paid.
In requesting a change of address, give the old address as well as the new one.
If your REPORTER does not reach you promptly and regularly, notify the publisher *at once*, so that the cause may be discovered and corrected.

☞ SUGGESTIONS TO CONTRIBUTORS AND CORRESPONDENTS:

Write in ink.
Write on one side of paper only.
Write on paper of the size usually used for letters.
Make as few paragraphs as possible. Punctuate carefully. Do not abbreviate, or omit words like "the," and "a," or "an."
Make communications as short as possible.
NEVER ROLL A MANUSCRIPT! Try to get an envelope or wrapper which will fit it.
When it is desired to call our attention to something in a newspaper, mark the passage boldly with a colored pencil, and write on the wrapper "Marked copy." Unless this is done, newspapers are not looked at.
The Editor will be glad to get medical news, but it is important that brevity and actual interest shall characterize communications intended for publication.

EXTIRPATION OF TUMORS OF THE BLADDER.

The general adoption of the operation of supra-pubic cystotomy in Europe has led to much more frequent attempts to remove tumors of the bladder than were made a few years ago, when only the difficult and uncertain route through the perineum was open to surgeons. At present no tumor is permitted to make serious advances or to do serious harm to a patient under the observation of a surgeon without an effort to remove it; and nowhere is this more true than in Paris, where the supra-pubic operation is practised almost to the exclusion of other methods.

An illustration of the scope of this operation is furnished by a case described in a recent lecture by Dr. Bazy, at the Hôpital Beaujon, which is reported in the *Bulletin Médical,* January 16, 1889. In this case, after the usual history of a papilloma of the bladder, the patient came under the care of Dr. Bazy, who opened the bladder from above the pubes, and removed a tumor about two and one-half inches in diameter, situated on the right side of the bladder and encroaching a little upon the *bas-fond.* After describing the operation—in which he unwittingly cut off the lower end of the right ureter—Dr. Bazy states his opinion that excision of tumor of the bladder is preferable to enucleation, or scraping, or cauterization. Total ablation is, he thinks, the only way of dealing with these new growths, and that this should be practised as early as possible and made as thorough as possible. The line of excision, he says, should pass through the healthy mucous membrane, and it may even include the opening of one or both ureters, if necessary. In case this is necessary, he thinks the stump of the ureter should be attached to an opening in the bladder-wall, made to receive it. Of course, in such an operation the wound in the bladder and abdominal wall would not be entirely closed, and a suitable drainage-tube should be left in the bladder.

These views are radical, but we believe entirely sound. Tumors of the bladder are dangerous, not only on account of their local and immediate effects, but also on account of their influence upon the kidneys and their proneness to recurrence. It is rational to remove them—as Dr. Bazy advises—as early and as thoroughly as possible, and we think he makes a good point when he prefers excision to the easier methods of scraping or cauterization.

EXPULSION OF FOREIGN BODIES FROM THE ALIMENTARY CANAL.

It is now well understood that very many foreign bodies which have been swallowed will pass through the alimentary canal without giving rise to disturbance, if they are left to nature, and especially if a full vegetable diet is recommended and the use of purgatives is avoided. But it remained for Dr. Cameron, of Glasgow, to propose, for the management of cases of this sort, a formal method which is called the "potato-cure." It consists simply in getting the patient to eat large quantities of potato, which are expected to surround the foreign body and conduct it innocently through the intestines. This plan has worked admirably in a number of cases, and many foreign bodies, both sharp and of irregular form, have been successfully expelled from the alimentary canal under its working.

The subject was brought before the Royal-Imperial Society of Physicians of Vienna, January 11, 1889, and Dr. Cameron's method was warmly endorsed by several distinguished men who had tried it. The general opinion was that it might often obviate the necessity for laparotomy; and a case was reported by Dr. Hochenegg, in which by this means a foreign body had been removed in nine days precisely similar to one which had been removed by laparotomy by Prof. Albert four or five years before.

Such a showing certainly justifies calling attention to this method, although—as stated above—its underlying principles are well enough understood by most medical men.

DEATH CAUSED BY COCAINE-HABIT.

It is reported from Cincinnati that a physician of that city died recently from the effects of cocaine which he had formed the habit of taking frequently. It is said that he began experimenting with the drug a few years ago, and that he soon became a hopeless victim to its influence.

This is a sad story, and one which has a moral. Every now and then it happens that a physician becomes engaged in the toils of alcohol or a narcotic; and the result is usually the same as with men who have no medical training to protect them against delusion in such matters. Under such circumstances the spirit of kindness to the erring generally prompts those who comment on the occurrence to seek out its mitigating circumstances, and to dwell upon them, so as to shield the reputation of the victim as much as possible. This, however, we believe to be more creditable to the hearts of those who discuss so unfortunate an event than to their heads. It would be more likely to prevent the repetition of careers of this sort if a little wholesome truth followed each one. The fact is that physicians, of all men, ought to understand that it is a shame and a disgrace to yield to the seductions of stimulants or narcotics. They know, better than any other class in the community, the peril of trifling with such things, and they have no excuse for indulging a dangerous taste for them. It is probable that men who fall victims to the cocaine, or opium, or alcohol habit are men of weak will, although they may disclose their weakness only in this way. But no medical man can be excused who begins the "easy descent to Avernus," for medical men who do this sin against light; and such errors would probably be less numerous than they are, if the plain truth were told about them. The adage "*nil nisi bonum de mortuis*" has something very attractive in it; but it ought not to stand in the way of truth.

CAMPHORATED NAPHTHOL.

It has recently been found that naphthol, which is very insoluble in water, can be combined with camphor so as to form a liquid. It is only necessary to rub up one part of naphthol with two parts of dry camphor, to obtain a creamy liquid. This product is of a pinkish color if the naphthol is not pure. It has been found to be an excellent antiseptic application to wounds and ulcers, and is said to clean off the false membrane in diphtheria.

IMPOSING ON A PHYSICIAN.

It is almost incredible, but what was printed as a joke in the REPORTER some months ago has been actually put in practice in France. According to the *Gazette Hebdomadaire*, Feb. 1, 1889, a physician in a town in France was called up from his bed on a stormy winter night and implored by a peasant to come to see his child, who was suffering with an affection of the throat which threatened strangulation.

To the hesitation of the doctor to go a distance of five or six miles, he replied that he had come all the way on foot, and it was not too much to ask the doctor to go to such a desperate case. Reluctantly the doctor yielded to his sense of duty, had his carriage made ready, and then, taking his summoner with him, drove to a little village six miles away to see the patient. Arrived here, he gained access to the house with difficulty and found a child with no appearance of illness whatever. The father professed great astonishment, and protested that when he left the child it appeared about to die. With thanks to the doctor, and imitation of the symptoms of the child at an earlier hour, he allowed the physician to make his way home.

A few days later the doctor learned that just before he called him, the man had been in the town on a drinking bout, and had made a bet with a companion that he would not walk home. He won his bet at the expense of the doctor.

It is hard to believe a story of this kind, and yet it is not absolutely beyond belief. The correspondent who communicates it to the *Gazette Hebdomadaire*, couples it with another, to indicate the trials which may meet a physician in the discharge of his duty, and asks what can be done to punish those who could thus impose on the sense of duty and humanity of physicians? Some punishment a wretch of this kind ought to have; but he might better receive it from his fellows than from anyone else, for they would probably find whom the trick hurt most the next time one of them really needed medical aid at night.

The story is mainly interesting as showing that the experience of physicians is pretty much the same all the world over, and that they must expect to make certain sacrifices, for the sake of their calling, not only to the needs of their patients, but also to their ignorance or even their baseness. It is in the face of just such imposition as this story illustrates that the nobility of the medical calling shines brightest.

THE PHILADELPHIA COUNTY MEDICAL SOCIETY.—The members of the Philadelphia County Medical Society are informed that any member who has an appointment to read a paper before the Society will have it set up in type and two galley-proofs furnished him on or before the day of the meeting, provided his copy is placed in the hands of the Editor of the Transactions at least a week before the time it is to be read. This regulation must prove of great convenience to the authors of papers.

PUBLISHING LECTURES WITHOUT PERMISSION OF THE AUTHOR.—On January 7, 1889, Judge Allison made a decree in Court of Common Pleas No. 1, making perpetual the injunction which restrains Walter B. Saunders, a publisher of Philadelphia, from publishing and selling books on general and medical chemistry made up of condensations from lectures delivered at the University of Pennsylvania by Dr. Theodore G. Wormley, Professor of Chemistry and Toxicology in the Medical Department of that institution. The defendant is ordered to pay the costs of the suit. The action of the Court was based on the fact that the defendant failed to plead answer or demurrer to Dr. Wormley's bill of complaint. This decree of Judge Allison may be accepted as finally settling the question of ownership of oral lectures, and will doubtless hereafter deter anyone from publishing lectures without the owner's permission.

BOOK REVIEWS.

[Any book reviewed in these columns may be obtained upon receipt of price, from the office of the REPORTER.]

HANDBOOK OF THE DIAGNOSIS AND TREATMENT OF DISEASES OF THE THROAT, NOSE AND NASO-PHARYNX. BY CARL SEILER, M.D., Instructor in Laryngology and Lecturer on Diseases of the Upper Air Passages in the University of Pennsylvania, etc. Third edition, thoroughly revised, and greatly enlarged. Illustrated. Small 8vo, pp. 373. Philadelphia: Lea Brothers & Co., 1889. Price $2.25.

The fact that Dr. Seiler's manual of the diseases of the throat and nose has reached a third edition may be taken as an indication that its value as a clear and trustworthy treatise on the subject has been appreciated by the profession at large. The present edition has been fully revised so as to make it conform to the advances in laryngology during the last ten years, and it is an admirable representative of the present standing of this department of medicine. The author's style is interesting and attractive, and his book furnishes abundant evidence of his ingenuity and practical skill. It is so written as to be comprehensible to general practitioners as well as to specialists, and, indeed, it seems to be intended rather for the former than for the latter.

It is handsomely printed, abundantly illustrated, and well bound, and as a book is as creditable to the publishers as to its author.

PAMPHLET NOTICES.

[Any reader of the REPORTER who desires a copy of a pamphlet noticed in these columns will doubtless secure it by addressing the author with a request stating where the notice was seen and *enclosing a postage-stamp.*]

217. FUNCTIONS OF A SCHOOL FOR FEEBLE-MINDED. BY A. C. ROGERS, M.D., Faribault, Minn. From the *Proceedings of the Fifteenth National Convention of Charities and Correction,* July, 1888. 5 pages.

218. NEW SERIES OF METRIC TEST-LETTERS AND WORDS FOR DETERMINING THE AMOUNT AND RANGE OF ACCOMMODATION. BY CHARLES A. OLIVER, M.D., Philadelphia. From the *Transactions of the Amer. Ophthalmological Society,* 1886. 3 pages.

219. CANTATORY PARESIS. BY J. SOLIS-COHEN, M.D., Philadelphia. From the *Medical News,* Oct. 6, 1888. 4 pages.

220. SYPHILIS OF THE LARYNX, TRACHEA AND BRONCHI. BY J. SOLIS-COHEN, M.D., Philadelphia. From the *Transactions of the Philadelphia County Medical Society,* Sept. 12, 1888. 24 pages.

221. INEBRIATE ASYLUMS AND THEIR WORK. BY T. D. CROTHERS, M.D., Hartford, Conn. 16 pages.

222. WHY ELECTROLYTIC TREATMENT OF STRICTURE DOES NOT SUCCEED IN ALL HANDS. BY G. C. H. MEIER, M.D., New York. From the *International Journal of Surgery and Antiseptics,* Oct., 1888. 18 pages.

217. Dr. Rogers's paper is one of great interest to all good citizens, and especially to medical men who have so much influence in determining the treatment of those who are sick or maimed in mind as well as in body. He regards idiots and imbeciles as practically incurable, and recommends placing them in homes where they may lead a happy, harmless and measurably useful life in assisting to care for their fellows.

218. Dr. Oliver's pamphlet is somewhat belated in coming to our table; but it deserves attention because it describes a series of tests for accommodation founded upon careful and accurate study of the conditions essential to accurate determination of the range of this function, which we believe have met the approval of other laborers in the field to which he is specially devoted.

219. Dr. Cohen describes the symptoms and treatment of a condition which is familiar to most persons who sing much, and in which attempting to make a given musical note is accompanied with a sense of weakness or even of pain.

220. This paper of Dr. Cohen's is an elaborate and able review of the subject of syphilitic manifestation in the larynx and lower breathing passages. In it the author discusses the pathology, etiology, diagnosis, prognosis and treatment of the various morbid conditions coming under the classification of his title, in a manner which might be expected from his long study and experience in diseases of this region.

221. Dr. Crothers's pamphlet contains part of a lecture delivered before the Young Men's Christian Association of Toronto, Canada, Oct. 2, 1888. It reviews the history of asylums for inebriates—which we have compunctions about calling "inebriate asylums," and makes a special plea for their usefulness and efficiency in curing the alcohol habit. As the superintendent of a well-known establishment of the kind, and as the Editor of the *Journal of Inebriety,* Dr. Crothers speaks with authority on this subject, and his pamphlet will prove interesting and suggestive to those who have the care of any of that unfortunate class for whom such institutions are provided.

222. This is another pamphlet written to defend Dr. Newman against the reflections of his critics, some of whom have classed him with charlatans, and otherwise indicated undisguised contempt for his methods. According to the old maxim: "*Audi alteram partem,*" those who have not done so already might well learn what Dr. Newman and his friends have to say in regard to the comments and experiences of those who think his claims extravagant and his method worthless.

LITERARY NOTES.

—B. Westermann & Co. announce the appearance of the *Microphotographischen Atlas der Bakterienkunde,* edited by Privatdocent Dr. C. Fraenkel and Stabsartzt Dr. R. Pfeiffer. The atlas is to appear in 12 or 15 parts, each containing 10 photograms, and costing $1.50.

—Dr. J. J. Mulheron announces in the *Medical Age,* Feb. 11, that the duties of the chair of Gynecology in the Michigan College of Medicine and Surgery, to which he has been appointed by the Trustees of that institution, added to the cares of private practice, have made it impossible for him longer to edit the *Medical Age.* Dr. B. W. Palmer succeeds Dr. Mulheron as Editor.

CORRESPONDENCE.

Are Medical Witnesses to Be Subjected to New Tests?

To the Editor.

Sir: The report of the treatment of a medical witness by an attorney in a court in Chicago, as published in the editorial in the Reporter of February 16, calls us as physicians to be very cautious when we occupy the position of a witness. It is not probable that a respectable lawyer would imitate the conduct of the one referred to in the case reported; but a question concerning the bearing of a quotation from a medical work may be asked by a lawyer in such a way as—unintentionally to him—to lead a medical witness into error, because the attorney has mistaken the sense of the author. Some years ago, the writer was present in court when an important case was on trial. The prisoner was on trial for his life, being charged with poisoning some of his family with arsenic. His lawyer attempted the defense by taking the position " that the persons who died were affected by cholera morbus, a disease in which there are bloody stools.' The following symptoms were read from a popular medical author on cholera morbus: " The vomiting and purging are almost incessant; everything taken into the stomach is promptly rejected, the discharges being often brown or blackish, acid, or even bloody." This was read to medical witness after witness, and the question asked each one: " Is the author good authority? Is it as stated?' The question specially included the supposition that bloody evacuations from the bowels were meant by the author.

The writer was not satisfied with the nature of the defence, as he had never observed bloody stools as characteristic of cholera morbus. On his return to his office, he consulted the author. On reading the quotation, it will be observed that, after the semicolon, the purging is not referred to, but the author speaks only of the vomiting. The writer repeated this to the prosecution on the following day, with the statement that the author quoted said nothing about bloody stools. The writer was then called to testify and read the passage quoted, pausing after the semicolon and saying "*semicolon*"; then read the remainder of the sentence, when the attorney said : " That is the way in which *you* read it !" " Yes," was the reply, " and so everybody reads it who reads English correctly." Nothing more was heard of the bloody stools during the trial or in the address to the jury.

The writer was called later during the trial to certify to the correctness of passages from medical writers on epilepsy, etc., etc., but he always asked for the book, that he might read the passage referred to for himself.

The moral learned from this and the late trial at Chicago is, Testify to the truth of no printed or written statement before reading it. Yours truly,
Easton, Pa., Traill Green, M.D.
February 21, 1889.

Treatment of Ichthyosis.

To the Editor.

Sir: I have a case of ichthyosis in a colored girl 8 years old. She is otherwise healthy, and has been affected with the disease three years. The whole cutaneous surface is affected, and the feet often crack so that she cannot walk. I have tried all the usual remedies without avail, or only temporary effect. I should like to ask you or the many readers of the Reporter if there is any reliable treatment for this most troublesome affection? An answer will greatly oblige,
Yours truly,
E. I. Persinger, M.D.
Campti, La.,
Feb. 4, 1889.

[It is presumed, in the attempt to answer the inquiry of our correspondent, that his diagnosis is correct; although the statement that the affection began when the patient was five years old throws some doubt on that point, as the disease is usually noted at the second year. Still the error may have been in the statement of the patient.

Ichthyosis is, so far as our present knowledge goes, an incurable disease. The condition may, however, in almost all instances, be kept under control by judicious management. Internal medication is of no value, although it must be stated that the fl. ext. of jaborandi by promoting the perspiratory secretion appears in some cases to have a slightly beneficial effect. The essential treatment of the disease, however, consists in the use of baths and emollient applications. In the milder cases simple soap and hot water baths, or baths made alkaline by the addition of sodium carbonate or borax, will serve to keep the skin in a comfortable condition. After the bath, which should be taken daily or every second day, a mild ointment should be gently rubbed in. For cases of a more severe type, hot water baths with the use of sapo viridis as the soap are useful, supplemented by the application of one of the several well-known ointments advised in the text-books. An ointment especially to be recommended is one consisting of lanolin with ten to fifty grains of salicylic acid to the ounce. In those rare cases of ichthyosis hystrix, operative measures may be demanded.—Editor of the Reporter.]

Removal of Gunpowder from the Face.

To THE EDITOR.

Sir: In reading the REPORTER of February 2, I was much interested in a communication from Dr. John Gray, having reference to the removal of gunpowder from the face. Last Fourth of July, I treated a similar case, partly by removing the individual powder-grains with a cataract-knife, partly by rubbing the face with moistened surgical gauze, but without waiting for suppuration to occur. The latter method proved, in the aggregate, less painful to the patient and more effective than the use of the knife. The result was very satisfactory, but not so perfect as in the case reported by Dr. Gray.

Yours truly,

Philadelphia, A. L. BENEDICT, M.D.
Feb. 11, 1889.

Good Form in Professional Cards.

To THE EDITOR.

Sir: In the REPORTER, February 2, "Country Doctor" asks for a "good form" of medical card. Permit me to offer my country *confrère* the following clipping, not from the *Arizona Kicker*, but from an Arizona weekly of respectability. I do not give the name.

J. E. ——, M.D.,

PHYSICIAN AND SURGEON.

Health Officer, City of ——; for five years
County Physician —— County; Medical
Director Department of Arizona, G. A. R.;
Late Surgeon U. S. Army; for 20
years U. S. Examining Surgeon;
the largest Medical Practitioner
in Arizona, and charges fees
in proportion to his size.
His patrons will find
it to their advan-
tage to keep
healthy.

Office and Dispensary, - - —— Street,

Corner of ——,

——, - - - ARIZONA.

Yours truly,

PELLET.

——Mr. Henry C. Lea has offered to give $25,000 to the Department of Hygiene of the University of Pennsylvania, provided that an equal amount is raised from other sources.

NOTES AND COMMENTS.

The Disposal of Garbage.

The Philadelphia *Ledger*, Feb. 19, 1889, states that the city of Buffalo has in practical operation a method of disposing of garbage which seems to be entirely unobjectionable, and may be made to pay more than the expenses. The system is known as "the Merz" system. The garbage is hauled to two dryers, each of which receives about 5000 pounds at one charge. Each dryer consists of a double-walled metallic cylinder, between the walls of which steam, at a pressure of about eighty pounds, circulates. Within the driers, rakes made of steam pipes revolve. These also contain steam at 80 pounds pressure; but no steam is admitted to the garbage. That which arises by the drying of the mass is carried off by means of a fan to a chamber, where it is condensed by sprays of water and passes off in an inodorous and harmless stream of water. The heat to which the garbage is subjected acts as a disinfectant, if disinfection be needed. Sixty per cent. of the weight of the garbage is thus removed as water. The dried garbage is afterward put into an extractor, which removes all the grease and oil it contains by the liberal use of benzine. The latter is used over and over again without appreciable loss.

The plant in Buffalo disposes of 30,000 pounds of garbage daily, from which about 1800 pounds of grease is recovered. The dried product is screened, and what is removed is sorted out and finds a ready sale, much of it as a fertilizer. There is only a small residuum, which has to be carted away to serve as filling.

It is said that this method of treating garbage pays a good interest on the investment required. If this is true there should not be much difficulty in having it introduced in all large cities, much to the relief of the health authorities.

At the meeting of the Board of Health Feb. 19, the committee to which had been referred the matter of the proper disposal of garbage presented a report to which was appended a resolution that "it is the opinion of the Board of Health that destruction of garbage by fire is the best plan of disposing of this waste material in the cities," and that the "department having charge of the matter be requested to adopt this method as the one best adapted to Philadelphia, and most conducive to the health and comfort of the community."

Hypodermic Injections of Ergot in Facial Neuralgia.

Dr. J. T. Stewart writes to the *Peoria Med. Monthly*, Jan., 1889, that for the relief of facial neuralgia, hypodermic injections of ergot are incomparably superior to either aconite or gelsemium. He says he has used it during the last six years and has only had it fail in one case, in which there was evidently organic disease. Ordinarily, he says, one injection relieves the pain permanently. Sometimes two, and in one very severe and obstinate case which had gone through the hands of several physicians without relief, it required three. After the third injection, the patient never had a twinge of pain. The injection was made as nearly over the seat of pain as convenient. He uses the plain extract, and has it made on purpose for hypodermic use, so that one minum represents two grains of ergot. Of this solution he uses from eight to twelve minims, blood-warm, at one injection, and without further dilution.

In order to make this treatment a success, he says two things are essential. One is, to have a fresh and pure article of ergot to make the extract from, and the other is, to have the extract reasonably fresh. If kept long, it is not only worthless, but is irritating. When properly prepared and fresh, the injection produces more or less pain for ten or fifteen minutes, and when the pain from the injection subsides the neuralgia is usually gone, and does not return.

He has also used this treatment for sciatica and other forms of neuralgia, but not with very satisfactory results.

Action of Peru Balsam in Buccal Leucoplakia.

Dr. Siegfried Rosenberg communicates to the *Therapeutische Monatshefte*, II, 10, 1888, a paper on the action of balsam of Peru upon idiopathic leucoplakia and other epithelial opacities of the mucous membrane of the mouth. He has employed it locally in different affections of the mucous membrane of the mouth and has found it good. When there is great pain and in persistent rhagades the balsam is painted on with a fine pencil, in the thick insensitive plaques with a bristle-brush, from one to three times a day. Care must be taken to have a pure, good preparation, to admonish the patient to hold the balsam some minutes in the mouth, and not to abandon the treatment too soon— especially in leucoplakia the result is at times somewhat long delayed. Dr. Rosenberg communicates a number of histories of patients, and concludes with the following words: Peru balsam acts as an anodyne in the painful affections depending upon tissue alterations of the mucous membrane; in loss of tissue it hastens skinning over and healing, and causes epithelial opacities to disappear.—*Schmidt's Jahrbücher*, Jan. 15, 1889.

Camphoric Acid in Catarrhs of Mucous Membranes.

Dr. Max Neisel states in the *Deutsche med. Wochenschrift*, XIV, 40, 1888, that he has employed, in Mosler's clinic, camphoric acid in one-half to one per cent. glycerine or alkaline solution in the form of gargles, applications made with a brush, or inhalations, and has obtained good results in slight catarrhs of the larynx, throat, and bronchi. The action of washings of a twenty per cent. alcoholic solution diluted with luke-warm water to one-half or one per cent. was especially favorable in two cases of chronic cystitis.

Given internally, camphoric acid seems to be of advantage in the night-sweats of phthisis. It may be given in capsules containing fifteen or twenty grains.—*Schmidt's Jahrbücher*, Jan. 15, 1889.

Anemone Pulsatilla in Gonorrhœal Orchitis.

Dr. Martel has employed anemone pulsatilla for some years in gonorrhœal orchitis with success. In 1885 and 1886, he reported a series of cases which he had cured with this agent, in doses of thirty drops of the tincture in twenty-four hours. The drug has the advantage of mitigating the pains and enabling the patient to walk. Dr. Bazy has taken up the experiments lately in the Hospital Midi, Paris, and communicates to the *Sémaine Médicale*, No. 2, an account of forty-eight cases so treated. In thirty-five cases, recovery was complete; in ten, there was marked improvement; in two, recovery is uncertain; and in one case, the drug had no effect.

Bazy employs the drug in the following formula:

℞ Tinct. anem. pulsatillæ . . . gtt. xxx
    Syrupi . . . . f ℥ iv
M. Sig. Dessertspoonful every two hours.

The remedy is willingly taken and well borne by the patients. Treatment must be continued until complete recovery occurs. The average time required for cure is eleven days.—*Wiener med. Presse*, Jan. 20, 1889.

Disagreeable Effect of Sulphonal.

Dr. J. M. Loebl writes to the *Wiener med. Presse* that his advice was sought by a woman who complained of having been affected with sleeplessness for a long time. The patient looked anæmic, but he found nothing else to account for her sleeplessness. He prescribed thirty grains of sulphonal in two doses, with the direction to take a powder in warm soup or milk one hour before bed-time. When he was called two days later he found the patient in a lamentable condition. She stated that after the first powder she did not obtain much sleep, and on the following day was somewhat deaf. In the evening she took the second powder. After a restless night, in the morning she felt intense headache, dizziness, nausea, sensations of heat and cold. Every effort to rise induced nausea. The skin was cool, the pulse 55. After the patient had taken tea and rum the pulse rose gradually to 70, though the remaining symptoms lasted the whole day and a great part of the night. On the following morning she was able for the first time to resume her household duties, though she still felt giddy. It was then learned that the patient was menstruating, and to this Dr. Loebl was inclined to attribute the whole disturbance, but the patient declared positively that she had never been so affected before, and attributed the condition to the hypnotic.

The author suggests that this case shows that sulphonal can give rise to disagreeable symptoms in some persons—probably in anæmic patients—and that it has a cumulative action.

Fatal Case of Corrosive Sublimate Poisoning After a Surgical Operation.

Professor Wilhelm Weiss communicates an account of a fatal case of corrosive sublimate poisoning after a surgical operation in the *Casopis lékaru Ceskych*, Nos. 1 and 2, 1889. At his clinic on October 19, 1888, a strong woman, 53 years old, had a lipoma weighing twenty-seven and a half pounds removed from the inner surface of the left thigh, and the wound washed with two quarts of a one per cent. corrosive sublimate solution, the wound then appearing to be covered with a fine white coating. The wound was dressed with sublimate gauze bandages. Some hours after the operation collapse and frequent vomiting of a greenish fluid occurred. In the night there were pains in the abdomen, repeated vomiting, and involuntary passage of fetid stools. Opium clysters and stimulants were administered. On the following day there were frequent evacuations with tenesmus, and collapse. Death occurred on Oct. 22, at six o'clock in the morning.

At the autopsy were found acute gangrenous inflammation of the ileum and colon as the result of corrosive sublimate poisoning; also acute parenchymatous degeneration of the kidneys. Weiss thinks that the occurrence of poisoning in this, as well as in most of the cases of corrosive sublimate poisoning occurring in surgical operations, must be attributed to a special idiosyncrasy toward mercury; and he mentions a case seen by him in which, after a single insufflation of a small quantity of calomel, violent stomatitis and other pronounced symptoms of poisoning had occurred. He regards the inflammation of the ileum and colon in corrosive sublimate poisoning as conditions secondary to the primary parenchymatous nephritis, and therefore urges the necessity of being assured before every surgical application of corrosive sublimate that the kidneys are perfectly healthy.—*Wiener med. Presse*, Jan. 20, 1889.

Eschscholtzia Californica: a New Hypnotic.

Ter - Zakariantz speaks highly in the *Semaine Médicale*, No. 52, of a new hypnotic—eschscholtzia californica. It belongs to the family of the papaveraceæ, and he declares it to be both a valuable hypnotic and a very useful anodyne, and, being harmless, preferable to morphine. It can be administered in the form of a potion, of a syrup, or in pills in daily doses of thirty-seven and a half to one hundred and fifty grains. Several formulæ are given by him.—*Wiener med. Presse*, Jan. 6, 1889.

Munificent Gift to the Presbyterian Hospital.

Mr. John H. Converse has about perfected arrangements for the erection of a building, to be given by him to the Presbyterian Hospital, of Philadelphia. This intended gift was referred to in the REPORTER, Feb. 16, p. 215.

The new structure is to be called the Administration building, and will cost between $60,000 and $70,000. It will be an ornamental structure of stone and brick, and will be supplied with all the improvements adapted to a building of the kind. It will be four stories high with a large basement. In the basement there will be offices, dining rooms for servants, kitchens, pantries, etc. The first floor will contain the office of the superintendent, a surgical clinic room, operating rooms, an apothecary shop, a room for the meetings of the Board of Trustees and the offices of the physicians in charge of the hospital. The second, third and fourth floors will contain the various sleeping apartments for the physicians and nurses.

The Minnesota Medical Act.

Dr. Perry H. Millard, of St. Paul, Minn., writes to the *Journal of the Amer. Med. Association*, Feb. 2, 1889, concerning the work accomplished by the State Board of Medical Examiners of Minnesota in the brief period of its existence, working under the provisions of the present State Medical Practice Act. The statistics are presented with the hope that they may direct the attention of the profession anew to the benefit to be derived, by both the public and profession, from efficient medical legislation, and trusting that they may further stimulate the profession in securing, at the hands of the respective legislatures, now in session, such legislation as is required to protect both the public and the profession. The present Act regulating the practice of medicine in Minnesota, became operative, July 1, 1887, and succeeded the old Act that had been in successful operation for a period of four and a half years. The old Act was a verbatim copy of the present Illinois Act, excepting that the exemption clause was five years instead of ten, which is the period of exemption of the Illinois Act. Through the operations of the old Act the profession of the State had experienced some of the benefits of medical legislation, and was therefore disposed to aid and support the present Act in every way possible. The Minnesota Act has been enforced in a quiet, conscientious and determined manner, by a board composed of the leading representative men of the profession of the State. The Act has received no mention by the medical press of the country, notwithstanding the fact that it is the best Act in existence in any State, and is as ably enforced as any of the various State Medical Acts. The present board has held seven quarterly meetings, at which eighty-six physicians have applied to be examined. Of this number six were refused admission to the class, not having taken three full courses of medical lectures of six months duration each. Of the eighty entering the various examinations, fifty-one were licensed. Some of this number under-

went several quarterly examinations before being successful. Twenty-nine were rejected, not possessing the knowledge of medicine required by the board. Of those who passed, forty-nine are Regulars and two Homœopaths. Of those failing to pass the examination, eighteen were Regulars, eight were Homœopaths, and only three were electic physicians. Those passing the examinations of the board were mostly graduates of McGill, Harvard, Chicago Medical, and the University of Michigan. Students who were graduates of the two-term schools and those having sessions of less than six months duration, are of course prohibited the privilege of practice in the State.

American Medical Association.

The Fortieth Annual Meeting of the Association will be held in Newport, R. I., June 25, 1889, under the Presidency of W. W. Dawson, M.D., of Cincinnati, Ohio.

The Chairman of the Committee of Arrangements is H. R. Storer, M.D., of Newport, R. I.

Those who intend to read papers are requested to send word as soon as possible to the chairman of the proper section. The sections and officers are as follows:

Practice of Medicine, etc.—F. C. Shattuck, Boston, Mass., Chairman; G. A. Fackler, Cincinnati, O., Secretary.

Surgery and Anatomy.—N. P. Dandridge, Cincinnati, O., Chairman; W. O. Roberts, Louisville, Ky., Secretary.

Obstetrics and Diseases of Women.—W. H. Wathen, Louisville, Ky., Chairman; A. B. Carpenter, Cleveland, O., Secretary.

State Medicine.—J. Berrien Lindsley, Nashville, Tenn., Chairman; S. T. Armstrong, U. S. Marine Hospital, New York, Secretary.

Ophthalmology.—Geo. E. Frothingham, Ann Arbor, Mich., Chairman; G. C. Savage, Nashville, Tenn, Secretary.

Laryngology and Otology.—W. H. Daly, Pittsburgh, Pa., Chairman; E. Fletcher Ingals, Chicago, Ill., Secretary.

Diseases of Children.—J. A. Larrabee, Louisville, Ky., Chairman; C. J. Jennings, Detroit, Mich., Secretary.

Medical Jurisprudence. — W. Kiernan, Chicago, Ill., Chairman; T. C. Evans, Baltimore, Md., Secretary.

Dermatology and Syphilography.—L. Duncan Bulkley, N. Y., Chairman; W. T. Corlett, Cleveland, Ohio, Secretary.

Oral and Dental Surgery.—F. H. Rehwinkle, Chillicothe, O., Chairman; E. S. Talbot, Chicago, Ill., Secretary.

NEWS.

—The Swedish government has permitted cremation under certain medical and clerical restrictions.

—Fifteen hundred physicians attended the third Russian Medical Congress held at St. Petersburg Jan. 15.

—Hiram Vandusen, of New York City, asserts that he has lived for sixty-five days on Vichy and Croton water.

—The will of the late Alexander Murray, of Montreal, bequeaths to the Montreal General Hospital the sum of $750,000.

—The son of Dr. Jacoby, a boy 11 years old, was recently cremated in Paris. This is the first cremation that has taken place there.

—The *Lancet*, Feb. 9, announces that Dr. H. Frémy has been sent by the French Government to Colorado to study its climate.

—The Moral Reform Union of England has been exerting its influence to prevent the employment of children of a school age at theatres.

—The deaths in Philadelphia for the week ending Feb. 23, numbered 347. There were 11 deaths from scarlet fever, 18 from typhoid fever, and 7 from diphtheria.

—The *Lancet*, Feb. 16, says the Russian Government has found it necessary to issue a regulation forbidding female medical practitioners to attend adults of the male sex.

—Dr. William Pepper, Provost of the University of Pennsylvania has announced that during the coming year it is proposed to put up a dormitory building for the accommodation of the University students.

—The *British Med. Journal*, Feb. 9, states that Dr. Fancourt Barnes's "Manual of Midwifery for Midwives" has been translated into Burmese by order of those in charge of the Countess of Dufferin's Fund.

—An extensive epidemic of a scarlatinal character is said by the *Lancet*, Feb. 16, to prevail in and around Macclesfield. Upward of a hundred cases have already occurred, and some deaths have been reported. The milk supply is suspected to be the source of the poison.

—A state vaccine institute has been established in Italy by Royal decree. It will be under the direction of the Department of Public Health and of the Ministry of the Interior. The Committee of Management consists of Professor L. Pagliani, Dr. Felice Baroffio, and Prof. Davide Toscani.

HUMOR.

It is doubtless a knowledge of the fact that every one can see through it that causes the window pane.—*Life.*

Needed a Change.—Doctor—"What your husband needs, Madam, is change of scene."

Mrs. De Temper—"Do you think he should go off for his health?"

"Well, it doesn't matter which goes—you or he."

"The editor down the street," writes a Kansas editor, with withering scorn, "should go to school during the winter months, so that the teacher can learn him something about grammar. We have seen bad writers before, but we never seen one who could crowd so many grammatical erratum into a single sentence."—*Kansas City Star.*

A Wise Medicine man.—Dr. Ebbonie—"Dat chile o' yours am lookin' poo'ly, Mrs. Yallerby. What's he done gone an' swallowed this time?"

Mrs. Yallerby—"A bit ob lead-pencil, docto'."

Dr. Ebbonie—"H'm! What he wants now, ma'am, am an erasive remedy. I recommend him ter chew a piece ob Injy-rubber half an hour afore each meal."—*Puck.*

A placard placed on the window of a shoemaker's shop near Cripplegate, London, many years ago, is said to have read as follows:

Surgery
performed on aged
Boots and Shoes
broken Legs sett and bound upright
disordered feet repaired
the wounded heeld, .
The whole Constitution mended
and the Body supported
by
a new Sole. By T. T.

OBITUARY.

WILLIAM WEIGHTMAN, JR., M.D.

Dr. William Weightman, Jr., died at his residence, Falls of Schuylkill, Feb. 10. Dr. Weightman was born in Philadelphia October 10, 1845. After a thorough school education he studied medicine at the University of Pennsylvania, from which he was graduated with honors. Immediately after graduating he entered the employ of Powers & Weightman, manufacturing chemists, and was admitted into the firm in 1884, soon afterward taking charge of the works at the Falls of Schuylkill.

MEDICAL AND SURGICAL
REPORTER

No. 1671.   PHILADELPHIA, MARCH 9, 1889.   VOL. LX.—No. 10.

CONTENTS:

LECTURE.

ANÆSTHETICS.[1]

BY J. WILLIAM WHITE, M.D.,

PHILADELPHIA.

DEMONSTRATOR OF SURGERY; CLINICAL PROFESSOR OF GENITO-URINARY DISEASES; SURGEON TO THE PHILADELPHIA, GERMAN AND UNIVERSITY HOSPITALS.

Gentlemen: The various methods of producing anæsthesia for surgical purposes at the present day are deserving of the most careful study and consideration. The number and variety of surgical operations have so enormously increased under the influence of the discovery of antisepsis that the problem of how most safely to produce unconsciousness has become one of correspondingly increased importance. I shall try to review the subject as well as can be done within the limits of an hour, confining myself to the fundamental principles involved and

[1] A lecture delivered to the Graduating Class of the University of Pennsylvania, Session 1888-1889.

using freely such teachings and writings as are considered authoritative.

The agents employed as anæsthetics may be included under the following heads: 1. Alcohol. 2. Chloroform. 3. Ethers. 4. Methylene. 5. Nitrous Oxide.

The first four in all probability act in a somewhat similar manner in producing anæsthesia, *i.e.*, they directly affect the nerve centres; but their secondary effects are altogether different.

ALCOHOL may be dismissed in a few words. The narcosis which it produces when swallowed is unfortunately familiar by observation to almost every one, in the shape of profound intoxication, but it may also be brought about by inhalation as is the case with the other anæsthetics. Alcoholic narcosis, however, is much more persistent and consequently much more dangerous than that of the more volatile anæsthetics which are absorbed and eliminated with greater rapidity. Unconsciousness can be produced in this way only by a much greater expenditure of time. The preliminary period of excitement is vastly more prolonged, the patient is far more uncontrollable, and the resulting narcosis will sometimes persist for hours. The drug is therefore not used at the present time as an anæsthetic, and requires no further consideration.

CHLOROFORM.—In this country chloroform is employed as an anæsthetic, by the great majority of surgeons, only in those cases in which the other anæsthetics have failed, or in those exceptional operations, such as staphylorraphy, in which it is especially desirable to prevent coughing and the hypersecretion of bronchial and laryngeal mucus. It is still used largely in obstetric practice, and is said to be far safer when given to children than when employed with adults. So far as I know no satisfactory explanation of this fact, if it be a fact, has yet been advanced.

Chloroform undoubtedly has certain advantages over ether. It is cheaper, it acts in smaller quantity, its local anæsthetic action is greater than that of ether, and hence there is not so much mucus thrown out from the throat and lungs; it is not so apt to be followed by nausea and vomiting; being less volatile it does not so completely fill the pulmonary spaces with its vapor, and there is less of the suffocating feeling which most patients have when they take ether.

These are, I believe, all the advantages that can possibly be claimed for chloroform. To counterbalance them we have the one all-important fact, that chloroform has killed about one person out of every 2600 to whom it has been administered. The individuals to whom it is safe to give it cannot with any certainty be selected beforehand. In many cases the autopsies have disclosed no evidence of disease of any sort. The patients have simply died "poisoned."

We have, as yet, no conclusive evidence or statistics to enable us to balance the merits of the different anæsthetics in a perfectly mathematical manner. We know that between the years 1870 and 1885, 184 deaths have been published in England as occurring under chloroform, which is slightly over 12 in a year. The number of times that chloroform has been administered in the same period is not known. At Saint Bartholomew's from 1875 to 1880, chloroform had been used 4810 times with two deaths. Mr. Williams has recorded, as his personal experience, 208 cases of chloroforming with one death. On the other hand, between 1870 and 1885, 28 cases of death from ether in England alone have been recorded. Saint Bartholomew's tables give 6440 cases with two deaths; Mr. Williams 1050 cases with one death.

Of course, in giving any anæsthetic it is highly important that the lungs, the heart, and the kidneys should be sound. But this is far more important or essential in giving chloroform than in giving any of the others. It has so high a boiling point and is therefore volatilized with such comparative slowness that it is probably never eliminated entirely by the lungs, but only with the aid of the excretory organs generally.

If the lungs have a smaller area than usual on account of disease, just so much more strain is thrown on the kidneys, and if in addition they are contracted or fatty, the danger is greatly increased. It is, however, usually by its depressant action on the heart that chloroform kills, and it seems highly probable that it often does this by the property which it has been shown to have, of destroying the contractile power of the cardiac muscle when it reaches it in a sufficiently concentrated form.

Various circumstances may greatly affect the degree of its concentration in the lungs and circulation, and thus increase, or decrease, the danger of its employment. Of these the most important are those connected with the character of the respiration of the patient and the circulation through the lungs. For example, a given quantity of chloroform, say one drachm, will exert its greatest effect when the respiration is deep and quick, because the vapor is then carried, in any given moment of time, in larger quantity into the air spaces of the lungs. If, at the same time, the patient, being only partially anæsthetized, stops suddenly after breathing deeply, i. e., closes his glottis and strains, he increases the rapidity of absorption of the chloroform vapor into the blood; or if the movement of blood through the lungs is exceptionally slow as shown by a dusky or congested appearance of the face, the opportunity for absorption will likewise be greater, and the blood will reach the heart overcharged with chloroform, and possibly produce its poisonous effect. A low temperature of the blood of the patient, as in cases of shock, seems to act in the same manner, probably by hastening the condensation of the chloroform vapor in the pulmonary tissues and favoring its absorption into the blood.

A combination of these conditions therefore should put the anæsthetizer, especially one who employs chloroform, on his guard. And, during the preliminary stages of chloroformization, at least, it may be said that a patient who is shocked by injury or accident, who is only partially anæsthetizéd, whose face is dusky or congested, whose breathing is quick, and who is struggling against the anæsthetic, is in the greatest danger. Many deaths have occurred from chloroform under these circumstances and in this first, or so-called stage of excitement. The second stage is the period of true anæsthesia, during which consciousness and sensibility are abolished, the muscles relaxed, the pulse weak, the breathing often shallow and feeble; it is during this stage that operations should be performed and great care observed to limit the quantity of chloroform used to the least amount necessary to continue the condition without causing it to pass into the third stage, or that of narcosis in which there is increasing weakness of the pulse, stertorous breathing, complete abolition of the reflexes and other indications of profound involvement of the nerve centres. This is still more dangerous than either of the other stages. There may be no premonitory symptoms of danger, or it may be indicated by either great paleness or congestion of the face, or by marked irregularity and failure of the pulse.

It seems probable that the position of the patient during chloroforming has much to do in increasing or diminishing the risks of perspiratory or cardiac failure. It is said that during gynecological and obstetric operations, in which the patients are kept lying on the left side, the pulse and respiration have been more satisfactory during anæsthesia from chloroform than when the patients have taken it in the usual position. A celebrated surgeon is said to have noted the fact that all of his patients who, when in danger of death from chloroform, were rolled upon the left side recovered, while those kept on their backs or placed in other positions not infrequently died. It may be that the view which attributes special safety to the drug in obstetrical cases took its origin in the fact that the customary obstetrical position in England is upon the left side. Dr. Buxton thinks that the influence of position is unquestionably important and is due to the fact that the condition of the heart, lungs, tongue, and larynx is more nearly correct physically and physiologically when a patient is placed in the left lateral position instead of on the back. He mentions as corroborative the circumstance that during sleep and in all conditions in which respiration is shallow and is carried on at a disadvantage, most persons instinctively assume the lateral position. He adds that

the difference in the condition of the pulse and respiration of patients chloroformed in the dorsal and lateral positions has been so striking as gradually to force on one the lesson of placing every patient where it is possible on the left side before chloroforming him.

Various apparatuses have been devised for the administration of chloroform, most of them too complicated and expensive for practical use. In my opinion the safest and therefore the best way of giving it is by pouring a few drops at a time upon the surface of a folded towel or napkin and, holding it at first two or three inches from the nose of the patient, gradually lessening the distance as its effects begin to be produced. It should always be given while the patient is in a reclining or recumbent posture, being especially dangerous on account of the tendency of heart failure if it is given to persons in an erect or semi-erect position. During its administration certain indications should put the anæsthetizer immediately upon his guard. These are, in the order of their danger, first, failure of the pulse; second, sudden change in the color of the face, extreme pallor denoting a tendency to syncope while a dusky or purplish face indicates obstructed respiration; third, stridulous breathing; this if very marked may indicate spasm of the glottis either from direct irritation by the chloroform vapor, or from reflex action caused by the operation which may have been begun; or the same breathing may be produced by the falling backward of the tongue and epiglottis, which thus cover more or less completely the aperture of the larynx.

These conditions, while more likely to occur during anæsthesia from chloroform, may also be produced by ether and other anæsthetic agents. The duty of the anæsthetizer should be the same in every case. He should promptly take the following precautions:

1. Remove the anæsthetic and secure a plentiful supply of fresh air about the head and face of the patient.

2. Place the fingers back of the angles of the inferior maxilla and press it strongly forward, thus carrying with it the tongue.

3. Seize the tongue near its tip and draw it forward.

4. Lower the head of the patient or, if the case is a grave one, raise the lower limbs, pelvis, and trunk higher than the head and shoulders.

5. Begin the movements of artificial respiration, catching the arms at the elbows and carrying them outward and upward

until they almost meet in a line above the head, then bringing them down again until they touch the sides of the chest ; at each movement moderate pressure should be made upon the lower portion of the sternum These motions should be repeated not oftener than 16 or 18 times per minute. This time honored method of artificial respiration has never been improved upon, and a large quantity of air can be made to pass through the lungs with each of these movements.

6. Dash alternately hot and cold water on the front of the chest.

7. Give hypodermics of strychnia.

8. Rub the extremities strongly toward the heart.

9. Compress the abdominal aorta.

The last two methods are intended to keep the blood in the region of the heart and great nerve centres where, at least during the period of shock, its presence is vitally important.

10. Faradize the diaphragm, placing one pole on the pit of the stomach and the other over the root of the neck.

11. Small lumps of ice, or " ice suppositories," inserted into the rectum, will sometimes by reflex action bring about deep breathing.

12. As soon as swallowing returns use diffusible cardiac stimulants—alcohol, ammonia, and possibly digitalis. The majority of these directions apply also to difficulty arising during the use of ether, which we may now consider.

ETHER.—Ether is the chief anæsthetic employed in practical surgery in this country. It produces when inhaled a succession of conditions very like those described as caused by chloroform, but with important differences.

1. A stage of excitement preceded by a feeling of strangulation or of suffocation, with a burning sensation in the fauces, lachrymation, often more or less coughing, accompanied by excessive secretion of laryngeal and bronchial mucus. In other words, we have during this period of excitement the evidences of the local, irritating action of the ether upon the mucous surfaces with which it comes in contact. The patient may at this time pass into a condition closely resembling natural sleep, often mistaken by inexperienced etherizers for one of true anæsthesia. During this condition the patient can easily be aroused and is sometimes quite conscious of all that is going on about him. Indeed, during the whole of this stage the special senses are often almost preternaturally acute, and a remark made by the surgeon or his assistant will often be responded to promptly and intelligently by the patient.

2. This passes after a variable interval into a period of unconsciousness, at first accompanied by some degree of muscular rigidity, but soon followed by relaxation. The complexion should be unaltered ; the pulse is usually increased in force and volume.

3. If the etherization is pushed and a large quantity of the anæsthetic employed a stage characterized by stertor and profound coma follows, the pulse being still strong and full but the face becoming flushed or purplish. This stage should only be occasionally and accidentally reached during etherization, and should be the signal for the temporary withdrawal of the anæsthetic and immediate inspection of the respiratory conditions with careful attention to the mouth and throat and watchfulness to see that the tongue is well forward, and the movements of breathing deep.

It cannot be said that ether is absolutely safe and harmless under all circumstances, as there have been a number of deaths reported from its use or, at least, during its use. In the great majority of these cases the exact responsibility of the anæsthetic itself has never been determined.

In 1861, a committee of the Boston Society for the Improvement of Medical Science reported that after a labored search they had learned of no case which was unquestionably and unavoidably fatal from the breathing of pure sulphuric ether. They considered two conditions essential to placing the responsibility of any case of death upon the anæsthetic: 1. That the event should occur while the patient is actually anæsthetized. 2. That the circumstance of its occurrence should be inexplicable by any phenomena of disease or by the operation. Very few, if any, reported cases comply fully with these conditions.

The deaths recorded by Turnbull and Lyman in their treatises, and by Jacob (*British Med. Journal*), are either uncertain in their relation to etherization, or were caused by asphyxia, or more rarely by syncope.

Druet (*Des Contraindications de l' Anæsthesie,* 1880) and Kappeller (*Deutsche Chirurgie,* 1881) give no new light on sudden deaths occurring during anæsthesia, and accompanied by cessation of respiration. The cases of Hunt, Morton, Levis, Hutchinson, Norris, Sims, Emmet, and others, are all instances of death after anæsthesia, at periods ranging from two hours to eighteen days, and possibly associated with nephritis.

One reported by Allier and two by Post occurred during operations for tumors of the neck. In connection with these the observation of Schiff should be remembered, that when animals are anæsthetized, pinching the skin of the neck will at once arrest both respiration and the action of the heart.

In several recorded cases, while herniotomy was being performed, the patient vomited and died. Mr. Marcus Gunn has suggested that as the vomiting of acute intestinal obstruction results from a powerful descending impulse of the vagus, and as sudden arrest of the heart's action in diastole is also known to be produced by such an impulse, we may expect to meet with this association of vomiting and sudden heart-failure during as well as before and after anæsthesia. The same result has occurred even more frequently under other anæsthetics.

Warrington Hayward records a death during etherization from the sudden failure of respiration owing to the occurrence of an epileptiform spasm of the respiratory muscles, whereby the chest was fixed in the position of expiration. Nothing was discovered either at the time or at the autopsy, which gave any clew as to how the fatality could have been avoided.

The doctrine of cerebral inhibition advanced by Brown-Séquard should not be overlooked in its application to the few cases of sudden death during etherization in which the autopsies failed to explain the accident. He has shown that there is an arrest or suspension of function in the nerve centres, muscles, and nerves, taking place without demonstrable organic change, and following immediately upon irritation of the nervous system at some point more or less distant from the part in which the effect is observed. He attributes to this cerebral inhibition the cases of sudden death and "death without agony" which are analogous to the loss of intellectual activity that occurs in epilepsy. Such death may be produced in animals by a prick of the ventricle of Arantius in the floor of the fourth ventricle.

But one instance of death during etherization has come under my immediate notice. A middle-aged man, apparently healthy, came to Philadelphia from the northern part of this State to have an operation for the relief of hemorrhoids performed by Dr. Agnew. After the customary prep-

arations, the administration of ether was begun, and progressed until the second stage was reached, muscular rigidity not having entirely disappeared. Sensation having been abolished, however, the operation was begun and one hemorrhoid was ligated, when the patient suddenly ceased to breathe. Every effort was made to bring about natural respiration, but without success. The entire quantity of ether given did not exceed four ounces. The autopsy showed that death had resulted from an apoplexy into the fourth ventricle, a small coagulum being found in that position and resting upon the respiratory centre. The vessels of the circle of Willis were brittle and atheromatous, as were also the vessels of the entire brain. The increased vascular tension produced by the ether was probably the immediate cause of death in this case, but of course the anæsthetic should not be held accountable for the death, as any other condition which would have increased the blood-pressure would have produced the same accident.

Dr. Fritz Feuter has recently published an elaborate article upon ether anæsthetization, recording his experience in a large number of cases. He has always employed a large face mask, around the edges of which a folded towel is laid to prevent evaporation of the drug.

The following four points were separately dealt with, as being of most importance: First, the time from the beginning of anæsthization until anæsthesia is produced. Second, the quantity of ether necessary for this. Third, the total quantity of ether used; and fourth, the duration of the anæsthesia. His method of administration is as follows: From a graduated bottle about 50 Ccm. is poured upon the mask (for an adult, for children half this quantity is sufficient). The mask is then slowly brought down to the face so that the patient gradually becomes accustomed to the fumes; this does away with that painful choking which always occurs if the mask is abruptly placed upon the face. So soon as the mask is well over the face a folded towel is placed around it, and the mask is not removed again until there is complete relaxation of the extremities. In this way the patient is continually inhaling ether fumes, for even his exhalations are partly reinhaled, and assist in producing anæsthesia. With these precautions carefully adhered to, the author has invariably found that complete anæsthesia could be induced within two minutes. More than this, the amount of ether subsequently required to maintain unconsciousness is remarkably small. Often in operations of over a half hour's duration, and even longer, no addition of ether was necessary.

In his opinion the two most important points upon which the success of etherization depends are the concentration of the fumes and the non-removal of the mask. The nausea following etherization he believes to be due to the swallowing of saliva which is filled with ether, the secretion being greatly increased by the drug; naturally, therefore, the less ether used the greater probability that nausea will not be produced; and indeed his experiments seem to justify this conclusion, for in one hundred and fifty cases vomiting only occurred in ten, and in two of these the patients had taken a meal immediately before the operation. In quoting the statistics of other clinics, he states that out of five hundred and fifty-three cases vomiting occurred in one hundred and forty-eight. Feuter continues by giving a list of personal observations which differ but slightly from those of other practitioners. One fact, however, deserves special notice, viz., he has observed in several cases that when the patient had taken a moderate quantity of alcohol just previous to the operation that the anæsthetization was greatly accelerated; indeed, in one instance hardly a minute passed before the patient was in a complete stupor. Emmet was the first to point out the danger of etherizing patients affected with nephritic troubles. He claims that it is absolutely necessary to examine carefully the urine of such patients before operating, and holds that the presence of albumin is a positive contra-indication for the use of ether, and direct indication for the use of chloroform. Other authorities are of the same opinion. In direct contradiction of the above statements, Feuter declares that he has frequently etherized patients with albuminuria without dangerous symptoms resulting.

Dr. Robert Lovett has reported lately some careful observations in a series of sixty consecutive cases at the Boston City Hospital. He used two methods; one, which he calls the gentle method, in which the ether was given slowly and cautiously; the other the "forcible" method, in which the cone was at once applied closely to the nostrils and mouth of the patient. The former method required an average time of 9.3 minutes and an average amount of 2.5 ounces for complete anæsthesia. The latter only required 4.4 minutes and 1.5 ounces, but the choking sensation was very much aggravated and the patients were very apt to react and struggle violently if they got only a breath of air.

I may say that this experience about corresponds with that of Dr. Agnew and myself in the use of a rapid method by which the ether contained in a bottle was dropped into a bucket of hot water by the bedside of the patient, the vapor being conveyed by a long flexible tube to a mask placed tightly over the mouth and nose of the patient. Our average time for producing insensibility in some dozens of cases was considerably less than a minute—about 43 seconds, and was often within a half-minute; but the condition was rather one of asphyxia than of true anæsthesia; the distress of the patients was very great, and the evidences of excessive increase of vascular tension were so unmistakable and sometimes so alarming that after a fair trial we gave up the method, believing that no economy of time or of ether would compensate for the slightest increased risk to the patient.

On the whole, it may be said that there is no perfectly satisfactory evidence that ether *per se* ever kills, and although it undoubtedly may do so by producing asphyxia, in the vast majority of cases it will do this so slowly and give such marked evidence of its threatening action that every opportunity will be afforded the etherizer to avoid or prevent it.

There is hardly a case in which ether can not be given with safety, but there are certain classes of cases in which there is special danger. These are: 1. Very old people with emphysema, fatty heart, hypertrophy or valvular disease of the heart. 2. Persons with marked tendency to weak heart action or syncope. 3. Persons with extensive lung disease, or with lungs greatly tied down by old pleuritic adhesions. 4. Habitual drunkards. 5. Persons who as the result of alcohol, syphilis, gout, rheumatism, or old age have marked evidences of extensive atheromatous disease.

In the presence of any of these conditions ether should be given very slowly with a large admixture of atmospheric air, and with great attention to the pulse, complexion, and the movements of breathing. The following rules, many of them almost self-evident but all of them important, apply to the preparation of a patient not only for etherization but for the administration of any anæsthetic.

1. The stomach should be empty. No hearty meal should have been taken for at least six or eight hours before the operation.

It is a good rule to insist that all nourishment taken on that day shall be liquid or nearly so, and in many cases it is well to limit the patient to a glass of milk taken early in the morning. This precaution lessens the risk of solid morsels of food being drawn into the air passages during vomiting; makes vomiting less frequent and severe; and diminishes subsequent nausea. In addition, it may be said that the presence of any large quantity of food in the stomach may embarrass respiration by interfering with the action of the diaphragm.

2. Loosen all garments that could in any way impede the movements of respiration or those, such as tight collars or neckbands, which could obstruct the flow of blood through the great vessels of the neck.

3. Remove false teeth or plates from the mouth. Never neglect to inquire as to their presence, no matter what may be the apparent age of the patient.

4. Keep the room at a temperature of at least 68° F. or 70° F., or if the operation is to be a prolonged one at 72°. Practically this is an excellent rule because patients often take cold by exposure during etherization. There is also an additional theoretical basis for it in the fact that when the blood and pulmonary tissues become saturated with ether, evaporation takes place from the surface of these tissues, causing a rapid loss of heat. If the air inspired is warm this supplies the heat necessary to volatilize the ether; if the air is cool the heat of volatilization is taken from the surrounding tissues, quickly chilling them, producing violent contraction of the capillaries, prolonged stasis, engorgement of the right side of the heart, and asphyxia.

5. Have the room perfectly quiet. The preliminary stage of etherization is, as has been said, one of acute sensitiveness to external impressions, and may be greatly prolonged by noise, bustle or excitement in the room.

6. Always examine the heart and lungs, and if the operation is to be severe or prolonged, examine the urine previously.

7. See that no light or flame is near the ether, especially on a lower level.

8. Quietly tell the patient in advance what to expect. Explain the suffocative feeling, mention that it is of almost invariable occurrence and is of no importance; describe the proper method of breathing through both the mouth and nostrils; caution the patient against struggling and resisting. Do this quietly and gently, and it is astonishing how often it will secure such intelligent co-operation on the part of the patient as will make the etherization rapid and easy.

9. Have an assistant ready to render whatever aid may be required, and, if inexperienced, caution him against the use of unnecessary force.

10. Of the various apparatuses employed for the purpose but two need be considered. One of these, that devised by Dr. Allis of this city, consists of a wire frame work, large enough to cover the lower part of the face and through which a strip of bandage has been passed to and fro so that numerous folds are exposed to the wetting action of the anæsthetic. These large evaporating surfaces, the thorough admixture of air, and the economy of ether are the three most definite advantages of this excellent little apparatus. An ordinary towel if folded into a cone, an aperture being left at the apex large enough to insert a finger, answers every purpose in private practice and obviates the necessity for carrying the more cumbrous inhaler.

11. The etherizer should watch three things —the breathing, the complexion, the pulse. When the breathing is regular and full without snoring, there can be little if any danger; if it is shallow and interrupted, watchfulness should be redoubled and a plentiful admixture of air given with the ether. If it ceases, the anæsthetic should be instantly removed and the tongue drawn forward; if respiratory movements do not begin, artificial respiration should be employed. If the face is very pale and the skin cool, the head should be lowered; if the complexion is livid or purplish, the head should be raised slightly, a freer supply of air given and the tongue and lower jaw brought forward. In case of failure of the pulse the head should be rapidly lowered, the ether immediately withdrawn, and hypodermics of whiskey and digitalis administered. Occasionally in patients who have been etherized after having eaten heartily, a condition may be noticed which includes to all appearances several of these elements of danger, but which is precedent to the act of vomiting; the breathing becomes irregular and interrupted, the face cold and pallid, the pulse almost indistinguishable. In the vast majority of cases this is followed by an expulsion of the contents of the stomach and then by the disappearance of these alarming symptoms. It should not be forgotten, however, that in exceptional cases death may occur during vomiting, possibly, as has been mentioned above, from the

descending excitation of the pneumogastric arresting the heart's action in diastole. This affords an additional reason for forbidding the taking of food for some hours previous to the administration of an anæsthetic.

A recent suggestion of Dr. Benjamin Howard, as to the cause of death in certain hitherto unexplained cases of fatality during anæsthesia, seems to me worthy of the most careful consideration. His views are founded upon his own observations and upon those of Dr. R. L. Bowles, made many years ago in conjunction with Drs. Fox, Hunter and Marshall Hall. Dr. Bowles claims precedence, I believe, for his work, but agrees in the main with Dr. Howard's views, which are as follows: A certain number of cases of apnœa and death are due to falling backward of the epiglottis, a condition often unrecognized, and almost surely fatal if unrelieved. There are many reasons for believing that traction on the tongue or pushing the jaw forward, while of the utmost value when the tongue itself is the obstructing body, do not affect the position of the epiglottis in these exceptional but equally dangerous cases:

Traction on the tongue is ineffectual because:

a. The tractile force supposed to be exercised upon the epiglottis is arrested chiefly by the frænum linguæ, and through the muscular fibres within it is expended upon the inferior maxilla into the genial tubercles of which they are inserted.

b. The surviving force is expended almost entirely upon, and intercepted by, the anterior pillars of the fauces.

c. For any tractile force which may survive, a continuous and sufficient medium for its transmission to the epiglottis is wanting.

Extension of the head and neck is the only sure means of causing instant and complete elevation of the epiglottis, because: by a three-linked chain, in which the hyo-epiglottic ligament is the lower link, the body of the hyoid bone the central link, and the combined genio- and mylo-hyoidei muscles the upper link, the epiglottis is so connected to the body of the inferior maxilla, that above a certain point, as the body of the lower jaw is moved upward, the epiglottis instantly, irresistibly, and inevitably moves upward exactly in unison till it is erect. The violent wrenching asunder of the clenched teeth, in proportion as it depresses the body of the inferior maxilla, antagonizes a distinct effort of Nature to maintain the elevation of the epiglottis.

Having, by bringing the patient to the edge of the table or bed, or by elevation of the chest, provided that the head may swing quite free, with one hand under the chin and the other on the vertex, steadily but firmly carry the head backward and downward. The neck will share the motion, which must be continued until the utmost possible extension of both head and neck is obtained. Assuming the mouth to be shut and the inferior border of the inferior maxilla to be at a right angle with the cervical column, as in the average recumbent posture, the head must be continued to be extended from thirty to thirty-five degrees more before it is possible for the epiglottis to be affected at all. Not until after the skin from the symphysis to the sternum is quite tense do the relaxed muscles in question beneath it become tense at all. These being tense, from this point the elevation of the epiglottis begins.

In a nut-shell: Make the line of skin from the chin to the sternum as straight as it can be made, and the complete elevation of the epiglottis is assured.

By extension of the head and neck carried to the utmost, the remaining obstructions from the backward-fallen tongue, the velum palati, and uvula, are also simultaneously removed, and the entire pharynx is enlarged throughout. Because: *a.* The tongue, the dorsum of which before fell by gravitation upon the then horizontal posterior wall of the pharynx, falls upon the now horizontal arch of the palate. *b.* The velum palati, by means of the great tension of the palato-pharyngei muscles, is pulled away from the posterior wall of the pharynx, the entire membrane being stretched tightly forward and downward, behind part of the dorsum of the tongue, helping to complete the shutting of the tongue out of the pharynx and into the mouth, and together with its dorsum forming a partition—the anterior wall of a new air-way, thus created and maintained. *c.* The pharynx, anteriorly, from the base of the tongue to the cricoid cartilage, is stretched strongly forward by the extreme tension of the sterno-thyroidei muscles.

Dr. Howard summarizes his interesting paper as follows:

1. Contrary to universal belief, traction of the tongue cannot raise the epiglottis.

2. By sufficient extension of the head and neck, whether by volition, instinct, reflex action, or by the effort of another, whether in the healthy, the dying, or the dead, the epiglottis is instantly, and beyond preven-

tion, made completely erect. 3. By complete extension of the head and neck the tongue and velum are as respiratory obstructions, simultaneously with the epiglottis, removed; and without a moment's delay the entire air-way can be straightened, enlarged, and be made free throughout by the nearest person. 4. If syncope happens to be the chief factor, or only incidental, this also gets thus the quickest and best corrective.

He expresses the hope and confident belief, that the facts above submitted will be found to be permanent additions to our means of averting death.

In the *British Medical Journal*, Jan. 26, 1889, Mr. Frederic Hewitt calls attention, one, to the occasional impossibility of adopting Howard's suggestion, on account of tonic spasm of the muscles of the neck, jaws, etc.; and two, to the danger of trusting to a post oral (or nasal) air-way which might so readily be occluded by tumefaction of the mucous membrane, by mucus, or by morbid conditions. Drs. Martin and Hare, in the *Medical News*, March 2, 1889, reaffirm this latter statement, recommend moderate instead of forced extension of the head and neck, so that space may be left between the tongue and palate to permit of breathing through the mouth, and the simultaneous pushing forward of the hyoid bone and the lower jaw. If obstruction to breathing still persists, the tongue should be at once drawn or pushed forward by force exerted upon its dorsum posterior to the anterior half arches of the palate. The subject is an extremely interesting one, and will bear further investigation; but it would seem now to be fairly well established that in the main Dr. Howard's conclusions are justified, and that his method in the majority of cases and in the absence of nasal obstruction is at once the simplest and the most efficient.

12. The etherizer should attend strictly to the anæsthetic, and unless of long experience and perfect self-possession, to nothing else.

13. Etherization is complete when the arm raised from the side drops helplessly, and when the orbicularis palpebrarum fails to respond when the conjunctiva is touched.

14. After this time the ether should be given in small quantities and with plenty of air.

15. With the completion of the operation the responsibility of the etherizer does not end, although it is not uncommon to see him walk away from the operating table or bedside to inspect a tumor or look at a wound, or aid in washing and cleaning instruments. He should only leave the patient when his place can be taken by a trained and experienced nurse, and should even then for some little time be within call in case of emergency. The vomiting which frequently follows etherization is itself distinctly dangerous if any food has been taken. The patient, incapable of intelligent movement, can readily perish from asphyxia caused by the inspiration of solid portions of the ejecta, and should be carefully watched with this possibility in mind. Then, too, during the intoxication and excitement, which often constitute a distinct stage preliminary to a return of consciousness, he will require careful supervision to prevent him from doing himself harm.

The pain or smarting of the wound will at once draw his attention in that direction and he is very apt to attempt to remove the dressings. The records of surgery show many distressing cases in which this has occurred. One of them, which always seemed to me to be peculiarly horrible, is that of a patient who, being left alone immediately after an operation for strangulated hernia, tore off his bandages, opened the wound and actually pulled out yards of his own intestines.

METHYLENE.—With this anæsthetic we have had but little experience in this country and I believe that has not been very favorable. It was introduced to the profession twenty years ago by Dr. Richardson, of London, who, after a long series of experiments, concluded that its action was more rapid than that of chloroform and that it produced a more prolonged and profound narcotism, but rapidly escaped from the system, and was accompanied by an equally rapid return of consciousness. Deaths have been recorded from its use both here and abroad, as well as from the use of the methylene ether, a mixture of methylene dichloride and absolute ether, also introduced by Dr. Richardson. I have recently seen this anæsthetic administered by Dr. Day, one of the physicians to the Samaritan Hospital in London, who has given it in between 1200 and 1300 cases without difficulty of any kind. He has reported the interesting fact that twelve drachms is the largest quantity he has ever administered in an operation lasting one hour. This agrees with curious accuracy with the statement made by Dr. Richardson as long ago as 1867, when he reported the quantity used in surgical operations as averaging about one drachm every five minutes. In the case which I saw there was no apparent period of excitement, the patient coming rapidly under the influence of the anæsthetic and almost as rapidly recovering consciousness. Dr. Day watches particularly the color of the face and the character of the respiration, paying little or no attention to the pulse; although experiments on the lower animals seem to show that when methylene kills it does so by paralyzing equally the circulation and respiration. I have had absolutely no personal experience with this anæsthetic, but am disposed to reject it as somewhat more dangerous than ether, and without sufficient advantages to counterbalance the increased risk.

NITROUS OXIDE.—This is made by heating nitrate of ammonium in a retort until it decomposes into watery vapor and the so-called laughing gas. The latter collected in a rubber bag or other proper receiver may then be administered as an anæsthetic by inhalation. It would seem from chemical considerations, nitrous oxide being a stable compound at the temperature of the body, and from experimental observation, dogs dying in it in precisely the same time as when put in nitrogen, that nitrous oxide acts by producing asphyxia, or at least by preventing oxidation of the blood. There is, however, no doubt, a primary effect of specific stimulation of the nerve centres as shown by a period of exhilaration, from which it derives its familiar name. There are a few reported cases of death during, or after the inhalation of nitrous oxide, but, not more than three, I believe, and even these are more or less doubtful. In one of them there was found extensive fatty degeneration of the heart; in another no autopsy was made; and in the third only two inhalations of the gas had been taken when the patient died after the extraction of teeth, probably from syncope produced by nervous shock. In this city at the rooms of certain dental operators enormous numbers of persons (nearly one hundred and forty thousand) have taken the gas without a single death.

The stages produced by this anæsthetic are two: 1. Exhilaration, or the development of the peculiar mental excitement, which is usually cheerful and often boisterously so. 2. Unconsciousness, lasting from two to four minutes, during a portion of which time there is a period of muscular relaxation which is, however, never so complete as under the other anæsthetics. The most common danger associated with the administration of this gas is that arising from a spasm of the muscles leading from the base of the tongue to the hyoid bone and pharynx, producing a condition known as "swallowing the tongue." This sometimes occurs with great suddenness and if unrelieved threatens death from asphyxia. The tongue should of course be immediately drawn forward by forceps and held there until the spasm disappears or the patient recovers consciousness. In cases of extensive heart disease the danger of fatal syncope should be borne in mind, and similarly the risk of asphyxia should be remembered in cases with grave pulmonary troubles. On the whole, however, nitrous oxide may fairly be said to be the safest of all known anæsthetics within the limitation of its present use, which is chiefly in the performance of such trifling operations as the opening of boils, abscesses or felons, the removal of small epitheliomata, the division of fissures of the anus, or the extraction of teeth.

In *résumé* I may formulate the following conclusions:

1. As a rule ether, as the safest of the more powerful anæsthetics, is to be preferred; the lessened risk to life more than counterbalances its minor disadvantages.

2. Chloroform may be employed when ether has failed, or cannot be procured, or when there is a distinct record of serious trouble during a previous etherization. It is possibly safer in children than in adults, and it is said to be exceptionally adapted for administration in obstetrical cases. It has some distinct advantages over ether in cases of stenosis of the larynx or trachea, and may be considered in those cases of emergency in which an operation has to be performed a short time after a solid meal.

As secondary indications for its employment the following may be mentioned:

a. Protracted operations about the mouth, jaws, nose, or pharynx which necessitate the mouth and nose being uncovered.

b. Operations needing the employment of the actual cautery, in the vicinity of the mouth.

c. Severe bronchitis, emphysema, or asthma.

d. Extensive renal disease.

e. Marked atheroma.

3. Nitrous oxide should be employed in operations which can be completed in from two to five minutes.

4. Methylene, methylene ether, and the various anæsthetic mixtures, such as that of alcohol, chloroform and ether, are not so safe as ether alone, and have no decided advantages to compensate for the increased risk.

COMMUNICATIONS.

PRACTICAL ASEPTIC SURGERY.[1]

BY J. W. LONG, M.D.,

RANDLEMAN, N. C.

(Concluded from p. 261.)

Having discussed the various prerequisites of modern surgery, and the object of this paper being purely practical, I will now ask you kindly to examine these bags, which you will find contain every thing that aseptic surgery really demands. Take the smaller bag first. You will observe that it is only an ordinary leather satchel, about twelve inches long; that it is carried by the handle or a strap thrown across the shoulder. On opening it, we find a leather strap sewed in loops along the sides, and containing the following articles, to wit: Gerster's iodoform box; a two-ounce bottle of chloroform, with a notched stopper tied to the neck; a two-ounce bottle containing the corrosive sublimate mixture; two ounces of carbolic acid; a half-ounce of Churchill's tincture of iodine—the iodine and acid bottles have a bit of cotton about the mouth and are wrapped in protective; a half-ounce of four per cent. solution of cocaine, and a small pipette; hypodermic syringe, tablets of morphine, and a small exploring-needle; a stiff nail-brush; litmus paper; and two ounces of glycerine, with twine tied around the neck of the bottle for making vaginal tampons. A plain sack or cover made of rubber sheeting about 6 by 8 inches holds one or two ample pieces of protective, a yard or more of corrosive sublimate gauze, and a large piece of borated cotton. In the bottom of the bag is a narrow Esmarch and several cotton bandages. There is also a plain cloth case containing such instruments as one may wish to carry. A little side-pocket holds needles, silk, pins, and safety-pins, the former two wrapped in protective.

This arrangement of the various articles enumerated is very simple and convenient; besides, it leaves the body of the bag for extra instruments, an unusual amount of dressing, or anything else. This bag soon paid for itself over and over again. Now I could not get along without it. With it any minor operation may be done after the style of modern aseptic surgery. I will give some examples by way of illustration.

Case I.—March 1, Mrs. ——, while picking up clothes for the wash, ran a needle deeply into the upper part of the palm of the right hand. It gave her great pain. Her husband immediately telephoned for me, and the operation was conducted as follows: Pulling off my coat and rolling my sleeves above the elbow, I first thoroughly washed my hands and arms in hot water and soap; then I washed the patient's hand and wrist. Next, the instruments needed were laid in a small dish containing a three per cent. solution of carbolic acid—an ordinary goblet will answer every purpose for holding the small instruments necessary in such operations, and two fluid drachms of acid solution to a goblet of water approximates a three per cent. solution. Twenty minims of a four per cent. solution of cocaine were injected into the proposed line of incision. While the cocaine was being absorbed, my hands and the patient's hand and wrist were washed in a 1 to 1000 solution of corrosive sublimate. The application of a rubber bandage rendered the hand and wrist bloodless. A short deep incision was made directly over point of entrance of the needle. The bloodless condition of the parts enabled me to see the needle passing upward and backward beneath the annular ligament, and it was easily extracted. The wound was washed in the sublimate solution, iodoform freely dusted over it, sublimate gauze applied, and snugly held in place by a roller bandage; after which the rubber bandage was removed. The entire operation was painless and bloodless. In a few days, the dressing was removed—the wound had healed by first intention, without a drop of pus. Some one may say that extracting a needle is a trivial matter and not worthy the consideration of this society; but do you think that any one who can not extract a needle aseptically should be trusted to do a laparotomy or a herniotomy?

Case II.—Geo. A., about thirty years old, white, had a tumor the size of a marble on the inner side of the left ring-finger. It had been growing four years, since the finger had been hurt in a scuffle. The preparation of hands, patient, and instruments was as in the first case. Cocaine and the bandage were used. A longitudinal incision displayed a dark looking mass, having the appearance of malignancy. The tumor extended through the lower end of the first phalanx and seemed to spring from the medullary canal; the bone had evidently been fractured in the scuffle four years ago. The mass was torn and trimmed out with forceps and scissors, leaving a healthy look-ing cavity. This was packed with iodo-form gauze, and the whole finger thickly covered with sublimate gauze and absorb-ent cotton, held in place by a roller band-age. The wound rapidly filled up by granulations, the dressing being changed as often as it became soiled.

Now, kindly notice this larger bag, which is specially gotten up for major operations. It is a leather satchel about 17 inches long, with a stout handle. On the outside are strapped a nest of four oblong tin pans, the inner one holding Dr. Kelly's surgical pad and a piece of rubber sheeting, three by four feet. On opening the satchel you will observe that the partition has a side pocket containing two ample pieces of protective, and several envelopes holding respectively, silver wire, pins and safety pins, silk and needles wrapped in protective ; and another containing several powders for making Theirsch's solution. The other side of the partition presents loops for the following articles : razor, shaving brush, nail brush, test tubes, bottle (in tin case) of bone drains, a four ounce bottle (in tin case) of carbolic acid, a two ounce bottle (also in tin case) of Churchill's tincture of iodine, a four ounce bottle of whiskey, bottle of cat-gut in oil of juniper, a bottle of corrosive sublimate tablets, and a box of iodoform ointment. The body of the bag con-tains in . one side a case (five yards) of corrosive sublimate gauze, an ordinary rubber syringe, a fruit jar holding sponges and rubber drainage tubes in a five per cent. solution of carbolic acid ; a four ounce bottle of Squibb's best chloroform protected by a box of wedge-wood ; three shallow tin basins ; two or three pie pans ; two quarter-pound cans of ether ; a wide rubber bandage ; a cake of soap ; and a number of cotton bandages. A fountain syringe to be used as an irrigator is rolled up and placed in the pans. On this side is also a chloroform inhaler, which is simply a wire muzzle covered with coarse cloth. These articles are covered by two or three towels (take plenty of towels with you) all held in place by two transverse straps. The other side of the bag holds a half-pound or more of absorbent cotton rolled in a clean towel. Also an ether inhaler, which is a plain lamp chimney with a soft rubber face-piece. Both inhalers and the fountain syringe are kept in bags of rubber sheeting, as they are apt to get soiled and contaminate other articles in the bag. This leaves a large space for instruments, which are selected for

each operation and placed in a cloth case or wrapped in a clean towel and stowed away in the bag just beneath the roll of cotton, which keeps them from jostling about and becoming injured. Some extra towels are in this side also.

Of course the arrangement in the bag of the various articles enumerated is entirely arbitrary and must be made to suit the con-venience of each operator. The large bag contains no iodoform, cocaine, hypodermic or exploring needle, and no bandage or scis-sors, as they are all carried in the small bag ; but might easily be added to the large bag.

Case III.—On Feb. 14 I was called by Dr. S. Redding to remove a tumor the size of a large orange from the hepatic region of Miss Hinshaw, white, about 26 years old. The tumor had a history of ten years' dura-tion, and recently had begun to suppurate at its most prominent point. It was causing the patient and family a great deal of uneasi-ness. We proceeded as follows : A dining-table was covered by a thick quilt and oil-cloth. Upon a small table near by several of the pans shown in the large bag were placed and filled, one with five per cent. carbolic solution for instruments, one with 1 to 1000 sublimate solution for sponges, and two with clear water, one being to drop instruments in as they became bloody, and the other for washing soiled sponges in before being returned to the sublimate solu-tion. A strong sublimate solution coagu-lates the blood in a sponge and makes it hard to clean ; besides the solution soon becomes turbid with blood. Therefore, during an operation, the sponges should be washed first in a vessel containing plain water and then replaced in the sublimate solution before being handed to the oper-ator. An observance of these precautions in regard to the sponges and instruments will prevent confusion and add much to the orderly management of an operation. Another pan contained needles in a three per cent. carbolic solution ready threaded with silk, while another held the dressing—sublimate gauze, iodoform gauze, absorbent cotton, and roller-bandages. The iodoform pepper-box was near ; a hypodermic syringe charged with whiskey, and a glass of whis-key were also convenient. Our hands and arms having already been scrubbed in hot water and soap, I proceeded to wash the field of operation, while Dr. Rudding administered ether. After using soap and water on and around the tumor, the parts were sponged with a sublimate solution; 1 to 1000, after which towels soaked in a similar solution were arranged around the parts to be operated on. A small tub had been placed under the edge of the table to catch the water and blood during the operation, and a large pitcher was filled with 1 to 2000 sublimate solution for irrigation. Every thing being in order, my hands were placed for one minute in a 1 to 1000 sublimate solution, and a bowl of the same placed near by on a chair in which to dip the hands during the operation. The tumor was surrounded by two long elliptical incisions, and rapidly enucleated. Quite a quantity of blood was lost owing to the fact that the tumor, while of a fatty nature, was channeled in every direction with sinuses filled with blood. After the enucleation one or two spurting arteries were tied with very fine silk, the wound irrigated thoroughly from the pitcher, and the sides approximated with numerous silk sutures. The parts then presented a simple straight line of incision about eight inches long. No drainage was employed except a strand or two of silk carried beneath the sutures and projecting from either angle of the wound. While the patient's shoulders were gently raised her back was cleansed of blood and water. Iodoform was freely dusted over the parts, iodoform gauze laid along the line of the incision, sublimate gauze and absorbent cotton thickly applied over this; the dressings were held in place by a wide roller bandage. At the end of two weeks the dressing was removed and the wound found healed throughout, except about an inch in the middle where the sutures had cut out—a retentive suture should have been used. The parts were sweet and healthy, and in a few days were entirely healed.

The dressing employed in this case is a typical example of the dry dressing, and the results of the case—no suppuration and no fever—show what may be expected from aseptic surgery. Below I append a case illustrating the moist dressing.

Case IV.—Dr. W. A. Woollen asked me to see the following case, occurring in his practice. Sam S., black, 7 years old. The patient gave a history of acute inflammation of the right tibia, which commenced last November. Some time before I saw the patient his leg had been lanced for the escape of matter by Dr. Stanton. The left femur was enlarged and tender, but no sinus existed from it. The affected tibia was discharging freely from three or four sinuses, the probe readily detected dead bone. May 2, with the kind assistance of Drs. Woollen, Fox and Walker the following operation was done. The room having been previously scoured—floor, walls and ceiling —and all unnecessary furniture removed, a dining table and a small one were prepared as in Case III; a bed was also prepared. A quantity of boiled water and a number of towels and bowls were provided. The hands of operator and assistants were washed as heretofore described, our coats being first removed and a clean apron pinned around the waist of each. The instruments and dressings and solutions with basins of clear water were arranged as usual. A fountain syringe was filled with 1 to 2000 sublimate solution and suspended from a nail near the ceiling. The edges of oil cloth covering the table were doubled so that the bloody water would be carried to a tub under the edge of the table. The little patient having had a general bath early in the morning was laid on the table and anæsthetized. His leg was thoroughly scrubbed with soap and water, followed by the sublimate solution, 1 to 1000. The limb was elevated to the perpendicular for five minutes to allow the surplus (?) blood to gravitate into the body. It was then surrounded by a sublimate towel and an Esmarch bandage applied from the toes to near the hip; the lower end of the bandage being unwound, the ends were tied in a bow-knot above the knee. This rendered the limb bloodless and should never be omitted in operations upon the extremities, unless positively contraindicated. The operator's hands were again dipped in the sublimate solution and the leg douched from the irrigator. An incision through all the tissues down to the bone and extending from one sinus to another displayed abundant dead bone, pus, and detritus. Thinking to chisel and scoop out the diseased parts and leave a trough of healthy bone, we proceeded cautiously with chisel and gouge. But the further we went the more dead bone we found; finally we discovered that the tibia was honey-combed with dead tissue from joint to joint. This left us with only two alternatives—amputation or exsection of the bone in its entirety. The latter plan was quickly decided upon, in the hopes of giving the little fellow a tolerable limb. The periosteum was easily stripped from the bone and the lower end of the bone broken loose from its attachments, a triangular piece of the lower end adhered to the cartilage and was broken off. In trying to remove this the ankle joint was inadvertently opened, and it was thought best to remove the tibial cartilage in order to insure better drainage.

The upper end of the tibia was loosened from its cartilaginous covering by means of a sharp chisel, and the remnants of bone scraped away with Volkmann's scoop ; the knee joint was left intact except an insignificant nick in the synovial sac. During this time a stream from the irrigator had been playing upon the parts every few minutes. The wound, which was very extensive, being again thoroughly irrigated, was snugly packed with iodoform gauze freshly wet in corrosive sublimate solution, 1 to 1000. Over this successive layers of sublimate gauze were laid in an orderly manner, and wet throughout from the irrigator. The entire limb was now enveloped in a thick layer of borated cotton, and this in turn covered by protective extending from the perineum to the tips of the toes. A roller bandage applied rather tightly held the dressing in place and controlled hemorrhage by pressure. Splints were adjusted to insure immobility of the joints and to keep the parts at rest. The last thing was to remove the rubber bandage and see that the blood returned to the toes.

In spite of this terrible operation—compared with which amputation of the parts would have been a comparatively small matter—this child's temperature never reached 102°. His appetite improved and he began gaining flesh almost from the day of the operation. On the ninth day the parts were dressed, using the same precautions as to hands, dressing material, irrigation, etc., as in the operation itself. A little chloroform was given. The wound was found fresh and sweet and rapidly filling up with healthy granulations—"new inflammatory formation" of Billroth. The limb has been dressed once a week since and is now entirely healed, except a short, wide hole at the ankle and the knee.

I show you the tibia removed from my little patient. This case strongly illustrates the triumphs of aseptic surgery. Where is the surgeon who would undertake to save a limb under just such circumstances—after the old ways of surgery?

It may be objected that this paper contains little that is new or original. My answer is, that I do not come with untried theories and impracticable suggestions, but only with those methods proven by actual experience—the only crucible in which the dross is consumed and the gold purified.

—The chemical and pharmaceutical laboratory of the Ohio State University was destroyed by fire Feb. 12.

THE INFLUENCE OF SEXUALISM IN REFLEX OCULAR NEUROSES.

BY GEORGE M. GOULD, M.D.,
PHILADELPHIA.

It has been a matter of frequent observation with me that, prior to the age of puberty, the young, as the result of eyestrain, are troubled a great deal with conjunctival and blepharal congestions and inflammations, and much more than after puberty; that boys, both before and a longer time thereafter, are troubled in this way somewhat more than girls; that girls and women, after puberty, are far more prone to have headaches and neuroses than boys and men. However frequent the exceptions I think the rule is that, with irritational eye-strain, the male sex is more apt to show ocular evidences of the same than the female, that both have these ocular symptoms more before than after puberty, and that after this period girls and women have far more headaches than men. It is a matter of not uncommon observation that vernal conjunctivitis, to which young girls are peculiarly subject is almost incurable, but that it disappears, as if spontaneously, at the age of 13 or 14. Styes are frequently seen in young girls and boys but seldom in young ladies and men. Many other palpebral or conjunctival derangements have been noticed to follow this law. A practitioner of great experience and fine observation, Dr. O. P. Rex, of Philadelphia, tells me he has noted very many such facts in his practice.

I do not at all deny that it is possible to explain certain of these cases as due to some inherited dyscrasia that is conquered by the growth, or whose poison is eliminated by the development of the organism and the power of yet stronger inherited tendencies coming into their destined inheritance of the organism. It may also be said that men often avoid the natural consequences of eye-strain by change of occupation and by freedom from the sewing and the house life that in women necessitates work at short range. Many other explanations might be found that would satisfy an easy-going logic, but I believe the facts are too numerous and the law too general to be satisfied with such a solution. There must be a more profound law running beneath that will bring the facts into a better consonance with evolution and life.

No student of Wallace and Darwin and the facts of the evolution of form and beauty both in the animal and the human race, can fail to have been struck with the preponderant influence of sexualism (with its ideals of beauty) upon the life and appearance of all animals and men. To that unconquerable instinct everything, except perpetuation of the species itself, is unhesitatingly and ceaselessly sacrificed. And this is not a whit less true to-day of the social animal, the young man and woman of whatever land or language. My present thesis is therefore this: 1. The natural result of an irritational eye-strain is (in harmony with the physiological law of a return of the reflex to or near the organs primarily irritated) to induce inflammations of the conjunctiva, lids, etc., with the necessarily consequent congestion and despoiling of the beauty of the eyes. 2. To the flowering sexual being, this of all things is most detestable, and all the arts of conscious and unconscious life conspire to prevent it. 3. The methods by which these things are prevented are either (*a*) by means of an inhibition of the return of the eye-strain reflexes to the eyes; or (*b*) by deflecting and derouting the reflex discharges to other organs. In the first case, by withholding, storing and diffusing in the mass of the cerebral centres the incoming irritational stimuli, there is produced the great modern female complaint, headache. In the second case, when inhibition becomes no longer possible, and where, through weak ganglia and irregular associate fibres, the overflow spends itself upon innocent organs, we find the great family of reflex neuroses. It is a matter of great regret that peripheral irritations as a cause of headache are too often ignored, and that reflex neuroses are too often considered as idiopathic affections of the complaining organ.

I have elsewhere tried to emphasize, what is, indeed, sufficiently patent and well-known, that the law of all physiological function is that peripheral stimulus of whatever kind normally results in a reflex or return discharge, motor, vaso-motor, secretory, trophic, etc., to the point, or so as to correspond to, or answer, the peculiarity of the stimulus. Pathology begins when the return discharge is not correspondent to the stimulus. If, by disease of the ganglia, or because of irregularity of commissural fibres, the return discharge is sent by wrong centrifugal routes to innocent organs, we find resulting irritational choreas and reflex neuroses of all kinds. If such reflexes and *débordements* are inhibited, more serious cerebral and mental mischief may result. There are good grounds for believing that headache is often but the first stage or symptom of a hierarchy of functional derangements due to retention and overflow of persisting uncured peripheral irritations. When inhibition begets such tension that *débordement* must take place, it may occur by single or several outlets (choreas, irritabilities, gastric neuroses, etc.); or the discharge may be explosive and general (epilepsies, spasms, etc.); or, again, the outflow may exhaust itself upon intellectual centres and result in monomanias and insanities. It is a good rule of social life and minor morals that a man should, so to speak, burn up his own smoke (extinguish within himself his own personal faults of temper, etc.) without offending his neighbor's nostrils therewith. It would certainly be a great desideratum if the physical brain had the power of neutralizing and consuming those irritational stimuli whose sources it cannot quench. But it seems to have only a limited power of this kind, and the inhibition of irritational stimuli for but a short time results in such surcharge that it is manifested by headache, or in a wretched vicarious overflow upon other organs. We may have toothache in the ear, the stomach, or even in the hip,[1] and eye-strain may be manifest only in the brain, the heart, or the stomach. It is evident that some nervous organizations have more power than others of setting bounds to the unregulated overflow to innocent peripheral organs; some have better smoke-consumers than others. But, in most organizations, the penalty of such power, is headache. All these questions have a dynamic aspect as mathematically exact as thermo-chemistry or gravitation. Give the brain a power of estoping persisting irritational stimuli from their physiological reflexes, and you must supply means of dissipating the inhibited discharges. Such inhibitions and would-be dissipations are the (probably) vaso-motor cerebral disturbances manifested by headache. Intercurrent with the headache there is frequently gastric derangement. It is not clear just what the mechanism of this "sympathy" may be, but there can no longer be any doubt that eye-strain, with headache, may also produce such gastric troubles as dyspepsia, flatulence, emesis, gastralgia, anorexia, etc. Perhaps the gastric irregularity may be an early symptom of the impossibility of longer inhibition and denotes the first relief of tension by this overflow along the line of least resistance. At least,

[1] See, Brubaker, The Reflex Neuroses of Dental Pathology, Lea's American System of Dentistry.

in cases of extreme eye-strain, I have hardly ever failed to find some and often great gastric derangement coexisting with the headache. In other cases this point of weakest resistance is through the motor centres of the extremity-muscles, whence chorea. Should all the gateways present a watchful and firm barrier against the egress, the general tension may perhaps find relief only in that general explosion of many surcharged centres, that goes by the name of epilepsy—after which the brain is drained to a temporary condition of dynamic sanity.

We may now seek an answer to the question, What is the cause of the retention and inhibition of the ocular irritational stimuli, that results in so many evils? It must be a powerful force that can thus reverse the universal law of physiology whereby pain and congestion result in the organ irritated. What is the force that vicariously subjects the brain to injury and headache rather than the offending eyes? Or that, *comme dernier ressort*, will viciously wreak its vengeance upon innocent centers and organs by a reflex neurosis? I can imagine no power or motive strong enough to produce such a preposterous illogicality and injustice, except the all-penetrating and all-powerful one of sexual selection and sexual beauty. To put it brutally, a chemotic and blear-eyed girl would not be the beaux' favorite, and nature has purchased the clear conjunctiva and limpid beauty of the eye at the frightful expense of headaches and innumerable neuroses. It is no fallacy of sentiment that makes the eye the silently speaking exponent of the soul's deepest thoughts and emotions. To mar its beauty and travesty its expressiveness is a sin against the future and against the species, that deserves and receives nature's most solicitous care. The cerebral centers are compelled to inhibit the reflexes eyeward at whatever cost. The clear-eyed girl chooses, is chosen, marries, and begets clear-eyed daughters—clear-eyed, but, alas! they, all and several, are cephalalgics! If this seem mystical and far-fetched to conservative medical science, it may be urged that our profoundest naturalists and philosophers have not thought similar logic too weak to account for the evolution of the most profound morphological and psychological characteristics of a continental and a cosmic fauna. Before puberty the irritation-reflexes return to the eyes according to physiological law; after puberty, in women almost never, in men perhaps more frequently, but even in men the law is felt, though occupation and a robuster nervous

organization prevents the disastrous consequences so often seen in women.

In this sexual factor may be found the chief reason for the fact that ocular strain is by a hundred fold the most fertile source of headache and neurotic disturbance in the otherwise physiologically well-conducted organism. If, according to man's experience, the burthen of love-song and history has been the wound of heart by beauty's eye-glance, the weapon has been two-edged and its polishing has injured the fair possessor quite as frequently as her captive. Add to this the almost equally important fact that eye-strain arises chiefly from subjecting the naturally and normally hyperopic eye to the short-range work demanded of every servant of civilization, and we at once have another potent reason for the astounding frequency of eye-strain. From these two causes we realize why eye-strain is so common, and also why it is so subtilely hidden away under the masks of headache and neuroses. Were still another premise needed for our logic it might be found in the fact of the imperial and transcendant importance, intellectually, emotionally and physically, of the organ of vision above all the other senses, and that disturbances of its mechanism must speedily and intimately injure the coordinations and harmonies of every part of our being.

Why do other peripheral irritations so much less frequently set up headaches and neuroses than eye-strain? For many reasons: Because no other organ is to a thousandth part so intimately bound up with our every act and thought and emotion, and so necessary to them all[1]; because no other organ at the end and completion of its development has unwarned had thrust upon it a strain so unusual and of a kind so wholly different from that experienced in its evolution; because no other organ is so complex, so delicate, so easily thrown out of adjustment; and, lastly and chiefly, because to other organs the reflexes may generally return, according to physiological law, in such a way as to answer the stimulus, without running counter to such a profound

---

[1] I cannot conceal the thought that, conspiring with the law of sexual selection and beauty there may also have been this of the profound utility and importance of this sense-organ to the welfare of the *individual* organism. Even as a unit (apart from race-instincts) it might be better that other organs, and even the brain itself, should vicariously suffer the punishment of ocular sins, rather than its most important function should be impaired and endangered by the inflammations that would result from the warnings and danger-signals of the properly returned reflexes.

law of the organism as that of sexual selection based upon sexual beauty and perfection.

Next to the eyes, perhaps the teeth are the most frequent source of reflex neuroses. Professor Brubaker's essay contains a highly interesting gathering of such instances. But in the reflex neuroses of dental pathology, the centripetal stimulus seems to be checked and reflected back, or derouted by subordinate ganglia that like the lymphatics act as outposts or advance guards to protect the higher centers from injurious attacks. The intimate and direct cerebral connections of the ocular mechanism render impossible such ganglionic skirmishers and pickets. In childhood, the ear seems to bear the brunt of the derouted dental reflexes, and many a case of deafness is due to impacted or carious teeth. Irregularities of the nasal functions and, to a greater degree, of the genital organs, may occasion cerebral and reflex neurotic phenomena, but far less frequently than those of the eye. All of these, however, are of sufficiently frequent occurrence to put the careful diagnostician upon his guard, and warrant a scrutinizing inquiry where functional derangements do not present their own explanations, do not yield promptly to treatment, and where eye-strain is certainly excluded by the mydriatic examination of a competent person.

These, then, are the practical lessons to be gleaned from the preceding pages:

1. In headache *always* suspect eye-strain, and especially in women in the years between puberty and middle age.

2. In functional gastric derangements, not quickly to be explained otherwise,[1] suspect eye-strain, and especially if headache coexist.[2]

3. In other functional derangements such as chorea, nervous heart, extreme irritability of temper, hysteria, etc., that do not yield to treatment, or that are not idiopathically or otherwise explainable, exhaust the possibility of a reflex neurosis from eye-strain or other peripheral irritation.

4. Have the refraction estimated, under a mydriatic, and the coordination of the external ocular muscles proved, by a scientific authority, *in the case of every child, before or by the age of puberty.*

119 South Seventeenth St.

[1] I have always wondered if Carlyle were ametropic.

[2] I have seen a case in which a monocular rhythmical ptosis lasting for ten days alternating with ten-day periods of persistent emesis, had kept up for two years, the whole due entirely to eye-strain, and disappearing with the relief of the same.

SOCIETY REPORTS.

NEW YORK ACADEMY OF MEDICINE.

Stated Meeting, February 21, 1889.

The President, ALFRED L. LOOMIS, M.D., in the Chair.

DR. CHARLES MCBURNEY read a paper on

The Treatment of Inguinal Hernia with Reference to Radical Cure,

in which he first mentioned a procedure adopted in three cases for radical cure of hernia, and accounted for the return of the tumor by the fact that, in addition to securing a dense cicatrix in the canal, he had failed to remove redundant peritoneum, and thereby to carry out an essential step in the operation, namely, to restore, at the point where the hernia begins, a tense, smooth internal surface of the abdominal wall. It is well known, he said, that in laparotomies where large drainage tubes are used for a considerable period, subsequent appearance of ventral hernia is more likely than where no drainage tube is employed. Where the walls are equally brought together and no drainage tube is used, a smooth, tense peritoneal surface lines the cicatrix, and hernia seldom occurs. In inguinal hernia the loose connective tissue which accompanies the cord and fills the inguinal canal, forms no formidable backing to the peritoneum. Thus to cure hernia radically one must radically remove the predisposing causes, namely, peritoneal laxity at the internal ring, and give sufficient support to the peritoneum at this point.

Having abandoned irritative injections, operators then began to devote most attention to sewing up the external ring with various kinds of sutures, ignoring the fact that a hernia coming down into the canal is quite capable of breaking any suture or cicatrix that might lie before it. Macewen's operation does not reproduce the desired smooth peritoneal surface at the internal ring; besides, the operation is extremely difficult, if not totally impracticable, in many cases. Objections also obtain against other operations referred to. It has seemed to him clear that to reach and operate upon the extreme upper part of the neck of the sac with certainty and safety, the surgeon should expose it fairly, and Dr. McBurney thought he had devised a plan of doing so, but afterward learned that it had been done years before. When the anterior wall of the canal is split up to and a little beyond the internal ring one can make use of one of two methods: tying with a strong ligature; or cutting away the sac, and sewing the neck neatly and smoothly. In this way it is easy to restore the smooth condition of the peritoneum at the ring. This should now have a backing. Some operators are satisfied to have the support at the external ring, entirely ignoring the canal. This is obtained by sewing together the pillars of the external ring. But such sutures must either give way or cut through the dense pillars of the ring. Other surgeons pass the finger up the canal and trust to more active reparative formation following breaking up of the connective tissue to close the canal directly. Others pass sutures from one side of the canal across to the other, thus endeavoring to narrow it. The only certain measure for obtaining complete closure of the whole inguinal canal, except the portion occupied by the cord, is by the open treatment. But even this is uncertain. To insure firm and dense cicatricial tissue throughout the length and depth of the canal one must carefully pack by some dressing down to the transversalis fascia in the lower, and to the peritoneum in the upper, part of the canal.

Before operating, most careful antiseptic precautions are taken, especially in cleansing surrounding parts. The incision begins a little outside the inguinal ring, and extends sufficiently downward over the sac. This is rapidly deepened over the whole length of the canal, thus freely exposing the aponeurosis of the external oblique muscle. The superficial layers of the sac are now cleared away, and the two pillars are completely exposed the entire length. The sac is still covered below the external ring by fascia, which is now opened. The scissors are pushed under, and the canal is split a little beyond the outer edge of the internal ring. The deeper coverings of the sac are now cut off, this being best and most rapidly accomplished with the fingers. If now the transversalis is removed high up in the canal, it is quite easy to separate the cord from the sac. The cord now being separated from the sac a little within the abdomen, the whole sac is dissected out and lifted up. In some cases, as in congenital hernia, the sac must be cut away from the cord. The sac is now opened, and if intestinal contents are present they are reduced; if omentum, it is ligated, and cut away. Adhesions are broken down if any are exposed. The sac being now held up from the internal ring, the operator inserts one or two fingers through the neck a little way into the peritoneal cavity, to guard positively against return of a piece of omentum or intestine into the sac during the placing of the ligature. The ligature is placed about the neck of the sac at the highest point, the level of the peritoneum, drawn very tightly, and the part cut away. There is then a wound, the upper wall of which is formed by the edges of the skin, superficial fascia, external oblique aponeurosis and conjoined tendon; while the lower wall is formed by skin, superficial fascia, and a strip of aponeurosis or Poupart's ligament, including the outer pillar. The aim being to secure granulation to the bottom, it is not sufficient simply to pack the wound. Stitches are inserted, from four to eight in number, according to the size of the wound, to bind together the tissues which form the upper wall, and two or more tension sutures carried across the wound. The wound is now carefully irrigated, and dusted with iodoform throughout, and iodoform gauze is firmly packed the entire length down to the posterior wall. The scrotal or labial wound is sewed up without packing. Proper dressing is applied to prevent soiling of the wound. The dressing is changed once in four or five days. A clear scar forms in from five to six weeks, and is very strong. The patient is not afterward allowed to wear a truss or support of any kind, as pressure by a truss is regarded as injurious to scar tissue.

Dr. McBurney has done the operation thirty-six times in inguinal hernia. One patient, an old drunkard, died in delirium tremens. In only one has there been a relapse of the hernia, and that can be easily accounted for by a defective operation. The first operation was done only two years ago, consequently the time may not be long enough to convince some that the cure is permanent.

The paper was discussed by Drs. L. A. Stimson, A. G. Gerster, Abbe, McCosh, Hartley, Syms, Gibney, and Murray, most of whom had performed the operation and preferred it to any other.

———————

—The *Journal of the Amer. Med. Association*, Feb. 23, says that the Chief of Police of Berlin has ordered the hospital authorities to note the numbers of the carriages in which patients are taken to the hospitals, and the nature of the diseases of the patients. When the patients are suffering from infectious or contagious diseases the carriages are to be disinfected.

REPORTS OF CLINICS.

PHILADELPHIA HOSPITAL.

CLINIC ON DISEASES OF WOMEN—DR. MONT-
GOMERY.

Dr. Montgomery, in speaking of oöphorectomy for the arrest of growth of uterine
fibroids, said the removal of the ovaries and
even of the tubes also does not necessarily
arrest menstruation. In some women the
menopause is delayed one or two years
after the removal of these organs.

In diseases such as growths in the uterine
walls, in which the menstrual flow is found
to be continuing for years after the period
at which it would be expected to cease, it
is not unreasonable to fear that the removal
of the appendages will fail to control the
hemorrhages, and a second operation be
necessary for removal of the growth. From
this standpoint he advises removal of myoma-
tous growths, where it is possible, in preference to oöphorectomy.

Remains of Extra-Uterine Pregnancy.

While upon the subject of abdominal
surgery, he related the history of a patient
upon whom he had operated a week before.
The patient was married, the mother of
four children, and had had several abortions
from chronic metritis. Dr. Montgomery
was called in December, the patient thinking she was again pregnant, and about to
abort. She believed herself about five
weeks pregnant. She had a free discharge
of blood, but there was no enlargement of
the uterus and the cervical canal was contracted. The discharge continued for over
a week, and was attended with some pain
and the throwing off of some membranes
resembling decidua. He saw her again in
January, when she was complaining of pain
in the uterus and rectum, with a return
of bloody discharge. Examination now
revealed a fluctuating tumor posterior to
the uterus, which pushed the uterus forward,
and in this tumor could be felt a more solid
mass.

The sudden appearance of the mass within
a month, the symptoms of pregnancy, the
bloody discharge containing decidual membrane, led him to believe an extra-uterine
pregnancy present, with the foetus in active
growth. A few applications of electricity
were made, but pain continuing and the
tumor increasing in size, he was induced to
advise operation.

The sac behind the uterus was formed by
the matting together of the uterus, ovaries,
and broad ligaments. It contained nearly
a pint of fluid blood and a firm clot, in
which was found some characteristic membrane. The cavity was thoroughly flushed
out and both ovaries and tubes removed.
These organs were removed, not only
because of their being involved in the
adhesions of the sac, but for ovarian and
uterine distress from which she had been
suffering for months. The subsequent progress of the patient had been exceedingly
satisfactory.

Retroflexion.

The next patient was a woman forty-two
years old, the mother of seven children,
who had suffered pain in the pelvis for eight
years and since the birth of her last child
had menstruated every three weeks. An
enlargement was found behind the cervix,
which might be due to a number of conditions, viz: pelvic exudation, prolapsed and
enlarged ovaries, fibroid tumor, and retro-
flexed uterus. The presence of exudation,
Dr. Montgomery said, might be excluded
by the fact that the mass was movable,
smooth in outline, and could be readily
raised up; that it was not an ovarian
enlargement was evident from its close connection with the uterus; it was harder and
more dense than would be expected in an
ovarian growth, and there was absent
the sense of fluctuation, and the marked
tenderness characteristic of enlarged ovary.

The fact that the angle existing between
the mass and the cervix could be erased by
upward pressure against the fundus, and that
the uterus could not be outlined by conjoined
manipulation confirmed the suspicion of
retroflexion of the uterus. If there was any
doubt of the condition it might be still further confirmed by the use of the sound. If
in spite of the presence of this mass the
sound had passed forward in the normal
direction and the fundus could be felt
through the abdominal walls, it would
be an assurance that the retrouterine
mass was a fibroid growth. In the present case, however, the sound passed backward.

The uterus is frequently retroverted or
retroflexed shortly after parturition, from
the pressure upon the heavy organ by a
tightly applied bandage. If one is called
to a woman suffering from hemorrhage two
or three weeks after confinement, let him
examine with special reference to the presence of a retro-displacement.

In the treatment of retroflexion, Dr. Montgomery impressed upon the students the fact that the organ is not replaced by means of the pessary. The pessary serves a valuable purpose in retaining or supporting the replaced organ, but it is worse than useless before it has been replaced.

There are three principal methods of replacing the organ. 1. With the fingers. With the patient in the dorsal position, introduce two fingers into the vagina, with the middle finger in the posterior fornix push up the fundus, while the index is placed in front of the vaginal cervix and pushes backward. In this way the organ is acted upon as a lever. 2. With the uterine sound. The instrument is curved to pass the canal, is passed to the fundus, and then its external end moved through an extended arc in order not to injure the uterine membrane, and the fundus is thus carried upward. 3. By the genu-pectoral position and Sims's speculum, in which case we have the influence of gravity. In the latter course, it is usually necessary to draw down upon the cervix to secure replacement.

Now, the pessaries are of value, but a number of considerations are important. First, the pessary must be well adapted to the individual and fit so that its presence can give only comfort. Second, where retroversion or retroflexion has been of long duration it may be necessary to elongate the surface by the pressure of tampons preparatory to the introduction of a pessary. Third, there is a class of cases in which the displacement is redeveloped as soon as the restraining power is removed, in which the wearing of a pessary is very painful. There are cases in which there are bands more or less long between the posterior surface of the uterus and the anterior wall of the rectum. Relief is here obtained only by tearing the rectum from the uterus by introducing two fingers into the rectum above the uterus and dragging the anterior wall down while the uterus is pushed up by the thumb in the vagina.

Dr. Montgomery also spoke of the advantages claimed for electricity by Apostoli and others, who say that the uterus is supported by muscular filament running out between the folds of peritoneum ; displacement indicates more or less paralysis of these filaments ; hence electricity, through the restoration of the muscular power, holds the organ in position. This treatment has not done accomplished all its enthusiastic advocates claim for it.

As to Alexander's operation, he said that the ligaments become atrophied in marked displacements. The ability to draw them out is frequently restricted by attacks of cellular or peritoneal inflammation, so that the usefulness of the operation must necessarily be limited.

Where patients have suffered long and continually from an obstinate retrodisplacement, the abdominal incision and hysterorraphy seems to be the most feasible method of procedure.

MEDICAL CLINIC—DR. TYSON.

Bright's Disease.

Dr. Tyson introduced the first patient, a German, forty-six years old. He spoke of his having had small pox, scarlet, remittent and typhoid fever, but that he denied having had syphilis. When he came to the Hospital he had swelling in the elbows and wrists, albuminuria and purpuric spots. Three weeks later tube-casts we seen. He was now greatly improved, and, to the unaided senses, his disease would not be apparent. Examination of the urine, however, showed it to be a little turbid from flocculi which had to be filtered out, lest they might conceal a small quantity of albumin. Dr. Tyson said that if filtering does not separate the precipitated alkalies and bacteria, potash could be added and the urine warmed when they would be so thrown down with the phosphates that they could be easily filtered out.

After showing the albumin test and speaking of how acid albumin might not appear, though present, he showed the contact method, overlaying nitric acid with albuminous urine in a narrow tube. He spoke also of the methods with picric acid, for the successful working of which the alkaloids—especially quinine—must be absent. The ferrocyanide of potassium solution does not throw down the alkaloids and is a little more delicate than nitric acid. The mere presence of albumin is not sufficient to establish the presence of Bright's disease, for it might be due to pus or blood. The former is generally visible to the naked eye when in sufficient quantity to give the albumin reaction ; the latter may be invisible, so that the microscope must be used to detect it. We may not *find* the casts, and still have Bright's disease ; the amount of albumin may also be very small, and we fail to demonstrate its presence. In such a case, if there were no pus or blood corpuscles, we would have to fall back on general symptoms, to detect the disease. If albumin and casts are present, it means more or less kidney disease; although after a patient has practically recovered a few casts may often be found for awhile.

But the term chronic Bright's disease includes not only the chronic form of parenchymatous inflammations, but also interstitial nephritis producing the chronically contracted kidney, and the amyloid kidney. In chronic parenchymatous inflammations, the tubules are at least the primary seat of attack, though later, the interstitial connective tissue is also involved.

The finding of albumin and typical epithelial casts in the urine, with the presence of dropsical swelling, indicate the existence of acute Bright's disease. Other symptoms are the presence of blood, rendering it smoky, a diminished quantity of urine, and uræmic convulsions or other nervous phenomena dependent on retention of urea and other constituents of the urine.

In the treatment of acute Bright's disease he advised: 1. Rest in bed, which is often sufficient. 2. In the beginning determination of the character and quantity of urine. 3. To act thoroughly on the bowels, after which we will get a better effect from diuretics. 4. Diuretics, of which the best is digitalis, in the shape of the tincture in fifteen drop doses three or four times a day, or the infusion, a half ounce as often; but these large doses are not to be continued long. 5. If the case is very bad, cause sweating by (*a*), hot water cloths and bottles of hot water—a steam bath which is better than (*b*), the dry hot-air bath, which can often be rendered more efficient by slightly wetting the patient first; (*c*), if uræmic convulsions are present hypodermics of one-fourth to a third of a grain of nitrate or hydrochlorate of pilocarpine may be used, and if the patient does not soon sweat, one-fourth of a grain more may be used. 6. In severe cases it is desirable to apply counter irritation to the region over the affected kidneys. Wet cups may be used, and then a flaxseed meal poultice with mustard, the patient being always warmly covered in bed. Even blood letting may be done in convulsions, and in case of convulsions from puerperal nephritis it should always be employed.

—Dr. B. Alexander Randall has been elected Professor of Diseases of the Ear, and Dr. Edward P. Davis Professor of Obstetrics and Diseases of Children in the Philadelphia Polyclinic and College for Graduates in Medicine.

NEW YORK CORRESPONDENCE.

What Prof. W. Gill. Wylie Thinks of Pessaries.—Dr. Bulkley's Clinic.—Annual Address before the Alumni of Bellevue Hospital.—Dr. Carpenter's Treatment of Tapeworm.

NEW YORK, Feb. 18, 1889.

Dr. Wylie, Professor of Gynecology in the New York Polyclinic, gave a lecture and clinic on displacements of the uterus on February 14. He considers anterior displacements of little importance; it is usually only in posterior malpositions that treatment is called for. This treatment in his opinion should *never* be by pessaries. In his hospital, for the past several years, he has known only one to be used. They simply support the uterus without reaching the cause of the displacement. Furthermore, they are dangerous, because of their liability to infect the patient. They abrade the mucous lining of the vagina and, opening up the canal, allow free entrance of the air to the abrasion. He has often found women wearing the instruments for months and years without relief, whereas they have been quickly cured by curetting and the use of boroglyceride tampons. The tampons are a favorite method of treatment of many diseased conditions of the vagina and uterus with Prof. Wylie, and he uses them continually to support the uterus in displacements. The tampons are made by cutting sheet borated-cotton into strips, an inch and a half or two inches wide, and rolling them up, with medium firmness, until they are of the desired diameter, preferably about half an inch or a little more. They are then wet with the following :

℞   Boroglyceride   . . . . . f℥j
      Glycerine   . . . . f℥xiv

Mix and add a saturated solution of alum, containing ℥ss–j of the salt.

Prof. Wylie also thinks Alexander's operation of shortening the round ligaments rarely necessary, for, if the cause of the displacement is treated, the malposition can, in most cases, be cured.

Prof. L. D. Bulkley, at his clinic in New York Hospital, February 13, exhibited a case of leprosy. The patient was a woman, 21 years old, a native of Antigua, West Indies. Her family history revealed nothing, the father having died at the age of 74 and the mother and two brothers are still living and healthy. The patient came to this country three years ago. A year earlier a measly rash had appeared on her body and, in March, 1886, it was replaced by a papular rash on the arms, hands and scalp, with intense itching. Since then the disease has advanced steadily, until now the face, ears and lips are swollen, white and infiltrated. The voice is husky and the mouth very sore, with fissures on the lips. The arms and forearms are infiltrated and anæsthetic. There is hyperextension of the last two phalanges of the fingers, though the patient sews without difficulty and the sense of feeling is not greatly impaired. The feet and toes are also infiltrated, and there are ulcers and scars on the legs. Dr. Bulkley does not consider the disease contagious, and he cited the case of a priest in a leprous settlement in the Sandwich Islands, who did not contract the disease for seven years and, at last, had his scalp infected by flies. The doctor has had two cases in which he used eucalyptus and chaulmoogra oils, but without effect. This patient not being under his care, no treatment was recommended.

The second patient was a woman 19 years old. She was always well until three years ago, when a small tubercle appeared on the left side of her nose. Since then many more have grown on her face, hands and arms, while the one on her nose has increased to the size of a filbert. The diagnosis, which was confirmed by microscopical examination, was diffuse fibro-sarcoma. Four years ago the patient had an ulcer of the cornea. Iodide of potassium has been used and one growth was scraped, which caused it to disappear. Dr. Bulkley decided to try arseniate of soda by hypodermic injection.

The next patient was a man, 63 years old, who gave the history of being a moderate drinker. When he was 22 years old, his nose began to enlarge and an acne rosacea appeared on it. It developed into a syphilitic process and grew gradually, till now it is exceedingly large and bulbous, red, soft and pulpy to the touch, and the seat of some ulceration. Dr. Bulkley proposed, after thorough syphilitic treatment, to make an incision in the median line, down to the cartilage, scrape away the hypertrophied tissue and removing a wedge-shaped piece. Then by uniting the flaps he expects a respectable-looking nose. The process he diagnosed as rhinophyma.

The annual address, before the Alumni Association of Bellevue Hospital, is to be delivered, in April, by Dr. William Osler. The address will be followed by a banquet.

The late Prof. Wesley M. Carpenter had a favorite treatment for tapeworm, which is as follows: The patient is to eat his breakfast as usual and then eat no more till after delivery of the worm. At 6 A. M., on the second day, he is given Epsom salt ℥j; at 9 A. M., calomel gr. x; at 9.30, decoction of pomegranate f ℥ vj; at 10.30 A.M. f ℥ iv of the same, and then "look for the worm." The treatment is perhaps a little severe, but it brings the worm, head and all. The decoction of pomegranate is made by adding eight ounces of the *fresh* bark to one quart of water, and boiling down to ten ounces.

PERISCOPE.

Influence of the Electric Light on the Eyesight.

Dr. Dubinski of Kronstadt has had an opportunity during the last ten years of observing thirty cases of a peculiar ophthalmic affection occurring in young sailors whose duty had obliged them to remain in the vicinity of electric lights. The symptoms of this affection, which he proposes to denominate "photo-electrical ophthalmia" may occur during sleep. The patient is awakened by profuse lachrymation associated with intense peri-orbital pain. Photophobia is extreme. Nothing, however, can be seen upon examination except palpebral œdema and pericorneal injection of a very marked character. With the ophthalmoscope hyperæmia of the papilla is found, and sometimes a venous pulse in the retinal vessels. After a time varying from an hour and a half to three hours these symptoms subside and the patient is able to go to sleep, and the next morning he awakes quite well, with the exception of a certain amount of ocular fatigue such as is caused by reading late at night. Sleep appears to be an indispensable condition for the manifestation of photo-electrical ophthalmia. Thus, in the case of men who have been exposed during the morning to the electric light, when they take a midday nap the disagreeable phenomena wake them up at that time, and not during the succeeding night. Although the patient, when awake, suffers slightly from phosphenes, he is quite able to read and write during the evening. The pathological cause of the symptoms above described would appear to be a hyperæmia of the optic nerve and some lesion of the nervous filaments of the cornea.—*Lancet*, Feb. 9, 1889.

THE
MEDICAL AND SURGICAL
REPORTER.

ISSUED EVERY SATURDAY.

CHARLES W. DULLES, M.D.,
EDITOR AND PUBLISHER.

The Terms of Subscription to the serial publications of this office are as follows, payable in advance :

Med. and Surg. Reporter (weekly), a year, **$5.00**
Quarterly Compendium of Med. Science, - 2.50
Reporter and Compendium, - - - - 6.00
Physician's Daily Pocket Record, - - 1.00
Reporter and Pocket Record, - - - - 6.00
Reporter, Compendium, and Pocket Record, 7.00

All checks and postal orders should be drawn to order of

CHARLES W. DULLES,
N. E. Cor. 13th and Walnut Streets,
P. O. Box 843.   Philadelphia, Pa.

☞SUGGESTIONS TO SUBSCRIBERS:
See that your address-label gives the date to which your subscription is paid.
In requesting a change of address, give the old address as well as the new one.
If your REPORTER does not reach you promptly and regularly, notify the publisher *at once*, so that the cause may be discovered and corrected.
☞SUGGESTIONS TO CONTRIBUTORS AND CORRESPONDENTS:
Write in ink.
Write on one side of paper only.
Write on paper of the size usually used for letters.
Make as few paragraphs as possible. Punctuate carefully. Do not abbreviate, or omit words like "the," and "a," or "an."
Make communications as short as possible.
NEVER ROLL A MANUSCRIPT! Try to get an envelope or wrapper which will fit it.
When it is desired to call our attention to something in a newspaper, mark the passage boldly with a colored pencil, and write on the wrapper "Marked copy." Unless this is done, newspapers are not looked at.
The Editor will be glad to get medical news, but it is important that brevity and actual interest shall characterize communications intended for publication.

PRESCRIBING OPTICIANS.

The competition between opticians in American cities has grown so keen that the newspapers contain many seductive advertisements, bidding for the trade of individuals suffering with defective vision. Not satisfied with attempts to attract customers by the bait of asserted reductions in prices, many opticians add that at their shops eyes are examined without charge. But this ought not to be. Since ophthalmology has grown into a positive science, it is a grave mistake for opticians to take upon themselves the responsibility of prescribing glasses without the scientific knowledge necessary for this work. Prescribing glasses can only be done correctly with a positive knowledge of the anatomy and physiology of the eye, and day after day oculists are brought into contact with patients who are wearing glasses entirely unfitted for sight. Not only this, but itinerant venders of "crystals" even go so far as to prescribe glasses for headaches, pains, and failing vision, with an assurance that would startle an educated physician. It is within our knowledge that an optician of this city advised a patient, who had been most thoroughly and scientifically examined by a competent oculist, to discard the glasses given by this physician and to wear glasses to which the optician gave a high sounding name, stating that it was not glasses for seeing that he required, but simply "rest glasses."

The observation of careful ophthalmologists indicates that many individuals are given glasses which are worse than useless, and that in some instances so much valuable time is lost that subsequent intelligent treatment is of no avail—some of these are cases in which, if a proper ophthalmoscopic examination had been made and suitable drugs had been prescribed, the patient would have retained vision.

Such a case recently occurred in this city, where a young woman found her vision failing, and, on the advice of her friends, went to an optician, who examined eyes without charge, sold her a pair of glasses, and sent her home with the assurance that all she needed was "rest-glasses." A few weeks passed by, during which her vision grew gradually worse. Another consultation with the optician was held, and another pair of glasses was prescribed. This performance was gone through with twice more, with four changes of glasses in six months; and by this time the patient's vision was reduced to counting fingers at a distance of five feet. At this time an ophthalmoscopic examination revealed the unfortunate fact that the patient has post-neuritic atrophy of both optic nerves. Another case that might be cited is that of a little girl who was found wearing myopic glasses, given her by an optician, when an examination showed that she was exceedingly far-sighted.

It would not be hard to multiply illustrations of the injurious effects of the practice we have been commenting upon. It does not extend to all opticians; for there are a few honorable exceptions who refuse to furnish glasses when they discover visual defects. But too many dealers in spectacles have no compunctions about usurping the province of ophthalmologists, and yield to the temptations of profit and the unwise solicitations of their customers to do what they have no right to do. In acting thus they sometimes screen the first of these motives behind the second, and affect an air of philanthropy as they exclaim against the high charges of the skilled oculists. But this is a shallow subterfuge; for the charges of oculists vary with the circumstances of patients, and those who cannot pay them can get their eyes examined for nothing if they wish. And, while we may pity the ignorance of persons with defects of vision, who for mere motives of economy prefer to consult dealers in spectacles rather than physicians who make a specialty of treating these defects, we can only condemn these dealers who, knowing the risks their customers run, encourage their error for the sake of gain.

The time will yet come, we hope, when the practice of treating eyes without proper fitness for such delicate work will be punishable by law as other unwarranted assumptions of medical practice are now punishable.

Indeed, we believe that the laws now in force in the State would cover this case, and that a person who could show that his eyes had been maltreated by an optician would have little difficulty in recovering damages How far the rights of a dealer to sell his wares would protect an optician who combines with his business the custom of examining the eyes and otherwise imitating the regular methods of legally qualified practitioners of medicine, it is hard to say; but it would be interesting to have a test case brought before one of the courts.

DELIVERY OF THE PLACENTA.

Only a few years ago there was a fairly general agreement among obstetricians concerning the proper method of managing the third stage of labor. Nearly all agreed that nature should not be trusted fully in any case, and that art should always be employed in conducting this stage of labor. The method that was in such favor, as is well known, was that of Credé. Of late, quite a change has come about; the teachings of Credé are by no means so universally accepted, and have even been most strongly assailed in the country of their origin.

The methods of placental delivery which have strong champions at this time are: the method of Credé, the expectant method of Ahlfeld, the method of Berry Hart, and the ancient method of traction on the cord.

The method of Credé practically consists in following down the uterus with the hand, placed on the abdomen, as the child is delivered; making gentle friction with the hand to excite the uterus to contraction; during the height of the contractions compressing the uterus, using all gentleness so as to separate and expel the placenta from the uterus; and then to making downward pressure to expel the placenta from the vagina. The placenta may be delivered during the first or second, or not until the tenth pain. According to Lusk delivery is completed by one skilled in the method in from five to ten minutes after the birth of the child. According to Credé the time for expressing the placenta should depend upon the conditions in the individual case; and the operator should have three different objects in view: 1, the removal of existing dangers; 2, the avoidance of threatened dangers; and 3, the saving of time. The propriety of the first object is universally admitted. The second object is to be accomplished by efforts at expression, as already described. Usually from fifteen to thirty minutes are consumed in the process. There can be no objection to the third object, if in its accomplishment the woman is not injured.

The most prominent opponents of the method of Credé are Ahlfeld, Hart and Charpentier, the objections offered being that it is brutal, that it interferes with the normal mechanism of labor, that it produces increased loss of blood, and that it is the direct cause of the retention of pieces of membrane and placenta. The first objection is founded upon a failure to understand the way in which Credé's method should be carried out. To the second it is difficult to reply, since the nature of the mechanism of the third stage of labor is in dispute, and the evidence supports the view that there are several normal mechanisms. The third objection assumes a result of the method which is contrary to the experience of those who have used it most frequently. The last objection is unquestionably well founded; and it seems safe to assert that a direct relation exists between the percentage of cases of retention, and the rapidity with which the secundines are delivered.

The method of Ahlfeld is called the expectant method, although without entire justification. It consists in attending to bleeding wounds after the birth of the child; and in cleansing, drying, and making comfortable the patient. At intervals of five minutes the cloths applied to the vulva are inspected to see if the discharge of blood is normal. In most cases the cloths need not be changed for one and a half hours *post partum.* Then the urethra is cleansed, the urine is drawn, and the placenta is expressed.

When continuous hemorrhage ensues—not due to injuries—massage is performed. If the hemorrhage is now arrested the expect-ant method is resumed; but if massage fails to arrest the hemorrhage the placenta is expressed at once.

The semi-expectant method of Ahlfeld does not seem destined to wide adoption. The practitioner loses the guaranty against *post-partum* hemorrhage, which an earlier delivery ensures, and especially the knowledge which is gained by keeping the hand over the uterus until, and for some time after, labor is completed. He also loses the extra time which this plan demands of him.

Hart's method of conducting the third stage of labor is as follows: When the child is born the accoucheur must ascertain that the fundus uteri stands at or below the level of the umbilicus, and that the uterus does not contain a second fœtus. Then an ergotin injection is given in multiparæ, especially if labor has been slow. The cord is not tied until the child cries freely, and then only one ligature is applied, on the placental side of which the cord is cut; the fetal end being allowed to drain thoroughly of its contained blood, after which a second ligature is applied to prevent soiling the bedding. The second ligature must be applied at once in case of twins. Before attending to the cord it should be ascertained by abdominal palpation that the uterus is not so relaxed as to bleed. The hand must be kept over the uterus; nothing is to be done when a good contraction comes on, and the uterus is to be allowed its normal relaxation after the pain is over. Should bleeding from the uterus come on, or the pains be feeble, the uterus must be grasped so as to bring on a contraction and to arrest the hemorrhage. Nothing farther is done in a normal case until the lessening bulk of the uterus shows that the placenta is separated and being expelled; then the expulsion may be aided by expression. One can tell when the placenta is separated but not driven down by noting that gentle expression drives it down.

While not passing upon the theoretical

views upon which this practice is founded, the method appears to have much to recommend it. The hand rests over the uterus, so the practitioner is not appalled at sudden hemorrhage. The uterus is allowed to cast off the secundines—and this appeals to the physiologist. We are as yet however in want of full information regarding the method; more especially in regard to the time required for the natural separation of the secundines. The propriety of using ergot until labor is completed is questionable.

The ancient method of delivering the placenta, by traction on the cord, recently championed by Charpentier, opposed as it is to the natural method of delivery, and having inherent dangers possessed by no other method, must be regarded as obsolescent if not obsolete.

The renewed interest in, and the differences of opinion concerning, the proper management of the third stage of labor should prove instructive. 'The principal objection which is urged against Credé's method is, that it is too meddling. Many obstetricians who are supposed to accept Credé's teachings practically admit this, for they advocate waiting some fifteen or twenty minutes after the birth of the child before resorting to efforts to deliver the placenta. This may prove to be the solution of the problem. By it the patient is ensured against hemorrhage because the attendant's hand rests on the womb; the uterus is given an opportunity allowed to separate the placenta; and the practitioner's time is not unduly taken.

THE MEDICAL EXAMINER'S BILL.

Some of our readers may have been surprised to hear a rumor that the Faculty of the Jefferson Medical College was opposed to the passage of the Bill to appoint a Board of Medical Examiners which is now before the Legislature of the State of Pennsylvania, and to which we have already referred editorially a number of times. It is pleasant to call attention to the fact that this rumor is incorrect, and that it has been officially denied by the Dean of the Jefferson Medical College, as will be seen by reference to the letter published in the columns for Correspondence in this number of the REPORTER.

We think no respectable medical school in this State could be silent when classed with those who are inimical to this bill, and we hope that the influences which are now said to be working in secret to bring about its defeat may not prove successful on account of any lukewarmness on the part of those who ought to be found among its active and earnest supporters.

BOOK REVIEWS.

[Any book reviewed in these columns may be obtained upon receipt of price, from the office of the REPORTER.]

TRANSACTIONS OF THE ROYAL ACADEMY OF MEDICINE IN IRELAND. VOL. VI. EDITED BY WILLIAM THOMSON, M.A., F.R.C.S., General Secretary, Surgeon to the Richmond Hospital, Dublin. 8vo, pp. xxxvi, 482. Dublin: Fannin & Co., 1888.

In the opening pages of this Volume we learn that the Academy of Medicine in Ireland has, since its Transactions were last published, asked for and received authority from the Queen of England, to add the word "Royal" to its title; and so this distinguished body has testified its loyalty to the government of Great Britain and received a recognition which is highly prized on the other side of the Atlantic. But it needed no such patent to recommend it to scientific men; for it has long been the source of medical and surgical papers of great value, and its Transactions are equal in scientific worth to those of any medical body in the world.

The present volume fully maintains the standard of its predecessors. It is a matter of regret that the limits of our space forbid a detailed notice of the papers it contains; but we may say that every department of medical science is ably represented in its pages, and that the powers of observation, the skill and the judgment of our Irish *confrères* are abundantly illustrated in it. The Volume is a mine of information, and would be a valuable acquisition to any studious physician or surgeon.

LITERARY NOTES.

—B. Westermann & Co. announce the intended publication of an *Internationaler Centralblatt für die Physiologie und Pathologie des Uro-genital-Systems.* There will be one volume a year, issued in about 8 parts, and the list of editors contains the names of some of the most eminent surgeons in Europe.

CORRESPONDENCE.

Treatment of Locomotor Ataxia by Suspension.

To THE EDITOR.

Sir: In the REPORTER, February 23, 1889, there is a very interesting and practical editorial on "Treatment of Locomotor Ataxia by Suspension," in which you say: "The method of Motchoukowsky is simply suspension, as usually practised when a plaster jacket is applied for disease or deformity of the spinal column." If it is not asking too great a favor, will you kindly inform me whether the suspension is by the chin and occiput and the armpits, or by the chin and occiput while the patient draws on the rope with his own hands.

Yours truly,
STANTON ALLEN, M.D.
Brooklyn, New York,
March 2, 1889.

[The suspension is by the chin and occiput and the arm-pits.—Editor of the REPORTER.]

The Medical Examiners' Bill and the Jefferson Medical College.

To THE EDITOR.

Sir: The following letter explains itself, and I would be glad if you think it proper to publish it in the MEDICAL AND SURGICAL REPORTER.

Yours truly,
LAWRENCE F. FLICK, M.D.
Philadelphia,
March 6, 1889.

FEB. 25, 1889.

Lawrence F. Flick, M.D., Chairman of Committee.

Dear Sir: In reply to your letter of the 18th inst. I beg to state that the rumor of opposition to the medical bill on the part of our faculty is incorrect. We have not considered the matter formally.

The members of our faculty are not opposed to any medical bill that is favored by the general profession of the State.

Respectfully and truly yours,
J. W. HOLLAND, M.D.,
Dean.

—The *Chemist and Druggist*, Feb. 16, states that a statue of Gay-Lussac is to be erected in August, at Limoges, when the French Society for the Advancement of Science is to hold its annual meeting at the date mentioned.

NOTES AND COMMENTS.

Cure of a Case of Leprosy.

In the case reported (*Monatshefte für praktische Dermatologie*, No. 23, 1888) by Dreckmann, the disease was fairly advanced, had lasted four years, and presented numerous nodes, tubercles, and patches of infiltration. There was also marked anæsthesia of the feet, legs, and hands. The mucous membrane was also involved; swelling of the conjunctivæ, a discharging ulcer in the nasal septum, whitish patches on the larynx posteriorly, thickening of the left vocal cord, a small tubercle on the point of the epiglottis, and hard nodular infiltration of both tonsils. The patient, a Brazilian, forty-two years old, was at this time, thin, pale, and weak. The treatment, by means of pyrogallic acid, chrysarobin, and salicylic acid, together with the internal use of ichthyol, as suggested by Unna, was instituted; and finally, in the course of several months, all vestiges of the disease had disappeared, and the patient had grown stout and strong.

The pyrogallic acid was applied mainly to the hands, feet, and legs, in the form of a ten per cent. salve ; upon the other parts a salve of chrysarobin, of the same strength ; these were applied twice daily. To obstinate nodules and patches of infiltration the same remedies were used in the form of plaster-mulls. To the face a salicylic acid and creasote plaster-mull was applied, once daily. Discrete and sharply circumscribed nodules, when conveniently situated, were excised. The conjunctival swelling disappeared spontaneously. The ulcer in the nose, the nodules on the tonsils, etc., were successfully treated with the actual cautery. The constitutional treatment consisted mainly in the administration of ichthyol, beginning with six grains daily, and gradually increasing to forty-five grains. Under the use of these measures, the writer states, an apparent cure resulted—the general health being restored, and all evidence of the disease dissipated.

As incidental points of interest in the report, may be mentioned that the patient's wife had developed the disease eighteen years before ; the wife's brother was also affected. The children, four in number, from fifteen to twenty-one years old, showed no sign of the disease. The patient's parents and six brothers, all living in the same neighborhood, were also healthy.— *American Journal of the Medical Sciences*, March, 1889.

Ignipuncture of the Tonsils.

Dr. Wilhelm Roth, of Fluntern, finds that in order to reduce the size of the tonsils without risk of troublesome hemorrhage, which is not uncommon, especially in young subjects, the best plan is to employ igni-puncture, as has been recommended by Krishaber, and more recently by Verneuil. The tonsils and neighboring parts are first brushed over with a ten to twenty per cent. solution of cocaine. The finest point of the thermo-cautery, heated to redness, is then inserted to a depth of about five millimetres in three or four spots a few millimetres apart from one another on the tonsils. The instrument is not allowed to remain more than one or two seconds in the tissue. The whole operation, including both tonsils, can be performed in a very few minutes without any bleeding, and with scarcely any pain. It must be repeated four or five times at intervals of two or three days, and this is usually sufficient to cause the tonsils to return to their ordinary condition.—*Lancet*, Feb. 16, 1889.

Hysteria in the Russian Army.

According to Dr. Ozeretskofski, of Moscow, the existence of hysteria amongst Russian soldiers is by no means an exceptional occurrence. The affection presents the same diversities of form that it does amongst women. Frequently men suffering from this affection are put down as malingerers. Other cases are looked upon as instances of serious but somewhat obscure organic disease, the true nature of the case being nearly always overlooked, because it is not generally supposed that soldiers are liable to hysteria. So real, however, does Dr. Ozeretskofski consider the existence of this male hysteria, that, having had an opportunity of studying no less than thirty-eight cases in the Moscow Military Hospital, he is convinced that hysteria ought to be recognized as one of the affections which entitle the subject of it to exemption from military service.—*Lancet*, Feb. 16, 1889.

Round Ulcer of the Stomach.

Dr. Cherbakoff, of Moscow, in order to study the conditions under which gastric ulcers occur, injected a solution of chromate of lead into the gastric arteries of dogs, with the result that ulcers were produced which bore a considerable resemblance to ordinary round gastric ulcers in the human subject. These experimental ulcers, however, evinced a great tendency to heal rapidly and com-pletely. This tendency could be combated by increasing the acidity of the gastric juice. Indeed, by this means it was found possible to cause the ulcers to become deeper and deeper until they perforated all the coats of the organ. Clinically speaking, these results would appear to be not devoid of significance, as it is well known that round ulcer of the stomach is frequently associated with hyper-acidity of the gastric juice.—*Lancet*, Feb. 9, 1889.

Iso-Nitroso-Antipyrin.

Reference has already been made in the REPORTER to the alleged toxic effects of the salt (iso-nitroso-antipyrin) which results from the addition of antipyrin to sweet spirit of nitre. Dr. H. C. Wood and Dr. John Marshall have recently investigated the truth of the asserted toxicity of this salt, and they report the results of their investigations in the *Therapeutic Gazette*, Feb. 15, 1889. It was found that the crystals changed in color from green to brown, and developed a very distinct hydrocyanic-acid odor after standing a few hours. The quantity of cyanogen produced in this decomposition, however, is not large, and therefore, they say, could hardly be a cause of serious trouble.

In determining whether the iso-nitroso-antipyrin possesses toxic properties or not, it was administered under various conditions to dogs and rabbits, but in no case, as their experiments show, were the slightest untoward effects observed.

A New Tænicide.

M. Thiel (*Journ. de Méd. de Paris*) has examined the bark of a tree known as the "moussena," the *Acacia anthelmintica* of Baillon, growing principally in Abyssinia, and having a high reputation as a destroyer of tapeworm. It is said to be more active than koussoo, and to have a less disagreeable taste. The bark is the only part of the tree employed medicinally, and this is taken in the form of powder in doses of from one ounce to two ounces, alone, or mixed with honey and stirred up in milk. The Abyssinians mix the powder with flour, and make bread with it, and take a sufficient quantity of the bread with butter or honey three hours before the first meal in the morning. The same evening or the next day the worm is generally expelled in fragments. M. Thiel has found in the bark a substance whose chemical characteristics resemble saponine, and he calls this "moussenine."—*Chemist and Druggist*, Feb. 9, 1889.

Extraction of a Foreign Body from the Uterine Cavity.

At the last meeting of the Imperial Royal Medical Society of Vienna, Dr. Herzfeld reported the following interesting case: On December 30, a woman came into the clinic of Prof. G. Braun, of Vienna, stating that she had washed her vagina in the morning, and that the mouth-piece of the syringe was left behind; vaginal examination showed that no foreign body was present in the vagina. A sound was introduced into the uterine cavity, and the foreign body was then detected. The cervix uteri was dilated, and the foreign body extracted; it proved to be the handle of a crochet-needle. Answering the question as how this foreign body had found its way into the uterine cavity, the woman stated that she was twenty-five years old, and had already been confined of four children. As she did not wish to have more children, she was accustomed, at the instance of her midwife, to wipe her uterine cavity after each sexual intercourse. For this purpose, she used to press down the uterus through the abdominal parietes, and to introduce into it a crochet-needle around which was wrapped a piece of cloth; on one occasion the handle of the needle was left behind in the uterine cavity. Dr. Herzfeld remarked that usually such manipulations are only undertaken for onanistic reasons or for causing abortion; two similar cases had been reported by Prof. M. Hofmann, of Vienna. Such occurrences are important from a medico-legal point of view.—*Medical Press and Circular*, Jan. 30, 1889.

Prize Essays.

The following prizes are offered by the Academia Médico-Quirurgica Espanola: 1. For the Academy Prize: a critical estimate of antiparasitic remedies in medicine, surgery and obstetrics. 2. For the Morales Prize: a critical estimate of lithotrity, lithotomy, litholapaxy, and perineal and suprapubic cystotomy. The Academy Prize is a sum of 250 pesetas (about $50) and the title of Corresponding Fellow; the Morales Prize is a sum of 750 pesetas (about $145), with the same title. Essays may be written in Spanish, Portuguese, French, Italian, English, or German. Fellows of the Academy are excluded from competition. The essays, bearing a motto, and accompanied by a sealed envelope containing the name of the author, should be sent to the President of the Academy, Montera, 22 *bajo*, Madrid, on or before September 15, 1889. Every essay sent in shall remain the property of the Academy.—*British Med. Journal*, Feb. 9, 1889.

International Congress of Dermatology and Syphilography.

An International Congress of Dermatology and Syphilography is announced to take place in Paris, in connection with the Universal International Exhibition of 1889, on August 5 to 10. It will take place in the Museum of the Hôpital Saint Louis. The Presidents are Dr. Ricord and Professor Hardy. Dr. Colcott Fox and Mr. Malcolm Morris are Secretaries for London; Dr. Feulard, Chef de Clinique de la Faculté à l'Hôpital Saint Louis, is the General Secretary. The subscription is 25 francs, which entitles the subscriber to the volume of reports of the Congress. The subjects arranged for discussion are *A* the constitution of the group lichen: 1. Should the denomination of lichen be preserved for a number of affections which modern authors consider to differ one from the other? 2. If not, which affection should be separated; and if a new group of lichens be constituted, what forms should be admitted into it? *B* Pityriasis rubra and generalized primary exfoliating dermatitis: 1. What are the characters proper to pityriasis rubra, and how should those various types be distinguished? 2. Is pityriasis rubra pilaris a species of pityriasis rubra, or a special affection, or a variety of psoriasis? 3. What are the relations between scarlatiniform erythema and generalized primary exfoliating dermatitis? Other questions relate to pemphigus, trichophytic dermatoses, the treatment of syphilis, and the relative frequency of tertiary syphilis. Suggestions are also made as to voluntary papers. Members proposing to take part in the Congress and send communications are requested to communicate with the Secretary before May 15, and to forward a brief summary of their papers. The summary will be printed *in extenso* or in part in the general programme, which will be distributed before the opening of the Congress. This programme, which will be issued at the beginning of the month of July, will contain the names of members who have signified their intention to be present and have paid their subscription before May 15, the order in which they are down to speak on the subjects announced, the order of the day, and promised communications.—*British Med. Journal*, Feb. 9, 1889.

NEWS.

—Dr. Carey A. Evans died in Delphos, Ohio, Feb. 16, at the age of 60 years.

—Dr. H. G. Norton, of Imlaystown, N. J., will remove to Trenton, N. J., about April 1.

—In a suit recently in Boston to recover damages for the extraction of a sound instead of a decayed tooth, the plaintiff has been awarded $150.

—A building on West Forty-third Street, near Fifth Avenue, has been secured for the new academy and library of the New York Academy of Medicine.

—Dr. Loomis, of New York City, has been sued by the widow of the late Dr. Miller to compel him to pay for literary work said to have been done for him by Dr. Miller.

—At a recent meeting in London, presided over by the Lord Mayor, Mr. Algernon Coote suggested a plan for collecting 500,000 pence weekly—about $500,000 annually—to relieve the London Hospitals of debt.

—The Trustees of the William F. Jenks Prize Fund have made arrangements with Messrs. P. Blakiston Son & Co. to publish the successful essay on the "Diagnosis of Extra-Uterine Pregnancy," which, as announced in the REPORTER Feb. 23, has been awarded for this year to Dr. John Strahan, of Belfast, Ireland.

—The Executive Committee of the Medical Society of Virginia has appointed the following physicians to fill vacancies in the Medical Examining Board of Virginia: Drs. James W. Tankard, Dr. Paulus A. Irving, and Dr. Leigh Buckner. The *Virginia Medical Monthly* speaks highly of these men. The physicians whose resignations created the vacancies are Drs. W. W. Douglass, J. Herbert Claiborne, and Oscar Wiley.

—The Philadelphia *Ledger*, Feb. 16, says that the morphine habit has become so prevalent in San Francisco as to give rise to a peculiar slang applying to it and its votaries. The latter are called "morphine fiends," and the process of hypodermic injection is called "taking a shot." Hospital surgeons say that the morphine habit is increasing rapidly, and that most of the victims were initiated in Chinatown. One of these officials estimates that 60 per cent. of the petty offenders sent to the receiving hospitals of the city prison are victims of the morphine habit. Cocaine is so expensive that few acquire the "habit."

HUMOR.

MRS. HAYSEED—So young Wiggins is dead. I wonder what he died of?

Alonzo Hayseed (from college)—I heard it was pulmonary phthisis.

Mrs. H.—Land o'Goshen! and me thinkin' all the time the fellow had the consumption.—*America.*

NOTING a particularly healthy-looking child the other day, a lady asked the nurse, who had it in charge:

"Is that a nursing baby or a bottle baby?"

"Sure it's nayther, Ma'am; it's a condensed milk baby."—*Exchange.*

PHYSICIAN (arousing a tramp one morning from a nap on his doorstep)—Here, what is the matter with you? Can't you move more lively?

Tramp—I'm feeling pretty bad, boss, and can't be expected to move in a hurry.

P.—What's the matter?

T.—I've been at death's door all night.—*Boston Budget.*

A BANGOR lady was very ill a few days ago, and a physician was called, who prescribed for her. The prescription was given to a servant girl, who was directed to take it to a drug store and have it filled. She went to the drug store, but, instead of carrying out her instructions, bought a postage stamp, placed it upon the prescription and dropped it into the post office. In a short time it returned to the physician who gave it. It may be well to add that the lady did not die from the delay in receiving the medicine.

OBITUARY.

D. WILLARD BLISS, M.D.

Dr. D. W. Bliss, of Washington, D.C., died Feb. 21. He had been in poor health for several months, and two days before his death was stricken with paralysis from cerebral hemorrhage. Dr. Bliss was born in Auburn, N. Y., in 1825, and was graduated from the Western Reserve Medical College in 1850. Until the outbreak of the late war he practised medicine in Grand Rapids, Mich. In 1862 he was placed in charge of the Armory Square Hospital, the largest in Washington during the war. It held at times as many as 12,000 to 15,000 soldier patients. In 1865 he resigned this position and engaged in general practice in Washington. Dr. Bliss was present at the death bed of President Lincoln, and, as is well known, was the attending physician during President Garfield's long illness.

MEDICAL AND SURGICAL
REPORTER

No. 1672.　　　　　PHILADELPHIA, MARCH 16, 1889.　　　VOL. LX.—No. 11.

CONTENTS:

COMMUNICATIONS.

EUPHORBIA PILULIFERA IN ASTHMA.

BY M. GRAHAM TULL, A.M., M.D.,

VISITING PHYSICIAN TO BAPTIST ORPHANAGE, PHILA-
DELPHIA.

In connection with the use of euphorbia pilulifera for asthma I have had the following interesting and instructive experience. I will go somewhat into details with the hope that they may prove of value to the profession.

In the spring of 1888 I was called to attend a man, 55 years old. The patient was a man of means and occupied a position of great trust and responsibility. He was suffering from a severe attack of asthma, brought on in this instance apparently by indiscretion in eating, as it was attended by a severe attack of indigestion. When I saw him he was sitting up in bed, breathing with difficulty, with whistling expiration which could be heard all over the room.

He stated that he was subject to such attacks, probably four or five times a year. This one had come on at Atlantic City a few days previous to my visit, and the physician who was called had given him a hypodermic injection of morphine, which had been followed by such severe vomiting that the patient begged me not to repeat it except as a last resort. I then gave him a mixture containing fluid extract of euphorbia pilulifera, potassium iodide, potassium bromide, and tincture of belladonna. I also ordered three drops of amyl nitrite to be taken by inhalation, and that half an ounce of glycerine should be given by injection, as his bowels were very much constipated. I saw him again the following day, and found that he had refused the mixture, after two doses, on account of the intensely disagreeable taste ; so that later in the day I found it necessary to give him a hypodermic of morphine gr. $\frac{1}{4}$, and atropine gr. 1-60. This was followed by the happiest results, the patient dropping into a quiet sleep in about ten minutes.

After this I explained to him the importance of treatment in the periods between the attacks, ordering him a laxative pill and a stomachic, and telling him to pay special attention to diet and hygiene; and also advised him to spend the following August, when he was liable to an attack, in the mountains.

Although from time to time seeing other members of his family professionally I saw nothing of this patient for some months; but heard indirectly that he desired to see me, as he had been cured of the asthma by the "Buffalo Asthmatic Institute," to which he had been sent by a friend. Finally, about Christmas, I met him, and he at once told me that he had only been waiting a few months to see if his cure held out to tell me about the treatment, and that he now felt he could reasonably feel cured, and that a number of his friends had also been treated with wonderful success in the meanwhile. He cited the case of a cousin who had been unable to lie down for years, but who was now able to sleep in the normal position.

I then went home with him and he showed me the following drugs: The box he had received contained a box of pills, a box of capsules, and three bottles, also a couple of pamphlets with directions, etc. The pills were to keep the bowels regular; the capsules contained quinine (gr. ii) to be taken when catching cold. One of the bottles contained a stomachic to be taken before meals for the avowed purpose of keeping the stomach in good condition; one of the other bottles held the "Asthma Cure," and was to be taken over a period of about two years (with intermissions) in bad cases; in addition to these a thapsia plaster was sometimes ordered.

Upon examining the "Asthma Cure" I was at once convinced that it was the Euphorbia Pilulifera, and taking a sample of it I went over to Mr. Geo. E. Dahis, the druggist who had obtained the euphorbia for me, and without informing him of my reason asked him to compare the sample I had with his fluid extract of euphorbia pilulifera. This he did, and at once pronounced them the same. I then went back to Mr. A. with the two bottles, and he agreed that the taste, smell, and general appearance of the two were identical, except that the fluid extract seemed less clear.

He had been taking thirty drops in a wineglassful of water after meals. He had not recognized it, as I had given it in combination with potassium iodide, potassium bromide, and tincture of belladonna. The third bottle was evidently nitrite of amyl in glycerine. His directions were to take thirty drops at the beginning of an acute attack and not to repeat it but once without consulting the "Institute." The odor was that of amyl nitrite. This in the pamphlet goes by the name of the "clincher."

It happened, oddly enough, that on going home that evening I found a new patient who was suffering from an acute attack of asthma, from which he said, he had suffered since boyhood. This was on Saturday night, and I prescribed fluid extract of euphorbia pilulifera, thirty drops in a wineglassful of water every four hours, telling him to report to me the following Monday evening. I did not see him on Monday, but met him on Tuesday, when he said the reason he had not been around the night before was that the medicine had had such a wonderful effect that he had been able to go to work. The patient told me a month afterward that he had never breathed so freely before in his life. He was a brakeman on the railroad, and was much exposed.

A third patient, a photographer, has given me the same brilliant results since then. I am fully convinced that the euphorbia pilulifera is the key note to the undoubted and remarkable results obtained by the "Buffalo Asthmatic Institute" in the treatment of asthma. Only a few nights ago a friend of large experience in practice told me that one of his own patients was under their care, and that he is now able to sleep in a recumbent posture for the first time in months. My patient tells me the "Institute" has prospered to such a degree that it has opened offices in New York City, and that whenever he goes over he finds the offices filled with patients, and he says they all bear testimony to the wonderful good done them. The head of the affair is Dr. P. Harold Hayes, a graduate, I understand, of one of our leading schools. Now of course he gets his results by natural means, as it is not an age of miracles, and I feel confident that I have indicated above what his specific is.

I have learned that euphorbia pilulifera is a very common weed in Australia, and that it has a great local reputation there in the treatment of asthma and chronic bronchitis. Dr. J. P. Crozer Griffith very kindly sends me the following abstracts connected with the drug. "W. Jayes, in the *Ceylon Med. Jour.*, Aug., 1888, describes the plant known in Sinhalese as Boordada-Keeriya. The children use the juice to tattoo their arms. The author reports a case of asthma and one of chronic bronchitis, both very obstinate and of long standing, greatly relieved after a few doses of two fluid ounces of the decoction, taken three times a day. Thomas Christy in ' New Commercial Plants and Drugs' Nos. v and vii, 1888, gives an account of the plant and a history of its introduction into medicine. He says it was first used for asthma and other bronchial affections in Australia. He describes the method of making the decoction. I have now under my care an old lady with chronic bronchitis who is doing wonderfully well upon thirty drops of [the fluid extract of] euphorbia pilulifera, t. d.''

I trust that this may be the means of stimulating the profession to using what the above experience has led me to feel may prove a specific for this most troublesome affection.

4807 Woodland ave.

THE TREATMENT OF CATARRHAL DISEASES OF THE NOSE AND THROAT AT THE UNION DISPENSARY.

BY E. BALDWIN GLEASON, M.D.,
PHILADELPHIA.

Acute coryza is treated by first spraying the nose with "antiseptic solution" until all secretions are removed. The following is the formula for this solution, which has been found superior to Dobel's solution for use in the atomizer as well as for a nose wash for the patient to use at home.

> ℞ Sodii bicarb. . . . .
> Sodii bibor. . . . . āā ʒ viii
> Sodii benzoat. . . . .
> Sodii salicylat. . . . . . . āā gr xx
> Thymol.
> Eucalyptol . . . . āā gr x
> Menthol . . . . gr. v
> Ol. gaultheriæ . . . . gtt. vi
> Glycerini . . . . Oz. viiiss
> Alcoholis . . . . Oz. ii
> Aquæ . . . . q. s. ad Oxvi

Several of our Philadelphia druggists have combined the solid ingredients of this formula into a compressed tablet, and, for convenience, these are used at the dispensary instead of the original formula of Dr. Seiler given above. After the nose and throat have been cleansed by spraying with the "antiseptic solution," a pledget of cotton wool saturated with a 4 per cent. solution of cocaine is placed in each nostril; and, after the lapse of a few minutes, the nose is sprayed with a 4 per cent. solution of antipyrin. The effect is to control excessive secretion and the turgescence of the nasal mucous membrane, and this

effect lasts, as first pointed out by Dr. Hinkel, for six or eight hours, when the application may be repeated. In this manner, a "cold in the head" may be aborted; or, at least, speedily cured. In very severe cases, however, it has been deemed advisable to administer a saline cathartic as well; and, sometimes, also, small doses of atropia frequently repeated.

Simple chronic nasal catarrh is usually treated at the dispensary by ordering "antiseptic tablets" used at home by the patient as a nose wash, night and morning. Twice or three times a week he is required to present himself for treatment; and, after the nose and throat have been thoroughly sprayed with the antiseptic solution, the following solution is applied through the inferior meatus to the post nasal space by means of a cotton applicator, the parts immediately afterward being sprayed with cosmoline:

> ℞ Iodi . . . . gr viii
> Potas. iodidi . . . . gr. xxiv
> Glycerini . . . . f ʒ ss

If the patient is otherwise in good health, an uncomplicated attack of simple chronic nasal catarrh may get well in six weeks; but the antiseptic tablets must be used for some time longer, and an occasional application of the iodine solution should be made to prevent a relapse.

Hypertrophic nasal catarrh is treated as simple chronic nasal catarrh until the discharge has markedly diminished and all signs of active inflammation have subsided, when the anterior hypertrophies may be burned with the electro-cautery and posterior hypertrophies removed by the Jarvis snare. The preparatory treatment for these operations is deemed essential, as otherwise the reaction from them is very severe and recovery delayed, while the ultimate results are not as good. Antiseptics other than the "antiseptic solution" are now employed. In applying the electro-cautery to an anterior hypertrophy, rather a thick wire is used, made as described in my paper on "Galvano-cautery Electrodes," published in the REPORTER, August 11, 1888, page 174. The cautery knife is carried down through the hypertrophied tissues until the periosteum is reached. If this is not done there will be but little effect from the burn, and the operation will probably have to be repeated to secure a good result. A 4 per cent. solution of cocaine is used as an anæsthetic, because it has been found that, while anæsthesia from a stronger solution appears a little more quickly, yet it is not more thorough, and does not last as long as that produced by a 4 per cent. solution. Ecchondroses and exostoses of the septum might be classed among the hypertrophies, as they have been proven by Seiler to result from the catarrhal inflammation described by him in a paper published in the *Medical Record,* February 18, 1888. These growths are chiselled off from the septum, Seiler's chisels being used for this purpose. Here again a 4 per cent. solution of cocaine is found to give almost complete local anæsthesia, if it is allowed to remain for some time within the nose on a pledget of cotton. Cocaine has been used very freely in the noses of the dispensary patients operated on, and no untoward effects have ever been observed. I am convinced that many of the cases of so-called cocaine poisoning reported have been simply cases of fainting caused by the shock of the operation, rather than the effects of the cocaine employed as an anæsthetic.

In atrophic nasal catarrh "antiseptic tablets" are prescribed for the patients to use at home, as a wash, two or three times a day, so as to secure perfect cleanliness. As often as possible such patients are seen at the dispensary; and, after all plugs of inspissated mucus have been carefully removed, the following powder is applied by the insufflator:

℞   Argenti nitrat. . . . . gr. v
    Amyli . . . . ℥ iiss
M.

This application is followed by a slight smarting sensation, which, however, soon subsides. Should this smarting not occur, the powder is not irritating enough, and its strength should be increased, and as much nitrate of silver as eighteen grains to two and one-half drachms of starch, has been used by insufflation, with the best results. After the application of the nitrate of silver powder, a tightly rolled pledget of cotton is inserted upon the floor of each nostril and allowed to remain there; the patient being instructed to renew it as often as necessary. The silver nitrate probably acts simply as an irritant; but the plug of cotton, by the constant irritation of its presence; not only causes renewed growth of the atrophied parts, but also a watery discharge is at once established, which washes away inspissated and fetid mucus, producing an effect at once noticeable in the changed character of the exhaled air. The cotton, moreover, filling up partly the enormously dilated nares, brings the inspired air more directly in contact with the nasal tissues; so that the nose

at once resumes its function of warming and moistening the inspired air, and the chronic laryngitis, usually present in this form of catarrh, gets well almost without treatment. Pharyngitis sicca so soon disappears, probably on account of the increased secretion from the posterior nares, or the altered character of the air breathed; for it is well established that this condition is generally the result of breathing air not sufficiently moist, either through the mouth when the nares are not patulous, or through the enormously dilated nares of atrophic catarrh. There is one patient now at the dispensary, who, with this treatment during the past three months has nearly recovered from rather bad atrophic nasal catarrh; but ordinarily in such cases it takes a year or so to bring about a condition resembling health.

Perhaps the most interesting of all cases are those of ethmoiditis involving the middle turbinated bone. Many stages of this affection may be observed, from a simple polypoid degeneration of the mucous membrane of this region of the nose to large granulations or polypi overlying dead bone; and even in the final stage of cure, in which the dead bone having exfoliated, a large cleft may remain in the middle turbinated bone at the site of the former disease. If the disease is seen in the stage of polypoid degeneration, ethmoiditis is treated at the dispensary by snaring off all redundant mucous membrane from the middle turbinated bone, and by the application of the electro-cautery; when ordinarily the process is checked. When the case is first seen in what might be called the second stage of the disease, and large granulations or polypi are present, underneath which the probe detects dead and exposed bone, the polypi are first removed by means of the Jarvis snare and then the dead bone scraped away with the nasal curette. Ordinarily this is easily accomplished, the dead bone being like so much sand imbedded in soft granulations; but when the probe penetrates deeply before coming in contact with exposed and roughened bone, it has seemed best to introduce a fine electro-cautery knife along the sinus until the dead bone is felt. The cautery knife is then quickly heated. In this manner a slough is produced which brings away the dead bone with it. When polypi are simply snared off, they almost invariably return, but when the ethmoiditis which underlies the whole trouble has been treated and cured, the cause of nasal polypi having been removed the polypi do not return. No case of nasal polypi is considered cured as long as dead bone can be detected .by a fine probe at the spot whence the polyps grew.

Granular pharyngitis, pharyngitis sicca, and chronic pharyngitis being simply the result of nasal disease, get well as the result of treating the nasal trouble; and no applications have been made to the throat at the dispensary in such cases.

Acute tonsillitis is treated by the application of a sixty-grain solution of nitrate of silver to the inflamed structures once or twice a day. A gargle, or still better, a lozenge containing potassium chlorate, chloride of iron and bromide of potash is ordered for the patient to use every two hours. If the patient is seen early this treatment almost invariably aborts the disease. To do good the silver solution' must be of the strength of at least sixty grains to the ounce. If a weaker solution is used, its application is painful, but if a sixty-grain solution be employed, there is no pain whatsoever attending its use and the patient immediately experiences a sense of comfort. When seen a few moments after such an application the tonsils no longer appear of a bright red color, but are paler and seem to have shrunken somewhat. Of some thirty cases of acute tonsillitis treated in this way, not one went on to suppuration.

Chronic hypertrophied tonsils are divided into three classes; the soft, the hard, and the ragged. The first, if the anterior pillars are not adherent to them, are removed by the tonsillotome. When adhesion of the pillar is present, however, an attempt should be made to break down the adhesions with a probe and free the anterior pillars from the tonsils; for a branch of the tonsillar artery lies in the anterior pillar which, if wounded, gives rise to troublesome hemorrhage.

Hard, fibrous tonsils also are very apt to bleed profusely when cut, and are, consequently, removed either with the Jarvis snare or by repeated applications of the galvano-cautery, used in the following manner: The cautery knife is introduced cold into a crypt of the tonsil to be removed; and, being heated, is made to burn its way out through the tonsil. As this procedure is entirely painless it is not necessary to use cocaine. From five to ten such applications at intervals of a week are necessary to cause an hypertrophied tonsil to shrink to its normal dimensions: and during the progress of the treatment, little if any pain or inconvenience is experienced by the patient.

The so-called ragged tonsil, whose irregular shape is the result of frequent attacks of tonsillitis and consequent abscesses, is generally treated in the same manner as the hard, fibrous tonsils, unless it is large enough to be grasped by the tonsillotome or snare.

An hypertrophied pharyngeal tonsil and adenoid vegetations have always been removed by the finger-nail of the operator. The patient is seated crosswise on his lap, and the left arm of the operator being drawn tightly about the patient's body, all struggling is prevented. The right hand is now introduced into the patient's mouth and the fore-finger carried behind the palate, when such growths are easily scraped away with the finger-nail, if it be long and strong. As such growths are rare except in children, it has not been found necessary to employ any other method; the oldest case so operated on being that of a young woman sixteen years of age. Adenoid vegetations have also been observed to disappear after removing the fauceal tonsils; and, as the result of frequent applications of the iodine solution to the vault of the pharynx.

1346 Spruce St.

REFLEX, OR THE SO-CALLED USE-LESS, COUGH.

BY STANLEY M. WARD, M.D.,
SCRANTON, PA.

The subject of reflex cough, that is to say, of cough in which, in the words of A. A. Smith, the primary seat of irritation is outside of the respiratory tract, is one that seems to have attracted little attention from writers on medical subjects. In a paper recently read before the New York County Medical Society, Dr. Wm. H. Thomsen (*see* REPORTER, December 15, 1888, p. 750) stated that there are fourteen varieties of useless cough, and among the causes of it he enumerated worms in the intestinal tract, undigested food anywhere along the same canal, the cause of whooping-cough, foreign bodies in the auditory canal, a misplaced uterus, aneurisms in certain localities, and malaria.

During the spring of 1886 there came under my personal observation a typical case of reflex cough. I was satisfied that the cause of the cough was outside the respiratory tract, but to find out just where it was proved extremely difficult. At that time I consulted what literature I had access to, and especially the files of all the prominent medical magazines published in this country, but with little success except in one instance. A reprint of an article by Dr. A. A. Smith on reflex cough, which appeared in the *American Journal of the Medical Sciences*, came under my notice and was of valuable assistance, especially as it convinced my patient that after all she might not be a victim of "hasty consumption" or pneumonia, as her friends had declared. Dr. Smith in this article narrates the history of eleven patients who came under his own observation, and quotes one from *L'Union Médicale*. As a matter of interest I give an epitome of his cases.

Case I.—Male child, four weeks old. "Began to cough violently, one night, suddenly, and to cry each time he coughed." Had been perfectly healthy. He failed. to account for the cough and ordered a teaspoonful of castor oil. Seemed worse next day. A "most careful examination of heart, lungs and throat" failed to reveal a cause for the cough, which continued unaccompanied by fever until the fourth day, when the Doctor had the child stripped to the skin and noticed that every time the child coughed there was an "umbilical protrusion." A compress put over this stopped the cough, but when removed the cough returned. Thus having the key to the trouble the treatment was simple and a compress was fitted over the protrusion, which stopped the cough entirely and completely relieved the child.

Case II.—Female child, two and one-half years old. Always healthy and well until two days before being seen. Symptoms: loss of appetite, some nausea and vomiting, restless at nights, cough and abdominal pain. Examination of heart and lungs negative, but on the posterior wall of the pharynx was "a collection of mucus, and the tonsils were enlarged." Treatment of this condition availed nothing. Two days after the patient was seen with constant cough, temperature 103°, pulse 120, "restless and uneasy." Again a careful examination failed to reveal anything of importance. For three days more the child remained in about the same condition, "despite all my treatment," when on having a movement of the bowels a large peach stone passed in the stool, with a cessation of all bad symptoms.

Case III.—Female child, four years old. Two days before being seen the patient had developed some bad symptoms, prominent among which was cough. She was "anæmic, digestion poor, tongue coated, restless at night." There was no febrile movement. "Thinking I discovered evidences of periodicity in the attacks of coughing I ordered quinia and an anodyne cough mixture." At the end of two weeks there had been no material change. Another examination suggested the possibility of worms in the intestinal canal, and santonin and calomel were given. These had the effect of dislodging an "enormous quantity" of worms, and with their escape the bad symptoms vanished and did not return.

Case IV.—Female child, six years old. Never had been considered a healthy and robust child. "As a baby the patient was subject to attacks of indigestion." During the preceding summer she had been seen by Dr. Smith. The patient then had some peculiar attacks characterized by "pain in the abdomen, distension and diarrhœa, and violent cough and sometimes vomiting." In November she was first seen. For three months before there had been almost constant cough, loss of flesh and appetite, night sweats, pains in the chest, etc. The cough was unaccompanied by expectoration. An examination failed to reveal anything of note. "Treatment availed but little." Two weeks after she came under his care she passed spontaneously several sections of tape-worm. Appropriate treatment was instituted, and the expulsion of the worm was followed by complete cessation of all her disturbances.

Case V.—A woman 25 years old. The patient was first seen in September, 1875. She had had a cough for a month while in the country. Consulted the Doctor immediately on her return. She had been troubled with malarial symptoms the year before, and finding on examination no disease of heart, lungs or throat, he thought this cough might be malarial in its origin. In a month there was no improvement and there were added to the cough these other symptoms: loss of appetite, of flesh and strength, disturbance of digestion, anæmia, headache, and on the left side especially there was thoracic pain. By Nov. 1, all the symptoms were progressing except the cough, which remained "about the same." There was no expectoration. "She had lost since the middle of August about sixteen pounds." Another careful examination of every organ of the body failed to discover the cause of these bad and advancing symptoms. The next day she passed some segments of a tape-worm and treatment therefore with tonics, etc., was followed by such marked improvement that in two months more she had regained all that she had lost. Dr. Smith remarks in connection with this case that he could not feel convinced that the parasite was the cause of the trouble until he saw the rapid and marked improvement following its removal.

Case VI.—The patient was a woman in whom a cough seemed to take the place of that peculiar condition known as the "vomiting of pregnancy." Instead of having this latter she developed a cough which lasted through two and a half months of her pregnancy and then ceased. This had been noted in two pregnancies, which were all she had had at the date of the observation.

Case VII.—Female child, three and a half years old. The patient was attacked in the early morning with what was supposed to be "croup" by the mother, who knowing the effect that an emetic sometimes produces in this disease administered a teaspoonful of the syrup of ipecac. Prompt emesis followed but the "croupy cough" was seen to depend on the presence of undigested material in the stomach of the child—at least the emetic dislodged a mass of food and among the rest a quantity of meat eaten thirteen hours before, but not a particle digested, and the cough ceased.

Case VIII.—A man forty-five years old, of rather a nervous temperament; a good liver. He had been subject to asthmatic attacks for twenty years. He had a small growth on his back "situated about two inches to the right of the spinous process of the second dorsal vertebra." It was about the size of a split pea, and was not painful to the touch. It was not a neuroma. Scratching this would cause him to cough and to suffer from dyspnœa. This condition could be brought about at any time by stroking or rubbing the growth. The physical signs present on auscultation and percussion of the chest did not change during the time the cough was being forced upon him.

Case IX.—A young woman 19 years old, suffering with "a retroverted uterus and spinal anæmia with all its accompaniments." Electricity was one of the agents used for her relief, and it was noticeable that when one pole was placed on the cervical spine and the other was passed on either side of the spinous processes of the last dorsal and first two lumbar vertebræ she would cough, faintly at first, "but violently if the application were continued." This phenomenon occurred regardless of the kind of current used, but did not happen if either were applied elsewhere than at the points mentioned.

Case X.—A woman, 36 years old, mother of one child. The patient had had a cough for over a year, the cause of which an examination of the chest and throat failed to discover. For three months she was under treatment and though her general condition improved the cough persisted. At the end of this time she made an unusual muscular effort and completely or nearly retroverted her uterus. Her cough at this time is described as being "almost continuously paroxysmal." She also said that at the time of the menstrual flow the cough was aggravated. "An Albert Smith pessary was introduced in a few days, with the effect of . . . entirely curing the cough."

Case XI.—Female child, seventeen months old. After two days of restlessness, loss of appetite, etc., the patient began to cough. There was some febrile movement. She was seen on the morning of the third day by Dr. Smith who, on examining the throat and thoracic viscera, failed to account for the cough. An examination of the gums showed them to be much swollen and "very tender over the upper canines." They were freely lanced and the relief "seemed to be immediate." In a few weeks Dr. Smith was again called to see the child, which presented the same symptoms; this time an examination revealed a similar condition of the *lower* canines, and again an incision relieved the child of the cough.

An analysis of these cases shows that in over fifty per cent. the cause of the reflex cough was at some part of the alimentary tract. The large number of children affected, some with a rise of temperature, and the difficulty which all recognize of examining these little patients satisfactorily, might easily lead some less careful diagnosticians to find cases of pneumonia where a cherry-pit or a tape-worm was in fact the cause of the trouble.

My own case is as follows: The patient, Mrs. L., mother of two children, the youngest still at the breast, was accustomed, in order to increase the flow of milk, to drink two bottles of porter daily, and from a pint to a quart of milk. She had done this when her first child was a nursling and had experienced nothing except benefit. One night during the latter part of April, 1886, she began to cough violently and in paroxysms. The cough was dry and harsh but not "croupy." In spite of chloral, the bromides, etc., she kept cough-ing at irregular intervals for nearly twelve hours, when there was a complete cessation for an hour or more. Her temperature was normal. Physical examination of the chest and throat disclosed nothing. She was cheerful and bright and joked considerably about her condition. During the afternoon the cough began again, and with the excep-tion of the times during which she was stupid from the effect of narcotics, it raged with redoubled fury for the next six or eight hours. During the morning of the second day there was a little rest, but it was only momentary. The paroxysms came on and lasted from four to six hours in spite of anodynes freely administered, spraying the throat, blistering the chest, and doing every-thing that reason or fancy could suggest. Finally, having on the fourth or fifth day exhausted my materia medica, I decided to attack the complaint in another way, and administered a scruple of sulphate of zinc in lukewarm water, and followed it with a half ounce of the syrup of ipecac. I had a rather vague idea that the revulsion which would follow the emesis might have some effect on the cough. After rather longer than usual emesis began, and the stomach ejected mass after mass of coagulated casein. Some of the pieces were several inches in extent and had to be pulled forcibly from the mouth and pharynx to prevent choking. The cough immediately lessened. The patient slept some without hypnotics. The milk and porter were prohibited, and a full dose of pepsin administered, and afterward a brisk cathartic. The patient coughed no more after this except at long intervals, when she would "bark" a little; but practically the cure was complete.

I have no doubt that the cough was pro-duced by the irritation which the undigested casein produced on the gastric filaments of the pneugastric. I do not think the "reflex" cough can be invariably distinguished by its characteristics. Dr. Smith, in the article I have referred to, does not think so. Dr. Thomsen says that is always non-expectorant, and that the sound is always single. It is a question with me whether or not after a variable time the reflex cough may not be so irritant as to set up a pharyngitis and bron-chitis with their accompaniments.

—The *Bulletin Médical*, February 27, states that Mlle. Cattani is about to be named *privat-docent* in general pathology in the Faculty of Medicine of the University of Turin.

SECRETION OF MILK FOLLOWING OVARIOTOMY.

BY CHARLES B. PENROSE, PH.D., M.D.,
PHILADELPHIA.

The appearance of the milk secretion following ovariotomy is a rare phenomenon, and one of which I have found no mention in medical literature. It is doubtless a reflex disturbance similar to other well-recognized reflex mammary symptoms, such as pain and swelling, which often accom-pany diseased conditions of the reproductive organs in women.

The two following cases which have occurred in my experience are of interest in this connection.

Case I.—The patient, M. C., had had four children, but had not been pregnant for seven years. She was operated on for extra-uterine pregnancy, of about ten weeks duration, in February, 1888. The fœtal sac, which was on the left side, was removed along with the ruptured left tube and the ovary. The right appendages, which were diseased, were also removed. Convales-cence was slow. Eleven weeks after the operation both breasts became large and painful; the areolæ became dark and swollen; and the secretion of milk appeared, at times so abundantly that it was necessary to milk the breasts in order to obtain relief from pain. This secretion continued with-out interruption for eight months. Its first appearance corresponded to what would have been about the fifth month of pregnancy if the course of fœtal development had not been interrupted. The woman insisted that she was pregnant for several months after the opera-tion, not only on account of the mammary changes, but also because she recognized other signs, such as morning sickness, which she had had in previous pregnancies. At no time after the operation did she suffer with pelvic pain or any uterine disturbance.

Case II.—The patient, B. S., has never been pregnant. The uterine appendages were removed in December 1888 for left ovarian cyst and double salpingitis. While recovering from anæsthesia she withdrew the glass drainage tube from her abdomen during the inattention of the nurse. The tube was not replaced. Convalescence was uninterrupted. Three days after the opera-tion the breasts became large and painful, and an abundant secretion of milk appeared in them. The patient got up in eighteen days; the secretion of milk, however, con-tinued for two months after the operation.

She has not suffered since the operation with any uterine disturbance. In both the cases reported the milk presented the appearance of the same secretion in a woman at full term.

In the first case it seems possible that the secretion of milk may have been connected with the pregnant state: the cycle of mammary changes continuing, even after the product of conception had ceased to exist. This view is strengthened by the fact that the milk appeared about the same time as in her previous pregnancies, that is, at about the fifth month; and also by the fact that other signs of pregnancy continued to be present for several months after the operation.

In the second case, however, the mammary secretion immediately followed an operation in a non-pregnant woman, and must have been a reflex manifestation caused by the operative interference with the nerve relations of the reproductive organs.

1331 Spruce St.

WIRING THE FRAGMENTS IN SIMPLE FRACTURES OF THE LOWER EXTREMITIES.

BY CLAUDE A. DUNDORE, M.D.,
ASHLAND, PA.

ASSISTANT SURGEON STATE HOSPITAL FOR INJURED PERSONS OF THE ANTHRACITE COAL REGIONS OF PENNSYLVANIA.

The subject of wiring in treatment of fractures has been pretty freely debated during late years, and there has been a great deal said against it; but I think its value has been greatly underrated, especially in fractures of the lower extremities. I think there can be no reasonable doubt that in compound fractures of the leg the fragments should be immediately wired, when there is the slightest tendency toward displacement. It decreases the danger which is always present in compound fractures, by giving support to the leg and holding the fragments in good apposition, and in this way causes bony union to take place in a much shorter space of time than when such fractures are treated in the ordinary way.

Every surgeon has seen cases of compound fractures of the leg, which were difficult of reduction and in which the fragments were very often displaced, and consequently had to be brought into apposition again just as often. Now this causes a high degree of inflammation, and a tendency to suppuration if the most thorough antiseptic treat-ment is not followed, and often even when all antiseptic precautions have been taken. The operation of wiring the fragments obviates these difficulties, and, if it is done carefully, the above mentioned unpleasant symptoms are almost certainly avoided. The inflammation generally abates very rapidly and there is little or no suppuration, if perfect antiseptic treatment is carried out.

But what I particularly desire to advance in this communication is the advisability of cutting down to the fragments in simple fractures of the leg and wiring them. Of course, in fractures in which there is little or no displacement, or when reduction is not difficult, this measure is uncalled for; but there are many cases in which reduction is difficult or impossible, and the number of crippled limbs is the best evidence of it. The fragments are often of such a shape that it is impossible to bring them into apposition or to be able to ascertain what causes the displacement, without laying the seat of fracture open to view. If we do bring the fragments into good apposition we are often at a loss to keep them so, for the ordinary treatment does not prevent displacement. By cutting down to the seat of fracture we are enabled to see exactly what we are about, and after wiring the fragments there can be no displacement.

Dr. Biddle, of the Anthracite Hospital, is an advocate of this method, and the results we have had are the best proofs of its efficacy.

We have a case in the building at present in which Dr. Biddle wired the fragments four weeks ago, and the patient now has a plaster dressing on the leg, and puts his entire weight upon it.

This method is the only one which gives us satisfactory results in fractures of the patella, for there are no other means by which we can get good apposition of the fragments and bony union. All other appliances give us evil results too often for us to adopt them. In cases of fracture of the patella Dr. Biddle cuts down and wires the fragments, dresses the incision antiseptically, and places the limb on the ordinary straight splint with the heel elevated. By the time the first dressing is removed the incision has healed by first intention and we have a simple fracture for treatment, in which we have good apposition.

—The American Association for the Advancement of Science will meet in Toronto, August 27 to September 3.

SOCIETY REPORTS.

PHILADELPHIA COUNTY MEDICAL SOCIETY.

Stated Meeting, February 13, 1889.

The President, W. W. KEEN, M.D., in the chair.

DR. JOSEPH PRICE read a paper on

Gonorrhœal Diseases of the Uterine Appendages.

The attitude of numbers of professional men who express either incredulity or absolute disbelief in the causative relation between gonorrhœal disease in women and pyosalpinx and abscess of the ovary, is sufficient justification for a still further discussion of this subject. My views upon the matter are based neither upon theory nor upon microscopic examination. They are from surgical experience only, or from confessions of men whose wives have been diseased by them. From the time that Noeggerath first formulated his belief upon this subject it has been smiled at, contradicted, or controverted, but never in its essentials disproven. In his earlier paper, Noeggerath fell into the common error of enthusiasts, that of attributing too much to his discovery. This, without doubt, led many otherwise fair-minded men to pass over his paper as unworthy of attention, thus impeding the progress that otherwise would have followed its discussion and the observations based upon its claims. In taking up most later surgical works we find the etiology of ovarian and tubal disease considered from this standpoint omitted—a missing link—or differentiated out of sight. This is wrong. As early as 1877, Mr. Lawson Tait and others insisted upon the relation existing between gonorrhœa in man and tubal disease in women. Noeggerath antedated him about five years. Mr. Tait also insisted on its causative relation to perimetritis, this as late as 1883. Schroeder, in the early editions of his *Gynecology*, insisted upon gonorrhœa as bearing a causative relation to ovarian and tubal troubles. In the very latest edition he says: "Gonorrhœa, in the highest degree, appears as a causative disease in women." Sänger also is an ardent advocate of the same belief. He is wrong, however, I am persuaded, in holding that the gonorrhœal infection is always late in revealing its presence in the woman when transmitted by the man. To this subject I shall refer later.

Without further collation of authorities upon this subject, I shall proceed briefly to its discussion. Whether or not the presence of the disease can be diagnosticated absolutely by the presence of the gonococcus of Neisser, is of small importance, if by the chain of common evidence we can connect the presence of one disease with the other in their sequence. If, on discovering tubal disease in a woman who has never aborted nor had any of the diseases incident to childbed, who has been healthy up to a time when vaginitis has occurred, contracted from her husband, after which the woman from time to time experiences increasing pelvic pain, losing strength and weight—the case, it seems to me, is made out, save as quibbling may dispute it. This history occurs in most of the cases I have handled. Of the many cases that have come under my observation, I choose the following as illustrative and typical:

A young married woman, one child. Her recovery from childbed excellent: no gonorrhœal infection of the child at birth. Some months afterward the patient had inflammation of the vulvo-vaginal glands, with suppuration. Later she appeared with the abdomen tense and painful, enlarged tubes and ovaries, tender and painful on the slightest movement or pressure; she had lost in weight and strength. Her husband confessed to the infection of his wife. The diagnosis was made of gonorrhœal pyosalpinx, and operation proved the correctness of the opinion. Both tubes contained pus, were cheesy and friable—the ligatures cutting through all but the vessels. The abdomen was full of fluid, and the intestines gave evidence of acute peritonitis.

The history here is complete, leaving no possible doubt as to the origin of the disease. The early infection here exhibited is at variance with the views of Sänger, and shows that his statements are not necessarily correct, or are accidentally correct, if at all so. There is no sufficient reason why this infection should not be early. I incline to the belief that the disease originates early, but may be slow in its progress, and thus escape attention and discovery.

DR. J. WILLIAM WHITE, in opening the discussion, said : I had not intended to take part in the discussion, but as you have kindly asked me, Mr. President, I will say that neither the paper read this evening, nor anything else that I have heard or read, has convinced me of the frequent relation between tubal disease in women and gonorrhœa in men. I believe that such cases as

Dr. Price details are defective in some important point. They assert that the occurrence of suppurative disease of the tubes is a consequence of preëxisting disease in the husband, or of the individual with whom the woman has had connection. It seems to me that by a similar process we could demonstrate the relation between gonorrhœa in the male and mitral disease, cataract, or other ailment in the woman. This is another instance of the *post hoc ergo propter hoc* line of argument. It is carrying a theory, which has an undoubted basis in fact, to great extremes, and, as regards the views of Noeggerath, to ridiculous extremes. His sweeping assertions in regard to the persistence of latent gonorrhœa in the male, and his theory that women having connection with men who had ever had gonorrhœa, are constantly rendered barren, or if they do conceive do so only to abort, and that such women are the constant subjects of ovarian and tubal disease, are, I believe, contradicted by the practical experience of every surgeon and of every general practitioner.

I have had rather exceptional opportunities for examining cases of gonorrhœa in the male. Many of these patients have married, and the majority of them had, and still have, healthy wives and healthy children. While there is undoubtedly some foundation of truth in regard to this matter, and while there are undoubted instances of this form of infection, and while gonorrhœa in the male may produce vaginitis, cervicitis, endocervicitis, and pyosalpinx, yet it seems to me that these occurrences are exceptional, by no means so frequent as is claimed, and certainly not the rule. Dr. Price does not assert his belief in these views, but I am surprised at the favorable tone of his comments upon them. I have always regarded the theories of Noeggerath as examples of the extremities to which an enthusiast may be led, and only to be fitly characterized by the somewhat strong terms of absurd and ridiculous. Certainly in my personal experience I have never seen anything to warrant a belief in the relation of these two conditions, as cause and effect, in any very large proportion of cases.

The pathological side of the subject, to which Dr. Price merely alludes, is, after all, the one of greatest importance. If gonorrhœa in man is, as Noeggerath describes it, latent in a majority of cases, it must be that it depends on a peculiar microörganism, and the invariable association of the gonococcus, or some other low form of animal life, with gonorrhœa, must be demonstrated.

In this "latent" gonorrhœa, described by him, there may be no symptoms, and nothing which would enable the practical specialist in venereal diseases to recognize the presence of the affection. There must then be demonstrated at least that some microbe is present which belongs to gonorrhœa and produces the disease whenever it develops in the urethra. In order to demonstrate the relation between latent gonorrhœa and these diseases of the tubes and ovaries, some such microörganism should also be found in these latter cases. I believe that in certain persons the nidus for the multiplication of the organism is exceptionally favorable. In such cases it rapidly multiplies and tends to spread, and increases the severity of the disease. These are the cases, I doubt not, in which tubal disease follows infection. That it is frequent, or that there is demonstrated any invariable relation between the existence of the microörganism and such diseases in women, I do not believe has been proven. The clinical relation of the two conditions being, therefore, to my mind at least, not established, and the pathological evidence being entirely wanting, I am compelled to reject as unproven and unfounded the theories which so closely associate an antecedent gonorrhœa in the man with so many forms of disease of the uterine appendages. I believe those theories to have been harmful in their influence upon gynæcological practice in having given apparent justification to a large number of operations, a fair proportion of which I do not doubt will be shown within the next ten years to have been unnecessary and injudicious.

DR. WILLIAM S. STEWART: I am much interested in this subject, which is so much agitated at the present day. I am interested in the fact that so many tubes and ovaries are being removed. It seems to me an alarming thing that at the present time this should be the prevailing disease of women. I think, therefore, that it is a matter of great importance that we should come to some pathological determination as to the nature of the contagion of this disease, and whether its prevalence is due entirely to gonorrhœal infection, or to other causes.

I have had some little experience recently in exploring the tubes. I was anxious that some of the specialists who make removal of the tubes and ovaries an every-day matter, should have witnessed the treatment of a case. I succeeded in passing an aluminium applicator through the diseased tube, and in permitting the escape of the pus which the tube contained, and the patient, who I feared was going to die, recovered. The diminution of the enlarged tube was a matter of great satisfaction to me, as I feared that my previous treatment of the case had been the cause of the development of the disease..

I have passed the probe into the tubes in two other instances, and the results which followed—diminution of the inflammation and liberating the pus—have been a matter of great gratification as well as surprise.

DR. HOFFMANN: Dr. White's remarks show how two persons interested in the same subject may arrive at entirely opposite conclusions. Dr. White has had abundant experience in dealing with these cases, especially in the almshouse, in a class of people where he would be supposed to see the relation between gonorrhœa in the male and certain diseases of the female, especially in the uterine appendages. He, however, fails to connect the two in any marked degree. Bernutz has written a very remarkable work, appearing in the New Sydenham Society publications a few years ago, and the conclusions which he reaches are diametrically opposed to those of Dr. White. Bernutz, in examining 99 cases of pelvic peritonitis in women, concluded that 28 were distinctly attributable to gonorrhœa; 43 were traced to childbirth, and 8 of the childbirths were abortions. If you take away the 43 cases, due probably to infection from some incidental cause, we have remaining 56 cases, of which 28, or 50 per cent., were traced not only theoretically, but by a post-mortem examination, to gonorrhœa, all other causes being eliminated. Taking his statistics of the 28 cases which he considered analogous to orchitis in the male, we have 20 menstrual and 8 traumatic. The causes of traumatism were, in 3, venereal excesses; 2, syphilis of the cervix; 2, the introduction of the sound; and 1, the use of the cold douche during menstruation.

I have myself seen this condition so frequently that I cannot regard it as an unusual accident, and all the less after reading the remarkable record of which I have here a note, can I think that it is accidental. So far as Noeggerath's views are concerned, I think that Dr. Price sounded their value. His views are extreme, and we may as well, now as ever, regard them as extreme. There is no use in laying down the principle that only one cause can produce the disease. The original paper of Bernutz, published in 1857, antedating the publication of Noeggerath, is to me convincing.

Whether or not we always find the gono-coccus of Neisser is to me a question of indifference, and not always decisive. We know very well that one microbe will, by its presence, crowd out another. When we open the abdomen and find the tubes filled with stinking ˜pus, in which putrefactive changes have taken place, I am not surprised that the gonococcus is not found, its place being taken by some other form of micrococcus. In such cases I do not believe that the gonococcus is diagnostic.

·DR. WHITE: The statistics of Bernutz and Goupil, to which reference has just been made are quite familiar to me, although it was my impression that they were published in 1861, not 1857. This is quite a different question from the one I was discussing. These were prostitutes of the lowest class undoubtedly infected with gonorrhœa. The proportion of these cases in which pelvic peritonitis occurs is considerable. This is entirely distinct from the cases in which the history of a previous and often a long distant gonorrhœa in the husband is depended upon to explain ovarian and tubal disease in the woman, but in which there is no consecutive history of true gonorrhœal infection of the woman. It is to this that I object, not to the assertion that pelvic peritonitis and pyosalpinx *may* occur in some cases of gonorrhœa, especially in women of the lower classes. Dr. Hoffmann has missed the point of my remarks. I have quoted the statistics of Bernutz in a paper which has been accepted by the *British Medical Journal*, although not yet published. They simply present the records of two of the French hospitals to which the lowest class of French prostitutes are admitted, women broken down in health, and the subjects of virulent forms of gonorrhœa. This is entirely distinct from the proposition of Noeggerath, which connects not only existing disease in the man, but also precedent disease of which all active symptoms may have disappeared, with certain conditions of the woman—barrenness, tendency to abortion, and disease of the uterus and appendages. It is to that I object, and not to the assertion that in a large proportion of cases these complications occur in prostitutes with well-marked gonorrhœal infection.

DR. M. PRICE: In regard to the statement of Dr. White that these diseases are more peculiarly connected with these hospitals and these women of low character, I would say that all the cases that I have had in private practice, six or eight in number, have been not only of the better class, but among the best women of this town. The specimens from one of these cases I should like to show to the Society. This pair of tubes is unquestionably gonorrhœal. I treated the man some ten years ago. I afterward treated his wife for old-fashioned cellulitis and peritonitis. She has had five attacks during the last eight years, in every one of which there was high temperature and quick pulse, with the pelvis filled with inflammatory masses. These inflammatory conditions were cured about as the electrician cures pelvic abscess and pyosalpinx. The health and vigor of the woman were sufficient to cause absorption of the liquid portion of the pus, and for a time the disease was kept in abeyance. Four or five days ago I removed from this woman's pelvis a pint of pus of the most offensive character. This was her last struggle, her last effort to get rid of it. She was unequal to the task, and was slowly dying of a septic condition. The symptoms were of such an urgent character, that I opened the abdomen and removed both tubes. There we have a marked case of pyosalpinx unquestionably of gonorrhœal origin. Out of the eight or nine cases of pelvic trouble, I have had occasion to operate on, in all but one I could distinctly trace a gonorrhœal origin. In every one I had treated the man for gonorrhœa. From that day not one of these women bore a child. They always complained of symptoms of pelvic trouble, pain on pressure, pain on movement, and pain on slipping or jarring. The trouble in these cases was just as certainly gonorrhœal in origin as that any trouble existed.

The cases that Dr. Hoffmann has referred to as occurring after labor, have, I believe, in many instances a positive gonorrhœal origin. I recall one case of abortion where there was for a year previous unquestionable evidences of tubal trouble on one side. The abortion was followed by acute tubal inflammation, sepsis, and death. An attempt was made to relieve her, but it was too late. My impression is that a perfectly healthy woman, who has never been inoculated with gonorrhœal poison, is very slow to take on pelvic inflammatory trouble. It probably does exist, but there is usually a poison which has produced the condition, which these other incidental accidents aid and help.

Dr. White: I should like to ask Dr. Price what symptoms of gonorrhœa these women presented in addition to those which he has mentioned. To my mind, the argument, as I said before, seems to be entirely of the *post hoc ergo propter hoc* style, and it would apply just as well to a series of cases of goitre. It would not be difficult in a large number of these cases occurring in the best society, to demonstrate that ten years previously their husbands had gonorrhœa, but it is evident that in both series of cases there would be a missing link in the chain of evidence.

Dr. Price: A man comes to me stating that he is in trouble, and that he fears that his wife has been inoculated. I treat the husband for unquestioned gonorrhœa. In the course of ten days or two weeks, I treat the wife for unquestioned gonorrhœa. I think that is sufficient evidence as to the cause. I do not see any relevancy in the reference to goitre or heart disease. We know why these come in some instances. It is as plain to me as the nose on Dr. White's face that these conditions come from gonorrhœa, and from no other cause.

Dr. James Collins: I wish to ask one question. I have seen something of practice in my life, and I should like to hear something said with reference to the proportion of cases in which this trouble occurs. Taking the cases of gonorrhœa in men, I should like to know in what proportion of cases these sequelæ occur?

Dr. Hoffmann: I do not wish to cross fire; but it seems to me that as Dr. White has suggested that I have missed the point of his remarks, I might say that he has missed the point of what I said. I do not absolutely accept Noeggerath's views, which I consider extreme. I do not believe that a man who has once had gonorrhœa and has been completely cured, will necessarily transmit the disease. Dr. Price did not advocate that view. The only question is this: whether or not in the absence of any other proven cause, such as abortion, exposure to cold, the introduction of the sound, or the like, and gonorrhœal infection proven, the disease may be caused by the gonorrhœa? I think that when that is proven by experience with low-grade prostitutes with the same anatomy and physiology as the high-born ladies, we may apply our experience with the former to the latter. The whole thing is, therefore, narrowed down to this: whether or not we are justified by the exclusion of all other causes in saying that gonorrhœa is the cause. This brings us to a rational consideration of the question, and not the extreme views suggested by Noeggerath. The trouble is that in considering these matters men are apt to go to extremes, and to say that one condition or another is the invariable cause of the disease. I have seen tubal disease come from all the causes enumerated by Bernutz. The treatment of the disease must of course modify the condition as propagated from one sex to the other.

DR. J. M. BALDY: The views of Noeggerath, Burnutz, Sinclair, and others, including the author of the paper of to-night, are very extreme, and grossly misrepresent the facts. Venereal disorders in man are not so frequently the cause of pelvic inflammatory diseases in women as these men would have us believe. I think with Dr. White, that in order to settle this question, we must have more than mere clinical evidence; we must also have pathological research and experimentation. So far as the clinical aspect of these cases is concerned, I may say that the vast majority of them coming under my observation are not women who have never been pregnant. There is almost always a history of abortion or labor, with septic trouble at that time. Sinclair has demonstrated that most of these patients have the gonococcus present in the secretions of the vagina and uterus, and for that reason he has considered the disease to be of specific origin; in some cases where the gonococcus was not found he still believed the disease to be of specific origin, supposing that the gonococcus had been crowded out by other forms of micrococci.

The question arises whether the gonococcus causes gonorrhœa. I think that it has been positively settled by the experiments of Sternberg that the gonococcus is not the cause of gonorrhœa, and that it may exist in other discharges. He made pure cultures of the gonococcus and inoculated the eyes of animals with negative results. The vaginæ of animals were inoculated with these cultures, with the same result. He then secured three hospital patients who were under observation in bed, and inoculated the urethras of these men with the pure culture of gonococcus. The results were absolutely negative. The only observations opposed to this are those of Bokard, made at Buda Pest. He submitted the urethras of half a dozen medical students to experimentation. At the end of a week three of the students were found to have well-marked gonorrhœa. At first sight these experiments seem as conclusive as Sternberg's; but when we recall the fact, that these patients were medical students, and had a week's liberty before and after inoculation, in a city with the moral tone of Buda Pest, the experiment is absolutely worthless.

Sternberg found a microörganism in urine which had undergone alkaline decomposition so like the gonococcus that the two could not be differentiated. He has also found it in the pus taken directly from a whitlow. I think that in view of these observations, we can consider that it is proven conclusively, that the gonococcus is not the cause of gonorrhœa, and therefore whether the gonococcus is present or not, it makes little difference; its presence is not proof that the condition is due to gonorrhœa. In accepting this view we can plainly see that the conclusions drawn by Martin, Sänger, and other Germans, from the presence of gonococcus, are erroneous.

In regard to cases of chronic gonorrhœa or gleet, where, following gonorrhœa, there has been a stricture for years, with a little discharge, either mucous or pus, observed in the morning: such cases will no more cause gonorrhœa than will the gonococcus. Up to the present time no experiments have been made on this subject. I am at present engaged in investigating this matter, but am not yet ready to give the final results, as my observations are not yet completed. I will, however, say this: I have taken the discharge from the cases that I have mentioned, and inoculated the eyes of rabbits, with entirely negative results. Not satisfied with taking these discharges, when the urethra was in a quiescent state, I have irritated the parts by the passage of sounds two sizes larger than the men had been accustomed to use, and the next morning inoculated the eyes of rabbits, but still with negative results. Then fearing the criticism that Sternberg did, that possibly animals were not susceptible to this infection, I secured a man and inoculated his urethra with this discharge, and so far with just as absolutely negative results. If we prove that these cases of gleet and chronic gonorrhœa will not cause gonorrhœa, that the gonococcus will not cause gonorrhœa, and that the gonococcus is found in other discharges as well, we come down simply to the acute cases of clap as the cause of these pelvic inflammatory diseases in women. This is exactly where we stand. That a man with acute gonorrhœa will inoculate a woman is beyond peradventure true; and that the inflammation so set up will travel along the mucous membrane of the vagina, uterus, and Fallopian tubes, causing pelvic inflammatory trouble, is beyond cavil. That we can prove more than this I think is impossible. Pathological research and experimental investigation are against it. There remains nothing but the clinical facts. And here again we have illustrated how two different minds will approach a subject from the same standpoint, and yet draw different conclusions. In many of the cases in which I have seen Dr. Price draw the conclusion that the trouble was due to gonorrhœa, I could find no proof of that fact to satisfy my own mind. To me the history of gonorrhœa was most eminently unsatisfactory, while the history of puerperal septic infection, which he chose to ignore altogether, was perfectly plain and clear. I think that in many of these cases of pelvic inflammatory trouble, the origin is of a septic character, puerperal, or from dirty instruments. I should say that three-fifths of the cases that have come under my observation, were of septic origin, and that one-fifth was of gonorrhœal origin, leaving one-fifth for all the other causes.

DR. GEORGE STRAWBRIDGE: Are we to understand that the inoculation of mucous membranes with gonorrhœal pus is negative?

DR. BALDY: No, sir. I refer to the discharge from gleet, where the discharge has been present for years. Such discharges produce no effect when inoculated.

DR. STRAWBRIDGE: Some of the worst cases of conjunctivitis that I have seen have been due to the inoculation from chronic gleet. In some of these cases the entire eyeball has been destroyed in the course of forty-eight hours. In these cases the acute attack had passed over one or two months before. I have seen dozens of such cases in my own practice. I am quite amazed that the gentleman could use this pus without trouble following.

DR. WHITE: I think that Dr. Baldy and Dr. Strawbridge are talking about different conditions. I have never seen gonorrhœal conjunctivitis from gleet. The cases seen by Dr. Strawbridge have been in the later stages of acute gonorrhœa. He speaks of one or two months. Gonorrhœa will often retain its infective properties for that length of time. Gleets, depending as they commonly do on strictures of large calibre and on catarrhal conditions of the mucous membrane, are attended by discharges largely mucoid in character, only under exceptional circumstances mucopurulent, and are not contagious except in rare instances. A creamy or milky discharge is apt to be infectious, while a mucoid discharge is, as a rule, innocuous.

DR. ARTHUR V. MEIGS: I wish to say a few words bearing upon the purely pathological side of the question. As yet I have only made a thorough examination of two specimens, and these were given me by Dr. Penrose. In neither was there what could properly be termed pyosalpinx. In one there was no trace of pus, but extensive inflammation and thickening of both tube and ovary, with adhesion of the tube to the ovary. In the other specimen there was a pocket of pus extending from the fimbriated extremity of the tube, its other attachment having been broken in the removal. There was, however, no pus within the tube, but as in the other case thickening, inflammation and adhesions. I think that it is still an open question whether or no nature could remove such a degree of inflammation as was present in the first specimen, though there is every reason to believe that nothing but operation could have removed the adhesions.

DR. PRICE: I am not surprised that Dr. Strawbridge is amazed at Dr. Baldy's remarks. At the present time we are in possession of sufficient clinical evidence to prove what Dr. Strawbridge has said in regard to the causal relation between gonorrhœa and gonorrhœal ophthalmia. Years ago Dr. Agnew said that he dreaded to see a case of chronic gleet of two weeks' or two years' standing come to his office; and it is just these cases that can destroy the eye. The records of eye hospitals abundantly prove this.

We now care nothing, or next to nothing, about what Noeggerath wrote, for we possess sufficient clinical material in our own surgical experience to prove that gonorrhœa, and nothing but gonorrhœa, is responsible, except in rare instances, for the pathological conditions with which we surgically daily deal. Dr. Deaver and Dr. White have proven this in their own daily experience by sections for pus tubes due to gonorrhœa.

Dr. Baldy has alluded to my cases, but he heard only the history of the patient in front of him; but in every case, I subsequently obtained the history of gonorrhœa and stricture from the husband. The question of the influence of gonorrhœa in the production of pelvic diseases in women is one not necessarily dogmatic nor mathematical, but involving probabilities. As to the influence of this disease in producing a serious train of sequelæ in men, there seems to be no dispute; why there should be such a disparity between cause and effect with only sex to influence the condition, is a question that I do not believe the sceptics will attempt to explain. I have certainly no explanation for gratuitous disposition.

In the class of patients met at the almshouse, among the men there is no question as to the great prevalence of gonorrhœa. Among the women it exists about as often. In his description of a case, in the MEDICAL AND SURGICAL REPORTER, December 15, 1888, Dr. White says: "Two small patches of ulceration existed on the floor of the membranous urethra, each measuring about two lines in diameter." This case may be taken as a type of the many cases of which no microscopical examination can be made, or at least is made. Further on in this same paper, a troublesome case of gleet is noticed, having existed for several years. That the presence of gleet is a real source of infection is no longer doubted. Why then dispute that an existing cause of trouble must stop short and lose its virulence as soon as it touches the female organs? Among the complications of gonorrhœa in men, noted and admitted by good authorities, are peritonitis, subperitoneal abscess, perinephritic abscess, together with the only too frequent lesions of the bladder, prostate, and kidneys. Now, if peritonitis can occur with gonorrhœal origin through the roundabout road of the vasæ deferentes and seminal vesicles, how much more likely is it to occur in women by the direct route from the vagina, through the uterus and Fallopian tubes to the peritoneal cavity? Sinclair, in his little book, faulty and full of short-comings as it is, proves without doubt that most of the cases of pelvic peritonitis attributed by him to gonorrhœa are rightly so ascribed. Out of fourteen cases cited, in three the diagnosis is not proven and may be regarded as doubtful. It is the danger of every enthusiast to see too much in his theory. This was the cause of the slow reception of the theory advanced by Noeggerath. Noeggerath's view is not a new one; it is only the wide application that causes it to differ from opinions held long before. I can readily understand why the profession should be practically ignorant of the ravages of this disease. Nothing short of a rigid special training will enlighten the profession in this field. Again, it is additionally strange that in this age of boasted progress the profession should question the great prevalence of gonorrhœa in women, knowing it to be so very common in men.

Many important investigations have been made by Bumm, Sänger, and Oppenheimer. Donné, in 1844, discovered a parasite in the urethral discharges which he named trichomonas vaginalis. It is folly here to allude to the numerous small beasts that have been found in genital discharges—forerunners of Neisser's gonococcus. The latter presented his researches just at a time when the world was prepared to accept anything in the shape of a small beast. Clinically it is not necessary to determine the presence of the gonococcus to establish the infective virulence of gonorrhœal pus, and this I believe is in accord with the many researches on the subject. Considering it from a pathological and surgical point of view, a clear history of recent impure sexual contact, in the presence of certain well-known clinical features, ignoring the presence or absence of the gonococcus, will be accepted as sufficient evidence of the vice, and responsible for a large number of grave pelvic diseases, a much larger number than puerperal fever or syphilis is responsible for.

I think that I could easily prove my position by using the clinical evidence from my own college mates. I have taken pains to look them up, and investigated their histories, that I might draw some conclusions in that way. I think that I can prove a causal relation in that way, having personal knowledge of their contamination.

REPORTS OF CLINICS.

UNIVERSITY HOSPITAL.

GYNECOLOGICAL CLINIC—PROF. GOODELL.

Case of Oöphorectomy.

The patient was a woman thirty-eight years old who had been married nineteen years, during which time she had had seven children. Three years ago she had a miscarriage, followed by a septic fever keeping her in bed seven weeks; since then she had had pain in both groins, especially in the left, walked with pain, and could not work. Besides she has had a leucorrhœa appearing in gushes, which points to tubal disease.

Dr. Goodell said that the patient had an enlarged left ovary and tube, and as she was in pain all the time, and wholly disabled, he felt justified in operating. He stated further that since he had begun the new departure of performing all the laparotomies in the crowded amphitheatre, there had been over a dozen in all with but a single case of septicemia, and that in a woman with two exceedingly offensive and purulent cysts which were universally adherent.

Making a longer incision than usual on account of the large amount of fat, in the abdominal walls, he cut between the recti muscles. After tearing apart the preperitoneal fat, and after pinching up a fold of peritoneum to feel whether it had omental or intestinal adhesions, he raised it up by two catch-forceps and divided it between them. Upon the right ovary was found a corpus luteum. The Fallopian tube, which was occluded and thickened, was, together with the ovary, divided just above the ligature, which had been applied as near the uterus as possible, by the Tait knot. The left ovary, unlike the right, had adhesions which had to be broken up. It was doubled up under the broad ligament, and had to be unfolded. Dr. Goodell put in a sponge before dividing its attachments so as to collect any blood, and then, after ligating, removed it and the left Fallopian tube, also as close to the uterus as possible. The cavity was syringed out with warm *water* which had been boiled ; and as it came out clear, no drainage tube was introduced.

Dr. Goodell remarked that he used the following method for cleansing sponges: They were washed, taken home and put in running water for a night ; then soaked for twenty-four or forty-eight hours in a solution of washing soda ($\mathfrak{z}$ j to a pound of water) which is better than sulphurous acid, as it does not injure the sponges, although it discolors them. They are then, after being rinsed, put in a five per cent. solution of carbolic acid in water. By this process he is enabled to use them over and over again, and he prefers them to new ones. When a sponge has been used in pus cases, and has become saturated with purulent matter, he does not use it again for abdominal work, but reserves it for cases of cancer of the cervix.

After counting the sponges and instruments which had been used in the operation, the wound was dressed with the iodoform dressing, which he directed should remain on for a week.

The Danger of the Forceps.

The second patient he showed was a woman upon whom he had operated in the amphitheatre three weeks before by his own method, for a bad tear through the recto-vaginal septum. It extended one and a half inches up, leaving her wholly unable to control the sphincter. The patient was ready to leave the Hospital in a week, the operation having proved a success. The tear had followed the use of the forceps, and the reasons why he brought the patient before the class were to show the result of the operation which they had witnessed, and to impress upon them, that as young men who had not attained the requisite skill which long years of practice alone gives,

they should remove the forceps as soon as the perineum is well distended by the head, and should leave the subsequent delivery to nature. For otherwise they would be liable to turn out the head too soon, that is to say, before the parts had become sufficiently dilated. In his experience he had found that fully nine-tenths of all complete tears of the perineum were due to the use, or rather to the misuse, of the forceps.

SURGICAL CLINIC—PROF. D. HAYES AGNEW.

Hip Joint Disease.

The patient which I introduce is a girl four years old, and is a pale delicate child. Sometime back, her mother noticed that she had a very distinct limp when walking, always growing worse toward evening, and less noticeable in the morning after a night's rest. Recently, however, her nights have been passed with much less comfort, her sleep being interrupted by spasmodic starts of the affected limb. In order to examine the joint I shall place the patient on the table, the object being to ascertain the mobility of the articulations. When the affected limb is adducted and abducted the pelvis is seen to move with the leg. When the leg is flexed on the thigh and the thigh upon the abdomen, the same effect on the pelvis is produced, as seen in the raising of the buttock. When similar movements are made on the sound side the pelvis remains unmoved. In this fixedness of the articulation, we see nature's attempt to immobilize the joint, a most suggestive fact to guide the surgeon in the treatment of coxalgia. Pursuing the examination further, I next ask you to look at the change which has taken place in the buttock of the affected side. It has lost its normal rotundity; is lower than its fellow of the opposite side, and passes into the femoral region, with no sharp defining line, in striking contrast with the gluteal mass on the sound side where the boundary between the two is marked by a deep crease. Let the child now stand up and you will observe something peculiar in her attitude. The entire weight of the body is seen to rest on the sound limb, while the diseased limb is advanced, slightly flexed at the knee and somewhat rotated outward. No pain, I believe, is complained of at the knee, though this symptom is often present. The case, therefore, is a plain one, admitting of no uncertain diagnosis. It is a typical instance of coxalgia, or hip disease, in its first stage.

The seat of this form of articular disease is located in a large number of cases in the superior epiphysis of the femur—an epiphysitis, and has a tubercular origin. The treatment consists first in fixation of the joint, in order to lessen the blood supply, and thus combat the inflammatory element of the disease ; and second to relieve the muscles of a very irksome duty, that of immobilizing the articulation—both important antiphlogistic measures. These ends may be accomplished by placing the patient on the back and applying extension to the limb in the way we treat fractures of the thigh ; or, if the child is old enough to use crutches, by placing my modification of Thomas's splint to the posterior part of the pelvis and limb, elevating the sound leg by means of a high shoe, and then allowing the patient to go about on crutches. If the disease is early detected and treatment adopted at once, in many patients it will abort, and they will recover with movable joints.

Where the tuberculous diathesis is pronounced, constitutional treatment should not be neglected—cod liver oil and iodide of iron, nutritious food, and exercise in the open air.

Carcinoma.

Six months ago I removed the breast and axillary glands of this patient, who is forty years old. She comes back to-day with a little nodule on the axillary border of the pectoral muscle. There is no trace of disease elsewhere, the old cicatrix being entirely healthy. In excission of the mammary gland for carcinoma, the axillary glands should always be removed, even when no signs of involvement can be discovered by the touch. Until the axilla is opened it is impossible to form any just appreciation of its contents. Infection may exist in this region, and not be recognized by the eye or the finger. In exposing this little mass of induration, I find it lies in the fiber of the pectoral muscle and appears to be perfectly isolated. I believe in repeating operations on any recurrence of carcinoma, for while we may not succeed in conquering the enemy, we can greatly retard the progress of the disease. The exception to such a course will be in cases where the cachexia has become pronounced.

Chronic Cystitis.

This patient is sixty years old. He looks haggard and worn by suffering. ·He complains of frequent micturition, pain along the course of the urethra, the urine containing a large amount of muco-pus, all of which are signs belonging to inflammation of the bladder. I hope the examination may disclose some cause which will not only explain his trouble, but may at the same time be susceptible of removal. I shall examine for stricture ; no urethral narrowing is found. I next search for stone, and find no evidence of calculus, therefore we may eliminate stricture and stone from the rôle of causation. Possibly there may be an enlarged prostate. His age would naturally suggest such a condition. A finger in the rectum fails to discover any hypertrophy of this body, and consequently we have a case of vesical catarrh. Rich as are the resources of surgery it has no remedy for the cure of vesical catarrh. Much may be done, however, to palliate, and with this object in view, I shall direct that the bladder be washed out every second or third day with a solution of borácic acid (eight grains to the ounce of warm water) using three or four ounces for flushing the organ ; and as an internal diluent and food, the free use of milk. Benefit will be derived from the administration of capsules of balsam copaiba or of sandal wood, especially when the water after standing deposits a gelatinous mass which adheres to the bottom of the vessel. A large number of diluents are at our command in these bladder troubles, as the decoction of triticum repens, of the trailing arbutus, and of uva ursi. Creasote often proves useful in drop doses 3 or 4 times a day. A certain number of cases do well under drainage, by opening the bladder either through the perineum or above the pubes, and keeping the viscus empty with a rubber tube.

COLLEGE OF PHYSICIANS AND SURGEONS—VANDERBILT CLINIC.

SURGICAL CLINIC—PROF. BULL.

Sarcoma of the Skin of the Neck.

Case I.—The patient was a man 45 years old, who presented a superficial indolent ulceration on the right side of the neck just behind the ramus and angle of the jaw. The ulceration was situated on an indurated bluish-red base, and was of an area of about one by two inches. It had existed for five years, beginning as a small yellow pimple, which was cut off in shaving and which afterward scaled over. The scales were picked off from time to time, but were soon replaced by others. The lesion gradually grew in size and became indurated. At no time did it heal, nor did it heal in one place and extend in another. Sometimes it would appear to be smaller than at others, but for the past year there has seemed to be little variation in its size.

The patient had a chancre 22 years ago, followed by alopecia and an eruption on the body, but he gives no other syphilitic symptoms. Examination of the ulcer shows that it involves the skin, cellular tissue, and perhaps even the muscle ; it is not painful, and its hard base is well pronounced.

These forms of chronic ulceration, said Prof. Bull, are usually dependent on some blood dyscrasia ; they may be caused by syphilis, tuberculosis, lupus (which is now held to be a local tuberculosis), a carcinoma or epithelioma breaking down, or a sarcoma breaking down. The history of the present case does not aid much in diagnosis. It is not that of a gumma, which would come as a swelling, then soften and break down as an abscess ; nor is it that of lupus, which usually commences in red spots, not elevated, gradually increasing and coalescing ; and it is not that of epithelioma, which begins as an elevated or warty growth. Besides, in syphilitic ulcerations there is almost always noticed a disposition to heal in certain places and to extend in others, which is very characteristic. The throat, moreover, shows no evidence of cicatrices. Lupus is very rare in this location ; and in carcinoma or epithelioma the ulceration would be more excavated and the edges more elevated. And if of such long duration the lymphatics would most certainly be involved ; but they are not in this case.

The diagnosis therefore rests between syphilis and sarcoma, and is vastly in favor of sarcoma. The patient will, however, be put upon small doses of mercury and large doses of the iodide of potassium to give him the benefit of the doubt. Later a piece of the growth may be removed for microscopic examination ; this should settle the question. Sarcoma of the skin is not a distinct pathological condition, but it has certain special clinical features. It is doubtful if simple removal of this growth will cure the disease. Its antagonism by erysipelas has been too often noted to be merely a coincidence. Erysipelas seems to produce a condition of the tissues which is unfavorable to the growth of the sarcoma, and thus it cures it.

Dr. Bull recalls a case of sarcoma of this form on which two operations were performed in one year ; the wound would heal but, shortly after, the disease would break out afresh in the same spot. He operated for the third time and contemplated a fourth operation, but decided that the deep relations of the growth were too vital to admit of its complete removal by the knife without danger, and was satisfied with a thorough scraping out of the slough.

Shortly after the patient had two attacks of erysipelas, after which the ulceration began to heal, and the patient got well and has remained well since.

Chronic Rheumatic Arthritis.

Case II.—The patient was a man, thirty-five years old, a printer. He had a left elbow swelled, stiff and painful, which condition had lasted about one year. The motions of the joint were restricted by pain. An examination showed the left arm somewhat atrophied above the joint ; there was no pain on pressure ; but severe pain on an effort to flex the arm. On rotating the fore-arm a crepitation was noticed. A hypodermic needle inserted into the joint showed entire absence of fluid.

The patient has a clap ; can this be gonorrhœal rheumatism ? No ; because this form of rheumatism consists almost always of a chronic or subacute serous swelling of the joint, with no involvement of the bone, no atrophy of limbs, and is very seldom so acute as to be painful. The diagnosis is chronic rheumatic arthritis. There is here thickening of the synovial membrane and cartilage, and finally of bone, and the inflammation is a dry one. We would expect to find involved, also, some of the other joints, and notably the fingers. We do find one finger that has recently become stiff and without any apparent cause.

Tubercular Osteitis.

Case III.—The patient was a man, ten years old, who also had a left elbow joint enlarged, hot, painful, and with motion much restricted by pain. Six years ago the joint became inflamed and one year ago some operation was performed upon it, the scar of which is to be seen. The left arm is much atrophied. The amount of inflammation in the part, at present, is considerable.

This, said Dr. Bull, is evidently a case of tubercular osteitis ; but we can go further and find the part of the joint involved. We discover, by careful palpation, the greatest tenderness to be over the head of the radius, and this corresponds with the incision of the former operation.

The patient is probably suffering from a recurrence of the tubercular disease in the head of the radius.

It is of importance, in reference to treatment, to know whether or not the joint has been previously excised ; this can be readily determined by measurement and comparison with the sound limb.

FOREIGN CORRESPONDENCE.

LETTER FROM THE SAMOAN ISLANDS.

·(FROM OUR SPECIAL CORRESPONDENT.)

LEONE, TUTUILA ISLAND, Feb. 1, 1889.

The Samoan islands are especially interesting just now by reason of the war among the natives that is drawing Germany and America somewhat into the controversy. This is not the place to write of the political aspect of these interesting islands of the South Seas, but a few of the social and medical features may be of interest to the profession.

The Samoan Islands are known by geographers as the Navigator Group, and lie in latitude 12° to 15° south, and 172° longitude west. The climate is about the same as in all tropical islands, a dry and a wet season, just the reverse as regards the months, of course, of those found in lands north of the equator. It being now midsummer here we are in the midst of the rainy season. But rain does not bother the Samoan. He has no fine clothes to spoil. His dress is nature's own—except a small waist-cloth. This is true of women and children as well as of the men. The latter are fond of dressing the hair of the head in most fantastic styles—with oil, stiffened with lime and adorned with fancy wooden combs. During a rain his only concern is lest his hair become wet; and until he can seek shelter, he will hold over the head a large banana leaf, or wrap one carefully over and about the hair.

Of all the South Sea Islanders these people are the finest in form and feature; stalwart, strong, with even lips and bright eyes, and a complexion pleasantly browned, they present a fine appearance; and it is said that they are far more intelligent and bright than the Maori of New Zealand, the Papuas of New Guinea, or the Kanakas of Hawaii.

The island of Tutuila is one of the ports of call of the Oceanic Steamship Company of San Francisco, running to New Zealand and Australia. Sixty miles to the westward may be seen the mountain peaks of Upolo island, on which is situated Apia, and where the chief fighting is being done. Being rather warm in more ways than one there just now for an American, your correspondent contented himself with simply a view of the mountains of Upolo from the safe distance of Tutuila.

The Samoan islands are noted for being the home—natural habitat—of elephantiasis. It is endemic here. The inhabitants of Tutuila and the most eastward of the five islands constituting the group suffer most with it. Strange to say it is uncommon in other groups quite near, as, for instance, in the Tongalabu, Society, Friendly and Fiji Islands. I can find no satisfactory explanation for this fact. The natives say it is due to being in the sea water so much; but Samoans are not exposed this way more than the other islanders. Some of the cases now in Leone are sights indeed. One tumor weighs seventy-six pounds, another forty-eight pounds, besides the frightful enlargement of the legs and arms. A woman has a labial tumor of this kind weighing fifty-six pounds. Many of the cases are among aged people, who have been affected for very many years. The natives occasionally operate on each other, using either a razor or a prepared bamboo stick, which is said to cut equally well. As a rule, however, the operations are performed by naval surgeons who may be in port on some man-of-war. Conjunctivitis is also very common among persons of all ages and in both sexes.

There are no native doctors. The natives have learned to know the value of many of the native herbs. About one hundred and twenty-five remedies are in vogue and a few of these I learned. For rheumatism the oil expressed from a plant they call Feetan is used externally, and apparently is of much value. They practise massage, and this oil is rubbed in with a prolonged "*Lumi-Lumi*" (massage) which may have much to do with the cure. This *Lumi-Lumi* is not only a medical but a social practice. It is the method of treatment holding first rank in their eyes, and one is most luxuriously rubbed and kneaded for all complaints, from ennui up to the direst fevers ; and a part of the hospitality of the wigwam is to offer a visitor a *Lumi-Lumi*. If one comes in from the bush tired and overheated, he is prevailed on to put a towel about the loins in lieu of the unnatural European dress, lie down on a cocoa mat and have a skillful girl expertly knead the body ; to refuse is to be uncivil, a boor. There is no thought of there being any impropriety in this massage, and there is no immorality connected with it.

Another remedy is the expressed juice of the root of the Ivi tree. The tree bears edible nuts. This medicine has a reputation among the whites as well as the natives as being most prompt in curing dysentery—a disease not uncommon in the Islands.

The Pawpaw-tree flourishes in Tutuila and the fruit is used by the natives as food, and the milky juice of the unripe fruit as a digester of meats, etc. It is a veritable vegetable pepsin. If fresh meat is suspended in the tree, so that it can absorb the exhalations of the tree, the toughest meat will become tender. So powerful is the softening action of the juice that it must be used with caution, or the meat will drop to pieces. I find that some interesting experiments were made in 1879 upon this subject at the Royal Agricultural Museum, Berlin. A portion of the juice was dissolved in three times its weight of water, and this was placed with fifteen pounds of fresh lean beef in one piece in distilled water and boiled for five minutes. Below the boiling point the meat fell into several pieces and at the close of the experiment it had separated into coarse shreds. Hard boiled albumen, digested with a little juice at a temperature of 20 degs. C., could, after twenty-four hours, be easily broken up with a glass rod. The juice can be dried without losing its effect, but its efficacy in this respect does not appear to have been tested over a longer period than six months.

The Samoans have no regular meal hour. When anything comes in, or the cooking is ready, they eat. They will work all day in the bush on a young cocoanut as a diet. If there is plenty in the hut, they often will arise at midnight to eat most heartily. Like American Indians, they have a feast while food is about, even if it is a famine for days to-come. Their appetite is something frightful. With the aid of some pawpaw one man will eat a sucking pig at a meal. Fish they like rare, and especially a small species—something like a sardine; only a hundred at a time will make a satisfactory meal. They sleep on cocoa mats, with a bundle of bamboo sticks as a pillow. These are hung from the beams of the hut during the day. During rough weather cocoa mat curtains can be let down around the sides of the hut, which in shape is like a large field tent, but made of a thatched roof, supported by bamboo sticks, with no flooring. No chairs are used, the position of etiquette being a squatting one, with the legs drawn underneath. If you stand while conversing with them in the "house," you must apologize, saying that you being a white man can not easily learn their graceful postures. Fashion is as strong an autocrat in the South Seas as in Paris.

At daybreak the entire village, men, women and children go to low water mark at the ocean beach, and defecate. In case of need one may go there at any time, but the great exodus from house to "habit" is the earliest hour of morning. A stone is used as water-closet paper. Women always urinate in a standing position; men squat. They are cleanly in their habits—wash the body after any work, first in sea water then in fresh. Soap is used when they can get it. Lime juice is a favorite application with the bath. A bark, similar to soap-bark used with us in America, is used by the natives for lathering their body, as well as for general washing purposes.

Puberty begins at eleven or twelve years of age. Parturition is short and attended with but little pain. The patient is attended by neighboring women. No prevention of conception is even thought of. Not even for cleanliness sake is a wash indulged in after connection. Children are loved, and a large family honored. Even what they are able to do on their own account in child bearing does not satisfy many families, and child adoption is common, and the child adopted becomes the special pet of the household. Criminal abortion and infanticide are almost unknown. Family and marital relations are strict; prostitution is unknown in Samoa. I have the testimony of officers who have spent many months among these people that the women, both married and unmarried, are most wonderfully virtuous. It is candidly admitted by even the enemies of mission work that this has been so only since the teaching of the missionaries has begun. Those thoroughly able to judge say that secret vice has been on the increase in direct proportion to the improvement in promiscuous connections. This vice is performed in the most disgusting manner, one sex practising it on the other with hand or mouth. Twin births are very rare. I should have mentioned that the woman after confinement is about in a few hours, and in a day or two at her usual occupations. Great care is taken to preserve the flow of milk; large amounts of cocoanut milk are drunk to favor a full supply.

A curious custom is for each sex to remove all hair from under the arms and around the pubes. The hairs are plucked and whatever still persists in growing is shaved off. The shaving utensil is a piece of broken bottle. It is looked upon as slovenly for men to wear whiskers, though much pride is felt in owning a handsome mustache. The bottle "razor" is also used for the face, and I understand that even the white people often get shaved by the natives in a most dexterous manner with this odd shaving utensil.

Tattooing is begun in early youth, first about the thighs, then legs and arms, in both sexes, but is more thoroughly and extensively performed on boys. The operation is so painful that usually it is extended over a number of years. The boy is not a man, however, until all the regulation amount of fashionable tattooing is completed. Quite often the tattooing sets up an undue amount of inflammation, with the result of immense sloughing sores, that leave huge ugly scars. Hope is an important element in the issue of any disease the Samoan may have. During the war, men with only slight wounds would die if they were badly frightened, and, on the other hand, brave men would be shot through the body, come into camp to have the wound dressed, and be back to the battle within an hour, and finally recover.

The usual food of the natives is breadfruit, bananas, cocoanuts, fish, fowl, and swine meat. They have a curious custom of burying a cooked biscuit made from bread-fruit, to use in case of famine, and for posterity to use in the same emergency. Some was recently unearthed near Leone, said to be fifty years old. Its smell was quite similar to that of Limburger cheese. Another remarkable custom is the religious rite of circumcision. This was found to be an established custom when they were first visited by white men.

And what do you think of the nude Samoan belle with the latest American craze of the chewing-gum habit? But in the case of the Samoan, it is her tooth-brush. The bread-fruit exudes a gummy material, which is used by the natives as a tooth-cleaner, by chewing the gum and working it about over the teeth.

It was laughable beyond measure to see the odd and delighted pranks the men and women made in looking in some small mirrors I presented to them. A partly worn-out jersey was given to a family—*pater familias* confiscated it, put it on, and then looked approvingly at himself in the looking-glass. Naked as father Adam, except a crushed-raspberry colored jersey! Can you imagine his appearance?

They are very fond of perfumes, and they have discovered a number of plants in the bush which yield scents. They use them chiefly in dressing the hair. They seem to be fond of the taste of kerosene oil, as they will drink a little of it; and their method of filling a lamp would seem to confirm this.

To transfer oil into a lamp, either from a bottle or another lamp, it is first put in the mouth, and then squirted into the lamp which they desire to fill. Most of the oil comes from America. Our country is lighting up the rude huts of the savages in faraway South-land. In many other ways civilization is leaving traces of its contact with these people, and many of the most curious old customs are being modified or are passing away.

Their dead are buried in the garden adjoining the hut, close by the house, so that the lights in the house may shine out on the grave and cheer the spirit of the one lying there. The grave is marked all around with pieces of broken bottles, or stones.

The old are honored; grey hairs are respected, though baldness is looked upon as a disgrace.

I know no part of the world that possesses so many interesting features as Polynesia. Here is the spot for the tired doctor and for his patient. It will give me pleasure to answer any communication relative to this part of the world.

C. C. Vanderbeck, M.D.

PERISCOPE.

A Case of Reinfection with Syphilis.

The case is recorded in the *Giornale delle Mal Ven*, of a woman, 46 years old, who had contracted syphilis when a child from a schoolfellow. The patient suffered very severely at the time, and had the characteristic eruptions, tibial pains, sore throat, and subsequent abortions. Ten years later she had well-marked tertiary manifestations, which gained for her the soubriquet of *fistolosa*, in her village. While she was still in the same deplorable condition she was reinfected by her husband, who had a chancre on the penis and was covered with a roseolar eruption. She came to the hospital, and was found to have a typical indurated chancre on the labium with corresponding glandular enlargement, and a confluent rose-colored papular eruption all over the body. She also complained of general malaise and pain in the shoulders and knees. These symptoms promptly yielded to treatment, and there would not seem to be any reason to doubt the accuracy of the diagnosis in both instances. Indeed, that exceptions should exist in the protection afforded by a prior attack of syphilis is only what a study of other specific diseases would lead one to expect.—*Medical Press and Circular*, Feb. 6, 1889.

THE
MEDICAL AND SURGICAL
REPORTER.

ISSUED EVERY SATURDAY.

CHARLES W. DULLES, M.D.,
EDITOR AND PUBLISHER.

The Terms of Subscription to the serial publications of this office are as follows, payable in advance:

Med. and Surg. Reporter (weekly), a year, **$5.00**
Quarterly Compendium of Med. Science, - 2.50
Reporter and Compendium, - - - - 6.00
Physician's Daily Pocket Record, - - 1.00
Reporter and Pocket Record, - - - - 6.00
Reporter, Compendium, and Pocket Record, 7.00

All checks and postal orders should be drawn to order of
CHARLES W. DULLES,
N. E. Cor. 13th and Walnut Streets,
P. O. Box 843.   Philadelphia, Pa.

☞SUGGESTIONS TO SUBSCRIBERS:
See that your address-label gives the date to which your subscription is paid.
In requesting a change of address, give the old address as well as the new one.
If your REPORTER does not reach you promptly and regularly, notify the publisher *at once*, so that the cause may be discovered and corrected.
☞SUGGESTIONS TO CONTRIBUTORS AND CORRESPONDENTS:
Write in ink.
Write on one side of paper only.
Write on paper of the size usually used for letters.
Make as few paragraphs as possible. Punctuate carefully. Do not abbreviate, or omit words like "the," and "a," or "an."
Make communications as short as possible.
NEVER ROLL A MANUSCRIPT! Try to get an envelope or wrapper which will fit it.
When it is desired to call our attention to something in a newspaper, mark the passage boldly with a colored pencil, and write on the wrapper "Marked copy." Unless this is done, newspapers are not looked at.
The Editor will be glad to get medical news, but it is important that brevity and actual interest shall characterize communications intended for publication.

THE DIAGNOSIS OF PREGNANCY BY EXTERNAL EXAMINATION.

In connection with the editorial in the REPORTER, November 24, 1888, on early signs of pregnancy, it is interesting to note that Dr. E. S. McKee, of Cincinnati, in a paper read before the Cincinnati Obstetrical Society, recently called attention to the value of external methods of examination for the diagnosis of pregnancy, in regard to which our country is behind the European practice. The art of diagnosticating pregnancy by external examination is best taught and practised in the immense hospitals of Dublin, of Germany and of France. In a recent work Credé teaches that a woman in labor and in the lying-in-state is diseased only through infection from fresh wounds. His maxim is: "He who does not examine a woman does not infect her." From the most careful digital examination some wound may occur, and therefore examinations should be limited to the fewest possible, or dispensed with altogether. Digital examinations are omitted for weeks together in the lying-in-hospital at Leipsic, especially if the health of the patient is not good. Credé teaches that the external examination should be given preference, and that internal examination should be employed only when demanded by the peculiar conditions of any case.

To follow this plan intelligently all the external means of diagnosis must be wisely and scientifically employed.

Inspection shows pigmentation of the face; the pigmented areola or the tubercles of Montgomery of the breasts; the size of the abdomen; and the brown line extending down the linea alba; the state of the umbilical cicatrix; a transverse furrow when the ring of Bandl has contracted; the striae on the abdomen; movements of the abdominal wall from activity of the fetus; and the height of the uterus.

Palpation proves the presence of the fœtus in utero and the number of fœtuses; the presentation, position, approximate size, and general conditions of the fœtus, and the relations of the uterus. Alternating pressure can produce *ballottement* by displacing the solid body, after carefully exploring and outlining of the uterus. If the abdominal walls are thick and the amniotic fluid abundant, and the points of diagnosis are difficult to determine, the examiner may seize the fundus of the uterus in the hand and force it down against the symphysis pubis, thus bringing the back of the fetus more in the range of palpation.

Abdominal *ballottement* may be made

with one or both hands. It is one of the most reliable signs of pregnancy. The sensation produced has been described as like the sensation produced by a lump of ice floating in a vessel of water and striking against the sides. When the placenta is placed anteriorly it can sometimes be detected by palpation. It is to be recognized as a fleshy mass which raises the palpating fingers from the fetal surface. The death of the fetus can often, though not always, be determined by palpation. The fetus can be measured by means of calipers. Applying them to the head and breech gives one half the length of the fetus, and consequently its age and the size of the uterus. The cord has even been detected passing over the back. Dr. McKee considers intermittent uterine contractions almost infallibly peculiar to the pregnant uterus. These contractions, which were first brought to notice by Braxton Hicks, are constant and not simulated by any other sign. Fetal movements may be sensible or visible. Extra-uterine fetation can only be detected when a distinct lateral tumor is palpable, which is quite distinct from the uterus, and auscultation must be practised before palpation, because manipulation disturbs both mother and child, increases the frequency of the heart beat and seriously modifies the auscultatory signs.

Percussion is the least valuable of the means of external diagnosis, and it is hardly possible to admit the claim that pregnancy can be made out in the second month by percussion. The amount of distension of the bladder is the most important thing that percussion can disclose at this period.

Auscultation is one of the most important of the methods of external diagnosis. In most cases the unaided ear is better than the stethoscope. Auscultation enables the examiner to hear the umbilical or funic murmur, the placental murmur, the pulsations of the abdominal aorta and the gurgling noises caused by the fluids and air in the intestines. A splashing noise due to the movements of the fetus in the liquor amnii may be heard occasionally, the fetal shock, muscular susurrus—the sound due to the friction of the uterus against the abdominal walls; and most important of all, the fetal heart sounds. The auscultator must not listen with the head lower than the body, for he thus causes an increase of the cerebral circulation and hears imperfectly.

It is a good thing for all medical men to know how much it is possible to learn in regard to the existence of pregnancy without making a vaginal examination; for occasions not infrequently arise when it is very desirable to avoid the latter, if it can possibly be avoided—sometimes for the sake of the patient, and sometimes for the sake of the physician. It is also good to know that a careful external examination may altogether obviate the necessity for more than a single vaginal examination when a woman falls in labor.

We say more than a single vaginal examination, because we think most obstetricians would like to make at least one such examination in order to ascertain the condition of the genital passages. But while we thus express our appreciation of the method advocated by Dr. McKee, we do not think it can ever take the place of vaginal examination in obstetrical practice, for the reason that many women would object to the investigation of their lower abdomens by sight, by palpation, by percussion and by auscultation with direct contact of the physician's ear. In most confinement cases a single and rapid examination with the finger *per vaginam* reveals to the experienced accoucheur all that he needs to know until the head reaches the perineum, and this is less formidable to the patient than the method described above.

None the less, it is well for medical men to be familiar with all the resources of their art, and external examination of pregnant and parturient women is a very valuable method, and, in certain cases, might be indispensable.

THE INFECTIOUSNESS OF PHTHISIS.

Ever since the discovery and isolation of the tubercle bacillus by Koch, those who accepted his theory that the bacillus has an etiological relation to the disease have spent more or less time in looking about for evidence that tuberculosis is an infectious disease, and contagious when circumstances favor the conveyance of the specific micro-organism from a diseased to a healthy individual. This evidence has not proved easy to get—at least in such quantity as one might expect from the assumptions of the theory and the almost universal prevalence of phthisis. Still, medical records and unpublished experiences of intelligent observers indicate that cases of phthisis sometimes follow each other in a way which · it is almost impossible to explain, except on the theory that the disease is both contagious and infectious.

In regard to the latter point, we may refer to the painstaking investigations of Dr. Lawrence Flick, of Philadelphia—to which we called attention in the REPORTER, Feb. 4, 1888—who discovered what seemed to him indubitable evidence that phthisis pulmonum is in a very marked degree an infectious disease.

An apparent confirmation of Dr. Flick's views may be found in a paper by Dr. F. Engelmann, of Kreuznach, in the *Berliner klinische Wochenschrift*, Jan. 7, 1889. In this paper, Engelmann describes with commendable directness and accuracy a series of cases of pulmonary tuberculosis developing in persons who in succession occupied the same apartment in a large lodging for glass-blowers. The facts in regard to the inhabitants of this apartment are the more significant in view of the comparative infrequency of phthisis in the occupants of adjoining and similarly conditioned rooms. As narrated by Engelmann, the developments of the apartment referred to point strongly to its infection with the cause of tuberculosis of the lung, and to the influence of this infection in communicating the disease to previously unaffected individuals.

There are certain vulnerable points in the temperate argument of Engelmann that the cases are to be explained only in this way; but no matter what conclusions may be arrived at by those who read it, it cannot be denied that taken together the facts stated make his conclusion a reasonable one. We can heartily commend his paper to the attention of men interested in investigating the contagious and infectious nature of phthisis, as a model of what contributions to the literature of the subject should be. His facts are stated with great clearness, and his inferences with thoroughly scientific moderation; and such evidence as he produces goes a great way toward establishing the opinion that the cause of tuberculous phthisis is particulate and may infect a given locality for a reasonable length of time.

THE TREATMENT OF ENLARGED PROSTATE.

With the careful study of disease of the genito-urinary apparatus which has been made in the last ten years, a number of methods of treatment which were formerly rare, or even unknown, have come into vogue, and the surgeon of to-day has a very different duty from that which devolved upon his near predecessors. This is peculiarly the case in regard to the treatment of hypertrophy of the prostate. Until within a few years palliative treatment was almost exclusively applied to this disorder; but of late years a great variety of operative methods have been proposed or discussed, such as perineal drainage, electrolysis, and the division or partial excision of the prostate through the perineum or from above the pubes. For these purposes the knife, electricity, and the galvano- or thermo-cautery have been recommended, and it is not easy to decide what method has the greatest claim to general adoption.

In an able paper read at the last meeting of the Association of American Genito-

Urinary Surgeons, and published in the *Annals of Surgery*, January, 1889, Dr. Francis S. Watson, of Boston, attempts to bring order out of the existing confusion and to lay down rules to guide surgeons in deciding what they should do in treating cases of enlarged prostate. After citing a number of opposing opinions, Dr. Watson studies his subject from, first, the anatomical standpoint; and, second, the clinical. From the anatomical standpoint he classifies prostatic enlargements according to the distance from the junction of the membranous and prostatic portions of the urethra to the furthest point of the median enlargement, the form of the enlargement, and the capacity and distensibility of the bladder. He finds that in twenty-eight out of thirty specimens which he has examined, a median enlargement constituted the chief obstruction to urination, and that—contrary to the opinion of Prof. Guyon—the great majority of cases are amenable to operative treatment. In twenty-one of the specimens the median enlargement was within reach from the perineum; in ten cases a supra-pubic operation would have been impossible; and in seven a perineal operation would have been impossible. In other words, neither of these methods is applicable to all cases, and either must be adopted or rejected according to the peculiar condition of any case. So far as immediate danger to life is concerned Dr. Watson believes that radical operations are not worse than palliative operations—puncture and drainage, but that perineal puncture and drainage are much safer than supra-pubic puncture with retained catheter. He thinks that many more cases die from unskilful catheterization than from radical operations performed by competent surgeons. For this, and because radical operations *are* radical he prefers them to palliative operations or catheterization. Of radical operations, he thinks the perineal preferable to the supra-pubic, because it is applicable to about two-thirds of all cases, and because it is safer.

His conclusion is one in which we entirely concur, namely, that the best plan in cases of hypertrophied prostate requiring operation, is to open the membranous urethra and explore the obstruction, and then to incise or excise as may be required or possible; and if the obstruction cannot be relieved by this route, to perform a supra-pubic cystotomy and complete the operation, following it with drainage through the perineum.

THE MEDICAL EXAMINERS' BILL IN PENNSYLVANIA.

With this number of the REPORTER we send to each subscriber a *Supplement* containing the names and addresses of the members of the Senate and House of Representatives of the State of Pennsylvania, and we urge all those who favor the passage of the bill to see or write immediately to the members of the Legislature with whom they have influence or acquaintance, or in whose district they reside, as the fate of the bill may be decided next week. We beg our subscribers to bear in mind that nothing is so likely to lead to the defeat of the bill as evidence of lukewarmness in regard to it on the part of the medical profession, and nothing is so likely to secure its passage as marks of interest in it by those who are supposed to know most about its merits.

As our readers well know, we regard this bill as one of great importance to the community, and hope that it will pass. We believe that it meets with the approval of the best members of the profession, who have no private or school interest to subserve. Its career is being watched with deep interest in remote parts of the United States, and other communities will gather encouragement for the work of reforming the methods of studying and practising medicine if it passes, and will be disappointed—and perhaps discouraged—if it fails to pass.

So let its friends lose no time in doing what they can to secure its passage; for those who oppose it will not be idle or slow.

BOOK REVIEWS.

[Any book reviewed in these columns may be obtained upon receipt of price, from the office of the REPORTER.]

HANDBOOK OF MATERIA MEDICA, PHARMACY AND THERAPEUTICS, COMPILED FOR THE USE OF STUDENTS PREPARING FOR EXAMINATION. BY CUTHBERT BOWEN, M.D , B.A. Small 8vo, pp. vi, 366. Philadelphia and London : F. A. Davis, 1888. Price, $1.40.

This is another of the books which reviewers are apt to condemn on principle ; but, like some to which we have referred of late, it is so excellent of its kind that we cannot but give it its meed of praise. Critics, or no critics—it is clear, from the steady production of such aids to the memory, that there is a demand for them ; and, as the demand is often met by men who know what students need as well as what they want, it is a pure assumption to decry them as usurping the field of better sources of knowledge. Many books of this sort are capital manuals. The one before us is such. It is not perfect, but it contains a great deal of useful information, which could be appropriated with great advantage by many practitioners as well as students of medicine. In going through it, we have been favorably impressed by the plain and practical suggestions in regard to prescription writing, and the metric system, and the other things which must be known in order to write good and accurate prescriptions. The discussion of individual drugs and preparations follows the usual classification according to their effects.

SKIN DISEASES OF INFANCY AND EARLY CHILDHOOD. BY C. M. CAMPBELL, M D., C.M., Edin. Small 8vo, pp. 202. London : Baillière, Tindall and Cox, 1889.

This small volume discusses briefly, but with clearness, the various skin diseases incident to the earlier years of life. Additional value is given the book by including the exanthematous fevers. The salient features of each disease are presented. although in a work of this compass much that is valuable must of necessity be omitted, or very briefly passed over. In some respects the author's experience is not in accord with American observation. Thus, for instance, in recommending (p. 61) the oleate of mercury for inunction in the treatment of syphilis, with the statement that " the oleates certainly are more readily absorbed than any other preparation applied by inunction." The discussion on the oleates at a recent meeting of the American Dermatological Association, embodying this point, was practically unanimous in the negative. Dr Campbell modifies this statement, however, by adding, " but the ordinary mercurial ointment has always been satisfactory in my hands " Moreover we do not see, in this country at least, cases of *pemphigus contagiosus*, other that can be more properly classed under the head of impetigo contagiosa. The author accords a separate description to each, and evidently considers them as distinct. This being the case, the following (p. 38), if true, is to us more than curious : " It is a very curious fact that the next disease (impetigo contagiosa) which we have to consider . . . appears to be caused by the very same micrococcus as pemphigus (contagiosus)."

Although presenting, from a strictly dermatological standpoint, some misleading, if not erroneous views, such as the above, this small manual contains much that the general physician will find of service.

PAMPHLET NOTICES.

[Any reader of the REPORTER who desires a copy of a pamphlet noticed in these columns will doubtless secure it by addressing the author with a request stating where the notice was seen and *enclosing a postage-stamp*.]

223. DESCRIPTION OF A CASE OF COLOBOMA OF THE IRIS, LENS AND CHOROID : WITH A STUDY OF THE VISUAL FIELDS. BY CHARLES A. OLIVER, M.D., Philadelphia. From the *Transactions of the Amer. Ophthalmologica: Society,* 1887. 6 pages.

224. NYSTAGMUS IN CONNECTION WITH DISEASES OF THE EAR. BY CHARLES J. KIPP, M.D., Newark, N. J. From the *Transactions of the Amer. Otological Society,* 1888. 18 pages.

225. THE PRESIDENT'S ANNUAL ADDRESS. BY ROBERT BATTEY, M.D., Rome, Georgia. From the *Gynecological Transactions,* 1888. 15 pages.

223. This is a most interesting pamphlet, illustrated with a beautiful phototype of the appearances of the eye, describing the condition of a woman whose peculiarities seem to have escaped attention until she was admitted to St. Mary's Hospital for typhoid fever, and came under Dr. Oliver's notice.

224. Dr. Kipp describes those cases occurring in his own practice—and incidentally refers to a number of others—in which increased tension in the middle ear produced marked nystagmus. In one case there was an exacerbation of a chronic purulent otitis media, and the nystagmus came on while the patient was walking in the street ; in a second case there was a purulent mastoiditis and nystagmus came on while an abscess cavity communicating with it—and probably originating from it—was being syringed out ; in the third case, nystagmus was produced by pressure on the mastoid process in a case of acute purulent otitis media.

The production of nystagmus under these circumstances is an extremely interesting occurrence, deserving the attention of pathologists, physiologists, and practising physicians ; to all of whom we can heartily recommend Dr. Kipp's pamphlet as a very valuable contribution to the literature of this subject.

225. The first half of Dr. Battey's address is interesting, as it describes the present condition of the admirable society which is one of the most distinguished exponents of the art of gynecology in the world. The second part of his address is much less interesting because it brings to the front a private grievance, and introduces a suggestion which is utterly impracticable. From the first part, we infer that the American Gynecological Society is ready for some new members, if they are made of good stuff. This may interest a number of the readers of the REPORTER.

LITERARY NOTES.

—G. Masson, of Paris, announces the publication of a work entitled *Traité des Maladies du Testicule et de ses Annexes,* by MM. Charles Monod and O. Terrillon, two very well-known surgeons of Paris. The work will be issued in one octavo volume ; price sixteen francs.

—Dr. Budin has been elected a member of the Academy of Medicine in the Section of Obstetrics.

CORRESPONDENCE.

Formula of Basham's Mixture.

To THE EDITOR.

Sir : Please give me through the REPORTER the formula for Basham's mixture. I am not able to find it.

Yours truly,
W. C. EUSTIS, M.D.
Farmington, Minn.

[The formula for Basham's mixture is given as follows in the last edition of the U. S. Dispensatory:

Tinct. of chloride of iron . . . ℞ lxxxiii
Dilute acetic acid . . . . f℥ ii
Sol. acetate of ammonium . . . f℥ xiv
Elixir of orange . . . . f℥ vi
Syrup . . . . f℥ i
Water . . . . ad f℥ viii

Add the dilute acetic acid to the liquor ammon. acetatis, and then the iron, elixir, syrup and water.— Editor of the REPORTER.]

Mistura Acaciæ.

To THE EDITOR.

Sir : As several readers of the REPORTER have written to me asking for the formula for *mistura acaciæ,* it will probably be well for me to say that this preparation of gum Arabic is not known to the United States Dispensatory, but is officinal in both the Edinburgh and Dublin Pharmacopœias. The Edinburgh process for making it is as follows:

Take of mucilage . . . . three fluid ounces.
Sweet almonds . . . . ten drachms.
Pure sugar . . . . . five drachms.
Water . . . . two pints.

Steep the almonds in hot water and peel them; beat them to a smooth pulp in an earthen ware or marble mortar, first with the sugar, and then with the mucilage; add the water gradually, stirring constantly; strain through linen or muslin. The Dublin process is similar. This mixture is known by the English names, "Gum Arabic Mixture," and "Gum Arabic Emulsion." As a menstruum for medicines for children, it is more agreeable than the Mucilage Acaciæ of the United States Dispensatory.

Yours truly,
J. B. JOHNSON, M.D.
Washington, D. C.,
Feb. 15, 1889.

Case of Meningocele—Correction.

In the article of Dr. Baum on a Case of Meningocele, published in the REPORTER, March 2, p. 265, the word "gramme" in the second column, twelfth line from the bottom, should read "grain."

Allopathy.

To THE EDITOR.

Sir : Why the general practitioner should have submitted so long to the epithet "Allopathic," must seem strange to the right thinking mind. There is no such body of physicians, so far as I am aware of, nor ever has been. It is a name that has been forced upon us by Hahnemann and his followers, and should have been discarded long ago, as it puts the general practitioner in a false light before the public. He is not the exponent of a particular theory or dogma, and therefore the term "Allopath" is entirely inappropriate. Let it be known to the public that we are the exponents of Scientific Medicine, and not dogmatists, and the intelligent and educated laity will see more plainly where we stand as a scientific body. Let every practitioner be scrupulously clear of using the term as applied to himself, and at the same time try and educate the general public that they may have a right and just understanding in reference to our position as compared with the different 'pathies and 'isms.

There seems to have heretofore been an indifference on the part of general practitioners to the effort to settling upon *us* that which places us in a false light before the world. The Homœopath, in referring to the regular physician designates him as an Allopath, in contradistinction to h;mself. Let us disabuse the general public of this understanding, and educate it to see our position as medical men : that we are a body holding to no particular system, theory or dogma; that we are a scientific body, endeavoring to advance our knowledge in the healing art, collecting wisdom from whatever source it may be found.

If the intelligent public could be made to understand our position as compared with that of the dogmatists. the 'pathies and 'isms would soon become extinct.

Yours truly,
W. L. MARTIN, M.D.
Rancocas, N. J.,
3d mo., 4th, 1889.

—It is officially announced that the Trustees of the University of Pennsylvania have appointed Dr. De Forest Willard Clinical Professor of Orthopædic Surgery, and Dr. George A. Piersol Professor of Histology and Embryology. These appointments were indicated in the REPORTER, Feb. 9. Dr. Samuel G. Dixon has also been elected Professor of Hygiene.

NOTES AND COMMENTS.

Treatment of Sweating Feet and Hands.

Dr. Unna (*Mon. f. prakt. Derm.*) recommends the treatment of cold, sweating feet with hot foot baths, which should be taken at night with some stimulating substance, such as spirit of camphor, mustard, or vinegar, thereupon drying the hands and feet and rubbing with a stimulating ointment, for example: ichthyol and turpentine, of each five parts; zinc ointment, ten parts. In the morning, after washing, the feet should be rubbed with cold water and exercise taken, the cold rubbing being continued until a condition of hyperæmia and warmth is produced. The stockings are to be powdered with starch powder, mixed with a little mustard. In the treatment of warm, sweating hands and feet, he recommends ichthyol, but without the warm water at night and the cold water in the morning. In the evening he recommends lukewarm water and rubbing with a simple ichthyol ointment (ichthyol, water, of each 5 parts; lanolin, 20 parts). In the morning the feet are to be washed with lukewarm water and ichthyol soap, and the lather rubbed off with a dry towel so that some remains on the hands and feet.—*N. Y. Med. Abstract,* Jan., 1889.

Inebriate Asylums.

Dr. T. D. Crothers, of Hartford, Conn., in an address on "Inebriate Asylums and their Work," delivered at Toronto, Can., draws the following conclusions as being supported by the latest teachings of science and experience: 1. Inebriate hospitals must take the place of jails and station-houses. Such places are dangerous in their mental and physical surroundings, by intensifying the degeneration, and removing the patient beyond hope of recovery. They are in many cases literal training-stations for mustering in armies of chronic maniacs that never desert or leave the ranks until crushed out forever. 2 Inebriate hospitals should receive the incurable inebriates, and make them self-supporting, and build them up physically and mentally. They would relieve the tax-payer, and relieve society of untold burdens of sorrow and misery. 3. Inebriate hospitals should receive the recent cases, and place them in the highest conditions of enforced health and vigor, and thus return a large number to health and sobriety again. 4. Inebriate hospitals can and should be self-supporting when once estab-lished. They should be managed on scientific business principles, like military training-schools. 5. Inebriate hospitals should be built from the money raised by taxes on the sale of spirits, on the principle that every business should be obliged to provide for the accidents which grow out of it. 6. These are the realities which every inebriate hospital is approaching, and which all experience points out as practical and literal in the near future. 7. The inebriate hospitals of to-day are only in the infancy of their work, contending with great opposition and prejudice, misunderstood, condemned, and working against innumerable obstacles. 8. The work of the present inebriate hospitals, notwithstanding all the difficulties and imperfections, has the grandest promise for the future, and encouragement for further effort in this field, along the line of scientific research. 9. Lastly, there is an intense personality in inebriate hospitals to each one of us. They may bring salvation and restoration to some one near and dear. They may be fountains of healing whose influence shall cross and influence our pathway in many ways. 10. Inebriate hospitals and their work are the great new land which only a few settlers have reached. They are calling to us to come up and occupy, and thus help the race on in the great march from the lower to the higher.—*Science,* Jan. 4, 1889.

Albuminuria and Yellow Fever.

Dr. Emilio Martinez, writing in the *Revista de Ciencias Médicas,* of Havana, on albuminuria in yellow fever, gives it as the result of his experience that his usual recommendation to judge of the gravity of the disease by the amount of albuminuria is untrustworthy, as he has met with cases, of one of which he gives details, in which the amount of albuminuria was very considerable, even though the disease ran an exceptionally mild course. In the case in question it appeared as if the poison confined its virulence almost entirely to the kidneys, the liver and other organs being but very slightly affected. A much more important point than the amount of albumin is, in Dr. Martinez's opinion, the amount of urea excreted per diem. This forms a guide to the activity of the oxygenating processes which are going on in the body. If these latter are retarded by the disease the amount of urea is very sensibly diminished. Its quantity thus stands in an inverse ratio to the gravity of the disease, and in this way forms a fairly reliable guide in prognosis.—*Lancet,* Feb. 2, 1889.

Treatment of Ingrowing Toe-Nail.

Dr. Theodore Clemens of Frankfort strongly recommends the employment of tinfoil in the treatment of ingrowing toe-nail. He first has the toe thoroughly washed with soap and carefully dried. He then envelops the whole nail with tinfoil, putting a strip between the portion that grows in and the raw surface caused by it. The tinfoil is fixed by means of a very thin layer of common wax, and the patient told not to wash ' the part, but to use dry bran for rubbing off the dirt. Of course the toe has to be repeatedly dressed with tinfoil; but, if the operation is carefully performed, it is surprising how long the tinfoil will remain intact, even when the patient is, as was usually the case in Dr. Clemens' hospital practice, very poor and very badly shod. The results are stated to have been most satisfactory, and are ascribed by Dr. Clemens not merely to the mechanical action of the tinfoil, but to the effect of the permanent contact of a combination of metals comprising iron, copper, arsenic, molybdenum, wolfram, and bismuth, with a moist and growing portion of flesh. This, he says, brings about in a few weeks the complete healing of the sore, and causes the nail to grow more slowly and in a more healthy manner.—*Lancet*, Feb. 16, 1889.

Case of Poisoning with Citrate of Caffeine.

T. Geraty reports a case of poisoning with caffeine in the *Lancet*, Feb. 2, 1889. At 9 A. M. before breakfast, a lady suffering from migraine took a dessertspoonful (equal to 200 grains) of pure citrate of caffeine, in mistake for the granular effervescing form of the drug. Mr. Geraty saw the patient immediately after the accident; the only complaint she then made was · as to the nauseating taste. She was encouraged to eat a little porridge before having an emetic. As soon as the porridge was eaten, faintness and nausea came on; and a quarter of an hour after the reception of the poison there was semi-unconsciousness, grave depression, extreme pallor, complete relaxation of all the muscles and a decided inclination to sleep; pulse slow, soft, and very compressible; respiration slow and sighing. The treatment adopted was an early emetic (one-twelfth of a grain of apomorphia), which acted at once and very completely; the administration of small quantities of brandy; keeping the patient in the recumbent position, and the application of warmth. There

was a well-marked rigor about an hour after the caffeine was taken. Consciousness was recovered about an hour and a half after emesis, and the faintness passed gradually away.

A Druggist Censured.

The Coroner of New York City concluded an inquest on March 5, in the case of Mrs. Storch, the victim of an overdose of morphine, purchased of a druggist. A thirteen-year-old sister of the victim testified that she was in the habit of getting morphine for the latter to the amount of 60 grains three times a week at the establishment of the druggist in question, and had never shown any prescription there, but said she had always taken the half-ounce bottle in which the drug had been originally procured by Mrs. Storch. The jury, in their verdict, censured the druggist for his carelessness and recommended that the statutes be strictly enforced and additional safeguards be provided.

American Physiological Association.

A regular meeting of the American Physiological Association was held in the rooms of Jefferson Medical College, Philadelphia, on Dec. 29, and at the University of Pennsylvania on Dec. 31. A number of interesting communications were read. Professor Reichert recounted experiments showing that the anterior columns of the spinal cord possess no irritability of their own, or that the power of excitability is confined to the posterior sensory columns He also showed that the rate of transmission of a nervous impulse differs under different conditions. Dr. J. W. Warren described some recent experiments showing that a sensory impulse, such as the explosion of a torpedo, reenforces the knee jerk, and drew the curve showing the variation of this reenforcement with the interval between the sensation and the knee jerk. Dr. Donaldson showed specimens from which it could be seen that the effect of a long electrical stimulation is to decrease the size of the nuclei of ganglion-cells, and that the amount of this shrinkage is roughly proportional to the duration of the stimulation. Professor Martin in one paper gave the determinations of the minimal and maximal temperatures consistent with life that the blood supplied to an isolated heart could undergo, and in another showed that the variation in the amount of carbonic acid given off by a normal frog and one kept in the dark is due to the optical and not the psychic differences of the two states; because a frog deprived of its cerebral hemispheres acts in this respect just like a normal frog. All of these papers led to interesting discussions; and the discussion of Dr. Reichert's paper induced Dr. S. Weir Mitchell to place at the disposal of the society two hundred dollars, to be devoted toward aiding research upon the rate of nervous transmission, especially in man. The society was hospitably entertained, and found much pleasure in visiting the laboratories of the Jefferson College and the University of Pennsylvania. The members of the society were invited to participate in the International Congress of Physiologists to be held in Basle in 1889.— *Science,* Jan. 4, 1889.

Medical Examiners Bill and the Medico-Chirurgical College.

At a meeting of the Faculty of the Medico-Chirurgical College of Philadelphia, held March 5, the following minute was passed:

"Believing that every reasonable advance of the standard of medical education is to the advantage of medical institutions and the profession, and feeling that the present State Registration Law imposes an onerous and unpleasant duty upon the medical colleges,

"Resolved that we, the Faculty of the Medico-Chirurgical College of Philadelphia, give our sincere and hearty support to the effort now being made to pass a bill for a State Board of Examiners, to whom shall be referred all applicants for license to practice medicine in this Commonwealth.

"Resolved that a Committee, consisting of Profs. Shoemaker, Pancoast, Waugh, and Keyser, be appointed to represent the College in influencing a favorable sentiment."

Appointment at Haverford College.

The Board of Managers of Haverford College, on March 1, 1889, appointed Dr. W. S. Hall Instructor of Physical Training at the college. He will be resident physician, general hygienic adviser of the students and sanitary adviser of the college, lecturer on physiology and hygiene, have charge of all the gymnasium exercises and of the physical questions that arise in connection with the games of the students.

Dr. Hall is a graduate of the Northwestern University and of the Chicago Medical College, in which latter institution he is now demonstrator of histology. He has been connected for two years with the Chicago Athenæum Gymnasium.

NEWS.

—The removal of Dr. Aby as quarantine officer of New Orleans has evoked vigorous protests from his medical and political friends.

—The Board of Managers of Swarthmore College have established a department for the direction of physical education, and have appointed Dr. J. K. Shell Director.

—Dr. John Guitéras, who has recently been elected Professor of Pathology and Morbid Anatomy in the University of Pennsylvania, sailed for Europe March 9, intending to spend the summer there in pathological studies.

—Prof. Kahler, of Prague, has been appointed to the Chair of Medicine at the University of Vienna, made vacant by the death of Prof. von Bamberger. Prof. Schrötter, the well-known laryngologist, has been charged with the establishment of a third clinic.

—The Pennsylvania College of Dental Surgery held its thirty-third annual commencement in the American Academy of Music, March 1, 1889. Dr. S. W. Gross presided and conferred the degree of Doctor of Dental Surgery on ninety-one graduates. Dr. Henry Leffmann made the valedictory address.

—Final experiments were made March 12 by the New York State authorities to satisfy themselves as to the best means of executing condemned criminals by electricity. Several dogs, four calves and a horse were experimented upon. In every case death was instantaneous and without sound or struggle. The experiments were under the charge of Dr. Carlos F. MacDonald, of the Auburn State Asylum, assisted by Mr. A. E. Kennelly, Mr. Edison's chief electrician, and Harold P. Brown, the electrical engineer.

—An epidemic of diphtheria is reported to exist at Gallitzin, Pa., since November, and about 100 deaths from this disease alone have occurred during that time in a total population of 2000. The disease is attributed to the disregard of the common rules of sanitation.

A malignant form of diphtheria has also become epidemic in Cranberry township, Venango county, Pa. Nine children have died within four days. In St. Petersburg the schools are closed and no public meetings are allowed.

—The Philadelphia *Ledger,* March 11, states that an autopsy was held March 10, on the body of a Mrs. Houckler, of East

Providence, Rhode Island, who died March 6, after nine days' illness, under the care of a "Dr." Etienne, who advertised himself as "a seventh son and a natural physician." He diagnosticated her trouble as "a combination of inflammation of the bowels, pneumonia and diphtheria." The autopsy showed that the patient had had none of the complaints named. This case may have an important bearing on the bill to regulate medical practice in Rhode Island, which was defeated in the Legislature during the previous week, but is to be reconsidered.

HUMOR.

"AND THAT IS SILVER ORE, is it?" said Mrs. Snaggs, as she examined a piece of curious looking mineral. "Yes, my dear," said her husband. "And how do they get the silver out?" "They smelt it." "Well, that's queer," after applying her nose to the ore. "I smelt it, too, but didn't get any silver."

A GOOD STARTER.—Old Mrs. Bentley—"When d'ye s'pose, Joshua, they're goin' to git these telegraph wires under ground?" Old Mr. Bentley—"I dun know; I see there's a prominent telegraph official died two or three days ago, an' is to be buried to-morrer." Old Mrs. Bentley—"Well, Joshua, that ain't much, but it's suthin'."

CONCENTRATED.—A Vassar graduate, out in the country, went into the stable of a farm-house. "Dear me; how close the poor cows are crowded together!" she remarked. "Yes, mum; but we have to do it." "Why so?" "To get condensed milk, mum." The sweet girl-graduate went off relieved and enlightened.—*Bristol Med.-Chir. Journal*, Dec., 1888.

PECULIAR ASSAULT AND BATTERY.—A queer case was recently adjudicated by the correctional tribune of Lübeck. An old family physician — a man past sixty-five years of age—was arraigned for assault and battery upon a patient. It appeared from the evidence that the latter was a girl in her teens, whom the doctor had ordered to take certain medicines. On making his next visit he found that she had failed to do so, and without more ado he turned down the bed-clothes and spanked her soundly, *propria manu!* The tribunal sentenced him to nine months' imprisonment and a fine. It is likely that the former portion of the sentence will be remitted, as his many patients have petitioned the court to this effect.—*National Druggist.*

OBITUARY.

RUFUS STANFIELD HARWELL, M.D.

Dr. R. S. Harwell was born in Robertson County, Tenn., February 22, 1820. He was graduated in medicine at the University of Pennsylvania in the spring of 1843. He began the practice of medicine in McNairy County, Tennessee, and remained there for three or four years. He then moved to Oxford, Mississippi, and practised there for five years. Thence he moved to Ouachita County, Arkansas, where he was an acceptable and successful practitioner to the day of his death, Oct. 6, 1888. He suffered for many years from asthma, which greatly crippled his usefulness. He was universally respected as a Christian, an honest man, and an excellent physician.

He leaves two sons and one daughter, living near Camden, Arkansas, and two half brothers, John V. and Marcus J. Wright, who reside in Washington, D. C.

ELWOOD HARVEY, M.D.

Dr. Elwood Harvey died at his home in Chester, Pa., March 3, of pneumonia, after a brief illness. He was born in Birmingham township, Delaware county, and was about 62 years old. He was graduated from Jefferson Medical College, and many years ago held a professorship in the Woman's Medical College of Pennsylvania. He was a prominent member of the Delaware County Medical Society and, with Dr. George Martin, of Concord, took the preliminary steps in May, 1850, for organizing the society in Chester.

During the war he was an assistant surgeon at the Soldiers' Hospital, Upland.

His wife and two sons survive him.

WILLIAM J. FLEMING, M.D.

Dr. William J. Fleming died in Philadelphia March 1, of Bright's disease of the kidneys. He was born March 19, 1828, and was graduated from the University of Pennsylvania in 1851. Shortly after this he went to Europe, where he visited the principal hospitals, returning after a two years' visit. He entered the army at the breaking out of the war as a surgeon and served throughout the war. At the close of the war he returned to Philadelphia and resumed and continued in practice up to the time of his last illness. He was a member of the College of Physicians and of the County Medical Society.

MEDICAL AND SURGICAL
REPORTER

No. 1673.   PHILADELPHIA, MARCH 23, 1889.   VOL. LX.—No. 12.

CONTENTS:

CLINICAL LECTURE.

TRAUMATIC CROSSED SPINAL HEMI-PARAPLEGIA; POISONING WITH BISULPHIDE OF CARBON.[1]

BY PROFESSOR J. M. CHARCOT,

PARIS, FRANCE.

Traumatic Crossed Spinal Hemiparaplegia.

Gentlemen: The patient who will serve for to-day's demonstration is a young man, twenty-four years of age, a slater by occupation. In appearance he is tall, thin, has a very agreeable face, and woman-like behavior. Notwithstanding this, he seems to have been very early in his life attracted by persons of the opposite sex; and it was in some affair with a woman that he became a victim of the accident the consequences and remains of which we shall study together to-day.

[1] Delivered at the Salpêtrière, Paris.

The accident, to which I have just now alluded, seems to have made a deep impression on his mind; so much so, that to keep the remembrance of this fact he had himself tattooed, at the upper and internal part of his left forearm, with the words "Death to unfaithful women." To the unfaithful women alone does he address himself; hence he seems to be still less pessimistic than the great poet, who generalized too much when he said, speaking of woman in general, that she was "false as water."

After this short digression, let us return to our subject. It was in March, 1880, when this man was only sixteen years old, that he had a quarrel with Italians, and at that time was struck from behind with a knife, which seems to have penetrated very deeply into the upper portion of the trunk, at the base of the neck; there still remains to-day, opposite the second and third dorsal vertebræ, a linear cicatrix about an inch in length.

You are probably all aware of the results of wounds of the spinal cord, especially those of the kind exemplified by our patient.

A man is leaning forward, when his adversary strikes him from behind in the line of the spinal column, and more often opposite the third and fourth dorsal vertebræ—as shown by the histories of the cases of Müller, Salmon, Joffroy—very rarely further down, as in the case of Viguès, in the dorso-lumbar region. The knife penetrates the intervertebral space, and, strange to say, the spinal cord is more often wounded by a hemi-lateral section on the side opposite to that at which the knife penetrated the skin. In this patient, the knife penetrated on the right of the spinal column, and according to the symptoms presented the lesion has reached the right lateral half of the spinal cord; you all know that such lesions are very dangerous, and usually end fatally in from eight to fifteen days after the traumatism. Our patient, as you see, seems to have been very fortunate, but I believe that in his case there has not been a complete left hemi-lateral section of the cord, but only a puncture; the knife probably penetrated only the middle of the left half of the cord by its point; and if at the beginning the symptoms pointed to an hemi-lateral section it is because a limited inflammatory process rapidly developed around the sectioned part—a true left transverse hemi-lateral myelitis—equivalent, as regards the production of a paraplegic form, to an absolute section. You will soon say to me, when I demonstrate to you the paraplegic phenomenon, that the spinal symptoms have immediately been carried to their maximum, with all their special characters, and hence one is entitled to think that a consecutive inflammatory process necessitates some time for its developing?

This is all true. My answer will be to refer to Brown-Séquard, who has shown that in hemi-lateral lesions of the spinal cord a simple puncture in one of the halves of the organ is equivalent, as regards the symptoms immediately observed, to a complete section; the logical difference being that the symptoms produced by the puncture are of a more transitory character; while those resulting from a section are permanent.

In our patient the first symptoms observed must be attributed to the puncture, while the later ones are to be attributed to an hemi-myelitis consecutive to the traumatism. As to the immediate effect of the injury, we have to rely on the testimony of the patient; he says he remained conscious for a long time, and did not immediately know that he had received a wound in the back; he remembers that he fell immediately, his left leg felt as if broken, as if it had disappeared. He was helped to get up, but his left leg could not hold him up, and he fell again.

From this account, the motor hemi-paraplegia was instantly produced, as a consequence, according to our hypothesis just stated, of a puncture of the cord. The patient was soon after his accident taken to the hospital, and then for the first time he became unconscious. He mentions the fact that he suffered at the time from retention of urine, which necessitated the use of the catheter for several days in succession. This is corroborative of our statement as to the existence of a myelitic process, which at one time had probably extended beyond the limits of the left lateral half of the cord; for this symptom does not belong to simple traumatic hemi-lateral section of the cord. An established fact is that when the patient awoke the left lower extremity was completely inert, paralyzed, while the right lower extremity had perfectly free movements, except that the sensation was entirely gone; this condition is Brown-Séquard's syndroma. The patient also remembers the diagnosis which was often repeated by the attending surgeon, namely, lateral hemi-section of the spinal cord.

Let me refer to what is called "Brown-Séquard Syndroma" by most physicians, while a very few call it Brown-Séquard's disease. I much prefer the term syndroma, because we have to deal not with a disease, properly speaking, but with a series of symptoms which can belong to different varieties of diseases. For instance, besides hemi-section, syndroma will present itself in myelitis, in intra- or extra-spinal tumors, syphilitic or otherwise; in tuberculous meningitis, affecting a lateral half of the cord, or producing a compression of the same.

In animals, our illustrious friend Brown-Séquard has shown that a complete hemi-lateral section of the spinal cord produces invariably a syndroma, the clinical characters of which have been well described by him under the title of spinal hemi-paraplegia with crossed hemianæsthesia. He has also later demonstrated that the same occurs in man, precisely in the same manner as it does in animals. Let us now examine the symptomatology of the affection under consideration, and let us suppose, as in our case, that the left half of the cord has been sectioned.

On the left side, which corresponds to the spinal lesion, we observe, first, a complete motor paraplegia of the lower extremity, a fact already described by Galien; second, the skin of the left extremity is in a state of hyperæsthesia, and this hyperesthesia varies, going up toward the abdomen, according to the height of the spinal lesion, and is limited on this same side by a horizontal line—there is also a loss of muscular sensation; third, there is a certain increase in the temperature; fourth, more or less rapid muscular atrophy, with degenerative reactions; fifth, sometimes there are trophic articular changes, such as arthritis of the knee joint.

On the right side, the one opposite to the section, we observe first, cutaneous anæsthesia of the whole lower extremity, going up the trunk or abdomen, where it is limited by a more or less straight horizontal line; second, there is no increase of the temperature on that side; third, no traces of motor paralysis, of atrophy, or of increase in the reflexes; fourth, there are sometimes observed some cutaneous trophic troubles, such as an eschar in the gluteal region, a bed sore.

No vesical symptoms are manifest—this is the description of a recent case, of course; if the disease has been allowed to run its course for some time, we must anticipate a certain variability in the symptomatology, especially in those cases in which the patient has nearly entirely recovered the motor function in his paralyzed limb, such as will be encountered in those who have only suffered from a punctured wound, or from a temporary compression of one side of the cord; for it is clear, that only a temporary trouble would admit of the retrocession of these different symptoms, and a return to the normal state.

*In our patient we still observe to-day the following state: On the left side, no trace of motor paralysis of the inferior extremity is to be found. This paralysis is said to have been a complete one for the first fifteen days following the accident; after which the motor power gradually returned; when he left the hospital, eight weeks after the accident, he felt a certain annoyance in that extremity, which lasted for nearly three years, but which now has entirely disappeared. As regards the temperature of this extremity, to-day it is even somewhat lower than the other; there is no cutaneous hyperæsthesia. The knee jerk is now quite exaggerated; there is no ankle clonus. The left extremity is very much atrophied, as is shown by the following figures: the middle of the left thigh gives a circumference of 39 centimeters (about 12 inches), while the same region of the right

thigh gives us 43 centimeters (about 13 inches); the middle of the left leg gives us 26 centimeters (about 8 inches), while the right measures 33 centimeters (about 10 inches); no reaction of degeneration has been observed by Dr. Vigoroux, the medical electrician of the Salpêtrière, hence we must admit that this atrophy has been the consequence of the extension of the myelitic process to the anterior horns of the gray substance on the side of the lesion, yet has not produced complete destruction of these nerve cells.

On the right side there have never been observed any disturbances of motion. The reflexes are normal. There is no change in the muscular sensation, but there exists a great change in the sensibility of the skin. True anæsthesia is not really found in these cases, it is only an equivalent disturbance due to the existence of a spinal compression or of an organic lesion of the posterior columns. This I have called the phenomenon of dysæsthesia, which is noticed as follows: if you pinch your patient, he will feel it but will record the sensation after a striking delay, and even then without locating precisely the place where the excitation was applied. Moreover, the sensation becomes diffused above and below the excited point. Heat and cold when applied are also not recognized as such, but give rise to this diffuse sensation just mentioned. Let me remark here that this phenomenon of dysæsthesia, as far as we know, belongs only to organic spinal lesions and is not combined with the anæsthesic of hysterical patients. You see how easy it is, by the aid of an hypothesis, to interpret the existence of the remains of a spinal hemi-paraplegia with crossed anæsthesia.

One point, however, must have struck you, and that is that the line which limits the diæsthesic anæsthesia does not extend as high as we might expect, the wound having been inflicted opposite the third and fourth dorsal vertebræ.

In the case of Müller, which is very similar to our case, the line went up as far as the level of the axilla; while in our patient it extends only to Poupart's ligament in front and to the lumbar region behind; this is certainly a singular anomaly; yet we must remember that Müller's case was a recent one, the patient having died in fifteen days, while our patient was injured eight years ago, which makes us admit that with time, there has been a progressive restoration of the injured parts of the spinal cord.

In our patient there is a very interesting example of spinal hemi-paraplegia with crossed anæsthesia, as a result of a traumatic lesion of the spinal cord. I would stop the examination of this case here, but I cannot overlook the fact that this patient was addressed to me by one of my ablest students in neuro-pathology, as an example of traumatic hysteria. The reasons put forward for this opinion by our colleague refer to the anomalies presented by this man, as regards, for instance, the spinal hemi-paraplegic syndroma; or again the limit of the anæsthesia on the right side, too low for an injury of the cord opposite the third or fourth dorsal vertebra.

In our lesson to-day, I have explained to you the reasons for these anomalies. Our colleague thinks that all the phenomena of spinal hemi-paraplegia have developed in this man as a result of suggestion, while he was in a peculiar mental state just after his accident, which could be compared to the somnambulistic period of hypnotics. He thinks that the lesson made before his bed on the syndroma of Brown-Séquard by the attending surgeon, was the origin of the suggestion. This we cannot admit. You all know that in cases of hystero-traumatic epilepsy, paralysis with or without anæsthesia following a local injury does not appear on the spot, does not present itself immediately; this fact is very important; in our case, however, the observation which was taken at the hospital at the time of his admission for the injury mentions the fact that the patient was already in a state of paralysis.

Although I reject absolutely the intervention of hysteria in the production of the syndroma of Brown-Séquard in our patient, I would not say that he is absolutely free from hysterical phenomena, for he has certainly shown traces of this affection; he even to-day, has applied to the hospital, not for his nervous trouble, but for coughing and spitting of blood. A careful physical examination showed him to be in a perfect condition, and we have admitted that these hemorrhages belong to the class of neuropathic hemorrhages so common amongst hysterical subjects. In respect to his neuropathy, we must not overlook his hereditary tendencies; his father is actually in an insane asylum, and his grandmother on the maternal side was subject to hysterical attacks.

Poisoning with Bisulphide of Carbon.

Most of you have probably heard of the manufacture of bisulphide of carbon; you know that the manufactures in which this preparation is used furnish us a certain number of patients who present symptoms of a nervous character.

Duchenne de Boulogne and Bouchardat a long time ago called attention to this intoxication; yet Delpech, in 1863, is the one who has correctly defined the train of symptoms which characterize the sulphide of carbon neurosis.

This poor man before us is a typical example of this intoxication; he is sixty-three years of age, has been a very vigorous man, but lately he has failed in strength. The symptoms which bring him before us have appeared for the past six weeks or two months. His family history shows no traces of nervous inheritance; he also seems to have been a sober man and is leading a regular life.

During his youth he lived in the country as a shepherd; he never learned to read, hence it is not intellectual work which has injured him. I have just said, a moment ago, that he was a sober man; we have a proof of that, for he has been working for a very long time in a factory where bisulphide of carbon is prepared, and in this business no drinking man is taken as a workman; and, in addition, we find no signs which would indicate that he drinks.

He has been in his present occupation since 1872, but he has not worked steadily, and occasionally he returned to his first occupation, that of digging. Still he had continuously worked in the factory for four months, when one day, while cleaning a bucket which was to contain the bisulphide of carbon, he presented the following symptoms: After having felt a sensation of suffocation, he had a feeling of heat in his scrotum, and fell without uttering a cry, as if he had had a cerebral apoplexy. His colleagues thought him asphyxiated, and they assert that during his unconsciousness, which lasted half an hour, no convulsions were observed. Finally he came to himself again and was able to walk home. The first two days after this accident, which he spent in his room, he does not remember anything of; on the third day, however, he felt a sensation of numbness, and on the following day, a well-marked paralysis had developed. That same day the right upper extremity was taken in the same way, but in a less severe degree.

Gentlemen, this hemiplegia which rapidly followed the apoplectiform attack was the first revelation of his nervous affection, the character of which we shall now define.

I shall ask our patient to stand up and to make a few steps before you, but do not forget that his hemiplegia dates back six weeks. Remark that while the patient walks, he drags after him his paralyzed lower extremity, as if it were an inert body. Note well that the paralyzed extremity always touches the ground, the patient does not attempt to lift it up at each step he makes You will find no trace of the movement of circumduction, which always exists in an old hemiplegia of organic origin ; this fact will not be overlooked by those of you who are acquainted with it. If we now turn our attention toward the left upper extremity, we find that it is hanging powerless, very weak, and slightly deformed, probably because the fingers are extended straight, producing a right angle with the palm of the hand. We have here a spasmodic contraction, for we encounter an elastic resistance when we try to move the fingers in one way or the other, in flexion or in extension. We have here a spasmodic rigidity, but it is not the attitude of the hooked fingers which is observed in the hemiplegia of organic origin accompanied by contracture. By the dynamometer we obtain, for the paralyzed left hand, a pressure of 11 kilogrammes (29 pounds 4 ounces Troy), while the normal right one gives us 60 kilogrammes (160 pounds Troy). No increase of the reflexes is observed either in the upper or lower extremities, which already shows us that we have not to deal here with an ordinary hemiplegia of organic origin.

The next symptom observed is that cutaneous sensation is deeply affected, all along the paralyzed upper extremity, and also all along the corresponding lower extremity ; you already know that this symptom is very rare in ordinary hemiplegia, we only find it when the lesion involves the posterior portion of the internal capsule, and even then sensation is never so much reduced as it is in this man. There is also a remarkable contrast between the cutaneous sensibility which is deeply involved and the motion, which, on the contrary, is not completely abolished ; this again is not found in organic hemiplegia. Anæsthesia is not only present in the paralyzed extremities but is also found over the left half of the body, in front and posteriorly, and on the half of the head and face ; and this anæsthesia involves not only the skin but also extends to the deeper portions, for the articulations can be twisted and pulled upon most energetically without the patient feeling it ; he also is not aware if we displace his limbs,

and cannot determine what position is given to them.

With these different facts just developed, those of you who are expert in the matter will not fail to recognize that we have to deal here with a case of hysterical hemiplegia. Is this man, who appears broken down, quiet, prostrated, showing signs of precocious senility—is he an hysterical patient? Yes, gentlemen, and those who are acquainted with the patients we see in this clinic, will not doubt it one moment.

Let us now establish the diagnosis of hysteria. I shall not return to the symptoms already mentioned : total deep and cutaneous sensitive hemi-anæsthesia, paralysis of the upper and lower extremities with loss of muscular sensation, absence of rigidity and absence of increase of the reflexes, while this hemiplegia is already more than a month old—these phenomena are already sufficient, but we have other additional symptoms.

In the first place, we remark that the inferior facial nerve is not involved ; hence we have not a true hemiplegia, but an associated monoplegia. The convulsive movements of the right upper lip are not due to facial paralysis, but to facial hemispasm, which corroborates the diagnosis of hysteria. A remarkable fact is that you will find the facial hemi-spasm well indicated in several observations of poisoning with bisulphide of carbon, and especially in two observations of Mr. Delpech ; but certainly the hysterical nature of these spasms has not been suspected. To the glosso-labial spasm we can add other strengthening symptoms ; there is a well-pronounced contraction of the visual field on the right—the paralyzed side, while on the left the visual field is normal. Remark this fact of the contraction of the visual field on one side only, as it is rare. I have just said "permanent contraction," because such contractions are alone characteristic of hysteria in certain diseases. No dyschromatopsia, but a well-marked monocular diplopia is observed in this case ; also an insensible pharynx ; hearing power on the right side is very much reduced ; taste is absent on the right side of the tongue. After all these classical symptoms of hysteria, it is not necessary to hunt further. Certainly our man has no convulsive attacks ; we find no hysterical or hyperæsthetic spots ; but these symptoms are not necessary to constitute the hysterical disease.

One word on the mental state of our patient. If I do not admit that there are as many distinct kinds of hysteria as there are different origins giving rise to the affection, yet I admit that hysteria presents different forms, different varieties. A certain quantity of alcohol will produce a different drunkenness in different individuals; one will become very bright, full of fun; another, on the contrary, will remain very quiet, stupid. Our patient was very bright before his accident, and since then he has become quiet, morose, thinks himself worthless, and is quite discouraged. In hysterical men you will often find a condition of mental depression, and will also hear of their having most terrific dreams. This fact is also observed in our present patient; he is pursued nearly every night since his accident by lions, wolves—all sort of imaginary animals; his last dream, of which he spoke to us this morning, was that he found himself on the top of a mountain, and water was coming up gradually on all sides to drown him; he awoke in a state of great anxiety. If I insist upon these frequent psychical changes observed in hysteria in men, it is because some persons have been tempted to consider it as belonging to a traumatic neurosis, and having even a character separating it from true hysteria. This is not so. These same characters belong absolutely to the hysteria of man, and are found not only when the disease originates from a traumatism or nervous shock, but also when the affection' is developed in consequence of the action of a toxic cause, saturnine or sulpho-carbon—or even under any cause. This particular mental state does not belong to a special form of hysteria, but is found in every variety of hysteria.

Having shown you that all the symptoms presented by our patient belong to hysteria, shall I say that hysteria is the disease observed by Delpech in so many patients, workmen in bisulphide of carbon factories? This would be going too far; yet we find in all his observations certain undeniable symptoms of this neurosis, such as the glosso-labial spasm, suffocation, *globus hystericus*, peculiar sensations in the genital organs, anæsthesias, hyperæsthesia, contractions, etc.

From our present knowledge we can safely say that most of the authors who have written on the sulpho-carbon intoxication have observed hysteria in some of its manifestations; hence hysteria would be the disease originating most frequently as a result of intoxication by the vapors of bisulphide of carbon. Hereafter then we must study more closely the relation exist-

ing between such a disease and hysteria. Amongst the observations recorded, there are manifestly certain symptoms which do not belong to hysteria; such are the acute and sudden pains which patients complain of as being located in their extremities, while at the same time the walking is uncertain. These patients have been looked upon as suffering from locomotor ataxia (sulpho-carbon ataxia); but I think we most likely have to deal with a peripheral neuritis, similar to the one observed in other intoxications, such as those in beri beri, or those arising from the use of alcohol; and that the motor troubles of the extremity resemble much more those resulting in the walk of the "stepper,"[1] than those of the tabetic patient. I am certain these troubles have no relation to hysteria.

Finally, we can say that there exist certain affections of the nervous system, which are due entirely to the action of vapors of bisulphide of carbon. Hereafter we must try to be more careful in our observations, so as to be able to differentiate correctly the symptoms belonging to hysteria from those which belong to the intoxication. Now that the patient has left the room, let me say one word in regard to the prognosis. This man will be cured with difficulty, this being the rule in hysteria of the male adult. This disease will last, notwithstanding our most careful treatment, several months, even several years. Suggestion after having produced the hypnotic state, cannot be employed on this patient, he not being capable of hypnotization; but suggestion in the awakened state (*état de veille*) can be employed with success against his paralysis. In addition to this treatment, the general tonics can be recommended; and finally, we must ask our patient to give up his occupation in a bisulphide of carbon factory.

————

—The commencement exercises of the Meharry Medical Department, and the Dental Department, of Central Tennessee College were held at Nashville, Feb. 22. The exercises marked the thirteenth anniversary of the Medical Department and the third of the Dental. This is the only Dental school for colored persons in the United States, and the Medical College is one of two in the country.

[1 Prof. Charcot probably means by the "walk of a stepper," a gait in which the feet are raised high off the ground (as in locomotor ataxia), but in which there is no exaggeration of their lateral or outward sway, and no irregularity in their rise and fall.—Editor of the REPORTER.]

COMMUNICATIONS.

HEADACHE IN INEBRIETY.

BY T. D. CROTHERS, M.D.,

HARTFORD, CONN.

SUPERINTENDENT OF WALNUT LODGE.

Recently I have seen several cases of inebriety, in which a history of early paroxysmal headache was prominent. The frequency of this symptom, in widely differing cases, has attracted my attention, and is evidently of much clinical importance in the prognosis of such cases The clinical histories of some cases will make this fact more apparent.

Case I.—John B., a steady drinker of twenty years' duration. His parents were both temperate, but his grandfather on his mother's side was a chronic inebriate. When about six years old he suffered from severe headaches lasting several hours, and reappearing every few weeks. They continued for many years, and resisted all treatment, becoming more and more severe in intensity and duration. At puberty they disappeared for two years, then returned. They seemed to follow from the exhaustion of overwork as a bank-clerk. From this time down to the age of twenty-four, he had constant recurrences of these attacks. Often they would be preceeded by great exhilaration and buoyancy of feeling, then suddenly merge into severe frontal headache, and later the entire top of the head would be sensitive, painful and very hot. This condition would last for eight or ten hours, then subside within a few hours and be followed by a profound slumber.

At twenty-four years of age, he began to use wine on the table, and within a year drank strong liquors. The headaches ceased altogether from this time and the use of spirits was kept up until he came under my care. Three weeks after admission he complained of great depression of both mind and body, lasting for several hours. These attacks of depression continued, only growing less in intensity, until he was discharged. His history since then has not been obtained.

Case II.—William H., a periodical inebriate, began to use spirits while in the army. His father drank to excess at long intervals up to his death. His sister was hysterical and died of consumption early in life. The patient began to suffer from severe headaches soon after puberty. These attacks came on unexpectedly and without any apparent cause, and after several hours of agonizing pain, ended in sleep, from which he awoke free from headache and well. They were called "bilious" attacks, and were variously treated, but with no results. In the army the surgeon ordered large doses of spirits and quinine, and from this time the headaches disappeared. He became an inebriate, and twenty years after came under my care and recovered and was discharged a year later.

Case III.—B O., an irregular inebriate, who had been a lawyer, politician and active man of the world. He drank to excess at irregular times and places. His mother died of consumption soon after his birth. His father was a nervous, passionate man, who died of apoplexy. He had headaches from infancy; sometimes they were severe and he had to go to bed, at other times he could keep at his business.

At twenty years of age these headaches were so severe that he was confined to bed for a week after the attacks. They came on several times every year, and resisted all treatment. He had been an abstainer, for the reason that beer and spirits produced intense nausea. When about twenty-four he was given large quantities of brandy for this headache, and ever after he could use it. When the pain subsided he used spirits largely. As he became more addicted to spirits the headaches died away, and for twenty years before admission had not been noticed. A few weeks after coming under my care they returned, but were less severe and continued while he was under treatment. They seemed to be preceded by mental and muscular irritation for several hours, and were followed by great exhaustion.

These three cases are more prominent types of nerve paroxysms preceding inebriety. In many cases there are histories of irregular periods of headaches, occurring before inebriety appeared. In some cases headache appeared first at puberty and was very intense for a time, and then subsided. In others, severe headaches of childhood disappeared at puberty or broke out again in later life, and merged into inebriety. The presence of headache in early life is always a grave symptom of brain exhaustion and neurotic disturbance from heredity. In such cases there is a strong probability that some neurotic disease will appear in later life, from the slightest exciting causes. When these headaches come on later in life, some conditions of profound exhaustion and nerve disturbance are present. It may be stated as a general fact that a history of severe headache in a case of inebriety is a hint of serious nerve and brain disorder, requiring constitutional treatment. When they appear after inebriety is established, in cases in which there is a possibility of syphilitic infection, specific treatment is required.

When they disappear from the use of spirits the prognosis is grave, especially in those cases in which they return when the alcohol is withdrawn.

In some cases these headaches resemble epileptic seizures, in the suddenness and intensity of the paroxysm, and the irritation and depression which follow. They may be most aptly called "nerve storms," or discharging lesions, of the higher centers. A practical point would be never to use spirits in these cases of paroxysmal headaches, for fear of fixing and developing the graver disorder of inebriety, or some allied insanity.

Moreover, when headache is found to be prominent in the history of inebriety, the case is more serious, and requires more careful study and treatment. In all probability the presence of headache preceding inebriety is only a hint of brain degeneration that may or may not merge into inebriety, depending on some special exciting causes. When headaches follow inebriety, the conditions and causes are complex and grave.

Medical art and skill can do much in both cases. In a case under my care in which the inebriety began with the use of spirits to relieve these paroxysms, Turkish baths broke up these attacks, and the inebriety disappeared as the health improved.

In another case of inebriety in which severe headaches followed the drink storms, rest, improved nutrition, and general tonics, baths, and constitutional remedies resulted in permanent recovery.

Paroxysmal headaches in childhood and following puberty should always attract attention, and receive careful medical treatment. Narcotics of all kinds are both dangerous and uncertain. The only safe remedies are tonics, nutrients, and all means to build up and strengthen the organism.

—*Science*, Feb. 15, says that Professor Ruata of Perugia is authority for the statement that there are annually in Italy nearly 300,000 cases of typhoid-fever, of which number 27,000 prove fatal. One-third of the persons in Italy who reach the age of forty-five have the fever, and in some districts more than three per cent. of the population die from this one cause.

THE SEGMENT TREPHINE AND AN ASEPTIC TREPHINE.[1]

BY JOHN B. ROBERTS, M.D.,
PROFESSOR OF ANATOMY AND SURGERY IN THE PHILA-
DELPHIA POLYCLINIC.

The frequency with which operations are now done upon the skull and brain has made apparent the need for improvement in our instruments for opening the skull. Seven years ago I published[2] an account of my experiments with the surgical engine, as a means of making openings in the skull; and I still believe it an excellent and safe means of effecting access to the cranial contents. The chief disadvantages are the expense of the engine and its liability in ordinary hands to get out of order. This latter objection held good at least in one hospital with which I have been associated.

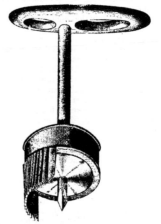

The ordinary trephine, either cylindrical or conical, will probably be used much more frequently, therefore, than the surgical engine; hence suggestions to improve its character are not inadmissible. The "segment trephine," described in the *Operative Surgery of the Human Brain*,[3] is, I think, a valuable instrument with which to deepen any portion of the groove surrounding the button of bone to be removed, without cutting along its entire circumference. The skull is often very much thicker in some parts of the area of operation than in others,

[1] Read at the meeting of the Philadelphia County Medical Society, February 27, 1889.

[2] *Philadelphia Medical Times*, 1881-82, xii, p. 206.

[3] Page 78.

and the ordinary trephine has to be tilted to avoid injuring the cerebral membranes at the points where the skull is thinnest. Tilting is not always easily done when the trephine is large and deeply imbedded in the bone. A "segment trephine," having the same radius of curvature as that with which the operation was begun, enables me to cut more deeply and with great care at any selected part of the groove. The accompanying illustration renders a detailed description of the instrument unnecessary. The cutting edge extends one-third of the circumference, and the centre-pin, not requiring retraction, may be immovably fixed to the head of the trephine. The instrument has no groove in the stem or handle to collect septic matter, and is readily cleaned.

A serious objection to the ordinary trephine is the fact that it is almost impossible to get assistants and nurses to keep the centre-pin, and the tubular stem in which it slides, perfectly aseptic. Indeed, it is difficult, with every intention of perfect cleanliness, to keep the hollow stem of the instrument absolutely clean. I have endeavored to remedy this objection by making the stem solid, and substituting for the ordinary sliding centre-pin a circular block of metal, accurately fitting into the crown of the trephine, with a point upon its lower extremity.

As soon as the surgeon has cut a groove deep enough for the teeth of the trephine to be maintained in position upon the skull, the central block is taken out of the crown of the trephine, and the operation continued as with the ordinary instrument, after retracting the centre-pin. Upon the upper surface of the block is cut a shallow slot, into which fits a slight projection from the upper part of the trephine crown. This compels the block to rotate with the rest of the trephine when the operator is making the first incision into the bone. The trephine itself is made as thin as possible, in order that the groove between the disc of bone removed and the rest of the skull may be very narrow. The button of bone, when replaced, can then be held in position more readily than if the groove is a wide one. I believe that after using a thin trephine, such as this, it at times will be well to stitch the button of bone into position by catgut sutures passed through the periosteum, which may be allowed to remain upon the surface of the disc of bone, and upon the skull adjacent to the trephine opening.

The crown of the trephine must not be too conical, because such a trephine in cutting through the thick skull makes the outer portion of the incision a very wide one. I am inclined to think that a surgeon of even moderate skill never needs a conical trephine to prevent his plunging the instrument into the brain; a cylindrical one should be just as safe in his hands as a conical one. An advantage in having the crown of the trephine slightly conical, when a large instrument is used, is that the instrument is less liable to become jammed in the groove. This annoyance not infrequently occurs on account of irregularities in thickness of the skull, especially when a large surface is included in the trephine. It is more apt to take place, I think, when the groove is made by a cylindrical instrument, which does not make the external aspect of the incision wider than the internal.

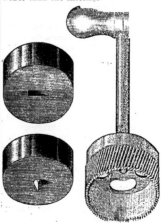

The weight of the metal handpiece can be minimized by fenestræ, or by making the handle hollow. It is best to attach the handpiece to the stem eccentrically, as suggested by Horsley, since the hypothenar portion of the palm needs a longer lever than the thenar.

This aseptic trephine, it will be seen, is somewhat similar to the safety trephine of Hopkins,[1] who suggested the use of a cylindrical block instead of a centre-pin, because of the possibility of the surgeon forgetting to withdraw the centre-pin, and, therefore, wounding the dura mater. His device contained a spring to keep the block thrust forward, and was therefore very difficult to clean. In fact, it was not constructed with an idea to facilitate asepsis, but to prevent careless puncture of the dura.

[1] *Annals of Surgery*, July, 1885.

SOCIETY REPORTS.

MEDICAL SOCIETY OF THE COUNTY OF NEW YORK.

Stated Meeting, February 25, 1889.

The President, ALEXANDER S. HUNTER, M.D., in the chair.

By special order, the discussion opened at the last stated meeting by a paper by DR. SIMON BARUCH, on

The Value of Water in modern Therapeutics,

was continued by a paper sent by DR. A. JACOBI and read by the Secretary. In this paper Dr. Jacobi reviewed his writings, some dating back over twenty years, recommending and describing the use of water for stimulating the circulation, reducing the temperature, and for its influence on local inflammatory swellings. Among the diseases in which he had given it especial attention, were typhoid fever and diphtheria; he had also used it extensively in various other affections some dozens of years, and twenty years ago succeeded, he said, in getting himself expelled from an institution because he was found guilty of using cold water in the treatment of sick children.

DR. HENRY DESSAU had found water as necessary in the maintenance of the health of children as of adults. There is still a tendency to overfeed infants, and not to allow the stomach time for rest between meals. The use of water as a drink would often allay the thirst of the child and its demand for too frequent feeding. In diarrhœa it relieves dryness of the mouth, and supplies a want arising from loss of intestinal secretions. Some have said it increases the diarrhœa, but such has not been Dr. Dessau's experience. He has also found a plentiful use of cold water as a drink in the nephritis of scarlatina a benefit because of its gentle diuretic and cleansing effect on the kidneys. The bath, he said, is the best tonic we have, and should be used regularly every day in infants four or six months old. In strumous and rachitic children the cold bath daily employed is one of the best protectives against catarrh from sudden changes of temperature. Cold sponging of the chest and spinal column is the best remedy for laryngismus stridulus. He also employs the bath in convulsions in children, usually the cold bath if the convulsions are a part of a fever, and the hot bath when they are due to peripheral irritation, such as an overloaded stomach, dentition, etc. He also employs cold water in the treatment of chronic diarrhœa in infants.

DR. DESSAU said he had formerly published an article in the *New York Medical Journal* on the endermic use of water for allaying pain, and said that it seldom failed. It seems to be best adapted, however, to the relief of pain of nerurotic rather than of inflammatory origin.

DR. AUGUST SEIBERT demonstrated the ease with which the stomach of the infant can be washed out. He uses a soft rubber tube, of small size, allows the water to run in from a graduated measure, say half a pint, and empties the stomach by siphon action. The temperature of the water should be about 102° F. The three disorders in which this treatment is especially useful are, cases of deranged stomach from simple overfeeding; chronic gastro-intestinal or enteric catarrh, and cholera infantum. One washing is usually sufficient in the first class, several in the second combined with proper feeding, and as a rule patients of the third class are also thus cured, Dr. Seibert having saved twenty-six out of twenty-eight cases last summer. No medicines were employed.

DR. VINCENT ZOLNOWSKI read a communication, and first emphasized the importance of a careful inquiry into the patient's previous history, the present condition of his urine, thoracic and abdominal organs, and general health, before applying hydropathic therapeutics. The treatment, he said, varies according to the condition of the circulation, temperature, age, and vital resistance of the person. Water can be used as an antiphlogistic, sedative, excitant, tonic, derivative and solvent, but the two general methods to be observed are its use as an excitant on the one hand, and as a depressant on the other. As an excitant it must be used quickly, the degree of temperature proportioned to the irritability to be overcome—the less the irritation the lower the temperature employed. The depressant method is of two qualities, antiphlogistic and sedative. In the former the heat is withdrawn slowly; but moderate temperatures are used in these cases only until the excitement is allayed. The sedative method is recommended when the nerves are greatly excited. Water used internally as a drink and by enemas acts mechanically.

Dr. Zolnowski cited, among other interesting cases, one pronounced schleroderma by some of the most eminent physicians of New York City, who thought the progress would be rapid to a fatal issue. The use of water, however, in the form of baths, half-baths, douches, packs, local application of wet cloths, etc., for two years or more, have now overcome the rigidity and pain which had existed in all the muscles of the body, until at present there is stiffness only in the fingers. He also cited a marked example of the morphine habit in a physician, overcome by hydropathy; likewise some neurotic affections due to the lithæmic habit.

DR. RALPH PARSONS gave his experience with water in the treatment of mental and nervous disorders, and said he has found the hot bath of special benefit in maniacal excitement, and uses the warm bath at bed time to overcome insomnia, following it by inunction of the skin. The cold bath should be used with care in the insane, and should not be employed by surprise, for while it has been claimed that some are restored to reason by the unexpected cold plunge, he believes much more harm has been done than would counterbalance the few cases of favorable issue.

DR. VAN VALZAH gave the conclusions he has arrived at after seven years experience with hydropathic treatment, especially in gastro-intestinal disorders, such as gastritis and dyspepsia. The use of the water internally in these affections should always be guided by judgment. Cold water promotes upward peristalsis, while hot water produces downward peristalsis. Hot water before meals should be sipped, and taken an hour and a half before. Special caution should be taken when there is a tendency to hemorrhage or during menstruation. A moderate amount of hot water stimulates thirst more than the same amount of cold water in diabetes. The safest general rule to be guided by in the administration of water is the condition of the urine, which should be kept, if the use of water will do it, at from 1.016 to 1.018, and of not too high color.

DR. WALLIAN spoke of the principles involved in the use of water in fever and other affections, and remarked that an intelligent treatment would not be adopted until physicians recognize fever as a symptom instead of as a disease. Instead of paying so much attention to the cure of disease by drugs, one should remember that the cause of all diseases is unhealthy surroundings, improper food and drink, or excessive or deficient function of parts of the economy; and the physician should restore the normal circumstances. A most important indication is to prevent accumulation of waste and poisonous products. The use of water will do more than anything else to stimulate the functions of the skin. He deprecates the tendency to rely upon antipyretic drugs in fevers. He thinks cold water will not replace hot water in the treatment of typhoid fever.

DR. HOLCOMBE gave an account of his own case, that of Bright's disease, supposed to have been far advanced, and of gastric disturbances, and his restoration to health, after unsuccessful trial of various other measures, by the use of flesh diet largely, and of water.

DR. HUNGERFORD, of Connecticut, said he had had a different experience with the treatment related by Dr. Holcombe, he himself having been a sufferer from gastritis, and was made much worse when he tried the meat diet and water.

DR. SIMON BARUCH made some closing remarks, among others that he had found the warm bath of little use in the convulsions of children, for by the time it was ready the convulsion would be over or prove of a nature not to be remedied by the bath. In convulsions due to hyperpyrexia, however, nothing equals the graduated cold bath as a preventive measure.

NEW YORK ACADEMY OF MEDICINE.

Stated Meeting, March 7, 1889.

The President, A. L. LOOMIS, M.D., in the Chair.

DR. FRANCIS DELAFIELD read a paper on

The Treatment of Acute and Sub-acute Nephritis,

which, he said at its commencement, was not intended to bring forth any new drug or method, but to determine how plans of treatment and drugs already employed may be applied intelligently in individual cases. A review of works by German, French, and American authors show that there is a disposition at the present time to direct treatment to the symptoms of nephritis rather than to the nephritis itself, and he proposed to view the subject from the opposite standpoint.

It is necessary at the outset to separate acute from subacute nephritis. After a brief review of the pathological changes present in acute nephritis, a disease most frequently seen after scarlatina, diphtheria, and some other acute inflammatory affections, he based on these his views regarding appropriate treatment. In mild cases, he said, no treatment is necessary further than to keep the patient in bed and give fluid diet.

In the more severe cases other treatment will be required—and the first condition to be met is the nephritis itself—and besides that, arterial tension should be lessened. In treating the nephritis itself it is to be observed that although the quantity of urine is small, its quality is good ; that the secretion of urine relieves the congestion, and therefore it is better that the kidneys should be active than at so-called rest. It should also be remembered that as long as the congestion continues the quantity of urine will be diminished, and a considerable diminution for several weeks is often well borne ; and it is not necessary always to try to get the skin and intestines to do the work of the kidneys. It is wiser, by relieving congestion of the kidneys, to get them to do their work, for the moment this takes place the congestion will still further diminish. To relieve the congestion, cause the blood to collect at the surface of the body by the application of heat to the entire skin ; use dry or wet cups over or heat over the lumbar region ; use empirically calomel or sulphate of magnesia in small doses repeated at short intervals until the bowels begin to move ; use also such drugs as will decrease the arterial tension. It is not expected to bring the urine up to the full quantity as long as congestion continues, but only to the point of securing safety. The febrile movement requires no treatment. Prostration, nausea, and vomiting call for rest in bed and fluid diet. Anemia can be successfully treated only after convalescence sets in.

Cerebral symptoms have received most attention. They accompany contraction of the arteries with increased tension and labored heart action. To overcome the arterial tension, aconite, chloral hydrate, and opium are suitable, and are preferably given in small doses, so that their use can be continued for some time. When arterial tension exists it should be reduced, without waiting for the development of cerebral symptoms.

In opposition to the condition present in acute nephritis, there is, in subacute nephritis, long continuance of the inflammation, but no congestion ; the exudation is of the profuse, almost dropsical character met with in other subacute inflammations, as in pleurisy with effusion ; and there are permanent changes of the stroma and glomeruli of the kidneys. The interference with the renal function consists in diminution of the solid constituents of the urine. The quantity of the fluid is often increased. The symptoms of the disease are largely due to the effect upon the blood and nutrition of the body. The anemia, dropsy, and loss of strength are prominent features. Contraction of the arteries is absent, or present only at intervals, and the cerebral symptoms are chronic rather than acute. The symptoms of acute nephritis may be present during exacerbations. Only very few patients seem to recover permanently. The conditions requiring treatment are the subacute nephritis, the changes in nutrition and in the composition of the blood, the dropsy, the condition of the arteries, the cerebral symptoms, and the acute exacerbations of the inflammation.

For the nephritis the patient should reside in a warm climate and lead an out-of door life. If his home is in a cold climate he will have to stay in the house much of the time. Except during the exacerbations he should take as much solid food and fats as he can digest. The excessive use of milk and mineral waters is to be avoided. It is possible that opium and bichloride of mercury favorably affect the nephritis. The anemia is a most important symptom, and requires iron and oxygen, together with massage and relief of constipation. The dropsy may be only an inconvenience, or it may be a most distressing symptom. It often reaches its greatest development with low arterial tension and large excretion of urine. In some cases the treatment of the anemia and regulation of the diet answer also for the dropsy. It is not wise to increase the urine more than is sufficient to enable the patient to excrete his five hundred grains of urea a day. The fluid taken should not exceed the urine passed. In extreme cases of dropsy it is necessary to purge, sweat, puncture the skin, or tap serous cavities.

High arterial tension, should it exist at any time, may be controlled with nitroglycerine, chloral hydrate, or opium. To avoid cerebral symptoms one must watch the amount of urea excreted and the condition of the arteries. The acute exacerbations are to be met as in acute nephritis.

Dr. T. E. Satterthwaite sent a communication, expressing his views on treatment, which were modified in different cases according to the pathological condition existing in the kidney and the lesions elsewhere in the body, which the renal affection might accompany.

Dr. A. Jacobi disapproves of the use of caffeine for cerebral symptoms when high arterial tension exists. Bichloride of mercury, he said, is useful in cases of nephritis when one is unable to distinguish between the subacute and chronic form; and it should be administered in small doses and continued for months. Subacute nephritis in men who have reached the age in which the arteries become changed is much benefitted by bromides, given in doses of not more than fifty grains a day, and combined with general treatment.

Dr. KINNICUTT laid stress upon the value of vaso-motor dilators in arterial tension, such as the nitrites, and said that on theoretical grounds at least he preferred not to give digitalis.

Dr. J. WEST ROOSEVELT pointed out the source of danger in arterial tension, and said it is direct only when the arteries are diseased, and acts indirectly by causing a strained heart to do still greater work, and by causing anemia of the tissues through contraction of the arterioles and capillaries. Digitalis in this condition is objectionable, and vasomotor dilators can be used only to tide over temporary great danger. Real treatment consists in reestablishing the function of the kidneys.

Dr. J. E. WINTERS regards the amount of albumin in the urine in subacute nephritis as the chief indication of the progress of the case, and he regulates the diet so as to reduce its quantity, giving little albuminoids.

Dr. LAURENCE JOHNSON spoke of the excellent results obtained in uremia, manifested in coma and convulsions, from the use of pilocarpin, and said no evil effects had followed in patients of good general condition.

The PRESIDENT said he always took into consideration the age, predispositions, and habits of his patient before commencing treatment. The management called for in children manifestly differs from that called for in adults. In acute Bright's disease the rule calls for rest in bed, room of even temperature, regulation of the diet, moderate purgation. Arterial tension should be reduced by drugs acting on the vasomotor system. This is best effected in his experience by calomel in small doses, accompanied by salines. Further measures consist of irritation over the kidneys and stimulation of the surface of the body.

In subacute nephritis the patient should not be depleted by any method whatever. The nutrition should be improved. Iron in these cases seems to be of little value. If digitalis increased the urinary excretion it would prove of value; otherwise, it would do harm. It is contraindicated in arterial tension. Small doses of opium are of marked value, and can be long continued in patients with weakened heart from accumulation of poison in the system.

Dr. DELAFIELD remarked that iron might prove of benefit, and the benefit be manifest not in reduction of dropsy or effects on the quantity of urine, but in an increased number of red blood cells and of hæmaglobin.

The PRESIDENT stated that the Academy had secured a plot of ground, seventy-five by one hundred feet, just west of Fifth Avenue on Forty-third Street, and that it was proposed soon to commence the new building.

REPORTS OF CLINICS.

PENNSYLVANIA HOSPITAL.

MEDICAL CLINIC.—PROF. LONGSTRETH.

Diabetes. Fallacies of Some of the Tests for Sugar. Remarks on Diet and Methods of Treatment.

This young woman, 20 years old, was admitted to the wards three days ago. She is a seamstress. In her family history we find that kidney diseases occupy a very prominent place. Her father and two uncles were afflicted with Bright's, and her mother, also, seems to have been a victim of that disease. The patient says that she herself was fairly healthy until within a year ago. She then began to complain of pain in her back, her bowels were sluggish, and she had some uterine trouble. The commencement of her present illness dates from last July. At that time she first noticed that there was a large increase in the quantity of urine she passed. Thirst was somewhat more frequent and her appetite became enormously sharpened. Five or six meals in the twenty-four hours were barely sufficient to satisfy it. In spite of this heavy consumption of food, her strength rapidly declined. She did not lose much in weight, but she became unequal to even ordinary exertion. Her eyes then gave her some pain, there was a dimming of vision, and she was compelled to relinquish her sewing. These eye symptoms have now, however, passed away. There was a moderate evening rise of temperature and marked flushing after meals. Sleep was disturbed. She did not complain of pain at any time, but there was a more or less constant sense of fulness in the epigastrium.

On admission the girl seemed well nourished. There was no perceptible dryness of the skin. The tongue was clean, but abnormally red. Pulse rapid. No organic lesions could be discovered, examination of the lungs, heart, liver, etc., being negative. The abdomen was full, but not tympanitic. She has now been under observation three days. Immediately after her admission she passed 32 ounces of urine, and during the ensuing twenty-four hours 120 ounces. Its specific gravity was 1042, slightly acid. The acidity of urine varies with its degree of dilution. If, with a normal proportion of salts, we have a largely increased bulk of fluid, the acidity will naturally be much lessened. An alkaline diabetic urine is of unfavorable significance. It indicates as a rule the occurrence of extensive tissue changes, these being principally located in the liver.

In carrying out the various tests for sugar, grave errors, unfortunately, are by no means infrequent. The reduction tests are often rendered unreliable by the fact that urea or urates are sometimes capable of reducing both copper and bismuth. There will form a dirty yellow precipitate which is frequently mistaken for the brighter brick red precipitate which is characteristic of the presence of sugar. Many cases are treated as diabetes which have been falsely so diagnosticated. Some years ago the late Prof. Wallace sent me for examination several specimens of urine which, I found, were free from any trace of sugar. Yet the patients from whom these specimens came, had been placed upon a diabetic treatment on the testimony of a chemist who erroneously thought that he had discovered in them a greater or less quantity of sugar and had so reported to Dr. Wallace.

Of the different tests for sugar, I think that by fermentation is the best. Several apparatuses have been devised for conveniently carrying it out. This one that I show you is very simple and sufficiently accurate (Einhorn's saccharometer). It consists of a bulb connected with an upright tubular arm, one side of which is graduated to the volume of carbonic acid gas in cubic centimetres, while the other shows the percentage of sugar. Its capacity is 10 c.c. A gramme of compressed or any other variety of yeast is added and with a little heat fermentation quickly occurs. With regard to the treatment of these cases, an accurate knowledge of the amount of sugar given off by a diabetic, whether large or small, is not of so much importance, as is a knowledge of the rate by which it is being reduced from day to day. This will indicate most clearly whether the measures you have adopted are or are not proving effective.

In taking up the treatment of diabetes, I wish to call your attention to one of the newer of the many remedies that have been proposed for that disease—nitrate of uranium. It has been used in this case with apparent good effect, the amount of sugar passed having been consideraly reduced. It is given in the dose of one grain three times daily, in pill or powder. An addition of nitric acid is required to effect its solution, and, therefore, this is not a desirable form in which to administer it. I have not instituted as yet any change in the patient's diet. Personally, I disapprove of the very abrupt changes of diet to which these patients are commonly subjected. The diet lists usually prepared for diabetics, are much too rigid, I think, for sudden enforcement. A gradual reduction of the hydro-carbonaceous elements of the food is much more likely to be favorably borne than a sudden deprivation of them. The system suffers more or less shock when it is abruptly deprived of such an important class of materials as these. It is more prudent to strike out the sugars and the purer starches first, and then by degrees to cut them off, if necessary, altogether. Instead of immediately forbidding all kinds of bread, let the patient limit himself for a time to the bran breads. While eliminating the starches it is a good plan to add the fats. These are especially useful when there is any tendency to constipation. Butter and cream may be used in such cases with benefit. The human body requires a certain amount of variety in food. We are not made up of bread and butter, for example, and we can hardly expect, therefore, to maintain a man's health and capacity for labor on any such slender supply of nourishment My first order, generally, to victims of this disease is, that they shall eat only such vegetables as grow *out* of the ground, and give up those that grow *in* it. Of course, such articles as rice and beans are excepted from this rule, which, I think you will find, is a fairly good one.

Now, let us, for a moment, ask ourselves why this woman should have diabetes. What has occurred to give rise to it? This disease may be dependent upon a variety of causes. In this case, where we detect some digestive disturbance, I think the liver is chiefly at fault. For some time previous, the bowels were inclined to be inactive, digestion was imperfect, and, through defective assimilation, the normal proportion of sugar in the blood became gradually increased. While, in treating these cases, it is well enough to endeavor to reduce the amount of sugar appearing in the urine, still it must not be supposed when that point is gained, that the disease itself is conquered. Our chief object should be to bring about such a state of the assimilative functions that our patient, with ordinary attention to the special rules of health operating in his or her case, may live comfortably without provoking a return of the disease. The first symptoms complained of by this patient drew our attention to the condition of the abdominal circulation. It was inactive. The liver was too fully charged with blood to perform successfully its secretory functions. In time we should have had obstinate constipation with a marked deficiency of biliary salts in the stools. To avoid this, and, at the same time, to prevent the occurrence of any permanent change in the liver, the portal circulation must be stimulated. The intestinal evacuations should be as carefully examined as to the presence of sugar and bile salts, as are those from the kidney.

In studying the treatment of diabetes in this country we have largely confined our attention to the regulation of the diet. In doing this we have overlooked the claims to consideration of certain natural and easily obtained remedies. In England and on the Continent the waters of some of the springs there, are used almost exclusively in the treatment of this disease. The Carlsbad waters are probably the most efficient of those in common use. We no longer however have to send our patients abroad in order to obtain them. We now receive the natural water in glass, and, in addition, the Sprudel salt in powder form. The Carlsbad water on cooling throws down an excess of salts which it contains when drawn directly from the springs. By artificially warming the water and adding a sufficient quantity of the Sprudel salt, we can restore to it its original proportion of saline constituents. This water should be consumed in moderate quantities only. The best effect upon the liver is not to be obtained by the production of violent catharsis. A comparatively gentle action will quickly show beneficial results in the improved character of the stools. The most valuable constituents of the various laxative mineral waters, are the chlorides. It is when these are present in large quantity that a water acts most vigorously as an hepatic stimulant. The treatment already instituted in this case will be continued.

One of the chlorides, if necessary, will be added to the uranium, and the diet will be gradually reduced to the requisite degree of rigidity.

[A few days later, without premonitory symptoms, the specific gravity and the quantity of sugar showed unusual oscillations without the quantity of urine secreted daily changing to a marked degree. A microscopic examination of the urine showed blood corpuscles, and blood and granular epithelial casts, which were not present on the patient's admission.

The terminal symptoms were ushered in by violent abdominal pain, especially in the lower epigastric region. The relief was with difficulty obtained by anæsthetic inhalations and morphia. To this condition succeeded gradually increasing stupor and finally coma, with reduction but not complete suppression of urine. No amelioration was effected by hot-air baths or by pilocarpine hypodermically administered. Death came by respiratory failure.

The *post-mortem* examination showed a swollen fatty liver, much congested, and thick dark green bile in the gall-bladder; the kidneys swollen, with the tubular epithelium opaque and granular; no other organic disease.]

BELLEVUE HOSPITAL, NEW YORK.

GYNECOLOGICAL CLINIC—PROF. POLK.

Pyosalpinx.

Prof. Polk operated for pyosalpinx in a patient, 35 years old, whose chief symptom was persistent pain. The disease was of several years standing,

On opening the abdomen the uterus, tubes and ovaries were found matted firmly together in a circumscribed mass. The left tube and ovary were adherent to the pelvic floor, and also to the rectum. The left ovary was enlarged and contained pus; and the tube was also distended with pus. On the right side, the ovary was very tightly attached to the rectum; the tube was twisted on itself, enlarged from pus, and adherent to the ovary.

By slow dissection with the fingers (the assistant pressing up the uterus with the fingers in the vagina), familiarizing the touch as well as possible with the different tissues, Prof. Polk isolated the left ovary and tube and removed them. The right ovary was so firmly adherent to the bowel that its removal meant almost certain laceration of that viscus; it was, moreover, hard and evidently contained no pus; it was therefore allowed to remain. The corresponding tube, which was distended with pus, was separated with considerable difficulty from its plastic relations, and removed.

The seat of the operation was flushed with carbolized water; the peritoneum sewed with continuous catgut sutures; a glass drainage-tube inserted in the inferior angle of the wound (to be removed in 24–48 hours, if possible); the fascia, together with the abdominal wall, sewed with interrupted silk sutures; iodoformed lint and gauze laid on, in layers; and a wad of antiseptic cotton applied under a binder.

Prof. Polk remarked that these were the sort of cases he would formerly have refused to operate upon. But of late his views have changed in this regard. And, although the operation had lasted nearly two hours, he believed the patient's chances of recovery about as good as after an ordinary oöphorectomy. He said it would surprise him very much if the patient were to die.

The operation could have been much more quickly performed had the old method of procedure been followed; namely, a longer incision, and the removal of the intestines from the pelvis and placing them upon the abdomen (there covered with hot wet towels), to permit of inspection as an aid in separating the adhesions. But the result would be, almost certainly, a fatal termination to the case. It makes a vast difference whether adhesions are of years' or of months' standing. Old adhesions, such as were present in this case, bind the viscera so closely together that it is almost impossible to distinguish one tissue from another. And it is only by the slowest and most careful procedure that separation may be safely accomplished. Had the right ovary been found to contain pus, he would, nevertheless, not have attempted its removal, but would have laid it open, washed it out, and inserted a drainage-tube into it.

———

—The *Boston Med. and Surg. Journal*, Feb. 28, says: From a report laid before the Dominion Parliament, it appears that there are at present nineteen lepers confined in the Dominion lazaretto at Tracadie, New Brunswick—eight males and eleven females. During the year two new patients were admitted from the surrounding country. Last year one of the male lepers escaped from the institution to the United States, where he has been located by the Dominion officials.

BOSTON CORRESPONDENCE.

(FROM OUR OWN CORRESPONDENT.)

Progressive Muscular Atrophy.—Supra-pubic Prostatectomy.—Chronic Arsenical Poisoning, especially from Wall-Paper.

BOSTON, March 11, 1889.

At the last meeting of the Boston Society for Medical Improvement, Dr. Philip Coombs Knapp showed a case of progressive muscular atrophy, the most interesting feature of which was the man's age, viz., sixty-eight years, since it is a very rare thing to find this disease coming on so late in life. Reference was made to Gowers, who says that progressive muscular atrophy may come on at various periods until seventy years of age; but during this latter period it is surely very rare. In the case exhibited, the appearance of the disease dated back only about six months. It commenced with a wasting and numbness of the hand. The reaction of the muscles showed the ordinary changes of degeneration. There was no sensory disturbance to be made out, and the probable onset of bulbar disturbance made the case quite clear. There was no difficulty of swallowing and no exaggeration of the reflexes.

Dr. F. S. Watson reported a most interesting case of profuse hæmaturia, in which the operation of supra-pubic prostatectomy was performed, followed by recovery. The patient, whose age was sixty-nine years, had been in excellent health until ten years previously, when symptoms of urinary obstruction due to hypertrophied prostate appeared. The use of a catheter kept him comfortable until about three years ago, when there was blood in the urine due to profuse hemorrhage into the bladder. During the next two years he had two or three other attacks of bleeding, since which they have been more frequent, occurring latterly about once in two months. The attacks were characterized by the loss of a large quantity of blood at the onset, then there was a diminution in the quantity during the following days, until, at the end of about a week, the urine was quite clear. The hemorrhages were independent of exertion and there was no pain, excepting from the retention of clots and over-distention of the bladder. The patient thought he had noticed fleshy bits in the urine, and he stated that an eminent physician in New York had told him that a villous growth could be plainly seen through the cystoscope.

When the patient first visited Dr. Watson he was very anæmic and weak from the effects of a hemorrhage that occurred about a month before. Although examination of the urine for several days failed to detect any positive evidence of a bladder tumor, the hemorrhages were undoubtedly of bladder origin; and, moreover, they were increasing in severity and occurring at diminishing intervals, so that they pointed to a fatal termination. On this account an operation was determined upon, and as the patient had an hypertrophied prostate, together with a large and distensible bladder, it was decided to open the bladder above the pubes. The cystotomy was performed in the manner recommended by Petersen. When opened the inner surface of the bladder was found to be entirely smooth and no villous or other growth was present, except the projecting lateral portions of a greatly enlarged prostate. They were connected by a less prominent median ridge, which, sometime previously, had been perforated by an instrument about half way from its base, and, about this hole were flabby and exuberant granulations. The lateral lobes of the hypertrophied prostate were divided into halves by a blunt bistoury, and each portion was removed to its base by a wire écraseur. The median portion was then removed with scissors and the curette, thus clearing away the granulating surface. The wounds were left open and a large, double, rubber drainage tube was placed in them, reaching to the bottom of the bladder. There was little hemorrhage, either during or after the operation, and it ceased on the fourth day.

This operation was performed three months ago—and there has been no hemorrhage since. With the exception of one or two attacks of heart failure the patient had a good convalescence, and went home at the end of six weeks from the date of the operation. The peculiarity of this case is that the hypertrophied prostate simulated in its symptoms bladder growths.

Dr. Watson thought that an attempt at removal by operative procedure should be made if a diagnosis of a bladder tumor, probably benign, is made. If, however, the tumor is believed to be cancerous, it had better be left to itself if it is not attended with pain ; but when there is much pain associated with it, palliative measures by drainage should be attempted. Quoting from his own writings, Dr. Watson said that advice as to operative interference in cases of prostatic hypertrophy should be based upon the following indications: "Necessary, frequent (once an hour), painful catheterization, or urination without the catheter, especially when accompanied by a foul or hemorrhagic cystitis; attacks of retention; and failure to relieve such condition by palliative treatment."

The notes on twenty-five cases in which arsenic was found in the urine formed the basis of a most interesting contribution on chronic arsenical poisoning, especially from wall-paper, by Dr. James J. Putnam. In this paper he said that the time has nearly gone by when fair-minded persons, who have taken pains to investigate the evidence, need to be convinced that arsenical wallpapers and fabrics may be a source of poisoning. The problems of chief importance at present are : how we may learn to recognize with greater confidence the less typical cases ; how we may persuade our legislators to give us due protection against this widespread public danger. It has been asserted by our chemists that the dangers from these sources are by no means so great as formerly, but it is evident that they are still far from being obviated. Acute arsenical poisoning has long been familiar to toxicologists, and the subacute form is usually easily recognized ; but in the chronic varieties we have only the shadows of these characteristic symptoms to guide us ; and, moreover, we may be led astray by the fact that the arsenic may only act by bringing out the latent weaknesses of the patient. The most convincing symptom is neuritis of a sufficiently advanced degree as to cause changes in electrical reaction, diminution of cutaneous sensibility, and impairment of motor power or of coördination. Another important physical sign is a peculiar browning of the skin, especially of the face. Still another important sign is albuminuria, with casts and sometimes blood in the sediment. Cerebral symptoms, such as vertigo, impairment of memory and mental endurance, and rarely epileptiform seizures, are met with in cases of chronic arsenical as in lead poisoning ; and they may be suggestive, if not characteristic, if other causes can be excluded.

Dr. Putnam then gave in detail the history of certain cases that had come under his observation, and especially the case of a woman forty-three years of age, naturally of good health and habits. The symptoms pointing toward possible chronic arsenical poisoning, the wall-papers were examined and a large quantity of arsenic was found in two of them, which covered the walls of three rooms. The largest amount was found

·in the room used by the patient as a bed-room. A month later the urine of the patient, on analysis, was found to contain a very large quantity of arsenic. After various vicissitudes in cleaning lodgings and wall-papers there was, some months later, a marked improvement in the symptoms; but the continued presence of arsenic in the urine rendered it probable that the poison was still given off from sources still accessible.

A most interesting discussion followed this paper, and among other speakers Dr. Edward S. Wood, the expert in toxicology, said he thought the only way we shall ever be able to get a law restricting the sale and manufacture of arsenical wall-papers, is by being able to bring forward a large number of accurately reported and well-authenticated cases of arsenical poisoning, in which there is no doubt whatever as to the presence of arsenic in the system, and when we are able to state accurately, or at any rate within narrow limits, the amount of arsenic in a wall-paper which has proved dangerous. Dr. Wood thinks it is very difficult to make any accurate statement in regard to the time of elimination of the arsenic. There are certain cases which seem to show that it requires six or eight months for arsenic to be entirely eliminated from the system. The number of sources for the absorption of arsenic is so great that it is very difficult to say when all of the sources of poisoning have been entirely removed. This seems to him a fair explanation of the continuation of the arsenic in the economy in some of these long-continued cases.

PERISCOPE.

Three Remarkable Cases of Actinomycosis.

Bertha reports from Wöfler's Clinic at Graz to the *Wiener med. Wochenschrift*, No. 35, 1888, three cases of actinomycosis, which are interesting both from the seat of the disease and the mode of infection. It is highly probable that in all three a direct infection of the person was received through the actinomyces clinging to grain, while we are usually accustomed to consider animals affected with actinomyces as the agents of the infection.

In the first case, a laborer, 52 years old, in the act of drinking, swallowed the beard of an ear of corn, which stuck in his pharynx. An inflammatory affection of the throat resembling an abscess developed, but apparently healed after surgical treatment; after three years, however, it relapsed and was recognized as actinomycosis. In both the other cases, there was an actinomycotic affection of the hands in persons who handled grain.

Such localized actinomycotic affections on the hand and leg have been described only once hitherto in literature, but in Bertha's opinion are not so very rare; they have often been erroneously regarded as lupoid or tuberculous.—*Centralblatt f. d. med. Wissenschaften,* Jan. 12, 1889.

Relation of Purpura to Malignant Disease.

The causation of the purpura which has been noticed in connection with malignant disease, especially sarcoma, has not yet been satisfactorily determined. With the view of throwing some light on the obscure subject, Dr. Thomas Harris communicates to the *Medical Chronicle*, Feb., 1889, an account of a case in which he had occasion to make an autopsy. The patient was a young man who had died a few hours after admission to the Manchester Royal Infirmary. The body, a fairly nourished one, was markedly anemic. All over the trunk and limbs were a large number of petechial hemorrhages into the skin. In the mediastinum was a tumor the size of a goose-egg, apparently a firm lymphosarcoma. The right pleura showed signs of what appeared to be acute inflammation, and the cavity was distended with a quantity of thin blood. Petechial hemorrhages were present in the stomach, intestine, peritoneum, and pericardium. The spleen was increased in size, weighing eight ounces, and was of a pale-red color. No growth except the one in the mediastinum was evident to the naked eye, and the chief change from the normal presented by the organs throughout the body was one of anemia.

After giving some of the cases observed by the late Dr. Hilton Fagge, he discusses the theories as to the causation of the purpura, especially in his own case. He rejects the view that there might have been minute developments of sarcomatous tissue, with growths made up of embryonic cells at points which became the seats of the petechiæ. He also is disinclined to believe that the malignant disease had caused a profound alteration of the blood, analogous to that found in pernicious anemia, and that the hemorrhages were due to this. For a microscopical examination of the liver, and especially of the kidneys, showed that in those organs there were emoboli, composed of minute masses of tissue similar in appearance to that composing the mediastinal growth. Although he found no emboli in the vessels of the skin, he nevertheless regards the purpura that occurred in his case as due to emboli lodging in the small vessels.

___

Prevention of Phthisis.

Dr. J. E. Squire read a paper on prevention of phthisis before the Epidemiological Society of London, January 9, 1889. He said that phthisis took its place with bronchitis as one of the most frequent causes of death in this country, and its importance is the greater as it carries off its victims during adolescence and adult life. The discovery of the bacillus tuberculosis allows us to place phthisis in close relation to infectious diseases, toward the control of which preventive medicine has already done so much; and experiments have proved that tubercular disease can be communicated from affected to healthy animals. That consumption can be communicated from person to person has long been a popular belief, and cases were referred to by Dr. Squire which seemed to prove it. Phthisis depends primarily upon the reception into the body of an infective particle or micro-organism; but a lowered vitality of the tissues places them in a more favorable condition for the development of the bacillus, and thus constitutes in the individual a predisposition to the disease. The bacillus may gain entrance into the body (1) by inoculation through a cut or scratch; (2) by means of the genito-urinary mucous membrane; (3) by the product of conception, and by direct hereditary transmission; (4) by the mucous membrane of the alimentary canal; (5) by the mucous membrane of the respiratory tract, and by the air-cells of the lungs.

The possibility of infection through the alimentary tract assumes importance from the prevalence of tuberculosis in animals which are used as food, and from the experimental proof of the infectiveness of the milk of tuberculous cows. The necessity for careful inspection of cattle kept for dairy purposes and for precautions in using the milk, and possibly also the flesh of diseased animals was pointed out. But as infection through the respiratory system is more potent and probably more frequent than by any other means, and as the risk of infection is intensified by close contact and by the crowding together of sick and healthy, the necessity for free ventilation is apparent, and becomes more so when the predisposing causes are considered. These are: (1) hereditary predisposition; (2) influence of air and sunlight; (3) age and sex; (4) effect of certain occupations; (5) influence of locality and habitation, which includes the consideration of climate, temperature, altitude, nature of the soil, density of population, and the condition of dwelling-houses, both as to their construction and the overcrowding of the inmates; (6) influence of certain diseases, local and general. Indoor and sedentary occupations, as well as those in which much dust is inhaled, largely influences the prevalence of phthisis. Much of this amongst persons following such occupations is preventable. Here again the basis of all preventive measures is found in efficient ventilation. The home-workers—for example, tailors—are more difficult to deal with than the factory hands; but public workrooms, in which men can find conveniences for their work, may lessen the evils of the present state of things. With regard to climate, its influence in the causation of phthisis is probably infinitesimal as compared with the effect of density of population. Overcrowding is of two kinds: the aggregation of buildings on a confined area, with insufficient open space around and between houses, and the crowding together of persons within the houses.

By-laws should be enforced regulating the width of streets, the amount of open space around houses, the minimum height of rooms and size of windows, and efficient inspection of new houses should be carried out before they are allowed to be occupied. Tenement houses might be licensed to hold a certain number of inmates, and be liable to inspection. As many diseases producing general debility thereby predispose to tuberculosis, general sanitary and hygienic measures, framed for the control of these, tend to diminish the amount of phthisis in a community; and seeing that insufficiency of food, of fresh air, and of exercise, continued anxiety and mental depression, and dissipation, must be reckoned amongst the predisposing causes, the philanthropist might assist the sanitarian. The fundamental principles which must form the basis of any successful attempts to diminish the prevalence of phthisis are (1) to provide a sufficiency of fresh air in and around dwellings and workplaces; and (2) to endeavor to improve the resisting power of the individual by physical training during the period of growth and development, and by exercise and recreation alternating with the work of maturer age. As the effects of phthisis are handed down by hereditary transmission from parent to child, any causes which tend to increase tubercular disease amongst the adult members of a population must be regarded as tending to produce a progressive deterioration of race. It is, therefore, to the interest of the community to allow no time to be lost in commencing a systematic attack against the preventable causes of phthisis.—*British Med. Journal*, Jan. 26, 1889.

Spinal Hemorrhage with Pyrexia.

Before the Staffordshire Branch of the British Medical Association, Nov. 30, 1888, Dr. Arlidge related a case of hemorrhage within the sheath of the spinal cord, attended with high temperature. The patient was a well-built and well-nourished man, but of drunken habits, 44 years old. He was admitted into the North Staffordshire Infirmary on September 19 last, having four days previously been suddenly seized with complete loss of power over his legs. The attack was preceded for a day or two by a slight feeling of *malaise*, but he had never been laid up with serious illness, and never had syphilis or rheumatism, nor had he suffered any hurt to the spinal column. There was complete motor paralysis of the legs, and some weakness in the arms, where too formication and numbness were experienced. Sensation was normal, and the legs were painless and their reflexes abolished. His only complaint was of dorsal pain. The bladder was distended, and, prior to admission, had been emptied by the catheter; but there was no dribbling of urine. Some rhonchi were noted in the upper part of the left lung; heart healthy; bowels confined for four days; the cerebrum undisturbed. The first temperature taken was 103.6°, but the next day it fluctuated between 105° and 106°, and rose to 107.4° the day preceding his death, on September 26, and was accompanied by some delirium. A post-mortem examination revealed a copious hemorrhage within the meninges of the spinal cord, extending downward from the last cervical vertebra for about six inches. The blood was coagulated. No ruptured vessel was found in the cord itself, and no cerebral disease, although the dura mater was very adherent to the skull. There was no fracture of the spine, and no caries of any vertebra. Dr. Arlidge called attention to the suddenness of the onset of the paralysis and the high temperature, the former phenomenon being characteristic of spinal hemorrhage, whilst the latter was an altogether exceptional occurrence. Other points of interest were the stillness of the paralyzed limbs, their freedom from spasm, and likewise from hyperæsthesia and anæsthesia alike; and, lastly, the absence of any physical injury, or of evident antecedent spinal lesion, to account for the production of the hemorrhage.—*British Med. Journal*, December 22, 1888.

An Unusual Cause of Asthma.

Professor Leyden had recently under treatment a young woman who suffered from extremely irritable cough, with some pain in the neck. The diagnosis he made was that of bronchial catarrh combined with asthma. The remedies he prescribed were of little use. He then sent the patient to Schwalbach, but this also proved of no avail. It was then proposed that she should spend the winter in a warm climate, when she appeared one day with the gratifying intelligence that she was now quite well. Upon drinking a cup of tea that morning she was seized with an exceedingly violent fit of coughing, so that she thought she would have been choked. Suddenly, however, she coughed up a small portion of bone, and having got rid of that her cough was at an end. It seems that some eight or nine months previously she swallowed a piece of bone while eating, which caused a most violent attack of coughing. She immediately sought the aid of a medical man, who passed a probang, but found nothing. Ever since that time she had suffered from the cough and from severe pains in the throat, for which she ultimately consulted Professor Leyden. It is impossible to say exactly where this splinter had lodged, but having sharp points, these were probably embedded in the mucous membrane of one of the bronchi. A somewhat similar case is mentioned as having occurred under the care of Professor Bardeleben in the Charité, Berlin, where a case of persistent hoarseness was found after death to be accounted for by the lodgment of a coin (a one-mark piece) below the right vocal cord.—*Lancet*, Feb. 16, 1889.

—Diphtheria is prevalent in the neighborhood of Macungie, Pa.

THE
MEDICAL AND SURGICAL
REPORTER.

ISSUED EVERY SATURDAY.

CHARLES W. DULLES, M.D.,
EDITOR AND PUBLISHER.

The Terms of Subscription to the serial publications of this office are as follows, payable in advance:

Med. and Surg. Reporter (weekly), a year, **$5.00**
Quarterly Compendium of Med. Science, -   2.50
Reporter and Compendium,   -   -   -   - 6.00
Physician's Daily Pocket Record,   -   - 1.00
Reporter and Pocket Record, -   -   -   - 6.00
Reporter, Compendium, and Pocket Record, 7.00

All checks and postal orders should be drawn to order of

CHARLES W. DULLES,
N. E. Cor. 13th and Walnut Streets,
P. O. Box 843.   Philadelphia, Pa.

☞SUGGESTIONS TO SUBSCRIBERS:
See that your address-label gives the date to which your subscription is paid.
In requesting a change of address, give the old address as well as the new one.
If your REPORTER does not reach you promptly and regularly, notify the publisher *at once*, so that the cause may be discovered and corrected.
☞SUGGESTIONS TO CONTRIBUTORS AND CORRESPONDENTS:
Write in ink.
Write on one side of paper only.
Write on paper of the size usually used for letters.
Make as few paragraphs as possible. Punctuate carefully. Do not abbreviate, or omit words like "the," and "a," or "an."
Make communications as short as possible.
NEVER ROLL A MANUSCRIPT! Try to get an envelope or wrapper which will fit it.
When it is desired to call our attention to something in a newspaper, mark the passage boldly with a colored pencil, and write on the Wrapper "Marked copy." Unless this is done, newspapers are not looked at.
The Editor will be glad to get medical news, but it is important that brevity and actual interest shall characterize communications intended for publication.

HEAD-DOWNWARD PRESENTATION.

The remarkable fact that in about ninety-six per cent. of cases of labor the fœtus is born head first has attracted attention since the days of Hippocrates, and doubtless long before. Nor is it less striking that in about seventy-five per cent. of labors the child should assume one relation to the mother— that the fœtal occiput should be in relation with the left anterior segment of the mother's pelvis. The oldest known theory in explanation of these facts is that of Hippocrates, which supposes that the fœtus is originally head uppermost in the uterus, where it is held by bands proceding from the umbilicus until the seventh month, the legal time of labor, when these bands break, and the fœtus, from its own weight, turns a somersault, and so places itself head-downward. Ambroise Paré asserted that the fœtus instinctively placed itself head-downward because delivery is easiest in that position. Paul Dubois, after satisfying himself that the fœtus does not present head downward because of gravity, since the centre of gravity of the fœtus is not situated in the head, but at a point in the trunk near it, returned to the theory of Paré, that the fœtus, by instinctive or voluntary determination, makes certain movements until it finds the position most favorable for its sojourn in the uterus, and for its delivery from it. Simpson denied that the fœtus is able to make voluntary movements; and declared that the attitude of the fœtus is produced by reflex movements induced by a lack of relation between the contour of the fœtal ovoid and the containing uterine walls; that after the seventh month of pregnancy both the fœtus and womb are ovoidal in form, the wide end of the fœtal ovoid being at the breech, the wide end of the uterine ovoid at the fundus; and hence that irritation and reflex movements ensue until corresponding diameters of each come into relation with those of the other, when irritation ceases and the presentation becomes fixed and definite.

Matthew Duncan still insists that the attitude of the fœtus *in utero* is produced by the laws of gravity, and he offers elaborate explanations of various facts which apparently conflict with this view. Credé, Kristeller and others attach much importance to the intermittent contractions of the uterus throughout pregnancy, as a cause of the attitude of the fœtus. Pajot considers the form of the matured ovum, the dimensions of the uterus, and the fact that it is alternately in a state of motion and repose, as the determining causes of the attitude of the fœtus.

Other and less celebrated theories have

been offered, until, as Charpentier says, there are explanations enough, but unfortunately there are objections to each.

In the *Edinburgh Medical Journal*, September and October, 1888, Dr. James Foulis contributes an interesting and elaborate paper on the cause of head-downward presentation and the first cranial position. He reviews the theories of Simpson and Duncan, points out the objections—more especially to the theory of Simpson—and rejects them both. The principal objection which is urged against the theory of Simpson is his assumption that the uterus has a fixed and definite form independent of the form of the fœtus—spheroidal before the sixth month, and ovoidal after that time.

Dr. Foulis asserts that the head-downward presentation of the child *in utero* is the necessary and ultimate consequence of the continued extension of the child's lower limbs against the most resisting parts of the uterine sac. Before the seventh month, and to a certain extent after this time, when the fœtus has a considerable amount of mobility within the uterus, extension of the child's legs must drive the head along the surface of the uterine wall; and since the feet meet with the firmest resistance from the maternal pelvis, the ultimate consequence of the movements must be to bring the head downward, which position is maintained in the later weeks either by the straitened room of the fœtus limiting its mobility, or by the head entering the true pelvis as a ball in a cup.

Dr. Foulis maintains that the first cranial position is produced by the continued extension of the child's lower limbs against the most resisting part of the uterine sac at its upper part—namely, that which lies in the right hypochondrium, under the liver—after the child has assumed the head-downward position.

The arguments of Dr. Foulis are certainly ingenious, and are apparently based on that foundation of medicine, anatomy; but we are not convinced that his explanations are truer or his arguments better than are those which he seeks to overthrow. It seems plain that the attitude of the fœtus in its relations to the mother, is produced by no one cause, but that it is the result of the combined action of several causes; these are: the form of the matured ovum, the dimensions (its shape being variable) of the uterus, gravity, the intermittent contractions of the uterus, the varying amount of liquor amnii, and the movements of the fœtus—all of which usually act in harmony to bring about the head-downward presentation of the fœtus. Other presentations occur under unusual conditions, as when the relation of the diameters of the uterus is altered by flaccidity of its walls, or by deformity of the pelvis; when its axis is altered by relaxation of the abdominal parietes; when the form of the fœtus is abnormal, as in hydrocephalus; or perhaps when an ill-timed, vigorous, extension of the child's legs produces other than a head presentation, which altered presentation becomes permanent owing to the straitened room of the fœtus, which limits subsequent mobility.

The writer's argument that the first cranial position is most frequent because the child's lower extremities meet with more resistance, in extension, in the right upper segment of the uterus—owing to its location under the liver—than in the left upper segment, and hence that the dorsal region of the child is pushed over to the left, is not so happy. How on this ground can it be explained that the position second in frequency is the very reverse of this—occiput to the right and posterior? The usual explanation is more satisfactory.

But while his conclusions may not be accepted, Dr. Foulis has presented an ingenious explanation of the result of the movements of the child in utero; and his scholarly paper has called the attention of the profession anew to the subject of the accommodation of the fœtus—one of the most interesting problems in physiology.

HOSPITAL TREATMENT.

There is an impression, quite general among the poor, that entrance into a hospital as a patient involves the risk of becoming the subject of experimentation by the physicians and surgeons connected with the institution. This is especially the case in regard to hospitals connected with medical schools; and very recently an English writer who takes the name of Æsculapius Scalpel has done what he could, in a book called "St. Bernard's," to confirm this impression where it exists, and to create it where it has not already taken root, by describing the experiences and observations of an assistant in a large hospital. The scenes described in this book are too real and too like the truth to be scoffed at as wholly untrue, although the way in which they are used is unfair and unjust. There can be no doubt that the author is one who has walked the wards of an English hospital, and has witnessed occurrences which seemed to him cruel and unfeeling. No one who has seen much of hospitals in any land can deny that operations are sometimes performed in them with apparently less regard for the good of the patient than the eagerness to seize opportunities for demonstration. Nor can any one who has studied physical diagnosis much have failed, we believe, to have seen cases in which persons weary and worn with disease have been subjected to examinations too repeated and too prolonged for the benefit of students.

It is not altogether amiss, then, for those who pursue science ardently to be reminded that those whom they find interesting subjects of investigation have feelings and rights which ought to be respected; but it is far from right for an author to sanction the idea that hospital doctors, as a rule, disregard these feelings and rights. In this country, certainly, the men who have charge of hospital patients are not generally unfeeling; and those who are under their care usually enjoy the blessing of skilful treatment combined with humane consideration to an extent which more than counterbalances the unavoidable disadvantages of their situation.

BEQUESTS OF ISAIAH V. WILLIAMSON TO MEDICAL CHARITIES.

In the will of the late Isaiah V. Williamson, of Philadelphia, who died March 7, 1889, leaving an estate valued at about ten millions of dollars, the following bequests of interest to medical men were made: To the Pennsylvania Hospital $100,000; $50,000 each to the Episcopal Hospital, the University of Pennsylvania and the University Hospital; $40,000 each to the Children's Hospital, the Women's Hospital, the Orthopædic Hospital, and the Woman's Medical College. The testator expressed the desire that these sums should be invested by the recipients, and he directs that the income shall be expended for the establishment of free beds only. By this it is probable he meant the maintenance of free beds, as the invested funds would serve to establish them.

One of the items of this will directs the investment of $300,000 by trustees, who are directed to pay five per cent. of the income —which would be about $500 annually—to the Philadelphia Lying-in Charity. Three per cent., or about $300 a year, is to be paid to the Philadelphia Dispensary. Two per cent., or about $200 a year, is to be paid to the Northern Dispensary, and a like amount to the Howard Hospital (a dispensary) and to the Church Dispensary at Southwark—a portion of Philadelphia.

These bequests, with others to non-medical charities, make up a principal sum of a million dollars, and within a few months Mr. Williamson established a trust for a training school for boys, with a gift of $3,000,000.

In this way it will be seen that he has furnished another striking example of the way in which wealthy men in this country often use their wealth for the good of their fellow-men—a thing which has no adequate counterpart in any country in the world.

MEETING OF THE AMERICAN MEDICAL ASSOCIATION.

The Local Committee at Newport, R. I., decided some time ago, after consultation with some of the officers of the American Medical Association, to change the date of the next meeting of the Association, to be held at Newport, to June 25–28, because that date offered better opportunities for the entertainment of the members. Dr. Horatio R. Storer, Chairman of the Committee of Arrangements, has issued a notice stating that the general Sessions will be held at the Music Hall, Bellevue Avenue, adjoining the Ocean House, and those of the Sections at the Newport Casino, which is also close at hand, and which, for the first time in its history and as an act of courtesy, is permitted by its Governors to be occupied for other than the purpose for which it was built.

The hotels at Newport are, in order of their nearness to the place of meeting, the Ocean House, the Clifton House, the Germania Hotel, Pinard's, Hartmann's, the Aquidneck, Brayton's, the Kay Street House, the Perry House, the Park House, the Sherman House, the Cliff Avenue Hotel, and Bateman's.

The approaching meeting of the American Medical Association occurs nearly synchronously with the two hundred and fiftieth anniversary of the settlement of Newport. The city authorities, Dr. Storer says, will probably fittingly recognize the presence of the National Medical Convention at such a moment, the more cordially since the virtual founder of the colony, certainly its principal leader, John Clark, was a physician. The Mayor of the City was one of the incorporators, in 1879, of the Newport Sanitary Protection Association.

Members of the Association or others who intend to be present may get any information they may desire from any member, preferably the Chairmen of the various sub-committees, which are constituted as follows:

Of *Finance*, Drs. F. H. Rankin, H. G. MacKaye and G. D. Hersey; of *Reception*, Drs. H. E. Turner and G. M. Odell; of *Halls and Accommodations*, Drs. C. F. Barker and M. E. Baldwin; of *Entertainment*, Drs. S. H. Sears and T. A. Kenefick; of *Invitations*, Drs. W. C. Rives and G. T. Swarts; of *Registration*, Drs. H. Ecroyd, Jr., and W. S. Sherman; of *Exhibits*, Drs. C. A. Brackett and E. P. Robinson; of *Transportation*, Drs. P. F. Curley and W. H. Palmer; of *Section Work and Programme*, the Chairman, Dr. H. R. Storer, and the Local Secretary, Dr. Valentine Mott Francis. All of these gentlemen may be addressed at Newport, R. I., except Dr. Hersey, Dr. Swarts and Dr. Palmer, who live at Providence, R. I.

Members of the Association desiring to read papers should address the Chairman or Secretary of the various Sections, who were named in the REPORTER, March 2, p. 287.

It is hoped that the next meeting of the Association, which will be its fortieth annual meeting, will be a large and successful one, and that it will serve to cement anew the bonds of sympathy which ought to unite the profession in all parts of the United States.

PRESERVATION OF CHLOROFORM.

As many of the accidents which follow the administration of chloroform as an anæsthetic, are believed to be due to impurity, it is important to know the best means of preserving it from change after it has been manufactured. This subject has recently been discussed by M. Marty, in the *Archives de Médecine et de Pharmacie Militaires*, and he suggests that chloroform should be kept in bottles of yellow glass, with ground glass stoppers, which have been thoroughly cleaned and dried, and that to the chloroform should be added one thousandth part of its weight of pure and absolute ethylic alcohol.

—John L. Adams, who was undergoing a long fast, died March 13. He had entered upon his twenty-seventh day of fasting, and was greatly emaciated.

BOOK REVIEWS.

THE YEAR BOOK OF TREATMENT FOR 1889. BEING A CRITICAL REVIEW OF THE PRACTICE OF MEDICINE AND SURGERY DURING 1888. 8vo, pp. viii, 344. Philadelphia: Lea Bros. & Co., 1889. Price, $1 25.

Those who are familiar with the admirable predecessors to this little book will be glad to know that the volume for 1889 is now issued. It contains a brief summary of the progress in therapeutics during 1888 and appears very promptly after the conclusion of the year it covers. If it were nothing but an uncolored summary, it would have its advantages, but it is far more; for the articles are prepared by men well known in this profession, and specially fitted for the task; and they bear the stamp of the individuality of each. In regard to the book before us, it is enough to say that it is calculated to maintain the excellent reputation of the series to which it belongs, and we wish it success equal to its merit.

EXPLORATION OF THE CHEST IN HEALTH AND DISEASE. By STEPHEN SMITH BURT, M.D., Professor of Clinical Medicine and Physical Diagnosis in the New York Post-Graduate Medical School and Hospital, etc. Small 8vo, pp. xiii, 206. New York: D. Appleton & Co., 1889. Price, $1.50.

The author of this book, in his preface, states that it has been prepared in response to requests from members of his classes for a work which should embody his views; and his book indicates his familiarity with the wants of persons studying physical diagnosis. It is plain, practical and sensible The style is pleasant, the teaching is sound, and the whole is beautifully illustrated with wood-cuts and photo-engravings. In looking over the book, we note with satisfaction that the author does not fall into the error of speaking of heart murmurs as if they were pathognomic, taken by themselves. This is a point of great importance in physical diagnosis; for serious and damaging blunders can be made if heart murmurs are not studied in connection with other signs of disease or health

In other respects this book will be found a trustworthy guide, and it may be heartily commended to the attention of our readers.

PAMPHLET NOTICES.

226. BELOW SEA-LEVEL. NATURE'S PNEUMATIC CABINET – HIGH ALTITUDES OF SOUTHERN CALIFORNIA. By WALTER LINDLEY, M.D., Los Angeles, Cal. From the *Medical Record* and the *Southern California Practitioner*. 12 pages.

227. DOUBLE CHORIO-RETINITIS WITH PARTIAL DEGENERATION OF THE OPTIC NERVE, ETC. By CHARLES A. OLIVER, M D., Philadelphia From the *Trans. of the Amer. Ophthalmological Society*, 1887. 6 pages.

228. THE RADICAL CURE OF VARICOCELE, ATTENDED WITH REDUNDANCY OF THE SCROTUM, DEMONSTRATED BY TIME. By MORRIS H. HENRY, M.D, New York From the *Journal of the Amer. Med. Association*, Nov. 10, 1888. 12 pages.

229. THE HISTORY OF THE FILARIA SANGUINIS HOMINIS, ETC By WILLIAM M. MASTIN, M.D., Mobile, A a From the *Annals of Surgery*, November, 1888. 42 pages.

230. INFLATION OF THE STOMACH WITH HYDROGEN GAS IN THE DIAGNOSIS OF WOUNDS AND PERFORATIONS OF THIS ORGAN. By N. SENN, M.D., Milwaukee, Wis. From the *Medical News*, August 25, 1888. 11 pages.

226. Dr. Lindley's first paper calls attention to that part of San Diego County in California known as the San Felipe Sink, or the Conchilla Valley, a basin about thirty miles wide and one hundred and thirty miles long and depressed below the sea-level, at its lowest point, about three hundred and sixty feet. This he thinks would be a sort of natural pneumatic cabinet and good for phthisical or asthmatic persons. Dr Lindley's second paper describes the natural advantages of the San Jacinto Mountains in Southern California as a resort for persons affected with diseases of the lungs The descriptions of the beauty and grandeur of these mountains are interspersed with incidental allusions to persons who have been benefited by residing among or on them.

227. The case described by Dr. Oliver was that of a boy, 12 years old, who in addition to the trouble indicated in that part of the title given above, had very curious lymph extravasations upon the retina of one eye and floating free in the vitreous humor of the other. The excellent description of these conditions is very much enhanced in value by two beautiful chromo-lithographs prepared from water color sketches made by Dr. P. N. K. Schwenk.

228. Dr. Henry is well known as an earnest advocate of excision of a portion of the redundant scrotum for the cure of varicocele—an operation first proposed by Sir Astley Cooper, revived by Dr. Edward H. Dixon, in this country, and adopted by Dr. Henry about 30 years ago. Dr. Henry has now operated in this way fifty-nine times, and thinks as highly of the operation as ever.

229. Dr. Mastin's pamphlet contains a full and scholarly summary of our knowledge of the filaria sanguinis hominis, with especial reference to the observations in regard to it which have been made in the United States, and its relation to chylocele of the tunica vaginalis testis. It is illustrated with three woodcuts, contains a table of thirteen cases seen in this country and concludes with a full bibliography of the literature of the subject.

230. Dr. Senn's pamphlet describes his experiments to prove that the method of inflating the intestines, which he demonstrated so brilliantly at the last meeting of the American Medical Association, could be applied to the stomach, to detect perforations, together with the account of a case in which he successfully applied it to the human subject. This paper is not only very interesting, but a so a valuable and instructive contribution to the literature of surgery.

CORRESPONDENCE.

Compound Fracture of the Skull.

To THE EDITOR.

Sir: Burton Unkerfer, 13 years old, was kicked by a horse on the left side of his forehead over the eye. The wound was one and one-half inch long by three-fourths of an inch wide, and extended through the skin, bone and brain - membranes. The edges of the bone around the wound were almost as smooth as if they had been cut with a sharp instrument. The fragments of bone were driven through the membranes into the brain, and were completely covered with clotted blood and pulpified brain matter. The wound looked as though the bone had been removed. I began to examine the wound, and soon found that I could not do so satisfactorily without the use of an anæsthetic. I therefore called in consultation Dr. J. N. Ketcherside, who administered chloroform; and we then proceeded with great care to explore the wound and remove the fragments of bone. We did not quit until we were perfectly satisfied that every piece of bone had been removed. In all we removed seven pieces, the largest of which was about three-fourths of an inch long by one-fourth of an inch wide. All clots and contused tissues were carefully removed. We then allowed the patient to rally from the anæsthetic, dressed the wound with a solution of chlorate of potash, and left it open for twenty-four hours, covered constantly with cloths wet in the solution. I left bromide of potash and ergot to be taken every two hours, aconite to control fever if it should arise, and opiates to control pain if any should be felt. I visited him next day and found him doing well. The wound was therefore closed. At the time of closure the brain and edges of the membranes were protruding considerably, but I pressed them back and closed the wound up entirely, except one small place left open for drainage. Nothing of any morbid nature interfered after this except a small fungus growth, which was removed by gentle washings.

The patient entirely recovered, and at this time, two years since the accident, has all his former characteristics unmodified. All that is left to show that he was once hurt is the cicatrix. I attribute the success obtained in this case to the thoroughness with which the fragments of both bone and flesh were removed, and also to good after-treatment. One object should always be in view in such cases, viz., to leave nothing in the wound to irritate the parts, and not be in a hurry to get through.

Yours truly,
S. M. HUNTER, M. D.

Hope, Kansas,
March 9, 1889.

Abortion, with Placenta Previa.

To THE EDITOR.

Sir: At 9 o'clock on the evening of Feb. 10, 1889, I was called to see Mrs. S., 19 years old, five months advanced in a second pregnancy. During the preceding two weeks she had been troubled with feelings of general discomfort, but no symptoms of a definite nature occurred until the day on which I saw her, when irregular pains in the back and pelvis, accompanied with moderate hemorrhage, had been going on for several hours. Without making an examination, I informed her of the threatening miscarriage, and ordered one quarter grain of morphine, to be repeated in forty-five minutes if the pains and hemorrhage persisted. Cold compresses were applied to the hypogastrium, and the thighs were raised on pillows.

At 2 o'clock the following morning I was hastily summoned to see her, and found her experiencing hard expulsive pains with a small amount of hemorrhage. Examination revealed a bag of waters of considerable dimensions, low in the vagina. Having no suspicion of anything being abnormal, I ruptured the membranes without attempting to diagnosticate the presentation, and was considerably surprised to find nothing presenting, although an effort was made to crowd the womb down by external pressure, with negative result. Feeling assured that a continuance of the contractions would force the fœtus down sufficiently to enable me to diagnosticate the presentation in a short time, I sat down to await results. In less than three minutes blood began dripping from the bed. A hasty examination now disclosed an os dilated to the size of a silver dollar, with a placenta centrally implanted over it. A small portion was detached, and through the aperture I could distinguish nothing, owing to the high position of the womb. The pains were weak, but sufficient to produce severe flooding at each contraction, and the patient was rapidly losing strength, being almost pulseless in five minutes from the time when the membranes were ruptured. I hastily administered alcohol, ammonia, and ergot, and sent for assistance, meanwhile making pressure on the cervix with my fingers in the vagina, thus checking flooding to a considerable extent. On arrival of assistance, in the person of Dr. Smith, the vagina was tamponed with good results; the flooding ceased, strong contractions set in, and in fifteen minutes an 8-inch fœtus was extruded. The placenta was delivered almost immediately afterward, and the case has since progressed well.

The peculiarity in this case was the large bag of waters low in the vagina in front of the presenting placenta.

Yours truly,

WILLIAM S. CARY, M.D.

Gothenburg, Nebraska,

Feb. 21, 1889.

NOTES AND COMMENTS.

Treatment of Scabies.

In a paper on the Increasing Prevalence of Scabies, with Remarks on Treatment, Dr. James C. White, Professor of Dermatology in Harvard University says that in sulphur, styrax or Peruvian balsam, and naphthol we have three effective, sufficient parasiticides. The action of the other substances employed so generally in combination with them, the alkalies, tars, gritty powders, etc., is simply auxiliary, and addressed to the solvent or mechanical removal of the epidermal coverings, or crusts, which protect the animals and eggs in the burrows and pits against the active agents; or these agents are intended for the relief or prevention of the inflammatory processes, which always accompany the disease, or may be provoked by the injudicious use of the remedies employed in its cure. It is in a proper knowledge of these latter, most essential, points of treatment that the successful management of scabies chiefly consists. It should never be forgotten, he says, that every case of advanced scabies is mainly an eczema, developed, in extent of surface affected and intensity of lesions, by individual peculiarity of the cutaneous tissues under the influence of scratching; and that the changes in the skin due to the direct action of the parasite are always but a small practical part of the same. The mere destruction of the animal in all its phases may be, therefore, only a part of treatment, although always the first and essential step. It is important therefore, first, that in the choice or combination of remedies those should be selected which shall destroy the animal with certainty and quickness, and yet shall not aggravate the existing inflammatory changes in the skin; and second, that they should not be used too long.

Dr. White says he generally employs in dispensary practice the following method, and that it is applicable in every case, however extensive or severe may be the accompanying inflammatory processes. He prefers a mixture of the three active agents (a scattering shot), and combines them in this way.

$$\text{R} \quad \text{Flowers of sulphur} \ldots \ldots \ldots \ \text{ʒ ii}$$
$$\beta\text{-naphthol} \ldots \ldots \ldots \ldots \ \text{ʒ i}$$
$$\text{Balsam of Peru,}$$
$$\text{Vaseline} \ldots \ldots \ldots \ldots \text{aa } \text{ʒ i}$$

M.

This quantity, he says, is generally sufficient for the cure of a single case. The patient is directed to rub a third of this mixture into the whole surface of the body, from the neck downward, at bedtime. He is especially told to rub it between the fingers and upon the penis, and that it must be applied to the back by some other person. He is to sleep in old garments, that the bedclothes may not be soiled. In the morning the skin is to be thoroughly washed with soap and water. The use of the bath in this class of patients is of course out of the question, nor is it essential. The ointment is to be used in this way for three consecutive nights. Generally the itching ceases almost wholly on the first application. The patient is also told not to use it after the third night, unless, after waiting two more nights, there should be a decided return of the pruritus here or there, in which case the salve is to be rubbed into such parts only, and only for two nights running. For very young children he omits the naphthol in prescribing the ointment, on account of its occasional irritating properties.

In cases in which the accompanying eczema is severe, it is well to require an inspection of the patient again on the sixth or seventh day, when it will sometimes be found necessary to direct a course of treatment addressed to this residuary condition. He warns the physician that a very frequent mistake at this stage is the conclusion that the appearances, or accompanying itching, are signs of the continued activity of the original affection, and the consequent renewal of the use of the stimulating parasiticide, which only aggravates the existing process. He has often seen cases of post-scabietic eczema in dispensary and private practice, which have been kept going for months by such errors of judgment. It must also be remembered that in prolonged cases of itch the cutaneous nerves have acquired, as it were, the habit of demanding to be scratched, and seem to require it for a long time after every visible sign of the disease has disappeared, and these cases of surviving pruritus are often mistaken for remaining evidence of the original affection, and mistreated accordingly.

Directions are always given that on the first night of the treatment all the clothes which have been worn next to the skin,—shirts, drawers, and socks, and the 'sheets and pillowcases last slept in,—shall be thoroughly boiled before being used again. Gloves should be baked or destroyed. It is to be assumed that every bed-fellow has the disease also, and requires treatment as much as the patient. Every member of the family should, he says, also be inspected and treated in the same way, however slight in character or extent may be the indications of the affection. He says he has seen the disease keep up a continued and alternating existence in a large family for a year, during which period nearly all its members underwent treatment one or more times, simply because they were not treated simultaneously. He has recently directed five members of a private family to be thus generally treated, although only two of the household at that time presented any positive indications of the presence of the disease.

As to the more general control of the affection in its well-nigh epidemic state of prevalence, it is only by drawing the attention of the profession to this activity, and to the best methods of destroying it in individual instances, that it may be hoped to accomplish anything.

The Microbe of Diphtheria.

The announcement of the discovery of the microbe of diphtheria by MM. Roux and Yersin of the Pasteur Laboratory, has led somewhat prematurely to sanguine hopes that the disease will now be amenable to prophylaxis by inoculation. The micro-organism of diphtheria, however, has been before now discovered by such investigators as Oertel, Klebs, and Loeffler. Nevertheless, but little fruit in the direction of successfully combating this highly fatal disease has yet accrued from these researches. We await with interest the full details of this latest inquiry, and shall be glad to see to what extent MM. Roux and Yersin have advanced beyond the stages reached by their predecessors in this field.—*Lancet*, Feb. 9, 1889.

Parasites and Monkeys.

At the last meeting of the Academy of Natural Sciences, of Philadelphia, Mr. Ives stated that, while examining a specimen of a monkey, the sooty Mangabey, which recently died in the Zoological Garden, he had found in the omentum and distributed through the lungs, peritoneal cavity and elsewhere a curious parasite, allied to the mites and ticks. It had also been found in the mandril, the Macaque and the Chacma baboon. The animals present curious modifications, fitting them for their parasitic existence. The monkeys in which these parasites occur are all old world species, and it becomes an interesting question whether they were developed in the Zoological Garden or before the capture of the infested animal.

In answer to an inquiry the President stated that there is no marked correspondence between the parasites of man and those of the higher apes. As far as he is informed the same species of tape worm does not occur in man and monkeys, although Trichocephalus dispar and the round worm Ascaris lumbricoides have been found in both.

New Amber Beds Near Dantzig.

The district of Heubode, near Dantzig, has suddenly become the scene of considerable speculation and of a good deal of activity in consequence of recent discoveries of amber made there. The main region of the shores of the Baltic, where amber has hitherto been found in paying quantities, is between Pillau and Grosz Hubenicken, some distance to the east of the present find. The attention of the authorities was first called to the matter some years ago by a person who offered 1,800 gulden (about $720) annually for the exclusive privilege of mining amber in the district. For some reason it was not accepted, and the matter was dropped until very recently, when the offer was renewed, the sum being increased to 6,000 gulden. It was accepted, and the parties have gone to work on a three years' lease at these figures. After the lease was executed the authorities received an offer, from another person, of 1,000 gulden monthly for a period of six years, or a cash in hand price of 72,000 gulden for the same privilege. These figures indicate that somebody is confident of finding amber in large quantities in the new field.—*National Druggist*, March 1, 1889.

The Bacillus of Diphtheria.

Dr. George M. Sternberg, in a lecture delivered at the Hoagland Laboratory, Brooklyn, Jan. 26, reviews the investigations made by different bacteriologists to determine whether or not there is a specific bacillus of diphtheria. In conclusion, he says that the experimental evidence, with reference to the etiological *rôle* of Loeffler's diphtheria bacillus is rather more satisfactory than that which has been adduced in favor of the relation of Eberth's bacillus to typhoid fever, or Koch's "comma-bacillus" to cholera; and that most conservative bacteriologists seem inclined to the view that it is in fact the specific infectious agent in this disease.—*Brooklyn Med. Journal*, March, 1889.

Cocaine in Angina Pectoris.

Professor Valerian G. Lashkevitch, of Kharkov, tried (*Novosti Terapii*, Dec. 1888, p. 440) hydrochlorate of cocaine internally, in the dose of one-third of a grain, three or four times a day, in sixteen cases of angina pectoris associated with cardiac or vascular disease, or, as in some of the patients, angina apparently caused by excessive tobacco smoking. The results obtained justify the author in regarding cocaine as a genuine specific remedy for the affection. The attacks of angina were invariably relieved even on the second day of the treatment, and ceased altogether and permanently in the course of a few days. Recovery takes place still more rapidly, when inhalations of oxygen gas are simultaneously employed.

A Fatal Prescription.

The recent death in Germany of a child as the result of taking a prescription containing an incompatible and dangerous compound, viz., chlorate of potash and iodide of iron, deserves the attention of all practitioners. The iron was precipitated in the form of the sesquioxide, and all the iodine liberated. The following formula will illustrate the chemical changes which took place in the medicine: $2FeI_2 + KClO_3 = Fe_2O_3 + KCl + 4I$.

Creasote with Cod-liver Oil and Saccharin.

Dr. Seitz gives the following formula in the *Therap. Monatshefte*, 1889, No. 48:

Creasote	2.5 parts
Cod-liver oil	200 "
Saccharin	1 "

Dose: A tea to tablespoonful, 1 to 3 times daily for adults; for children the amount of creasote should be less.

Bill for Adulteration of Food Defeated.

The House Judiciary General Committee of the Pennsylvania Legislature decided on March 8, to report negatively the bill advocated by the Society to Prevent Food Adulteration. The bill was aimed to prohibit harmful and deceptive and regulate harmless and necessary adulteration of food and drugs. Ex-President Kline, of the Philadelphia Drug Exchange and of the National Wholesale Druggists' Association, and Dr. Robbins, President of the Pharmaceutical Board, were before the committee in opposition to the bill so far as it related to drugs. They said it would cause heavy and unnecessary expense, and admit inspectors to rooms where they could learn valuable business secrets. Besides, they thought there was already enough law on the subject to protect the people, although it might be well to increase the penalties for violation. President Ammerling, of the Anti-Adulteration Society, vainly tried to convince the committee that the bill ought to be passed.

Athletic Sports and Gymnastics at the University of Pennsylvania.

It is stated that the opinion has prevailed among the medical students of the University of Pennsylvania that it is impossible for them to devote any time to athletic exercise without lowering their class standing and failing in their examinations. But a number of medical students who are in training for the crews have formed an "Oarsman's Quiz Club," and every day, after they have taken their pull, they meet and quiz each other on the subjects which they must prepare upon for examination.

There has been some difficulty experienced in having the department of physical education established on an equal basis with the other branches as regards compulsory attendance and ranking in class. When the department was first introduced at the University it was said that hours would be assigned for gymnasium work just as for recitations or lectures. An attempt was made to introduce this feature into the regular curriculum, but it never succeeded for lack of interest and support in different quarters. Dr. Leuf, the Director of Physical Education, has now succeeded in having regular gymnasium hours assigned to the two lower classes, and it is said that the Trustees are endeavoring to secure a permanent instructor, so that the gymnasium may be open regularly for several hours every day.

NEWS.

—The Trustees of the University of Pennsylvania have just purchased from the city three properties, amounting in area to nine and a quarter acres, in the vicinity of the University, paying $149,800.

—Dr. S. Weir Mitchell, of Philadelphia, has written a story of life in the lumber regions, which the Lippincotts will publish. Its title is *Far in the Forest.* The work is said to be an outcome of personal observations among an interesting class of people.

—The Philadelphia *Ledger*, Feb. 23, 1889, reports that a young woman died in a dentist's chair in Norwalk, Ohio, on Feb. 21. She had taken chloroform preparatory to having teeth drawn, and it caused her heart to cease beating. It is thought she was affected with heart disease.

—The Woman's Medical College of Pennsylvania held its thirty-seventh annual commencement March 14, and conferred the degree of Doctor of Medicine upon 36 graduates. Dr. Clara Marshall, Dean of the College, presided, and the address to the graduates was delivered by Dr. James B. Walker.

—At the meeting of the College of Physicians of Philadelphia, March 6, a report of a committee, setting forth the importance of "a rigid inspection of meat and milk," was adopted and a committee was appointed to act with other bodies with the view of obtaining legislation to accomplish the desired ends.

—The *British Med. Journal*, Feb. 9, publishes the conclusions arrived at by the physicians who made the autopsy on the late Crown Prince Rudolph, of Austria. There seems to be no doubt that he shot himself, and the conditions of his brain and skull justify the supposition that he was mentally deranged.

—Dr. Alvan Talcott, of Guilford, Conn., who has given $25,000 to endow a professorship of Greek at Yale, is one of the oldest alumni of that university, having been graduated in 1828. He is past eighty years old, still practises medicine, and reads Homer daily with far more earnestness than ever in his undergraduate days.

—On March 4, Dr. A. L. Loomis was examined in New York City in the suit brought against him by the widow of the late Dr. Miller, which was referred to in the REPORTER March 9. The manuscript of the essay said to have been written by Dr. Miller was in Dr. Loomis's handwriting, and Dr. Loomis testified that Dr. Miller's work on the essay had consisted in engrossing some tables and copying them afterward for publication; he did not revise or do any original work upon the essay.

OBITUARY.

AUGUSTUS F. TAYLOR, M.D.

Dr. Augustus F. Taylor, an ex-Mayor of New Brunswick, N. J., and one of its oldest residents, died March 6, at the age of eighty years. He was educated at Rutgers College, and was one of the oldest graduates of that institution. He studied medicine and began its practice nearly sixty years ago. He sailed for California in 1849, and amassed a fortune. On his return he resumed the practice of his profession, and continued it until eighteen years ago, when he lost his eyesight.

PHILIP D. MARSHALL, M.D.

Dr. Philip D. Marshall, of Reading, Pa., died March 5, of pneumonia, at the age of fifty-six years. He was a graduate of Jefferson Medical College, Philadelphia, and was a surgeon for a number of years in the United States Army, having been stationed for a long time at Jefferson Barracks, near St. Louis, Mo. He was an intimate friend of Dr. Joseph Pancoast, and was the first surgeon to perform the operation of tracheotomy in Reading. He was prominent in his profession, and was the author of many valuable papers on surgery.

CHARLES E. L. WAGNER, M.D.

Dr. Charles E. L. Wagner died in Hanover, Germany, Thursday, March 7, 1889. Dr. Wagner was born in Hanover in 1823, was graduated at the University of Göttingen in 1847, and entered the Hanoverian army in the same year. During the Schleswig-Holstein war, of 1848–1849, he served as surgeon in the army, and in 1855 he entered the British army as surgeon of the Third Regiment — British German Legion—serving during the Crimean war.

In 1860 Dr. Wagner came to the United States and took up his residence in Wilkes-Barre, Pennsylvania, where he remained, practising medicine, until 1874, when he retired from active practice and spent most of his time abroad, returning however to this country every few years. He had already engaged passage for his return from Germany to this country when he was stricken with apoplexy and called away suddenly to a better and everlasting home.

MEDICAL AND SURGICAL
REPORTER

No. 1674. PHILADELPHIA, MARCH 30, 1889. VOL. LX.—No. 13.

CONTENTS:

CLINICAL LECTURE.

CÆSAREAN SECTION FOR CARCINOMA OF THE CERVIX UTERI: THE NEW SÄNGER OPERATION.

BY WILLIAM GOODELL, M.D.,

PHILADELPHIA.

PROFESSOR OF GYNECOLOGY IN THE UNIVERSITY OF PENNSYLVANIA.

This woman, 32 years of age, was married before she was 15. She has had eight children at term and four miscarriages. A year ago last February she began to lose blood per vaginam. This was neglected until some time later when an examination revealed the existence of cancer of the cervix. In October last this was curetted and the hemorrhage ceased. At that time the fact that the woman was pregnant escaped notice. About two weeks later, however, the fœtal movements apprised the mother of her condition. This is a very scant history, but it is all that we are possessed of. By a rough reckoning, I conclude that the pregnancy is now within about ten days of its normal duration. Now, why am I going to operate on this woman? I shall do so because the whole vagina is blocked by a dense, scirrhous mass that is impassable. In its present condition it would be impossible for the cervix to dilate sufficiently to permit of the passage or extraction of the child. If we allowed the case to proceed to labor, it would probably prove fatal both to the mother and to the child. I think it wisest to operate now while the woman's morale is good and her strength is fair, because the hemorrhages have returned, and because we can select the time of the operation. The sole objection, and not a very important one, to this immediate operation is the absence as yet of canalization of the cervix. The period of election for the Cæsarean section is after the beginning of labor when the cervical canal has dilated sufficiently to permit of the escape of the waters and of the subsequent drainage of the lochia. On the other hand, such an amount of dilatation in this case would probably require many hours of exhausting labor for its production, and I shall, therefore, produce it artificially. We have here, according to my diagnosis, a breech presentation. The body of the child is lying in the left half of the uterine cavity, and yet, which is somewhat singular, we hear the sounds of the fœtal heart much more distinctly over the right side of the mother's abdomen. As to the statistics of this operation, the old Cæsarean section was very fatal. It was generally undertaken too late, after the forceps had been tried for a long time, and when the woman was almost or quite in extremis. Sänger, of Leipsic, has recently devised an improved method of operating, the results obtained by which have been much more satisfactory. Our great statistician, Dr. R. P. Harris, who has honored us by his presence to-day, tells me that thus far there have been in the whole civilized world 163 operations by the Sänger method, with 45 deaths—viz., a mortality of 27⅝ per cent. In this country the showing is not so good, there having been 26 operations with 16 deaths. This larger mortality is probably due to the fact that the woman was not operated upon until every other means had been tried, and she had become exhausted by the delay, and injured by the efforts made to deliver her per vaginam.

There is one thing to be said concerning my patient. She has displayed a wonderful amount of nerve and pluck, and, while she appreciates the danger to which she will be exposed, she yet feels much confidence in the result. One reason for this is, I think, that since she has been here she has seen many women recover from operations which have been performed for the removal of tumors, etc. Since the beginning of this session my son and I have performed twenty-three such operations in your presence, and with but three deaths. Only one of these was from septicæmia, the patient's death being almost a foregone conclusion. The tubes and ovaries were distended with rotten pus, and were everywhere so adherent that they burst and deluged the belly with putrid matter; nor could the ovaries be wholly removed. The second death was due to shock, after the removal of a large uterine sarcoma by supra-vaginal hysterectomy. The patient was very feeble and had been bed-ridden for many months. The third death took place in the fourth week after the removal of pus tubes and ovaries, and was in no wise due to the operation. The patient had paralysis of the

lower extremities and displayed a mental hebetude which I deemed hysterical. But my diagnosis was evidently incorrect, for her subsequent history plainly showed some obscure but serious cerebro-spinal lesion. For over a week after the operation she did extremely well, then symptoms of general paresis developed themselves, the sphincters gradually lost power, and death finally resulted from the advance of the cerebrospinal disease.

Our patient lying before us has shown wonderful pluck. With the prospect of death before her, she has displayed no fear, but she has made a last request of me which I have promised to fulfill. It is that her child be baptized as soon as it shall have been delivered.

And now, with the statement that all the external parts involved have been antiseptically cleansed, and the vagina disinfected by a bichloride of mercury solution, I shall begin the operation. Having opened the abdominal cavity, and exposed the pregnant uterus, I may proceed in one of two ways. I may either lift the womb and bring it out through the opening that I have made in the abdominal wall, and then incise it and extract the child, or, I may open the womb *in situ*. By this latter method some of the fluid contents may enter the abdominal cavity, but the abdominal incision will be much shorter. (The uterus was now opened, *in situ*, and the child delivered; shortly afterward the placenta was detached and removed with the membranes.) I now bring the emptied womb out on the abdomen, and control the hemorrhage by an elastic tube thrown around its lower zone. You will notice that the womb was raised up and the abdominal cavity was packed with sponges to catch any fluids that may have escaped from the womb. I shall first introduce the deep sutures into the walls of the uterus. These are inserted in this way. The needle enters the uterine wall a half inch from the edge of the womb and is carried obliquely downward and inward till it emerges just above the edge of the mucous lining of the womb. It is not allowed to penetrate this inner membrane for the reason, that a communicating channel might be established along the course traversed by the suture, and through this some of the fœtid and septic contents of the uterus might escape into the peritoneal cavity. After all the deep sutures have been inserted, the closure of the wound is completed by the insertion of a number of Lembert sutures. By these latter stitches we secure the turning in of the cut edges of the serous investing membrane of the uterus and their maintenance in close contact. Why does the present technique (Sänger's) yield better result than the old operation? It is, I think, because of the great care that is now exercised in the closure of the uterine wound. It is upon the careful introduction of the deep and the superficial Lembert sutures and the adoption of rigid antiseptic precautions, that the increased success of the operation seems to depend. You may ask why I did not perform the "Porro" operation here. For two reasons. First, it is slightly more fatal than the Sänger operation; and, secondly, I found that it would be impossible to remove the womb in its entirety. If I could have succeeded in removing the whole womb, I should have done the "Porro," but I found the walls of the bladder and rectum so infected by the disease, so hardened and massed together, that complete hysterectomy was quite out of the question. You saw that the child presented by the breech, thus verifying my diagnosis. The woman has had two such presentations before. She has been a very prolific mother, one of her four miscarriages having been with twins.

We have now completed the closure of the uterine incision, and, on counting our stitches, we find that we have put in fourteen deep and seventeen superficial or Lembert sutures. These, with the natural contraction of the womb, effectually control any hemorrhage. The parts are now thoroughly well cleaned, the womb is sponged off, and the space between it and the bladder carefully examined and cleaned. Although this has been a very clean operation, I shall take the additional precaution of thoroughly irrigating the peritoneal cavity previous to closing it. We shall use ordinary water that has been boiled. The cutaneous sutures will be first introduced and the irrigation then performed before they are drawn tight. In placing these sutures we should endeavor to secure such a union of the divided abdominal wall as shall prevent the occurrence of a subsequent ventral hernia. We want to bring forward as much tissue as possible. It is particularly necessary to draw the rectus and its tendon well into the line of union and get them in accurate apposition, and if there should be any difficulty in doing this we may resort to traction on the tendon by a pair of forceps. In spite of our best care, however, these hernias will sometimes occur, and I should like very much to know of some method by which they can be wholly avoided. I am going to cut her navel out. It is a dense mass presenting a very hard and narrow surface, which is liable to give way and cause hernia, so I shall excise it. The anæsthetic that has been used during this operation is chloroform. Whenever pressure is exerted either upon the respiratory organs or the kidneys by the presence of a tumor, and we can certainly call the pregnant uterus by that name, I prefer the administration of chloroform to that of ether. I use it altogether in my private laparotomies. When the renal vessels are subjected to any pressure and ether is used as an anæsthetic, the kidneys may suddenly become congested and stop work, with resulting uræmia and death. Ether is also strongly contraindicated where albumin is present in the urine, and in the aged who have bronchial affections.

Now that all our abdominal sutures have been introduced, we shall irrigate this abdominal cavity. Again, I say, we shall use only plain boiled water. This manner of paddling about with my hand among the loops of intestine may look like rough work, but it does no harm. I now draw the omentum down over the intestines and the womb and proceed to close the cavity. (The abdominal sutures were drawn tight, tied, and the redundant ends cut off. All soiled linen, towels, etc., were then removed from the woman and she was sponged perfectly clean. The wound was freely dusted with iodoform, a layer of iodoform gauze (50 per cent.) laid over it, on this a layer of carbolated gauze, and then a broad, thick mass of baked cotton, which was firmly held in place by strips of adhesive plaster. Over all a flannel binder was applied.)

Now that we have completed the operation and the dressing, the last thing that I shall do will be to pass my finger within the vagina and clear a channel through the cervix that shall permit the escape of the lochia. I might have done this from above before I closed the uterus, but I was afraid of contaminating my fingers with the cancerous juices, and so I postponed it till now. I wish to avoid as far as possible the use of opium in the subsequent treatment of this case. If much pain should be complained of, of course, we cannot withhold it altogether. The woman will now be removed to her bed, she is in good condition, and I think she ought to recover. In looking back over the operation I do not think we have omitted anything that might have added to the patient's chances of recovery.

I may, possibly, have made one mistake in delivering the child by the head instead of the feet, thus necessitating a somewhat larger opening in the womb, but the child presented with the breech, which placed the feet at a distance from the incision, and it was easier to deliver by the head. Nor do I think that this will militate in any perceptible degree against a favorable result.

[Twelve days have now (March 25) elapsed since the operation, and the patient is apparently out of danger. She is eating and sleeping well, and she has an abundant supply of milk for her infant, which is thriving.]

COMMUNICATIONS.

THE INFLUENCE OF STOMACH DIGESTION ON THE HEART'S ACTION, AS A PROXIMATE CAUSE OF HEART FAILURE.

BY WILLIAM H. BURR, M.D.,

WILMINGTON, DEL.

On the night of Nov. 18, 1888, I was called up at 12 P.M. to visit a man who was said to be very ill. I reached the patient's house in about fifteen minutes, and found that he had been dead ten minutes. I found him on his knees, with his head bent over on the pillow where he had dropped it in the act of vomiting. His face and neck were deeply congested. When the patient's head was lowered a small quantity of bloody fluid oozed from his mouth.

History of Attack.—At about 11.30 P.M., shortly after retiring, the patient complained of fulness of the chest, was deathly pale, and began to rift and belch up quantities of gas, which somewhat relieved him for a time. The fulness and oppression increased, and with them there was agonizing pain over the whole region of the chest, especially over the left side, and extending to the bowels. His wife went into another room to procure some remedy and on returning found the patient on the vessel purging. He got into bed again, but immediately rose to vomit, bringing up with great effort and straining a small quantity of partially digested food, accompanied with a little dark, bloody fluid. He now complained of being intensely cold—"freezing to death," as he expressed it. His extremities were cold and clammy. He attempted to vomit every few minutes, leaning over the foot of the bed and pressing on his chest and stomach, each attack being accompanied with agonizing pain. He then sat up in bed and begged the assistants to bathe his limbs in hot water as they were freezing to death. He put his hand over the region of his heart, and wondered if it was his heart that was troubling him. Suddenly he got up on his knees for the last time, in an uncontrollable attack of vomiting, his wife supporting him, and while in the act, he fell forward with his head almost in the basin, gave one or two gasps, and was dead.

Post-Mortem.—The lungs were apparently healthy, but much congested, containing blood of arterial hue. The heart presented marked signs of fatty degeneration; the left ventricle was hypertrophied, the right dilated, thin, and tearing easily; the valves were healthy, with no atheromatous change. Liver much enlarged. Bowels, congested. The stomach was well filled with partially digested food. The kidneys were apparently healthy, except that the left had an adherent capsule and showed signs of old inflammation. All the internal organs except the lungs were filled with an immense quantity of uncoagulated blood, black, and tarry-looking. All the blood in the body seemed concentrated in the internal organs.

Previous History.—The patient had for several years been troubled with occasional attacks of indigestion, at which times he would eructate quantities of bitter fluid, have a bitter taste in his mouth, all of which would disappear under appropriate treatment. He had been treated eight or ten years before for enlarged, torpid and painful liver.

Twenty-five years ago he had an attack of acute nephritis, which confined him to his bed for six weeks and from which he suffered for three years afterward, apparently recovering, with the exception of occasional attacks of congestion of the kidneys since. Three years ago we removed a large sarcoma of the left testicle, which disease had developed in an undescended and undeveloped testis and was of ten or fifteen years' growth. It had showed a decided malignant tendency for the last six months before we operated. There was never any indication of return. The patient's wife reported that, though he had never consulted a physician for the trouble, he had had occasional dyspeptic attacks, as he called them, the first one of which we have a record being twenty years ago, the last one being the attack which resulted in his death, previous to which he had not had any for a long time. The symptoms at each attack were exactly similar, though not so intense as during the fatal attack. He would have fulness, oppression, and pain, only relieved by retching and rifting, with never any vomiting, but with congestion of the veins, and sometimes distension of the bowels with gas, and œdema of the tissues over the abdomen.

The patient had always been a hard-working man, lifting and straining in his work from 5 A.M. to 11 P.M. He was a slight man, weighing about 130 pounds, and had the facial appearance which is described as being found in cases of fatty heart, i. e., the veins of the neck being habitually distended, and the countenance looking dusky and anxious.

In a second case of this sort which came under my observation, a large portly, full-fed man, noted for mental acuteness and application, on a warm summer day, after eating a full meal, started to walk to his place of business. About half the distance had been traversed when he became deathly sick, complained of great pain through the chest, had an attack of vomiting, and died in a few minutes.

Post-Mortem.—Every organ in the body was perfectly sound and without disease. The stomach contained almost all of the large dinner he had taken. No evident attempt at digestion had taken place.

In a third case a young man, in the evening, shortly after eating, was taken with vomiting. Upon the arrival of medical aid he was almost pulseless, his heart was acting tumultuously and irregularly, his surface was cold and clammy, his respirations diminishing. A prompt emetic of mustard and water was administered, and the patient vomited immense quantities of hard lumps of curdled albumen, some of them as large almost as an adult fist, so large that it seemed incredible that they could have passed through the gullet.

With the vomiting the symptoms improved, and from a condition of collapse bordering on death the patient became convalescent. A slight amount of low grade of pneumonic inflammation developed, but it was successfully treated and the patient recovered.

These cases are not entirely similar. The last two belong more especially to that class of cases denominated paralysis of the stomach. But they all show very decidedly the effect of suspended or difficult digestion on the action of the heart and lungs. They show, what is seldom adverted to in the books, that a nerve storm may develop in the stomach and bowels which shall overwhelm and bring disaster on the circulatory apparatus and lungs, and cause death. There also seems to be a lesson to be drawn here directly from nature, for does she not in these cases undertake to rid the system by purging and vomiting of those matters which are causing its death? And if, by assisting nature to throw off the *materies peccans*, we can tide the patient over such a danger it is adding much to our therapeutic resources. Hlasko has investigated the question of the cranial center for the stomach movements with results which lead him to conclude that the center for the constrictor fibres of the cardia lies in the corpora quadrigemina, and that it is connected with the stomach chiefly through the vagus, but partly by the spinal cord and sympathetic system. The center for the dilator fibres, and for those that control the movements of the stomach walls also, are supposed to lie in close proximity. Another author believes that the center for vomiting lies in the corpora quadrigemina.

The *par vagum* is composed of both motor and sensory filaments, and, besides other organs, supplies the stomach and heart with motor influence. The stomach and heart, as every one knows, are intimately connected through the cranial and sympathetic systems. Would it be strange then if that much abused organ of digestion, the stomach, were to refuse to act, it should inculpate with itself the organs most important to life with which it is so intimately connected, which organs stop not day or night and know no rest except it be the rest of death? That this is due to nervous sympathy and not to mechanical pressure is clearly demonstrated, as the heart can be bent into almost any position by effusions, and be more or less cramped, without complaining seriously of such distortion.

Vomiting itself in a healthy person will often induce faintness and almost a state of collapse. When the heart is already crippled it falls an easy prey to even a slight sympathetic disturbance.

There are several questions which might be considered in regard to the treatment of these cases. Almost nothing is written in the various text books in regard to the symptoms portrayed above and their proper treatment; so that when the practitioner is brought for the first time face to face with such a case, hovering on the brink of the grave, he is without advice and without weapons. There are but a few moments to do anything. Something must be done, and that quickly. ·The balance, which for years has been ready to go up or down at a moment's notice, has turned the wrong way.

What shall we do? Are there no means to whip the tired organs into renewed activity, to tide the patient over the terrible crisis until we may bring such slower agents to bear as change of occupation and general attention to building up the health?

The first case was undoubtedly one .of cardiac failure, due to fatty heart, which was itself largely caused by the anæmic conditions and mode of life of the patient. The circulation was so weakened that the act of vomiting itself was almost enough to cause collapse. The treatment here, based upon the symptoms taken with the result of the *post-mortem* examination, would seem to have been to stop the vomiting immediately, to strengthen the weakening circulation with morphia and atropia administered hypodermically in *hot* solution, and the administration of hot whiskey and ether hypodermically, with the use of hot bottles and hot bathing.

In the second case there was no history of heart disease previously, and here death was obviously caused by the paralyzant action of the large masses of food which the stomach, unable to digest easily, had refused to act on at all. Here it would seem that the first object should be to empty the stomach and at the same time, or afterward, to stimulate the flagging circulation. In the third case, the same line of action would seem to be indicated, and was adopted with the result of saving the patient's life.

To conclude, it might be asked : are the vomiting, retching, pain and discharge of fermented gasses in fatty heart due to passive congestion of the stomach and bowels, which congestion is the first act in the tragedy of failing circulation?

Again, does that congestion occur unavoidably, or is the presence of undigested or difficultly digested food the cause of the trouble, producing first .congestion of the internal organs, then the pains and irritative symptoms, crippling of circulation and death? Lastly, in the paralyzant cases there seems to be no doubt but that death is caused by direct nervous paralysis, sympathetic in its nature.

—A number of the crew of the bark Fannie Skalfield, which arrived at Jersey City from Calcutta March 13, were affected with scurvy. One of the crew died and two were reported to be likely to die.

CROWDED HOSPITALS FOR THE INSANE.

BY JOHN CURWEN, M.D.,

SUPERINTENDENT OF THE STATE HOSPITAL FOR THE INSANE, WARREN, PA.

The consideration of the overcrowded condition of the different State Hospitals for the Insane of Pennsylvania has been a matter of serious concern to the trustees and officers of the institutions, and on the part of some of the hospitals action has been taken which follows too closely the English plan to be acceptable to the majority of the people Without entering into a full statement of the manner in which the crowded state has been brought about, it is sufficient to say that an effort has been made by the Committee on Lunacy to remove all the insane from the almshouses, while there was not room in the State Hospitals for their accommodation without unduly and improperly crowding them, and rendering all uncomfortable and more liable to disease from the effects of such overcrowding.

Among those thus removed to the hospitals were a large number of imbeciles and very many quiet and demented insane, for whom only simple custodial care was needed. The law is express in its requirements that recent cases shall have preference over those of long standing. Every one familiar with hospitals for the insane knows that for recent cases quiet and freedom from unpleasant surroundings are essential to the obtaining of that rest and sleep which are a first requisite in treatment. How can this be properly secured when the rooms are all occupied, and to give proper accommodation some one must be crowded out into closer quarters to give even a measure of the accommodation demanded?

Crowding, and worse, overcrowding is a serious bar to all proper classification, and without proper classification, so as to separate the quiet from the excited, the restless ·and fretful from others over whom they may exert an improper influence, the requisite treatment cannot be fully and advantageously carried out. In confirmation of this statement the following resolution of the Association of Medical Superintendents of American Institutions for the Insane may be quoted: " That this Association regards the custom of admitting a greater number of patients than the buildings can properly accommodate, which is now becoming so common in hospitals for the insane, in nearly every section of the country, as an evil of great magnitude, productive of extraordinary dangers, subversive of the good order, perfect discipline and greatest usefulness of these institutions and of the best interests of the insane.''

It is not with recent curable cases that the hospitals are crowded, but with those classes which have been gradually accumulating in the almshouses, or have been kept in private families until the families have found it impossible longer to bear the strain.

In the State of New York twenty years ago it was thought that the establishment of the 'Willard Asylum for the chronic insane would in a large measure relieve the other hospital and also remove the insane from the county poorhouses. That institution has now in its charge about two thousand patients, but in the years since its establishment the hospitals at Buffalo, Poughkeepsie and Middletown have been built, and they are now crowded; the Inebriate Asylum at Binghamton has been converted into an asylum for the chronic insane, and it is full, and another asylum to accommodate a large number of insane is in course of erection near Ogdensburg; while nineteen counties in the State have been authorized to construct buildings for the insane in connection with the poorhouses. In the above enumeration no account has been taken of the insane of the city of New York and in the adjoining counties on Long Island, for whom provisions have been made in those localities.

In Pennsylvania the hospitals for the insane are all overcrowded, and the majority of the poorhouses which have accommodations for the insane are nearly empty. In many counties of this commonwealth there are very good accommodations for the insane, arranged specially for them; but notwithstanding this fact all the insane have been removed to the State Hospitals, overcrowding them, and impairing their usefulness and efficiency of treatment, without any corresponding benefit to those removed, but on the contrary rather placing them where they cannot have the amount of space they should have and adding to the discomfort and annoyance of those in the hospital before their admission. The taxpayers certainly have some rights to be respected in such cases, and in the counties in which large sums of money have been expended in the erection of accommodations for their quiet and demented cases, there is a general feeling of discontent that the accommodations erected at such cost should be practically useless.

Just here the plain practical question meets us: Shall we impair the ability and efficiency of the hospitals for the insane to take just and proper care of the recent cases so that they may be restored and returned to the community as producers and taxpayers to aid in relieving the burdens of the community? or shall we crowd the present hospitals with imbeciles and quiet demented patients who can be well taken care of in the almshouses, under proper regulations?

The Board of Public Charities has, in each county where there is an almshouse, a committee of visitors whose duty it is to visit the almshouses and jails regularly; then there is the General Agent of the Board and the Secretary of the Committee on Lunacy. With these means at command a careful and systematic visitation of the different almshouses can be made, and the manner in which they are kept and the inmates are attended to can be strictly observed, and all abuses can be prevented or corrected.

With such a system in full and regular operation the objection that the insane and imbeciles would not be properly taken care of would be obviated, and by careful selection of those to be removed from the hospitals, the overcrowded condition of the hospitals could be relieved and better accommodation given to the recent cases, to those who must be kept in the hospital on account of their excitable character, and to those from districts where no accommodations of any kind are now provided.

The theory that the State should provide for all the insane is correct and true, but in actual practice such a condition has not yet been realized; and, however much it may be desired, it is not probable for financial reasons that it can be realized for some years to come, and while laboring and waiting for such a desirable end, we must use the best means at command for the relief of those who are now to be cared for.

That such quiet, chronic cases can be made as comfortable in a hospital where they are compelled to sleep from fifty to one hundred in one room, as in an almshouse where each can have a room or where only three or four are placed in one room, the writer of this does not believe; nor does it seem in the nature of things reasonable and right. The present effort seems to be to treat the insane in masses and not as individuals, and that is a sure way to add to the already large number of chronic cases.

The more thoroughly individualized the treatment the greater the prospect of success in that treatment, and of restoration to sound mental health.

SOCIETY REPORTS.

PHILADELPHIA OBSTETRICAL SOCIETY.

Thursday, February 7, 1889.

The President, THEOPHILUS PARVIN, M.D., in the Chair.

DR. HORATIO R. BIGELOW through the Secretary read a paper on

Apostoli's Place in Gynecology.

After some complimentary remarks on Apostoli himself Dr. Bigelow went on to discuss the armamentarium necessary for carrying out the electrical treatment. He thought it necessary to have a galvanic battery, a Faradic battery, a collector, a galvanometer, intra-uterine electrodes for both currents—and one for carrying both the positive and negative of the induced current within the uterus—bulbous, charcoal-pointed electrodes of various sizes for galvano-caustic applications, intra-uterine platinum electrodes, and large bulbous vaginal and rectal electrodes. The belly-plate could be made of potter's clay, in which the metal plate could be buried; or better still is the plate devised by Martin, of Chicago. A good galvanic battery should have a slight chemical action and great constancy. The Leclanché cells or those of Daniell he thought the best. With 36 Leclanché cells, without a rheostat, a strength of from 300 to 350 milliamperes can be had. He thought the collector invaluable, and that to measure the dosage exactly is an absolute pre-requisite of success. The best galvanometer is that made by Gaiffe. The best Faradic battery is that of Gaiffe with a chloride of silver-pile, and the induced current of high tension from the long thin wire the one to be generally used, within the uterus.

"The induced current penetrates the tissue profoundly by reason of its high tension, but contrary to physical laws, the continuous current of low tension, has a longer and more profound action. We have proved the diffusion of the electric currents and that the galvanic current propels itself through organic tissues, its influence being felt at remote points; the current *never remains limited between the two poles.*" (Onimus.) "If we now consider the difference that exists between continuous and induced currents during their constant passage we find that it is not difficult to distinguish between them, as the line of demarcation is clear. The induced current acts for an exceedingly short time during its passage. It produces at each instant of passage a greater or less excitation and causes molecular shock. The induced current acts mechanically as an excitant, but the continuous current penetrates more gradually the tissues but more profoundly, acting chemically in such a way as to produce molecular orientation and chemical combination" (Onimus).

The induced current traversing the liquid, semi-liquid, or solid substances that go to form the human body, produces no chemical action whatever, simply a mechanical molecular disturbance. The continuous current however not only produces its chemical action at the poles, but this molecular disintegration and orientation is propagated throughout the zone between the poles. Just what the galvano-caustic action is that dissipates a tumor is not yet known—whether it coagulates the albuminoids or creates interstitial inflammation, Dr. Bigelow says he does not know; *it does reduce the tumor* and it remains for us to find out the *why.* He believes that time will demonstrate a change of *cell life* in addition to the purely chemical action, which takes place around the poles. In Apostoli's clinic the induced current is not often used. It has a wondrous effect, however, upon the ovarian pain in hysterical women. Dr. Bigelow has now seen twenty cases of this kind and every woman received immediate relief after a *séance* of ten to fifteen minutes. He has seen a large number of bleeding fibroids, but has as yet to see one that failed to respond immediately to the continuous current, the positive pole being within the uterus.

Apostoli often carries the current up to 350 milliamperes without any discomfort to the patient. It is most important that every part of the lining membrane of the uterus should be treated, and every hemorrhage, no matter how severe it may be, will resist. Dr. Bigelow affirmed that the treatment would also very appreciably diminish the size of fibroids and at times entirely dissipate them. He quoted cases to prove this point. Punctures were made into the tumors to the depth of from one to three centimeters, with a lance-pointed steel needle, the galvano-*negative* caustic being used, usually. Everything was religiously clean and antiseptic. None of the patients had any bad symptoms. He affirms that Apostoli's method arrests hemorrhage, diminishes size, relieves pain, and improves nutrition without endangering life, and does this better and more surely than any other method; and he asks why then resort to Tait's operation of excision of the appendages?

The catarrhal forms of salpingitis yield kindly to the simple action of the continuous current, one pole in the uterus. Dr. Bigelow is not yet ready to offer any decided opinion in regard to pyo-salpingitis. He however cited several cases in which negative puncture of the tube relieved or cured the case. In metritis the galvanic or Faradic current should be used according as one or the other agrees with the patient. Apostoli says that "this treatment, applied according to his double or bi-polar method, is an excellent and sometimes sovereign remedy in certain cases (recent subinvolution, chronic metritis in its first stage); inefficacious, or at least very insufficient, in others (such as chronic metritis in its latter stages), and endometritis in any form." In endometritis the continuous current and the positive pole within the uterus are used. He cited some cases of fungoid endometritis which had been cured. Dr. Apostoli Faradized every woman, even when under an acute attack, who was suffering from periuterine inflammations, observing certain rules which he has laid down. In the subacute stage, he uses first bi-uterine Faradization with a current of tension. When the inflammation begins to give way he uses the intrauterine continuous current, beginning first with the positive pole and following with the negative as soon as he is sure that the patient can bear it. In the chronic stage he uses the continuous current and galvano-puncture (negative), making the puncture in the diseased part itself. In old cases of perimetritis with much tenderness around the utero-sacral ligaments, much relief may be obtained by the vaginal electrode in the posterior fornix, while the negative pole is on the abdomen, using the induced current of high tension.

Dr. Joseph Price read a paper on

A Year's Work in a Maternity Hospital.

In making this report I desire briefly to call attention to the amount of work done, the routine treatment of patients, and a few alterations which have taken place in the building. During the year 1888 there were 184 deliveries in the Preston Retreat. Of these patients, 69 were primiparæ. There were 186 children born, including two sets of twins; 9 of these infants were still-born; 102 were males, 84 were females. There were 13 forceps deliveries. Labor was induced in 2 cases in the eighth month, for, in one case, a contracted pelvis and in the other, the presence of a large uterine tumor. There have been no deaths of mothers in the Retreat for a period of nearly five years, furnishing a series of 540 deliveries without a death, the last death being from puerperal convulsions in a patient suffering from chronic Bright's disease, who had had convulsions in five previous labors. Since this death there has not been a case of puerperal septicæmia in the institution.

The great success attending the work of this Maternity is due to the strict enforcement of the law of cleanliness. Every thing and every body in the house is clean, and jealously kept so. This system was enforced by Dr. Goodell and has been carried out on the lines laid down by him. The routine treatment of patients is as follows: the patient on entering the house is given a hot soap bath, dressed in clean underclothing and given a clean bed in the waiting ward. If necessary a laxative is given and the bowels kept open during her waiting period. Thereafter, until her confinement, she is obliged to take at least two hot soap baths per week, and to wear clean clothes. She is allowed to do such light work about the house as the physician may deem advisable, and is encouraged to take as much open-air exercise as circumstances will permit. Every effort is made by the officers and *employees* of the institution to make it as cheerful and homelike as possible. When ready for the delivery room, the patient is again given a hot soap bath, and an enema and a vaginal injection of 1 to 2000 bichloride of mercury solution. She is clothed in clean night-robe and drawers and placed upon a new, clean, delivery bed. Scrupulous cleanliness is observed in all manipulations of the patient, and after delivery a second vaginal injection is given and a vaginal suppository of iodoform is introduced. The patient's person is carefully cleaned and all soiled clothing removed, the binder applied, a clean set of night clothes put on, and the patient placed in a new, clean bed in the ward. All of the soiled articles are immediately removed from the delivery room and a new bed made up for the next patient. The patients in the ward are carefully observed by the nurses, but no unnecessary handling or interference is indulged in. The patients remain in the ward until they are able to be up, when they are removed to the convalescent ward. As the ward is emptied, the beds are burned and all the bedding most carefully cleansed. No soiled linen (as draw-sheets, diapers, napkins, or other articles of clothing) is allowed to remain in the ward; but when soiled it is immediately placed in a covered receptacle and removed from the ward and building. No sponges, wash-rags or absorbent cotton are used in the house. Corrosive jute supplies the place of these articles, being clean, soft, remarkably absorbent, and cheap; it is destroyed immediately after use. The pads used to absorb the lochia are also composed of jute and are likewise destroyed after use. The beds in the wards are of new straw. All discharges from the delivery room are immediately burned. All bedding soiled beyond cleansing or contaminated by purulent or specific discharges are likewise burned. In short, every effort is made to keep the house perfectly pure and sweet. The arrangement of the house permits of rotation in the use of the wards, so that a ward once emptied is not again used until three others have been filled. In the meantime it is most carefully and scrupulously cleaned and thrown open to the atmosphere. A similar system is pursued in the convalescent wards and delivery room.

A few alterations in the building have very markedly increased the effectiveness of the institution and the comfort of its inmates. In the first place, the bath-room and water-closets have been removed from the building proper and placed in the towers in the rear. The plumbing is as nearly perfect as modern sanitary science can make it. The verandas have been enclosed in glass, forming large, light, airy corridors about the rear of the building, and furnishing a distinct, circulating atmosphere between the house proper and the wards and the water-closets. The ventilation of the entire building is simply perfect. The capacity of the house at present is about 50 patients per month and, when a few contemplated changes are made, the capacity will be doubled and the institution rendered as nearly an ideal maternity hospital as is practicable.

Dr. Wm. Goodell said it had always been a matter of great regret to him that he did not adopt this system a year or a year and a half before he did. He supposed that his delay was partly due to the conservatism of old age and partly to a series of some 40 deaths from bichloride of mercury poisoning he had collected. Tarnier's reports of the results following the use of this agent so impressed him, that he was led to make the change. Before he adopted the system which has just been detailed by Dr. Price, he had once as many as five deaths in about 150 cases, four of these due to septicæmia. Latterly hardly a year would elapse without the occurrence of one or two deaths. When he first started everything about the institution was new and clean, and for several years he had the best record of any maternity hospital in the world. After the building and articles had become old, deaths began to occur. He tried carbolic acid, but it proved of little value. After beginning the use of corrosive sublimate injections, iodoform suppositories and antiseptic pads, he did not have a death from septicæmia. The only death was one from Bright's disease of the kidneys. During this time he had been consulted perhaps a dozen times in the course of a year to see women dying from puerperal septicæmia. He thought that in private practice it would not be needful to follow out so strictly the details of the method as it is practised at the Preston Retreat. For instance, the antiseptic pad and the iodoform suppositories might be done away with. He believed however that every practitioner should syringe out the vagina both before the birth of the child and after complete delivery, with a bichloride solution of 1-2000. The hands should also be disinfected. He was called in consultation by a physician in the country who had had four or five deaths from sepsis in a short time. Dr. Goodell found he had been treating a case of phlegmonous erysipelas. He knew of another physician who had lost, he thought, seven cases, certainly five, from dressing a sloughing case of erysipelas. Antiseptic measures would probably have saved all these cases.

Dr. Henry Leaman called the attention of those who have the opportunity of observing the physiological processes of labor to one point, viz.: presentation. It is very difficult to determine accurately the presentation, especially of the face, brow and posterior presentations. These observations should be verified by examination of the abdomen previous to labor and by the location of the fœtal heart sounds. They should also be confirmed by observation of the position of the head in the act of delivery. A mistake is readily made in posterior presentations. Posterior presentations are, he thinks, more frequent than we are in the habit of considering them. Every case of labor is a case for the minutest observation. There is another point which he thought should be observed, that is, the hour of the day at which labor occurs. There is probably some connection between arterial pressure and the time of delivery. In recording the hour an allowance is to be observed in cases in which the forceps. are used. There is another point not mentioned, and that is the position of the succedaneum and its extent. These have to do with the natural process of labor and aid in determining the presentation.

DR. J. PRICE said he was as anxious about a labor as he was about a section. When he read reports of Maternity Hospitals with a mortality of from two to twenty-seven per cent., this troubled him not a little now that he controlled a large maternity hospital, one in which Dr. Goodell had left a record of 275 cases without a death. He sees a labor case as frequently as he does one of drainage after abdominal section. When this hospital was new, Dr. Goodell had a run of 250 cases without a death from any cause. This was the longest run of any institution at that time; after this deaths began to occur; later he adopted the gospel of cleanliness, and with what result he has just stated. The results are now precisely the same as he left them. In regard to Dr. Hirst's question as to whether the same results might not be obtained by simpler methods, Dr. Price said that they did not differ much in regard to the use of solutions and that portion of the treatment. The toilet of the house was perhaps just as systematically carried out at the Philadelphia Hospital as at other institutions. The pad which he had shown would hold a pint of fluid. It saved an immense amount of laundry work. It was now coming into use as a menstrual pad and was very convenient for women traveling. In private practice the mortality is greater among the rich than the poor. Among the poor he has had 700 deliveries without a death. He thought the difference was in the water-closets which the better classes have in their houses. The mortality throughout the country is large. In a small town in Ohio, with a high elevation and beautifully located, he had recently known of two deaths from septicæmia. Last summer he had been called to see puerperal cases nine times, and all the patients died.

—The Philadelphia Polyclinic has devised a scheme to accommodate physicians who are unable to leave home for a prolonged period. It now issues tickets, good in any department for one clinic weekly for three months, and at the usual fee for a six weeks' course of daily clinics. This should be a great convenience to practitioners residing within a day's journey of the city.

REPORTS OF CLINICS.

PHILADELPHIA HOSPITAL.

CLINIC ON DISEASES OF CHILDREN—DR. HIRST.

Method of Conducting Post-mortem Examinations of Infants.

Before beginning the *post-mortem* examination on the body of an infant that was three months old and was supposed to have died of congenital syphilis, Dr. Hirst remarked that the body should always be weighed first; he also said that the liver and spleen in congenital syphilis are not, as in health, one thirtieth and one three hundredth respectively of the whole weight, but bear a much larger ratio, the former reaching sometimes so large a ratio as one sixth of the whole body weight. There are certain anatomical peculiarities in an infant's body with which one should be acquainted. The bladder, sigmoid flexure, and vermiform appendix are much larger proportionally in infants, while the position of the stomach is vertical, thus rendering vomiting so easy as to be mere regurgitation.

Upon external examination of the child nothing noteworthy was found. On opening the abdomen, the spleen was found to be of normal size, as was also the liver, so that there proved to be far less ground for suspicion of congenital syphilis than had been looked for. The kidneys were, as usual, lobulated. The respiratory organs were examined from the mouth down, in order to detect a foreign body, as a curd of milk, in the trachea, if the child had during life inspired some solid substance. The lungs were healthy, thus excluding pneumonia, which is a very frequent cause of death in infants. The thymus gland was normal. Dr. Grawitz has reported two cases in which this gland was so enlarged as to choke the infant. The heart was normal. The ductus arteriosus was closed. Dr. Hirst has seen it open in an infant four weeks old, and again at the third month. The foramen ovale, which remains patulous for a few days in all cases, was found reduced to an opening the size of a pin. It is not rare to find an opening the size of a pin-hole at the site of the foramen ovale as late as the twelfth month. The dura mater being, as usual, adherent to the sutures, the cranium was hard to remove. A knife was passed down the coronal and sagittal sutures, and the frontal and parietal bones thus removed.

The brain was slightly congested, but not to a degree sufficient to have caused any serious symptoms.

Dr. Hirst thought that the cause of death in this child, which had had diarrhœa, was either an ulcerated condition of the mucous membrane of the large intestines or an inflammatory infiltration of their connective tissue, causing atrophy of the absorbent glands, which latter condition a microscopic examination would be necessary to show. He also referred to the common occurrence of *post-mortem* intussusception in young infants and remarked that the difference between *ante-* and *post-mortem* intussusceptions is that the latter are without signs of inflammation or congestion.

He regards sterilized milk as the great remedy to prevent diarrhœa in infants, and he has recently devised a cheap and efficient apparatus for its preparation.

CLINIC ON NERVOUS DISEASES—DR. F. X. DERCUM.

An Affection Allied to Myxœdema.

The first patient I bring before you is a woman, fifty years old. When first seen, twenty months ago, she was confined in bed and her arms were fixed. She complained then that the least movement gave her intense pain; and her face showed it. There was also noticed this tremendous swelling of the arms.

Her history shows nothing peculiar. She has been married and has had several children that were healthy. Two and a half years before coming here she noticed that her arms were swelling, and six months after pain in the right arm began to appear, along the nerve trunks. These pains were paroxysmal, lasting from two hours to several days. During the paroxysms the arms looked larger and lobulated. This appearance subsided as the pains left. In spite of tenderness over parts of the limbs, there existed areas of marked anæsthesia, which were found up to within a short time ago. Some anæsthesia still remains in the right arm and the left forearm. The trunk and leg on the right side were also anæsthetic in patches, associated with which there were peculiar pains Now there is some anæsthesia of the right side of the neck, but none has ever existed on the face. The visual fields are now contracted, especially on the right side. The tongue has suffered, as the organ of taste, and the sense of smell has likewise deteriorated.

The hearing on the right side is not as good as formerly.

The question for us to decide is : whether the case is one of local dystrophy, dependent upon some organic disease, or some general disease of nutrition affecting the body as a whole. I am inclined to the latter opinion, on account of the enormous masses of flesh upon the back, right thigh and knee, which have a nodulated feeling.

Myxœdema has been suggested. In this disease there is usually swelling of the connective tissue in all parts of the body, especially in the face and hands. This is not the case here. The skin is especially affected with hypertrophy. There is also in this case an absence of the dryness and hardness, as in myxœdema proper, from a deficient innervation of the sweat-glands. Some discoloration has been present and there was noticed a change of nutrition affecting the tissues beneath the skin. This change, however, did not extend to the muscles, which are not enlarged, nor to the bones ; but is found in the subcutaneous tissue, which is connective tissue. This is found out by introducing a Duchenne trochar and excising a small piece of tissue, which, under the microscope, is found to be largely mucous tissue and embryonal fat. The blood-vessels show an infiltration of their sheaths—a kind of sclerosis.

The nerve fibres—not the cerebro-spinal but the sympathetic—show a thickening of tissue and degeneration from inflammatory change, the connective tissue about the ganglia being much altered. Associated with these organic lesions, we must also bear in mind the curious pains and symptoms that we have mentioned.

It is not typical myxœdema, because the mental faculties are all right. It is true she is irritable, but no more than would be accounted for by her suffering. In myxœdema the thyroid gland undergoes lessening in size and marked change in structure. Here also we cannot feel the thyroid. In myxœdema there is hemorrhage from the mucous surfaces. Our patient has had hemorrhage from the throat, lungs and uterus. She has also vomited blood.

The prognosis in myxœdema is almost always unfavorable. One of the most favorable symptoms is great sweating. This woman at her worst did not sweat at all, but as she began to improve, the sweating commenced. She is not now getting any better. Her arms have increased an inch in circumference during the last six months.

As regards treatment, when the pain was

violent, she was given morphia. Now, as the pain is less, she is given antipyrin. Her general treatment has been tonic and symptomatic. She also has frequent cardiac dyspnœa, a symptom often found in myxœdema. This will be treated when necessary with cardiac sedatives.

UNIVERSITY HOSPITAL.

SURGICAL CLINIC.—PROF. D. HAYES AGNEW.

Fracture of the Clavicle.

This boy, eight years old, fell and fractured the right clavicle near the acromial end. Great care is to be used in the detection of such fractures in children, not only because they are less apt than adults to recognize them themselves, but also because they do not assume the position so characteristic in adults. This position consists in placing the forearm of the injured side across the chest and supporting it by holding the hand of the sound side beneath the elbow. The head also slightly inclines to the injured side. Children, too, also use their injured limbs remarkably well, because some fibres may not be broken, constituting a kind of green-stick fracture.

Fracture of the clavicle generally occurs, as in this case, near the acromial end, on account of the position of the curves and consequent distribution of force. The fragments in these fractures are more easily retained in position than if the fracture were at the sternal end.

In dressing such a fracture the loop of an adhesive strap is placed about the middle of the arm. Another adhesive strap, with a nick for the olecranon process, is placed beneath the elbow. The first is carried around the body behind and secured in position, not including the sound arm. The ends of the second piece are carried up over the shoulder of the sound side, one going in front of the chest and one behind it.

Pott's Disease.

This girl, eleven years old, has antero-posterior curvature of the spine, with a projection. She had worn a plaster-jacket for a year until a week ago, when she took it off as an experiment. Though the plaster-jacket interferes with development and should, therefore, be left off as soon as possible, yet as the reproduction of the disease would be such a serious matter, and as the reparative parts of the bone that have been thrown out are liable to

injury because they are still spongy, it would be safer to keep it on for six months more.

Multiple Exostoses.

This girl, twenty-five years old, has many exostoses, occurring upon the tibia, knee, left angle of the scapula, and ribs. One near the upper end of the femur was so large as to interfere with locomotion and had to be removed. The wound is now healing satisfactorily. The patient never had rheumatism.

These exostoses began to develop about the age of puberty, when the epiphyses and diaphyses come together, and near the ends of the bones where the osteogenetic function is most active. They are true bone, and may begin from a slight inflammation of the periosteum.

NEW YORK CORRESPONDENCE.

Prof. Winters on Constipation in Children.—Prof. Gibney on White Swelling and Pott's Disease.—Prof. Thomson on Jacksonian Epilepsy, Hammer Palsy, and the Treatment of Scarlet Fever, Typhoid Fever, and Diphtheria.—Dr. Holt on Chorea and Petit-Mal.

NEW YORK, March 19, 1889.

Prof. J. E. Winters, in a recent clinic on constipation in infants, said that if the constipation is in a nursing infant, look first to the mother's bowels. If she is costive (has a daily but not a free and full movement), give her belladonna or ipecac, with small doses of strychnia, as the costiveness is probably due to diminished secretions in the alimentary canal. Follow these drugs with a cold, salt-water abdominal bath, kneading the abdomen thoroughly. If the mother is constipated (does not have daily movements), add some mild cathartic to the above treatment; cascara sagrada and the mineral waters are good. The diet should not be restricted but should consist of a plentiful supply of vegetables, fruits, and farinaceous food. Excessive tea drinking by the mother is sometimes the cause of colic and constipation in the infant. In such a case, discontinue the tea absolutely and use milk, chocolate, gruel, and coffee in moderation. If the cause does not lie in the mother, turn your attention to the child, and begin treatment with the juice of fruits; that of oranges is preferable, and a child two days old can take the juice of one-fourth of an orange, twice daily; and this amount should be increased daily. If this is not effectual try grape juice, or the meats of stewed prunes and cherries. The latter are especially good. The cold, salt-water abdominal bath should be used for the mother in connection with this treatment of the infant. If it does not act, give an injection of glycerine (f℥ ss-j) daily at a definite hour. It acts on the circulation and increases the secretion of the bowel. In addition to the injection, to every bottle of milk add a fluid drachm of glycerine, or a piece of fresh, unsalted butter as large as a hazel nut. Never use castor oil or rhubarb. If drugs are necessary, begin with a small dose of ipecac (gtt. ij-v), especially when the movements are hard and dry. Also use small doses of nux vomica and belladonna. If a cathartic becomes necessary, cascara sagrada is good. It does not lead to constipation and does not lose its effect by continual use. Begin with a small dose and increase it until there is a good movement daily, and then decrease it until it can be discontinued. Use fruit and glycerine injections with it. The use of opium by unscrupulous nurses and mothers is a frequent cause of constipation.

At a recent clinic by Prof. V. P. Gibney, at the New York Polyclinic and Hospital, the first case was one of caries of the ankle, a tubercular osteitis or, as it is commonly known, white swelling. The patient was a child 3 years old who, up to eight weeks ago, was perfectly well, though malnutrition and weakness were written on every line of her face. In walking she gave the characteristic ankle limp, directing attention immediately to the right ankle. Examination showed the presence of swelling, tenderness, atrophy of adjacent muscles, heat, and reflex spasm. The last symptom is important and characteristic of joint disease. The foot could be flexed, extended or rotated only a slight distance; beyond that, movement was opposed by muscular spasm. Palpation showed tenderness only at the epiphyses of the long bones, and Dr. Gibney thought the tarsus not involved. The lesion is a softening of the bone with the presence of tubercle, the process working from the centre to the periphery. Formerly, said Dr. Gibney, it was thought, and many surgeons still hold the same opinion, that there are only two ways of dealing with this disease, namely, by amputation or by excision; the diseased bone had to be gotten rid of. Dr. Gibney is decidedly opposed to operation and thinks the expectant plan of treatment the only plan upheld by results. For instance, he would treat this child in the following manner: pad the sole of the foot thickly with cotton, and put on a plaster bandage, running it well up the leg. By this means excessive weight is kept off of the ankle, and jarring is prevented by the cotton pad. Then give the child cod liver oil and iron, look after her general health, and get her out into the air and sunshine. When she is ten years of age she will have as good an ankle as anybody, and will be able to walk, skate, or dance. Let her go into most hospitals, however, and an operation will be performed that will not only maim her for life, but which, in most cases, will fail to stop the disease. In support of these statements he gave a synopsis of fifty or sixty cases, which were treated expectantly, and with brilliant results. This treatment refers to children, for, if the patient is an adult, it is useless to spend so much time. The proper course in adults is either to scoop out the diseased bone, amputate, or do excision.

The second patient was a boy, 15 years old, with well-marked Pott's disease of the dorsal region of the spine. He is being treated by fixation of the spine by means of a corset with two iron bars in the back, one on each side of the bony column. The disease, said the Professor, comes on usually between the age of two and eight years, seldom later than that. It attacks tubercular subjects, and the tuberculosis may be either congenital or acquired—acquired usually after a disease with a tardy convalescence. This gives good soil for the bacilli, which give evidence of their presence by means of a running ear, an eczematous head, or a phlyctenular conjunctivitis, the so-called "strumous condition." With such a condition a slight fall may start up the disease, or it may start without apparent cause. When deformity exists the disease is easy of diagnosis, and there is no excuse for mistake. It should be, however, diagnosticated early in its history, before there is any deformity. The following are some of the symptoms: pick the child up by its arms or chest and it cries; it moans in its sleep, tosses and is restless; its cry is very different from the sharp cry of hip disease; it walks peculiarly, with short, careful steps, holding the spine stiff; there may be associated spinal curvature, and if in the lumbar region, it will cause a hip-limp; the pain is a constant symptom, and if the disease is in the lumbar region the pain will radiate down the anterior crural nerve; if in the cervical region up the occipital nerve; while if the disease is in the dorsal region there will be gastralgia.

Dr. Gibney's treatment of spinal disease includes not only fixation, extension, etc., as the case may require, but also the internal use of the iodide of potassium, on the efficacy of which he lays great stress.

At a recent clinic by Prof. W. H. Thomson, at the University Medical College, the first patient exhibited was a child three years old, who, when eight months old, had had a fit. The spasm was confined chiefly to the left side, the eyes being turned to the right. It left the patient with paralysis of the left arm and leg, and a high fever lasting for two weeks. At irregular intervals since then, especially when cutting teeth, she has had similar fits, affecting the same side and giving the same manifestations. At night she clenches her hand and grinds her teeth. The convulsions and paralysis are epileptic, there probably having been a fall or some injury, with hemorrhage under the dura mater causing some thickening over the motor area. There is every indication of meningeal irritation over this area, and the implication of the eye shows that the irritation extends back to the angular gyrus or occipital lobe. If the fits recur, the case is just the kind that is suitable for the operation of trephining, for the removal of the hyperplasia. It is the kind of epilepsy called Jacksonian, and has these characteristics: that the fits always begin on the same side of the body, in the same muscles, and recur frequently. There being paralysis, and the fits being comparatively rare, the case might be mistaken for infantile paralysis, or anterior poliomyelitis. In the latter, there is a peculiar reaction to electricity. The Faradic current has no effect, while the galvanic or constant current causes contraction, both when the poles are applied and when the circuit is broken. This peculiarity indicates organic disease of the spinal motor centers, and is called the reaction of degeneration.

The next case was one of a rare disease called hammer palsy. The patient was a man, 53 years old, and a tinner, which occupation necessitated the continual use of a hammer. Four years ago, his right arm began to grow weak and to shake. His trouble increased, until now he has a well-defined case of palsy. Placing his feet together and shutting his eyes increase his tremor, but his body does not sway. An effort of the will to stop the tremors increases the shaking. There is no tremor of the tongue. There is great pain in the arm and leg. The palsy is one due to injury of the nerves from over-exertion and is similar to writers' palsy. The tremor being aggravated by the will excludes paralysis agitans.

The following is Prof. Thomson's treatment of scarlet fever:

R Acidi carbolici . . . . gr. xvj
   Bismuthi subnit. . . . . . . gr. xl
   Pepsini sacch. . . . . gr. xl
M. Div. in pulv. viij. Sig. Take one every three hours.

This helps digestion and is antiseptic. Beef tea should be avoided and the diet consist only of milk. In the case of heart failure, heart stimulants must be used.

For other fevers, especially typhoid fever, he uses the following: Disinfect the alimentary canal with a calomel purge; a child three years old can take four grains. As soon as it acts use chlorine in the form of Labarraque's solution of chlorinated soda. Sweeten the milk and add this solution. A drachm can be given every half-hour if necessary. If the bowels are irritable use paregoric, etc.; but above everything else keep up the chlorine.

In diphtheria he uses Smith's solution of bromine, locally and internally, in some cases giving as much as a grain of bromine to a child one year old. When concentrated it produces strangury, hence it must be largely diluted. It does not cause vomiting as do the tincture of the chloride of iron and quinine. Diphtheria is a self-limiting disease, and all that a physician can do is to ward off complications. The greatest danger is septic poisoning, and Prof. Thomson thinks bromine the best remedy with which to avert this.

Dr. L. Emmet Holt, at one of his clinics on diseases of children at the Polyclinic, showed a case of chorea in a boy, which was interesting in showing the connection of chorea, heart disease and rheumatism. The patient's grandfather has heart disease; his father, heart disease and rheumatism; his brother, rheumatism; his sister, heart disease and rheumatism, and the patient himself chorea and heart disease. The boy had a phimosis, and he fell into the hands of a quack who operated upon him, giving the parents the assurance that the phimosis was the cause of the chorea and that upon its removal the chorea would disappear.

Another patient was a girl, 4 years old, whose parents have three other children in good health. When she was a year old she had eight or nine convulsions, and now, after an interval of nearly two years, they have returned. She falls; her face is pale, and the pallor is followed by cyanosis and dilated pupils; there is loss of consciousness; her jaws are closed. The fits occur in the daytime, are of short duration, and are followed by a sound sleep. In her sleep she clenches her hand. It is a case of epilepsy, *petit mal*, and interesting from the fact that like many epilepsies it can be traced back to infantile convulsions. Epilepsy is often associated with rickets, but in this child the teeth appeared at the fourth month, she walked at the eighteenth, and there was no evidence of rickets. Dr. Holt's treatment was with the bromides; he prefers bromide of sodium, as it does not disturb the stomach and is pleasanter to take. When this can not be used, oxide of zinc, hyoscyamus, chloral and antipyrin can be tried. The treatment should be kept up at least a year and a half, and should include tonics.

PERISCOPE.

Diabetes and Tumors.

Dr. Tuffier has recently published a monograph on this somewhat important subject in the *Archives Générales de Médecine.* The coincidence of diabetes and neoplasms, only noted hitherto in a few scattered publications, and entirely overlooked in standard text-books, does not appear to be rare. This coincidence is not surprising to the author. He accepts M. Verneuil's bold theory that both tumors and diabetes are related to the arthritic diathesis. Already almost every form of tumor has been observed in diabetic patients. Almost every form of diabetes has been found to attack persons already the subjects of tumor. As a rule, the constitutional disease comes first; the patient is diabetic already before the tumor makes its appearance. Malignant tumors, as a rule, advance without causing much pain, and somewhat slowly in these cases, but they proceed more rapidly than the diabetic symptoms. They are apt to be taken for innocent growths. The complication in question is very serious in respect to operative interference, as we all know. No surgeon should think of removing small, innocent tumors which are causing no trouble. Dr. Tuffier describes two instructive cases. In the first, death occurred forty hours after the removal of a small parotid tumor. The fact that the patient was diabetic had been overlooked. This was also the case in the second example of the dangers of operation under the circumstances. "A little hypertrophic

tumor of the skin of the cheek" was removed, at the patient's request. Phlegmonous erysipelas, followed by sloughing, set in and killed the patient within five days. Urgent operations must, Dr. Tuffier asserts, be undertaken with great caution. The safer are preferable to the most thorough, in his opinion. When an operation appears absolutely necessary, but not urgent, it is important to spend some time in reducing the diabetic symptoms by medical treatment. Should, however, all the sugar and polyuria disappear, the surgeon must still never overlook the nature of the patient's diathesis. Under the most favorable circumstances, in any case of that kind, deep operations and prolonged dissections, free division of vessels, and the formation of large flaps are to be avoided. The slow progress of tumors and the little pain which they produce are important facts, according to Dr. Tuffier. He has found that malignant tumors lie almost latent in diabetic subjects for a long period. Removal of a similar growth from a healthy subject would hardly insure him against so long an interval of time before recurrence. When an operation is thought advisable, the thermocautery is preferable to the knife. No attempt to insure union by first intention should be made if it involves the slightest traction on skin flaps. The wound must be laid open, but dressed with extreme antiseptic precautions.—*British Med. Journal,* Feb. 16, 1889.

The Formation of Hæmoglobin in the Spleen.

Dr. Krieuger, of Dorpat, has made a number of experiments on cats with the aid of Hüfner's spectro-photometer, for the purpose of discovering whether the amount of hæmoglobin contained in the splenic artery is greater than that in the splenic vein. He found that the quantity of blood in the splenic vein amounted to 9.52 per cent., while in the artery it was only 9.28 per cent. From these researches he came to the conclusion that hæmoglobin is actually formed in the spleen. The results are quite consistent with those obtained by different methods by Drs. Malassez and Picard in France and by Drs. Pashiutin and Vinogradoff in Russia. It is of course well known that there is a considerable quantity of iron in the tissue of the spleen, consequently there is no inherent improbability in Dr. Krieuger's theory.—*Lancet*, Feb. 16, 1889.

Nephrectomy for Floating Kidney.

Dr. W. Hager, of Wandsbek, in a paper published in the *Berliner klin. Wochenschrift*, Jan. 14, 1889, says that there is at present no subject in the whole of medicine upon which the opinions of authors differ so widely as upon the pathology and treatment of movable kidney. The explanation of this is found principally in the fact that the clinical pictures of floating kidney are so wonderfully different. While a degree of kidney dislocation may be borne in one woman with scarcely any discomfort, the same state of affairs will in others, for unexplained reasons, excite the most painful and serious symptoms.

The views in regard to the treatment of floating kidney differ still more widely than they do in regard to its pathology. While Keppler considered extirpation as the only possible cure, Landau and others reject every attempt at operative interference. For ordinary cases of floating kidney the bandage treatment is recommended by most authors. Dr. Hager, however, has been satisfied with it in only three out of the twenty-two cases in which he has used it. One of the patients had a protruding abdomen, and here the application of the bandage secured a highly satisfactory result, as it did also in a striking case of movable liver. Among the other cases, among which there were five nulliparæ, the bandages were very soon laid aside as useless, or even injurious In course of time, especially with careful regulation of the bowels, the discomfitures were lessened or the patients learned to become accustomed to them.

For the serious, though few, cases of floating kidney that require operation, there are two methods of operating :

1. Nephrectomy, first recommended by Keppler, of which, according to the latest statistics, there have been thirty-six cases, and 2. Nephroraphy after Hahn's method, which, according to the same statistics, has been performed in twenty-nine instances. The trial of both operations forces Lindner to the conclusion that in future he would rather himself assume the risk of nephrectomy than propose to his patients nephrorraphy, an operation which is never entirely without danger and the results of which are so doubtful, as former experience proves. He further states that in nephrectomy when it is a success, patients are without exception freed from their sufferings.

To decide this very important question as to whether nephrectomy is, indeed, the only legitimate operation and, if it is a success, always leads to recovery, the report of the following case may be of weight.

Miss —— was in good health till August, 1886, when, while sea-bathing, she violently struck her abdomen, which pained her very much for a short time. In September her appetite became poor, and nausea, dizziness and at times, shortness of breath developed. Upon going to stool, the patient felt as though she were being drawn forward. She was considered chlorotic and iron and quinine prescribed. In December she suddenly had a violent attack, beginning with severe abdominal pain and general numbness, partial paralysis of the tongue and opisthotonus. Such attacks occurred two or three times a week, lasting several hours, and were accompanied with vomiting, nausea, and constipation ; there was also marked anemia and emaciation.

Upon April 20, Dr. Hager was summoned to the patient, and found her in an attack which, at first, appeared to be tetanus. There was agonizing pain in the epigastrium and opisthotonus The attack lasted two hours. Examination the next day showed the heart and lungs to be normal, the epigastrium very tender, while the right kidney descended on deep inspiration. This movement was plainly perceptible ; the left kidney was normal. The urine, temperature and pulse were normal, so that only rest in bed and regulation of the bowels were ordered.

On April 27, a light kidney-shaped truss was ordered. A week afterward the patient was doing well, and then had a severe attack.

For a month all modes of bandaging were tried and failed, so that Dr. Hager felt forced to operate. He hesitated between nephrectomy and nephroraphy, and Dr. Wiesinger, of Hamburg, being called in, rejected nephroraphy as being at best uncertain and advised nephrectomy by Czerny's lateral incision, which operation he performed, tying the vessels with cat-gut ligatures. The wound was stuffed with iodoform lint and a bichloride dressing applied. The extirpated kidney was healthy. The pulse was fairly good after the operation. In the evening there were pain, vomiting and anuria ; the temperature was 97.7° F.

At three o'clock that night Dr. Hager found the patient apparently moribund from loss of blood, and, there being no bleeding vessel, he closed the wound with deep sutures, thus arresting the hemorrhage. The patient came to, June 6, passed a little urine and had great nausea. Both symptoms improved the next day. On June 7 a drainage tube was introduced and the wound from that time improved rapidly, though the patient had continual desire to pass urine, which was dark, but contained no albumin and no abnormal constituents. On July 2 the wound was perfectly healed, and at the end of the month the patient could sit up in a chair for several hours.

On August 29 the patient was worse, and confined to bed with pain in the left side of the abdomen, dysuria, weakness and giddiness. Two weeks later Dr. Hager found that the left kidney was movable and that the patient had passed several stones. The urine was acid and free from albumin. On October 5, there had been pain and vomiting, but lately and during the last few weeks about fifty stones the size of a millet-seed were passed. Dr. Kummel now performed nephrorophy by Czerny's method and the patient returned home nearly well by the end of the month. After staying in bed and dieting ten weeks the patient could get up, and eight weeks afterward could walk about. The stones lessened under the use of Lithia water.

On Oct. 8, Dr. Hager was called to the patient and found her suffering with anuria of sixteen hours' duration, accompanied with headache, vomiting, and swelling in the left side, which was very tender and showed an area of dulness the size of one's hand. Uræmia being threatened, the propriety of establishing a urinary fistula was considered, but this proved to be unnecessary, as the flow of urine returned the next day. A dislocation of the kidney could not be demonstrated. It is nevertheless safe to assume that anuria, whether caused by a stone or acute angle in the ureter or kidney degeneration, will finally cause death from uræmia, especially since neither the family nor patient can be persuaded to consent to another operation.

The above case, he says, requires no further commentary, for there seems no doubt but that, in a previously healthy patient, dislocation and lithiasis in the left kidney are to be regarded as the results of the removal of its fellow organ.

He endorses Landau's opinion that in future no one will think of the extirpation of a sound kidney. Sometimes an operation will be indicated, and then only nephrorophy should be considered, which in most cases will prove satisfactory. Should there be a relapse, the operation, under antisepsis, may be repeated without danger. It will be of great importance to keep the patient in bed a long time with good regimen; for not unfrequently the symptoms of floating kidney have been seen to disappear for a long time without any operation under the use of Dr. Weir Mitchell's method of treatment.

Immediate Correction of Deformities from Hip-disease.

Dr. V. P. Gibney read a paper on the immediate correction of deformities resulting from hip-disease before the New York Surgical Society, Oct. 24, 1888. In this paper, which is published in the *N. Y. Med. Journal*, Feb. 2, 1889, states that during the previous ten months he had employed the following treatment:

Under an anæsthetic, simple manual force is employed to pull the limb into position; the adductors and flexors are divided subcutaneously by means of the Adams fascia knife; the deeper flexors are cut by open incision; the femur is divided below the trochanter minor (Gant's operation); the plaster-of-Paris bandage is applied over a closely fitting stockingette or cheese-cloth bandage from the ankle to the free ribs; and rest in bed is required for a week or ten days.

He says he has made no attempt whatever to secure motion or to break up the adhesions. His aim has been to supplement the manual force with tenotomy, myotomy, or osteotomy—one, or all combined when necessary—and to secure parallelism of the limbs at one operation if possible. In many cases he states that the deformity has been so great and the resistance so obstinate that a second or third operation has been necessary to secure the object desired. The duration of the disease or the stage of deformity has not been taken into consideration. Where abscesses exist, or where numerous sinuses remain, he has freely opened the one and curetted the other.

The treatment subsequent to operation has been to continue the plaster-of-Paris dressing for a few weeks, and then to employ the long hip-splint for traction of the limb and protection of the joint. He asserts that in no single case upon which he has operated has any acute joint suppuration followed. Where abscesses or sinuses existed, the suppuration did not always cease; but the suppurative process has not been aggravated by the treatment employed. Friends of hospital patients have in a few instances complained that positive injury was inflicted. He gives in detail the histories of some of his cases.

Seventeen patients were between three and eight years of age, ten between eight and twelve, and three were over twelve years of age. The disease had existed as follows: Six months in one case, one year in four cases, two years in three cases, three years in six, four years in four, five years in four, six years in five, seven years in two, and eight years in one case.

In four cases there was double hip-disease. In six cases Pott's disease also existed, and in one of these osteitis of the knee was likewise present. Ten cases presented deformity in a moderate degree, in eighteen the deformity was great, and in two it was extreme. He states that in only three cases the result has not been as good as was anticipated.

Professor Sée on Heart Diseases.

The Paris correspondent of the *Lancet*, Jan. 19, 1889, says that in resuming his winter course of lectures on clinical medicine, M. Germain Sée began by a general review of the diseases of the heart. Diseases of the heart, said the Professor, are not distinct from one another. It is the same affection presenting itself under different aspects, and offering different types. Whether the case be one of subacute or acute endocarditis, ulcerative or vegetating, the disease is always parasitic, and this view leads to a no less revolutionary deduction, that of the negation of their inflammatory nature. Under the latent, and sometimes the remote, influence of a specific disease, especially of articular or choreic rheumatism, the endocardium is exposed to the action of the microbe, easily defined in this part, although not so readily recognized in the joints. At other times the cause is a typhoid fever, or an attack of diphtheria long forgotten, scarlatina, infectious pneumonia, or even syphilis. There is no exception to this rule of the parasitic origin of valvular or myocardial mischief, except in chronic affections of the aortic orifice of old people, which coincide and result from the fatty, atheromatous, and sclerous changes of the arteries. Like all other cardiac diseases, those of the aortic orifice in the young are parasitic. It is degeneration without a trace of inflammation that is found in all heart lesions, whether acute or chronic, and to this condition Professor Sée would give the name of "*endocardie.*" The same parts, the same elements, and the same spots are invaded, the permanent lesion consisting of a hyperplasia of the connective tissue. The disease is a continuation of the morbid process, which began in an acute or subacute form, perhaps unperceived by the patient or medical attendant. There is consequently but one cardiac disease, presenting two types—the endocardial and the valvular types. A third type is due to sclerous, atheromatous, and other changes in the arteries, comprised under the general term "arteritis," due to age, alcoholism, gout, diabetes, etc. The fourth type, and to which M. Sée assigns the most important place, is that condition of the heart which is caused by sclerosis of the coronary arteries, leading to degeneration and narrowing of the vessels, and ultimately to sclerosis of the myocardium—the fifth type. In the sixth class, Professor Sée places the hypertrophies and dilatations consequent upon primary valvular disease. The seventh class comprises the nervous troubles. Professor Sée does not think, however, that palpitation and acceleration of the heart's action ever leads to hypertrophy. A pulse of 140 may exist without producing this effect. Nor does exophthalmic goitre lead to the slightest lesion or fatigue. The eighth type is the pericardiac, the cause here being always parasitic. In the ninth and last category, come dilatation and aneurisms of the aorta.

Blennorrhœa in Women.

During the period of six years Horand has had under his care 5,090 women and 764 little girls suffering with blennorrhœa, and it is upon this large number of observations that he bases (*Lyon méd.*, 1888, lix, 251) the present study. He is a firm believer in the gonococcus as the cause of blennorrhœa, and teaches that where the gonococcus is not found there is no blennorrhœa. In the women the parts affected are, in order of frequency, the urethra, vagina, glands of Bartholin, uterus, and anus. In little girls the order is vagina, urethra, vulva, and anus. Urethral blennorrhœa in women causes little disturbance; it may give rise to slight itching or more frequent urination; cystitis is rare. It may continue a long time, months or years, and is apt to remain limited to the urethra. Inflammation of the vulva is rare in women, more frequent in girls. It is generally consequent upon mechanical irritation, want of care, direct contagion, attempts at rape, or is accidental from contact with objects soiled with blennorrhagic pus. It may exist alone or associated with elytritis or urethritis. The epithelium of the vestibule seems to offer a good deal of resistance to infection. Elytritis is more frequent—rather more so in girls than in women. Uterine blennorrhœa is very rare—

it was found only six times in four hundred and eighty-three examinations. It is the result of transmission from the vagina. Bartholin's glands are affected only secondarily. Anal blennorrhœa is more frequent in women than in men. It is the result both of mediate and of immediate contagion. Gonorrhœal rheumatism is very rare in women, as is gonorrhœal ophthalmia. For the treatment of urethritis the best means is nitrate of silver, a grain and a half to the ounce. For elytritis in a child, irrigations with a warm boric-acid solution of one-per-cent. strength should be used; in adults, the silver nitrate in stick applied directly every four or five days. The same treatment is also best for the disease when it affects the uterus, the anus, or the conjunctiva.—*N. Y. Med. Journal*, March 2, 1889.

Poisoning with Sulphocyanide of Mercury.

A patient was recently poisoned in Paris in a way that for some time remained undiscovered. The *Chemist and Druggist*, Feb. 14, gives the following explanation of it:

A sergeant, attached to the hospital, and chemically inclined, undertook one day to prepare Pharaoh's serpents' eggs. Being too much of a tyro to make the chemical himself, he purchased sulphocyanide of mercury from a dealer in town, and began to rub it to powder in a stone mortar in the hospital pharmacy. He was called away before finishing it, and, being unaware of the danger, left the stuff in the mortar. During his absence a nurse, sent, against the rules, by the sick officer for subnitrate of bismuth, took in lieu of it some of the sulphocyanide of mercury, which poisoned the patient, young De Carayon-Latour. As soon as trouble broke out, the sergeant threw away the contents of the mortar and said nothing. On investigation traces of a mercurial compound were found in the implement, and the cause of death was clearly traced to mercuric poisoning. But, as it was shown that the poison-closet had not been unlocked, it was impossible to conceive how the mercury could have been procured, until the sergeant confessed his fault. It may be interesting to note that the present is said to be the first instance of fatal poisoning by mercuric sulphocyanide recorded by French authors. An accident occurred in 1865 to a princely guest of one of the Paris hotels, who received immediate medical attendance, and speedily recovered. In the Carayon-Latour case, on the contrary, the patient, to save a comrade from punishment, concealed his state as long as he could, and received medical treatment too late to save his life. Considering the reckless use of the serpents' eggs by children and others, it must be conceded that the mercuric compound cannot be called a very violent poison. At the same time it cannot be considered the harmless insoluble combination that some pretend it to be. The treatment successfully resorted to in the older case was simple lime-water and reduced iron internally, and a warm poultice, with laudanum on the abdomen. The next day the patient was well, and the voiding of a tapeworm, hitherto unsuspected, was the only reminder of the internal commotion caused by the sulphocyanide.

Syphilitic Disease of the Cervix Uteri.

Dr. E. Rode, of Christiania, has observed three cases of ulcerating gummata of the vaginal portion of the cervix. They appeared from ten to twelve years after infection. In all these cases there was extensive œdema of the pelvic connective tissue. Diagnosis was based upon the distinct history of syphilis, which was readily obtained from the patient. There were, moreover, no symptoms of local cancer, tuberculosis, or simple erosion. The patients all recovered rapidly after the administration of iodide of potassium. No local treatment beyond simple cleanliness was thought desirable. Dr. Rode's experiences are of considerable interest. A good monograph on the ulcers of the uterus, written by a recognized authority, would prove of great utility to practitioners and specialists. The nature of so-called "ulceration" of the cervix and its innocuous character have been proved. The "ulcer" is hardly even an erosion; it is rather the replacement of the natural squamous epithelium of the outer part of the cervix by a layer of the columnar epithelium proper to the cervical canal. The severe symptoms once attributed to "ulcerated womb" are due to totally different causes. Nevertheless, there are such things as ulcers of the cervix, due to cancer frequently, to syphilis occasionally, to tubercle rarely. The practitioner, recognizing the truth that a formidable-looking erosion is of little or no clinical import, must take care not to mistake an incipient true ulcer for that relatively harmless pathological condition.—*British Med. Journal*, Feb. 16, 1889.

THE
MEDICAL AND SURGICAL
REPORTER.

ISSUED EVERY SATURDAY.

CHARLES W. DULLES, M.D.,
EDITOR AND PUBLISHER.

The Terms of Subscription to the serial publications of this office are as follows, payable in advance:

Med. and Surg. Reporter (weekly), a year, **$5.00**
Quarterly Compendium of Med. Science, -   2.50
Reporter and Compendium, -   -   -   -   6.00
Physician's Daily Pocket Record, -   -   1.00
Reporter and Pocket Record, -   -   -   6.00
Reporter, Compendium, and Pocket Record, 7.00

All checks and postal orders should be drawn to order of

CHARLES W. DULLES,
N. E. Cor. 13th and Walnut Streets,
P. O. Box 843.   Philadelphia, Pa.

☞SUGGESTIONS TO SUBSCRIBERS:
See that your address-label gives the date to which your subscription is paid.
In requesting a change of address, give the old address as well as the new one.
If your REPORTER does not reach you promptly and regularly, notify the publisher *at once*, so that the cause may be discovered and corrected.
☞SUGGESTIONS TO CONTRIBUTORS AND CORRESPONDENTS:
Write in ink.
Write on one side of paper only.
Write on paper of the size usually used for letters.
Make as few paragraphs as possible. Punctuate carefully. Do not abbreviate, or omit words like "the," and "a," or "an."
Make communications as short as possible.
NEVER ROLL A MANUSCRIPT! Try to get an envelope or wrapper which will fit it.
When it is desired to call our attention to something in a newspaper, mark the passage boldly with a colored pencil, and write on the wrapper "Marked copy." Unless this is done, newspapers are not looked at.
The Editor will be glad to get medical news, but it is important that brevity and actual interest shall characterize communications intended for publication.

THE TREATMENT OF DIPHTHERIA.

Notwithstanding the fact that the treatment of diphtheria is a subject which has been so frequently discussed that medical men are in some danger of being confused by the variety of opinions expressed in regard to it, there can be no question of the advisability of calling attention to new communications which seem calculated to aid them in dealing with this formidable and unhappily common disorder.

In the *Berliner klinische Wochenschrift*, February 18, 1888, there is a paper by Dr. Arthur Hennig, of Königsberg, describing a plan for treating diphtheria which he has used in the enormous number of ten hundred and fifty-four cases, with the best results. One might hesitate to accept these figures as credible, were it not that the whole of Hennig's article bears the marks of great carefulness in statement, and that he distinctly declares that he includes under the head of diphtheria only well-pronounced cases, with actual diphtheritic membrane, and no cases of catarrhal diphtheria or diphtheritic catarrh, which are so often seen in families in which a case of real diphtheria has appeared.

Hennig regards diphtheria as primarily a local affection, and the constitutional disturbance as being in the nature of an intoxication from the products of the local disease. His treatment consists chiefly in applying ice-bladders to the neck and lime-water to the fauces. For the former he employs a suitable piece of the œsophagus of a steer, cleaned, filled with ice, wrapped in a napkin, and laid across the neck from ear to ear. Its application is kept up continuously—the ice being renewed when necessary—day and night until the patient finds the cold uncomfortable, and complains of chilliness, stiffness in the neck and a burning sensation in the larynx. When this occurs the ice-bladder has done its work. The most important parts of Hennig's recommendations in regard to the use of ice are that it should be used continuously, and that the application should always be dry, and never wet.

The use of lime-water is by gargling, when this can be done, or by taking a large quantity into the mouth and holding the head back and shaking it from side to side. In addition to this—or as a substitute for it— Hennig orders large quantities of lime-water to be swallowed, a tablespoonful or two at a time, and often enough to make up as much as three quarts in twenty-four hours. This amount has no ill effect upon the general system. The administration of lime-water is continued until the membrane disappears and the fauces are plainly healed.

To avoid the slight cauterant effect of the lime-water on the lips, they should be smeared with vaseline occasionally. When the diphtheritic process invades the nasal cavity, this is washed out every half-hour with lime-water. For this Hennig uses a small rubber ball, with an elastic tube attached. When lime-water cannot be applied to either the throat or the nose in any of the ways already mentioned, Hennig employs a spray-apparatus for the purpose.

In some cases of diphtheria Hennig uses a solution of chlorate of potash—one to three per cent.—giving the patient from a teaspoonful to a tablespoonful every two or three hours, according to age. He warns especially against using large quantities of this drug, or giving it at all, if the patient's heart is weak; and when it is to be given, he chooses a time after food has been taken. In regard to nourishment, Hennig recommends cold boiled milk, with from two to four egg-yolks stirred in it in the course of each twenty-four hours, when the appetite is deficient; and when the appetite is good he adds to the milk-diet clear soup, meat, and other solid food. He thinks it important to keep the bowels open with mild laxatives, and has no fear of heart failure from allowing a patient to be raised up to have a stool. Pain in the throat he treats with small pieces of ice, or moderate quantities of ice-cream. He permits his patients, if they feel like it, to get up, and allows children to be out of bed and to play, if they wish to, and adults to go about in the open air.

The plan of treatment described above is one which—aside from the large and fortunate experience of Hennig—commends itself to our judgment as rational and likely to be successful. Especially can we endorse his strong recommendation of the use of lime-water, as a safe and efficient remedy in diphtheria, and his methods of administering it. The writer of this Editorial has for years employed lime-water in the treatment of diphtheria, in adults, in children and in infants, in exactly the manner recommended by Hennig, with the most satisfactory results. We can also heartily endorse the other recommendations of Hennig, which are practical and sensible, and show plainly that he is an exceptionally careful observer of the needs of children, who furnish so large a proportion of the cases of diphtheria. Those who can read his whole paper will find in it details which we cannot now repeat, but which add materially to its value. Enough has been said, however, to give the readers of the REPORTER a clear idea of his method of treating diphtheria, and we trust they may find it helpful in their practice.

PICROTOXIN AS AN ANTIDOTE TO MORPHIA.

The discovery of a comparatively safe antidote to morphia would be a great gain to medical men, and it is interesting to learn that Prof. Arpad Bókai, of Klausenburg, in Hungary, thinks he has made such a discovery by experiments with picrotoxin. He finds that picrotoxin in small doses increases the activity of the respiratory centre in the medulla oblongata, and stimulates the vaso-motor centre. For these and other reasons he hopes that picrotoxin will prove to be a useful drug to administer in opium poisoning, as well as to prevent chloroform poisoning.

It does not appear from the abstract of his paper which is to be found in the *Wiener med. Presse*, Feb. 10, 1889, that he has experimented to prove the effects of picrotoxin after administering opium; but his expectations do not seem unreasonable, and it may be that some investigators in this country will undertake the work of determining how far they will be realized when put to the test. It would certainly seem worth while to do this, in view of the difficulties sometimes met with in treating cases of opium poisoning, and of the great advantage it would be to multiply our resources in such cases.

THE TREATMENT OF OZÆNA WITH GLYCERINE.

At a recent meeting of the Society of Military Surgeons in Vienna, Dr. Sidlo strongly recommended the treatment of ozæna with glycerine. His method consists in daily washing out the nasal cavity with a two per cent. solution of chloride of potassium, to which ten per cent. of glycerine has been added. This is followed up with the insertion of rolls of cotton soaked in a mixture of one part of glycerine and three parts of water, the tampons being allowed to remain in place for an hour at a time.

Using this method he claims good success in the management of ozæna. The method requires some weeks to effect a cure; but no one who has treated ozæna often will think a few weeks too long to devote to any method which is likely to be successful. The one proposed by Dr. Sidlo is so simple and apparently so rational that it certainly seems worthy of further trial, and if other medical men can cure such cases as he has cured in this way, it will be a very useful addition to our therapeutic resources.

THE AMERICAN PUBLIC HEALTH ASSOCIATION AND THE NEW YORK HERALD.

The Secretary of the American Public Health Association, has issued a circular calling attention to the fact that the Association has been made a victim of a deception by the *New York Herald.* It appears that, soon after the Milwaukee meeting of the Association, Mr. H. Lomb received a telegram, signed by James Gordon Bennett, asking for the Lomb Prize Essay on Sanitary and Economical Cooking for Persons of Small Means. It was thought desirable to publish it in the *New York Herald,* as that paper was believed to be a good medium for the presentation of this valuable essay to the public. Mr. Lomb and the Secretary went to New York to interview the representative of Mr. Bennett, who offered to purchase the essay. The offer was declined, but it was agreed to let the *Herald* have a copy of the essay and the privilege of being the first paper to present it to the public, with the understanding that it would be published in full. This proposition was accepted. But when it appeared, it was found that the *Herald* had disfigured it by various alterations and omissions, and by inserting unscientific and striking headlines. The result was to convert a useful scientific paper into a comparatively useless and sensational article. The American Public Health Association feels that it has been bitterly deceived, and that great injustice has been done to it as well as to the author of the essay. It seems that the Secretary appealed to the *New York Herald* to do the Association and the author of the essay justice; but he has so far received no reply. He has, therefore, issued a circular, stating these facts, and desiring the coöperation of medical journals to set the matter straight. We extend our sympathy to the American Public Health Association, and to all who may have been injured in this matter. But we cannot feel the surprise which the Secretary of the Association expressed at the way in which the *Herald* carried out its part of the bargain. Judging from the general and long established reputation of the *New York Herald,* it could hardly be expected to let slip an opportunity to amuse and entertain its readers out of consideration for the tender feelings of scientific men. But the occurrence will serve to enforce the lesson that those who have scientific matter to present to the public had better send it to legitimate scientific journals, and not to run the risk of falling into such a trap as this case seems to illustrate.

RELATION OF THE EDITOR TO THE ADVERTISER.—In an Editorial in the New York *Medical Record,* March 23, the Editor states that a subject upon which he is frequently asked to advise the readers of the *Record* is one that concerns the reliability of advertisers and the relative merits of two or more houses dealing in the same class of goods. He states further: "Attentive readers of this journal cannot have failed to perceive that the advertising department .is distinct from the editorial department. The publishers exercise all possible care to accept advertisements from responsible parties only, and our readers must be content with this. The editor cannot personally endorse advertisers, nor can he undertake to decide upon the relative standing of two rival houses."

On turning the page on which these statements are made we find, at the conclusion of another editorial, the following: "In this connection we may refer to an article on 'Hydriodic Acid,' by Dr. William C. Wile (*Journal of the American Medical Association*). This writer speaks in high terms of hydriodic acid as a substitute for the iodides. He has used it successfully in chronic bronchitis, obesity, tertiary syphilis, chronic rheumatism, and in lead and mercurial poisoning."

The original paper of Dr. Wile in the *Journal of the Amer. Med. Association,* Jan. 26, 1889, concludes with the significant declaration : "It is scarcely necessary for me to state, that I have never used any other preparation than that of the originator of the unalterable syrup, of Mr. R. W. Gardner, of New York."

Turning now to the advertising pages of the *Record* we find that "Gardner's Syrup of Hydriodic Acid" occupies just half a page. It would perhaps be unkind to suppose that there is anything more than a mere coincidence in this association of publication ; but it a rather singular coincidence.

--------●◆●--------

—*Science*, Feb. 15, says that Dr. Schmelk of Christiania (*Centralblatt für Bacteriologie*) has found vast colonies of bacteria in the ice of the Jerstedalsbræ glacier and in the streams fed by it. They appear under the form of rods, and resemble the *Bacillus fluorescens liquefaciens*. During their period of growth these bacteria emit a fluorescent material. They multiply with great rapidity during periods of thaw.

BOOK REVIEWS.

[Any book reviewed in these columns may be obtained upon receipt of price, from the office of the REPORTER.]

INTESTINAL SURGERY. By N. SENN, M D., Ph.D., Attending Surgeon Milwaukee Hospital, etc. Large 8vo, pp. vii, 269. Chicago: W. T. Keener, 1889.

Dr. Senn's book contains three papers: the first was read before the Congress of American Physicians and Surgeons, in Washington; the second was published in the Annals of Surgery; the third was read at the last meeting of the American Medical Association. They are all marked by the thoroughness which characterizes Dr. Senn's literary work, and deserve to be collected as a monument to his labors in connection with intestinal surgery.

It would be impossible, in the space we can spare, to give any adequate idea of the contents of this book; and this is not necessary, for Dr. Senn's work in intestinal surgery is now very well known, and the statement that we have here the results of his wide study, ingenious experimentation, and ski ful practice, will indicate how valuable a contribution he makes to the literature of the subject.

We congratulate him upon the results he has achieved in this important fie d of surgery, and commend his book very heartily to the attention of the readers of the REPORTER.

THE THEORY AND PRACTICE OF OBSTETRICS By P. CAZEAUX, Adjunct Professor in the Faculty of Medicine, Paris, etc Remodeled and Rearranged by S. Tarnier, Prof. of Obstetrics and Diseases of Women and Children in the Faculty of Medicine, Paris. Eighth American Edition. Edited and Revised by ROBT. J. HESS, M.D., Physician to The Northern Dispensary, Phila. With an Appendix by PAUL F. MUNDÉ, M.D , Prof. of Gynecology at the N. Y Polyclinic. etc. Illustrated with Chromo-Lithographs, Lithographs, etc., and 175 Wood engravings. 8vo, pp. xxxii, 1221. Philadelphia: P. Blakiston, Son & Co., 1889. Price $5.00.

It is unnecessary to speak of those features of this book which have made it popular for so many years— they are well known to all. Cazeaux and Tarnier's obstetrics will always possess much historical value, not only because it contains the elaborated views of the authors upon the principles and practice of obstetrics, but also because it contains a very full *résumé* of contemporary and older obstetric literature.

But is the present edition brought up to date by its revision and by its appendix? Unquestionably not. To mention only a few of the many sections which need revision or entire recasting, we would note the sections on embryotomy, Cæsarean section, symphyseotomy, induction of premature labor, the forceps, version, ergot, artificial delivery of the placenta, hemorrhage, ante-partum and post-partum, extrauterine pregnancy, and placenta prævia—in fact about every subject of practical obstetrics. No mention is made of the improved Cæsarean section, its development, technique or results. We have simply a cut of Tarnier's forceps, but no account of the investigations which led to its invention or the principles upon which it works. Under "version" no mention whatever is made of combined internal and external version, as taught by Braxton Hicks and others—oftentimes an invaluable procedure, especially in the treatment of placenta prævia. No consideration is given to the modern methods of treating placenta prævia—the methods of Barnes, Hicks, and Murphy, which have effected such a great saving of life. Did our space permit, this list of omissions and failures in revision could be very much enlarged To a certain extent the appendix by Mundé corrects or supplements the text, but unfortunately the topics discussed in the appendix cover but a small part of the field of obstetrics.

There is no sign by which the additions and alterations of the Editor can be distinguished. This does not seem fair to the Editor, to Cazeaux and Tarnier, nor to the reader. Had the usual custom been followed, the Editor's notes would have added to the value of the book as a working guide, without detracting from its historical value.

The illustrations are, with a few exceptions, unusually poor. The printing is apparently done from old plates.

We have told the exact truth about this book, and we are very much surprised to find the unqualified endorsement of a number of our most celebrated obstetricians printed on one of its fly leaves.

PAMPHLET NOTICES.

[Any reader of the REPORTER who desires a copy of a pamphlet noticed in these columns will doubtless secure it by addressing the author with a request stating where the notice was seen and *enclosing a postage-stamp.*]

231. TWO CASES OF GUNSHOT WOUND OF THE ABDOMEN, ILLUSTRATING THE USE OF RECTAL INSUFFLATION WITH HYDROGEN GAS AS A DIAGNOSTIC MEASURE. BY N. SENN, M.D., Milwaukee, Wis. From the *Medical News*, November 10, 1888. 9 pages.

232. DISEASES OF THE NOSE AND PHARYNX, AND THEIR TREATMENT. BY W. CHEATHAM, M D, Louisville, Ky. From the *Virginia Medical Monthly*, December, 1888. 8 pages.

233. REPORT OF SURGICAL OPERATIONS. BY J. B. LUCKIE, M.D., Birmingham, Ala. 8 pages.

234. A CASE OF TUMOR OF THE CERVICAL REGION OF THE SPINE. OPERATION AND DEATH. BY JAMES HENDRIE LLOYD, M.D., and JOHN B. DEAVER, M.D., Philadelphia. From the *Amer. Journal of the Med. Sciences*, December, 1888. 7 pages.

235. ACUTE UNILATERAL OPTIC NEURITIS, WITH THE REPORT OF A CASE. BY G. E. DE SCHWEINITZ, M.D., Philadelphia. From the *Transactions of the Philadelphia County Med. Society*, October 10, 1888 7 pages.

236. RETROJECTION IN GONORRHŒA. BY E. R PALMER, M.D., Louisville, Ky. From the *New York Medical Journal*, December 1, 1888. 7 pages

237. MEDICO-LEGAL ASPECTS OF SOME INJURIES OF THE SPINAL CORD. BY JAMES BURRY, M.D., and F. W. ANDREWS, M.D., Chicago.
REMARKS ON MEDICO LEGAL ASPECTS OF SOME INJURIES OF THE SPINAL CORD. BY HENRY M. LYMAN, M D, Chicago. WITH DISCUSSION. From the *Journal of the Amer Med Association*, Dec. 15, 1888. 24 pages.

231. We have here an account of two cases in which he applied his now well known method for the detection of perforations of the intestine. Both of the cases demonstrated the great value of Senn's method and one of them the disadvantage of allowing much time to elapse before operating when the intestine has been perforated. In this case Dr. Senn first saw the patient twelve hours after he had been shot.

232. Dr. Cheatham advocates surgical interference for the relief of the effects of hypertrophied nasal tissue and bony ridges, and hypertrophy of the glandular structure of the nasopharynx. His pamphlet is interesting and instructive, and does not overlook one important fact — which is, that all deviations from what is often called normal do not require operative treatment.

233. Dr. Luckie gives accounts of a successful case of suprapubic lithotomy; of two cases of fracture of a cervical vertebra, with recovery; and of two cases of successful triple amputation after railway accidents These are all very interesting cases. The diagnosis in the cases of fracture of the vertebræ may be open to question; but certain of the symptoms undoubtedly point to the conclusion arrived at by Dr. Luckie.

234. This pamphlet consists of a medical report by Dr. Lloyd, and a surgical report by Dr. Deaver. The patient was a woman under Dr. Lloyd's care in the Philadelphia Hospital, in whom he diagnosticated a tumor of the spinal cord, and on whom he invited Dr. Deaver to operate for its removal. The operation consisted in removing the spinal processes and part of the laminæ of the third and fourth spinal vertebræ and passing an exploring needle through the dura mater. No tumor was found in the spinal canal; and the patient died on the fourth day.

The reports are interesting and instructive and the reporters are to be applauded for publishing a plain statement of the history of the case and the operation, although the result was so different from what they hoped for.

235. Dr. De Schweinitz, in this pamphlet, gives a clear and succinct account of the history of a case of optic neuritis, under his care, with some general remarks upon this interesting form of eye-disease and its proper treatment. His paper is instructive in pointing out the manner in which an attack of optic neuritis may begin and progress, and a careful reading of it might lead to recognition of such cases by general practitioners in time to secure for the patients the advice of an experienced ophthalmologist when it would be of the greatest service to them.

236. Dr. Palmer gives a remarkably fair and just review of the present status of the method of treating gonorrhœa by washing out the urethra from behind forward with an antiseptic solution He describes the method—not formally, but rather incidentally—gives the plan he finds most useful, namely, to combine the use of one of the usual injections with the "retrojection," and states the results which may be reasonably expected. His paper is very interesting and instructive, and may be heartily commended to the attention of our readers

237. This pamphlet contains the report of a meeting of the Chicago Medico-Legal Society in which the question of injuries of the spinal cord, such as are produced by railway accidents, was very fully and very ably discussed. An attempt was made to distinguish between the real and the false in cases of apparent injury in which no structural change can be detected. The paper and the discussion are both interesting and instructive and well worthy of careful study.

CORRESPONDENCE.

Artificial Stimulation of the Growth of Bone.

To THE EDITOR.

Sir: I am obliged to your kindness, which induced you to send me the number of February 16 of your distinguished paper, with an extract of my discourse in the Berlin Medical Society "on the artificial stimulation of the growth of bone in men." In this extract you do not mention another method, which I first employed in men, and which for this purpose and aim in men, before me was not yet used; that is, the application of thick, steel pins, or needles (of different sizes, mostly two millimeters thick and from three to five inches in length) in the ends of the long bones nearest to the cartilage connecting the diaphysis with the epiphysis—as we call it "*Intermediärknorpel*" or (with Volkmann) "*Fugenknorpel.*" These steel nails (which must be nickled—*vernickelt*) must be applied under *strongest antiseptic measures;* the limb is then fixed on an iron splint or in a plaster-of-Paris bandage (*gypsverbana*); ice is applied and small repeated doses of morphine given for the pains. After 6 to 10 days the nails *sive* needles are removed under the same strong aseptic measures. A week or two later I apply the constricting rubber tube, the massage, the exercises and the nourishment, in which especially must be avoided lactic acid and the formation of this acid out of the nourishment (to avoid the starch-meal - containing nourishments and those which contain lactic acid).

The application of the steel needles is best done with an special handle, in which the needle is fixed by a screw. I bore the needle in the bone, then unscrew the handle, leaving the needle in the bone. The removing of the needle is done with the same handle, after having fixed the free end of the needle in the handle by the screw. Thus this work is done in the most careful manner without any disturbance and shaking of the bone.

The combination of this operation with the treatment reported also by you, gives a very successful increase of blood and a moderate but sufficient irritation in that part of the bone from which comes the growth and lengthening of the bone in youth. Success is to be seen much more quickly than without operating. But *all must be done very carefully.* According to this plan I treated three patients, with the best success. These are also reported in my paper. Now I have some more patients under treatment. In one case I had a lengthening of the femora of 5 centimeters (nearly 2 inches) in half a year; in others 4 centimeters, etc. We have, I think, in this combination an especially good measure to stimulate the growth of the bone in men—a measure without any danger in careful hands.

Please give these lines also to your readers.

Yours truly,

PROF. D. MAX SCHÜLLER.

Berlin, Germany,
  March 4, 1889.

The Virginia State Medical Examining Board.

[A physician of this city who is very much interested in the passage of the bill to appoint a state board of medical examiners, which is now pending before the State Legislature of Pennsylvania, wrote to Dr. Dabney, Professor of Practice of Medicine in the University of Virginia, and Ex-President of the Virginia State Medical Examining Board, to learn the truth concerning certain charges of dishonesty and partiality made against that Board, which charges were contained in a letter to the *Medical Register* of Philadelphia, in its issue of February 23, from a Dr. E. L. Detwiler, and endorsed editorially by the *Register.* In reply to the inquiries made of him, Dr. Dabney sent the following letter, which shows that the Virginia State Medical Examining Board has endeavored to act honestly and impartially in all its examinations, and that the effort to have the graduates of Virginia Colleges exempt from the operations of the act was strenuously resisted by prominent members of the Faculty of the University of Virginia.]

MY DEAR DOCTOR:

Your letter and two extracts from the *Medical Register* were duly received. I had not seen these attacks upon the Virginia Medical Examining Board before, and I at once wrote to Dr. H. T. Nelson, who is now the President of the Board, to learn the facts.

I will take up the charges made in the *Medical Register seriatim.*

1. It is stated that the President of the Board (Dr. A. G. Latham, of Lynchburg, was then President) requested that a certain candidate be given "a nominal examination of ten minutes." Dr. Nelson tells me that the circumstances were as follows: a Dr. Blubaugh, who had practised in Virginia prior to January 1, 1885 (when our law went into effect), as *a member of a firm*

of physicians, asked whether he would have to stand an examination. The law was not explicit on this point, but Dr. Latham believed he was entitled to practise *without* an examination; but he advised Dr. Blubaugh to stand a nominal examination so as to comply technically with the provisions of the law. Subsequently, however, Dr. Latham reconsidered the matter and told Dr. Blubaugh that he must stand a regular and thorough examination.

2. It is stated that the returns "were altered" at a recent meeting of the Board. Dr. Nelson tells me that at the meeting in Norfolk in October last two negroes presented themselves, one a graduate of Howard University, Washington City, and the other a graduate of the Leonard Medical School for colored men, in Raleigh, N. C. One of these men had been registered three times before, and the other once before. At the meeting in Norfolk they did not reach the required standard (75 per cent.); but the Board made an exception in their cases, and licensed them to practise medicine in Virginia. The Board was induced to do this, Dr. Nelson tells me, by two considerations; one was that these men expected to practise in a section of country inhabited almost entirely by negroes, and where no white man could make a living; the second consideration was that they had spent all their means in acquiring what education they had, and therefore could not pursue their studies further at any medical school. It was the opinion of the Board furthermore that they were capable of doing substantial service to the persons among whom they proposed to settle.

3. It is stated that the object of the Medical Law in Virginia is to force students to attend the Virginia schools.

I am in a position to answer this question myself, without reference to Dr. Nelson, though the facts are familiar to him and any other member of the profession in Virginia who has taken any interest in the matter. I was the chairman of the committee of our State Medical Society appointed to present the "Medical Bill," as it was then called, to the Legislature. A proposition was made then by several members of the Legislature to exempt the graduates of the Medical Colleges of the State from examination, the argument used being that the number of students in attendance upon our State schools would thereby be increased. I opposed this proposition with all the energy I could command, and told my brother-in-law, Mr. Moon, who was the patron of the bill in the House, to have it defeated rather than to have such an "exemption clause" inserted. Subsequently, after the law had been enacted and the Board had been organized, a similar proposition was made. It was bitterly opposed by the Board, and I (as President of the Board) addressed a letter to Dr. I. L. Cobell, the senior member of the Faculty of the University of Virginia, and a similar letter to the Dean of the Medical College of Virginia at Richmond, asking if they desired the graduates of their respective schools to be exempt from the State examination. Both replied that they desired their graduates *to stand* the State examination ; and Dr. Cobell wrote so forcibly and earnestly on the subject that his letter was of immense value to us and has been used with telling effect since. As a further evidence that the Board shows no partiality to the Virginia Medical Schools, I may state that 33 of our graduates have stood the State examination and 1 (one) has been rejected ; and 57 graduates of the Medical College at Richmond have stood the examination, of whom 8 were rejected.

I do not know Dr. E. L. Detwiler, of Herndon, Virginia, who makes this charge of partiality toward the State schools as against the Board, but Dr. Nelson and I found, in looking over the Register kept by the Board the other day, that a man of that name and having the same post office, was rejected by our Board in April 1886, but passed his second examination some months afterward. Possibly it is the same gentleman.

I need not take up your time by giving Dr. Nelson's explanation of the apparent mistake in his tables; from which it appeared that three *different* graduates of the Medico-Chirurgical College had been rejected, instead of but one who was rejected three times. The apparent mistake was due to the way in which the tables were arranged.

I sincerely trust that you may succeed in getting the proposed law through your Legislature. The only way, it seems to me, to elevate the standard of medical education in a country like ours is to have in each State a Board of Examiners who shall *not be connected with any school* and who will *recognize no diploma.* This plan was proposed by Dr. I. L. Cobell of the University of Virginia more than forty years ago.

Very truly yours,

WM. C. DABNEY.

University of Virginia,
March 23, 1889.

NOTES AND COMMENTS.

A New and Simple Method of Estimating Per Cent. of Fat in Milk.

In a letter to the Philadelphia *Ledger*, March 16, 1888, C. B. Cochran, Inspector of Foods, Pennsylvania State Board of Agriculture, says: To creamery men at least, if not to others, the most valuable constituent of milk is the fat. Hence has arisen within the past few years the custom of paying for milk prices dependent upon the per cent. of fat it contains. In many creameries throughout the country this custom was adopted just as soon as it was made feasible by the discovery of a simple and practical method of estimating accurately the fat in milk. There are two methods now in use among creamery men. In the first method, the fat is separated from the milk by means of an instrument called the lactocrite, and the per cent. found by measurement of its volume. In the second method, the insoluble fatty acids of the milk fat are separated and their volume measured. From this measurement and from the specific gravity of the milk is calculated the per cent. of fat. This method is commonly known as Short's method.

The chief objection to the lactocrite is its cost, which, when complete, is about $250. The method of Short requires from three to four hours' time, and gives results not so reliable as the lactocrite.

The method which we now, in outline, bring before the public, will be found, we believe, to combine the following desiderata—cheapness, simplicity, rapidity of execution and accuracy. The necessary apparatus consists of one 10-cubic centimetre pipette, two 5-cubic centimetre pipettes, one 10-cubic centimetre lipped test-tube, and the analyzing flasks, the number of which will depend upon the number of samples of milk to be analyzed. These flasks taper at the top into long, narrow cylindrical necks, so graduated as to read both volume and per cent. of fat. To the above apparatus it is desirable to add a good lactometer or lactodensimeter.

The method of analysis is as follows: Into one of the flasks drop 10 cubic centimetres of the milk to be analyzed, add five cubic centimetres glacial acetic acid and five cubic centimetres sulphuric acid. Stand the flask in water boiling hot, or nearly so, for 10 or 15 minutes, shaking it once or twice in the mean time. Then remove the flask from the hot water bath, allow it to cool, add from the test tube 10 cubic centimetres of ether, shake thoroughly so as to mix the ether with the contents of the flask. Allow the flask to stand for three or five minutes, then boil off the ether. When the ether is all evaporated a layer of clear fat is found floating on the liquid.

By the addition of hot water this layer of fat is now raised into the narrow graduated tube, which constitutes the neck of the flask, and its volume and per cent. there ascertained. The water used for the last named purpose should be nearly boiling hot, otherwise there is a tendency for the fat to adhere to the sides of the tube, and thus produce too low a result. By the use of hot water, however, there is little or no danger of loss from this source. This process seems to effect a complete separation of the fat from the milk, and, furthermore, the fat is free from every trace of casein, and can be very accurately read.

The fat of eight or ten samples of milk can be estimated by this method in about one hour, and I hope to be able, by changing the shape of the flask somewhat, so that the ether can be boiled off more rapidly, to shorten this time. The matter of the shape of the flask is now under consideration and will be settled soon.

Results obtained by me in the above described process agree closely with results obtained by Hebner's formula and by the paper coil process. This last named process has been officially adopted by the English Society of Public Analysts.

Bacteria in Milk.

The Berlin correspondent of the *Lancet*, March 9, 1889, says that it is intended to establish a bacteriological laboratory for the investigation of milk. The idea is due mainly to Dr. Hueppe, of Wiesbaden, who has for several years made a special study of the bacteria that appear in milk. He has definitively proved that lactic acid fermentation is caused by a special fungus, and butyric acid fermentation by another. Prazmowski, Liborius, Fuchs, and Neelsen have discovered other bacteria in milk, and their purely scientific researches, undertaken solely with a view to widening the limits of bacteriology, are now bearing valuable practical fruit. It is known that infant mortality is due largely to unwholesome milk, which can now be rendered harmless by sterilization. Further practical advantages are certain sooner or later to accrue from these investigations.

Massage in Pelvic Inflammation.

Dr. Semianikoff has employed massage in twenty cases of pelvic inflammation of a chronic character which had resisted other forms of treatment, and speaks very highly of the results obtained. All the cases were in Professor Slavianski's gynecological clinic in St. Petersburg. The cases in which the most marked effects were produced were those in which there were peri-uterine effusions of moderate dimensions. Chronic ovaritis, too, yielded to the same treatment. It should be stated that in some of the cases daily sittings for about three months were required to effect a cure. Of course the treatment was intermitted during the menstrual periods.—*Lancet,* Feb. 9, 1889.

Fatal Case of Cocaine Poisoning.

The *Lancet,* Feb. 9, 1889, says that an inquest was held at University College Hospital on Jan. 31, by Dr. Danford Thomas, coroner for Central Middlesex, touching the death of Charles Sidney Fletcher, who at the time of his decease was an inmate of the hospital. Fletcher was admitted under the care of Mr. Berkeley Hill, for disease of the urinary organs. From the evidence of Mr. John Creswell, house surgeon, it seems that it was intended to wash out the bladder with a detergent astringent solution, and to deaden the sensibility to the pain a solution of cocaine was to be first injected. The two prescriptions, the one for the cocaine and the other for sulpho-carbolate of zinc, were written on the same paper. The former simply directed that twenty grains of cocaine were to be dissolved in one ounce of water, and to it was appended the word "*statim,*" without an accompanying verb to make the term intelligible. It was this defect which primarily led to the mistake which cost the deceased his life. The house surgeon wished to convey by the word "*statim*" that the solution was to be *dispensed* immediately. The dispenser, misled no doubt by the meagreness of the directions, misinterpreted it, and believing the solution to be a *draught* for the patient to take, put it in a measure glass and gave it to the nurse who waited for it. The latter administered it to the patient at once. It appears that upon writing the prescription the house surgeon put the paper on the table of the ward, and told the nurse to obtain from the dispensary the drugs ordered. When the nurse returned to the ward the house surgeon was engaged at an operation in another part of the building, or probably it would have chanced that he would have been consulted as to the correctness of the dispenser's reading of his prescription. Curiously, although the sulpho-carbolate of zinc solution was directed to be made into an *injection*, no intimation of the intended use of the cocaine solution was given. The fatal error was not recognized until the effects of the working of the cocaine became manifest. What the initial symptoms were is not known, for it was not until nearly an hour had elapsed that the nurse, hearing the patient making some unusual noise, had her attention drawn to him. It is said that there was some arching of the back resembling the opisthotonus of tetanus, and that there was a convulsive movement of the limbs. Consciousness was to some extent retained almost up to the fatal issue, since the patient, although apparently insensible, could be roused sufficiently to say, "I shan't," in answer to an injunction to do something. Death took place in about an hour after swallowing the cocaine solution.

The post-mortem showed tuberculosis of both lungs and of the right kidney. The left kidney had been entirely destroyed and its place occupied by the remains of the shrunken capsule.

Over-Pressure in Children.

In a note recently published by Professor Charcot on "over-pressure," the author asserts that intellectual or cerebral overwork does not exist in children under sixteen years of age. A child, he says, can make only the amount of intellectual effort of which he is capable. If he has programmes too overcharged to fulfil, he simply does not fulfil them; if one insists on cramming his memory with crude facts, no result whatever is obtained; but this does not in any way affect the brain of the child, the passiveness of which is complete, and the indifference absolute. On the other hand, according to the Professor, "over-pressure manifests itself only in youths above sixteen or eighteen years. It is characterized by a number of nervous troubles, principally by a pain in the occipital region, which extends down to the back of the neck, and goes up again in front of the ears. This over-pressure is seen in pupils of the superior branches of study, in men of letters who write much, in political men who are or who believe themselves to be overwhelmed with responsibilities, in men of business, etc., who lose their sleep, but never in the pupils of our *lycées* and colleges."—*Lancet,* Feb. 23, 1889.

Case of Chorea Major Associated with Formation of Fungi in the Pia Mater.

Prof. B. Naunyn reports this case from the medical clinic at Königsberg. The patient was a girl, 17 years old, who had had severe chorea since her eleventh year. On July 16, she died. At the autopsy there were found endocarditis and slight œdema of the brain and spinal cord. The pia mater in the neighborhood of the chiasm and in spots in the fossa (fissure) of Sylvius a peculiar brownish - red coloration as of deposited hæmatin. Microscopic examination showed that there were fine fibres in the pia, especially along the vessels, which proved to be fungi. According to Prof. Zopf, the fungus belongs to a kind between the *cladothrix* and *leptothrix.* Similar fungus-formation was found on the valves of the heart.—*Schmidt's Jahrbücher,* Jan. 15, 1889.

Therapeutics of Eczema.

Dr. Veiel, of Canstatt, says in the *Med. Correspondenz-Blatt d. würrt arztl. Landesver.*, that in acute eczema internal treatment is not indicated, while in chronic, widely distributed eczema arsenic is to be used simultaneously with external treatment. If chlorosis is present iron should be administered half an hour before meals and arsenic one hour after meals. Cod liver oil and regulation of the diet are very important in scrofulous eczema. For the itching of eczema, he uses chloral and bromide of potash internally.

The stage of the affection is of importance as regards treatment. In acute eczema all irritants are to be avoided. Where, as in children, baths are not entirely to be avoided, some mucilaginous substance should be added to them. All soaps are to be avoided. To diminish the burning and itching in acute, but not moist, eczema, Veiel recommends Unna's zinc paste:

R Oxide of zinc
   Gelatin . . . . aa ʒ iv
   Glycerine . . . . f ʒ viss
   Distilled water . . . . . f ʒ iss

To be warmed in a water-bath and applied with a bristle pencil.

After several days it is to be washed away with lukewarm water. In moist eczema the affected places are washed once daily and then the paste is again applied. If this proves ineffective, Veiel employs starch cushions, which remain cool and are often changed. If in universal eczema the paste is not borne starch is applied in powder, with which, if there is much itching, two per cent. of camphor is mixed. If this is of no service, the parts are washed with borax, or acetate of alumina, with some glycerine:

R Liquoris alum. acet. . . . . . . ɱ cl
   Aquæ destil. . . . . f ʒ iii
M.

or,

R Boracis . . . . gr. liii
   Acid. salicyl. · . · . . . . . gr. ivss
   Aquæ destil. . . . . f ʒ vss
   Glycerini . . . . f ʒ i
M.

For extensive weeping eczema ointment-mulls and pastes are employed. If the scurf is dry and scaly, a five per cent. tannin salve is used.·

In chronic eczema the crusts and scales are first loosened with soft soap, baths, or oil. The healing of the moist places is brought about as before. The addition of one or two per cent. of ichthyol is very serviceable. If the eczema still continues scaly, Lassar's paste is indicated, or tar with alcohol:

R Picis liquidi . . . . ɱ xv
   Alcoholis . . . . ɱ xlv
M.

or tar may be added in the strength of one or two per cent. to the salve above mentioned. The employment of the latter on the hairy parts of the face and pubes is contraindicated, as in these places inflammations resembling sycosis are easily developed. If the eczema does not yield to the tar, pyrogallic acid and chrysarobin (in an ointment, from two to ten per cent. strength) is at times attended with success.—*Wiener med. Presse,* Feb. 3, 1889.

Charcot's Opinion of Professional Women.

M. Charcot, one of the Jury of the Faculty of Medicine in Paris, in complimenting a young lady who had obtained her doctor's degree, said that "women pass their examinations, when they do pass them, even more satisfactorily than men; but what will be always a bar to their success is that they have no real love of their proposed profession. What they aspire to is the first rank, the most prominent posts, the most lucrative offices; and what they dislike is the humble and unpleasant, but necessary, service of humanity such as is given by the hospital dresser." Curious, but precisely the same thing might just as correctly be said of men.—*Chemist and Druggist,* Jan. 5, 1889.

Medical Practice in Michigan.

A bill to regulate the practice of medicine in Michigan has been introduced into the Legislature. It provides for the appointment by the Governor of a board of six physicians to be medical examiners. Two are to be of the homœopathic school, two eclectics, and two regulars. All are to be graduates, but none can be connected with a medical college in any capacity. Any person practising medicine without a license from this board may be fined $100 or sentenced to jail for ninety days. All persons are regarded as practising who append M.D. or M.B. to their names, or direct, or for a fee recommend, for the medicinal use of any person any drug. Every person licensed must have attended three courses of lectures of at least six months each, and must be examined in the fourteen standard branches of medical practice. The examination fee is $10, and the license must be filed with the county clerk. The board can revoke a license for unprofessional or immoral conduct.—*Medical Standard*, March, 1889.

Cocaine in Teeth-Extraction.

In the St. Petersburg weekly *Rüsskaia Meditzina*, No. 39, 1888, p. 623, Dr. I. S. Kolbasenko, of Kopal, writes that he resorted to Dr. G. Vian's method of local anæsthesia (*Therapeut. Monatschr.*, 1887, p. 502) in nine cases of teeth extraction, once in his own case. The method consists in injecting into the gum, both into its buccal and lingual surfaces, a solution of ¼ of a grain of cocaine in ten drops of a 2 per cent. aqueous solution of carbolic acid. The following noteworthy conclusions have been arrived at by the author. 1. In the presence of an inflammatory swelling of the gum, cocaine does not develope any pain-killing effects whatever, which may be explained by the well-known fact that infiltrated tissues lose their absorptive power more or less completely. 2. But when the gum is normal, *i.e.*, not inflamed, the injection is invariably followed in a few seconds by a local numbness, and in two or three seconds, never later than in four minutes, by a complete anæsthesia. The extraction performed at this stage remains always quite painless from the beginning to the end. 3. The injection, however, is constantly accompanied by a train of more or less pronounced general phenomena, such as giddiness, clouding of sight, acceleration of the pulse, and, later on, by a kind of drunkenness with talkativeness,

exhilaration, etc., the symptoms being especially marked in anæmic and nervous persons. In the latter a genuine hysterical fit, with clouded consciousness, tears, etc., may supervene. 4. Hence in those susceptible subjects a due caution is necessary. 5. The best means for preventing and weakening the general symptoms are these: (1) the injection should be preceded by the internal administration of a wineglassful of rum or strong wine; (2) After the extraction the patient should be placed in a horizontal posture with his head hanging down; (3) inhalation of two or three drops of amyl nitrite should be resorted to.

National Association of Railway Surgeons.

The Annual Meeting of the National Association of Railway Surgeons will be held at St. Louis, Mo., on Thursday and Friday, May 2 and 3, 1889. Dr. W. B. Outten, of St. Louis, is the Chairman of the Committee of Arrangements. Any desired information can be had by addressing the Secretary, C. B. Stemen, M.D., Fort Wayne, Ind.

Pennsylvania State Medical Society.

The Fortieth Annual Meeting of the Medical Society of the State of Pennsylvania will be held in Pittsburgh, on Tuesday, Wednesday, Thursday, and Friday, June 4, 5, 6, and 7, 1889, commencing on Tuesday, June 4, at 9 A.M. The appointments for 1889 are as follows:

Address on Practice of Medicine, Dr. J. C. Wilson, of Philadelphia; *address on Surgery*, Dr. J. B. Roberts, Philadelphia; *address on Obstetrics*, Dr. Frances N. Baker, Media; *address on Mental Disorders*, Dr. Alice Bennett, Norristown; *address on Laryngology*, Dr. W. H. Daly, Allegheny; *address on Hygiene*, Dr. T. J. Mays, Philadelphia.

The Chairman of the Committee of Arrangements is Dr. E. A. Wood, of Pittsburgh, to whom all applications to read papers at this session should be sent *not later than April 15.*

The Secretaries of County Medical Societies are earnestly requested to forward at once complete lists of their Officers and Members, giving the post-office address of each.

All who desire Excursion Orders should notify the Permanent Secretary, Dr. Wm. B. Atkinson, at an early date, stating which railroad must be used.

NEWS.

—The Eighteenth Congress of the German Surgical Society will be held in Berlin, April 24–27.

—Dr. Adolph Bardeleben, Professor of Surgery in the University of Berlin, celebrated his seventieth birthday March 1.

—Dr. Charles F. Stillman, of New York, has been elected to a chair of Physical Examination for Life Insurance, which has just been created in the University of Vermont.

—Dr. John G. Womble, a prominent physician of Baltimore, died suddenly in that city March 13. He was graduated from the University of Maryland Medical School in 1871.

—Dr. Thomas Fitch Perley, Medical Inspector General during the closing years of the war, and a noted entomologist, died in Portland, Maine, on Thursday, March 21. He was 73 years old.

—The *Lancet*, Feb. 23, states that yellow fever is said to have broken out at Versailles, and to have numbered thus far four victims. It has been suspected that the germs of the disease have been carried there from South America in the plumage of parrots

—Mr. Henry Carter died recently in England at the age of 92 years. He is believed to have been at the time of his decease the oldest member of the Royal College of Surgeons of England. His death was caused by a fall which fractured his left hip.

—The Faculty of Medicine of Paris, upon the report of a committee composed of Professors Potain, Jaccoud, Grancher, and Straus, have decided to give the Lacaze prize of 10,000 francs to M. Malassez, Director of the Histological Laboratory of the College of France, for his investigations upon tuberculosis.

—The *Memphis Medical Monthly*, March, 1889, says of its midwives: "There are twenty-one of these persons. Seventeen of the twenty-one acknowledge their signatures with an X. They are an old set, as evidenced by the time of service in the capacity of midwife claimed by each—the average being twenty-five years and eight months."

—Dr. William H. Ford, President of the Board of Health of Philadelphia, states that the bill to prevent the sale of adulterated and impure milk was negatively recommended, owing to the opposition to a prohibition of the sale of skimmed milk. He also said that the Board had now taken the matter into its own hands, and that a relentless war would be carried on against dishonest milk dealers. The Sanitary Committee of the board has been instructed to take further steps to promote the passage of a milk bill.

HUMOR.

WEAK EYES.—A Knoxville, Tennessee, doctor advised a patient to use whiskey on his forehead every morning for neuralgia. Meeting his wife a few days after the physician inquired as to her husband's health. "He's no better," replied the lady. "But I told him to rub whiskey on his forehead," said the doctor. "True," answered the lady, "but John never uses it higher than his mouth."—*Cincinnati Lancet-Clinic.*

FREE MEDICAL ADVICE.—"Doctor," said a citizen, as he overtook him on the street, "what do you do in case of a gone stomach?"

"Well," replied the doctor, thoughtfully, "I've never had such a case myself, but I would recommend you to advertise for it, and then sit down in a large easy-chair and wait until somebody brings it back."

WHAT DID HE MEAN?—"I hope, Mr. Templecourt," said the lady, as she rose from the chair which had vibrated with her voice for an hour and a half, "that I haven't been taking up too much of your valuable time." "Not at all, Mrs. Chatty," returned the lawyer, glancing wearily at the pile of letters on his desk: "I assure you that this time has been of no value to me whatever."—*Puck.*

A STORY is going the rounds concerning the absent-mindedness of Byron, the playwright. A new play was running through the dramatist's head as he was walking through Pall Mall, when a friend stopped him and said: "I am in grief." "What is it?" asked Byron mistily. "I lost my father last week," said the man. "Too bad, too bad," said Byron, with an air of absent sympathy; "very sorry." Then he walked on and continued to think about his play. Three weeks later he happened to be again in Pall Mall, when the same man came up to him and said: "More misfortune." "Eh?" said Byron absently. "I have just lost my mother," said the man lugubriously. "Dear me!" said the dramatist petulantly. "You lost your father only a little while ago. What an exceedingly careless man you are."

MEDICAL AND SURGICAL REPORTER

No. 1675.   PHILADELPHIA, APRIL 6, 1889.   VOL. LX.—NO. 14.

CONTENTS:

CLINICAL LECTURE.

NERVOUS DYSPEPSIA.[1]

BY EDWARD T. BRUEN, M.D.,

PHILADELPHIA.

ASSISTANT PROFESSOR OF PHYSICAL DIAGNOSIS IN THE UNIVERSITY OF PENNSYLVANIA, AND PHYSICIAN TO THE PHILADELPHIA AND GERMAN HOSPITALS.

I shall bring before you only one case this morning, not so much for the lessons which may be drawn from the study of the case in itself as for the purpose of describing the method of clinical study which should be pursued in the analysis of the symptoms, especially by means of certain chemical tests which have been recently suggested as very useful in such cases.

Dyspepsia, it is well known, is a term like albuminuria, or dropsy, or anemia; it is a name which may embrace very many totally different pathological conditions.

For our purpose we may divide dyspepsias

[1] Delivered at the German Hospital.

into three groups: (1) those in which there is a lack of secretion of hydrochloric acid; (2) those in which there is an increased secretion of hydrochloric acid; (3) those in which there is a want of nerve power, or a sympathetic nervous dyspepsia attended by the formation of a variable amount of hydrochloric acid.

Cases which belong to the first group are frequently those of gastric carcinoma; not because this process exerts any mystical influence to prevent the formation of HCl, but because the later stages of carcinoma of the stomach are attended with atrophy of the gastric follicles. The constant presence of HCl in anything like normal quantity is the best evidence which can be given that gastric carcinoma does not exist. There are, however, other cases of gastric disorder in which HCl is deficient. In the amyloid process, and in circulatory diseases which favor portal repletion the secretion of HCl is much reduced. In chronic gastric catarrh the same process of reduction in the elaboration of HCl occurs. The form of dyspepsia associated with chronic gastric catarrh must therefore be differentiated from malignant disease.

The dyspepsias of the second group include chiefly gastric ulcer. Indeed gastric hyperacidity is believed to be a predisposing cause of gastric ulcer. This hyperacidity may not only arise frcm the overproduction of HCl, but lactic acid, which exists in the stomach during the earliest stage of the digestive process, and is frequently formed during the digestion of food by fermentation, may also be a factor in causing the hyperacidity which so commonly precedes the development of gastric ulcer. Various other organic acids may be formed during the process of faulty digestion, but the presence of the others does not so commonly antedate gastric ulcer as does the excess of HCl.

The third class of dyspepsias includes the cases which are represented by the patient we have before us at this time. This form of the complaint is often met with in factory girls, or those who work in shops. These persons are apt to be confined too closely, have little out-door exercise, often eat improperly, and generally use tea and coffee to excess, or eat coarse food in large quantities, or hurriedly. Such persons are especially predisposed to dilatation of the stomach, which may render their dyspepsia really incurable.

This dilatation occurs because of the constant accumulation of gases formed during the process of fermentation of food in the stomach. This form of dilatation may be also traceable to regurgitation of gases from the intestine, in certain cases of intestinal indigestion, so that the stomachic indigestion is secondary. All the forms of dilatation of the stomach mentioned might be denominated functional, to distinguish them from the forms of dilatation secondary to pyloric obstruction directly dependent upon cancer, or chronic inflammatory pyloric thickening after ulcer, or obstruction dependent upon the pressure of some tumor adjacent to the pyloric orifice.

A chemical analysis of the gastric contents should be instituted when practicable at the outset of the examination. If possible the patient's stomach should be washed out in the evening, and on the following morning a test-meal should be given consisting of an egg with bread and butter, and some hot milk, water and sugar as the beverage. In an hour after the test-meal a soft flexible tube, eighteen or twenty inches long—that is, a tube one-third or three-eighths of the length of the body—should be introduced into the stomach. The tube may be lubricated with milk, and the patient can learn to assist in the introduction of the same by swallowing efforts. Light pressure over the stomach may then be made, and with the effort of regurgitation on the part of the patient about one ounce of the gastric fluid can be brought up. If this method of obtaining the contents of the stomach fail, the stomach-pump may be used. The introduction of the tube will often occasion vomiting. The gastric contents being obtained they should be filtered, and Uffelmann's test employed. This consists of a four per cent. solution of carbolic acid with four drops, or sufficient tincture of the chloride of iron to produce a steel blue color. The filtered gastric fluid should be dropped into the solution very slowly, a yellow color being produced by lactic acid, and decolorization in the presence of HCl. Since it is possible for decolorization to be caused by other acids than HCl, Uffelmann's test should be reserved for lactic acid, while for hydrochloric acid Günzburg's test should be used. This consists of fifteen grains of vanillin and forty grains of phloroglucin mixed in one ounce of alcohol. With a trace of mineral acid, it produces a yellowish-red color. By dropping some of the solution into the filtered contents of the stomach, the HCl present will form a precipitate of bright red crystals. If the proportion of mineral acid is very minute, equal quantities of the solution and juice should be employed, and it will be necessary to evaporate the liquid slowly in a porcelain crucible. A deposit around the edges of fine red crystals will then be obtained. Heat should be applied with the spirit lamp, care being taken that the liquid that is testing does not boil. When the gastric liquid contains considerable quantities of albuminates or peptones the isolated crystals are not observed; but the bright coloring persists and the crucible is covered with a mixture composed of albuminates and fragments of crystals.

For clinical purposes the phloroglucin-vanillin test is perfectly reliable, though Faucher[1] concludes from some experiments with eggs of various degrees of freshness—prepared by mixing their whites with a given weight of distilled water—that though new-laid eggs give a negative reaction with the phloroglucin-vanillin, eggs five days old become rose colored; three eggs of doubtful freshness gave an intense, dark-red color;

---

[1] *Journal de Méd.*, Paris, August 12, 1888.

in short, the intensity of the reaction was in proportion to the age of the egg, which contains an increasing quantity of sulphuric acid as it becomes stale. Dr. F. Spaeth has devised a very simple apparatus for .testing the presence or absence of HCl. He takes a small bullet (No. 6) and wraps about it a silk thread (No. 1), which he has previously soaked in a 0.015 per cent. watery solution of Congo red. To this is fastened also a small piece of elder-pith which has been soaked in blue litmus paper. The whole is attached to a long silk thread. The bullet and pith-ball are swallowed and allowed to remain in the stomach for a minute, and then drawn up. Any acid present turns the litmus pith to red, while if free HCl is present it turns the Congo-red thread a blue color. Acetic and butyric acids can be detected by the smell, especially after the fluid is shaken with ether, and the ethereal residue evaporated.

The patient whom I bring before you this morning is a woman, 28 years old, who complains of pain over the epigastric region, loss of appetite for the last two years; she has vomited blood once. The patient has lost forty-five pounds in weight, and is quite anemic—weighing now only one hundred and eight pounds.

Malignant disease may be set aside as unlikely to be present on account of the age of the patient. Gastric ulcer can be excluded because the pain is diffused over the whole stomachic region. Vomiting of blood has occurred only once. Localized tenderness is absent, and vomiting has been only an occasional not a constant symptom. But the analysis of the gastric contents shows a normal proportion of HCl, and such an analysis is a very helpful measure in the diagnosis.

I have prescribed for this patient:

R. Ext. belladonnæ . . . . . gr. i
Argenti nitrat. . . . . . . gr. ii *vel* iii
Fiant pil. No. xii.

Sig. One pill 15 minutes before each meal.

The diet should be Malted Milk, as made by the Racine firm, or Carnrick's Soluble Food. Very carefully watched these preparations may be used to represent milk, but the patient should be weighed every week, to note any gain or possible loss.

This treatment has been successful in the present case. We have cautiously added first slightly boiled eggs, then meat broiled, then well-baked bread. Milk itself can be very rarely used in these cases, since it is liable to cause vomiting. It is for this reason that the foods named are so valuable as *temporary* substitutes for milk. I say temporary, since I would never regard an artificial preparation as fully representing standard milk; but they are of great value in bridging over a certain period of time. When neither milk nor these substitutes I have mentioned can be tolerated, one may resort to broiled meats with *zwiebach*, or toasted bread. I have no doubt that attention to the diet will suffice to cure this patient; and it must be remembered as a cardinal point in these cases never to give more food daily than can be digested.

February 1.—This patient has been discharged, having gained in weight fifteen pounds and nearly regained her natural appearance as to complexion. At present the patient has no symptoms of gastric indigestion. It will be necessary for her to observe the injunctions to be careful of her diet for some months to come.

It will now be possible to begin with the series of remedies calculated to reestablish the crasis of the blood, such as arsenic in small doses, iron, and the like. I would simply remark that it is well to give these remedies for a long time, and therefore a small dose is very desirable. I usually give at this stage of the treatment some nux vomica, and possibly zinc as a nerve tonic, as in the following pill:

R. Acid. arseniosi . . . . gr. ss
Ferri sulph. exsic. . . . . gr. v
Zinci sulph. . . . . gr. iii
Ext. nucis vomicæ . . . . . . gr. v
Ext. gentianæ . . . . gr. xxx

M. Ft. pil. No. xxx.

Sig. One pill 3 times a day.

In closing, I would call attention to the fact that I employ pepsin but little, while I lay stress on the fact that dietetic treatment is all important. Pepsin may be used as an adjuvant to diet, but not as a principal mode of treatment. The effect of acids and alkalies is very doubtful in cases of chronic nervous dyspepsia. It is said by some that they precipitate the mucus and in the long run lessen the formation of HCl and the peptic ferment. Alkalies are said to dissolve mucus, and to promote the secretion of HCl and the peptic ferment. My own opinion is that both modes of medication are adapted only to temporary use, and that in cases of prolonged functional dyspepsia they may even be injurious.

—Prof. Wilhelm Henke has accepted the Chair of Anatomy in the University of Gratz.

COMMUNICATIONS.

FLAT-FOOT: A NEW PLANTAR SPRING FOR ITS RELIEF.

BY A. SYDNEY ROBERTS, M.D.,

FELLOW OF THE COLLEGE OF PHYSICIANS OF PHIL-
ADELPHIA, EX VICE-PRESIDENT OF THE
AMERICAN ORTHOPÆDIC ASSO-
CIATION, ETC., ETC.

Among the most distressing and painful deformities of the lower extremity, which the orthopædic surgeon is called upon to treat, cases of flat-foot stand foremost. I should not have ventured to speak of this very common deformity, did I not think that its importance is often overlooked, and that in many instances it is a source of much confusion regarding its etiology, diagnosis and treatment to those who have not had many opportunities for studying the disease.

As a rule the ordinary forms of club-foot are unattended with pain; this symptom entering only secondarily, either as a result of pressure from walking in the deformed position, or from the faulty mechanical appliances used to correct the deformity. In the form of talipes under consideration, however, pain plays an important part, and with this the disability produced is often so extreme as to render the patient unable to pursue his ordinary occupation. Thus, in addition to the usual end to be attained in the treatment of deformities of the feet, namely, the restoration to the normal form of the foot, we have another and more practical object, demanding our utmost attention and study, and that is the preservation of the means of livelihood to those who are unfortunately afflicted with flat-foot.

Like other forms of talipes, flat-foot, or talipes valgus, may be a congenital or acquired malformation, but it is very rarely found at birth to such an extent as to be considered pathological. On the other hand the acquired forms of valgus, taking all the varieties collectively—whether occurring as simple flattening of the. arch, as secondary to rachitis, as the result of infantile spinal paralysis, or those of the inflammatory type—talipes valgus probably occurs most frequently of all the distortions of the feet.

It may be well, in this connection, before proceeding to an account of the etiology of talipes valgus, to give a brief account of the normal mechanism of the foot and of the plantar arch. All of that portion of the lower extremity situated below the tibio-tarsal articulation enters into the construction of the foot, and in the adult has the form of an arch, with its convexity or dorsal surface above and its concavity or plantar surface below. At the highest point of this arch, which is formed by the astragalus, the weight of the body is received and transmitted; receiving the weight on its trochlear surface from the tibia, and transmitting it through the so-called pillars of the arch. Of these there are two, the anterior one composed of the scaphoid, three cuneiform and the three inner metatarsal bones, being the longer, less oblique and more elastic. The posterior pillar, formed by the os calcis, is shorter and thicker, its concavity being directed inward, and it is less elastic than the anterior one. The astragalus, therefore, may be regarded as the keystone of the arch, but it differs in certain respects from the keystone of the ordinary arch. Whilst its anterior surface by its opposition to the concave posterior surface of the scaphoid fulfils this requirement, posteriorly it rests upon and overrides the os calcis. Hence, this weak point in the arch has to be supplemented, so to speak, and this is accomplished by the soft parts, the interosseous ligaments, passing between, and binding together the bones, the calcaneo-scaphoid ligaments arising from the inferior surface and forepart of the os calcis, and passing to the posterior and under part of the scaphoid bone, thus giving direct support to the head of the astragalus. Again, we have a secondary arch, supporting the primary one. This is formed by the outer part of the os calcis, the cuboid, and the two outer metatarsal bones, this supplementary arch being supported by the calcaneo-cuboid ligaments, whilst the strong plantar fascia extends between and acts as a brace to the pillars of the arch. It must not be forgotten that while an arch has ordinarily to receive weight only in one direction, in the case of the foot the direction of the weight is continually changed by the various positions assumed by the body in its movements. Thus, while in the standing position, the weight would fall chiefly on the astragalus and be directly transmitted to the two pillars of the arch ; in walking, running, dancing, etc., involving as these movements do the different parts of the foot, the weight is constantly shifted, and consequently the ligaments and muscles of the foot are called upon to reinforce the arch by their action. Added to this there is the mobility of the tarsus, and this mobility is the greatest just where the greatest strain falls, namely, between the astragalus and scaphoid. The muscle principally called upon in this connection is the tibialis posticus, whilst the inner part of the calcaneo-scaphoid ligament is chiefly engaged in resisting all extra strain.

It will be easily understood then, that, associated with the different complex movements alluded to, involving as they do the raising (flexion) and placing of the foot on the ground (extension), that on the resistance offered by the tibialis posticus, and calcaneo-scaphoid ligament, and upon the help thus given to the arch, depend the conservation of the form of the foot. Again, the normal curves of the foot give a certain amount of mechanical advantage in the distribution of the superincumbent body weight. Thus, in flexion, the two curves of the foot, the larger with its concavity downward, and a lesser one along the inner side of the foot with its concavity outward, are increased. On the other hand, in extension, as when the foot is firmly planted on the ground, both these curves are diminished and the foot flattened. It is evident, therefore, that any cause operating to weaken those tissues, which, by their aid, serve to strengthen the arch, will cause a permanent extension of the foot, with obliteration of the natural curves. Thus, in occupations requiring continued standing or walking, or the maintenance of a given position for a long time, these structures become overtaxed, and as a consequence do not afford the proper accessory support to the arch; there exists a condition of permanent extension of the foot and sooner or later, depending on the constitution of the individual, flat-foot follows as a consequence of this abnormal strain.

The morbid anatomy of flat-foot, or spurious valgus, shows differences according to the etiology of the given cases. Thus, in the congenital variety very few pathological changes are noticeable. The external appearance of the foot shows a decided lowering or flattening of the normal arch, with the inner margin of the foot depressed and closer to the ground, whilst the outer border is raised, and the anterior part of the foot everted. Sometimes in these congenital cases there is a marked degree of equinus associated with the valgus, and when this occurs, there is decided contraction of the calf muscles. In the congenital form of valgus, there is not much displacement of the bones of the foot, the principal changes consisting of the elevation of the tuberosity of the os calcis, while the astragalus is pushed downward and forward, and is seen as a prominence on the inner side of the foot, with the rotated scaphoid bone, which is also prominent. There is a slight rotation outward of the cuboid bone, and the malleoli are depressed, being found on a lower plane than normal. The weight of the body coming on these disturbed relations is not properly received and transmitted, and, as a consequence, the strain becoming too severe on those tissues which serve to assist the arch, there is a resulting stretching of the ligaments on the plantar and inner side of the foot. Thus, the calcaneo-scaphoid ligament especially, which bears the brunt of resistance to displacement and is constantly called upon in this connection, becomes relaxed. In the congenital form, although the muscles show few changes, with the continuance of the affection there often ensues a marked contraction of the peronei and calf muscles, the foot then taking the form of an equino-valgus. With this there is often found a contraction of the extensor longus digitorum, the extensor pollicis, and the abductor minimi digiti, with slight alterations in the relations of all the tendons of these muscles.

The forms of flat-foot which deserve most of our attention will come under those found in the acquired variety, and these are the cases which, from the unusual suffering and disability they occasion constitute a large and important class. They have been variously called "splay-foot," "spurious valgus," "inflammatory flat-foot," "tarsalgia of adolescents," etc. In children the acquired form of valgus usually met with is the result of a poliomyelitis anterior, and in this condition the anterior tibial and adductor muscles are usually the paralyzed ones. At times, as in the congenital form, there is a coincident contraction of the calf muscles, rendering the deformity a compound one, and we have a talipes equino-valgus. It is also found very often associated with knock-knee and bow-legs, as a mechanical result of these deformities, especially in rachitic subjects. Rachitis itself is a very prolific source of this deformity, while as a symptomatic condition in ankle-joint disease, after injuries and burns of the foot, and following rheumatism, flat-foot is of frequent occurrence.

Each one of these causes must be made out and its relations to the deformity closely studied, but the limit of this paper is too short to give an extensive account of each variety. It is the condition variously named as already stated, that I wish to emphasize particularly.

While to the experienced orthopædist flat-foot is not especially difficult of detection, to one who has not seen many cases it frequently presents puzzling symptoms. Thus, it is frequently mistaken for neuralgia, rheumatism, and even for chronic osteitis of the tarsal bones, and I have had patients who have been treated for all these conditions before the real cause was diagnosticated. They are met with generally at the period of adolescence, although I have had several cases in which the patients were between forty and sixty years of age. In occupations necessitating long continuance of one position, as is the case in bakers, machinists, clerks, waiters, weavers, or in those vocations which compel constant and fatiguing motion, as in soldiers, the deformity happens frequently. Growing boys and girls, especially those of a languid disposition with an especial tendency to the accumulation of adipose tissue, are especially liable to this painful trouble. Certain races seem prone to this affection, namely, the negro and the Jewish races.

The gait and attitude of patients suffering with this trouble are characteristic and easily recognized. They have a heavy, dragging gait, the knees being bent, and the feet are placed in a careful, gingerly way on the ground, so that all the weight possible shall be kept from the tender part. When such patients step on an uneven surface the pain complained of is of an excruciating nature, and walking or standing is avoided as much as possible. The patients are easily tired and have an anxious expression of countenance, the general condition sympathizing to such an extent with the local trouble, that, in certain instances, the nutrition of the patient suffers very markedly. This is not difficult to understand when we reflect that, occurring as it does in young people generally active, and at a time of life when the desire for exercise and enjoyment is at its height, the enforcement of comparative idleness by the pain experienced prevents the proper completion of those functions which give the system at large its elasticity and tone.

The morbid changes found in the acquired form of flat-foot, are those which are found associated with the special etiological factors entering into the production of the deformity. For a long time it was supposed that the painful variety, in which we are especially interested, was due to an osteitis, but no absolute evidence of an inflammatory lesion, such for instance as that seen in the head of the femur in *morbus coxarius*, has been found. Still, I have seen cases in which, on rotation of the tarsus, marked reflex spasm of the abductor muscles was occasioned. If any osteitis be present, it would seem to me to be of the nature of dry, or caries sicca. In none of the cases that I have seen have there been evidences of suppuration, the local symptoms at times showing swelling, especially below the malleoli, with a semi-fluctuating feel; but heat is generally absent. On the contrary the feet of flat-footed people are, as a rule, cold, and have a peculiar, dark-blue look, as though the venous circulation was badly accomplished. The appearance of the bones is such that pressure in the deformed position would amply account for them. They are not especially altered in their relative positions, although, with the gradual falling of the arch, the astragalus becomes slightly displaced downward, the scaphoid and internal cuneiform bones being brought to a lower plane than normal, and nearer the ground. It is at the inner side of the foot where the astragalus and scaphoid show prominently, that, as a rule, the greatest amount of pain is experienced; but the location of the pain is by no means constant, the transverse tarsal joint, the metatarso-phalangeal articulation, and even the calcaneum being at times the seat. With the continuance of the abnormal pressure and the bony changes due to it, there is seen a gradual destruction of the normal arch. The abductor muscles begin to contract strongly, while the adductors are in a condition of functional paresis, and thus added to the flattening of the foot we have abduction, and a constant condition of extension; and if the contraction of the abductor muscles be maintained the outer edge of the foot is raised and does not touch the ground. In the extreme degrees of the affection the instep becomes totally obliterated through the loss of the convexity of the arch, and the internal malleolus especially becomes more and more prominent, and is seen with the protuberant astragalus and scaphoid bones as a prominence on the inner side of the foot.

In this condition, I have found, taking the medio-tarsal joint as a base line of measurement, and erecting upon this a perpendicular corresponding to the long axis of the os calcis, that the angle of internal deflection is reduced from twelve degrees in moderate cases to five degrees in severe ones. From an examination of severe cases I have ascertained the average deviation from the perpendicular to be about eight and two-tenths degrees.

The prognosis in cases of flat-foot depends in a large degree on the causes which occasion the deformity, the surroundings of the patient, and the time when he comes under treatment. In the congenital form of the disease, when it is not of great severity, the prognosis is usually a favorable one, but the severer cases, and those which have been allowed to go on for a long time, are usually more resistant, and often necessitate protracted treatment. In the acquired form, occurring as it usually does in the poorer classes, although the wealthy are by no means exempt, and being mostly met with in those who are dependent for their support on their vocation, the prognosis is not so favorable, many of these cases not coming under treatment until the pain becomes excessive, and the deformity far advanced. Still, where the hygienic and other surroundings can be improved and the patients placed under favorable conditions, and when the disease is not the result of incurable paralysis or of chronic joint lesions, I know of no disease in which so much can be done for the relief of pain, and in which such gratifying results can be accomplished, although much time and patience may be necessary for the removal of the deformity.

Concerning the treatment of flat-foot very little need be said regarding the congenital type of the deformity. When seen shortly after birth the patients may be successfully treated by manipulations alone, these having for their object the carrying of the foot to a more inverted position. To retain the advantage gained by these movements moleskin adhesive plaster (Maws), with a roller bandage may be employed to draw the foot into the varus position. When the deformity is more severe, and the child older, external splints of a simple character, composed of tin, gutta-percha, or hatters-felt may be employed. These are moulded to the part, and a gradual inversion of the foot accomplished. Should contractions occur, which cannot be overcome by the use of the simple means mentioned, tenotomy of the peronei and extensor longus digitorum becomes necessary. Should the tendo Achillis be contracted this will also have to be cut. These operations, however, are best divided into two stages, the peronei and extensor longus being tenotomized first,

and the tendo Achillis subsequently. Massage and electricity to the weakened tibial muscle may also be resorted to with the greatest advantage. When the child is old enough to walk, a simple support, consisting of two lateral uprights, connected with a band to encircle the calf, and with an inner pad corresponding to the axis of the astragalo-scaphoid articulation, and attached to the bottom of the shoe, may be used.

The forms of flat-foot which we shall be called upon to treat frequently are those which belong to the acquired variety. Here our treatment will, of course, be governed by the cause producing the deformity, and by the amount of pain and deformity. I have, already, in discussing the etiology of the disease given a brief account of the different causes operating to produce flat-foot, and will not dwell at length on the differentiation of these causes, but simply remark here that any constitutional causes or diatheses—whether strumous, rachitic or tubercular—should receive careful attention. Neither will it come into the province of this paper to discuss those extreme instances of valgus which, having been neglected for years, present so much deformity that nothing but exsections of the displaced tarsus will suffice for a restoration to a useful foot. The symptomatic valgus seen in the course of ankle-joint disease or osteitis of the tarsus, generally yields to the treatment employed for the primary lesion.

It is to the inflammatory form, so called, that I will place especial stress in the matter of treatment. I have already alluded to the difficulty of obtaining *rest* for these cases, owing to the fact that they for the most part occur in the working classes, where daily labor is necessary for their support. Where it can be done the removal of the patient from all employment suffices, especially, in beginning cases, to promote a rapid cure; but even in these cases some support to the weakened arch is called for. This has been accomplished in several ways, either by inserting pieces of leather, pads of different material and construction, steel-tempered bars, and springs on the plantar surface of the foot.

While relief can undoubtedly be afforded by these means, there are objections to their use; chief among these being the expense of especially constructed shoes and the introduction of these various contrivances. Of all those mentioned, however, I have had the best results from the use of tempered springs so made that the convexity of the spring shall be at that point where the arch of the foot is most flattened. These I have had made to extend from the middle of the os calcis to the base of the metatarso-phalangeal articulation, and their object is to supply an artificial arch for the foot. They have, however, to be inserted as a shank into the shoe, and this necessitates the construction of a special boot, and oftentimes the making of a special last for the patient. Again, being very narrow they do not, when there is extreme flattening, give the desired amount of support, patients often feeling the necessity for more pressure than can be given by them. I am indebted to Mr. Arthur H. Lea for an improvement on this spring, and it gives, undoubtedly, the best support of all the contrivances I have used, or am acquainted with.

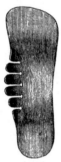

Fig. 1. Upper surface of spring.

The artificial arch illustrated in the cut is made of tempered steel. An outline of the patient's foot is first taken, on stencil-board, the tracing being extended upward on the inner side of the foot. The elevated portion, corresponding to the depressed arch of the foot, can be tempered to the extent required by the particular case. The lateral pressure brought to bear by the elevated flanges is such, that, whilst giving support to the arch to a certain extent, the artificial arch also prevents further displacement of the astragalus and scaphoid. Again, in place of giving only a limited amount of support to the inner side of the foot, this appliance supports the foot as a whole. The objection argued against the narrow spring is entirely avoided by the use of this one. It can be placed in any shoe and changed at pleasure. In most of the cases in which I have used it the spring is simply inserted into the shoe without any fastening whatsoever. The transition from absolute disability to comparative

freedom from pain which the use of this simple contrivance affords is surprising, and it is all the more gratifying from its simplicity and easy adaptability. Where the disease has lasted for a long time, I sometimes combine with it the ankle support

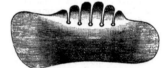

Fig. II. Under surface of spring.

mentioned, and it often serves as a valuable adjuvant in cases in which the muscles and ligaments are fatigued from long use in the deformed position.

I cannot close these remarks without enjoining the necessity of proper massage and electricity to the weakened parts. Much good also may be done at times by the use of rubber bands, especially in those cases in which the tibialis anticus is in a paretic condition. Concerning the use of plaster of Paris for the *redressment* of the foot, I would simply say that the chief objection against its use lies in the fact of its compelling the patient to keep his bed, and so depriving him of the benefit of fresh air and sunlight—both good adjuvants to the other treatment recommended.

COMPLICATIONS FOLLOWING ABDOMINAL SECTION.[1]

BY J. M. BALDY, M.D.,
PHILADELPHIA.

The attention of surgeons, in the past and at present, has so commonly and almost exclusively been called to the perfection of the different abdominal operations, that the possible complications which may follow have been lost sight of, or, if noticed at all, they are kept locked up in the bosom of the individual himself, and the profession at large hears and consequently knows very little about them. In consequence of this, medical men are continually running across these patients, and are having their faith in the value of the original operation shaken. Most men go into an operating room, see the operation, have a pathological specimen shown them, and then go away, satisfied as to the justifiability of the operation and confident as to the results. They may or

[1] Read at the meeting of the Obstetrical Society of Philadelphia, March 7, 1889.

may not see the patient several times during the treatment, but are generally satisfied with an inquiry as to how the patient is progressing, and finally have the satisfaction of hearing that she is well and has been discharged. The case is probably reported as cured to some society or medical journal, and thus the favorable statistics are swelled, and inexperienced and untrained men are led into attempting the operation, usually with the result of sacrificing several lives, before they are frightened off.

It is about time for surgeons to look at and seriously study some of the dark sides of abdominal surgery; for a dark side it certainly has. Our results, as far as removing disease is concerned, are about perfected; let us now turn some of our energies into preventing or alleviating some of the after-complications, which are in many cases as bad as the original disease itself. They do not probably cause such immediate danger to life, but produce symptoms just as hard to bear, as far as the patient is concerned, and to her belief, fully as bad at times, as her former trouble.

When I first began to give special attention to gynecological surgery, especially the abdominal variety, I was considerably worried that my cases did not always run as smooth and uncomplicated a course as I had been led to believe that those in the hands of my friends and others did. That they were not perfectly well when they got up, and came to me sometimes for weeks, complaining of one thing or another, was a source of great mortification to me. And finally, I began to find that troubles continued and others appeared, which it was extremely difficult to control. At first, supposing that I was the only one so afflicted, I thought there must be something radically wrong, either with my operations, or with my handling of the case afterward; and yet I could not reconcile these thoughts with the fact that I usually had the very best of assistance at the operation, and the constant advice of most competent men in the conduct of the after-treatment. Now I am constantly seeing and hearing of cases with troubles similar to my own, and also some with complications I have never personally met with. These cases are by no means confined to the practice of any one man, or any class of men, but represent patients of nearly every prominent operator in this city. Nor do I think that these results are confined to Philadelphia, but that they will be found wherever abdominal surgery is practised.

To consider fully the causes, prevention, and cure of these complications, is beyond the scope of this paper; my object being simply to call general attention to their frequency and to make a few remarks on the most common of them. Some of the subjects have been, from time to time, noted by other surgeons, and have been called to the attention of the profession, only to be dropped, almost as if they were subjects not to be handled and publicly discussed. Among the most frequent of these might be mentioned: hernias; simple fistulous tracks; fecal fistulas; pain, pelvic or abdominal; œdema of the lower extremities. I have seen many patients suffering from all of these troubles, and have had some of them follow in my own practice.

Holmes has found that he had thirty per cent. of hernias following his operations. Now as these cases were for the most part hospital patients, he could certainly not have kept track of them all, and so if the whole truth were known the per centage would be much higher. It would seem, at first sight, that a patient developing a ventral hernia would return for treatment; but not so, for in my own experience, with the exception of one patient, none of them ever reported, and I only discovered their existence from outside information. Thirty per cent. is, I think, a fair average of hernias following section. Most of the operators, with whose work I am familiar, have, I am confident, almost if not quite that proportion. I know of many cases in this city, of which the operator himself is not yet cognizant. Now a ventral hernia is by no means a harmless thing. I can recall women who suffer almost as much from the presence of the hernia as they did from the original disease—in fact more so; one case I know of had originally a small unadherent ovarian cyst, found in the course of a general examination, and which gave her few if any discomforts; she now has a good-sized ventral hernia, from which she suffers considerably. These hernias constantly tend to increase in size, and when the woman is one who must be on her feet constantly, carrying heavy burdens, lifting heavy weights, or in fact doing anything which will increase the tension at the abdominal opening, the result must invariably be a rapid enlargement of the protrusion, with all the accompanying distresses. There is no good reason why some of these hernias should not eventually, from various causes, become strangulated, and require a second and more serious operation; this has indeed actually occurred. The mere protrusion and displacement have caused so much trouble that an operation has been devised for the closure of the opening.

The causes of hernia have been somewhat a matter of dispute; some contending that the drainage tube is most at fault, while the advocates of the tube repudiate that idea. Then again improper suturing is charged with the results. Whatever the cause, the lesion is certainly a lack of union of the muscular tissues and of the deep fascias; the remedy is plainly that of securing perfect apposition of the edges of these tissues. Time is frequently a most important element in an operation, and there is no need of wasting it by passing a separate row of sutures, in the peritoneum itself, as has been advocated and practised in some of our neighboring cities. The peritoneum always unites, and does so in a very short time. As far as I know, it has never failed to do so, excepting in those cases in which the whole incision failed. The hernia is always found to have a covering of skin, superficial fascia and peritoneum. It seems to me that a continuous catgut suture of the muscles and deep fascia is all that is needed, beyond the usual all-the-way-through suture. I can recall a case in which the presence of a hernia, by demanding an operation for its closure, resulted in the death of the woman.

This city now contains a large number of women with fistulous tracks in their abdomens. Some of these have followed the use of drainage tubes and others have been produced by abscesses that have ruptured through the incision, leaving a track which has never closed. The extra-peritoneal method of treating the pedicle in hysterectomy is a very frequent cause of fistula. The length of time it takes the clamp to come away is often so great as to leave an opening, which constantly discharges pus— in small quantities it is true, but yet enough to be exceedingly annoying and uncomfortable to the patient. I have had two such fistulas following hysterectomy, and neither of them have I yet been able to cure; one, however, now gives fair promise of soon closing. I have, fortunately, had no other fistulæ following my operations.

One patient I know of was a few years ago operated on for some pelvic trouble, and after a few weeks she was sent to her home, with a drainage tube (rubber, I think) in her abdomen. The surgeon lost sight of her, and the tube being neglected, soon became most foul. The patient afterward drifted into one of our large general hospitals and there died.

Another patient was operated on for a pus

tube; the second tube and ovary, being apparently healthy, were left *in situ*, but these afterward took on disease and a second operation failed to remove them. A third operation was undertaken, by another surgeon, with what result was never known except by a select few; certain it is that a fistulous track followed, after a severe illness. This woman also finally found her way into one of the general hospitals, and was miserable enough to die, if she did not do so; what finally became of her I do not know.

A third patient had one side of a double tubal trouble removed, and the drainage track never closed. I saw this woman a year or more after the operation, on her death bed. The track was discharging pus freely, and always had done so; before her death, feces were also finding their way through the opening, a slough having evidently come away from the bowel.

A fourth patient, after everything else had been done without success, had a counter opening made into the vagina, by another surgeon into whose hands she had fallen. The operation, unfortunately, opened the bladder, so high up that it was impossible to repair it; she has now a vesico-vaginal fistula in addition to her other troubles, and at last report was in a dying condition.

And so I could go on with case after case, some as bad and some not so bad; but at its best, a fistula is a most miserable complication and too much attention cannot be given to its prevention. If the drainage tube is not responsible for the hernias, it certainly is for a large number of the fistulas; and although I am a firm believer in the great benefits to be derived from free drainage, I fully realize its disadvantages and often wonder if it could not be done away with oftener than it is. The great preventative of the formation of these fistulas is the prevention of abscesses and the necessity of their subsequent discharge; if they do form, it is better to go boldly in and empty them at once, than to wait and have them open by a slow, tedious and uncertain process, which may not be brought to an end before the patient dies; the avoidance of the unnecessary use of the drainage tube, and when it is used, the most careful attention to its cleanliness, and its early withdrawal. I believe a permanent track results oftener from an unnecessarily prolonged use of the tube, than from any other cause.

Fecal fistulas are not so common, and yet enough of them occur from time to time to be a warning of the danger of their production. When they do occur, they are usually so deeply seated and so bound around by inflammatory products that they cannot be reached, and if they are reached, as a rule, they require one of the most dangerous and difficult operations in the whole range of abdominal surgery. I can recall a number of these accidents: one could not be reached after an extended trial, and the whole incision was closed up in order that the patient might die as quietly as possible; this she did not do, however, but lived in spite of everything and the track afterward closed of its own accord. Another case required the most constant and careful irrigation, after an unsuccessful attempt had been made to reach it, to save the woman's life. And so they go; if an attempt is made to close them, a great risk is taken; if they are let alone and do not close spontaneously, the patient had better be dead. The usual cause, as far as I have been able to observe, is intestinal adhesions to diseased organs. After tearing a loop of gut loose, I have returned it in fear and trembling, lest a piece at the point of adhesion slough out and give me a fecal fistula. The prevention consists in the greatest care in tearing loose each adhesion, and a most careful attention to the after treatment. When fistulæ occur, they are best left alone.

A continuance of pain, or the appearance of a pain not before present, following abdominal section, is so common that every one engaged in this kind of surgery must have noted its frequency. This pain is usually not very severe, but is of a constant nagging character, such a one as so constantly to wear on a woman's nervous system that it soon renders life a misery to herself and makes her a burden to every one around her. At times, however, it assumes a severe character and becomes almost unbearable. I have known of a large number of such cases, some of which required an operation for their relief. In two cases of this kind the only lesion found was an omentum adherent to the abdominal incision, the freeing of which cured the pain. Many others are now going about, suffering as much as they did before the operation. Most of this pain is, I believe due to adhesions formed between the omentum or intestines and raw surfaces left by the operation, and the subsequent dragging on these points. This would seem to be true, as most of the cases which I have known of and which were operated on, and in which the adhesions were released, have been cured, or nearly

so. I also think that the adhesions in the original disease often cause most of the suffering; this is especially true in the pelvic cases. From these same adhesions, we have sometimes an obstruction of the bowels, either at once or later, after convalescence, which results in death. I can remember several cases of this kind, which could be explained in no other way and, in fact, some of which were demonstrated to be so by a *post-mortem* examination. The remedy for their formation and all their attendant dangers and discomforts, is to keep the bowels soluble, so that there can be no chance for adhesions to occur. The best way of accomplishing this is by purgatives, and by not using opium. Fortunately the indications for purgatives are so many and so constantly present, that they can almost always be used.

Œdema of the lower extremities, I have seen a number of times. Sometimes it is only temporary but at others it is of long enough duration and severity to be of considerable annoyance and worry to both patient and surgeon. In my own practice this has occurred several times, but has always eventually disappeared.

When every person, about to undergo an abdominal operation, must run the gauntlet of all these complications, as well as many more unmentioned, it becomes a serious matter in deciding for or against an operation. We have here to consider more than the immediate risks to life; we must think, if the patient has his or her present disease removed, will she be any better off, or may she not be the worse for the interference? At any rate, such a state of affairs should be a warning to inexperienced men not to be misled by the brilliant reports seen in the journals, and not to rush thoughtlessly into an operation, expecting to obtain the same perfect results. They should know that, as a rule, only favorable cases are reported, and that men do not like to publish to the world their bad work or misfortunes. Abdominal section is by no means the simple, easy procedure some men would make us believe, and such an operation should never be undertaken except after the most careful consideration of all the risks that must be run, the chances of benefit to the patient, and in the presence of actual demonstrable disease. Until the dark sides of abdominal work are well known to the profession at large, the *furor operandi*, which has been so justly complained of, will continue, and many women will succumb as the results of inexperience.

TREATMENT OF TAPEWORM.

BY TRAILL GREEN, M.D.,
EASTON, PENNSYLVANIA.

The treatment of tapeworm as given in the REPORTER, March 9, is doubtless very effectual when the remedy can be obtained in its active state, but, as stated, "is perhaps a little severe." Pomegranate has been used with very good results, but a decoction of ten ounces is a larger dose than many of our patients would be willing to swallow. You know I am fond of a palatable medicine. The active properties of pomegranate to meet the treatment of tapeworm can be put in less than an ounce of a liquid. I have used the remedy from the time of its introduction, and it has not failed in a single case. I introduced it to the members of our County Medical Society, who have used it with similar success.

Professor Laboulbene, member of the French Academy, who has made the cure of tænia a specialty, but who found it difficult to get good preparations of the medicines which are active in the recent state, wrote: "I wish that some one would discover and separate from the tænicide plants a sure alkaloid, always identical, and that would act with certainty; which is something we cannot obtain from pomegranate bark, or from old koossoo, which is nearly inert." (*Bulletin de Thérapeutique*, 1877.)

M. Tanret obtained the alkaloid from pomegranate bark, and named it pelletierine, in honor of Pelletier, the distinguished French chemist to whom we are indebted for so many valuable discoveries in organic chemistry.

The alkaloid has been used with great success in several of the Hospitals of Paris. Dr. Dujardin-Beaumetz has reported thirty-three cases, of which thirty-two were successfully treated. Professor Laboulbene treated fourteen cases and the tapeworm was expelled in every case. I have never used a tænicide which is so certain to bring away the whole creature—head and body. I very confidently tell a patient: "Soon after taking the medicine you will pass the tapeworm"; and my promise has not failed.

I write this that the members of our profession who have not heard of this remedy may have the pleasure of using that which will be satisfactory to themselves and grateful to their patients. I doubt not they meet with these cases frequently; I find that they are much more common than they were thirty or fifty years ago.

French physicians use with the pelletierine a French purgative, which is not official with us. I find an ounce of Epsom salt to act very well.

LYCOPODIUM DRESSING FOR ULCERS AND WOUNDS.

BY C. P. EDWARDS, M.D.,
GRANITEVILLE, S. C.

During the years 1862, 1863 and 1864 we, as Confederate medical officers, were in want of the usual antiseptic dressings to wounds and ulcers, and were thus taught to experiment with various articles of the materia medica in the hope of finding what would take the place of remedies such as the phenol preparations. Our supply of these accepted antiseptics was cut off by reason of the blockade; our hospitals were crowded with wounded, and our accommodations were tents, churches, and private buildings. The warm and moist climate attracted numerous flies which were nourished and fostered by suppurating wounds of every nature, and with all of our care we would sometimes find a nest of their larvæ in a wound, which would render our patients frantic with unrest.

These were readily routed by applications of oil of turpentine. But the important feature was to guard these wounds with a substance of a protective nature, which embodied the greatest amount of cleanliness. Hence the ointment made from our common elder flowers was adopted, but found objectionable from the unctuous matter used as a vehicle.

Having amused myself by covering water with a coating of lycopodium, and getting the ignorant to introduce their finger through this coating and to withdraw it from the glass in a dry condition, with the lycopodium covering the finger, as with the encasing of a kid glove, I suggested to my esteemed friend, Surgeon W. S. Meire, that we should adopt lycopodium as a dressing to freshly amputated stumps. That night we amputated twelve arms and legs, and having closed the wounds *secundum artem*, viz.: with sutures and adhesive straps, we applied lycopodium freely, and had the satisfaction of seeing eleven out of the twelve wounds heal by first intention.

Since then I have relied upon lycopodium as a dressing to all wounds, and in December, 1888, I was pleased with its application to a lacerated wound made by a cotton card to the forearm. During January, 1889, I used it twice—once in amputation of the thumb, with laceration of the back of the hand, the second time in a laceration of the palmar surface. Both wounds healed by first intention.

Let each surgeon now ask himself: What is lycopodium? Sulphur is death to insects. Lycopodium is a vegetable sulphur. In twenty-six years' use of it, I have never had any bad results in treating surgical wounds with it. I would therefore respectfully ask a trial of it by the other surgeons of our country, feeling assured that they will not be disappointed in the results obtained.

SOCIETY REPORTS.

OBSTETRICAL SOCIETY OF PHILA-DELPHIA.

Thursday, March 7, 1889.

The President, THEOPHILUS PARVIN, M.D., in the Chair.

DR. J. M. BALDY read a paper on

Complications Following Abdominal Section.[1]

DR. WILLIAM GOODELL, in opening the discussion, said he wholly agreed with the writer of the paper in regard to the stubborn nature of these fistulæ and to the impossibility of avoiding them. He had now three cases of fistula. One followed the removal of an intraligamentary cyst, in which he had reopened the wound for bleeding. The patient recovered, but a fecal fistula had made its appearance about the fifth day after operation and had never closed. He had to peel off the tumor from the rectum. It was now a year and a half since the operation, and the patient was in the hands of a competent surgeon in the country. The only annoyance to her is an escape of gas from the wound. The second case followed the prolonged use of the drainage tube, after abdominal section for pelvic abscess. He had not had charge of the after treatment, but the patient was in the hands of a skilful surgeon. It may be needful yet to make a counter-opening in the vagina. The third case was one of recurrent intraligamentary cyst. The fist-

[1] See REPORTER, page 420.

ula resulted from a previous operation, in which the surgeon used the clamp, many years ago. Dr. Goodell operated last November, and removed a recurrent cyst lying in a very large abscess cavity. A drainage tube was then used, which he still kept in, because he could not get the fistula to heal from the bottom. He had just made an application of iodine to the track, and told the husband to repeat it daily for a time. He has had cases of fistula when the drainage tube was not used, but they were due to non-encapsulation of the pedicle ligatures. In one while using the syringe the ligature was washed out. This gave him the cue, so in the others he fished the ligature out by means of a small hook on the end of a fine wire. On the other hand, in the case of an ovarian abscess, he had kept drainage up for several months, and yet the track closed. It is his intention in a third case to pass nitric acid to the bottom of the fistula, and see what can be accomplished in this way. In this case the patient menstruates through the track.

Dr. Goodell thought that if operators would wait some time after they have operated, before reporting their cases, they would find a number of hernias. He takes a good deal of pains to avoid this accident, and he closes the abdominal wound in an analogous way to that described by Dr. Price. The tendon when retracted he brings forward, as much as possible, with forceps, so as to bring it in contact with its fellow. He has had cases in spite of every care. In the official report of Imlach's cases, although these were all cases of oöphorectomy, needing a very short incision, the percentage of hernias was fifteen. Dr. Goodell keeps his patients in bed for two weeks, before allowing them to sit up. In two cases in which he removed the ovaries, in fibroid tumors, he has had the incision rupture, from too early taking out of the stitches. In these cases he sometimes leaves them in for two weeks. One patient went home nineteen days after operation, in spite of orders, and the train becoming derailed, the jarring forced the cutaneous part of the wound open. Stitches had to be put in.

DR. M. PRICE does not think with Dr. Baldy that abdominal surgery has anything to regret in these cases. He admits that much of the dirt and filth and many of the accidents which follow these terrible operations are actually due to the surgeon. He does not wonder at there being fistulous tracks, for the reason that in many of these cases the adhesions to the bowel are of such strength that their separation often removes everything down to the mucous coat. He has seen as many as six or seven sutures applied to such a case. Fistula is a repetition of the old, abscess, which finds its way to the surface through the drainage track. All of the disease has not been removed. In many cases the fistula saves the woman's life and gives the surgeon a path through which to perfect his otherwise imperfect work. Fistula is a proof that the case has not been properly cared for. He does not believe that thirty per cent., or even five per cent., represents the number of hernias. He has only seen two cases follow. Their closure is unattended with danger. If due care and cleanliness are observed, fistulæ will not occur.

DR. J. PRICE was a little surprised that one so deeply interested as Dr. Baldy, in this subject of abdominal surgery, should stimulate criticism of our present position. Dr. Baldy speaks of hernia. The position of the incision, the condition of the abdominal .walls, and the manner of introducing the sutures are of great importance. Death has followed tight sutures and he is satisfied that hernias often follow them. He always draws his sutures lightly. If three or four are used to the inch, tied lightly, with perfect coaptation, the results will, as a rule, be perfect. In introducing sutures he takes in half as much skin as fascia, and twice as much fascia as peritoneum. This gives better apposition to the centre of the wound. He has not had a suture-track abscess for more than a month, nor has there been any mischief about the tube. Nursing is of the greatest importance. The old nurses are meddlesome and dangerous, and he is glad to see them replaced by younger women. The tube can be dispensed with very often if the irrigation is thorough. Most surgeons are in too much of a hurry to get their patients up. Early rising is dangerous, and he has known surgeons to brag of getting their patients home in ten days.

In fistulous tracks, through which menstruation occurs, the only thing to do is to tie the tube and release it from the abdominal incision. A drainage tube resting against the torn bowel surfaces favors the occurrence of a fistula. A man who gets scared at a fistula or ventral hernia is not prepared to do good work; his work begins in doubt and ends in disaster. The operation for curing a ventral. hernia is not dangerous.

We cannot ignore the importance of precision in diagnosis. We must try to decide as to the probable nature of the lesion. Dr. Baldy calls attention to one point, that is, the necessity of recognizing something definite on which to operate. Savage and others are satisfied to operate for subjective symptoms only. This is not right. The other day Dr. Price refused to operate on a patient who had multiple abscesses in the lungs. Two weeks before he had gone to the house prepared to operate, but the family had refused. The time will come when operators will be most arbitrary in these cases. We shall have the right to say that if the general practitioner waits until the eleventh hour we will not step in. Last summer a patient refused operation, to-day she sent for Dr. Price and requested it.

Peritonitis is often due to an imperfect toilet. It is often of limited extent or localized, leaving adhesions to portions of the viscera. This is a common source of pain and discomfort. The only good remedy is to do the work over and release the adhesions. This past summer he had either done himself, or assisted others to do, eight of these operations over, and they had been the most difficult and trying of his whole experience. He wished to call attention to one case on which he had operated three times. Dr. Baldy saw the work. When he first saw the patient pus was escaping from the umbilicus. He opened the abdomen, but failed to remove anything. Drainage was followed by a good recovery, but the wounds did not close. A year later he re-operated, but a fistulous track was left. Again a year later he used a catheter made of coils of wire. He passed this along around the ileo-pectineal line, toward the region of the kidney. He dissected along the pelvic bones and irrigated through the catheter. Last week, the patient was delivered of a fine baby. In this case he could find the ovaries, and there was no lesion of them or of the tubes. This is the only case of pelvic abscess without tubal disease he has ever seen, in a long and rich experience.

He wished to speak of two of the cases referred to by Dr. Baldy in his paper. One case he had operated on early in his experience, and had removed only one side of a specific tubal trouble. This he would never do again. The patient went into other hands, and he did not care to refer to the surgery which followed. Another case of which he had personal knowledge, was a case of imperfect surgery. This was a large pus sac, which could have been removed but was drained. The woman died of psoas abscess. Skene has called attention in his book to the fact that pelvic abscess frequently causes psoas abscess. The incomplete removal of diseased tubes should be rectified. If an inch of tube is left it will most likely do mischief. He has curetted into the cavity of the uterus, removing a cone-shaped piece. The tubes should be tied hard on to the uterus, and the ovaries should be tied at a good surgical neck, and the results will be about perfect.

DR. MONTGOMERY said: We have become so enthusiastic in the field in which we are working as perhaps to overlook the dangers and difficulties, and in our desire to defend and possibly to push forward our own work, we sometimes fail to report our disasters. I think that Dr. Baldy has done us a kindness in dwelling on some of the disasters that may occur in abdominal operations. I am rather surprised to find that hernia is such a frequent lesion, in his experience. I have not found it so. The method of closing the wound suggested by Dr. Price, is the one that I have largely used, and unless Dr. Baldy has come across some case of which I do not know, I have never had a hernia in my experience. Fistulas with a constant discharge are exceedingly depressing and distressing. I have thought that drainage *per vaginam* might be preferable, where this accident is liable to occur. In such a case if fistula did follow, it would not be so bad as if it were in the abdomen. I operated last fall on a case in which half a gallon of broken-down blood was removed from a sac. The sac was drained, but death occurred in a few days. The *post-mortem* showed an abscess below the sac, which would have been opened if vaginal drainage had been performed. The after-treatment is exceedingly important in many cases. These results are no doubt due to the fact that there still remains some diseased tissue about the ligament or uterus. Where the tubal disease is gonorrhœal, it is very hard to tie close enough to the uterus to remove all the pyogenic membrane. Even when we do the inflammatory condition is still present in the uterus. The tendency of the extension of such inflammation to the pelvic tissues is in many cases the cause of after trouble.

DR. HIRST said that in three cases which he had lately to deal with, fistulæ directly followed laparotomy. One woman died a year after the operation in consequence of this complication. In one case of great interest a mass of ligature was fished up, but the fistula still remains. After waiting sometime he opened the vault of the vagina, behind the uterus, on the point of a sound passed into the fistula from above. He did not think he could have opened the bladder, but a vesical fistula must have already existed, for when he cut through the vault of the vagina, urine gushed out. A drainage tube was put through the whole track, but now four months have passed and the woman is dying. He would hardly think the use of nitric acid free from danger, used as recommended by Dr. Goodell.

DR. BALDY said: I did not bring these cases forward as an objection to abdominal surgery, nor would they, nor many more, stay my hand if I found a case which required operation. My desire was to call direct attention to such accidents as these and to stimulate our efforts to prevent their frequency. Nor is this by any means a complete list of all the cases on which I could put my hands. I could add dozens to the ones I have named. These cases have occurred in the hands of prominent men, men who profess to be teachers and who number their cases by the twenties, fifties and hundreds. If we see such accidents in the hands of such men, we shall have more serious results in the hands of those less expert. Many cases of fistula can be avoided by care in the use of the drainage tube. Few surgeons understand how to take care of a tube properly. I cannot agree with Dr. Price that fistulas always follow old fistulous tracks, and are caused by diseased tissue left behind. In the majority of cases that I have seen the diseased tissue has all been removed and the track occurs through what was formerly clean, healthy tissue. I think that one common cause of hernia is the use of hæmostatic forceps. These bruise the tissues and if allowed to remain on too long cannot help irreparably damaging the vitality of the parts included between the blades. The less we use the forceps the better union we will get. It is a rare occurrence that I have to use more than one or two pairs, sometimes three. These are always removed in a few moments—in fact, as soon as I open the peritoneal cavity. They are no longer needed and often, if we are working through a small incision, are in the way. The fewer foreign bodies in and about the abdomen and abdominal wound, the better for the patient and the easier for the operator. Cleanliness in all its details cannot be too strongly insisted upon.

NEW YORK ACADEMY OF MEDICINE.

Stated Meeting, March 21, 1889.

The President, ALFRED L. LOOMIS, M.D., in the Chair.

The Place of Electricity in Therapeutics.

The discussion on this subject was opened by DR. M. ALLEN STARR, the title of whose paper was,

The Physics and Physiological Actions of Electricity.

By electricity a new molecular state is produced in the body, but nothing is added to or subtracted from the body. Between the two poles this molecular change is more intense than elsewhere. He thought the term " current " responsible to a certain extent for the erroneous opinion prevailing regarding the action of electricity in therapeutics. The forms of electricity are frictional or static, voltaic or galvanic, and induced electricity or Faradism. He thought too much credence had been given to the therapeutic action of static electricity, for its effect is confined to the surface of the body, unless it acts reflexly ; it is only mildly stimulating, and serves this purpose no better than massage or other mechanically acting stimulants. Besides, this object can be as well obtained by means of galvanism, which can also be used for permanently charging the body and in producing catalytic, cataphoric, and electrotonic effects. For disintegrating the bodily tissues galvanism has but a limited application in therapeutics. It is used for the removal of hairs, but gives place to other surgical procedures in the removal of tumors, etc. As to its use for stimulating nutrition, as in paresis of certain forms, he knew of but one scientific observation, that of Dr. Thatcher, in a case of paresis of the upper extremities, in which galvanism hastened recovery, while Faradism produced no such effect, and massage did actual harm. He has never seen a case of organic disease of the brain or spinal cord which he could consider cured by the application of electricity. Some cases improved under the treatment for a time, then grew worse, while others did not improve at all.

Regarding the power of reaching the deeper tissues, it is to be noted that the body is homogeneous, and that the power of conducting electricity in different tissues is variable. But little of the current reaches, for instance, the brain or cord, in proportion to the amount applied to the surface. It is not impossible that favorable nutritive effects are produced by the increased circulation, and more rapid chemical changes brought about by the agent, as in lead palsy ; yet he has not been able to convince himself of definite benefit attributable to this remedy alone.

There is no doubt of the power of electricity to promote osmosis, and this quality has been made use of in introducing drugs to allay pain.

Dr. Starr's conclusions were as follows: 1. Static electricity offers nothing more than the interrupted galvanic current, and fails to furnish those effects which are most desirable in the treatment of disease. 2. The constant galvanic current can produce chemical changes which aid nutrition or destroy tissue according to the strength employed. 3. The constant galvanic current can transfer medicines within the body from without. 4. The interrupted galvanic or Faradic current can excite various organs to functional activity. 5. It is questionable whether the pathological state causing organic diseases can be in any way influenced by electricity. 6. If functional diseases are benefited it is in an uncertain manner. The agent, therefore, is used empirically, and the physiological indications for it are as yet uncertain. As a therapeutic agent its use is somewhat limited, and a careful weighing in the balance is required to establish its sphere.

He concluded by saying that after the constant use of electricity during the past ten years he must acknowledge to disappointment in the results obtained.

DR. LANDON CARTER GRAY read a paper on

The Effects of Electricity in Central Nervous Diseases.

He first made some remarks suggested by Dr. Starr's paper, and said that he would undertake as positively to obtain certain therapeutic effects from electricity in certain neuralgias and neurasthenic cases as he would from opium in other diseases. He did not claim, however, to cure the organic disease, and no more could be said of any drug in the Pharmacopœia. A great deal depends upon the way in which electricity is used. Electricity is useful in the functional insanities only in the period of convalescence. It is not considered in chronic and incurable forms. It is also beneficial in certain of the gross diseases of the brain, as in the early stage of cerebral syphilis, before hemiplegia has supervened. Meningitis of traumatic origin, producing hemiplegia, if slight, may be benefited by electricity, and if hemiplegia of vascular origin is not followed by contracture it can also usually be thus benefited. *Tic douloureux* is uncertain in its response to electricity.

The two currents which will answer every purpose of the physician are the galvanic and Faradic. The administration of electricity in diseases of the brain consists of cerebral galvanization and peripheral Faradization. Regarding the choice of poles, he could lay down no other rule than this: where one pole does not agree, try the other; and if that does not agree, stop using electricity. The question of the ascending and descending current has of late years been merged into the question of poles; although he thinks there is a difference, he knows no indication for one more than for the other. He said this in spite of the indubitable differences ˙chemically, physiologically, and pathologically between the negative and the positive pole.

Dr. W. R. Birdsall discussed

The Effect of Electricity in Spinal Cord Diseases.

He thought much of the disappointment of some persons in the employment of electricity is that they have anticipated too much of it. He agrees with Dr. Starr, that he has never seen it cure a case of organic disease of the spinal cord, but then he has never seen any other single remedy do this. Electricity, however, is beneficial in relieving certain symptoms attending these affections, as pain, anæsthesia, spasm, paresis, trophic changes. He regards its action as essentially stimulant, an excitor of living tissues.

Dr. A. D. Rockwell read a paper on

Effects of Electricity in Peripheral Nerve Lesions.

He has found the agent beneficial in several of the neuralgias, especially facial paralysis, in which the form of current to be used depends upon whether the intramuscular nerves have at the outset become completely paralyzed for the time being. If so, Faradic electricity, which exerts its influence chiefly upon them, would produce no response, while galvanic electricity would produce contraction because it influences principally the muscle fibre which is still intact. Electricity is useful in diphtheritic paralysis.

Dr. E. D. Fisher read a paper on

The Effects of Electricity in Functional Nerve Affections.

In the course of his remarks he said he would not discard static electricity quite so positively as it would seem Dr. Starr would do. He thought it had its uses in neurasthenic cases and in those functional affections characterized by errors in nutrition.

Dr. Putnam Jacobi summed up the statistics of uterine fibromata treated by electricity. They were not very extensive nor very definite. Those who had reported their experience with it had often seen relief from symptoms, and some diminution in the size of the tumor.

˙Dr. George W. Jacoby took much the same view of electricity as a therapeutic agent as Dr. Starr had done. The agent being used empirically, had been resorted to in every disease and symptom imaginable. Very frequently benefit was reported in cases which it is likely would have recovered without the electricity.

Dr. Leopold Putzell also thought those who attributed good results to electricity often overlooked the natural course of the disease. In facial paralysis, and diphtheritic paralysis, which had been referred to by Dr. Rockwell, this statement is true. The Faradic current applied with the brush over painful points in neuralgia often has a rapid effect. In one case varicose veins of the leg of twenty years' duration practically disappeared under Faradism.

Dr. J. H. Girdner had been experimenting to determine the electrical state of the human body in health and disease. Putting one pole in the mouth and the other in the rectum, a considerable difference in the electrical state was found under varying conditions. The variations were especially great between health and disease. This is not to be attributed to the fluid at the pole.

Dr. Peterson said he had lately been employing electricity in introducing a mixture of cocaine and aconite under the skin and at painful neuralgic points. He has thus been able to quiet pain for from five to eleven hours.

Dr. William H. Thompson distinguished between the influence of galvanic and Faradic electricity, and said that he had obtained much benefit from the latter in stimulating the arterial circulation of parts and thus overcoming paresis, and causing absorption of exudates in subacute affections, as articular rheumatism, pleurisy with effusion, etc.

Dr. Andrew H. Smith has found quicker and more positive benefit from static electricity than from any other form in stiffness and soreness of parts due to exposure to cold, as in stiffness of the hand and wrist of stage drivers, etc. He thought the electrical variations observed by Dr. Girdner were to be attributed to substances accidentally present in the body.

Dr. Starr, in closing the discussion, said, respecting the action of Faradism being directed more especially to the intramuscular nerves and galvanism to the muscular fibres, that there is no truth in this statement. The reason why Faradism does not produce a response is that the interruptions are too rapid. Make them slowly and the muscle will respond to it as well as to galvanism. He said the discussion had confirmed him in his view that electricity is of limited value in therapeutics.

REPORTS OF CLINICS.

PHILADELPHIA HOSPITAL.

CLINIC UPON OBSTETRICS, AND DISEASES OF CHILDREN—DR. PARVIN.

Death of an Infant from Hemorrhage from the Mouth.

Dr. Parvin first spoke of the death of an infant from hemorrhage from the mouth, a few hours after birth, and said: A most unusual case recently occurred in the Maternity. A woman was in labor, the presentation being pelvic; after the delivery of the body, and after the face had rotated posteriorly, the resident physician, anxious to keep the head well flexed and also thus facilitate delivery by traction, pressed upon the lower jaw with one or two fingers partly introduced into the mouth; the child was delivered living, but a short time after birth the nurse observed blood oozing from the mouth. Upon examination there was found blood coming from just beneath the tongue on one side. Various means to arrest the flow were tried, but they were unsuccessful, and the child died. It has been supposed that this child was a "bleeder," that is, suffered from hemophilia. The bleeding, whether traumatic or spontaneous in such a subject, is rebellious to remedies; such was the fact in this case, and so, reversing the familiar statement that the cure proves the disease, we might say the failure to cure may also prove the disease.

The point, however, to which I desire to call your special attention is as to the management of head-last labors with reference to assisting flexion and hastening delivery, when posterior rotation of the face has occurred after the expulsion of the body. The method most generally recommended is that known by the compound name Smellie-Veit. Two fingers of one hand are introduced into the mouth, care being taken to press only upon the alveolar processes of the lower jaw; at the same time two fingers of the other hand are passed over the nape of the neck; traction is now made, chiefly with the fingers pressing upon the lower jaw. But may we not produce safer and equally effectual pressure with two fingers upon the superior maxillary, while two fingers of the other hand press up the occiput, and thus secure the prompt expulsion of the mental end of the occipito-mental diameter?

Of course, a prompt delivery is imperatively necessary when this stage of labor is reached, for the child is liable to perish from asphyxia, the chief source of such asphyxia being pressure upon the cord, assisted by partial detachment or very great compression of the placenta when the uterus is so nearly completely emptied, provided its normal retraction has occurred. I cannot but think that pelvic deliveries are more liable to be attended by intra-cranial injuries, which, though not always mortal, may have a very injurious effect upon the child's condition. Cruveilhier has stated that of the children perishing in labor, one-third die from cerebral hemorrhage. In recently looking over some statistics of convulsions, or of paralyses following labor, and of defective mental development, I was struck with the relatively greater number of these unfortunates that had been born by a pelvic presentation, or after podalic version had been performed. If this be true the explanation probably is found in the necessarily rapid passing of the head, before time can be given for its molding, through the bony pelvis, and hence injurious compression made with consequent intra-cranial hemorrhage. The head must be delivered quickly, or the child dies: but this delivery may be secured by the sacrifice of the child's health—it comes into the world possibly to live only a few days, months or years, but at best living an imperfect, incomplete life.

Intra-Cranial Hemorrhage.

Seventy-two hours after its birth an infant in the Maternity was attacked with convulsions, and in twelve hours died. The autopsy revealed a hemorrhagic clot upon the right side under the dura mater. There was no external injury, and the labor had ended spontaneously and was not long. I mention this case to show you an example of intra-cranial hemorrhage caused by natural labor. The rule is that, if the effusion of blood be considerable, death takes place within twenty-four hours. The fact that this child lived so long before symptoms occurred and then for twelve hours afterward, shows that the rule must not be regarded as absolute. Where a diagnosis of hemorrhagic effusion has been made, it has been proposed to aspirate; but it seems to me that this would be very uncertain treatment, for it could not remove a clot, nor could it furnish any guarantee against a fresh effusion.

Induction of Premature Labor in Contraction of the Pelvic Inlet.

The measurements that have been previously taken, and which have now been again taken before you in order to give you an illustration of pelvimetry, prove that this woman, who is in her eighth month of pregnancy, has a pelvis of which the true conjugate is somewhat under four inches. You know that in the mechanism of labor in the simple flat pelvis, the fœtal head passes through the inlet with its biparietal diameter in relation with the true conjugate. When once the head has made this passage, cleared this strait, there is no more trouble in the labor. Now although in this woman, supposing the bi-parietal of the child's head at term to be three inches and a half, the true conjugate exceeds it by a small fraction of an inch; and although the former diameter may be reduced one centimeter, or about two-fifths of an inch, and therefore labor at nine months would probably be difficult, yet it is also probable that the woman could deliver herself, and it is possible her child might be born living, and without any intra-cranial injury such as has been referred to. It would nevertheless be safer to induce premature labor early in the ninth month. Bearing in mind that the increase of the biparietal diameter in the latter months of pregnancy is one centimeter a month, you determine, after having ascertained the degree of pelvic contraction, the time for the induction of premature labor, endeavoring to delay this as long as is safe for mother and child, so that the latter may have the best chance of living

after delivery. Many a child born prematurely perishes, but I confess I was somewhat startled by reading in Winckel's recent work upon obstetrics that the fœtal mortality after the induction of premature labor is 66.6 per cent.

The question as to the means of inducing premature labor may be asked. That method which most obstetricians employ is the one known as Krause's, that is, by the introduction of an elastic bougie between the ovum and the uterine wall. Quite recently I was reading in a French journal the history of a case in which such introduction, though attempted by an able hand, was impossible; the difficulty arose from a very marked anteflexion of the uterus: the operator then succeeded in bringing on labor by the use of tents.

Of course all antiseptic precautions must be used in this operation; the bougie must be clean, and dipped in an antiseptic solution—for example, in a solution consisting of 1 part of corrosive sublimate to 1000 of water; the vagina must be thoroughly cleansed with an antiseptic solution. The operator's hand, after careful and complete washing, must also be put in a similar fluid. Then the bougie is carefully passed into the uterus, made to feel its way, insinuate itself between the ovum and the uterine wall, always moving it in the direction of the least resistance, until it is quite within the uterus. Labor in the majority of cases begins within twenty-four hours; but in some it may be delayed for days. What is to be done in the latter case? Repeat the application of the bougie, only at each new introduction give the instrument a different direction from any that it previously had.

COLLEGE OF PHYSICIANS AND SURGEONS—VANDERBILT CLINIC.

CLINIC FOR GENITO-URINARY DISEASES— PROF. OTIS.

Gonorrhœa.

In the previous lecture Dr. Otis discussed acute gonorrhœa, but he said it would be improper to dismiss the subject without reference to those long-standing cases of acute gonorrhœa in which the inflammation is not confined, as usual, to the anterior part of the urethra, but extends to the membranous portion, and beyond; sometimes involving the bladder, ureters, and even the kidneys. The causes which tend to produce this condition are excessive exercise, bad living, alcoholic indulgence and, most decidedly, sexual indulgence, both in act and thought.

The first symptom that will call attention to the disease is frequent urination, which is a sign usually that the neck of the bladder is involved. For relief of this, rest is most important, together with suppositories of opium or enemata of hot water. It is most essential that the sound and catheter be not used during this stage. Even should there be retention of urine it is advisable first to employ other means of relief than the catheter, such as hot baths, hot enemata, and 5 to 10 drop doses of the muriated tincture of iron, every hour, in the hope of thus relieving the retention.

In cases of involvement of the deeper urethra there is danger when using instruments of pushing the contagion further on. But when the bladder is once involved there is no longer necessity for avoiding the use of catheters.

The treatment of the condition under consideration is by the injection of a few drops of a solution of nitrate of silver, 3 to 5 grains to the ounce, directly upon the membranous urethra. It is also one of the most reliable means of curing a beginning cystitis.

Chronic gonorrhœa is due to the fact that on the diseased spots the epithelium is not replaced because of the plastic material beneath. When endoscopy first came into employment it was supposed that its value would be very great, that these spots could then be exactly located and applications made directly upon them. But even after this treatment and after the patient had been discharged apparently cured, it was found that very frequently he came back, perhaps months afterward, complaining of a return of his discharge. In reality a stricture is at the bottom of most of these cases, and it is only when this is removed that we can expect a permanent good from the applications. Often the cure of the stricture will stop the discharge.

Case I.—The patient was a man 30 years old, who presented himself with chronic gonorrhœa. He has several strictures which will not now be located. By the endoscope we see evidences of these as well as patches of inflammation. The treatment now recommended in such a case as this would be the irrigation of the urethra after the following method. A syringe, holding several ounces of a medicated solution, is attached to a catheter and the catheter is passed down to the membranous urethra, not into the bladder. The syringe is slowly emptied through the catheter, the fluid passing along the deep

urethra into the bladder. The apparatus is withdrawn and the patient voids the injection, thus medicating the entire canal. The following solutions are recommended :

No. 1 Acidi Carbolici,
Zinci Sulphatis,
Alumenis . . . . āā 1 part
Aquæ . . . . 1500 parts
at first; then 1000; then 500 parts

No. 2 Potass. Permanganat. . . . 1 part
Aquæ . . . . 1000 parts

No. 3 Argenti Nitrat. . . . . . . 1 part
Aquæ Destil. . . . . . 1000 parts

To this method there is only one objection, namely, it may set up a prostatitis ; this is clearly due to the impact of the fluid against the prostatic urethra. The same complication sometimes occurs after the passage of a sound. It is an objectionable occurrence as it is liable to be persistent, not unfrequently lasting a year or more ; and being evidently due to the measures used by the physician he is pretty sure to be credited with it. So that although Prof. Otis has had most excellent results, especially from injection No. 1, employed in this manner in chronic urethritis, and also in cystitis, his advice would be not to use this procedure, but rather the ordinary syringe employed in the usual way. He decidedly advises against the use of a sound in these cases, previous to the large injection, for the purpose of ironing out the mucous membrane.

After the employment of these or similar injections, in many instances, the discharge continues. Then the endoscope may be used. But after all, though this instrument is of undoubted utility it is not a necessity. We can locate the diseased and tender areas as well with a bulbous sound, and in this manner as accurately apply our nitrate of silver as through the endoscope.

Stone in the Bladder.

Case II.—The patient was a man, 55 years old. For two years he has had trouble in urinating, micturition being frequent and but little urine passing at a time. He has had pain at the end of the penis. The urine has never stopped suddenly while being voided. This last is a valuable symptom, but it is well to remember that this and all symptoms may be frequently absent. Dr. Otis recalls a case in which a very large stone existed for many years without any symptom of bladder trouble.

In examining this man he first elevated the hips so that the stone fell to the upper part of the bladder. Passing in the sound he found a calculus, and applying the Billroth audiphone the click of the sound against the stone was heard 30 feet away. It was a large stone. If it had been found small, by measurement, it might have been crushed before the class, but he does not like to operate in such a case as this unless he is able to put the patient at once to bed. In this man there is some narrowing of the urethral canal as well as considerable spasm. The physician should always attend first to the determination of the condition of the urethra. Then before operating, he should make due preparation, by making the urethra large enough to facilitate the main operation.

The difficulties in litholapaxy are not from injuries to the bladder, but from irritation to the urethra. This point Dr. Otis was the first to make in 1881, and he believes it now fully proved by *post-mortem* evidence.

PERISCOPE.

To Avoid Corrosive Sublimate Poisoning.

In a communication to the *Amer. Journal of Obstetrics*, Feb., 1889, on the Puerperal Uterus, Drs. F. L. and John R. Haynes give the following advice:

1. Where intra-uterine irrigation is used in the absence of sepsis, use no sublimate, but plain hot water, or salt and water.

2. If the urine is albuminous and scanty, use no mercury.

3. If the urine is slightly albuminous and copious, or if the patient is profoundly anemic, do not use more than a pint of a solution of 1 : 8,000.

4. Always use tartaric acid and sublimate tablets or powders; dissolve thoroughly in a small quantity of water and mix carefully with a definite quantity of hot water in a pitcher, from which pour into the irrigator.

5. Always use a fountain syringe, and for the uterus a double tube, so as to insure the return of the solution. If for any reason the fluid fails to run out as fast as it flows in (if not through the reflux tube, by way of the channels at its sides), shut off the flow. The irrigator should not be raised more than three feet.

6. Precede by copious irrigation with hot water to wash out blood, etc., which may form with sublimate adhesive albuminous compounds, which may in time be absorbed. Follow by a quart or two of hot water to insure the evacuation of all the sublimate solution.

7. For the uterus, use a solution not stronger than 1 : 8,000 and not more than a quart, once daily.

8. For the vagina, use a solution not stronger than 1 : 4,000 and not more than a quart, twice daily.

Irrigation used in the above way is, they believe, a practice almost devoid of danger. They have made more than one hundred and seventy-five irrigations with the double tube and fountain syringe, with no untoward results, except in two cases an unimportant rise of temperature, and in one a severe but harmless chill; and even these slight accidents they are certain might have been avoided by greater care. Nevertheless they assert that irrigation of the puerperal uterus will always be a procedure requiring great care and judgment and some skill. They agree with Credé and Fehling, that both vaginal and uterine irrigations are attended with undoubted dangers, and should never be employed in the puerperal state unless to meet definite indications.

Chloroform Administration.

At the distribution of the prizes to the students of the Hyderabad Medical School, by their Royal Highnesses the Duke and Duchess of Connaught, on January 25, Surgeon-Major Lawrie, M.D., Principal of the Medical School, in a short address, referred to the commission appointed last year by the Nizam's Government, to make experiments with reference to the effects of chloroform. Dr. Lawrie said the experiments which had been carried out by the commission, consisting of Dr. Hehir, Mr. Kelly and Mr. Chamarette, were, in his opinion, the most important that had ever been made, and had conclusively decided a question which had been in dispute ever since chloroform was first introduced. There is no doubt, he said, that the anæsthesia produced by chloroform is best measured by its effect on the breathing, and that when the administration is pushed beyond a safe point, the breathing becomes embarrassed and then stops. The question in dispute is whether chloroform ever affects the heart directly or not; and this is important in its bearing on the way in which the administration of the anæsthetic should be conducted.

The following was the work performed by the commission, as described by Dr. Lawrie. They killed with chloroform 128 full-grown pariah dogs, averaging over twenty pounds weight each. This does not represent a tithe of the experiments they actually performed, which really amounted to several hundreds, as they varied the dose and the method of administering the chloroform in every possible way, and tested the value of artificial respiration in nearly every case by reviving the dogs over and over again after the breathing had stopped, and before the heart ceased beating. What they found was, that no matter in what way it was given, in no case did the heart become dangerously affected by chloroform until after the breathing had stopped. "This," adds Dr. Lawrie, "tallies exactly with my own experience. I have given chloroform as often, or oftener, than any man living, and have never had a fatal case; and I can state positively that in the 40,000 or 50,000 administrations I have superintended I have never seen the heart injuriously or dangerously affected by it. I take no credit to myself in this matter. I have simply carried out in India the principles Simpson and Syme practised and taught in Edinburgh." In the hospitals attached to their school, chloroform was invariably given with absolute, or with almost guaranteed safety, by students, and they were never allowed to examine the heart beforehand, or feel the pulse during its administration. In other places, and in London itself, deaths from chloroform constantly occur, but provided the administrator could swear he examined the heart and felt the pulse, they were always supposed to be accidental. Dr. Lawrie has no doubt deaths will go on occurring until the London schools, which of course influence the whole world, either entirely change their principles and ignore the heart in chloroform administration, or else confine themselves exclusively to the use of an anæsthetic like ether, which, with all its disadvantages, they know how to manage.—*British Med. Journal,* Feb. 23, 1889.

How to Preserve the Hands.

Dr. George Meyer, of Berlin, in a paper published in the *Berliner klin. Wochenschrift,* Jan. 14, 1889, says that in using the different methods of disinfection for the hands, which are at present considered necessary, the skin is always more or less affected. Reddening, eczema, and cracks of the skin are often the results of repeated washings and scrubbings with antiseptic materials, so that at times entire abstinence from the use of disinfecting fluids seems necessary. Fluid antiseptics contribute especially to roughening the skin of the hands, which results in the skin becoming cracked when the hands are subsequently exposed to the cold air and are not sufficiently dry.

There have been several methods, Dr. Meyer says, which have been proposed to keep the skin of the hands, especially physicians' hands, soft and pliable. He then speaks of a method recommended to him by Professor Liebreich, which is very easy to carry out. It has been of more use to him than all other formulas during the years that he suffered with red hands. It has nothing to do with the disinfection of the hands, but merely serves to keep their skin in a normal condition. His own hands, which for years were red and tender, have since its use become nearly normal in color. Moreover, he says he can use it with all disinfectants, without having to fear any further effects on the hands, since its use renders the skin smooth and soft.

After thoroughly washing the hands with a soap that makes a lather easily, they are well wiped and thoroughly dried; then the hands, especially the one most exposed to infection in the daily intercourse of life, is rubbed with a little lanolin, and any excess removed with a handkerchief. Other substances may be added to the lanolin, according to preference; Dr. Meyer uses the following:

> ℞ Lanolin Puriss. . . . . . 98 parts.
> Extract. Vanill. . . . . . 2 parts.
> Olei Rosæ . . . . gtt. j.

This, he says, is a salve for the skin which he has always found satisfactory. It has been shown that a smoother salve can also be made by the following formula:

> ℞ Lanolin . . . . . 79 parts.
> Liquid Paraffin . . 19 parts.
> Extract. Vanillæ . . . . . . 2 parts.
> Olei Rosæ . . gtt. j.
> M. et ft. terendo unguent.

For applying away from home the lanolin may be carried in small metal collapsible tubes. The ointment is to be reapplied after every washing, and each time in such a way that the lanolin will be thoroughly rubbed into the skin. This is especially recommended during the winter. In speaking of the favorable effect of lanolin, he mentions its power of mixing with water, by virtue of which, after washing the hands, any water remaining on the skin from imperfect wiping is absorbed by the lanolin, and the hands prepared for the cold with the least possible grease. By these two latter qualities the hands are prevented from cracking and reddening.

In practice he has used the method with good result for rubbing on the face, as in actors, whose skin had suffered from the use of paint.

THE
MEDICAL AND SURGICAL
REPORTER.

ISSUED EVERY SATURDAY.

CHARLES W. DULLES, M.D.,
EDITOR AND PUBLISHER.

The Terms of Subscription to the serial publications of this office are as follows, payable in advance:

Med. and Surg. Reporter (weekly), a year, $5.00
Quarterly Compendium of Med. Science, - 2.50
Reporter and Compendium, - - - - 6.00
Physician's Daily Pocket Record, - - 1.00
Reporter and Pocket Record, - - - - 6.00
Reporter, Compendium, and Pocket Record, 7.00

All checks and postal orders should be drawn to order of

CHARLES W. DULLES,
N. E. Cor. 13th and Walnut Streets,
P. O. Box 843. Philadelphia, Pa.

☞SUGGESTIONS TO SUBSCRIBERS:
See that your address-label gives the date to which your subscription is paid.
In requesting a change of address, give the old address as well as the new one.
If your REPORTER does not reach you promptly and regularly, notify the publisher *at once*, so that the cause may be discovered and corrected.

☞SUGGESTIONS TO CONTRIBUTORS AND CORRESPONDENTS:
Write in ink.
Write on one side of paper only.
Write on paper of the size usually used for letters.
Make as few paragraphs as possible. Punctuate carefully. Do not abbreviate, or omit words like "the," and "a," or "an."
Make communications as short as possible.
NEVER ROLL A MANUSCRIPT! Try to get an envelope or wrapper which will fit it.
When it is desired to call our attention to something in a newspaper, mark the passage boldly with a colored pencil, and write on the wrapper "Marked copy." Unless this is done, newspapers are not looked at.
The Editor will be glad to get medical news, but it is important that brevity and actual interest shall characterize communications intended for publication.

PALPATION OF THE KIDNEYS.

It is a curious fact that, within the last few weeks and almost simultaneously, two distinguished clinicians of Europe have published important communications in regard to palpation of the kidneys for diagnostic purposes. Both Guyon, in Paris, and Israel, in Berlin have recently cited their observations and experiences to show that the kidneys are not so inaccessible to touch as is commonly supposed. The former has described his methods of investigation in a lecture at the Hôpital Necker, reported in the *Gazette Hebdomadaire*, Feb. 8, 1889,

with great clearness and instructiveness, while Israel has published a very valuable article on the subject, in the *Berliner klinische Wochenschrift*, February 18, 1889.

Progress in treating diseased kidneys is now needed, as Israel states, more in the direction of finer methods of diagnosis than in that of the technique of surgical operations. The kidneys are situated upon the posterior wall of the abdominal cavity, upon the lowest dorsal and the three upper lumbar vertebræ. Their upper half is covered by the wall of the thorax, their lower half only by soft parts. Their diameter from hilus to convexity is directed obliquely, with the hilus presenting in front and toward the middle line. Their long axis is also obliquely placed, being nearer the spinal column above than it is below. The right kidney is placed at a slightly higher level than the left. If a line be drawn from the middle of Poupart's ligament, parallel to the linea alba, and a perpendicular be let fall from it two fingers' breadth below the point where it meets the lower border of the ribs, the perpendicular will meet the normal kidney. As Israel says, a correct understanding of these simple anatomical facts is of the greatest moment in examining the kidneys.

To utilize them certain favoring conditions are essential. The abdominal fat must not be too extensive, and the tension of the parietes must not be too great. To facilitate an examination, the bowels must always be emptied, and chloroform may be administered to relax the muscles of the abdomen, although anæsthesia interferes with voluntary deep inspiration, which is often of great assistance. Emptying the bowels not only diminishes their tension, but also removes the risk of mistaking fecal accumulations for the kidneys.

The best methods of examining the kidneys are these. First, by deep pressure with the fingers, gently and yet steadily following up the slight gain which can be made with each profound inspiration and expiration, taking care not to mistake any part of the liver or the spleen for the kidney. Second, by what Guyon calls *ballotement rénal,* which is effected by combining the first method with short taps or thrusts made with the fingers pressed firmly against the back, over the region of the kidney, by means of which it is propelled against the fingers pressing down in front. The third method is recommended by Israel, and consists in placing the patient on the side, with the knees and thighs slightly flexed, and making bimanual pressure very similar to that described by Guyon for *ballotement.*

A fourth method has been proposed by Glénard, of Lyons, which consists simply in palpating the region of the kidney between the thumb in front and the fingers of the same hand pressed up in the costo-vertebral angle.

In conducting these examinations all investigators agree that the rhythmic motion of the kidney with each inspiration can be detected, and alteration of its position, size, shape, consistency and sensibility. The detection of rhythmical motion in the kidney is a point in these examinations which it is important not to overlook, especially as the general supposition has been that the kidneys are immovable, and that motion in rhythm with the respiratory act serves to differentiate tumors connected with the intra-abdominal organs from those connected with or in the kidneys.

We cannot spare space at this time to point out all the valuable information in regard to the kidneys which may be gained by a successful palpation, as described above. But one extremely important point deserves mention. This is that, in any contemplated operation on the kidney, it must always be of great value to ascertain if the other kidney is present, and of probably normal size. Another point, which Israel has found extremely useful in practice, is that an erroneous diagnosis of floating kidney may

sometimes be corrected, and a useless operation avoided by finding the kidneys where they ought to be.

In conclusion, it may be noted that this valuable method of diagnosis is not practicable in every case, and that it should always be associated with every other known method of ascertaining the physical and functional condition of the kidneys. But, with this well understood, the methods we have described constitute a very valuable addition to our means of examining the kidneys, and one which deserves the widest dissemination among medical men.

FUNCTION OF THE COCCYX IN LABOR.

It is quite impossible to over-estimate the importance of thoroughly understanding the mechanism of the passage of the fœtus through the pelvis. This dominates the whole scientific practice of midwifery, and the practitioner cannot acquire more than a merely empirical knowledge, such as may be possessed by an uneducated midwife, or conduct the more difficult cases requiring operative interference, with safety to the patient or satisfaction to himself, unless he thoroughly masters the subject.

Thus appreciating a knowledge of the mechanism of labor, we have read with much pleasure a contribution to the study of the subject by Dr. Henry D. Fry, of Washington, entitled "The Function of the Coccyx in the Mechanism of Labor" (*Amer. Journal of Obstetrics,* Dec., 1888). Dr. Fry states that obstetricians in general attribute no function whatever to this little bone, except to get out of the way of the advancing head, and thereby to increase the antero-posterior diameter of the inferior strait. It is not even supposed to possess any obstetrical importance unless it rudely refuses to be pushed aside. He believes, however, that the coccyx has a distinct function to perform and that only after it has performed it does the bone recede before the advancing head. According to Dr. Fry, the function of the coccyx in labor is to cause extreme flexion of the head—in anterior positions of the vertex—at the inferior strait, whereby the escape of the occiput from beneath the pubic arch is facilitated, and the sub-occipito - bregmatic diameter of the head is brought in relation with the antero-posterior diameter of the pelvis, instead of the longer occipito-frontal, or occipito-bregmatic diameter. When the head reaches the inferior strait in normal labor it is not in extreme flexion. But as the head advances the brow meets with the resistance of the coccyx, its advance is arrested and the occiput descends. The resistance of the coccyx keeps up flexion until the occiput escapes from beneath the pubic arch and the nape of the neck becomes fixed against the symphysis pubis, when, since the occiput can advance no further, the force of the expulsive efforts is transmitted to the brow, overcoming the resistance of the coccyx and causing extension of the head with delivery of the brow and face.

While these views of Dr. Fry seem to be but a slight modification of the view that this last exaggerated flexion of the head is brought about by the resistance of the pelvic floor against the advance of the frontal region of the head—because the resistance of the normal coccyx must be equal to the resistance of its muscles—yet it is well to have the fact insisted upon that exaggerated flexion of the head does occur during the escape of the occiput, and prior to extension of the head. Because, while usually admitted, its bearing upon the proper management of the close of the second stage of labor is not generally appreciated. Having in mind the mechanism of passage of the head through the inferior strait and soft parts, the practitioner is enabled intelligently to manage this stage of labor, favoring flexion or extension of the head, and retarding or accelerating its advance by his manipulations as the circumstances indicate, all being done in accordance with, instead of in opposition to, the natural mechanism of labor.

HYSTERIA IN CHILDREN.

Typical examples of common diseases are easily and quickly recognized by general practitioners. It is in the diagnosis of rare diseases and of unusual manifestations of common diseases that mistakes are frequent. Thus a pneumonia of the apex has been mistaken for meningitis, and alcoholic delirium has been taken for acute mania. Such errors are often the result of carelessness rather than of ignorance; but it is at all times difficult, even for a well-read man, to keep such a comprehensive picture of a disease before his mind that he can at once recognize it, no matter how it may be obscured by unusual phenomena. This difficulty is increased when the disease in question is hysteria, in which the possible manifestations are limited only by the range of intelligence and degree of moral depravity of the patient.

Some of our readers may recollect a lecture by Charcot on Hysteria and Spiritism, which was published in the REPORTER, July 21 and August 25, 1888, and in which Charcot related in detail the histories of three children living in a penitentiary and developing hysteria under the influence of certain spiritistic exhibitions indulged in by their parents and others. There were three children, two boys and a girl. Hysteria developed in the latter in August, 1884, following a *séance* of spiritualism, in which the girl played the part of medium. At the end of the *séance* she was taken with convulsions, which were repeated from fifteen to twenty times a day, until both brothers followed the deplorable example set by their sister and developed fits of delirium associated with hallucinations.

Instances of hysteria in children, more or less similar to the one just quoted from Charcot, are not unknown in this country; but unfortunately they frequently fall under the notice of those who are unable to recognize the disease and who, perhaps, are ignorant of the fact that it may occur among children. What is perhaps a curious illustration of the statement just made may be found in the report, which comes from one of the Western States, that three children in one family, ranging from six to twelve years of age, were suddenly seized with "violent paroxysms," in which "they raved like maniacs and frothed at the mouth as if afflicted with hydrophobia." It is further stated that the children had to be locked in separate rooms and that at regular intervals they went into violent convulsions, which were so severe that two or three persons were required to restrain the patients.

These symptoms may or may not have been due to hysteria, but the fact that they developed suddenly and without apparent cause in three members of one family, and that the paroxysms were alike in each and occurred at the same hour each day, is strongly suggestive of hysteria. At least hysteria is the disease first to be thought of when the symptoms mentioned as occurring in these children appear, and the diagnosis of a more serious affection should not be made until the milder one has been excluded by careful examination. The important point, after all, is—not to know whether this or that instance of sudden explosion of nervous energy is due to hysteria or not, but rather to bear in mind the possibility that it may be, and to be able to recognize it when it is.

BOOK REVIEWS.

[Any book reviewed in these columns may be obtained upon receipt of price, from the office of the REPORTER.]

THE PATHOLOGY, CLINICAL HISTORY AND DIAGNOSIS OF AFFECTIONS OF THE MEDIASTINUM OTHER THAN THOSE OF THE HEART AND AORTA. By HOBART AMORY HARE, B.Sc., M.D., Demonstrator of Therapeutics, etc., in the University of Pennsylvania, etc. Large 8vo, pp. 150, with 6 photolithographs. Philadelphia: P. Blakiston, Son & Co., 1889. Price $2 00.

This book contains the essay to which the Fothergill medal of the Medical Society of London was awarded March, 1888. Dr. Hare, with great industry, has collated the statistics of five hundred and twenty cases of disease affecting the mediastinum, tabulating them carefully, and analyzing them so as to make them show just what diseases occur most frequently here, what are their symptoms, and how they should be treated. He concludes that cancer is more frequently found in the mediastinal space;

that abscess comes next in frequency; that sarcoma occupies the third place; and that lymphomata and lymphadenomata occur next, though they are much more rare than the other forms of disease named.

His work is one of great value, as it is the most important systematic study of mediastinal disease which has ever appeared. It is written in a clear and interesting style, and is beautifully printed.

COMPENDIUM OF THE LAWS RELATING TO PUBLIC HEALTH AND SAFETY OF THE STATE OF PENNSYLVANIA, TOGETHER WITH THE DECISIONS OF THE SUPREME COURT AND COUNTY COURTS RELATING THERETO. Compiled for the State Board of Health. Large 8vo, pp. 175. Harrisburg: Edwin K. Meyers, State Printer, 1888.

The title of this paper-covered book indicates its contents. It has been published by the State of Pennsylvania for the benefit of its own citizens, and it is a work of great value for all who wish to know the present state of the laws relating to public health and the practice of medicine. Five thousand copies have been printed, and any of our readers desiring a copy should apply to the Senator or Representative of his district, or to the Secretary of the Board of Health, Dr. Benjamin Lee, Philadelphia.

PAMPHLET NOTICES.

[Any reader of the REPORTER who desires a copy of a pamphlet noticed in these columns will doubtless secure it by addressing the author with a request stating where the notice was seen and *enclosing a postage-stamp.*]

238. THE PHILOSOPHY OF MEMORY. By D. T. SMITH, M.D., Louisville, Ky. From the *Practitioner and News.* 39 pages.

239. ZUR HEILUNG DER BACILLÄREN PHTHISE. (THE CURE OF BACILLARY PHTHISIS.) BY DR. LOUIS WEIGERT, Berlin. From the *Internationale klinische Rundschau*, No. 51, 1888. 4 pages.

238. As might be expected from the title of Dr. Smith's pamphlet, it contains a study of the nature and operations of the faculty called memory. These are matters hard to understand, and hard to explain. Dr. Smith regards memory as the persistence of vibrations of the part of the brain which is the seat of consciousness—a formula which will mean more to some people and less to others. He develops his argument in an interesting manner; but it would be too much to say that he succeeds in making his obscure and difficult subject very clear or comprehensible.

239. Dr. Weigert has made experiments (referred to in the REPORTER, November 3, 1888) which confirm the belief that the activity of certain microorganisms is diminished by the action of heat, and that human beings can inhale dry air, heated to 150° –180° Centigrade, or 292°–356° Fahrenheit, for hours at a time, without injury. Applying this to the treatment of phthisis he has found, in an experience of fifty cases, a marked improvement in the condition of his patients, and he recommends the inhalation of highly heated dry air as a formal method in this disease. His paper contains a description of the apparatus he uses, illustrated with engravings, which make its mechanism easy to understand.

The plan proposed is sufficiently striking to attract attention; and, if such results as he claims can be obtained by other medical men, his method will prove a valuable addition to the means of combating pulmonary consumption.

CORRESPONDENCE.

Treatment of Medical Witnesses.

To THE EDITOR.

Sir: The editorial in the REPORTER February 15, entitled: "Deception of a Medical witness," is exceedingly good and timely, and the infamous deception which was played on Dr. Kiernan should be a warning for medical experts in the future. While an honorable and upright lawyer would never descend to so base a trick, yet men who will are likely always to be found in the profession of law.

For many years I have, at times, been in the courts as an expert, yet there never was such an infamous thing attempted while I was in the witness-box. I am reminded, however, of a little episode which occurred some years ago in the trial of a case for malpractice. The late Prof. Hamilton's work on "Fractures and Dislocations" had been introduced, and admitted in evidence as a standard work previous to my entering the "box." A question was put to me, the answer to which I desired to explain, but the explanation was denied me. My opinion also was asked as to Prof. Hamilton's work being good authority, and I replied that it was. At this time the lawyer stood up and read a sentence which *appeared* to vitiate materially my testimony. He then said, "Dr., what do you say to that?" I replied: "that is not Dr. Hamilton's opinion on the point at issue." At once he stepped forward *and placed the book in my hands,* saying "read for yourself, and to the jury if you desire." Then, as the saying is, "I knew I had him." I began reading to the jury what the counsel had already read, and I continued to read. Soon he saw that the props were falling from under him, and he approached me and asked for the work. I declined, saying, that I had not yet quite fully corroborated my testimony. He then appealed to the judge (whom I knew to be very friendly with doctors generally), for an order requiring me to surrender the book. His honor declined, saying, "the counsel placed the book in the witness' possession, and asked him to read to the jury, and so long as his reading is confined to the treatment of this case, it shall remain in his possession, or until he voluntarily surrenders it." I did retain it until I was satisfied that, so far as the surgical testimony was concerned, the doctor was safe.

The expert must ever be on the alert.

He must not assume to possess more knowledge than he really does. Above all things he must be *cool, self possessed, and thoroughly posted.* I will relate an instance which occurred some years ago, and where eminent counsel were engaged upon both sides, and where damages to a large amount were claimed.

Without mentioning the particulars I will simply state that the question was whether or not pus could exist in the spinal canal, previous to death, without paralysis of any kind? I stated in my testimony, that "it had been found at an autopsy, and where there had been no paralytic symptoms previous to death." On the part of the defence was an expert, very distinguished in the profession, and one who occupied the highest position possible in one of the largest institutions of this State, who had fully endorsed a certain work which had previously been introduced, and admitted as authority, and who said he was familiar with it, yet swore positively that "no authority admitted the above facts." When the case was read to him, he could only say, "it don't seem possible." This was one of those cases where too much knowledge was assumed, and where very great humiliation was manifest to all in the court room.

Yours truly,
D. COLVIN, M.D.

Clyde, N. Y.,
March 4, 1889.

Retained Placenta; Removal.

To THE EDITOR.

Sir: About midnight of January 13, 1889, I was called to see Mrs. P., who, the messenger said, was bleeding to death. I found the patient nearly "bled out." She had been taken with flooding while in the parlor of a family that she was visiting. She had had one child, which is now six years old. On November 10, 1888, she aborted, at two and one-half months' utero-gestation, and since that event she had not had any bleeding except what she supposed was her regular monthly sickness, which occurred in December. I compressed the uterus through the abdomen, and the bleeding stopped. An examination with the finger revealed a slightly enlarged womb, a marked cicatricial line running from the anterior lip of the os uteri up the cervix, and a slightly patulous os. My diagnosis was retained placenta, although there was no dilatation of the cervix. The patient stated emphatically that such a thing was impossible, as the physician who had attended her in the miscarriage had seen and examined the fœtus and afterbirth and assured her that everything had come away, and that she might go about as she pleased, after the ninth day.

I packed the vagina with carbolized absorbent cotton, and gave, every three hours, suppositories containing ten grains of ergotin and a quarter of a grain of extract of opium. This treatment I continued for five days, being careful to remove the tampon and give a vaginal injection of a solution of corrosive sublimate—one to two thousand—every twenty-four hours. On the sixth day I dilated the cervix with dilators and removed the entire placenta—curetting the uterine cavity and washing it with a solution of bichloride of mercury. There was at no time any offensive discharge, and the patient had no pain and no fever. In two weeks after the operation she returned to her home in Atlantic City in good health.

Yours truly,
C. H. SHIVERS, M.D.
Haddonfield, N. J.,
March 5, 1889.

NOTES AND COMMENTS.

A Native Indian Doctor.

One of the recent graduates of the Woman's Medical College of Pennsylvania is a native Indian, Dr. Susan La Flesche, of whom Dr. Walker, in his address to the graduates, gave some interesting information. It seems that she commenced her studies of English at the school on the Indian reservation. Coming East, she continued them for a while at a boarding-school, and later at the Indian school at Hampton, Va., where she graduated in 1886, and then came at once to Philadelphia to study medicine. The impulse to a professional career was the result of a desire to see her people independent of the unskilled, and oftener indifferent, attention of the reservation doctor.

Anatomy of the Contortionist.

Dr. Thomas Dwight, in an article in *Scribner's Magazine*, April, 1889, says: What, then, is a contortionist? In the first place, it appears that a contortionist is a person who has preserved in his spine, and in some cases in his joints, the infantile condition which in most persons is merely transient. This implies a great flexibility of the spine in all directions, great powers of twisting it. It is also very likely that there are many small individual peculiarities all favoring uncommon freedom of motion. If a young boy without any of this special fitness should be trained for contortion, I think he probably would meet with some success, but never achieve distinction. So far as I am aware, children are not educated for this profession from their tenderest years, as they are for several kinds of acrobatic performances. Their capacity makes itself known by accident, from which it is fair to infer that it rests on an anatomical basis.

A Fight at the New York Maternity Hospital.

The Faculty of the College of Physicians and Surgeons of New York is investigating an exchange of blows which took place March 22, between the house physician of the Sloane Maternity Hospital and a student at the College of Physicians and Surgeons.

According to the statement of the latter and his friends, one day last week a patient was being attended by the house physician, when she clutched his arm. For this she was dealt a blow on the face. The student in question, who was standing by at the time, indignantly resented this treatment. A few days subsequently the house physician and the student met at the Maternity, and it is alleged that the former began the attack, which resulted in his getting a severe thrashing. The committee which has charge of the investigation will conclude its labors soon.

Convention for the Revision and Publication of the Pharmacopœia of the United States.

A call for a General Convention for the revision and publication of the United States Pharmacopœia, to assemble in Washington, D. C., at noon of May 7, 1890, has been issued by Robert Amory, President of the Convention of 1880. It is requested that every incorporated medical or pharmacal College, Association or Society desiring to be represented in the Convention send to Mr. Amory its corporate title and a list of its officers, addressed to the care of Dr. Edwin H. Brigham, Assistant Librarian of the Boston Medical Library, 19 Boylston Place, Boston, Mass , in order that Mr. Amory may prepare for publication, as directed by the Convention of 1880, a list of the bodies to be represented.

The Governor of Illinois on the Medical Practice Act.

In his message of January 9 to the General Assembly of Illinois, Governor Oglesby discussed the Medical Practice Act as follows:

During less than twelve years of its existence, this act has done much to protect the sick and the afflicted from charlatans and quacks; it has driven out of the State most of the ignorant, unqualified and unprincipled men who were preying upon the miseries of their fellows; and it is not too much to say that it has elevated and ennobled the practice of medicine, both in the State and throughout the country. The methods of medical education have been improved as a consequence, and the standard of attainments required of the physician who is to deal with the weighty questions of health and disease, and of life and death, is being steadily raised. The Illinois State Board of Health is now regarded as the pioneer in this work, and it is quoted as authority both in this country and abroad. Since the passage of the amended act—in force July 1, 1887—the Board has refused licenses to itinerant vendors of nostrums, with show accompaniments. The amount of these licenses would aggregate over $20,000, but the sum which the itinerants would fleece from the credulous would figure up hundreds of thousands a year.—*Indiana Medical Journal*, March, 1889.

Army Medical Board.

An Army Medical Board will be in session in New York City, N. Y., from May 1 to 31, 1889, for the examination of candidates for appointment in the Medical Corps of the United States Army, to fill existing vacancies, of which there are now seven, and an additional one will occur in July. Persons desiring to present themselves for examination by the Board will make application for the necessary invitation to the Secretary of War, before May 1, 1889, stating the place of birth, place and State of permanent residence, and enclosing certificates based on personal knowledge from at least two persons of repute, as to American citizenship, character and moral habits. Testimonials as to professional standing, from Professors of the Medical College from which the applicant graduated, and of service in hospital from the authorities thereof, are also desirable. The candidate must be between 21 and 28 years of age, and a graduate from a *Regular Medical College*, evidence of which, his Diploma, must be submitted to the Board.

Further information regarding the examinations and their nature may be obtained by addressing John Moore, the Surgeon General, U. S. Army, Washington, D. C.

The Medical Examiners' Bill.

The Philadelphia *Ledger*, April 1, 1889, refers to the remarkably fair and liberal bill providing for State examination of practising physicians, which was introduced into the Pennsylvania House of Representatives at the instance of the Medical Society of Pennsylvania, and quotes as follows from its issue of March 20 : "A claim is put forward by the doctors of several of the 'new schools' for minority representation in Examining and Licensing Board. That is a proper claim; it should be conceded and is conceded in the bill as it stands. But the trouble seems to be that, while the 'old school' doctors are willing to concede 'minority *representation*,' they are not ready to agree to minority *control*. They are right about this, for the amendment proposed by the 'new schools' of medicine might be easily made to give such a preponderance to less than *one-fourth* of the total number of medical practitioners in the State as would enable them or their representatives in the State Board to overrule the representatives of the other three-fourths." With reference to the amendments made to the Bill, which give an equal representation to all the schools, it says : "It will be observed that since the above article was published the Legislature has so amended the bill that the representatives of three-fourths of the doctors of the State cannot by any possibility be a majority of the Board, and that the representatives of one-fourth may, if united, control the Board. This is all wrong; yet so anxious are the leading physicians of the city to have State examinations that they have agreed to accept the amended bill, though it is unfair to them; but they ask in return that graduates of medical schools be required to attend a four years' term. This would force the higher education of physicians, and is a course which the better colleges would be glad to have made compulsory. But the Legislature, without regard to 'old school' or 'new school,' ought to make the bill a fair one by reconsidering the amendments made, and should certainly join heartily with the best physicians to raise the standard of doctors admitted to practice in the State so as to get rid of quacks and pretenders in all 'schools,' old and new."

NEWS.

—Scarlet fever is prevalent at Marlborough, a hamlet near Newburgh, New York.

—The Texas State Medical Association will meet in San Antonio, Texas, April 23–26, 1889.

—The Hospital Collection Fund of New York City amounted to $52,033.40 during the year 1888.

—Dr. H. C. Wood will deliver the annual address at the coming commencement of the Yale Medical School.

—Dr. R. P. Howard, Dean of the Medical Faculty of McGill University, Montreal, died in Montreal, March 28.

—The Alabama State Medical Association will meet in Mobile, Tuesday, April 9, 1889, and continue in session four days.

—The Nineteenth Annual Meeting of the California State Medical Society will be held at San Francisco, April 17, 18 and 19, 1889.

—The Thirty-ninth Annual Meeting of the Illinois State Medical Society will be held in Jacksonville, Tuesday, May 21, 1889.

—The Eleventh Annual Meeting of the Louisiana State Medical Society will be held in New Orleans, Tuesday, April 9, 1889.

—The Twenty-seventh Annual Meeting of the Mississippi State Medical Association will be held in Jackson, Wednesday, April 17, 1889.

—The Thirty-ninth Annual Meeting of the South Carolina Medical Association will be held in Charleston, beginning Wednesday, April 10, 1889.

—The Western Pennsylvania Medical College held its commencement March 28, and conferred the degree of Doctor of Medicine upon thirty-six graduates.

—Dr. Thomas J. Mays will deliver his third lecture on Pulmonary Consumption a Neurosis, Friday evening, April 12, 1889, at 8 o'clock, in the Philadelphia Polyclinic, Broad and Lombard Streets. Physicians are invited.

—The following numbers of infectious diseases and deaths were reported in New York City for the two weeks ending March 19 (*New York Med. Journal*, March 23, 1889): Typhoid fever, 18 cases and 5 deaths; scarlet fever, 728 cases and 95 deaths; cerebro-spinal meningitis, 4 cases and 1 death; measles, 425 cases and 40 deaths; diphtheria, 403 cases and 91 deaths.

OBITUARY.

EDWARD T. BRUEN, M.D.

Dr. Edward T. Bruen, of Philadelphia, Assistant Professor of Physical Diagnosis at the University of Pennsylvania, died March 31, of pneumonia, after an illness of less than a week.

Dr. Bruen was born in Philadelphia in 1851. In early life he attended private schools under the direction of his father, and later entered the University of Pennsylvania, from which he was graduated in medicine in 1873. In 1874 he was elected one of the visiting physicians to the Philadelphia Hospital, and has been a lecturer in the Spring courses at the University of Pennsylvania for a number of years. In 1880 he was elected Demonstrator of Clinical Medicine, and in 1884 was appointed Assistant Professor of Physical Diagnosis in the same institution. He was also a visiting physician to the German Hospital. His contributions to medical literature were numerous; his "Handbook of Physical Diagnosis of the Heart and Lungs," has passed through two editions. He was a member of the Association of American Physicians, of the American Climatological Society, and of the Philadelphia County Medical Society, and of other medical societies. He leaves a wife and two children.

Dr. Bruen's illness was sudden in its onset and proved fatal rapidly. Not long before he was taken sick he delivered the lecture on Nervous Dyspepsia, which appears in this number of the REPORTER, and it has a melancholy interest from the fact that it is probably the last manuscript that he revised before his death.

JOHN SWINBURNE, M.D.

Dr. John Swinburne, formerly Health Officer of New York City, died in Albany March 29, 1889. Dr. Swinburne was born in Denmark, Lewis county, in 1821, and was graduated from the Albany Medical College in 1846. He was soon made Demonstrator of Anatomy in the College, holding that position four years. In 1861 he volunteered, without pay, as an army surgeon, and served with distinction. In 1864 he became Health Officer of the Port of New York, and during his term he established the quarantine service which now exists there. While abroad with his family in 1870, he took charge of the American ambulance service in Paris during the Franco-Prussian war.

MEDICAL AND SURGICAL REPORTER

No. 1676.   PHILADELPHIA, APRIL 13, 1889.   VOL. LX.—No. 15.

CONTENTS:

CLINICAL LECTURE.

DIGITAL DILATATION OF THE PYLORUS.[1]

BY J. M. BARTON, M D.,

PHILADELPHIA.

SURGEON TO THE JEFFERSON COLLEGE HOSPITAL.

(Reported for the MEDICAL AND SURGICAL REPORTER.)

Gentlemen : The patient I bring before you is one who is slowly starving to death from obstruction to the pyloric orifice of her stomach. She now vomits nine-tenths of all the food she takes, and has lost more than one-third of her weight during the last year. She is 48 years of age, is a patient of Dr. Adams, of Vineland, New Jersey, and was in perfect health until five years ago.

During 1884, 1885 and 1886, she suffered with the symptoms of gastric ulcer—pain

[1] Delivered before the class of the Jefferson Medical College, February 16, 1889.

and vomiting immediately after eating, the vomiting occurring as often as six times in the twenty-four hours. She lost greatly in flesh and had two severe hemorrhages, vomiting at one time, she states, nearly a gallon of dark-colored blood ; this amount is probably greatly over-estimated. In 1887, all the symptoms of the disease left her, and for the greater part of the year she enjoyed excellent health, weighing, in January, 1888, one hundred and forty-three pounds, which was more than she had ever weighed in all her life.

During the last year, however, she has been very ill, with symptoms of pyloric obstruction, and she has lost flesh rapidly, weighing a few days ago only ninety-three and one-half pounds. She now vomits but once in twenty-four or forty-eight hours. This occurs when she lies down at night, and it is not accompanied by nausea. It is usually from one and a half to two quarts in quantity, and measures nearly as much and sometimes quite as much as all the nourishment taken since the preceding act of vomiting, twenty-four hours before. Many articles

443

taken during the day can be recognized when vomited at night; indeed, she states that she has occasionally been able to recognize articles eaten as long as two weeks before. As she takes her meals she feels that her stomach is becoming more and more distended, and when she lies down at night, gravity brings the contents of her stomach into her throat, and they are then vomited. Her bowels are obstinately constipated, acting only once in twelve or fourteen days, and then only after frequently repeated large injections; purgatives administered by the mouth produce no effect. She has lately been able occasionally to feel a small tumor about the size of a hazel nut, two inches to the right of the umbilicus.

Her stomach is greatly enlarged; we have determined its size by distending it with carbonic acid gas developed from half of a Seidlitz powder, giving the soda and the acid separately. Her stomach reaches as low as the umbilicus and as far as the small tumor, though we cannot say that the tumor is connected with the stomach. If the vomiting depended upon inflammation of the stomach or upon an ulcer, it would probably occur immediately after eating. If it depended upon indigestion, it would occur from half an hour to an hour after taking food; but when it occurs, as here, only when the stomach is fully distended, is influenced by gravity, is not accompanied by nausea, and when, moreover, the matters vomited consist of several preceding meals, and there is a desire for food immediately after vomiting—we may be sure that it is due to some mechanical obstruction situated at or near the pylorus.

Now this mechanical obstruction may be due to a new growth, as some form of cancer, or it may be due to stenosis of the pylorus from contraction following the healing of an ulcer, and the history points distinctly to this latter condition. For, during 1885 and 1886, her symptoms were markedly those of gastric ulcer; under proper treatment the patient not only recovered but increased in weight until she was heavier than ever before. After a year of perfect health, vomiting, of a totally different character, occurred, being now distinctly obstructive. The history is too long for the trouble to be cancer; the average duration of life in gastric cancer, according to Brinton, is one year; the maximum duration, according to Bartholow, is three years; in the present case it is now five years since the first hemorrhage. The complete recovery two years

ago and the subsequent return of symptoms is not the history of cancer. The size and mobility of the tumor, if the tumor has anything whatever to do with the stomach · and its symptoms, do not indicate cancer of five years' duration.

The character of the hemorrhage is also against the diagnosis of cancer. In cancer small amounts of blood are lost quite· frequently, whereas in ulcer the hemorrhages are large and occur at long intervals. The absence of diarrhœa caused by an ulcerating cancer, and her freedom from any hectic or cachectic appearance, are also points against the probability that the disease is cancer. ··

The diagnosis is, therefore, non-malignant stricture of the pylorus, due to cicatricial contraction after the healing of an ulcer. We must be prepared to treat the obstruction even if it should not be of the character. that the weight of evidence is in favor of. It might be a malignant tumor of the small bowel; if it should be so, and if it be far down, I shall excise that portion of the bowel as I did in a case I brought before you some time ago. After excising the bowel I shall make a temporary artificial anus and place Dupuytren's enterotome at once in position for its cure. If it be a tumor of the bowel high up, an artificial anus can not be made, as the patient would perish of inanition. I should then excise the bowel and growth and bring the divided ends of the bowel together, performing what is called a circular enterorrhaphy. If it should prove to be an extensive but non-adherent cancer of the pylorus, I might do a pylorectomy, excising the pylorus and growth and bringing the stomach and duodenum together. If it should be malignant and extensively adherent, I shall do a gastroenterostomy, making an opening in the stomach and in a contiguous layer of jejunum, bringing the two in apposition with the aid of these two decalcified bone plates, which I have here. If it be malignant, but of recent origin and still limited to the mucous membrane, I shall open the stomach and with the curette scrape away the mass after the method of Bernay's, of St. Louis.

But if it prove to be a simple stricture, as I hope and think it will, I will open the stomach and will then stretch the pylorus with these uterine dilators, these œsophageal forceps, and with my fingers. Will the pylorus stay dilated? Prof. Loreta, of Bologna, who first performed this operation, in 1882, has had a number of permanent successes; Mr. Hagyard, of England, reports upon a case fifteen months after operation, and states that the patient is still in admirable condition and there is no symptom of return. If it were not for these statements I should fear from analogy that it would re-contract, and I should then prefer the operation of Heineke, which consists in making a longitudinal incision, two inches long, through the pylorus, and in sewing it up transversely.

I shall slightly modify in two particulars the operation as performed by Loreta. He makes an incision five inches long on the right side of the middle line, from a point one inch below the xiphoid cartilage to one just below the cartilage of the ninth rib, and he makes the opening in the stomach close to the pylorus. In a case upon which I operated in this hospital about eighteen months ago I found a small median incision through the abdomen answer every purpose and possess many advantages. As the tissues close to the pylorus are apt to be, and were in my previous case, thickened and infiltrated with inflammatory deposits, I shall make the incision in the stomach several inches distant from the pylorus.

The abdomen of the patient was prepared yesterday by washing it with turpentine, soap and water, and corrosive sublimate solution; cheese-cloth wet in the latter solution was then bound over the field of operation, and it is still on. The patient's stomach was washed out this morning with a solution of biborate of soda; the fluid was pumped in and out a number of times until it came away quite clear. She is now under chloroform, which I prefer to ether, as there is much less danger of its causing vomiting, which would endanger the result of the operation.

The hands and instruments being prepared antiseptically, and the field of operation surrounded by towels wrung out of carbolized water, I make a small median incision about three inches in length terminating just above the umbilicus; the cavity of the peritoneum is soon reached, clamp forceps having been placed upon all vessels as they spurted. The stomach is directly beneath the incision; it is readily distinguished from the transverse colon by the thickness of its walls and by the fact that the omentum hangs from its lower edge. The pylorus even from the outside is markedly contracted and irregular on its surface; there is no tumor here. Passing my finger to the region occupied by the tumor that we felt from the outside, I readily find it and bring it to the wound; it is evidently a scybalous mass—indeed, the entire

colon is full of smaller ones; they need no attention.

Three inches from the pylorus the wall of the stomach feels quite healthy. I now fold the anterior wall of the stomach transversely, midway between the greater and lesser curvatures, and with a pair of sharp scissors make an incision about one and a half inches in length. I now introduce my index finger and feel for the pylorus; this movement produces some retching, which forces most of the stomach out of the wound. I will keep it here as it will be more convenient and there will be less danger of contaminating the abdominal cavity. With my finger in the stomach the pyloric opening is readily felt; it is about one-fourth of an inch in diameter, though its margins are quite hard. As I am unable to push my finger through it I introduce this small pair of uterine dilators beside my finger, and pass the blades through the small pyloric opening. By using considerable force I dilate the orifice until one finger enters, but the second will not until I again introduce the dilators and this long pair of œsophageal forceps, when I am able to introduce two fingers and to separate them slightly. This I will be satisfied with, though Loreta says he separated his fingers three inches. Mr. Hagyard, who had the first successful case in England, did not dilate the opening nearly so much, and McBurney lost one of his cases from hemorrhage following a rupture of the mucous membrane produced while stretching the pylorus.

There has been no bleeding from the wound in the stomach, though in several of the reported cases there was very free bleeding when the stomach was incised. The wound here being much further from the seat of the disease than it is usually made may account for the small amount of blood lost. I will now close it by first bringing the edges of the mucous membrane together by a continuous suture of fine silk, and then bring the peritoneal surfaces in contact by the continuous Lembert suture.

As there is no blood in the abdominal cavity neither irrigation nor drainage will be necessary. The stomach is now washed, the wound in it again examined, and it is returned to the abdominal cavity. The abdominal wound is now closed and dressed in the usual manner.

The operation of digital dilatation of the pylorus was first performed by Loreta, of Bologna, on September 14, 1882. Up to 1884 he had reported four cases with two recoveries and two deaths. Since then he and other Italian surgeons have performed a number of operations with varying success. It has been rarely performed in Germany, England or America. The first successful case in England was published in 1887. I have as yet found only four cases reported in America, including a previous one of my own; they all ended in death.

Note by Reporter.—The patient vomited about four ounces of blood, half an hour after the operation; but there has been no vomiting and no nausea since. She was nourished by the rectum until the fourth day; from then until the fourteenth day she was fed upon peptonized milk and broths; after the seventh day she took from forty-eight to sixty ounces of liquid nourishment in the twenty-four hours. Since the fourteenth day she has been fed upon a carefully selected solid diet. On the fortieth day after the operation she was able to eat eggs, mutton-chops, oysters (raw and stewed), beef, chicken, lamb, potatoes, cream toast, bread and butter, milk and coffee. Her temperature has never been over 99° nor under 98° Fahr., since the operation. The abdominal stitches were removed on the ninth day. The patient is now able to walk about, is much stronger, and weighs one hundred and sixteen pounds. For the first two weeks after the operation her bowels were moved every other day by the injection of one drachm of glycerine. They now move naturally every day.

SCURVY.[1]

BY FREDERICK P. HENRY, M.D.,
PHILADELPHIA.

PHYSICIAN TO THE PHILADELPHIA AND JEFFERSON COLLEGE HOSPITALS.

At the present day examples of this disease are rarely seen, and there can be no doubt that its frequency even in former times was much overrated. In the older medical works, the term "scorbutic" was very loosely employed, and the same criticism applies to popular works of fiction of the early part of this century. The writers of these books doubtless obtained their notions concerning this subject from the current medical literature. Readers of Dickens will surely recall the "scorbutic youth" who made himself so conspicuously disagreeable at Bob Sawyer's celebrated supper, and whose countenance was probably the seat of an eruption of acne. This and other skin eruptions were at that time supposed to be of a scorbutic nature; an opinion which is without scientific foundation.

I believe that I am acquainted with the entire literature of this subject for 1888, and it is exceedingly scanty. Besides three cases which I made the subject of a clinical lecture, published in the MEDICAL AND SURGICAL REPORTER, June 16, 1888, two have been reported by Variot[1] and one by Barkas.[2] An elaborate article on the "Occurrence of Scurvy among Troops and its Prevention," appeared in the *Practitioner* for May of the same year. In the course of it, its author, J. Hickman, remarks that the occurrence of a single case among troops "shows negligence, and is a reproach to the authorities." I cannot accept this statement without a word of explanation. A soldier, a prisoner, an inmate of an almshouse, or a hospital patient may be supplied with anti-scorbutic articles of food, and yet develop scurvy, because he does not eat them. Quite recently I was called to attend a rapidly growing boy, sixteen years old, who had gradually become weak and anæmic, and whose gums, on examination, I found to be decidedly tender and spongy. He had a comfortable home and was supplied with an abundance of nutritious food, but, as his mother told me in reply to my questions, he lived almost solely upon bread and meat.

The two patients I bring before you this morning owe their disease to the fact that they have steadily refused to eat potatoes, although abundantly supplied with them. The potato is one of the best of anti-scorbutics, and is believed to derive this property from the potassium which it contains in large amount. The opinion that potassium is a highly anti-scorbutic substance, and that its absence from the food is one of the causes of scurvy, was first announced about forty years ago, by Garrod, and was adopted by Liebig.

The diagnosis of a case of primary scurvy presents no difficulty to one who has closely observed a single well-marked case of the disease; but secondary cases, *i.e.*, cases occurring in the course of another disease, are very apt to be overlooked. The patient being already confined to bed, the pains on walking, so great in the primary forms, are unperceived, while the increasing feebleness is attributed to the primary affection. Lasègue and Legroux, who studied nearly one hundred cases of scurvy in the central infirmary of the prisons of Paris, during the

---

[1] Delivered at the Philadelphia Hospital, March 16, 1889.

[1] *Le Bulletin Méd.*, September 19, 1888.
[2] *Australian Med. Gaz.*, January 15, 1888.

siege of that city by the Germans in 1870, state with reference to their cases of secondary scurvy, that many of them would have been overlooked but for their daily careful search for its manifestations in *all the patients* under their care. The patients before you did not present themselves for treatment, but were recognized as cases of scurvy by one of the resident physicians, who systematically went through the "out wards" looking for signs of scurvy. The symptoms are well marked in both cases. In one, the gums at the time of admission were swollen to such an extent as almost to conceal the incisor teeth. In the other, the affection of the gums, though well marked, is not so extreme as in the first case. In both, as you observe, there are large subcutaneous extravasations of blood on the anterior surfaces of both tibiæ.

The influence of the mind over the body is often referred to in general terms, but seldom with special reference to the nutritive functions. Depressing emotions, whether by direct nervous action upon those functions, or indirectly by impairing the appetite, certainly predispose to scurvy. It is even believed by Barkas that the prevalence of scurvy among the Australian shepherds is in part due to their monotonous solitary lives. In their case, however, the diet, in my opinion, is all sufficient to account for it, for it is composed "solely of tea, salt beef, and 'damper.'" It is scarcely necessary to say that the emotions of an "out-warder" are depressing, for the very fact of his entrance here announces that he has abandoned hope.

The treatment of these cases will be almost exclusively dietetic. They will be supplied with onions, potatoes, and lemon juice—the best of anti-scorbutics. I can say this much with reference to their treatment, but no more, since neither of them is under my care. I am indebted to Drs. Tyson and Walker, in whose wards they belong, for the opportunity of showing them to you this morning.

They are both anæmic, and in one the precise degree of the anæmia has been ascertained by Dr. Hamill, who examined the blood with Gower's instruments. The corpuscles numbered about 4,000,000 per cubic millimeter (80 per cent. of the normal), and the coloring matter was reduced to 60 per cent. of the normal. Chalybeates are therefore indicated, and an excellent mixture in such cases is one containing the tincture of the chloride of iron and the fluid extract of ergot.

COMMUNICATIONS.

LAPAROTOMY FOR ·TUBERCULAR PERITONITIS, WITH REPORT OF ONE CASE.[1]

BY GEORGE ERETY SHOEMAKER, M.D.,
PHILADELPHIA.

The treatment of tubercular peritonitis by laparotomy has been attempted by many operators, but the cases are not yet sufficiently numerous, nor their after-histories sufficiently well recorded to make the chapter a closed one; and every case, if reported with its peculiarities, may help to clear up some obscure points. As will presently be pointed out, the results are probably not as absolutely certain as some writers apparently imagine, though they are remarkable.

The following case is reported at too early a date (five months) after operation to be called successful, except in one sense. To be sure, the patient was rapidly sinking; she made a prompt recovery from the operation, she considers herself well, and is working as a laboring woman; but there has been some return of fluid. This, however, is now apparently diminishing, and may disappear. It is tempting to put down operations as "recoveries" and "successes," but it is the after-histories which are important to the patients; while it is certainly exasperating to one who would study the truth of statistics, to find in so many reports the latest information dating from one or two weeks after the knife is used, with the indefinite word "recovery" following.

The case is as follows: Mrs. G., 23 years old; no tubercular family history; the patient has two healthy children, and another, of low vitality, still at the breast. She considered herself healthy until five or six weeks before coming under observation, the first irregularity noticed having been an enlargement of the right iliac region, which soon became bilateral. She never had noticed any hard tumor. When first seen she complained chiefly of abdominal distention. There was slight dry cough, and some pain in the back and in the right ovarian region, with a feeling of bearing down. She moved about freely and seemed fairly well, except for pressure symptoms; the temperature was 100.4° in the evening; there was slight loss of weight; no tenderness; bowels acted normally; menses had been normal, but

[1] Read before the Obstetrical Society of Philadelphia, March 7, 1889.

for two or three months they had appeared every two weeks, but were painless, increased in amount, with occasional appearance of blood in the intervals.

The examination showed the abdomen to be of the size of the belly in pregnancy at term; the walls were extremely tense, owing to the rapidity of the distention. No tumor was found; no coronal resonance; fluctuation was very distinct; dulness irregular in outline; there was a large external rectocele; the uterus was small, forward, fairly movable, independent as far as could be made out; nodules of the size of mustard seed were distinctly felt through the rectum in the peritoneum of the recto-uterine pouch. The urine was normal.

The probable diagnosis of ascites from tubercular peritonitis was made in the absence of heart and kidney lesion; pregnancy with hydramnios being excluded by the condition of the uterus; and there being no sign of liver disease. There was sufficient floating of the intestines, taken with other signs, probably to exclude the presence of a large ovarian cyst; though in some cases of extensive adhesion of the bowel and encysting of fluid, this differential diagnosis cannot be made. The short duration, about six weeks, did not favor, though it did not by any means exclude, a tubercular origin.

The history of an early unilateral swelling made it impossible to exclude absolutely a small malignant growth in the right side, but the absence of any sign of hardening accessible by vaginal touch made this unlikely. The presence of nodules in the peritoneum behind the uterus, first pointed out to me in consultation by Dr. H. A. Slocum, suggested three things: papilloma, tuberculosis, and malignant disease of the peritoneum. The presence of fever with loss of flesh was against the former; while the temperature, the slight, dry cough, the small, regular peritoneal nodules, pointed strongly to tuberculosis, especially in the absence of decided pain. As orthopnœa and insomnia from embarrassment of respiration rapidly developed, abdominal section was performed, although the patient was menstruating. The operation was performed for the relief or cure of tubercular peritonitis. A two-inch incision was made; the peritoneum where cut was one-quarter of an inch thick, and grayish-red; the fluid clear, highly albuminous, abundant. Everything in the abdomen felt as though plastered together with curdy exudate, while an enormous number of mustard-seed-like nodules studded the parietal and visceral peritoneum alike. Web-like adhesions were general but easily broken down, except in the right iliac region where denser adhesions and matting of the bowels had doubtless given rise to the patient's idea of early unilateral swelling. The Fallopian tubes were convoluted and slightly enlarged, but did not require removal; the ovaries and uterus were studded with tubercles, but not much altered in size. Nodules could, of course, plainly be felt behind the uterus, where they had been found before the operation. The visceral peritoneum was thickened, grayish-red, rough, injected. The point of the finger applied at any point would cover several nodules. Boiled-water irrigation was employed. No medicated application was made to the peritoneum; a glass drainage tube was used, and a plain absorbent-cotton dressing. Perfect cleanliness was maintained throughout by ordinary aseptic methods. Several pints of serum escaped from the tube during the first twelve hours; an annoying cough ejecting it so as to soil the dressing in spite of the nurse's care. The flow ceased and the tube was removed in forty-eight hours. Prompt recovery followed. The cough had disappeared by the thirteenth day, and the temperature, slightly elevated before the operation, remained normal after the fourth day.

Dr. J. P. C. Griffith kindly examined the lungs and confirmed the opinion that there was no definite sign of tubercular change there. About two months after the operation, there was some distention of the abdomen, probably from encysted fluid, though fluctuation could not be made out. This has since decidedly lessened in amount, and the patient has never been aware of its presence. Now, five months after the operation, she considers herself absolutely well. There is no hernia. It is the history of some cases that there is a temporary moderate reaccumulation of fluid, which is afterward absorbed. In other cases the belly refills rapidly and the case becomes as bad as before. At least one patient has been opened a second time for the ascites, without, however, effecting a cure.

The diagnosis of tubercular peritonitis is often very difficult, and in many cases it can not be made, especially in the absence of signs of tubercular trouble elsewhere.

Greig Smith,[1] referring to encysted effusions, says that it is "impossible to diagnose them with certainty." Again he says: "In

[1] Abdominal Surgery, p. 107.

many cases encysted dropsy of the perito-neum can not be diagnosed from ovarian cyst." The age of the patient is not significant, as it occurs from infancy to old age. Mr. Frederic Treves[1] operated on a child fourteen months old, death following in a few weeks.

The method of exclusion which must be adopted will not serve to eliminate some forms of pressure on the portal vein ; nor, as has been said, will it separate papilloma or malignant disease of the peritoneum with certainty.

As an aid to the diagnosis the examination of the peritoneum in Douglas's *cul-de-sac* should always be made. This is the only point in the body, in such cases (bimanual examination being impossible from distention), at which two peritoneal surfaces can be rubbed one upon the other by the finger. The cases must be very rare where a delicate examination, or indeed any, can be made by picking up the abdominal wall. Whether or not tubercles are always to be found, if anywhere, in the recto-uterine *cul-de-sac* is not known, for no records of examination of this locality have been observed. In one other case the writer has found them. It is suggested as a point worth noting in the future. Certainly if distinct nodules can be felt here the case is not one of ascites solely from mechanical causes, and exploratory laparotomy would be more than justifiable.

The statement sometimes made that exploratory incision is almost devoid of danger is not as true in tubercular peritonitis as in the cases in which the peritoneum is healthy; especially as these cases are too widely scattered to reach the few most skillful men. As far as the writer is able to learn eight patients have been operated upon in this city, and two have not recovered from the operation. Taking the whole of the United States together, 35 genuine cases with 6 deaths are known to the writer ; a mortality immediately following operation of 17.1 per cent. Excluding deaths in cases in which peritonitis was present before operation, the immediate mortality in exploratory operations (non-malignant) collected by Dr. J. M. Baldy,[2] is not quite 7 per cent.

The operations collected in Europe by Kümmell,[3] who has presented the most recent article on the subject, are 39.[4] He states distinctly that only two of these died as the result of the operation, though he is quoted by more than one American writer as reporting 6 deaths from operation on a previous occasion.

Fehling, of Basel, reports[1] 6 deaths among 29 cases operated upon. Another report[2] gives 28 cases, of which only 24 were operative successes. As the cases, though not all published in detail, are probably the same, the discrepancy in death percentage may perhaps be accounted for by a difference of opinion as to what constitutes a recovery from the operation.

In regard to the effect of operation on the condition of the patient, it may be said that there are a large number of carefully observed, *bonâ fide* cures reported ; while marked temporary improvement almost invariably occurs in cases which do not succumb to the operation. Improvement would naturally follow from evacuation of the fluid, with relief to the heart and kidneys. But it must also be said that too many cases are reported as "cured" at a very early period after operation. It is unfair to take only a portion of the world's cases for analysis, and the writer is fully aware of the unreliability of statistics ; but the following short analysis of American cases is offered as giving a fair general idea of the question of results : Of the 35 cases collected (reported and unreported) 6, or 17.1 per cent., did not survive the operation ; 4 died with recurrence within six months ; 14, or 40 per cent., are reported "cured" after periods ranging from *one month* to two and a half years. In other words, the "cures" known to exceed six months in duration are 11, rather less than one-third of the cases. Eight out of 29 cases studied by Fehling[3] lived one year.

The writer wishes to be understood as maintaining no argument against laparotomy in such cases ; he is a warm advocate of it ; the desire is to come nearer to the truth in probable prognosis, and to emphasize the fact that there are some cases in which no practical benefit can be looked for. Even if there were no hope of cure, other advantages justify operation. One writer on this subject has aptly said :[4] "The establishment of the diagnosis beyond question and intelligent treatment based thereon, together with relief of pain and freedom from opium,

[1] *Lancet*, November, 1887, p. 918.
[2] *Medical News*, April, 1888.
[3] *Arch. f. klin. Chir.*, Berlin, 1888, I, p. 39.
[4] Of his 40 cases one is American.

[1] Zur Laparot. bei perit. Tuberkulose. Vide *Centralblatt f. Gyn.*, No. 45, 715.
[2] *Nouvelle Arch. d' Obst. et Gyn.*, 1887, p. 519.
[3] *Centralblatt für Gyn.*, No. 45, 1887.
[4] McMurtry. *Annals of Gynæcology*, Sept., 1888.

are advantages of incalculable value; and give hope and comfort in a desperate, painful, and hopeless disease.''

Kaulich[1] has pointed out that cure is most likely to result in cases in which the onset is insidious, the progress slow, without much rise in temperature; and where ascites is abundant from an early period.

There are other cases of tubercular peritonitis, perhaps more correctly styled abdominal tuberculosis, in which there is no ascites, the belly is scaphoid, and intestines and organs are matted in one inextricable mass; where mesenteric glands have become large tubercular masses, and where every abdominal structure is studded with cheesy nodules from the size of a pea to that of an egg. Such a case, occurring in the male, died about six years ago under the observation of the writer. Laparotomy was not attempted, nor would it probably have been of the slightest service. At the autopsy the belly seemed almost absolutely dry, and there were no surfaces in contact which were not tightly adherent. Such patients if operated upon usually die soon afterward, but there are a few cases reported in which temporary comfort was derived in this way. Cases occurring in males are rare. Fehling (*loc. cit.*) speaks of two.

Cure may be anticipated where effusion is abundant and where there are no deposits outside the peritoneum. That the tubercles are real has been proved conclusively in a number of cases by microscopical demonstration and the cultivation of bacilli (Hartwig, Marcy). That they disappear absolutely from localities where they existed at the operation has been proven by autopsy in several cases (Hirshfield).

The reason for their disappearance is not known, and will not be until we know more of the life-history of tubercle. Some of the theories are: (*a*) That they become encysted or encapsulated and are absorbed; (*b*) that the hyperæmia of the peritoneum from withdrawal of ascites leads to their "strangulation"; (*c*) that the fluid is a source of irritation in itself [but aspiration is not as effective as laparotomy]; (*d*) that the majority of bacilli are drained off with the fluid and the remainder are overwhelmed by the vitality of the peritoneum.

This subject was discussed by Dr. Ely Van de Warker[2] before the American Medical Association in 1887. Hegar also has thoroughly considered the whole subject of

genital tuberculosis in women,[1] and has collected much material.

The following conclusions seem reasonable to the writer from data at present available.

1. The diagnosis is usually difficult and frequently impossible. Fortunately it is not always necessary.

2. The best known treatment is laparotomy, with simple water irrigation and drainage. The local use of iodoform, iodine, carbolic acid, etc., gives no better results.

3. The operation mortality is considerably higher than that of exploratory incision when the peritoneum is not diseased.

4. A considerable number of complete and permanent cures, anatomical and symptomatic, of genuine tuberculosis of the peritoneum, are on record. The reason for this cure is not known.

5. The most that can be looked for in more than one-half of the cases is temporary relief; but this is usually decided and far outweighs the risk of incision.[2]

3727 Chestnut Street.

CASE OF LARGE CEREBELLAR, AND SEVERAL SMALLER CEREBRAL HEMORRHAGES.

BY THEODORE DILLER, M.D.,

ASSISTANT PHYSICIAN IN THE STATE HOSPITAL FOR THE INSANE, AT DANVILLE, PA.

The following case is interesting viewed from several standpoints, and I think it is quite worthy of being noted. The history which accompanied the patient, though meagre and unsatisfactory, is still of value in the study of the case.

Mrs. D——, widow, admitted into the Danville Hospital, June 4, 1887; married 22 years ago; had one still-born child seventeen years ago; supposed cause of insanity, domestic troubles and money matters; prominent symptoms consist of incessant talk of a rambling sort. She is said to have had attacks of epilepsy or apoplexy several years ago. When irritated she has· threatened to jump out of the window. For more than a year there has been alternate mental depression and excitement. Various physicians have been employed and different remedies have been

---

[1] *Prager Vierteljahresschrift.*

[2] *Amer. Journal Obstetrics*, 1887, p. 935.

[1] Die Entstehung, Diagnose u. chir. Behandlung d. Genitaltuberculose des Weibes. Stuttgart, 1886.

[2] NOTE. The thanks of the writer are due to many gentlemen for late reports of operation cases, and also for several unpublished cases.

tried, but with no good result. When admitted her general health was impaired, for which a tonic was ordered. She had various erratic ideas concerning brain clots, her ideas being often disjointed and mixed.

On June 15, 1888—about a year after her admission to the hospital—her powers of locomotion were slowly becoming impaired. On her arrival here she was able to play some old familiar airs on the piano, but now she was unable to strike simple chords. Her language and power of expression had altered quite materially. She was very fond of creature comforts.

By Nov. 1, 1888, the patient had a peculiar gait, taking short steps, with her feet dragging on the floor. She had many symptoms which appeared to be of an hysterical character; for example, she asked if she were not fatally ill, and whether she would live until morning. She asked for a piece of brown bread, or a soft-boiled egg, with as much earnestness as though it were a matter of momentous importance. She spoke quickly, and in a jerky manner. She often stopped abruptly in the midst of a sentence and with a look of earnest appeal on her face would say: "What is it? What is it?" If the word was supplied, her face would at once light up, and she would be profuse in her thanks. She referred all her trouble to her brain, often saying: "There is a weakness" (indicating her head). Since June, 1887, nineteen convulsive seizures had been noted as follows: In 1887, June, one; July, none; August, two; September, none; November, none; December, two. In 1888, January, none; February, none; March, three; April, none; May, two; June, five; July, none; August, two; September, two.

Immediately after the occurrence of some, if not all, of the seizures, there was greater or less mental lethargy or confusion. The aphonia on one or two occasions, was complete. The ataxia usually increased while the general motor power decreased. The symptoms gradually lessened in intensity up to the date of the next attack; so that the patient had periods of great physical and nervous disturbance, alternating with periods in which the symptoms were much less pronounced. Her convulsions were not minutely noted, but they coincided with the description of none which follow a well-defined course. In one which I had a chance to observe she called out that she was dying, then, with her eyes rolled toward the ceiling, she was seized with a violent general convulsion.

It was the opinion of the writer at this time that she had many symptoms of hysteria—superadded to those resulting from some obscure, ill-defined organic trouble, probably a gross brain lesion.

On November 18, 1888, at five o'clock in the morning, the night nurse discovered that the patient was breathing very heavily and was unconscious, and at once notified me. The pulse was slow, full and strong (about 65); breathing stertorous; cheeks puffing out with each expiration, but regular in rhythm. The head and mouth were slightly drawn to the left side; pupils small, equal, and both responsive to stimulus of light. Tickling the soles of the feet and palms of the hands failed to produce any reflex action. Four drops of croton oil, with a little whiskey, were placed upon the tongue. An ice-cap was applied to the head, which was elevated. The oil failed to operate. The patient died at 8.50 A.M., the same day.

Autopsy.—26 hours after death. Rigor mortis well marked.

Brain-Envelopes.—On removing the calvarium, the dura mater which was presented to view was of a dark blue tinge in the lower or posterior half, the color being most marked along the longitudinal sinus. Upon cutting through the dura, this coloration was found to be due to a large amount of extravasated blood, partly clotted, between the brain proper and the membranes; but the pia mater and arachnoid were perforated at one point, so that the blood was directly beneath the dura. The convolutions of the brain were well marked, the sulci unusually deep, but the layer of gray matter rather thin. The vessels of the pia mater were somewhat engorged.

Cerebellum, left side.—Upon section, a cavity somewhat larger than a walnut was discovered, occupying the centre of the lobe. The walls of the cavity were quite ragged and at many points there were adherent to them small clots. These were mostly grayish or yellowish-white in color, and seemed to be well organized. At three or four points small fibrous bands (old blood-vessels) were joined to the clots from the cavity wall. The principal portion of the cavity, however, was occupied by a single, large, dark-red clot, apparently of recent origin. There was direct communication between the blood in this cavity and that upon the outside, already referred to, by means of a small ragged laceration in the gray matter of the cerebellum, which formed the posterior wall of the cavity.

Cerebrum, right side.—In the bottom of the sulcus between the first and second convolution, and midway between the anterior and posterior extremities of the frontal lobe, was a well organized, reddish-brown clot, of the size of a pea. It principally occupied the gray matter. In the centre of the Island of Reil, just beneath the gray matter, and occupying the greater portion of the island, was a large reddish-brown, or rusty colored, clot. Midway between the anterior and posterior boundaries of the parietal lobe, near the great longitudinal fissure, was a clot the size of a pea. It was situated partly in the gray and partly in the white matter, and was grayish-white in color.

Cerebrum, left side.—In the lower extremity of the ascending frontal convolution, a small reddish brown clot was found of the size of a pea. In the ascending frontal convolution, near the longitudinal fissure, was another small clot, well organized. In the occipital lobe, near the junction of the parieto-occipital and longitudinal fissures, on the outer aspect of the brain, a rusty-brown, moderately firm clot about size of a shellbark was found.

Base of brain.—The vessels were atheromatous in numerous places, this condition being especially marked in the middle cerebrals. It was thought that some of the immense cerebellar hemorrhage found its way into the fourth ventricle, although no means of communication between the two cavities could be demonstrated.

The principal points of interest in this case are as follows:

1. The immense cavity in the cerebellum, with the contained clot.

2. The large number of old clots on the cerebrum.

3. The obscurity and complexity of the symptoms which the case presented.

4. The fact that such extensive destruction of brain matter was compatible with life.

5. The possible confirmation of a theory, to be mentioned hereafter.

Almost all the white matter and the included *"arbor vitæ"* of the left cerebellum was disintegrated. Evidently some morbid process had been active here for a long time prior to the death of the patient. Most likely hemorrhages had occurred here from time to time. These. Clots were formed. These broke down into pus and were re-absorbed; but the process of disintegration had also involved brain substance. Hence the large extent of the cavity. This process of retrograde metamorphosis also involved the blood-vessels in this region. The large clot which was found in the cavity was evidently of recent origin and due to the rupture of a vessel of considerable size. This hemorrhage, with the pressure which it caused in this region—and most likely too in the floor of the fourth ventricle—was doubtless the immediate cause of death.

Some of the "attacks" which occurred at irregular intervals since 1886, were doubtless symptoms resulting from cerebral hemorrhage, while others were "motor explosions" or "pressure symptoms." It is not unlikely that several of them were principally or wholly of an hysterical character. It is interesting to note that the almost entire destruction of the function of one side of the cerebellum produced no train of characteristic symptoms, or symptoms by means of which the condition could have been diagnosticated.

That such extensive destruction of white and gray matter should produce as few disturbances as it did seems to me to be an argument in favor of the theory which Brown-Séquard recently advanced, that there are, for many, and perhaps all brain centres, supplemental centres. If the main or primary centre be destroyed the secondary or auxiliary centre is capable of taking upon itself a good portion of the work of the primary centre, and the extra work thrown upon the secondary centre tends to develop its capacity and power: just as we see unusual or compensatory development of a leg or arm when its fellow has been removed. At least this seems to me a very plausible theory by which to account for the gradual disappearing and recurrence of the aphasia from time to time in the case just described, when at the autopsy an almost entire destruction of the speech centre (lower part of left ascending frontal convolution) was noted.

The gradual lessening of the ataxia, the temporary increase in the muscular power, and the decrease and subsequent increase of the power of volition, would all seem to point to a confirmation of the theory.

—The *Lancet*, Feb. 16, says that the Queen of England has granted permission to those ladies in whose case illness, infirmity, or advancing years have rendered the usual costume unadvisable, to appear at the Queen's Winter Drawing-room in a high court dress. The term "high," unfortunately, is only a relative one, as the dress still leaves the front of the chest partly exposed.

THE TREATMENT OF SPINAL CARIES.

BY JAMES K. YOUNG, M.D.,

PHILADELPHIA.

INSTRUCTOR IN ORTHOPÆDIC SURGERY, UNIVERSITY
OF PENNSYLVANIA; ATTENDING ORTHOPÆDIC
SURGEON, OUT-PATIENT DEPARTMENT,
UNIVERSITY HOSPITAL.

The treatment of spinal caries may be divided into constitutional and local. The former includes the improvement of the general health and hygienic surroundings, a generous diet, with the exhibition of tonics and alteratives, such as syrupus ferri iodidi, lactophosphate of lime, cod liver oil, hypophosphites of lime and soda, with strychnia, etc. Recumbency is to be enjoined during the acute stage, with or without extension. In very young children the "*stehbett*," of Phelps,[1] or an ordinary fracture-box containing a pillow, will fulfil all the indications. If these become intolerable, after the accurate application of a spine-brace, the child if old enough should be encouraged to walk with assistance or be allowed to go about on all-fours after the plan of the Alaska Indians, who doubtless have copied it from the lower animals, in whom we are told vertebral caries does not occur. Davy[2] suggests that caries "is possibly one of the penalties we pay for walking in the upright position," while Albrecht[3] assumes that the upright position is the chief cause.

The local treatment is divided into mechanical and surgical. Local applications—such as counter irritation, heat, cold, etc.—are of greatest service where secondary lesions of the nervous system exist.

If the cases are diagnosticated early, their cure can be effected without deformity and with perfect flexibility, but as deformity has, in the majority of cases, occurred before the surgeon is consulted, all that can be accomplished by mechanical treatment is the fulfilment of the three indications:

1. To support the diseased spine.
2. To remove superincumbent weight.
3. To prevent increase of deformity.

The machines and appliances for the treatment of caries of the spine are innumerable, but they can all be classed in two groups: (a) the fixed jacket, of plaster of Paris and its modifications in silicate of soda,[1] poro-plastic felt,[2] leather,[3] woven-wire,[4] paper,[5] bamboo,[6] etc.; and (b) the spine-brace. The plaster-of-Paris jacket filled a long-felt want, and too much cannot be said in praise of the illustrious surgeon who popularized this useful appliance. The spine-brace of Dr. Taylor—the antero-posterior leverage spinal apparatus—has in my hands proved more satisfactory to the patient, has certain advantages which the other does not possess, and admits of frequent readjustment. For all cases of disease above the mid-dorsal region (6th dorsal vertebra) a chin-rest should be used to remove the weight of the head and neck.

The brace should always be applied with the patient lying prone on his face, in which position the spine is straightened out as much above and below the seat of deformity as if the patient were suspended. It is now recognized that the deformity itself cannot be straightened. In fact, attempts to accomplish this have been followed by immediate paraplegia and even death.[7]

The surgical treatment of spinal caries is yet in its infancy. It has been the habit of surgeons to treat the abscesses expectantly, to allow them to open spontaneously, to aspirate, or incise, and then allow them to close. These methods in many cases did well, but of late there is a growing tendency to do something in an operative way. Evacuation and hyperdistention of the cavity[8] with various antiseptic fluids has been much practised (Wood, Israel, Agnew, Treves, Dollinger and others) but the operation has not fulfilled what was anticipated from it, and Demours and Demoulin[9] have recorded a death from it.

Under strict antiseptic precautions openings and counter openings with insertion of drainage tubes have been tried, and some surgeons have freely laid the abscess cavities open, and thoroughly curetted the walls.

Dr. Rupprecht, of Dresden, who four years ago was an ardent advocate of this

---

[1] Schreiber, *Allg. u. Spec. Orthopäd. Chirurgie,* 1888, p. 93.

[2] *British Med. Journal,* 1885, ii. 8–10.

[3] Ue er den anat. Grund. der Skoliose, Hamburg, 1887. b

[1] Coover, MED. AND SURG. REPORTER, April 13, 1878.

[2] Cocking, *Med. Press and Circular,* 1879, n. s. xxviii.; Walsham, *Lancet,* 1885, vol. i., p. 619.

[3] Agnew's Surgery, vol. ii., p. 880.

[4] Roberts, *Intern. Journal of Surgery,* vol. i., No. iv., p. 207.

[5] *Med. Record,* N. Y., 1887, xxxii, 647. *New York Med. Journ.,* 1886, xliv., 261.

[6] Iji Slimshi, Tokio, 1884, No. 305, Feb. 2.

[7] Mr. Willett, St. Bartholomew Hosp. Reports;. Thos. Buzzard.

[8] Mr. Collender.

[9] *Progrès Méd.,* 1886, 2 s., iv., pp. 1029–1031.

heroic plan of treatment, informed me last summer that about one-half of the patients subjected to the treatment died of tuberculosis, the other half recovered, and that he had abandoned it. This is not as favorable as the experience at Volkmann's klinik,[1] where 20 patients died of tuberculosis subsequently, and in 23 the abscesses healed.

At present there is a desire on the part of surgeons to treat abscesses and sequestra of spinal caries just as in other parts.[2] Dr. H. L. Taylor,[3] of Cincinnati, has shown anatomically that "the bodies of all the vertebræ are accessible to the surgeon," and "that there is little danger of opening the pleural cavity"; and Dr. Thomas Lafflin suggested about the same time before the Royal Academy of Medicine in Ireland that this operation (sequestrotomy) should be extended to all the dorsal vertebræ. Doubtless these advances are all in the right direction and promise much, but it has occurred to me that the rule should be observed to operate in hospital cases where the disease is progressing in spite of appropriate treatment, but to avoid operation as long as possible in private practice, because in the latter patients are more apt to recover without operation.

The most common complication (aside from abscess) is paraplegia, and it is encouraging to know that so many recover from this distressing symptom. Taylor and Lovett[4] report out of 19 cases that 17 patients recovered; 1 recovered partly, and 1 remained paralyzed. Of 38 cases reported by Sayre either partly or completely paralyzed, 34 patients have recovered and 4 remain under treatment. The treatment consists in the application of a spinal support and in placing the patient in a recumbent position, with in some cases the administration of large doses of iodide of potassium, as suggested by Gibney.[5] These are tolerated even by children to a remarkable degree, but Ridlon[6] declares that "he (had used iodide of potassium and) had been convinced that it produced no effect upon the paralyzed unless there be reason to believe that hereditary syphilis is present"; and this has been my experience also.

·[1] Schreiber, *loc. cit.* p. 112.

[2] Pradrez, *Russk. Med.*, St. Petersburg, 1886, iv., 333. Treves, *British Med. Journal*, 1884, i., p. 58.
[3] MEDICAL AND SURGICAL REPORTER, 1888, lix, 136.
[4] *Med. Record*, N. Y., 1886, xxix, 699–702.
[5] *Med. Record*, N. Y., 1885, xxviii, 452.
[6] *Medical Record*, N. Y., March 26, 1887.

SOCIETY REPORTS.

MEDICAL SOCIETY OF THE COUNTY OF NEW YORK.

Stated Meeting, March 25, 1889.

The president, ALEXANDER S. HUNTER, M.D., in the chair.

DR. AUGUST SEIBERT read a paper on

The Etiology of Fibrinous Pneumonia.

Formerly pneumonia was regarded as due directly to cold. Only within the last twenty years, after the attention of medical men had been drawn to repeated observations of endemics and epidemics of pneumonia, and since the pathological changes during other processes could be traced to the division and growth of infectious material brought into the human body, and since the old ideas on inflammation and the formation of pus were modified by antisepsis, have prominent observers come forth with the theory that fibrinous pneumonia is an infectious disease. It was found by Leube, in 1877, that all the symptoms except the elevation of temperature were present in some cases; this certainly did not coincide with the prevalent idea regarding active inflammation. Gradually statistical reports concerning soldiers in the field and in barracks, Arctic expeditions, convents, boarding-schools, etc., were prepared, which went to show that persons leading an out-of-door life, often exposed to bad weather, were in less danger of pneumonia than those who lived indoors. They also showed that the tendency to get pneumonia was in exact proportion to the time spent in closed rooms.

Dr. Seibert cited numerous statistics of epidemics or endemics of pneumonia among persons confined in rooms which were warm, moist, and filthy. It was only natural that these manifold reports, mostly dated within the last twenty years, should stimulate some to experiments, others to statistical comparisons. Haidenhain attempted to produce pneumonia by forcing cold air into the lungs of animals, and failed; and others failed after him. A number tried to find the peculiar weather influence present in determining the frequency of pneumonia, and failed; but Poet, Seitz, Baker, and Seibert were more successful, and their results coincided very much, though differing in explanation.

In his first report on an investigation regarding pneumonia and the weather, published in the *American Journal of Med. Sciences*, in 1882, Dr. Seibert was able to prove that catarrh of the air passages and pneumonia showed similar lines of frequency. This view has since come to be generally admitted. In a collective investigation regarding pneumonia and the weather carried on by the Committee on Hygiene of the New York County Medical Society, in 1884-5, 44 practitioners of New York and Brooklyn and four hospitals took part, and gave the following results: 1. The origination of fibrinous pneumonia is greatly favored by certain meteorological conditions, thus explaining the difference in its frequency during the twelve months of the year. 2. Low and falling temperature, high and rising humidity, and high winds are each capable alone of exercising this influence. 3. If two of these weather conditions are found together there are more cases of pneumonia than when one is found alone. 4. If the three (cold, moisture, and high winds) are present, the frequency of pneumonia is great. Existing catarrh predisposes to fibrinous pneumonia.

In all his cases of endocarditis complicating pneumonia, Weichselbaum was able to cultivate Friedländer's pneumococcus from the pathological deposits on the endocardium. Emil Senger also found this organism, in all fatal cases of pneumonia, in the lungs as well as in organs involved in the complications, in cases of meningitis, pleurisy, endocarditis, nephritis and pericarditis.

On reading the article of Dr. Sternberg, in the *Medical Record*, March 16 and 23, Dr. Seibert was satisfied that Fraenkel's coccus, described by Dr. Sternberg as "micrococcus Pasteuri," would probably cause the more frequent form of pneumonia, known as the sthenic variety, while the pneumococcus of Friedländer was the usual agent for producing the asthenic, bilious, or typhoid variety. But to his mind the most important investigations regarding the germ origin of pneumonia are those of Rudolph Emmerich. In the State prison at Amber, where an endemic of pneumonia had attacked 161 and killed 46 out of a total of 1150 prisoners, Emmerich found Friedländer's coccus between the ceilings and below the floors of the sleeping apartments in great quantities, imbedded in very moist *débris* which had been used to fill up the spaces. White mice infected by injections of the coccus into the lung-tissue all died, and artificial pneumonia also occurred in some when they inhaled the microbe.

Secondary infiltrations in wandering pneumonia are to be explained, not by inflammation passing by continuity of surface, but by the presence of an infectious material. Central pneumonia, and cases lasting but one or two days, also favor the infection theory. Endemics and epidemics prove not alone that pneumonia is caused by specific poisons, but also that the germs are apt to thrive and grow in certain localities at certain times and under certain conditions. Whether or not pneumonia is contagious, so that the germ of the disease may pass directly from the patient to the attendant, as in diphtheria and scarlatina, has not yet been settled. It certainly is, if at all, contagious only to a very mild degree. Friedländer's pneumococcus appears to thrive best in warm, moist, dirty rooms and houses. This statement accords with observed epidemics.

Pneumonia is found oftener in old and very young persons than in the middle aged. Children under two years of age are attacked oftener than older ones; the explanation being that old people and children spend more time indoors.

Pneumonia not only frequently attacks persons suffering from bronchial affections, but it is also found complicating those diseases in which the pulmonary mucous membrane is usually in a state of congestion and hyperæmia, as in typhoid fever, measles, and pertussis. On the other hand, it is not often seen complicating scarlatina, diphtheria and meningitis. We are forced to conclude that the catarrh of the bronchi being absent in the one class of diseases, the opening in the mucous membrane necessary for the admission of the pneumococcus poison is wanting.

In conclusion, he said: fibrinous pneumonia is an infectious local disease, showing more or less general symptoms, the origination of which is greatly favored by existing bronchial catarrh, poor ventilation of rooms, moist and filthy condition of houses, and cold, moist weather.

DR. FRANCIS DELAFIELD opened the discussion, and stated that there is no other department of medicine in which so little advance has been made as with regard to the causation of disease. What advance has been made, however, is due to physicians no longer accepting general statements as to causation, but requiring more and more exact data. There is much yet to be learned with regard to the etiology of

456 *Reports of Clinics.* Vol. lx

pneumonia. It is known only in a general
way that pneumonia seems to belong to
the class of infectious inflammations, that is,
inflammations in which the inflammatory
process is always accompanied with the production and growth of pathogenic bacteria.
Such inflammations require for their causation three factors, any one of which in different instances may take the prominent
part, namely: (1) a pathogenic bacterium;
(2) some other exciting cause of the inflammation; and (3) individual susceptibility.
With regard to the pathogenic bacteria, all
we knew is that it seems pretty evident more
than one form of bacteria is capable of causing the inflammation of the lung.

Dr. L. E. Holt has been impressed with
the varying degrees of · susceptibility of
different patients to fibrinous pneumonia.
He has found this form of pneumonia more
common during the third, fourth, and fifth
years, than before the second. As to its
presence in measles, he has never seen it at
a *post-mortem* on a patient dead of measles
complicated with pneumonia; the pneumonia has always been of another form.

The discussion was continued by Drs. A.
F. Currier, Messenger, and the author.

REPORTS OF CLINICS.

COLLEGE OF PHYSICIANS AND SUR-
GEONS—VANDERBILT CLINIC.

MEDICAL CLINIC—PROF. DELAFIELD.

Cardiac Hypertrophy, Dilatation, etc.

The first patient was a woman, 48 years
old, who gave following history: she had
"malaria" six years ago; fourteen months
ago she had pneumonia on the right side,
and was in bed for two months, and then
began to improve slowly, and was in fair
health during the succeeding summer. Last
fall, she suffered from cough, and once
expectorated a little blood; with this she
had anorexia and vomiting, and was
extremely prostrated. About this time, on
October 29, she was examined at the Clinic.
The urine was found to be normal. The
heart extended from the right edge of the
sternum to the anterior axillary line; the
apex was in the sixth inter-space; there was
a presystolic thrill; and presystolic and
systolic murmurs were heard at the apex.
The patient was given chloral hydrate and
nitroglycerin, and was put upon fluid diet.
She improved. On November 14, the treat-

ment was changed to iodide of potash and
strophanthus, after which improvement was
so marked that the patient has remained
away until now. She says that since one
week she has had a return of her cough
and dyspnœa. She is so feeble as to be
scarcely able to be about, vomits after eating, and is unable to retain anything on
her stomach, and is suffering from general
pains throughout the body.

On examination the urine is found to
have a sp. gr. of 1,013, and shows a trace
of albumin. The patient's temperature is
98.8°; the skin ·is moist, the pulse quick
and very feeble. The heart's area is as
before noted: there are both hypertrophy
and dilatation; its impulse is more forcible
than that of the pulse—it is a laboring
heart. No murmur can be detected now,
but since it was observed at a previous
examination, there exists probably mitral
stenosis. Such a murmur is often missing.
The case is, therefore, one of old mitral
stenosis, with secondary hypertrophy and
dilatation of both ventricles and a disposition of the heart to take on rapid and
irregular action. This is the second
occasion on which this has taken place.
The cardiac condition present in this case
may occur apart from mitral stenosis, and
mitral stenosis can exist and the heart act
perfectly well; or, again, they may occur
together, as in the present case. As a
matter of 'fact, in these cases, we often have
a laboring heart and a feeble pulse.

With regard to treatment, ordinary drugs
do not aid much. The arteries are already
dilated, so that decreasing the tension will
not strengthen the pulse. And the heart is
working harder than it should, and yet does
not fill the arteries, so that digitalis, convallaria, strophanthus, etc., are harmful, as a
rule, though we sometimes find that under
the influence of these cardiac stimulants
the heart will not labor so much. Yet it is
not safe to try them experimentally. They
are liable to make the patient worse if not
given at the proper time.

Dr. Delafield recommended, first, complete rest in bed, not allowing the patient
even to sit up. This alone, he said, does
wonders in some instances.

There is one drug which may be of benefit, but whose exact scope is not as yet fully
defined, viz., the chloride of barium, given
in teaspoonful doses of a one per cent.
solution three times daily.

Dr. Delafield had showed to the class a case
similar to this one, a short time ago, at the
Roosevelt Hospital, in which the heart's

action was even more marked. Here, rest alone gave no improvement. Then the chloride of barium was used, and in two days marked benefit in every respect resulted. In some cases, he said, barium chloride will do no good.

The most reliable treatment is by absolute rest. This patient might fall dead at any moment; she is not safe while walking about. Even under treatment she may not improve.

Chronic Alcoholism.

The second patient was a man, 45 years old, a hard drinker. Two years ago he had pains across the stomach and loins, and "lightness of the head," and says he had an attack of unconsciousness lasting two weeks. He has had since several similar attacks, but they have been less severe. Three months ago he began to complain of dyspnœa and palpitation, with some œdema of the ankles, and he suffered with morning vomiting and flatulence, and swelling of the abdomen. An examination now shows that at present the urine is of a sp. gr. of 1,013, and has a trace of albumin. The radial pulse is very small—is felt with difficulty; in the temporal artery it is very feeble and quick. The pulmonary resonance all over the chest is of short duration, high pitch, and altered quality; expiration is prolonged, especially on the right side (emphysema). The apex beat of the heart to the left of the nipple is increased in area. The apex can be felt, but the impulse is not forcible; it gives evidence of considerable dilatation. The heart's action is feeble and irregular; there is no murmur. The left and right sides of the heart are both enlarged.

The liver is somewhat diminished in size. The spleen is not enlarged.

The diagnosis is in the first place chronic alcoholism. This has developed several conditions, namely, chronic gastritis, cirrhosis of the liver (without jaundice), atrophied kidney, emphysema (without bronchitis) and dilatation of both ventricles of the heart (probably secondary to the emphysema). This dilatation is apt to occur with emphysema and intemperance, especially in beer drinkers.

This man is well nourished and in a tolerably fair condition. He would not be suspected of having valvular disease, whereas the previous patient would be. Why? Because,—leaving the duration of the disease out of the question—of the character of the heart sounds. In this case they are good and clear cut, though not so strong as

they are normally. In the other, the reverse is true. The treatment here will be unsatisfactory because the patient will continue to drink.

Dr. Delafield recommended digitalis in moderate doses, kept up for a considerable length of time.

Chronic Constipation.

The third patient was also a man, 35 years old, a tailor. He was shown to the class four weeks ago, when he was complaining of feebleness, loss of strength and flesh, pains in the abdomen, and long continued and persistent constipation. The patient was then unable to do his work. The diagnosis of constipation was made, and it was believed no organic disease was present. The patient was admitted to Roosevelt Hospital and placed upon as liberal a diet as the Hospital afforded. He was given the following pill:

R Strychniæ sulphatis . . . . gr. 1-40
   Pulv. ipecac.,
   Ext. belladonnæ,
   Ext. colocynthidis co. . . . aa gr. ¼
   M.

At first he took four daily, then three, and then two. At once his constipation was relieved.

He is about to leave the Hospital and resume his work. At present, his appetite is good, he has no pain, and has gained and is still gaining strength and flesh.

He should continue with his pills, taking now one a day, and after a while they may be stopped and diet made to supply their office.

Some cases of this kind, Dr. Delafield remarked, are easily managed; others are not.

Pleurisy with Effusion.

The next patient was a man, 40 years old, a laborer. Up to four days ago was able to work. Then pains in the stomach, diarrhœa and vomiting set in. He now complains of neither cough nor dyspnœa nor pain in the chest. To-day his temperature is found to be 103⅓°; his pulse 140. The urine has a sp. gr. of 1,022, and contains considerable albumin. An examination of the chest shows dulness over the lower lobe of the right lung, and an absence of breathing and voice sounds.

The diagnosis rests between acute lobar pneumonia and pleurisy with effusion, being in favor of the latter from the patient's general condition; and yet from the data so far obtained it is impossible to decide positively. To be certain of the diagnosis we may either wait a day or so, when the signs will further develop, or we may use a hypodermatic needle.

The patient is exhibited to illustrate two points: first, the vague subjective symptoms of the pulmonary trouble, and second, the impossibility of differentiating in every case between these two diseases at a certain stage, relying alone on the physical signs.

Subacute Diffuse Nephritis.

The last patient was a man, 35 years old. Two or three years ago he had an attack of sickness, confining him to bed. He suffered, at that time, from pains and swelling in the hands, feet, and less generally throughout the body. After a while the swelling subsided, the patient improved, and he was able to leave the house in two months. Since this time there has been occasionally some swelling of the ankles; he has complained of headache, insomnia, and constipation. His appetite is fair and there has been no vomiting, and he is able to work.

On examination the urine is found to have a sp. gr. of 1,016, and to contain a large quantity of albumin. The pulse is good. Arterial tension slightly increased. The heart is normal in size, with no adventitious sounds.

The history is a straight one of subacute diffuse nephritis, beginning about three years ago. There has been no sharp attack since the first one, though the amount of albumin in the urine has varied probably in different weeks and months. The changes at first produced in the kidneys have remained— and even increased. The inflammation is both exudative and productive, more and more connective tissue has been formed, and the glomeruli have also undergone change and are less able to do their work. Hence the low specific gravity of the urine. We would find also that the urea excreted is less in quantity than it should be. The exudative part of the inflammatory process will probably lessen little by little, and finally stop; but the productive part will go on increasing more and more, perhaps not advancing much for many years to come, but certain to advance sooner or later. Sometimes these cases remain stationary for many years.

———————

—The Hahnemann Medical College held its forty-first Annual Commencement April 4, and conferred the degree of Doctor of Medicine on 65 graduates.

PERISCOPE.
———

Nature and Prevention of Urethral Fever.

Dr. James Bell, Surgeon to the Montreal General Hospital, in a paper read before the Medico-Chirurgical Society of Montreal, says that all surgeons, and in fact most general practitioners, are familiar with certain forms of constitutional disturbance which follow instrumental or operative interference within the urethra. In a certain number of such cases pre-existing disease of the kidneys, ureters or bladder, or of all these organs combined, or the setting up of a true sepsis (pyæmia or septicæmia), or the production of the disease known as surgical kidney, may explain these symptoms. But there still remains a large class of cases occurring in male patients of all ages, and often where no lesion of any organ can be discovered, even by post-mortem examination, in which instrumental or operative interference within the urethra is followed by the train of symptoms to which has been given the names urethral fever, urine fever, catheter fever, etc. These symptoms, he says, occur in one of four different forms: 1. Shock, collapse and death within a few hours after operation (9 to 24), with or without chill or fever, and with partial or complete suppression of urine. 2. A severe chill with high fever occurring a few hours after operation, and usually following the first act of micturition. Profuse sweating and prostration follow, but the whole disturbance lasts only from a few hours to two or three days. 3. Recurrent chills and high fever coming on at irregular intervals and lasting perhaps for weeks or months. 4. A moderate fever with slight chills or chilly feelings accompanied with great depression, low muttering delirium or semi-coma, dry, cracked tongue and anorexia, and usually ending fatally. Such cases occur only in old men with enlarged prostates, and in whom, as a general rule, attempts at catheterization with solid instruments have resulted in the formation of false passages just in front of the prostate and on the floor of the urethra. This form differs materially from the preceding ones, but clinical experience points strongly to its being identical in its origin.

Patients belonging to the second and third classes, he says, generally recover completely and satisfactorily. He then refers to three distinct theories which have been advanced as to its origin: (1) That it is a septic process; (2) that it is due in some obscure way to reflex nervous phenomena; (3) that it is due to uræmia.

After declaring these theories inadequate to explain the affection, he states that the discovery of the animal alkaloids known as ptomaines and leucomaines, and the experiments of Dr. Bouchard of Paris from 1882 to 1886 upon the toxicity of the alkaloidal substances found in normal urine seem to have given the key to a rational explanation of the origin of urine fever. From the amount of evidence which we now possess Dr. Bell thinks there can hardly be any doubt that this disease is due to the absorption of the products of decomposed or decomposing urine from cut, lacerated or abraded portions of the urethra. It is not a septic process, but a form of poisoning closely allied to uræmia and due to the absorption of a toxic alkaloid produced by or during the decomposition of the urine. The clinical facts pointing to this conclusion, he says, amount almost to a demonstration. They are as follows: 1. Urine fever is unknown after perineal lithotomy, external urethrotomy and internal urethrotomy in the pendulous urethra, and is far less frequent when the urethra is wounded on its roof than when it is wounded on the floor. 2. When, after internal urethrotomy, the urethra and bladder have been carefully washed out with an antiseptic solution, urine fever does not occur until some time after urine has been passed over the wounded urethral surface, and is then of a mild type and generally free from danger. 3. Operations upon the female genitals which wound or injure the urethra are not followed by any similar condition. 4. Mr. Harrison of Liverpool has shown by a number of operations that when the bladder is drained by a perineal wound after internal urethrotomy that urine fever never occurs, and he attributes its origin to the absorption of the products of decomposing urine from wounds of the mucous membrane.

· Dr. Bell then contributes his experience in support of this important observation and adds his testimony. in favor of the combined operation. He has records of five cases in which he has performed, within the past twelve months, the combined operation, and also of six cases of simple internal urethrotomy for stricture of the deep urethra performed within the same period of time. The 'five cases in which he drained the bladder by a perineal cystotomy were selected for this operation, because of specially bad features in each case. The six cases in which he did a simple internal

urethrotomy were, with one exception, not drained, because they were more favorable cases for operation. In the first series, in which he drained through the perineum, there was not in any case a subsequent rigor or rise of temperature, while in the six cases of the second series urine fever in a mild form followed in four cases, but only after micturition. Only two cases escaped, and in these he believes the result was due in great part to greater intelligence on the part of the patient in carrying out instructions.

After giving brief account of each of the cases referred to, he submits the following conclusions:

1. That urine fever is a consequence of the lodgment and decomposition of urine in contact with wounded urethral surfaces, the inference being that the absorption of the product of decomposition which takes place from the wounded surfaces, and which could not occur through the normal urethral mucous membrane, is the direct cause of this condition. Mr. Harrison has also shown that patients whose urine contains a diminished quantity of urea are less liable to urine fever after operations upon the urethra.

2. Urine fever is *absolutely preventable*, either by preventing the decomposition of the urine in contact with urethral wounds, or by providing a dependent drain so that it cannot lie in contact with wounded urethral surfaces long enough to decompose.

3. That a perineal cystotomy is a simple and easily performed operation, which does not materially add to the risks attending urethrotomy, and is not followed by unpleasant results if the drainage-tube or catheter be not too long retained in the perineal wound.

4. That decomposition of urine can be delayed for a considerable time by thorough cleansing of the urethra and bladder by injection of a weak antiseptic solution (salicylic acid or sublimate) after operation. This, with the precaution on the part of the patient of abstaining from passing urine for as long a time as possible, will greatly lessen the frequency of occurrence of urethral fever and diminish its risks. Repeated washings of the urethra in this way after each act of micturition for a few days would probably prevent the attack of fever altogether.

5. Quinine, aconite and other drugs may be of use when urine fever has occurred, but they are powerless in most cases to avert it.

6. Patients with enlarged prostate whose deep urethras have been lacerated by the passage of solid instruments should be

treated by perineal cystotomy at once in order to arrest urine fever (or sepsis), either of which is likely to occur as soon as the patient is able to evacuate a part of his urine without the catheter.—*Montreal Medical Journal*, Feb., 1889.

New Procedure in Anticipated Complete Rupture of the Perineum.

At the meeting of the Chicago Gynecological Society, Nov. 16, 1888, Dr. Edward B. Weston read a paper, entitled A New Procedure in Cases of Anticipated Complete Rupture of the Perineum, in which he said that on the fourth day of last October he was, for the fourth time, called to attend Mrs. H. in labor. The patient was a woman somewhat below the average size, and had rather a narrow pelvis, while her children were all large at birth. At the birth of her first child, a boy who weighed twelve pounds, a complete laceration of the perineum was received. The second child, also a boy, weighed nine and one-half pounds, and the perineum was torn to the anal sphincter. The third pregnancy was terminated in the sixth month by unknown cause. The child was of course small, but delivery took place very rapidly, and there was again a rupture, though not to the same degree as in the second labor. On visiting the patient at the beginning of her last labor, an examination showed a well-restored perineum, and a child seemingly very large, presenting in the first position.

On meditating over the situation, remembering what had taken place in her previous labors, Dr. Weston feared a complete rupture would again occur, however well he might apply the various methods or procedures for protecting the perineum. The thought came to him that it would be well to introduce a deep suture before the laceration occurred, and before the head began to press upon the perineum, so that if complete rupture did take place he would have one suture already in place, by means of which he could easily bring the parts into accurate apposition, and which could, in a measure, be used as forceps or tenaculum, and be of great service in whatever after-operation might be necessary. He therefore with a long curved needle introduced a silk suture a little more than half an inch to the right of the anus, and carried it up about an inch and a half in the recto-vaginal septum, and brought it out on the left side at a point corresponding to its point of entrance. Each end was left six inches long and then tied together. Again there was a lacera-

tion, though not a complete one. The child, a boy, weighed eleven pounds.

In the discussion that followed the reading of the paper most of the speakers agreed that the procedure instituted by Dr. Weston was a proper and valuable one as simplifying the primary operation for rupture of the perineum.—*Am. Jour. of Obstet.*, Feb., 1889.

Toxic Action of Edible Mushrooms.

It is generally supposed that edible mushrooms are under all circumstances a safe article of diet, but some recent observations made in Switzerland appear to show that there may be danger in at least one species, if it is preserved in the dry state. Some persons in Berne who had eaten the mushroom known as Helvella (or Morchella) esculenta, which had been purchased in the dry state, were seized with abdominal pain and vomiting a few hours afterward. It was at first thought that some poisonous species must have got mixed with the Morchella esculenta, but upon examination this was found not to be the case. A decoction of the dried plant was then examined by Professor Demme, with the result that it evidently contained a powerful poison, the behavior of which, when tested on cold-blooded animals, produced the impression that it was much more nearly allied to curare than to muscarin: the residue, when examined, was found to be inert. The toxic substance, whatever it was, appeared to have no connection with the Helvellic acid discovered by Boehm and Külz in Helvella. Trimethylamine was prepared from a watery distillate of the dried mushroom, and the watery and alcoholic infusions contained a base which presented all the chemical and poisonous characters of neurin ; the presence of other basic bodies also belonging to the group of ptomaines was suspected. The theory suggested by Professor Demme and Dr. Berlinerblau, who was associated with him in the investigation, is that the highly nitrogenous mushroom substance is capable, under special circumstances, of undergoing certain putrefactive changes which lead to the formation of products of a poisonous character bearing a close analogy to those formed during the putrefaction of animal bodies. Consequently there is a double source of danger in eating mushroom—viz., the chance of admixture of poisonous species and the possibility of the existence of ptomaine-like bodies arising from partial decomposition having set in.—*Lancet*, March 2, 1889.

THE
MEDICAL AND SURGICAL
REPORTER.

ISSUED EVERY SATURDAY.

CHARLES W. DULLES, M.D.,
EDITOR AND PUBLISHER.

The Terms of Subscription to the serial publications of this office are as follows, payable in advance :

Med. and Surg. Reporter (weekly), a year, **$5.00**
Quarterly Compendium of Med. Science, -   2.50
Reporter and Compendium, -   -   -   - 6.00
Physician's Daily Pocket Record, -   -   1.00
Reporter and Pocket Record, -   -   -   - 6.00
Reporter, Compendium, and Pocket Record, 7.00

All checks and postal orders should be drawn to order of

CHARLES W. DULLES,
N. E. Cor. 13th and Walnut Streets,
P. O. Box 843.   Philadelphia, Pa.

☞SUGGESTIONS TO SUBSCRIBERS:
See that your address-label gives the date to which your subscription is paid.
In requesting a change of address, give the old address as well as the new one.
If your REPORTER does not reach you promptly and regularly, notify the publisher *at once*, so that the cause may be discovered and corrected.
☞SUGGESTIONS TO CONTRIBUTORS AND CORRESPONDENTS:
Write in ink.
Write on one side of paper only.
Write on paper of the size usually used for letters.
Make as few paragraphs as possible. Punctuate carefully. Do not abbreviate, or omit words like "the," and "a," or "an."
Make communications as short as possible.
NEVER ROLL A MANUSCRIPT ! · Try to get an envelope or wrapper which will fit it.
When it is desired to call our attention to something in a newspaper, mark the passage boldly with a colored pencil, and write on the wrapper "Marked copy." Unless this is done, newspapers are not looked at.
The Editor will be glad to get medical news, but it is important that brevity and actual interest shall characterize communications intended for publication.

PHYSICIANS AND PROHIBITION.

At the present time the readers of the REPORTER in at least three States are no doubt thinking very seriously in regard to the attitude which they will assume or maintain in regard to the proposed amendments to their State Constitutions prohibiting the manufacture and sale of alcoholic liquors for drinking purposes.

Physicians know, perhaps better than any class in the community, the physical dangers of the improper use of alcoholic drinks and the risks involved in even a moderate use of them ; yet, while some physicians are bitterly and unreservedly opposed to the use of alcoholic liquors, even as drugs, we think the great mass of medical men are disposed to consider the relative claims of temperance and total abstinence without prejudice, and without any of the absurd and untenable assumptions which furnish the stock in trade of many well-meaning but illogical moralists. Facts, we believe, appeal to our professional brethren, and facts will determine what they shall think and say in regard to the proposal to prohibit the sale of alcoholic beverages in Massachusetts, Pennsylvania and Nebraska, and in any other States in which the matter shall hereafter come up.

This being the case we cannot do better than to consider how prohibition has worked in States where it has been in force for some time.

The three most conspicuous examples of the results of prohibition are Maine, Kansas and Iowa. After thirty-six years of thorough testing, the verdict of the vast majority of the citizens of Maine is unqualifiedly favorable to prohibition. Every declaration of opinion that comes from responsible sources, every deliverance on the subject in the public press, on the political platform, or from the lips or pens of those qualified to judge, affirms the benefit and effectiveness of prohibition. Official records verify the statement that, before the enactment of this law, distilleries, breweries and saloons were in operation day and night throughout the State. To-day, although drinking is not wholly abolished, not a distillery, brewery or open saloon is plying its vocation within the borders of that State.

In 1884 Iowa placed on her statute books a stringent prohibitory liquor law. At the time of its enactment the liquor traffic held undisputed possession of the field. Distilleries, breweries and saloons were conducting their business openly in every part of the State, and no successful effort had been made to restrict or restrain them. At the end of four years, Governor Larrabee, himself an opposer of prohibitory legislation

Editorial.

when first proposed, declared that in eighty-five of the ninety-nine counties of the State the law is absolutely effective, and in the remaining fourteen partially enforced, with a steady advance toward complete enforcement. More than half of the county jails are vacant; pauperism and crime are steadily decreasing; intelligence and morality are advancing; the resources of the State are rapidly developing, and prosperity is said to follow every department of trade and every branch of industry.

The effect of prohibition in Kansas is indicated in a recent article in the *Topeka* (Kansas) *Capital Commonwealth*, replying to questions in regard to the effect of the prohibitory liquor-law in that State and the sentiment of the citizens in regard to it. From this article we learn that drunkenness and crime have diminished eighty per cent. since the saloons were closed in Kansas; that pauperism has decreased very materially, while the welfare of the people and the prosperity of the State have improved in equal proportion.

In his farewell address to the Kansas Legislature last January, Governor Martin said that no observing and intelligent citizen has failed to note the beneficial results already attained. Nine-tenths of the drinking and drunkenness prevalent eight years ago has been abolished. Crime has diminished enormously; thousands of homes where vice and want and wretchedness once prevailed are filled with peace, plenty and contentment. Although the population has increased rapidly, the number of criminals in jail has decreased steadily. Many of the jails are empty, and all show a marked falling off in the number of prisoners they contain. In the capital city (Topeka), with 60,000 inhabitants, not a single criminal case was on the docket when the then present term of court began. The business of the police courts had dwindled to one-fourth of its former proportions, and in cities of the second and third class the occupation of the police courts is practically gone.

These facts cannot fail to interest our readers, and must be of service in helping them to shape their expressions and actions intelligently and conscientiously toward the very important question which is before them.

EARLY DIAGNOSIS OF CANCER OF THE CERVIX UTERI.

The relative frequency of cancer of the cervix uteri, the certain death of the patient unless it can be extirpated, and the probability of recurrence unless it is removed early, render the subject of the early diagnosis of this disease one of great practical importance. It has been taught in the past that the cardinal symptoms of cancer of the cervix are hemorrhage, pain, and offensive watery discharge; these symptoms are associated with loss of flesh, debility, and cachexia, and have been considered specially important when they occur in women over forty years of age.

In a short paper in the *Medical Record*, February 9, 1889, Dr. Henry C. Coe considers the value of these symptoms and others as aids to the early diagnosis of cancer of the cervix. Dr. Coe has found that more than one-fifth of the women suffering with this disease are under forty, and that they frequently present every evidence of robust health, even in cases of advanced disease. Pain has been a late symptom, and is often absent. Hemorrhage often has not been sufficient to deserve the name, and very rarely threatens life. Moreover, the foul, watery discharge has not been uniformly present, even when extensive ulceration has existed.

Dr. Coe considers bleeding as the most common symptom noted in connection with incipient epithelioma of the cervix. This may be merely an increase of the menstrual flow — especially in women near the climacteric — but the most significant form of hemorrhage is what the Germans call "atypical," *i. e.*, a slight show at irregular intervals between the periods. It may be simply a pinkish discharge. This is especially significant when it occurs in women after the climacteric. Bleeding after coitus is always significant, and calls for prompt examination, even if no other symptom is present. A profuse leucorrhœa in a woman who has passed the climacteric should awaken suspicion, even though no odor is detected. Pain, of the severe lancinating character present in the advanced stage, is absent in the early stage. Vague, shooting pains in the pelvis, in women previously free from them, are of suspicious import.

Upon physical examination at this early time the cervix is usually found lacerated, large, thickened, and having peculiar nodules along the edges of the everted lips. At a somewhat later stage, the cervix will feel more like a mushroom. Firm pressure is not painful, but may cause slight hemorrhage. No odor is noted on withdrawing the finger. The uterus is somewhat enlarged, but movable, and there is no evidence of perimetritis. As seen through the speculum, the cervix may present the ordinary appearances seen in erosion — the distinction between which and cancer can often be determined only by microscopic examination. If there is a sharp demarcation between the healthy and the diseased areas, this fact is suspicious. The cancerous nodules appear as glistening yellowish nodules, elevated above the level of the healthy tissue. General hardness of the cervix in connection with extensive erosion is a sinister sign. In order to make a diagnosis in doubtful cases, a section of tissue must be removed and submitted to microscopic examination.

This study of the early diagnostic signs of cancer of the cervix is timely. The practitioner who waits for the appearance of the symptoms heretofore considered necessary to justify a suspicion of the existence of cancer, waits until there is no longer hope of a radical cure by removal of the parts. It behooves us all to study the signs of the invasion of cancer of the cervix, that a vaginal examination may be insisted on, and a diagnosis made while there is yet hope of cure by a radical operation. If we wait for the full development of the classical symptoms our diagnosis is certain, and the doom of our patient is not less certain.

EXCISION OF THE GALL-BLADDER.

The effect of total excision of the gall-bladder has been carefully studied, a few months ago, by Dr. Oddi, who at the suggestion of Dr. Marcacci, removed this receptacle from three large dogs and observed what followed. According to an abstract in the *Centralblatt für Chirurgie*, Feb. 23, 1889, he found in all three cases bile-pigment in the urine, and the stools became liquid, intensely colored and mucous. The animals had an increase of appetite; but they lost flesh. After a month, of a month and a half, these conditions were all reversed. Dr. Oddi thinks that after excision of the gall-bladder bile flows continuously into the intestinal canal, causing a catarrhal condition of the mucous membrane and resorption of the bile-pigments. The wasting he explains on the supposition that smaller quantities of bile meet the chyme as it leaves the stomach, and that therefore its fat is imperfectly emulsified, and consequently less perfectly absorbed. This view seems to be supported by an observation in which he made a fistulous connection between the stomach and the gall-bladder and ligated the ductus communis choledochus. In this case bile-pigments appeared in the urine, but there was no diarrhœa nor loss of weight. On the contrary, the animal had an increase of appetite and gained flesh. This effect Dr. Oddi ascribes to the accumulation of bile in the stomach and its periodical discharge, with the chyme, into the duodenum.

One of the most interesting disclosures of Dr. Oddi's experiments was the fact that removal of the gall-bladder was followed in one case by dilatation of the biliary ducts, while in two of the animals, which were killed after two and three months respectively, the biliary ducts were not much enlarged, while the cystic duct was so dilated that it looked as if Nature were attempting to make a new gall-bladder. Dr. Oddi has already made experiments which lead him to believe that the ductus communis choledochus has a sphincter, and he thinks that after excision of the gall-bladder, the action of this sphincter together with the dilatation of the biliary ducts, may lead to renewal of the normal periodical discharge of bile into the duodenum, and reinstatement of normal conditions of intestinal digestion.

The results of his experiments are of very great interest, and have an important bearing upon the operations which are nowadays practised on the gall-bladder.

TREATMENT OF LOCOMOTOR ATAXIA BY SUSPENSION.

It is interesting to note that Motchoukowsky's method of treating locomotor ataxia by suspension of the patient with bands passing under the chin and occiput and under the arms—the method described in the REPORTER February 23—has been on trial in the nervous clinic of Professors Eulenburg and Mendel, in Berlin. The results obtained by these distinguished specialists in nervous diseases are stated by the *Berliner klin. Wochenschrift,* February 25, 1889, to be in entire agreement with those we have referred to from Charcot's clinic. The patients are at first suspended for one minute, and gradually the time is lengthened until the limit of three minutes is reached, the suspension being practised three times a week. About twenty patients have thus far been subjected to the treatment in the polyclinic in Berlin, and the distrust with which it was first regarded has given way, until now the patients look forward to it with eagerness and steadily growing confidence. Too short a time has elapsed to speak of cures or even of undoubted improvements, nevertheless they say it can be stated that a certain number of patients exhibit after the suspension an easier and freer gait, have less staggering, and com-

plain less of lancinating pains; in a few cases there has been also improvement in the bladder symptoms. Moreover, in their experience up to the present time the treatment has been free from bad symptoms, and is evidently well borne by women.

They are careful, however, to add that the actual value of the treatment is still in doubt, and that physicians should be warned against forming precipitate and exaggerated hopes of it. This last statement obtains support from the experience of the treatment which has been had in the Infirmary for Nervous Diseases in Philadelphia. Fourteen patients have thus far been subjected to the treatment in that institution. As a rule the suspension has been well borne, but care is required to have the pressure equable—not more in the neck than in the armpits. Patients after the suspension is over are found to be unsteady when first let down, so that they are not released for a minute or so. The only unpleasant effect observed occurred in a patient who fainted during suspension, and had convulsive movements; he recovered, however, in a few minutes after being let down. While it is as yet too early to speak of the results obtained at the Infirmary, it is significant that there has not been in any case marked improvement.

MORRELL MACKENZIE AGAIN.—In reply to the notification of the vote of censure passed upon Sir Morell Mackenzie by the Royal College of Physicians, his secretary replied as follows to Sir Henry Pitman, the Registrar of the College:

"SIR: I am requested by Sir Morell Mackenzie to express his surprise that you should have written to him on behalf of the Royal College of Physicians. I am further instructed to inform you that Sir Morell Mackenzie takes no interest whatever in the proceedings or opinions of the College of Physicians, and to request that as the representative of that body you will do him the favor to desist from all further intrusion."

This note is characterized by effrontery which would be surprising in most men, but which is not remarkable in a man who first disgraced his profession, and then in various ways affected indifference to the reprobation his conduct excited.

BOOK REVIEWS.

HANDBOOK OF THE DIAGNOSIS AND TREATMENT OF SKIN DISEASES. By ARTHUR VAN HARLINGEN, M.D., Professor of Diseases of the Skin in the Philadelphia Polyclinic and College for Graduates in Medicine, etc. Second edition, enlarged and revised. 8vo, pp. 410. Philadelphia: P. Blakiston, Son & Co., 1889. Price, $2.50.

"Good wine needs no bush," and a book like this one by Dr. Van Harlingen needs little recommendation when it comes to a second edition. It has already secured the approval of the medical profession because it is clear, succinct and interesting. It is admirably adapted to the needs of general practitioners, who are sometimes deterred from the study of dermatology, because the works devoted to it are too ponderous, and filled with elaborate details of which confuse those who are not specialists in this department, and make them despair of gaining a working knowledge of it. Dr. Van Harlingen has brought to the preparation of his book the knowledge gained by many years of faithful study, a large experience as a practitioner and a teacher, and a singularly conscientious method in all that he does.

Those who turn to his book will find it a thoroughly trustworthy manual, and one very convenient to refer to. The various subjects are considered in alphabetical order, so that an index is not needed—and none is given.

We can heartily recommend the book to our readers as one of the most sensible and practical works on diseases of the skin with which we are acquainted.

OBSTETRIC APHORISMS FOR THE USE OF STUDENTS COMMENCING MIDWIFERY PRACTICE. By JOSEPH GRIFFITHS SWAYNE, M.D., Consulting Physician Accoucheur to the Bristol General Hospital, and Lecturer on Obstetric Medicine at the Bristol Medical College. Ninth Edition. 16mo., pp. viii, 159. Philadelphia: P. Blakiston, Son & Co., 1888. Price, $1.25.

When a book reaches a ninth edition it is because of its inherent merits, and because it is well adapted to the end for which it is intended. Covering as it does the more practical part of obstetrics, instructing the young practitioner in the details of the conduct of the accoucheur toward his patient, laying down sound methods of treatment for easily managed puerperal cases, and pointing out the cases in which the beginner stands in need of counsel, the "Obstetric Aphorisms" supplies a want on the part of young practitioners which is not supplied by more comprehensive and systematic treatises. The author, however, should have revised in this edition the sections treating of the third stage of labor, the use of ergot, *post-partum* hemorrhage, diseases of the breast, and puerperal fever. While these sections contain much that is true and valuable, a careful revision would have eliminated some errors of principle and practice, and have introduced some more modern views. With these exceptions we have only commendation for the subject matter of the book, and doubt not that this edition will meet with the same approval accorded its predecessors.

PAMPHLET NOTICES.

240. EXPERIMENTAL RESEARCHES RESPECTING THE RELATION OF DRESS TO PELVIC DISEASES OF WOMEN. By J. H. KELLOGG, M.D., Battle Creek, Michigan. From the *Transactions of the Michigan Med. Society*, 1888. 22 pages.

241. LA TREPANACIÓN EN LA EPILEPSIA. (Trephining for Epilepsy.) By DR. D. ENRIQUE DE AREILZA. Triano, Vizcaya, Spain. 16 pages.

242. PROGRESSIVE MUSCULAR DYSTROPHIES. By B. SACHS, M.D., New York. From the *New York Medical Journal*, December 15, 1888. 44 pages.

240. This pamphlet contains an account of the result of a series of experiments to demonstrate the effects of tight lacing on the pelvic and thoracic organs, and it leads the author to believe that many ailments peculiar to women are directly traceable to her present style of dress. He, therefore, advises her to resort more to the physical activities characteristic of savage life, and to adopt clothing which secures freedom of motion to the whole body. Dr. Kellogg's experiments are extremely interesting and valuable, especially as they confirm the views in regard to the influence of clothing in producing the costal type of respiration in women which were published by Dr. Mays, of Philadelphia, nearly two years ago.

241. As indicated in our notice of a former pamphlet by Dr. Areilza, in the REPORTER, January 28, 1888, he is an enterprising practicer of cranial and cerebral surgery. In the pamphlet now before us he discusses the value of trephining in epilepsy, and gives the histories of two cases, in one of which he operated for the relief of true epilepsy, extirpating the cortical area presiding over the muscles affected in the convulsions, while in the second he trephined, opened the dura and removed a small fungous growth. The result of these operations was at least a temporary relief. He does not venture to say it will be permanent, although he hopes it may be.

Like his former essay, this paper bears the marks of courage in action and of careful study of the subject. It is very interesting, and deserving of the attention of all students of cerebral surgery.

242. Dr. Sachs defines progressive muscular atrophy as a form of disease in which a primary progressive wasting of some or all of the muscles of the body is the most characteristic feature, and in which this wasting (atrophy) may or may not be associated with true or pseudo hypertrophy of some muscles. In this classification he excludes muscular atrophy following cerebral, myelitic, or peripheral nerve-disease. His pamphlet discusses with great fulness and completeness the forms of disease covered by his definition, and leads up to a classification which he proposes as founded upon a correct understanding of them. His paper also contains a useful bibliography of the literature of this interesting and somewhat obscure subject.

—The *Memphis Journal of the Medical Sciences* is the name of a new monthly magazine published in Memphis, Tennessee. It has a corps of six editors, who have charge of separate departments. The first (March) number contains 32 octavo pages of reading matter, and makes a good showing. Price, $2 a year.

CORRESPONDENCE.

Death of a Fœtus from Knotting of the Umbilical Cord.

To the Editor.

Sir: I was called March 23, 1889, to see Mrs. T., white, 42 years old. I found her in labor at full term, the os well dilated, and the pains severe. There was an abundance of amniotic fluid, so much so, indeed, that I could not feel the child until my finger was introduced well up into the uterus. The child's head was found directly over the os. I then ruptured the membranes, and I believe a half-gallon of liquor amnii came away.

The child was born within fifteen minutes, with the umbilical cord around its neck; and the cord near its centre was tied in a firm knot. The child was dead and evidently had been for three or four weeks. It was quite dark in color, and so was the cord up to the knot; but above the knot the cord was healthy looking.

The patient stated that she had not felt the child move for four weeks. It weighed eight pounds when born. The death of the child was due, no doubt, to the fact that the cord was tied in a knot.

I report this case as I never heard of a similar one.

Yours truly,
G. G. Morris, M.D.

Washington, D.C.,
March 26, 1889.

Infectiousness of Tuberculosis.

To the Editor.

Sir: The Editorial in the Reporter, March 16, on the infectiousness of phthisis, reminds me of the photograph of a tuberculous finger on the hand of L. Barton, M.D., living some seven miles north of Essex, New York, which I saw in 1876, published in the Transactions of the Medical Society of the State of New York for 1871. The finger as represented was double its natural thickness, with tubercles all over it. The account says: "In June 30, 1840, in making an examination of the lungs thirty hours after death, of a subject that died of tubercular phthisis, I accidentally cut the middle finger of my left hand, over the first joint; the wound was slight, not penetrating through the true skin. The wound healed kindly, but remained somewhat red around the cut. In about two weeks inflammation set in, and a row of

hard tubercles appeared in the line of the cut, about the size of millet-seeds. In two weeks a second and more numerous crop appeared; in this way the disease progressed for two years in spite of all means suggested, till it had extended from the nail half way to the second joint, and half way around the finger, producing a fungoid thickening of the skin, which was removed with caustics. It was finally cured by the continued use of powdered nitrate of silver."

This is an abbreviated account as there published. After seeing the photograph from this case of inoculation, I concluded that the exhalations and expectoration from a patient with phthisis must be infectious; and soon afterward I was confirmed in this opinion by the death of a mother and daughter, who had been well and hearty when they began attending upon the husband and father, who was suffering with phthisis. The patient's free, thick expectoration covered a large surface of newspaper lying on the floor when I visited him. A few months after his burial, I was told that his wife had consumption; she soon died; and then it was announced that the daughter had it, and she too soon died. It was during our warmest weather when I witnessed this unpleasant spectacle; and that sad ending of mother and daughter seemed plainly to show that the bacillus was active in that fatal deed. Many other similar scenes recur to my memory.

Yours truly,
E. Vanderpoel, M.D.

New York,
March 22, 1889.

Alopecia Areata.

To the Editor.

Sir: The patient, A. S., 36 years old, was a man of seeming perfect health, and of a nervous temperament. He states that one morning in September last, as he was preparing to shave, he ran his fingers over his scalp for a loose hair and was surprised to find he had a handful. Having prided himself on his head of dark hair, his astonishment was profound when after about ten days he presented himself without a *hair on his body*. The scalp was as smooth as though it had been for years as bald as now. After about a month his head showed an occasional white hair, but even at this time, with the hair evidently coming in anew, there would be but little difficulty in numbering those upon the head and face. The patient has never had any constitutional disease nor any long sickness, and if he had not happened to have at the time a slight erythema of the chest he would have felt even better at the time of the accident than at any time for years.

Yours truly,
MILES D. GOODYEAR, M.D.
·Groton, N. Y.
March 21, 1889.

NOTES AND COMMENTS.

Professor Agnew's Farewell.

Professor D. Hayes Agnew delivered, on April 5, his last lecture as John Rhea Barton Professor of Surgery in the University of Pennsylvania, although he will continue to lecture in the Hospital. In honor of the occasion the students had filled the amphitheatre with tropical plants and cut flowers which encircled the space in which the lecturer was to stand. On a bank of roses was a small sheet of paper with this inscription:

"Professor D. Hayes Agnew, as a token of the love and respect of the members of the Class of '89, and with their wishes that he may 'live long and prosper.'"

Dr. Agnew, when he entered the lecture-room, was somewhat astonished at the flowers, and looked around for a few moments bewildered. The applause which signalled his entrance was loud and long continued. After a simple bow of acknowledgment the distinguished surgeon proceeded, without any flourishes, to deliver a brief lecture on tracheotomy. When he had finished, Dr. Agnew paused briefly, and then said:

"And now, gentlemen, I have delivered the last of the lectures that it has been my privilege and my pleasure to deliver to you. In taking my leave from the associations of nearly my whole lifetime, I cannot do so without dwelling for a moment on the reflections that this occasion gives rise to. I have been connected with this institution from its early days, through its rapid growth, to where it stands to-day in the front rank of the medical institutions of the country. With a feeling of satisfaction that I can thus behold this institution which we love so dearly, I turn to contemplate the retirement which I have sought. I feel like a galley-slave with the manacles thrown off and breathing the air of freedom.

"There comes a time in the life of every man when he wants to be free. For over forty years I have been—as they say in the-atrical parlance—on the boards, before the public, and as I glance back over that long period of almost a lifetime, three most delightful thoughts occur to me. The first of these is that, at no time have I ever been received by any act of discourtesy or unkindness by any of the gentlemen whom I have had the honor to address here. The second is that the post of responsibility which it has been my cherished privilege to hold here was one that I had never sought nor asked for. It came to me unbidden. And the third thought is that God has given me the sense, the good sense, to resign it while I feel that I am yet in the full enjoyment and possession of all my faculties. These I have endeavored to strengthen, to broaden, and to render useful in the sphere of my professional life, for I feel that I have lived to very little account if I have not lived to learn.

"In a few days we part, some of us, perhaps, to meet no more. You have chosen a profession which is one of the highest and noblest that a man can make his calling. See that by your faithful zeal and application you endeavor to maintain it in all the dignity that belongs to it. As we take this leave I wish that all of you may prosper; that it may be your aim to elevate your lives, and to round them off in the fulness of an undeviating regard for duty and a high purpose; that, in short, you may be good men and true, good physicians and pure, and good citizens and honorable. I trust, in the effort to attain these high marks in the life that stretches out before you that you may continue in a reverent regard for the faith that has sustained you, guarded you from the paths of evil."

At the conclusion of Dr. Agnew's farewell, the large lecture-room resounded with applause and cheers.

During the lecture and the farewell address, Professors H. C. Wood, Joseph. Leidy, James Tyson, T. G. Wormley, J. William White, E. T. Reichert, William Goodell, and other members of the faculty, occupied seats in the enclosure.

Antiseptic Saccharin Dentifrice.

Dr. Constantin Paul proposes the following formula for an agreeable dentifrice:

Saccharin	gr. cl
Bicarbonate of soda	gr. lx
Proof spirit	f ℥ iii
Oil of peppermint	gtt. xx
Tincture of cochineal	q.s.

—*Chemist and Druggist,* Jan. 5, 1889.

Treatment of Tapeworm.

The following from the *Boston Med. and Surg. Journal*, March 7, 1889, will be interesting in connection with the communication from Dr. Traill Green, published in the REPORTER, April 6, 1889:

Bérenger-Férand, who has written an authoritative book " On the Tæniæ of Man," has communicated to the *Bulletin Général de Thérapeutique*, February 15, 1889, an article in which he sums up the cases of tapeworm,—in all one hundred and ninety-one patients—at the Maritime Hospital of Toulon during the year 1888, and the results of treatment.

Of these 191 patients treated for tapeworm 112 were discharged cured, the worm being expelled head and all; in every instance the tænia was of the variety known as *Tænia inermis*. In 87 instances but one parasite was found; in 11 there were two; in four there were three; in one there were five; in two there were six; and in one unparalleled case seventeen heads were counted as the result of an anthelmintic.

As for the time during which these patients had been afflicted with the parasite, four had carried their tæniæ for three years; two for eight years; and one for eleven years.

As regards the treatment, Bérenger-Férand still gives the preference to pelletierine. This tænicide, which is the active principle of pomegranate bark, is by far the most successful of all remedies used. During the year 1888 pelletierine was employed one hundred and fifty-two times as a tænifuge at the Toulon Hospital. Of these cases one hundred and ten were successful, forty-two were unsuccessful, giving 72 per cent. of recoveries.

As for the manner of administration of the remedy, the patient takes nothing but bread and milk for supper the evening before; the next morning thirty centigrammes (five grains) of the sulphates of pelletierine and isopelletierine are administered in solution with fifty centigrammes (8 grains) of tannin (or half a bottle of Tanret's solution of the mixed pelletierines, the other half to be given in an hour); from 7.30 A. M. to 8 A. M. a full dose of a tablespoonful of the German tincture of jalap is given, or from an ounce to an ounce and a half of castor oil. A few hours after the ingestion of the medicine the patient experiences a slight vertigo, and the tapeworm is voided, as a rule, four hours after the dose is taken. In order to avoid breaking of the worm during its passage, and before the head is voided, it is advised that the patient shall sit at stool in a vessel nearly full of warm water. Bérenger-Férand has lately resorted to injections of a decoction of pomegranate bark to assist the expulsion of the worm, and claims that this is an improvement in the treatment.

It is needless to say that the above is now the favorite treatment of tænia in France, and Dujardin-Beaumetz affirms that " since we have established these rules of treatment, and wherever patients have scrupulously complied with them, we have had numerous successes, and in nine cases out of ten we obtain the worm with the head."

Bérenger-Férand finds in his last year's experience in the treatment of this painful malady gratifying confirmation of the results obtained in past years.

Sharpening the Section Knife.

The *St. Louis Med. and Surg. Journal*, March, 1889, says that judging from the number of queries which are made from time to time, and from the interest displayed by students and others on this point, sharpening the section knife, while simplicity itself to one who has learned the " knack," is one full of difficulties to the uninitiated. Giving in succession three or four students who complained that they could not succeed in getting the right kind of an edge on their blades, an old knife and a hone, and closely watching their manœuvres, what appears to be the prime cause of the trouble is seen to be an involuntary turn of the wrist upward at the end of each forward and backward motion of the knife on the hone, whereby the edge placed on the blade at the centre of the stroke is rounded off and worn away. There is another habit, also quite common, which has a similar effect on the edge, viz., the reversing of the blade at the end of a stroke on its edge, instead of on its back, as a fulcrum. The blade should be laid on the surface of the hone in such a manner that every part of the flat side is in contact at one and the same time, and this contact should be maintained throughout the stroke. On the hollowed side the cutting edge and the edge of the back should be kept constantly on the surface of the hone. The knife should be drawn over the stone *edge foremost* with a smooth, even stroke, from heel to point. Where the knife is very dull or hacked, most of the honing should be done on the hollowed side, for obvious reasons. As to hones: some difference of opinion exists as to the relative merits of the Turkish, the " barber " or " German razor," and the

Ouachita or Hot-Springs stones. Each has its merits. The Turkish hone cuts more rapidly than either of the others, but leaves a wiry edge that must be strapped off. The "barber," if a good specimen, leaves little to be desired on the score of either rapidity of cut or smoothness of edge; but for a perfect edge, requiring no strapping, the finer qualities of Hot-Springs hones are unexcelled. Other things being equal, the hone with the broadest bearing surface is the best. As a lubricator olive oil should be used with the Turkish stone, soap-suds with the "German razor," and pure glycerine with the Arkansas hones. As to "strops," unless they handled in a gentle and scientific manner they always do more harm than good, by rounding off the edge.

General Paralysis Associated with Locomotor Ataxia.

Dr. A. Strümpell communicates to the *Neurologishes Centralblatt*, No. 5, 1888, an account of a case in which he thinks that under the influence of syphilis general paralysis and locomotor ataxia developed together in the same person. The patient was a girl 13 years old, whose father had contracted syphilis two years before the birth of the child. The child had always been delicate and subject to skin eruptions. When thirteen years old it was attacked with transient paralysis of the whole of the right side. This paralysis disappeared in half an hour, but reappeared fifteen days later complicated with aphasia. Similar attacks recurred subsequently every three or four weeks for a year. After the first attack a decline in the intelligence of the child was noted. Subsequently, embarrassment of speech persisted; the gait became unsteady; and pain was complained of in the belly and in the side.

The chief symptoms noted by Strümpell at his first examination about twenty months after the first attack, were: Very pronounced enfeeblement of the intellect, entirely characteristic embarrassment of speech, shaking and trembling of the muscles of the face, when the patient spoke, difficulty in writing such as is manifested in patients with general paralysis—forgetting letters, syllables, or entire words—abolition of reflex movements of the pupil, trembling of the tongue, unsteady movements of the arms, very pronounced ataxia of the lower limbs, abolition of the knee jerk, blunting of the sensibility to pain.

Iodide of potassium seemed to improve the condition of the lower limbs and of the speech. Then the disease resumed its progress. Six months later the patient had a fresh and violent attack of paralysis which lasted half a day.—*Gazette médicale de Paris*, Jan. 12, 1889.

Scarlet Fever, Diphtheria and Measles in New York City.

The prevalence in New York City of scarlet fever, diphtheria and measles is shown by the statistics of the Board of Health for the month of March. The cases of scarlet fever numbered 1709, while for the corresponding month of last year they numbered only 613. Cases of measles have increased from 236 in March, 1888, to 800 in March, 1889. Diphtheria shows a much smaller percentage of increase, the number of cases for March, 1889, being 811, while in the corresponding month last year the number was 534.

The spread of these diseases is attributed in part to the neglect of disinfection by the attending physicians, and in part to carelessness in the matter of isolating patients.

Commencement of Jefferson Medical College.

The sixty-fourth annual commencement of Jefferson Medical College of Philadelphia was held April 3, 1889, and the degree of Doctor of Medicine conferred upon two hundred and twelve graduates. The following prizes were awarded:

A prize of $100, offered by *The Medical News* for the best thesis embodying original research, to Michael Valentine Ball, of Pennsylvania; a gold medal, for the best essay on a subject pertaining to the practice of medicine, to Joseph John Burke, of Pennsylvania, with honorable mention of the essay of Thomas Clinton Seright, of Ohio; a gold medal, for the best anatomical preparation, to Howard Roeder Swayne, of Pennsylvania; a case of instruments, for the best examination in materia medica, to Ellis Freedom Frost, of Rhode Island; a case of instruments, for the best examination in surgery, to Malcomb Wayland Everson, of Pennsylvania; a gold medal, for the best report of Dr. Thomas G. Morton's surgical clinic at the Pennsylvania Hospital, to Ross Parker Cox, of Georgia, with honorable mention to George D. Thomas, of the undergraduate class.

The valedictory address was delivered by W. S. Forbes, M.D., Professor of General, Descriptive and Surgical Anatomy.

NEWS.

—Dr. Wilbur P. Klapp and Dr. Lewis H. Adler, Jr., have been elected Resident Physicians at the Episcopal Hospital.

—The Training School for Nurses of the New York Hospital conferred diplomas on fourteen graduates on April 4.

—The thirty-second annual meeting of the Missouri State Medical Association will be held at Springfield, May 21, 22 and 23.

—At the eighth annual commencement of the Medico-Chirurgical College April 4, the degree of Doctor of Medicine was conferred upon 30 graduates.

—The mortality reports of the city of Philadelphia continue to be favorable, and the returns for the week ending April 8 show a smaller proportion than usual of deaths from such diseases as scarlet and typhoid fevers and diphtheria.

—The Dean of the Faculty of the Woman's Medical College of Pennsylvania has announced that the Faculty are prepared to advocate the proposed amendment to the Medical Examiners' bill, which makes the course of medical study four years.

—Passed Assistant Surgeon Hervey W. Whitaker, of the Navy, who is at present attached to the nautical school-ship St. Mary's, has been appointed clinical assistant to the chair of hygiene at the Post-graduate School of the College of Physicians and Surgeons, New York.

—The second annual address before the Society of the Alumni of Bellevue Hospital was delivered April 3, at the Academy of Medicine, by Dr. William Osler, Professor of Medicine in Johns Hopkins University. Dr. Osler's subject was *"Phagocytes."* After his lecture he was given a reception.

—Dr. George B. Loring, who has just been nominated as Minister Resident and Consul General to Portugal, was graduated in medicine at Harvard, in 1842. He was surgeon to the Marine Hospital, Chelsea, Mass., from 1843 to 1850, and a Commissioner to revise the United States Marine Hospital system in 1849.

—Dr. Benjamin Lee, Secretary of the State Board of Health of Pennsylvania, who represents the interests of the Middle Atlantic District, has gone to Florida to confer with a commission of sanitary officials, recently appointed by the Legislature of Florida, with reference to the proper means to adopt to prevent a recurrence of yellow fever in that State.

OBITUARY.

PROF. FRANCIS CORNELIUS DONDERS.

Prof. Francis Cornelius Donders, the well-known Dutch doctor and eye specialist died very recently at the Hague. Dr. Donders was born at Tilburg, in Brabant, May 27, 1818. He studied medicine at the Military Medical School at Utrecht, became military surgeon at the Hospital of The Hague and afterward professor at the Utrecht school. He was subsequently called to the university of the same city, and became successively professor of histology and physiology, and then of ophthalmology, to which was added the clinic of diseases of the eye. In 1863 he obtained from the Government the title of professor, and was voted a sum of money to construct a physiological laboratory corresponding to the needs of modern science, where many delicate and valuable researches have since been carried out.

Dr. Donders is, best known for his researches on the physiology and pathology of the eye, and for his works on Astigmatism and on Anomalies of Refraction. In them he treated the eye as an optical instrument, showed that it was liable to cause distorted images on the retina with corresponding defective vision, and concluded with profound researches on lenses, prisms and cylinders of glass as means for correcting these errors of refraction.

RESOLUTIONS ON THE DEATH OF DR. BRUEN.

At a meeting of the Medical Staff of the Philadelphia Hospital, held April 1, 1889, the following resolutions were adopted:

"Whereas another vacancy on our Staff has been created by death,

"Resolved: that by the death of Dr. Edward T. Bruen, who was an indefatigable worker, a clear thinker, and an able writer, the interests of scientific medicine have suffered severe loss.

"Resolved: that while this loss will be felt by every medical practitioner, it is but slight compared with that experienced by numerous personal friends to whom he had endeared himself by many amiable qualities.

"Resolved: that the sincerest sympathy of the Staff of this hospital be tendered to the family of their late colleague.

JAMES TYSON,
President.

L. W. STEINBACH,
Secretary pro tem.

MEDICAL AND SURGICAL REPORTER

No. 1677.   PHILADELPHIA, APRIL 20, 1889.   VOL. LX.—No. 16.

CONTENTS:

CLINICAL LECTURE.

DUODENAL ULCER; SUDDEN ENORMOUS HEMORRHAGE; DEATH [1]

BY WILLIAM PEPPER, M.D.,

PHILADELPHIA.

PROFESSOR OF THEORY AND PRACTICE OF MEDICINE IN THE UNIVERSITY OF PENNSYLVANIA.

The man from whom these specimens were obtained was about thirty-five years of age. He was a prominent athlete, had taken part in many contests requiring strength and endurance, and had distinguished himself on many occasions as a runner and an oarsman. He had been suffering more or less constantly for eight years. He was a man of generally careless habits, and this was especially noticeable in the irregularity of his meals and in the want of care he displayed in selecting his food

[1] Delivered at the Hospital of the University of Pennsylvania.

and drink. His first complaint was of epigastric pain. He had irregular attacks of this at first, and these gradually became more frequent, prolonged, and violent. They were partly relieved by firm pressure over the immediate seat of pain. His suffering was attributed to gastralgia, and his only remedy was this forcible pressure, to which he always resorted.

It was not long, however, before it became clear that something more was the matter than simple gastralgia. The existence of gastric catarrh was noted, and, in time, another symptom was developed: he began to vomit. At first this was occasional, then it occurred several times a week, and, finally, it became of daily occurrence and so continued for several years. For this trouble he sought medical advice, but with only temporary benefit. Among other things, a milk diet was directed for him. This, he thought, seemed beneficial. It afforded him some relief from his constant pain and he kept it up largely for this reason. He had a craving sense of discomfort and irritation, and, to allay this, he

471

drank prodigious quantities of milk. When the pain happened to be especially annoying he would drink a pitcher-full of cold milk at a draught. This did, indeed, give him some ease, but it was merely transitory and he was soon again in distress. Previous to his illness he had been addicted to the use of wine and tobacco, both in excess; but soon after the commencement of his gastric trouble he entirely abandoned them. We cannot know, therefore, in what manner the administration of stimulants would have influenced his symptoms. He preferred bland, cooling drinks, and these, as you see, he used in large quantity. He lived in this way for a long period, working hard, keeping up his exercise, and maintaining an appearance of good health. There was no emaciation.

Two weeks ago to-day, that is on Saturday, he went to his office in the morning and, on approaching his desk, suddenly fainted and fell to the floor, vomiting an enormous quantity of blood. Everything near him was deluged with the fluid, and he must have lost a quart at least. Immediate assistance was rendered him; he was removed to the house of a relative, and powerful restoratives administered. I saw him about noon and found him in a state of partial collapse, with cold extremities, a thready running pulse, and all his tissues blanched from the great loss of blood.

With the foregoing history that I then obtained and the sudden and violent hemorrhage, I confidently diagnosticated the existence of a gastric ulcer, and felt some surprise that it had not been recognized much sooner. There was no difficulty in excluding cancer, for the pain had been of much too long standing for that disease; there had also been no obstruction of the bowels, and there was no emaciation. It could not be an instance of rupture of an aneurism, for there had been nothing which would indicate the presence and growth of an aneurism. The man had been uninterruptedly pursuing his business and exercise, there was no arterial rigidity, and there had been no shortness of breath. The only other question was as to cirrhosis of the liver. I have before dwelt upon the fact that cirrhosis of the liver will not only frequently occasion a violent gastric hemorrhage, but that this sudden hematemesis is often the first *severe* symptom of that disease. This startling event may, indeed, be quickly followed by a long train of the commoner symptoms of the disease—disordered digestion, hemorrhoids, distension of the abdominal veins,

ascites, etc.—but until the occurrence of that hemorrhage, they may all have remained entirely latent. In this case we had a prolonged history of generous living and of a gastric catarrh extending over several years; but I found that the patient had not been in the habit of consuming strong spirits and it is only these, as a very general rule, that produce cirrhosis. Again, this man had for a long time experienced severe pain which was relieved by pressure and by the imbibition of cool drinks; whereas in cirrhosis the pain is not violent and is not mitigated by either of these measures. I did not attempt to make any careful examination at the time, but I satisfied myself that the liver was not materially diminished in size. Taking all the more striking features of the case into consideration, therefore, I determined that it was one of gastric ulcer.

The treatment adopted consisted of very simple remedies. The patient was kept completely at rest, ice bags were placed over the stomach, and, at intervals, small pieces of ice were swallowed. A pill of nitrate of silver and opium was given, and the nourishment consisted of small quantities of milk and lime water. Evening found the patient in better condition and quite cheerful. His only complaint was of constant thirst. During the night, however, he became restless, there was a return of epigastric pain and discomfort, and with the coming of dawn another hemorrhage occurred. Again the quantity lost was fully a quart. I neglected to mention that on the preceding day the patient had taken a few doses of Monsell's solution. In spite of this, however, the ulcer had either been bleeding continuously during the night, or else a vessel had suddenly given way in the morning and occasioned this abrupt gush of blood. I think the latter of these views is the more probable. The patient again sank into a state of profound collapse, and in the evening was barely living.

At this time I called Dr. White to see the case with me, with a view of employing transfusion to revive the rapidly ebbing life. From this time until the following Saturday evening, when death occurred, the patient was under continuous observation, Dr. Daland remaining with him day and night. During the seven days over which this acute illness extended, the thirst was incessant and insatiable. This is without doubt the most pitiable symptom in these cases. The sufferer cries in agony for drink and yet, in dread of provoking another hemorrhage, we can permit only the smallest quantities of liquid to be given. The supplies of milk and lime water were now alternated with small doses of champagne and Apollinaris water, mixed in the proportion of one part to three, and then partly frozen at a neighboring confectioner's. This proved very grateful to the parched throat of the patient. To support his strength the measures chiefly depended upon were nutritive enemas and the hypodermic administration of powerful diffusible stimulants.

Ether, digitalis, atropia, and morphia were given in sufficient amount to control the restlessness and distressing thirst and to stimulate the heart. It was only by the frequently repeated use of these potent remedies, that life was prolonged during the several days that followed the occurrence of the primary hemorrhage. I have no doubt whatever that had they been withheld for a few hours only, death would have promptly taken place. During the day following the second hemorrhage, on Monday, it became evident that something else would have to be done to rouse the patient from the state of fatal collapse into which he was sinking. It was decided to resort to transfusion. At one o'clock Tuesday morning a hot saline solution, an artificial serum, was injected into the left median basilic vein. This was accomplished without accident and its immediate effects were very gratifying. Unfortunately, however, they were maintained for only a few hours, the patient relapsed into his former condition, and the operation was not repeated. Nothing was now left us to depend upon but frequent supplies of concentrated liquid nourishment, and stimulants. The stomach had become quiet and a slightly increased quantity of fluid was permitted.

Now, however, an unfortunate complication arose. Fever made its appearance, and the temperature steadily rose to 102°, 102.5°, and 103°, Fahr., where it remained until the end. The proper explanation of this fever was difficult at the time, and it still remains somewhat clouded. It was probably due to a combination of several causes, and some of these I will detail. We found that if we wished to continue using the rectum as a medium for nourishing the patient, it would have to be emptied and cleansed. An injection given for this purpose procured the discharge of a great quantity of black, tarry, fetid blood, the stench of which was indescribable. It was diffused throughout the whole room in a moment. This evacuation was evidence that at the time of the discharge of blood from the stomach, a large quantity had made its way into the intestine, and, remaining there, had undergone decomposition. It was clearly necessary to rid the intestinal canal of this rotting mass, for it was acting not only as a powerful excitor of gastro-intestinal irritation, but also as a source of septic poisoning. These two factors were quite sufficient partly to explain the rise of temperature. As an additional explanation of this symptom, I thought it probable that some inflammatory action had been excited around the seat of the ulcer. The results obtained from the autopsy showed that all of these causes had been active in producing the febrile condition. Large enemas, to which Listerine was added, brought away large quantities of blood of a gangrenous odor, and subsequently, hot concentrated saline solutions were given in the same manner with the effect of causing still further evacuations of a similar character. But, notwithstanding the fact that at least four pints of this offending material were removed in this way, the *post-mortem* examination revealed the presence of certainly as much more.

It is clear, therefore, that coincidently with the profuse gastric hemorrhages, an enormous amount of blood passed downward into the intestines. We need but little besides these three conditions—the frightful loss of blood, the subsequent severe irritation of the gastro-intestinal tract, and the septic infection produced by the local changes in the effused blood—to account satisfactorily for the rise of temperature. In instances of gastric hemorrhage a certain amount of overflow into the intestinal canal is quite common — sufficient, usually, to produce one or two dark stools; but I do not think I have ever met with a case in which the quantity of blood entering the intestine was so excessive as it was here.

The patient's prostration gradually became more profound, and death finally occurred from heart failure and cerebral exhaustion, accompanied with persistent high temperature, but with no recurrence of hemorrhage. We could not tell positively whether or not some oozing into the intestinal canal had been continuing during the final days of the illness, but I did not think this probable. Two other points in connection with the case remain for consideration. First, there was a heart murmur. This was heard most distinctly over the left edge of the sternum and was systolic in time. It seemed plausible, in view of the great loss of blood, that this was anemic in character; but its position did not conform to that usually occupied by murmurs dependent upon that cause. The problem was as to whether or not it was the result of valvular change. The second and last point to be mentioned is, that the urine was albuminous. It contained no casts, however. It is not improbable that this abnormality was occasioned by altered conditions of blood-pressure, and possibly also, the operation of transfusion may have had some bearing upon it. The body was embalmed shortly after death and the examination then made.

Let us look at these specimens together, taking the heart first. We see at a glance that the murmur was organic—an aortic systolic murmur. The condition found here is remarkable for such a comparatively young man, and is suggestive of protracted and violent overstrain. The valvular flaps are fenestrated and there are several nodular elevations upon and around them. It is evident that they permitted some regurgitation. The walls of the aorta are slightly atheromatous. As to the kidneys, the considerable blanching of these organs by the fluid used in the embalming process, interferes to a great extent with an accurate recognition of their condition, but I venture the assertion that they are somewhat fatty. We now take up the viscera that will determine for us the cause of the hemorrhage. We have here a stomach that displays unmistakable evidences of frequent overdistension. It is enormously dilated, its walls are thickened, the rugæ of the mucous membrane are prominent, and it bears all over its mucous surface the lesions of a chronic catarrh. In some few places the mucous membrane has been thinned; *but upon no part of it is there a sign of an ulcer!* Let us pass to the duodenum. We find it, proportionately, as much dilated as is the stomach. It averages fully eight inches in circumference. Just here, about an inch beyond the pyloric orifice of the stomach, we find a loss of substance which completely encircles its inner surface. Within the limits of this breach of tissue we discover the ragged extremities of a branch of the pancreatico-duodenal artery, which has been ulcerated completely through.

Here, then, is the solution of the whole case. We were dealing with an extensive duodenal ulcer. This lesion is encountered much more rarely than is gastric ulcer, and it is, almost in the same degree, more grave. This is the most striking case of the kind that I have ever seen. There seems to have been no attempt at closure of the divided ends of the artery, by the formation of firm clots. It seems somewhat probable, therefore, that continuous bleeding may have taken place from the time of the last severe hemorrhage until shortly before death. Being only slowly effused, however, the blood passed quietly down into the lower bowel and there accumulated. It was only when the sudden and violent gushes of blood occurred, that the pyloric opening of the stomach was burst through and the excess of fluid ejected by the mouth.

This rather full recital of this man's illness and death, will doubtless impress upon your minds the difficulties of diagnosis and of treatment in such cases, and the very grave dangers which constantly threaten the patient. In looking back over my conduct of the case, I cannot think of anything omitted which might have added to his chances of recovery, nor do I think that anything was done which might have diminished what few chances he had. It was, of course, too late to have hoped to effect a permanent cure. The patient himself was largely responsible for his death, in that he constantly neglected the commonest rules of health, and postponed, until a hopelessly late day, submitting himself to the care of a physician.

COMMUNICATIONS.

OBSERVATIONS ON PUERPERAL ECLAMPSIA.[1]

BY B. F. RECORDS, M.D.,

SMITHVILLE, MO.

Gentlemen: I am aware of the magnitude of the subject I have undertaken to bring before you; also, that it may appear to you presumptuous for a mere country practitioner to attempt to write anything on a disease, the etiology and treatment of which have puzzled the closest observers, as well as having been the source of controversy amongst the ablest writers and thinkers in our profession. My only excuses for my presumption are: first, the rarity of the disorder: it being so rare indeed that the general practitioner sees but a few cases in a life-time, and hence the necessity of occasionally reviewing it, in order to be prepared to meet it when called upon as we generally are when least expecting it. Another reason

---

[1] Read before the Kansas City District Medical Society, March 14, 1889.

is, that as an old practitioner I have seen a good many cases, and formed my own conclusions; not, however, independently of the observations of others more able than myself; yet, they may be somewhat at variance with the opinions of the Fellows of this society—how much remains to be seen.

Etiology.—I see no reason to doubt that albuminuria is the prime cause of puerperal eclampsia. I believe from my own observation, and careful investigation of our best authors, that the mechanical interference with the circulation, occasioned by the enlarged uterus, together with the larger quantity of blood required for the nutrition and development of the fœtus, imposes a greater amount of work upon the heart, the left ventricle of which becomes hypertrophied to compensate for the extra work thrown upon it; thus placing the kidneys on a strain correspondingly, and by these combined forces, brought into and kept in continued action, the latter organs become irritated by overwork and the pressure of the gravid uterus upon the renal vessels, and so allow the superabundant albumin to escape. Dr. W. H. Parish, Obstetrician to the Philadelphia Hospital, in a communication published in the MED. AND SURG. REPORTER, vol. xxxv, said: "Physiologists tell us that the modifications in this (the puerperal state) consist in a lowered specific gravity, an increased amount of water, an increase in the entire bulk of blood, an increase in white blood corpuscles, an increase in urea and in fibrin, a deficiency in the number of red blood-corpuscles, and a deficiency in albumin; also, the disturbance in respiration permits the retention in the blood of more than the normal amount of carbonic acid. There is, in other words, a plethora, a fulness of the entire vascular system, but plethora of hydræmic blood, with a deficiency of those elements destined for nutrition, and a superabundance of those elements representative of retrograde tissue metamorphosis, as urea, fibrin, and carbonic acid. Associated with blood alteration there is an increase in the propelling force of the heart; an increased vascular tension incident to an hypertrophied condition of the walls of the left ventricle, this hypertrophy being an accompaniment of probably every case of advanced pregnancy. . . . Again, the nervous system undergoes a modification apart from its disturbed nutrition. . . . The low specific gravity of the blood, its increased amount, and the increased force with which it is driven through the vessels, all coöperate in greatly increasing the process of exosmosis. This is evinced in the tendency to general anasarca. The intra-cranial tissues partake of this general condition, and there is at first an engorged state of their blood-vessels, then, by the increased exosmosis, an œdema of the brain tissue occurs. If this œdema is marked at the central portions, or the base of the brain, then convulsions may be occasioned, especially if to this state of œdema is added an irritable condition of the brain centre incident to perverted nutrition, and if also, this increased intrinsic irritability is aggravated by irritation reflected from the peculiarly sensitive uterine nerves, or even if this reflected irritation originates in some part not included in the generative organs."

Œdema is not always present in women having puerperal convulsions. Two of my cases (Cases III and IX) had no sign of infiltration, yet the urine in both was albuminous, and by examining the urine of all pregnant women it will be discovered that many patients with albuminous urine present not a vestige of œdema. M. Blot found it in 23 out of 41 cases. It is also well known that there are many cases of Bright's disease without dropsy. "Freirich found that, of 220 cases of Bright's disease, 175 were accompanied with œdema, and 45 were free from it." (Cazeaux.)

The kidneys of women dying in puerperal convulsions have been found to present the characteristic anatomical lesions of albuminous nephritis, according to MM. Cazeaux and Rayner: and they found "in them the second, sometimes the third, and only once the fourth degree of alteration." M. Blot "regards puerperal albuminuria as generally unconnected with Bright's disease." So also, "M. Bach, of Strasbourg, thinks that it is only *sometimes* due to albuminous nephritis, and M. Imbert Goubeyre endeavors to prove that it is always a sign of Bright's disease." (Cazeaux.)

As to uræmic toxæmia being the true cause of puerperal eclampsia, as is frequently claimed, I beg leave—with due deference to the great men of the profession who so contend—to differ. That the convulsions and coma which are observed in uræmic intoxication and albuminuria are similar to some extent, I do not deny; but to my mind that is no sufficient reason for believing that it is due to the former instead of to the latter. I think it would be nearer the truth to consider that uræmia and albuminuria are so intimately connected that their combined influence is required to produce the convulsions and coma of puerperal eclampsia. Dr. Bourneville, in the *Archives de Tocologie*, for April, 1875, says: "1. In the eclamptic state the temperature rises from the beginning to the end of the attack. 2. In the intervals of accession the temperature maintains a high figure, and at the moment the mercurial column registers a slight ascension. 3. Lastly, if the eclamptic state ends in death, the temperature continues to rise, and attains a very high figure; if, on the contrary, the accessions disappear, and the coma diminishes or ceases definitely, the temperature progressively lowers and returns to the normal figure." He adds: "From the first we note a lowering of the temperature in uræmia, and an elevation of temperature in puerperal eclampsia. In the course of uræmia the temperature is progressively lowered, whilst in the course of the eclamptic state it rises more and more from the onset of the accessions, and that with great rapidity. These differences are accentuated at the approach, and even at the moment of death; in uræmia the temperature descends very low, even much below the normal figure; in eclampsia, on the contrary, it attains a very high figure." (*Ranking's Abstract.*) I suppose every one of us can bear testimony to the above evidence of Dr. Bourneville. If so there can be no longer a question as to the cause of convulsions, and the thermometer can decide for us. In the few cases of uræmic intoxication which I have noticed the low temperature and the slow pulse were not to be mistaken.

Whilst puerperal eclampsia is very rare, puerperal albuminuria is very frequent. "Dr. Lantos, of Buda Pesth, has recently made a series of observations on albuminuria of pregnancy in the wards of Professor von Kezmarsky. His paper was published in the *Archiv für Gynäkologie*, vol. xxxii, part 3," an extract of which I quote from THE MEDICAL AND SURGICAL REPORTER, Feb. 16, 1889: "In over 18 per cent. of 70 pregnant women he found albumin in the urine, whilst in nearly 60 per cent. of 600 newly delivered women the urine was albuminous. Albuminuria was detected in over 70 per cent. of 268 primiparæ, and over 50 per cent. of 332 multiparæ. The percentage was distinctly lower in premature labor, and 50 per cent. lower in abortion cases. . . . Out of 14,815 labor cases observed in the course of fifteen years, he noted 53 cases of puerperal eclampsia, a ratio of 278 to 1. Over 78 per cent. out of 42 cases of eclampsia occurred in primiparæ; 15 out of the entire 53 died."

"Pajot found puerperal eclampsia once in 350 cases; Hyernaux, 20 times in 6,370 cases. Its frequency varies with the period of pregnancy; in 200 cases of eclampsia, 60 during pregnancy, 100 during labor and delivery, and 40 during the puerperal state." (Verier.)

Prognosis.—There is no question but that puerperal eclampsia is a serious and dangerous malady. Mauriceau lost 21 out of 42 cases; Velpeau 8 out of 21; Pajot 12 out of 26; Hyernaux 8 out of 20. Madame La Chapelle states that one half of the cases of eclampsia die. In my own cases I lost 1 out of 6, whilst of the patients that I saw in consultation, three in number, *all* died. They were all in a comatose condition from the start, and apoplectic.

The fatality is determined I think by the greater or less quantity of albumin in the urine. Braun has a table of 36 cases which I take from Cazeaux's Midwifery, which is at least evidence of some value.

Albumin was very severe in 3 cases, 2 died.
"	"	"	consid'ble	7	"	4	"
"		"	only	"	14	"	5	"
"		"	"	moderate	8	"	1	"
" .		"	"	slight	4	"	0	"

There is another condition which may or may not be attended with severe albuminuria, and in my opinion is nearly always fatal; I allude to such cases as go almost immediately into what might be termed *apoplectic coma*. Cases IV, VII, and VIII, were such cases. All three were completely comatose, with stertorous breathing when I first saw them shortly after their first seizure, notwithstanding that they had each had the most approved treatment from the start. The cause of death in Case II, I attribute to the fact that the patient was severely albuminous, and had had eleven convulsions before treatment was begun, and was so completely overwhelmed by carbonic and uric acid as to be beyond medical aid.

There are cases of convulsions during and before labor, in which there is neither albumin nor uric acid. They are hysterical, and are not worth a notice in this place.

A strange feature in the cases that I saw, was that three of them occurred in six months of the year 1879, whilst the remaining six were scattered over a period of *twenty* years, from my first to last cases. Cazeaux met with but 3 cases in 2,000 deliveries at the Hôtel Dieu, and then saw 7 cases from July to October, 1846, at his clinique.

Treatment.—The urine of all pregnant women should be tested (if it can be obtained) frequently during the latter months of gestation; especially if there is œdema, or a falling off in the quantity of urine excreted daily, or if there is headache, or other evidence of failing health. Nine times out of ten, however, the physician in the country is not notified that his services will be required, or that the woman is *enciente* even, until he is wanted in great haste to attend her in labor. Many women are confined and "it is all over," when the doctor arrives. I have when engaged beforehand made it an invariable rule to inquire into the condition of my patient's health, and to prescribe if necessary for any deviation therefrom. I think in this way I have perhaps prevented a few cases of eclampsia; at least no case of eclampsia has occurred in my practice when the patient had submitted to prophylactic treatment. Where albumin is found during pregnancy, milk should be prescribed in large quantities; also such diuretics and tonics as may be indicated. It is a good and safe rule, when called to a case of labor, to inquire about the action of the bowels and kidneys. If necessary, draw the water and boil it; if there is albumin enough to endanger the welfare of the patient this rough test will show it. In such a case institute treatment at once. A large dose of sulphate of magnesia or other active cholagogue should be given, followed by acetate of potash, sweet spirits of nitre, buchu, or digitalis.

Supra-orbital pain is a danger signal not to be slighted, and it often precedes convulsions. Here the purgative dose must be followed by raising the head, applying cold cloths to the forehead, mustard to the nucha, and giving large doses of bromide of potash, with tincture of aconite, repeated every half-hour, or hour or two, as indicated. I believe in one case, at least, I succeeded in warding off a severe attack of eclampsia by following the foregoing plan. If I should meet such a case again, and there was apparent cerebral hyperæmia, with the other prodromata, I should, in addition to the treatment named, take blood until the head was relieved.

There are cases in which there is neither infiltration nor supra-orbital pain, and the first symptom noticed is that the patient becomes restless, tossing about without reason, then the eyes turn to the left, and the head follows the eyes, and instantly a horrid convulsion seizes the patient. In such a case the physician has no time for preventive treatment. What to do just at this time, is an important question. Of course nothing can be done during the convulsion. In most cases a hypodermic of one-quarter to one-half grain of morphine, with a dose of tincture of gelsemium, will give time to bleed if the case demands it, or to use whatever, in the judgment of the physician, is indicated. If the patient is hyperæmic, bleed. If she is hydræmic, administer a purgative, and follow with bromide and aconite, and diuretics between the doses of the latter. Then, if the patient does not become comatose, place her under the influence of an anæsthetic. If labor is fairly on the way, it is to be encouraged. If labor is not begun, the uterus should be let alone. If apoplectic coma sets in early, the case is desperate. A large venesection should precede everything else. It should be carried far beyond the amount usually prescribed, if it is to do any good. From two to four pints of blood, or more, must be taken. A decided impression must be made upon the arterial tension. This is the remedy *par excellence.* No patient with eclampsia who was a proper subject for venesection was ever lost by being too freely bled—or, at least, I think so; but numbers of them, I believe, have come to an untimely grave for the lack of a large bleeding. We have all witnessed the remarkably rapid restoration of women who have had post- or ante-partum hemorrhage until they were left exsanguine. Are we to learn nothing by witnessing the wonderful recuperative power of nature in such cases?

There is another and quite a different condition which we frequently meet. It is a hydræmic condition; just the reverse of the foregoing. Here there may be an appearance of plethora, but it is plethora of watery blood. The patient's skin is white, and infiltrated; the muscles soft; the pulse rapid, tremulous and small. In such cases I believe that the lancet is injurious; though I am aware that venesection has been resorted to without reference to the condition of the blood. I have myself been guilty of just such a lack of discrimination. If the patient survived, it was in spite of my foolish treatment.

The lancet will not cure all cases. Indeed I doubt if alone it will cure any. It is only one of the many means to be resorted to. Now I believe that so far as we are able, we ought to adopt a specific or rational treatment. By that I mean that the particular condition of each case ought to be taken into consideration, and the treatment based on the specific indications.

There should be no routine in the treatment of puerperal eclampsia. Routine treatment is a mark of ignorance, prescribing for a name, instead of for a pathological condition. See what the indications are, and meet them intelligently. If your patient's bowels were loose, and thoroughly emptied in a natural way, you would certainly not give her a quarter pound of salts, or five or six drops of croton oil. If she had lost a half-gallon or so of blood, as may be the case in post-partum convulsions, you certainly would not open a vein. By no means. If nature has already removed the red corpuscles from the blood, and replaced them with white corpuscles, you would certainly not assist nature in destroying the vital principle of the blood further by venesection.

The real remedies in puerperal eclampsia are few. In one case the lancet ; in another the hypodermic use of morphia and gelsemium. In another chloral, in twenty to sixty grain doses, by mouth or rectum. In all cases the bromides in forty, sixty or one hundred grain doses, with aconite, and with or without diuretics, purgatives, etc. Then, in some cases, chloroform is the remedy. I do not believe that chloroform or morphia either should be administered where there is deep coma. The reasons for this are self-evident, and need not be discussed. Here the pack should be used, preceded if possible by a bath; but in a country practice the bath is rarely obtainable.

Liebermeister's method is as convenient as any. "The patient is placed in a bath at 98° and the temperature is elevated as much as the patient will bear ; immediately after the bath (which should last until the patient perspires freely), the patient is enveloped in woolen wraps and so remains for several hours." A free perspiration is kept up for several hours. The patient frequently regains consciousness before leaving the bath, others in the course of a few hours, whilst still others become tranquil and go into a natural sleep from which they awake in a day or two conscious. If labor has not begun, it should not be urged, as in many cases eclampsia has preceded labor, coming on a month or so in advance of full term, and if the convulsions can be cut short and the albuminuria cured the patient may go to full term safely.

Dr. Brens, in the *Archiv. für Gynäk.* (as quoted in the MED. AND SURG. REPORTER, vol. xlviii, p. 328), believes that active diaphoresis alone, induced by a hot bath (40 to 45° Cent.) followed by the pack, is sufficient. The bath must not be prolonged over one-half hour, and two or three hours is sufficient for the envelopment in the pack. This treatment, according to Brens, will also cause the œdema and albuminuria to disappear without interrupting the pregnancy.

I have never been situated so as to give the foregoing plan of treatment a trial, yet it commends itself to my judgment as being the only treatment that promises good results in those desperate -cases of coma, either apoplectic or hydræmic. Even when we cannot use the bath, a pack, with the patient surrounded with bottles or jugs of hot water, might, I think, be tried with at least a hope of procuring an abundant perspiration and thus relieving the albuminuria without interrupting the process of parturition, if it be going on ; or labor may be brought on prematurely, in the hope of emptying the womb as a means of relieving the kidneys.

Jaborandi and its alkaloid, pilocarpine, have been by many considered as the foremost of all remedies for the removal of albuminuria, and the control of the convulsions. Where it has succeeded at all it has done so by its powerful diaphoretic action, and as a substitute for the bath and pack before-mentioned. It is to my mind a most dangerous substitute, however ; for, while it is capable of producing the needed diaphoresis, it also is liable to bring on a most dangerous bronchorrhœa which, so far as I know, is uncontrollable. Whilst unloading the blood by cutaneous transpiration, it is filling the lungs and bronchi with a viscid mucus, which the comatose patient is unable to expectorate. Dr. Fordyce Barker gave jaborandi a fair trial in six cases : *all died.* Dr. Barker does not use jaborandi now, I believe. The medical journals a few years ago were teeming with the cures made by the use of pilocarpin ; but like many other new things, it seems to be passing into oblivion—and very justly too, I think. There are many more deaths than cures reported under the use of this potent medicine.

Chloral hydrate should hold a conspicuous place as a remedy in puerperal eclampsia. In large doses, dissolved in mucilage or starch-water, and injected into the bowels, it has been sufficient to keep off the convulsions.

Bromide of potash or of soda, in large doses (30 to 60 grains), combined with aconite, veratrum, or gelsemium, as indicated, is always in order.

There are many other remedies, and expedients which may be resorted to in this malady; but there is no absolute specific for it. The important thing is to understand the specific indications and be governed accordingly.

I have seen and treated altogether nine cases of puerperal eclampsia. Four of them were my own cases. Two more fell into my hands by accident or in the absence of the family physician. The remaining three cases were in the hands of other physicians and I was in consultation. All of the nine cases had albuminuria, and all were œdematous except two.

INTRAPELVIC INJURY CORRECTED BY LAPAROTOMY.

BY N. F. SCHWARTZ, M.D.,
SHANESVILLE, OHIO.

On July 14, 1888, Ida N., 26 years old, unmarried, presented herself for examination and treatment. The patient gave the following history of her case, which I carefully recorded and from which the following is drawn. She has not enjoyed good health for about nine years, during which time she has been under medical treatment almost constantly, without deriving any permanent benefit.

The conditions for which she had been treated were various, all however relating to intrapelvic trouble. Her menstrual derangements have, according to her statement, been of every possible variety; for a long time no two menstrual fluxes have been alike. The patient complains of a feeling of great fatigue, which is intensified when she is in the erect position, or during even moderate exertion of any kind. Sleep is disturbed, and the appetite capricious, though she seems well nourished. She has constantly an indescribable pain in the left side of the pelvis, which at times becomes aggravated, and then she has pain in the back and groin.

The patient first menstruated late in her fourteenth year; menstruation continued easy and regular until the winter of her seventeenth year, when she had a fall, to which she refers the beginning of her present illness. The fall occurred in the following manner: She was carrying a heavy burden down a stone-stepped cellar-way, which was covered with ice; she slipped and, before finally falling, made vigorous efforts to recover her footing, during which she felt as if something had given way, causing her intense pain. She then fell on her left hip and lumbar region, striking with all her weight on a corner of a stone step. She was assisted to her room, and was confined to bed for some time, and from that time to the present there has been hardly a day that she has not had some painful reminder of the accident.

Physical examination yielded very doubtful results. The patient was generally well developed. The abdominal circumference measured twenty-eight inches. The most prominent part of the abdomen was about midway between the umbilicus and the left anterior superior spinous process of the ilium. Pressure over this point elicited some complaint; palpation and percussion yielded nothing of value. Digital examination *per vaginam* showed the uterus to be *in situ*, beyond which nothing was learned. Here, after careful interrogation and reinterrogation, I rested my examination; I was far from any conclusion as to the cause of the symptoms. I prescribed a cathartic, and requested the patient to call again on the 20th, which she did.

On July 20, the patient reported that her bowels had been freely moved by the cathartic. The abdominal circumference was found to be increased to thirty inches in the standing position; the prominence of the abdomen previously mentioned seemed more marked, and deep pressure upon this point communicated a peculiar sense to the touch; the spot remained tender, and all previous symptoms were present and intensified.

The symptoms were certainly so undefined that no opinion could be formed except that there was some intra-abdominal or pelvic trouble or some injury resulting from the fall many years before. No certain diagnosis was arrived at therefore, and of course my prognosis and therapeutics remained equally uncertain. I told the patient and her friends candidly of my inability to make a diagnosis, indicating time and its developments as the all important factor in clearing up the present uncertainties. I stated that, should the present conditions continue to grow worse with time, and destroy her comfort and usefulness, exploratory laparotomy alone would clear up the doubt, and lead to a recognition of her trouble, not omitting to lay before her the danger such a measure necessarily implied.

Several months were allowed to pass, during which some alterative and palliative measures were employed, without, however, checking the rapid increase of the abdominal circumference, nor failure of appetite and painful sleepless nights. One menstrual discharge in this time was profuse and painless, another was scanty and painful.

At this juncture at my suggestion, a practitioner of large experience, who had treated the patient during her failing health, was called in consultation. The consultation, however, resulted in nothing beyond a possible elimination of cyst development, which, on account of the rapid increase in the circumference of the abdomen, was reasonably suspected. Soon after this a consultation was held with another practitioner, who had previously had the patient in charge. The abdominal circumference was now forty inches. This consultant, after a most careful examination, found it impossible to unravel satisfactorily the perplexities surrounding the diagnosis.

Desiring still further to temporize, we determined to test the value of electricity. I accordingly resorted to the galvanic current, employing for this purpose a Harris battery, applying one pole over the sacrum with the other over the greatest prominence of the abdomen, thus continuing the static current for about fifteen minutes, the current being as strong as could be borne. This caused her much suffering for many hours following its use, and she objected to its repetition vigorously—but finally yielded to its application a second time. It however had the same result as before, causing much pain, and she would not again permit its employment.

The patient now demanded whatever there might be in laparotomy for her, as she was miserable and practically useless, desiring even to brave the hazard of surgical measures than to undergo longer the disappointment of experimental therapeutics and live a useless existence. The gravity of exploratory section was fully made known to her and to her family; the risks even, possibly, overdrawn; she, however, nothing daunted, desired the operation, not alone to have her trouble recognized and corrected, but also to silence the slimy tongue of scandal which was already wagging against her; and she preferred even to die if necessary, in vindication of her character.

I now acquainted Dr. John Homans, of Boston, with some of the salient facts in the case, and he very promptly suggested "a clean antiseptic exploratory laparotomy" as the proper thing to do to clear up any doubt in the case. And having exhausted the resources of even experimental therapeutics without benefit, I deemed it a duty to operate.

Every precaution, to the minutest detail, for complete antisepsis was observed, omitting the spray; and my patient and family yielded an intelligent obedience to every demand made upon them in carrying out the necessary antiseptic precautions before the operation, as well as in excluding the crowd of curious visitors afterward.

The rules as laid down by Prof. William Goodell, in Pepper's System of Medicine," governed my course throughout. The operation was done in a second story room of a large farm-house, with the assistance of my student Dr. J. G. Stucky, who assumed charge of the case for the three days next succeeding the operation, remaining with the patient.

The incision was made in the linea alba and was about three inches in length. The abdominal walls were found thick, and the recti muscles pressed fully an inch to the right side. In the pelvic cavity there was found left lateral flexion of the uterus, enlargement of the Fallopian tube on the left side. The tube contained fluid, but was not distended. The ovary was in front and under the tube, and was enlarged to the size of a large English walnut. The ovarian ligament was found overlying the tube near the uterus, and its terminal extremity about half twisting the tube upon itself. The parts were held in these different positions by adhesions.

There evidently had been a laceration of the posterior portion of the broad ligament at the time the patient had the fall, many years before, which alone could render such a displacement of the ovary possible; and the fall at the same time caused the tube to be held in such unnatural position as to render it almost impervious. I will not here attempt to say how the conditions described could act as a cause of long years of distress in an otherwise healthy patient. Suffice it to say, the correction of these different malpositions has relieved the patient *entirely*, and, since the fourteenth day after the operation, she has resumed her part in performing domestic duties with an ease and comfort not possible in many years. She now menstruates regularly and without pain, though somewhat scantily.

The recovery from the operation was prompt and easy, unmarked by a single unfavorable symptom. The only anodyne used was opium in a few suppositories.

Remarks.—In performing this operation I unfortunately overreached the limitations fixed by some of my neighboring fellow practitioners, exploratory laparotomy; and my operation, though as successful in its results as could be wished, is looked upon as a violation of a "time honored custom," and I am criticized for performing it out of season. I am also reminded that I "found no tumor"; and so, because I did not discover in my patient's abdomen a tumor as large as a prize pumpkin at a county fair, my undertaking is declared a failure, etc.

As general practitioners of medicine and surgery of the latter part of the nineteenth century, we are met at almost every turn by some new problem, and measures which for many years remained in the hands of specialists, powerful for good or equally potent for evil, are becoming proper for general practitioners. Their intelligent comprehension and proper use are necessary in meeting the growing demands of the present time.

To us the practical needs of humanity are best known, and the questions of the hour have become a part of each day's study; and upon their correct interpretation depends much of the happiness or woe of those placed in our care. Moreover, as the conservators of the lives and health of those in our care, our duties, under the explicit professional mandate, *to restore health and preserve life without hazard, when possible,* and, *at all hazards when necessary,* cannot be performed in a merely perfunctory way.

Eager haste in using dangerous resources should and will always be discountenanced by careful practitioners, but dogged prejudices against their use when necessary are also reprehensible. Exploratory section, though practised for many years by specialists, hospital staffs, and many surgeons of large cities, beyond these environments has hardly attained recognition, and remains relegated to the realm of *post-mortem* surgery.

In advocating or contemplating laparotomy as an available diagnostic measure in general practice, that healthy conservatism which should preside over all important surgical means placed in our hands for use, when necessary, should not be ignored. It is a double-edged weapon of undoubted keenness, and is to be used only when we are reasonably assured that the end will justify the means.

The gravity of the operation will, and should, always keep it out of the fascinating current of fashion which has brought valuable operations into undeserved disrepute; *e. g.,* Emmet's operation—an operation of undisputed merit—was practised by some surgeons to an extent bordering, if indeed not trespassing, on the ridiculous. Every woman who came under the care of these enthusiasts was found on examination to have one or more lacerations of the cervix uteri, and "must have an operation performed."

It is one of the great triumphs of modern surgery that general practitioners may now extend to those situated away from special skill the advantages of both exploratory laparotomy and ovariotomy, which were hitherto accessible to only a privileged few.

Abundant proof of the value and comparative safety of exploratory section, when it is done in accordance with the well-established rules of antisepsis, may be found in surgical literature of the present and past years; and yet there remain those who continue to refuse patients this means and will temporize until nature asserts her inexorable claims, when no time is lost to make an autopsy and *find the cause of death,* great pride being taken in exhibiting *post-mortem* trophies.

Another reason urged against the performance of exploratory laparotomy by some surgeons throughout country districts is the fear of criticism by an uneducated laity. Medical men must necessarily be their own missionaries; they alone are to blame if Voodooism and religious superstition continue to obtain among the persons with whom they have lived for any considerable time. Intelligent persons will naturally seek for information concerning the healing art, and its limitations, whilst the ignorant should be enlightened as to our powers—and who are more competent than we to do it?

It may be fairly maintained that the degree of intelligence of a community upon matters pertaining to the medical profession is a fair index of the qualifications of their medical advisers; therefore the plea of an ignorant laity is in a great measure only a reflection upon him who offers it. Public opinion cannot guide us in our choice of means when dealing with disease, but we should pilot public opinion in all matters of reform and progress within our profession.

Such a position alone can command the confidence of the people and lead them to accept eagerly and confidingly any measure, however hazardous, when it is required to supplement the strong hosts of the materia medica in the battle against disease and death.

———◆◆◆———

—The Indiana State Medical Society will hold its next annual meeting on Wednesday, May 1, at Indianapolis.

SOCIETY REPORTS.

NEW YORK ACADEMY OF MEDICINE.

Stated Meeting, April 4, 1889.

The President, A. L. LOOMIS, M.D., in the Chair.

An oil portrait of Ex-President A. Jacobi, M.D., was presented to the Academy by Dr. August Caillé and some of his colleagues.

Dr. T. GAILLARD THOMAS read a paper on

Acute Mania and Melancholia, or Hypochondriasis, as Sequelæ of Gynecological Operations.

His object was to place on record what he thought must be rather a remarkable experience as to the occurrence of these conditions. He stated at the outset that he did not announce these alarming conditions as complications or necessarily as results of operative procedure, but merely as sequelæ which may or may not be dependent upon the operation; and he did not assert that operations for the relief of diseases of women are more likely to be followed by them than other operations.

The author related six cases which had come under his observation, four of which were cases of acute mania, and two of melancholia. In four of the six there was evidence of eccentricity even before the operation, and in two of the four cases it was quite marked at times. In all the six, except one, there were distinct prodromal symptoms following the operation and antedating by some days the formal outburst. In the other the symptoms of acute mania came on rather suddenly, and resulted fatally within thirty-six or forty hours. In none could he discover an hereditary tendency to insanity. Of the six, four died, one completely recovered, one was still in progress. In all excepting one the urinary secretion was carefully watched and examined, and in none did the kidneys appear to be factors in the mental state. In four of the cases no iodoform at all was used, so that in them there could be no question of iodoform poisoning as a factor. In the two remaining cases the little that was used was along the line of external abdominal sutures, where absorption was almost impossible. His long experience with septicæmia barred that out as a factor.

In addition to his six cases, Dr. Thomas was able to find recorded in medical literature but twenty others, which would seem to show great rarity of the condition. Before concluding, he propounded the following questions:

1. Were these twenty-six cases of mania and melancholia really due to the operations which immediately antedated them, or did they follow as mere coincident states? 2. Any great mental strain may be followed by mania; is it at all remarkable that in the vast number of gynecological operations performed in the last quarter of a century in Germany and America that twenty-six cases of this malady should have occurred? 3. If the mania which followed the operations in the twenty-six cases was the consequence of them, how in the future is the tendency to this accident to be avoided? 4. Are the operations in gynecology any more likely than other surgical procedures to disturb the condition of the mind?

DR. J. B. HUNTER opened the discussion. He does not think gynecological surgery is more liable to the accident than other surgery. The condition does not seem so rare, for at a meeting a few nights before the surgeons present all related similar experiences. He has himself seen several cases. He divided the cases into four classes: 1. Those in which the condition is due entirely to the operation; these are few. 2. Those in which there is predisposition to nervous development, the operation acting simply as a torch. 3. Those in which the patient is already the subject of nervous disease, which simply progresses after the operation. 4. Those in which there is drug poisoning, as by iodoform, bichloride of mercury, carbolic acid, etc. He also thought ether in some patients who had a predisposition might bring on insanity. A psychological condition should not interfere with the operation unless it was incipient insanity. Then the operation was justifiable in as much as it benefited psychological patients oftener than it brought on the condition described in the paper. Operations exposing a large surface might possibly tend more to the condition by offering a better opportunity for drug poisoning.

DR. NICHOLS, Superintendent of the Bloomingdale Asylum, said only two cases of insanity following gynecological operations had been in the hospital in the past eleven years, one of which was in a patient of Dr. Thomas's. He thought long contemplation of an operation might place the mind in a favorable condition for insanity before or after the operation.

DR. P. F. MUNDÉ had had three cases of insanity following gynecological operations, his first patient, seven or eight years ago, dying in a maniacal state. He then supposed it was due to septicemia, but is now convinced that it was not. Another case was one of melancholia, of recent date, showing itself partly in refusal to speak for three or four days after the operation. In the third case the operation was Alexander's, with antero- and postero-kolporraphy for prolapsus. The patient remained maniacal two weeks after the operation, and recovered. He does not believe iodoform has anything to do with the condition, for in some cases wounds were packed full of iodoform and mania did not follow.

Dr. W. M. POLK thought it was only to be expected that mental disturbances were more likely to occur in gynecological operations than others, or in women than in men, for the female sex is more emotional, and once a month many women who at other times show the best judgment and greatest business ability, are so irritable as to be incapable of managing ordinary domestic affairs. He much prefers not to operate on women who beforehand show any mental peculiarity or eccentricity, for he has had three cases of insanity following operations on such patients, all of the patients dying. One of his patients had a sister who also was peculiar.

Dr. W. GILL WYLIE had had but one case of insanity following a gynecological operation, but he had operated on a number of patients who were already wholly or partly insane, sometimes with the result of curing the mental condition. The treatment of the rectum and colon which in such patients are often diseased has a markedly beneficial effect on the nervous disorder. His mind is not yet fully made up on the subject of the paper.

Dr. TOWNSEND, of Albany, related a case in which salpingo-oöphorectomy was performed during the past winter on a woman who, about seven days after the operation, became markedly melancholic and hysterical, and went on to develop acute mania. She died comatose, apparently from exhaustion, as was true in most of Dr. Thomas's cases. This patient showed marked hydræmia before the operation.

Dr. LANDON CARTER GRAY thought to Dr. Thomas belonged the credit of having described a new genus of insanity. His six cases corresponded to none of the described forms in all respects. They properly belong to delirium grave—most of the cases of which die—and to the form called post-febrile insanity. He would distinguish it as post-operative insanity, rather than as acute mania or melancholia following gynecological operations.

The PRESIDENT mentioned a case of his in which Dr. Lange removed one kidney, the operation being followed some days later by acute mania, from which the patient finally recovered and still remains perfectly well.

Dr. THOMAS, in closing the discussion, referred to some of the side questions which had been raised, among others that of iodoform poisoning, and said it was a serious question whether or not, if iodoform were capable of producing such grave symptoms as had been described, its use were justifiable at all. As to ether producing insanity, he thought from long experience that it was impossible, yet he had had such disagreeable results from its use after laparotomies, in the form of prolonged vomiting, etc., that he thought it a serious question whether American surgeons would not do well to abandon its use for that of chloroform in abdominal surgery. Regarding the influence on the patient's mind of long contemplation of the knife, he thought it was marked, and for that reason he advised his students always to remove tumors of the breast, of whatever nature and whatever size. It would do no harm. It might prevent cancer. It certainly would relieve the woman's mind. He left it for others to answer the questions which he had propounded.

—The committee appointed to investigate the discovery of M. Pasteur for the extermination of rabbits in Australia has made a report of the result of their inquiries, which states that upon experiment it has been found that rabbits which had been inoculated with the virus of chicken cholera, or which ate food which had been infected with the virus, died, but that the disease was not communicated by one rabbit to another.

—The *New York Tribune,* March 26, 1889, says that F. W. R. Waring, who has practised medicine under the name of "Dr. Thomas McGahan," was sentenced March 25 by Judge Cowing to five years in the New York State Prison for violating provisions of the Medical Code of New York State. The sentence is the most severe that has been passed under the code, but the defendant had been indicted for manslaughter in causing the death of a woman several years ago, and was twice tried on the charge.

REPORTS OF CLINICS.

PHILADELPHIA HOSPITAL.

CLINIC UPON OBSTETRICS—DR. PARVIN.

Inflammation of the Breast After Death of the Infant.

The first patient presented at Dr. Parvin's clinic, on February 27, was a woman, twenty-five years old, who more than three weeks ago had given birth to a child that died three days subsequently; a few days afterward inflammation of the breast was observed. There was a chill, and some continuous elevation of temperature succeeded it. The inflammation had extended so that suppuration seemed inevitable, notwithstanding that ice had been used, and then compression of the diseased gland with a bandage, the internal employment of quinine and of salines. Referring to this case Dr. Parvin said: Mammary inflammation occurs, according to Winckel's statistics, in about 6 per cent. of all lying-in women, and the vast majority of those thus affected are primiparæ. The disease appears most frequently in the second or third week of lactation; it usually begins with a chill, which is succeeded by fever, and, according to Schroeder, if the fever continues to the third day suppuration is almost inevitable. It has generally been held that the disease is in most cases a lymphangitis, and has its origin in disease of the nipple, such as fissures and excoriations, the infecting agent entering through these breaches of tissue. But now it seems to be well established that the infection may find its way not only through these wounds and the lymphatics, but also through the milk canals, for bacteria have been found in the milk in the yet undiseased gland. An interesting fact may here be stated, that these bacteria have the power of changing the normal alkalinity of the milk, and this fluid becomes acid: it would be well if the Resident having charge of this patient, would ascertain whether the statement can be verified in her case—that is, as to the milk having become acid. The staphylococcus is the one most frequently found in lobular inflammation; Cohn discovered in a non-suppurating parenchymatous mastitis a peculiar streptococcus. Further, it has been shown that in phlegmonous mastitis the streptococcus pyogenes is present. These facts as to the different bacteria present in mammary inflammation, are briefly presented in the last edition of Schroeder's work upon obstetrics.

Two remarkable things are to be noticed in this case. First, the inflammation occurred without any previous disease of the nipple, at least none was observed. Next, the little elevation of temperature the patient has had—it has seldom risen above 100°, F. Now the first fact can be explained only by admitting the hypothesis that the infection entered through a milk duct, and this view is further sustained by the statement that the inflammation began in one of the lobes of the gland. A question of some practical importance is, what effect if any has arrest of lactation upon inflammation of the gland; or, in other words, will the retention of milk be injurious? In the great majority of cases this question may be answered in the negative. Winckel makes the statement almost in this form; and he adds that he has never seen sudden interruption of lactation the cause of mastitis. So positive was I, indeed, in reference to this point that my axiom for many years was, milk does not make matter. It may, however, be now stated that in some cases it is possible that the entrance of microörganisms through the milk ducts into the milk may produce such changes in the milk that mastitis results.

In the treatment of mammary inflammation as you meet it in the nursing woman, the first thing is to take the child from the breast; next properly support the organ, and probably give a saline. Then you will consider the two methods which, as you know, have been vainly tried in this case—ice, and the compressing bandage. A few years ago a physician living near Philadelphia, whom all men honor for his many years, his faithful labors, and his useful life, Dr. Hiram Corson, wrote a paper strongly advocating the use of ice, stating that he had always had favorable results in mammary inflammation when the remedy was employed soon enough. Then again the bandage has been just as strongly advocated by others. And I must say that between the two my preference is for the latter. Schroeder recommends the ice treatment only in case the inflammation is superficial. But my preference may be a mistake; there are many things in medicine in regard to which we had better say, we believe, rather than we know. We are so eager for certainties that there is something very fascinating in positive utterances, in the declaration of what is claimed to be absolute truth, in dogmatisms. And here, without any reference to the therapeutic views which have been presented, but speaking in general, it seems to me that there is no class of men who need to have impressed upon their minds more strongly that one swallow does not make a summer, than young physicians and medical students. How often one hears physicians who have lived for some years veiled in their own vanity, and with very limited knowledge, endeavoring to set aside truths established by large inductions, because their experience is different. A man who imagines that the feeble light of his "tallow-dip" will reveal to him such vast knowledge that he need not care what others have discovered, and that he is in a position to contradict their discoveries, is one of the most dangerous of human beings, and at the same time he is one of the most useless in his vain boasting and self-glorification.

Returning to the treatment of this patient, I do not think any further continuance of the quinine is indicated, the elevation of temperature is so slight; the saline may be still used, and so too the bandage will be applied, for it gives the patient comfort; but it will hardly prevent the formation of an abscess.

Before leaving the subject of mammary inflammation, let me refer to a form of the disease which occupies only a superficial portion of the gland, and the presence of which does not require taking the child from the breast. This has been called sub-areolar inflammation; a tumor as large as a filbert, as a hickory nut, or even as a walnut appears, is sensitive, though not exceedingly painful, and soon suppurates: free exit for the pus being made rapid healing follows. This superficial mastitis need not interfere with nursing. In the graver forms of suppurative mastitis an early opening should be made, all antiseptic precautions being used, and a drainage tube inserted. In regard to the gravest form of mastitis, that which occurs as one of the manifestations of general septic infection, rare even in such infection—which itself is not frequent and is becoming still less so with the advent of physicians who believe in antiseptic obstetrics — I shall not speak to-day.

Striæ upon the Abdomen, the Hips, and Mammæ.

This woman is presented before you that you may see an unusually striking instance of the striæ gravidarum, which in her not only occupy two thirds of the anterior abdominal wall, but are also found upon the hips, and especially upon the mammary glands. She is now seven months advanced in her pregnancy, and the abdomen seems very greatly distended, though there is no reason for believing there is either plural pregnancy or polyhydramnios. Having in a previous lecture considered at some length the origin and significance of the striæ of pregnancy, I shall not speak of these topics to-day.

Pulmonary Tuberculosis and Pregnancy.

Two weeks ago there was brought before you a primigravida, seven months pregnant, who had tuberculosis, the disease involving both lungs. She had been married less than a year, and, a little before she became pregnant, as she said, "caught cold," and ever since has been losing flesh and strength. A few days ago this woman had premature labor, and her child died; the disease has been making rapid progress since, so that her death may occur almost any day. The case illustrates what you will too often be called to witness, the usually injurious influence of pregnancy upon so-called consumption; or if there is a temporary improvement while the woman carries her child, the labor is frequently followed by a more rapid progress of the disease. In many cases the pregnancy does not go to term, miscarriage or premature labor occurring: these accidents in some instances result from the violent coughing, in others from the death of the fœtus, and in still others possibly from the imperfect aeration of the blood, that is, accumulation of carbonic acid excites uterine contractility. The teaching when I was a medical student was different from that which I believe it my duty to give you; how well I remember that most courtly gentleman, that accomplished teacher and learned physician, the late Dr. George B. Wood, telling us that he had in many instances seen the disease kept at bay in women by marriage and childbearing. The investigations of the late Dr. Austin Flint have shown, on the other hand, that in a large proportion of women pregnancy and lactation are important factors in the development of the disease. Therefore it is best, so far as the woman herself is concerned who already has pulmonary tuberculosis, or has any decided tendency to such disease, not to marry; and if married it is fortunate for her if she do not become pregnant. Even if she escape the death penalty, she can not expect to bring into the world healthy children. Marriage is no more an infirmary for consumptive women than it is a reformatory for debauched and drunken men.

A Case of Justo-Minor Pelvis.

The patient now lying upon the table is said to have a justo-minor pelvis, that is, a pelvis which, theoretically at least, has all its diameters uniformly lessened. But, that you may properly appreciate the fact, her pelvis will be measured before you, and the measurements obtained contrasted with those of the normal pelvis, putting the two side by side upon the black-board.

The distance between the anterior superior spinous processes of the ilium are in this pelvis,

Twenty-four centimeters. In the normal pelvis, 25. Between the iliac crests, 25c. In the normal, 28c. The external conjugate is 19.5c. In the normal, 20c. Distance between the trochanters is 28c. In the normal 31c. The circumference of the pelvis is 83c. In the normal 90c.

But in order to complete the pelvimetry we should have the diagonal conjugate, by deducting 2 centimeters from which we have, in most cases pretty accurately, the true conjugate. In an effort to ascertain the diagonal conjugate it was difficult to reach the promontory, and in such case the usually just conclusion is that the true conjugate is not materially shortened. Still more, the measurements of the pelvic outlet must also be obtained before we can conclude that the pelvis presents all the characters required in the term justo-minor. But it is not necessary to carry this examination further, for while all the measurements made are less than the normal, yet the differences are not great, and it is quite probable that the labor will not require any aid from art.

Nevertheless a word or two upon labor and its management in the justo-minor pelvis. The descent of the head into the pelvic cavity, which occurs in the great majority of cases of primigravidæ in the latter weeks of pregnancy, is not observed, and labor begins with the head at the inlet; strong flexion is necessary to secure its entrance, and such flexion is the rule during the entire passage through the pelvis. The labor is longer than in the case of a woman with a normal pelvis, and the caput succedaneum of unusual size. Nevertheless you would not think of trying to shorten the labor before the head had been very completely moulded, by the application of the forceps. Further, you would regard it as fortunate that the vertex presented rather than the pelvis, for the delay in the passage of the head would in the latter case be so great that the child's life must be lost almost inevitably. It is hardly necessary to add after this statement, that podalic version is contra-indicated in the justo-minor pelvis.

An interesting fact in the history of this patient is, she had typhoid fever a few weeks ago, but as you see the pregnancy was not interrupted, nor was there any threatening of miscarriage during the illness. It has been claimed by some authorities that pregnancy in a good degree exempts women from typhoid fever; but such an opinion is not generally held. Very frequently the pregnancy is arrested by the disease—according to some statistics in more than one half the cases; but it is probable that these statistics are derived chiefly from hospitals in which cases of especial gravity are found, and that if we were to collect from a large number of physicians in private practice their results, the conclusion would be different. This opinion is based upon the fact that I so frequently read in medical journals, or hear reported in medical societies, cases of typhoid fever in pregnancy, and the latter pursuing its normal course. Various explanations of the death of the fœtus and the consequent interruption of the pregnancy, have been given. One of these is that high maternal temperature (the fœtal as you know being greater normally than that of the mother) brings danger and death to the fœtus. This conclusion was drawn from experiments upon pregnant animals, in which miscarriage was caused by subjection to very high temperature. But experiments made subsequently proved that if the elevation of temperature was gradual this result did not follow, but the pregnancy continued. Probably the most frequent cause of miscarriage or premature labor in the pregnant woman suffering from typhoid fever is hemorrhagic endometritis.

Accidental Hemorrhage.

If hemorrhage occurs in a pregnant woman, the placenta occupying its normal situation, the hemorrhage is called accidental. Recently one of the women, in the waiting-ward, quite far advanced in pregnancy, went out to visit some friends; the night after this visit she had severe hemorrhage, losing according to the statement of the Resident at least a quart of blood. There were bruises upon the abdomen, but the woman would not acknowledge that she had met with accidental or intentional injury. The treatment employed was successful in stopping the bleeding, and the chief part of that treatment was thorough tamponing of the vagina. After her recovery it was impossible to hear the sounds of the fœtal heart ; her pregnancy, however, went to term, when she was delivered of a dead child, the death having occurred at least several days before. The failure to hear the fœtal heart sounds in several trials, after having previously heard them distinctly, is quite conclusive evidence that the child is dead. Recently a new proof of the death of the fœtus has been brought forward, and this is the presence of peptones in the urine of the mother— that is, she has peptonuria. Now if a sufficient number of observations come to confirm this statement, the fact will be one of very great value, so that we will not need stethoscopic examinations to decide as to the death of the fœtus. Unfortunately this method of examination was not suggested in the case considered.

A word or two in regard to the treatment of accidental hemorrhage. The admirable paper by Dr. Goodell upon this subject, which was published some years ago, is a fountain of knowledge from which all who ever write upon accidental hemorrhage necessarily draw ; it proved how very dangerous this occurrence is to both mother and child. Yet I think that possibly those who advocate immediately emptying the uterus, as most obstetricians do, as the essential thing in the treatment of accidental hemorrhage, are too positive, too absolute in opinion, too active in practice. This case which has been narrated to you illustrates the fact that by the tampon the danger was averted so far as the mother was concerned—it is probable no treatment would have saved the child. Spiegelberg and others, who have opposed immediate delivery, take the ground that with the unruptured membranes you have most effective pressure for the arrest of the bleeding ; when those membranes are ruptured and the amnial liquor escapes, unless vigorous uterine contractions follow promptly, hemorrhage is invited, not restrained. Thus you will see that this is not as simple a question with only a single answer possible, as some think. There are comparatively few things, in obstetric therapeutics at least, in regard to which you may positively say, " This, and this only, is true."

I think that the course pursued in the case presented was wise, and the immediate induction of labor would have been most perilous to the mother : therefore the action of the resident physician is to be commended.

When to Interfere in Acute Intestinal Obstruction.

At the meeting of the Medical Society of London, Feb. 18, 1889, Dr. B. W. Richardson read a paper with the object of eliciting an expression of opinion as to the proper moment for resorting to surgical interference in cases of intestinal obstruction. He confined his remarks to acute attacks, leaving aside all cases of the chronic kind, from malignant stricture or hernia. He narrated a typical case which he said might serve as the base of his observations. The patient was a man who had gone to bed in apparent good health, but was awakened during the night by violent pain in his abdomen, and special symptoms pointing to mechanical obstruction high up. He was called to the case by Mr. Buckston Browne. Purgatives had been tried without effect, and a long tube was passed into the bowel and an injection used, but without affording any relief. There was no fever, but the conjunctivæ were tinged slightly yellow. There was an obscure history of gall-stones some years before. On making a careful examination of the abdomen, a well-defined hard substance could be felt in a line with the transverse colon, movable laterally but not in any other direction. They arrived at a diagnosis of obstruction caused by impacted gall-stone. The patient complained of nausea, but there was no vomiting. They injected a copious enema of oil, and soon after a fair-sized gall-stone passed from the rectum. This was followed by immediate relief, but some hours later the pain returned, and then there was vomiting with a fecal odor. They determined to try another injection of oil, and other mild measures, and to operate in the morning if relief was not obtained. During the night the symptoms recurred with such violence that the patient rapidly passed into a condition of collapse, and died before anything could be done. At the *post-mortem* examination they tried what could have been done by operation, and they found that they could easily have come upon a calculus fixed in the lower part of the small intestine, a little above the cæcum. This could have been pushed along the' gut and extracted without difficulty and without opening the intestine. Three other small calculi were found in the colon, and at the entrance to the common bile-duct there was some ulceration and adhesion, together with an abscess of the substance of the pancreas. He discussed the nature of the case and the chances that early operative interference would have been followed by relief to the symptoms. He summarized his conclusions as follows: 1. That in all cases of acute intestinal obstruction the use of milder measures, such as purgatives, enemata, massage, etc., may safely be carried out until the supervention of fecal vomiting. 2. That as soon as this is established an exploratory incision into the abdomen should be made without delay. 3. That obscurity of diagnosis, in the presence of this symptom, should not be allowed to stand in the way of an operation. 4. That clinical experience shows that there is very little chance of recovery, when once stercoraceous vomiting has declared itself, unless an operation is performed. 5. That fecal vomiting is a symptom of much more gravity than would attach to the mere mechanical effect of obstruction. 6. That symptoms of collapse are not a contra-indication to operative interference.

Mr. Edmund Owen observed, in regard to the question as to when to operate in acute intestinal obstruction, that some men would say, when the physician has done his best or his worst; as a general rule the surgeon is called in too late. He urged that the symptom proposed by Dr. Richardson as the test would not be applicable to a large class of cases in which the obstruction is high up, say in the jejunum. In such cases fecal vomiting can not take place, and if the patient is allowed to go on while they wait for that sign, his chances of recovery will be few.

Mr. Bryant urged that surgeons should be guided less by this or that sign than by the diagnosis of the particular nature of the strangulation. He objected to the term obstruction, as applying only to the cases in which the difficulty came from the inside, by far the least frequent source of mischief. In any case he thought that much valuable time would be lost if the advent of fecal vomiting were awaited; by that time a great deal of the mischief is done. He said that directly the surgeon was satisfied that there were symptoms of strangulation he should be prepared to operate.

Dr. Ruth protested against too speedy a resort to operative procedures. He said he had met with a great many cases in which recovery had ensued without operation, although stercoraceous vomiting had occurred. He advocated a freer use of antispasmodics, such as chloroform and belladonna.

Dr. Richardson, in reply, admitted that he had not mentioned the cases of obstruction high up. Such cases are very rare. He prefers the term obstruction as more comprehensive than strangulation. He doubts the ability of the surgeon to arrive at a differential diagnosis in a large proportion of the cases, and fecal vomiting is generally the first sign to impress the medical attendant with a sense of the gravity of the case. If the plan suggested by Dr. Ruth were confided in, the patients would often die, for want of more radical measures.—*British Med. Journal,* Feb. 23, 1889.

Symmetrical Gangrene.

In the *Medical Chronicle,* Feb., 1889, Joseph Collier reports a case of symmetrical gangrene, or Raynaud's disease, occurring in a single woman, 20 years old. After giving a full account of the case and of the results of the autopsy, he says that from the point of view of causation, the disease seems to fall into one of several groups:

1. Those due to a direct stimulation of the peripheric ganglia. In this group are the cases with gangrene dependent on vascular spasm, produced by some altered condition of the blood. Of course in these cases the production of gangrene will be partly due to mal-nutrition of tissue, and partly to action of the blood on the higher cerebro-spinal centres, as in cases of paroxysmal hemoglobinuria.

The gangrene of Bright's disease, and of diabetes mellitus, will be to some extent produced in this manner. The vaso-motor symptoms in alcoholic paralysis are probably also due to the circulation of impure blood.

2. Those due to irritation of prevertebral sympathetic ganglia, or vaso-motor nerves leaving them, as in the author's own case.

Probably pathological conditions of the large abdominal sympathetic ganglia are much commoner than is usually suspected, especially in anemic girls of the age of those generally attacked by Raynaud's disease. Dr. Donald has pointed out to Mr. Collier as an interesting fact in this connection, the frequency with which epigastric pain in anemic girls is associated with pulsating aorta, and a form of constipation due partly to anemia and partly, no doubt, to splanchnic spasm. Many vaso-motor fibres accompany the spinal nerves, and thus in those cases in which gangrene from neuritis approaches the paroxysmal form, it will be to some extent due to action of these fibres.

3. Those due to irritation of central origin, as in a case of gangrene of the

left hand recorded by Hochenegg, in which chronic hydrocephalus and syringomyelia were found at the autopsy. Cases more or less due to emotional origin would come into this group.

4. Those due to some peripheral stimulation acting reflexly through cerebro-spinal centres. Thus, cutaneous sensory fibres irritated by cold, or in the cases of symmetrical gangrene from sclero-derma. Here again part of the action of peripheral neuritis in producing arterial spasm will be produced in this manner. In the cases of the disease associated with syphilis, congenital or acquired, it is difficult to be positive that endocarditis, or some other arterial degeneration, has not been the main cause.

Case of Cerebellar Abscess.

Dr. George Buchan communicates an account of a case of abscess of the cerebellum in the *Glasgow Medical Journal*, Feb. 1889. The patient was a woman, a mill-worker, 63 years old, and was admitted into the Town's Hospital on May 15, 1888. She was a very healthy woman, and never had any very serious complaints, and was always at work until the illness to be described began.

About a week after New Year's she began to complain of symptoms resembling a severe coryza, but only on one side of the head, the right. There was running at the nose (right nostril), watering of the right eye, and at times an involuntary winking of the right eyelids. This continued for about a week, when a severe pain began in the right occipital region, which gradually extended all over the right side of the scalp and stopped at the right eye. The pain was not continuous, but came and went. A fortnight later she began to vomit occasionally a very bitter green stuff, which she thought was the bile, and at same time began to feel at times a giddiness in the head, and was languid and tired about her legs; to assist her when she was coming home from her work she would get between two of her fellow-workers, and, placing an arm in each, was thus steadied and helped very materially in the getting home. On account of the vomiting she consulted physicians, who prescribed for biliousness. The patient continued in this state for about a month or six weeks, still at work, but tired, languid, and feeble about the legs, with a sensation of swimming in the head, and always liable to fall; in the house, if she was bending down for anything, she would fall down altogether, and she got

many a fall that way. She then had to take to her bed. She was restless in bed—one time at the head and another time at the foot of the bed; she also became very irritable in her temper, and her niece could not put up with her any longer. She applied to the Parochial Board, when she was visited by the district doctor, who said the trouble was nervous debility, and ordered her removal to the hospital.

On examination in the hospital she was found to be fat and well nourished, lungs and heart normal, abdominal organs normal, no albumin in the urine, and the quantity of urine normal. She complained of diarrhœa and slight vomiting; and on examination it was found that the stools were loose, but the bowels were not frequently moved. The tongue was clean; there was no nausea; and the vomiting, even in the worst attacks, occurred quite mechanically. She took her food fairly well, but as a rule for some time after her admission she vomited always a little of the food. On looking at her face, there was a peculiar leer about the right eye, which reminded Dr. Buchan of the look of one trying to make fun of another. Pupils were regular and responsive to light, and there was no complaint about her eyesight; she could see as well as ever she did; her hearing also was quite good, and there was no history of her ever having had suppurating ears. There was no paralysis anywhere; the reflexes were normal. In bed she lay principally on her right side with her legs drawn up, her head drawn a little backward and to the right, boring into the pillow. She could turn herself any way, and draw up and put down her legs. On being assisted out of her bed and asked to walk along the floor, she could do so as long as she was holding on by the bed, but no farther. Dr. Buchan on the one side and the nurse on the other tried to help her along, but she was just like one miraculously drunk. She tried to steady herself but could not—her legs bent under, her feet slid away from her. Thus reeling backward and forward, she would have fallen backward and to the right had she not been kept up. By a process of exclusion he came to the opinion that this case was one of cerebellar disease, as the characteristic symptoms of this lesion—staggering gait, vomiting, giddiness, drawing back of the head, and to the right in this case, and severe occipital pain—were present. The pain, however, was not at the seat of lesion, as some authorities state, but at the opposite side. The patient continued in this state quite happy and contented and taking her food well, when about three weeks before death she 'began to complain of a numb feeling in her lip and arms, her speech became thick, and there was a slight difficulty in swallowing. This continued for a week, when paralysis of the lip and arms set in, and she could no longer feed herself. There were no rigors or sweatings at any time. Four days after this the temperature rose a little (99.6°), and paralysis of the sphincters set in, and two days before death there was stupor and coma.

At the autopsy the membranes of the brain were found fairly healthy, with here and there evidences of old slight inflammatory adhesions between the dura mater and the arachnoid. The left lobe of the cerebellum had a soft, pulpy feel, and on turning upward the base of the brain, there were found five or six openings on the posterior inferior lobule of the cerebellum, out of which a yellowish, glairy fluid was oozing. Dr. Buchan describes it as having just the appearance of a discharging carbuncle before the slough separates. On cutting two or three of the divisions and tearing up the part, a ruptured encapsuled cavity was displayed, as large as a medium sized egg. This ruptured cavity explains the symptoms noted thirty-six hours before death.

Hernia of the Parturient Uterus Through the Linea Alba.

In a paper read before the Medical Society of the District of Columbia, October 31, 1888, Dr. Charles E. Hagner said that in July, 1884, he delivered a primipara, after a prolonged labor, of a full-term female child. Forceps were used, with slight laceration of the perineum, which was immediately stitched up and healed perfectly. The patient made a good recovery, and showed no signs of ventral hernia. In March, 1886, Mrs. B. was delivered of a second full-term female infant without forceps, the perineum remaining intact, the labor being a short one (six hours), and perfectly normal. Within three months the patient called his attention to a "lump" about the umbilicus. Upon examination he found an umbilical intestinal hernia, about the size of an egg, which was readily reduced, the opening being large enough to permit the introduction of the end of the finger. An abdominal truss was ordered which retained it perfectly. The patient wore this until she was taken in labor with her third child, in Feb. 1888.

On Feb. 8, 1888, he was called to see Mrs. B., and found her in the first stage of labor, the os dilating and the pains frequent. He remained an hour, when, everything progressing normally, he left her for an hour and a half. Upon his return he found the bag of waters ruptured, the patient in bed and in active labor; the os fully dilated, the head engaging L. O. A. The labor progressed normally and actively for about an hour and a half, examinations being made from time to time. Suddenly the patient, after a very violent pain, called out and said: "Oh doctor, I am tired out, I can no longer bear down." It had been about ten minutes since Dr. Hagner's last examination. On approaching the bed, he observed that the abdominal tumor, heretofore perfectly normal, presented a peculiar appearance, being much more prominent, and seeming to project at right angles to the patient's body, who was lying on her back. Upon lifting the sheet, he was startled to find that the uterus had left the abdominal cavity, and was covered only by the skin, which was very tightly stretched, and seemed as thin as tissue paper. The uterine vessels were clearly seen, also the contractions, when a pain came on. The head at this time was in the vagina, and he immediately saw that the woman was correct in saying that she could make no expulsive effort. Notwithstanding the uterine contractions, which were regular and strong and visible, the head made no advance, and the patient becoming exhausted, Dr. Hagner immediately applied the forceps and delivered the child. There was no difficulty in applying the forceps, as the head was well down, but the impossibility of restoring the uterus to its normal position, and its tendency to fall to one side or the other, made it necessary to have the nurse support it in the median line until the child was extracted. It proved to be another fine healthy girl. The placenta was quickly extracted by the hand, as the patient seemed exhausted, and Dr. Hagner was most anxious to terminate the labor.

As soon as the placenta was removed there was little trouble in replacing the uterus through the opening in the walls of the abdomen, it having thoroughly contracted and reached its proper size. A suitable bandage was applied, and the woman made a good recovery. It is surprising, he says, to find how small an opening there seems to be in the abdominal wall at present. The woman is wearing the abdominal bandage she wore before her last pregnancy, and says she suffers no inconvenience.—*Jour. of Amer. Med. Association*, March 2, 1889.

THE
MEDICAL AND SURGICAL
REPORTER.

ISSUED EVERY SATURDAY.

CHARLES W. DULLES, M.D.,
EDITOR AND PUBLISHER.

The Terms of Subscription to the serial publications of this office are as follows, payable in advance:

Med. and Surg. Reporter (weekly), a year, **$5.00**
Quarterly Compendium of Med. Science, - 2.50
Reporter and Compendium, - - - - 6.00
Physician's Daily Pocket Record, - - 1.00
Reporter and Pocket Record, - - - - 6.00
Reporter, Compendium, and Pocket Record, 7.00

All checks and postal orders should be drawn to order of
CHARLES W. DULLES,
N. E. Cor. 13th and Walnut Streets,
P. O. Box 843.   Philadelphia, Pa.

☞SUGGESTIONS TO SUBSCRIBERS:
See that your address-label gives the date to which your subscription is paid.
In requesting a change of address, give the old address as well as the new one.
If your REPORTER does not reach you promptly and regularly, notify the publisher *at once*, so that the cause may be discovered and corrected.

☞SUGGESTIONS TO CONTRIBUTORS AND CORRESPONDENTS:
Write in ink.
Write on one side of paper only.
Write on paper of the size usually used for letters.
Make as few paragraphs as possible. Punctuate carefully. Do not abbreviate, or omit words like "the," and "a," or "an."
Make communications as short as possible.
NEVER ROLL A MANUSCRIPT! Try to get an envelope or wrapper which will fit it.
When it is desired to call our attention to something in a newspaper, mark the passage boldly with a colored pencil, and write on the wrapper " Marked copy." Unless this is done, newspapers are not looked at.
The Editor will be glad to get medical news, but it is important that brevity and actual interest shall characterize communications intended for publication.

THE STATE BOARD OF MEDICAL EXAMINERS.

Since our last Editorial in regard to the proposed law to establish a State Board of Medical Examiners in Pennsylvania, the bill before the House of Representatives has been amended by adding a proviso that at no time shall a majority of the members of the Board belong to any one school of medicine. This proviso has been inserted on the recommendation of the homœopaths, who protest that if the old school were in possession of a controlling power in the Board it would sooner or later use it to oppress practitioners belonging to other schools. This fear is not unnatural, although we believe it to be unwarranted. Our hope has been that the establishment of a State Board of Medical Examiners would tend to obliterate the distinction between those who practise according to the dictates of common sense and sound reasoning, whether they are openly attached to the school which holds this to be the only proper method or are called by a name which implies that they follow some other and more restricted one. In this way, we have hoped—and see no reason to conceal the fact—that before long the title of physician would come to be sufficient for all who practise medicine, and that medical schools would have no other ambition than to teach their students thoroughly the nature and effects of disease and the means which experience has shown to be the best for curing it. In regard to these points men have differed in all ages, and it may be long before the wisest are of one mind; so that there is room for honest variance in theory and in practice, and there ought to be tolerance between those who differ, while yet all are pressing forward toward the same goal. Of oppression there ought to be no question, and we regret that the homœopaths have so little confidence in the sincerity and fairness of those who make up the overwhelming majority of the medical profession.

At the same time we are so convinced of the desirability of having the right of licensing men to practise medicine taken from the medical schools, that we would rather have a Board constituted after a concession to the unreasonable fear of the minority than no Board at all, and we feel sure that the result of its operations would be to secure for our fellow-citizens a better class of physicians than can be secured so long as each medical school may fix the grade of attainments for its own graduates and have its diploma stand as well before the law as that of any other.

So far, then, as the amendment referred to

is concerned, we trust that it may not prove an obstacle to the passage of the proposed law in Pennsylvania.

Another amendment has been proposed by the active supporters of the bill, which is intended to make it more beneficial to the community. This amendment requires that those who apply for a license to practise shall have passed through a four years' course of study in a chartered medical school. The effect of this amendment, would be to compel all the schools in this State to adopt a four years' course, and to incite all the schools in the Eastern States to do the same, as otherwise their graduates would be disqualified for practising in Pennsylvania.

If this amendment be adopted it ought to be developed, so as to define what a year of study is to mean. Without such a development, it might soon prove a farce.

CONFERENCE ON YELLOW FEVER IN FLORIDA.

The epidemic of yellow fever in Jacksonville, Florida, last year impressed upon the State the necessity for the creation of a State Board of Health, and one was called into existence, too late to be of service in that epidemic but with the hope that its counsel might aid the citizens and physicians of the State in the attempt to prevent a repetition of the sad experiences they had recently passed through. The State Legislature at its last session adopted a resolution inviting a commission of sanitary officials to visit Jacksonville and other points in Florida exposed to outbreaks of yellow fever, and to confer with the State Board of Health as to the best means to prevent a recurrence of the epidemics of previous years. In response to this invitation, a number of gentlemen, representing the sanitary authorities of different sections of the country, started from Washington April 1, and the result of their mission will be looked for with much interest.

It is to be hoped that the visitors will succeed in giving the aid, by counsel and moral support, which is looked for by the newly created State Board of Health in Florida. If they make a careful inspection of Jacksonville, and if they confer with men who feel that it is better to heal a sore than to clap a plaster on it and say it is well, they will undoubtedly find opportunity to make suggestions which that city might wisely adopt. At the present time it is in a condition which falls far short of the standard of cleanliness which prudence dictates, and its sanitary arrangements are by no means what they ought to be. These matters will no doubt attract the attention of the visiting sanitarians, to whom a rare opportunity for useful work is open.

It is to be hoped that this year no serious outbreak of yellow fever will occur in the South; and, if it does, we hope that its management will not be in the hands of men whose recommendations reflect the ignorance and senseless fear of the middle ages. Cleanliness, calmness and intelligent views as to the nature of yellow fever would banish it almost wholly from the Florida peninsula; and we trust the conference which has just taken place, and the coöperation which will doubtless follow it will contribute materially toward the attainment of these conditions in regions where yellow fever has heretofore occurred.

DENTAL FISTULÆ.

The recent report by the *Deutsche Monatschrift für Zahnheilkunde*, December, 1888, of a remarkable case of dental fistula, in which an opening near the nipple of the left breast was found to be caused by disease of the roots of the first left lower molar tooth, furnishes an illustration of the importance of bearing in mind the possibility that disease of the teeth may manifest itself in comparatively remote lesions. One who is sufficiently impressed with this fact may often find a way to cure sinuses or fistulæ which otherwise would baffle treatment.

It ought to be a rule with physicians and surgeons to examine the teeth of their patients whenever there is the slightest reason to believe that they may be a cause of obscure disorders. This rule applies obviously to fistulous openings upon or near the face; and the case cited shows that what seems an almost incredible distance may be traversed by the products of a diseased tooth. It also applies to other disorders, such as neuralgia, and affections of the ear, which are not infrequently dependent upon disease of the teeth. Various specialists have called attention to this matter at different times; but there is still some propriety in directing the attention of general practitioners to it, and in suggesting to them that they may often find an educated dentist a valuable colleague in the management of their patients.

LABOR IN WOMEN WITH FLAT PELVES.

The disputed question as to whether it is best in cases of labor complicated by minor degrees of flattening of the pelvis—in which the natural forces are incompetent to effect delivery—to render assistance with the forceps or by version, is still awaiting authoritative settlement. The impossibility or undesirability of applying the forceps to the sides of the head when it is arrested at the brim in the flattened pelvis, on the one hand, and on the other the fear that by applying them to the sides of the pelvis over the sinciput and occiput, the cross diameters —bi-temporal or bi-parietal—which are engaged in the contracted conjugate, may thereby be increased, tend to cause the obstetrician to select version rather than the forceps. Since the invention of Tarnier's forceps, however, the tide of opinion which was setting in favor of version under the conditions named, has been checked, and the forceps are now in greater favor.

Several points bearing upon this question are brought out in a paper by Dr. R. Milne Murray, in the *Edinburgh Med. Journal,* Nov., 1888. He reports two cases of labor in women having flat pelves of minor degree, in which he effected delivery with Tarnier's forceps, as modified by himself. One woman had been delivered once prematurely, and once by turning after the failure of the classic forceps. He delivered her with surprising ease with Tarnier's forceps. The second woman was a primipara, and she also was delivered with comparatively little difficulty. After referring to the general belief that the application of the forceps over the brow and occiput causes an increase in the transverse diameters of the head, he points out that the effect of compression with the axis-traction forceps must be the same as with the classic forceps. To permit of traction a certain amount of compression must be applied, and consequently the locking of the transverse fœtal diameter in the maternal conjugate diameter, if it occurred with the older pattern must likewise occur with the new; and yet delivery is effected generally with the axis-traction forceps with comparative facility in the minor degrees of contraction. This fact throws doubt upon the theory that increase in the transverse diameters does result from the application of the forceps over the brow and occiput.

To settle this point nine recently delivered fœtuses were taken for experiment. A cephalotribe was placed with its blades accurately applied over the occiput and sinciput and the compression-screw then turned until the bones began to show signs of giving way under the compression. At intervals the occipito-frontal, bi-mastoid, bi-temporal and bi-parietal diameters were carefully measured. The occipito-frontal diameter was reduced from an inch to an inch and a half, yet in spite of this very great reduction the transverse diameters underwent hardly any change, although the compression used was far greater than can be made with the forceps. This shortening of the long occipito-frontal diameter without corresponding increase of the transverse diameters, is explained by Dr. Murray by the fact that the occipital and frontal bones, under the compression of the forceps slide under the borders of the parietal bones—the head "telescopes" from before backward—while at the same time the vertical diameters of the head become elongated. Dr. Murray also considers the effect of applying the forceps obliquely—one blade over one side of the brow, the other over the opposite side of the occiput—and concludes that it is far less advantageous than the application directly over the brow and occiput, since the "telescopic adjustment" is entirely lost, and since the compression of one oblique diameter of the head tends to produce a lengthening of the free oblique diameter.

The experiments of Dr. Murray are of great interest from their bearing on the question of the application of the forceps at the brim of the pelvis. They will go far to do away with the fear of increasing the transverse diameters of the head by applying the forceps over the occiput and sinciput. The experiments are the more interesting as being made in Edinburgh, the home of Simpson, the father and great exponent of the doctrine that, when the head is arrested at the superior strait by contraction of the conjugate diameter of the pelvis, the proper obstetric procedure is version rather than the use of the forceps.

TAMPONNING FOR POST-PARTUM HEMORRHAGE.

There has been considerable discussion of late in Germany in regard to the value of a method of treating *post-partum* hemorrhage which was warmly recommended by Dührssen in the *Centralblatt für Gynäkologie*, No. 35, 1888. This method consists in tamponning the uterus with a long strip of iodoform-gauze, so as to promote contraction of the uterus and to stop the bleeding, partly in a mechanical way, and all with a material which might safely be allowed to remain in the cavity of the womb.

Notwithstanding the successful employ-

ment of the method by Dührssen, it has been opposed as dangerous as well as unnecessary, if other well-known methods were used. On the other hand, Dr. Becker, of Hamburg, in the *Berliner klinische Wochenschrift*, Feb. 18, 1889, comes to the support of Dührssen, and by argument and by citing his own experience maintains that the method of the latter is a very valuable procedure, and that it may be relied upon in cases which seem to baffle every other resource of the obstetrician.

In this we believe that Becker is right, and that tamponning the uterus with iodoform-gauze for post-partum hemorrhage is a safe and excellent method. It has never yet—so far as we know—given rise to iodoform poisoning, and it has certainly checked hemorrhages which had resisted other measures faithfully tried before it was employed. There is much in its favor theoretically, and practically it has accomplished about as much as could be asked of any claimant for professional approval.

Of course it will be understood that no such heroic method as this should be employed where a simpler one will do. There are few cases in which intrauterine injections of hot water, and especially hot water with a little vinegar added, will not control post-partum hemorrhage ; and, as a clean and convenient method, which leaves no foreign body in the uterus, it is preferable to any other. But, if simple measures fail, one must have more powerful ones, and a careful packing of the uterus with antiseptic gauze might prove of the greatest utility.

—The *New York Medical Journal*, April 13, says that during the four weeks ending Tuesday, April 9, the following numbers of cases and deaths from infectious diseases were reported to the Sanitary Bureau of the Health Department of New York City : Typhoid fever, 32 cases and 10 deaths ; scarlet fever, 1,710 cases and 228 deaths ; cerebro-spinal meningitis, 12 cases and 8 deaths ; measles, 678 cases and 66 deaths ; diphtheria, 739 cases and 189 deaths ; small-pox, 1 death.

BOOK REVIEWS.

[Any book reviewed in these columns may be obtained upon receipt of price, from the office of the REPORTER.]

A TREATISE ON HEADACHE AND NEU-RALGIA, INCLUDING SPINAL IRRITA-TION AND A DISQUISITION ON NORMAL AND MORBID SLEEP. By J. LEONARD CORN-ING, M.A., M.D., Consultant in Nervous Diseases to St. Francis Hospital, New York, etc. 8vo, pp. viii, 231; illustrated. New York: E. B. Treat & Co Price, $2.75.

The title of the book gives a good general idea of its contents. The first part of the book is taken up with a consideration of headache and neuralgia. In the treatment of the latter he lays great stress upon the value of antipyrin and cocaine. His method of using cocaine is deserving of mention. An instrument is first employed which at one stroke makes a number of needle-point punctures in the skin of the affected area; a sponge electrode saturated with a five per cent. solution of cocaine is placed over the punctures and connected with the positive pole of a three or four cell galvanic battery; another electrode saturated with warm water is placed on the skin near, but not in contact with, the first, and connected with the negative pole of the battery. The current is then passed for ten or twenty minutes, and it causes the absorption of the cocaine solution. To prolong the contact of the anæsthetic with the affected nerve, he has devised the following procedure: a piece of wire gauze, cut to fit the affected area, is firmly pressed into the skin and held there by a suitable compress. This checks the flow of blood in the part and so prevents the anæsthetic from being washed away.

The book is stamped strongly with the individuality of the author. Some exception might be taken to the freedom with which he uses cocaine, for it is by no means free from danger. The book would also be the better for more careful proof-reading. But it is full of useful hints upon treatment, and will well repay the time spent in reading it.

FIELD'S MEDICO-LEGAL GUIDE FOR DOC-TORS AND LAWYERS. By GEORGE W. FIELD, LL.B. 6¼ x 4¾ inches, pp. viii, 291. Albany and New York: Banks and Brothers, 1887. Price, sheep, $2.00; cloth, $1.75.

This is an interesting little book, and one which may be useful to many a physician. It is written, we believe, from the standpoint of the State of New York, but it contains valuable information, applicable in all parts of the United States, in regard to the status before the courts of medical witnesses, the decisions in regard to expert testimony, the legal view of insanity, the nature of privileged communications, of abortion, of liability for neglect or malpractice, and the rights of physicians to compensation.

Questions are often asked of the Editors of medical journals which are fully answered in this book, and physicians familiar with its contents would be saved from errors which are sometimes committed through ignorance of the way in which the law looks at subjects which physicians often consider quite differently. Nothing in it is of more interest than the discussion of the physician's liability for malpractice and his claims for compensation; and we would advise any of our readers who are engaged in actions, or suits, involving either of these matters to learn what the book before us teaches, as it may help them very materially.

PAMPHLET NOTICES.

[Any reader of the REPORTER who desires a copy of a pamphlet noticed in these columns will doubtless secure it by addressing the author with a request stating where the notice was seen and *enclosing a postage-stamp*.]

243. THE INFLUENCE WHICH THE DISCOVERY OF COCAINE HAS EXERTED ON OPHTHALMIC SURGERY. By SAMUEL THEOBALD, M.D., Baltimore, Md. From the *Transactions of the Medical and Chirurgical Faculty of the State of Maryland*, 1888. 3 pages.

244. IS ASTIGMATISM A FACTOR IN THE CAUSATION OF GLAUCOMA? By SAMUEL THEOBALD, M.D., Baltimore, Md. From the *Amer. Journal of Ophthalmology*, October, 1888. 7 pages.

245. PULMONARY CONSUMPTION CONSIDERED AS A NEUROSIS. By THOS. J. MAYS, M.D., Philadelphia. From the *Therapeutic Gazette*, November 15 and December 15, 1888. 63 pages.

246. DOES SPECIAL MEDICAL LEGISLATION IMPROVE AND ELEVATE THE PRACTICE OF MEDICINE? By G. W. PICKERELL, M.D., Indianapolis, Ind. From the *Indiana Eclectic Medical Journal*, October, 1888. 11 pages.

243. Dr. Theobald's paper describes very briefly the advantages of cocaine anæsthesia in operations for cataract, and in the application of agents such as sulphate of copper and nitrate of silver to the eyes, as well as in the treatment of strictures of the nasal duct.

244. Dr. Theobald answers the question which heads his article in the affirmative. In his experience astigmatism—and especially that form of astigmatism in which the meridian of least refraction is vertical, or nearly so—is a very frequent concomitant of glaucoma, and he is disposed to think it has a causal relation with it. His pamphlet contains a brief account of the history of twelve cases which he has studied in a comparatively short time, and which seem to support his opinion.

245. In an editorial in the REPORTER, January 26, 1889, we gave an outline of the contents of this pamphlet by Dr. Mays, which indicated the views which it advocates, and our reflections upon them. It will suffice here to say that Dr. Mays states the reasons which have led him to look upon pulmonary phthisis as a neurosis of the pneumo-gastric nerve—an opinion which is curious enough to attract considerable attention, and which he supports with considerable ingenuity.

246. It is not surprising to find a professed "eclectic" arguing against legislation to regulate the practice of medicine, and any one who reads this pamphlet will not be surprised that its author should undertake the task. He objects to such legislation for various reasons, one of the most amusing of which is: " 5. I object, because it places the medical profession under police regulation and servililaip (sic), ignobling the noblest calling of man to that of the criminal code. '*Registration*, smile at it as we may, implies baseness, criminality, the tendency of which is to cast suspicion and dishonor upon him who is required to register.'"

It is painful to observe, also, that he regards the "sickening cant about 'protecting the dear people'" as a mere "subtifuge" (sic). This is too bad; and men like Dr. Pickerill can hardly be expected to take kindly to anything which would bear so hard on them.

NOTES AND COMMENTS.

Medical Examining Boards.

The Alabama *Medical and Surgical Age,* February, 1889, says that the necessity for Medical Examining Boards for different States has been thoroughly discussed by the press of this country during the past year. Those who have taken the position that a diploma from a reputable medical college should entitle the holder to practise medicine anywhere in the United States, and that said parchment is sufficient protection for the people, would profit by seeing the written examinations of a number of graduates who have been examined by the County Boards in Alabama. They can form a meagre idea of some of these examinations by reading in the Transactions of the Medical Association of the State of Alabama the criticisms of the State Board of Censors. These criticisms are as fair and free from prejudice as is possible for any criticism to be; for the State Board of Censors had nothing to do with making the examinations, and in a large majority of instances knew nothing of the applicants. This board reviews the examination papers sent up by the County Boards, and then makes such criticisms upon County Boards and applicants as are thought to be deserving and expedient.

A few of the criticisms made by the State Board of Censors, and published in the Transactions of the Medical Association of the State of Alabama for 1887 and 1888, are then quoted. In making these criticisms, the Board of Censors gives the name of the applicant and the college at which he graduated, but for prudential reasons the *Age* does not give the names.

In reviewing the examination of a graduate of a Tennessee college, the Board says: "Applicant is utterly ignorant of both medicine and English, and the wonder is how any college could graduate, or board license such a man."

The same board says of another Tennessee graduate: "He ought to have been rejected on his spelling, though there was sufficient reason without that. His answers are not only incomplete in every case, but are often incorrect.

Of two Georgia graduates, the board says: 1. "The applicant exhibits a lamentable ignorance of medicine." 2. "He answered almost nothing."

It says of the examination of one of the graduates of a Kentucky college: "Applicant shows the most astonishing ignorance of medicine, and if he carries into practice some of his ideas of treatment, will materially diminish the population of his community."

These are only a few of the many criticisms of a similar nature. They show not only the necessity for a board to examine graduates, but the absolute necessity of a law requiring a preliminary examination to the study of medicine.

Chronic Cocaine Poisoning.

M. Magnan, at the Société de Biologie, lately (*Progrès Médical,* No. 5) described three cases of chronic poisoning with cocaine characterized by marked mental and sensory disturbance. The first case was one in which cocaine had been substituted for morphia in the relief of renal colic. After two months' use of the drug the patient began to suffer from illusions of sight and hearing and neuro-muscular irritability. He discontinued the cocaine for six months, resorting to morphia; but on again resuming cocaine the delusions recurred, the patient feeling imaginary blows on the body, or something under the skin, together with a certain degree of analgesia. At the end of a short time he had an epileptic seizure. In the second case (one of hepatic colic) the same substitution of cocaine for morphia had been effected, and produced very similar effects, also terminating in an attack of epilepsy. The third patient also presented hallucinations of sight and hearing, sensation of foreign bodies beneath the skin, and slight analgesia. M. Magnan pointed out that in its action on sensation and the sensory organs cocaine seemed to resemble the alcohols and absinthe rather than morphia, with this difference, that whereas the influence of cocaine poisoning seemed to operate on the cerebral cortex from the occipital lobes forward, alcohol and absinthe appeared to affect the cortex in the reverse order.—*Lancet,* Feb. 9, 1889.

Insanity and Sex.

The Medico-Legal Society of New York City has sent out circulars containing questions to be submitted to those in charge of insane patients, with a view to finding out what proportion of the insanity in this country is the result of sexual causes. The chairman of the committee in charge of the inquiry is Edward W. Chamberlain, 120 Broadway, New York City, who will be glad to hear from any one having facts on the subject in question to communicate.

Dr. Holmes and His Books.

Dr. Oliver Wendell Holmes, in the course of an address delivered to the Boston Medical Library Association, at the formal presentation of his medical library, said: "The most interesting parts of a miscellaneous medical library are its oldest and its newest portions. Between these is a long, dreary interval, filled up by books not old enough to be curious or even rare, and not new enough to represent the existing state of knowledge. I am thinking especially of works on practical medicine. We care nothing, or next to nothing, for the speculative notions of such writers as Forestus and Fernelius. The theories of Stahl and Van Helmont, of Hoffman and Boerhaave, the conflicts of the Brunonians and the adherents of Cullen, mean as little to the physician of the present as the farrago of remedies with which they puzzled the astonished and indignant viscera of their patients. Still, something may be gained from these obsolete and utterly neglected writers. They were not all fools because they had not the wisdom which comes with the knowledge of a later day. There were, and are always, men of common sense—good, strong, coarse common sense—in the medical profession. Sydenham was one of these. I believe I have hardly ever delivered a medical address in which I have not referred to the 'roast chicken and pint of Canary' which he prescribed for a patient affected with what a Dublin physician might probably call 'male hysteria.' I have always thought it a stroke of genius in Dupuytren—if the idea was original with him, but I have an impression that it was borrowed from an earlier authority—when he ordered a patient to drink the milk of a goat which had been rubbed with mercurial ointment, the patient having a dread of mercury as commonly administered. That was a kind of infinitesimal dosing, and I have no doubt that the patient got as much good from the mineral in the goat's milk as the Sultan did from the drugs in the handle of the bat with which he exercised every day until he was in a free perspiration. But Sydenham's prescription was the best lesson the over-drugging doctors ever got, unless it may be from watchful mothers and keen-witted, observant nurses.

"As I have referred to the infinitesimal dosing business, let me remind you that if you wish to understand the pseudo-scientific vagaries of to-day you will find more instruction in the 'Ortus Medicinæ' of Van Helmont than in any other old work with which I am acquainted. The infinitesimal, or make-believe, dosing is to be found in the chapter entitled 'Butler.' Butler was an Irishman in a Belgian jail, where Van Helmont found him. He had a pebble which he used to dip in oil, then take a teaspoonful of that oil and add it to a small flask of the same oil and apply one drop of this to the ailing part. Then he would give his pebble a lick with his tongue, and clap it in his waistcoat pocket. This whole chapter, 'Butler,' should be read by the student of Hahnemann and by all intelligent students of medical history. The doctrine of the 'mind cure' is abundantly illustrated in other chapters of the 'Ortus Medicinæ,' the date of which in my copy, now yours, is 1652."—*Boston Med. and Surg. Journal,* February 6, 1889.

Clairvoyant "Physicians."

The Legal News quotes the opinion of the Supreme Court of Wisconsin, by Lyon, J., holding that a clairvoyant physician is liable for failure to exercise the ordinary skill and knowledge of a physician in good standing, practising in the vicinity, and not merely to the ordinary skill and knowledge of clairvoyants. If he holds himself out as a medical expert and accepts employment as a healer of diseases, but relies for diagnosis and remedies upon some occult influence exerted upon him, or some mental intuition received by him when in an abnormal condition, he takes the risk of the quality of accuracy of such influence or intuition. There are so many persons now who assume to act as physicians and take the lives of people in their hands that this decision holding them to a strict liability may perhaps be timely.—*Journal of Amer. Med. Association,* April 13, 1889.

Disinfection of Cities and Towns after Yellow Fever.

The *Atlanta Med. and Surg. Journal,* April, 1889, says that the Quarantine Conference which met at Montgomery early in March, refused by a decided vote to endorse the proposition that it is necessary to disinfect a town or city, in which yellow fever had prevailed, but in which there had been no cases for several months, and after the place had been subjected to the frosts and freezings of winter; deeming that the use of disinfectants, under these circumstances, was not only useless but tended to breed unnecessary terror and distrust, not only among the people of the place, but among those of surrounding States.

Brain Softening from Thrombosis.

Renvers (*Deutsche med. Wochenschrift*, Nov. 17, 1888) reports the case of a man 55 years old, who was deaf from bilateral suppurative otitis media from his youth, and who for several years had had a paralytic weakness of the left extremities, as well as left-sided homonymous heminanopsia, with the light reflex intact. This patient developed left-sided hemiplegia and deafness of the left ear after an apoplectic attack. After a few weeks there was a second attack with coma, in which the patient died.

At the autopsy extensive yellow softening was found in the right hemisphere, which had been brought about by arterio-sclerotic thrombosis of different terminal branches of the artery of the fissure of Sylvius. The middle halves of the anterior central convolution and a part of the first and second frontal convolutions were also softened, and a strip of the first parietal gyrus and the whole of the second parietal gyrus, from which the softening extended into the middle gyrus of the temporal lobe and upon the second occipital gyrus. The remaining parts of the brain were intact. In the motor and frontal region the softening was confined to the cortex, while in the other places it stretched to the white matter. In the pyramidal paths there was secondary descending degeneration.—*Centralblatt f. d. med. Wissenschaften*, Feb. 2, 1889.

Case of Colocynth Poisoning.

Dr. Jansen communicates to the *Therapeutische Monatshefte*, No. 1, 1889, a curious case with symptoms of poisoning attributed to colocynth. It seems that a healthy woman, 44 years old, was suddenly taken sick on September 6, after she had brewed as a bug-killer about twenty-five colocynth fruits, which had been purchased at a shop, in a pint of urine. The patient asserts that she poured the fruit whole, without touching it, from the paper in which it came into the vessel, and that in doing so she neither noticed dust nor was conscious of a bitter taste. At noon she complained of severe dizziness, loathing of food, but no vomiting. On the following morning there was violent diarrhœa, which continued two days. At this time there was moderate pain in the abdomen, headache, thirst, loss of appetite, nausea, coated tongue. In the evening she was somewhat chilly. On the third day the throat and face were swollen and painful, but there was no difficulty in swallowing; there were also œdema of the feet which continued fourteen days, and a moderate amount of albumin in the urine. On September 20, the patient was emaciated and complained continually of dizziness on movement, headache, loss of appetite, oppression after eating, belching of wind, weakness and faintness, moderate constipation. Examination showed nothing abnormal in the different organs; the urine contained no albumin; free hydrochloric acid was continuously absent from the stomach for weeks.

How the poison in question could have penetrated into the body seems doubtful. It would be plausible to suppose that it passed into the stomach in the form of a light powder, although the occurrence of a bitter taste in the mouth was denied. It might also have been a volatile poison inhaled in the vapor and so entered the circulation. The hitherto isolated active principles of colocynth—colocynthin, colocynthidin, as well as citrullin—are of course not volatile.

This and similar cases, he says, indicate the need of precaution. The sale of substances such as colocynth, whose highest dose is four and one-half grains, should be governed by more stringent regulations than have heretofore been imposed upon it.— *Wiener med. Presse*, Feb. 3, 1889.

Influence of Eruptive Fevers upon Syphilis.

Marius Auriel, in a recent Paris thesis, expresses the opinion that in the influence of eruptive fevers upon syphilis two different modes of action may be considered. The first is a general influence profoundly modifying the organism and substituting itself for the diathesis so as to cause its disappearance. Except, perhaps, in the case of variola, this curative action is problematic. The second mode of action of dermatoses upon syphilis is purely palliative. "It is limited to causing the disappearance, by a kind of local revulsion, of atonic ulcerations and malignant eruptions which treatment is unable to overcome." Without going as far as Garrigues, who, with Hardy, does not hesitate in a similar case to advise inoculation with small-pox, Auriel admits that this happy local influence exists. Diday has reported one observation in which a rebellious syphilide was seen to retrocede and disappear. The favorable influence of erysipelas in analogous cases has been attested by numerous observations. The truth of the fact is therefore beyond doubt. —*Gazette médicale de Paris*, Jan. 19, 1889.

Case of Eruption from Rhubarb.

At the meeting of the Berlin Medical Society, January 30, 1889, Dr. Litten exhibited an interesting case of drug eruption which had occurred in the patient for the fifth time. On the 23d of January the patient received a prescription for infusion of rhubarb (8 parts to 200) with bicarbonate of soda, and also a solution of chloral to be injected into the rectum. As the patient had before repeatedly had an eruption after taking rhubarb, he at first refused to take it, and indeed received only a teaspoonful instead of a tablespoonful. A half hour afterward, before the chloral had been injected, the exanthem appeared. This consisted of large-sized hemorrhagic maculæ, and of a severe pemphigus, which was accompanied on its appearance with severe chills, and developed especially on the elbows, hands, feet, scrotum and penis. The whole mucous membrane of the mouth, tongue, hard and soft palates was likewise covered with elevations of the epidermis. The separate dark-red spots the size of the palm of the hand remained unchanged under pressure, and had their seat especially upon the trunk, the extremities, the throat and the face. Since the 27th of January the hemorrhagic spots had gradually faded and the pemphigus blisters dried.—*Deutsche med. Wochenschrift,* Feb. 7, 1889.

The Contagiousness of Tuberculosis in Man.

At a recent meeting of the Board of Health of the Health Department of the City of New York a resolution was passed to the effect that Dr. T. M. Prudden, Dr. H. M. Biggs, and Dr. H. P. Loomis, the pathologists of the department, be requested to formulate a brief and comprehensive statement regarding the contagiousness of tuberculosis in man, stating the evidence of the same, and recommending in the briefest possible manner practicable the simplest means of protection from its influence.

Blue-Black Writing Ink.

A correspondent of the *Scientific American* submits the following formula:

Tannic acid	gr. cc
Gallic acid	gr. l
Protosulphate of iron	℥ i
Indigo carmine (neutral)	gr. cccxx
Powdered cloves	gr. v
Water	Oi

Dissolve the tannic and gallic acids in the water. To this solution add the iron salt, and filter through cotton. Then add the indigo carmine, and lastly the cloves. One good copy can be obtained from this ink.

NEWS.

—The Governor of Pennsylvania has signed the bill to regulate the practice of veterinary surgery in the State of Pennsylvania.

—The Memphis Hospital Medical College held its commencement March 29, and conferred the degree of Doctor of Medicine on 62 graduates.

—On April 7, the temporary hospital building of the U. S. Marine Hospital Service, at Cape Charles, Va., was destroyed by the surf during a severe storm.

—The Governor of Iowa has issued a proclamation revoking the cattle quarantine against States other than Connecticut, New York, New Jersey, Delaware and Maryland.

—Dr. E. L. Keyes has resigned his position as Professor of Genito-Urinary Diseases, Syphilography and Dermatology in Bellevue Hospital Medical College, and has been succeeded by Dr. Samuel Alexander.

—At the Semi-annual Conversational Meeting of the Pathological Society of Philadelphia, on April 25, Prof. Roswell Park, of Buffalo, will read a paper entitled: A Study of Acute Infectious Processes in Bone.

—The Trustees of the Chicago Medical College at a recent meeting decided to lengthen the college term to seven months, and to recommend an *optional* four years' course. Dr. G. W. Webster has been elected Professor of Physiology.

—A bill prohibiting the sale of tobacco to minors under seventeen years of age, without the written consent of their parents or guardians, has passed to third reading in the Michigan Legislature. It will be followed by an iron-clad bill prohibiting the sale of cigarettes in any form, which bill, it is stated, has many advocates.

—*Daniel's Texas Medical Journal,* March 1889, says that under the laws of Texas the State University has been required heretofore to give medical and law education free. The Twenty-first Legislature, however, has just passed a bill repealing the objectionable clause, and authorizing a charge of $80 per session for instruction in law, and $150 for instruction in medicine.

—The *Journal of the Amer. Med. Association,* March 23, says that an American Hospital is one of the features of the City of Mexico. All English-speaking persons that apply are admitted. Regular contributors to the Hospital, who subscribe not less than $1 monthly, and Americans without means of support, are entitled to attendance and medical treatment in the general ward, free of all charge. Other persons may enjoy the privileges of the Hospital on equitable terms, and private rooms are provided for such as desire them.

—The Medical and Chirurgical Faculty of Maryland will hold its ninety-first annual session in Baltimore on April 23, 24, 25, and 26. Professor William Osler, of the Johns Hopkins University, will deliver the annual address, on "The License to Practise, with special reference to State Boards."

—The *New York Tribune*, April 4, says: "In the examination of jurors for the trial of Krulisch the fact was developed that a number of the men summoned objected strongly to the hanging of convicted murderers, but could easily reconcile themselves to the thought of executing them by electricity. This is proof in confirmation of the general belief that the new method of execution is more humane than the old. In fact, the substitution of a silent, powerful current of electricity for the gallows, with all its attendant horrors, marks a distinct step forward in our treatment of criminals."

HUMOR.

IT IS WHEN LANDED in the scales of Justice that the weigh of the transgressor is hard.—*Texas Siftings.*

A BOLOGNA BANK CASHIER has absconded. We suppose the detectives will collect evidence against him link by link.

TWO LITTLE MOBILE BOYS were fishing from a wharf the other day, when one of them fell into the water. The other rushed up to a deck-hand, exclaiming: "Save him, mister! He's got de bate!"—*Burlington Free Press.*

NURSE—"We ought to have a piece of soft old linen to bind up Master Rupert's bruise.'

Young Mother (anxiously)—"Ought we, Barker?" (To under-nurse) "Jane, go right out and buy three yards of the finest old linen you can get."—*Epoch.*

WHAT WAYS!—"Mamma!"

"Well, my dear?"

"What awfully queer ways these Western folks do have, don't they? I have been reading an article in 'The Stock Breeders' Gazette' that papa brought home, and it says that cows should have their corn fed to them in the ear!"—*Drake's Magazine.*

WASTED EFFORT. — Charitable Visitor *(about to leave the hospital)*—"I never saw such a cold-hearted person as that patient near the window. I read one of Heber Newton's sermons to him fully ten minutes, and he didn't show the least emotion." Attendant—"I'm sure he didn't mean to hurt your feelinks, Mum; he's as deaf as a post."—*Puck.*

OBITUARY.

SAMUEL W. GROSS, M.D.

Dr. Samuel Weissel Gross, Professor of the Principles of Surgery and Clinical Surgery in Jefferson Medical College, died of pneumonia in Philadelphia April 16, in the fifty-third year of his age.

Dr. Gross was a son of the eminent surgeon, Samuel D. Gross, and was born in Cincinnati, Ohio. He received his early education at Shelby College, Kentucky, and subsequently studied medicine in the medical department of the University of Louisville and at the Jefferson Medical College, graduating from the latter institution in 1857. Soon afterward he began delivering lectures on surgical anatomy and operative surgery, and later, on genito-urinary diseases in Jefferson College, and on surgical pathology before the College of Physicians of Philadelphia. For some time he was surgeon to the Howard and the Philadelphia Hospitals, and for a number of years was a member of the surgical staff of the Jefferson Hospital. On April 1, 1882, he was elected one of the Professors of Surgery at the Jefferson College, which position he held until his death.

During the civil war Dr. Gross was a brigade surgeon, with the rank of Major of volunteers, and at its termination he was brevetted Lieutenant Colonel. He was a member of various medical and surgical associations, in whose discussions he always was an active participant, while for a number of years he was a leading contributor to prominent medical journals. He was well known as an author, and was an acknowledged authority on genito-urinary diseases and on tumors of the female breast.

Dr. Gross was a man of warm and generous impulses, a learned and skilful surgeon, and a bold operator. His untimely death removes one of the ablest surgeons of Philadelphia at the height of his usefulness, and will be heard with sorrow by all, especially by those who listened to his instruction at Jefferson College.

MEDICAL AND SURGICAL REPORTER

No. 1678   PHILADELPHIA, APRIL 27, 1889.   VOL. LX.—No. 17.

CONTENTS:

CLINICAL LECTURE.

SCURVY IN A HEMIPLEGIC. PULMONARY PHTHISIS.[1]

BY FREDERICK P. HENRY, M.D.,

PHILADELPHIA.

ATTENDING PHYSICIAN TO THE PHILADELPHIA AND JEFFERSON COLLEGE HOSPITALS.

Scurvy in a Hemiplegic.

Dr. Henry began his lecture by showing another case of scurvy which, he said, was at least as interesting as either of the two exhibited on the previous Saturday, an account of which was published in the REPORTER, April 3.

Dr. Henry then said: the gums are still swollen, spongy, and tender, and at the time of his admission, a few days ago, they were the seat of spontaneous oozing of blood. The anterior surfaces of both tibiæ contain patches and spots of extravasation so numerous as to leave but little healthy

[1] Delivered at the Philadelphia Hospital, March 29, 1889.

skin between them. The arrangement of these patches is remarkable for its symmetry, which is so great that every large ecchymosis and small petechial spot seems to have its counterpart on the opposite side. This symmetrical arrangement of the cutaneous lesions, together with another fact to be presently alluded to, leads me to exclude any participation of the nervous system in the pathogeny of scurvy. Nervous affections, such as neuralgia, and the cutaneous lesions dependent upon them, such as herpes, are generally asymmetrical; whereas dropsy and other symptoms of blood dyscrasia are, as generally, symmetrical.

The mention of dropsy calls to mind certain experiments of Ranvier, which prove that the nervous system may take part in its production. This well known pathologist was unable to produce œdema in the lower extremities of a dog by tying the inferior vena cava. If, however, in addition to tying this vein, he divided the sciatic nerve, œdema made its appearance on the side of the nerve section. The effect of cutting the nerve was to add the dilatation

501

of vaso-motor paralysis to that of passive congestion. While these facts are not wholly, they are undoubtedly in part, applicable to dropsy in the human subject; for œdema resulting from vaso-motor paralysis—acute congestion—is a well-recognized pathological condition. Such a form of dropsy may properly be called neurotic. These remarks are by no means irrelevant. On the contrary, they have a marked application to the case before us, for one patient is hemiplegic on the left side. In such cases, vaso-motor disturbances on the paralyzed side are very common. Whether they are invariable or not cannot be determined, because their presence or absence is not always noted in the reports of cases of hemiplegia. The probability that they are always present seems so great as to amount almost to a certainty.

The paralysis in the case before us has lasted many months and the patient's intelligence is so much impaired that his contribution to the clinical history amounts to little if anything. It cannot be ascertained from him whether the paralyzed leg has been at any time red or swollen. Increase of temperature on the paralyzed side has been often observed in cases of hemiplegia, and Fagge mentions a case in which dropsy, of renal origin, was limited to it. Speculation is needless, in the absence of any positive data concerning the existence of vaso-motor paralysis in this case; but the interesting fact remains that, in a case of hemiplegia, the manifestations of scurvy have been remarkable for their symmetry.

Pulmonary Phthisis.

In this patient, a man 35 years old, there is dulness over the base of the right lung, as may be perceived in any part of the room. In the same region there are bronchial breathing, increased vocal resonance, and sub-crepitant rales, the whole being indicative of a consolidation of the lung which is just beginning to soften. With the aid of the valuable data derived from the clinical history, the diagnosis of pulmonary phthisis is established beyond doubt.

Basal phthisis, as compared with apical, is a comparatively rare affection. According to one authority, the proportion of basal to apical phthisis is as 2 to 1000; according to another as 1 to 70. These figures naturally excite the question why the apex of the lung is such a favorite nidus of the tubercular process, a question which is usually answered by the statement that the proper nutrition of an organ demands that it be functionally active, and that the respiratory movements, which are the chief gauge of the functional activity of the lungs, are least active in the apices. Other reasons for this localization of the tubercular process are derived from a study of the effects of cough. In coughing, the lungs are compressed, and the air containing the irritant exciting the cough is driven into their upper portions. That a certain amount of air in the act of coughing enters the apex of the lung, is plainly proved by observing this act in emphysematous patients whose lungs bulge upward into the supra-clavicular region at each expiratory effort. With this air, as a matter of course, there may be carried into the apex mucus or other foreign substance, and once lodged in this part of the lung its exit may not be easy. Such foreign bodies may excite inflammation which, by lowering the nutrition of the lung, renders it a suitable soil for the tubercle bacillus.

The diminished movement of the upper part of the chest, and phthisis resulting from it, has been attributed to the weight of the arms. This explanation is purely fanciful and is not borne out by clinical experience. James, a recent writer on phthisis, mentions three cases under his observation, in which the arm had been amputated close to the shoulder, and in which phthisis developed years afterward on the side of the amputation.

Cough.—A symptom of phthisis invariably present in greater or less degree, is cough. Theoretically, cough, which is a muscular action intended to expel an offending substance from the air passages, should not be interfered with. Practically, it is found, in most cases, to be altogether out of proportion to the urgency of such requirements. Its frequency and violence depend not only upon the amount of secretion to be removed, but also upon the irritability of the nervous system. This is greater in the young than in the aged and, therefore, in the former, the cough is more distressing. In the insane affected with phthisis, cough is said to be much less prominent as a symptom than in the sane. It is very common for a phthisical patient to have a violent fit of coughing at two or three o'clock in the morning, after which he may sleep until six or seven. This is explained by the fact that during sleep the respiratory centre is blunted and the secretions accumulate until the irritation of their bulk is so great as to rouse it to action. The offending matter having been expelled, the patient again falls asleep, to be awakened by the same cause a few hours later. On rousing a phthisical patient from sleep an attack of coughing will be excited almost invariably. The amount of bronchial irritation which was insufficient to excite cough while he was asleep, immediately does so when he is awakened.

A certain amount of cough is beneficial in phthisis, and should not be interfered with. That which awakens the patient from sleep during the night, and that which occurs at the hour of rising, are of this nature. The offending substances have at such times accumulated in large amount, and must be expelled. If, however, the violence and frequency of the cough are out of proportion to the amount of expectoration—a point which can be decided only by observation and experience—some measures must be adopted for its relief.

Cough is injurious in several ways : 1. By its succussion, it interferes with any possible healing process. 2. It may rupture blood vessels in the walls of cavities or in the trabeculæ traversing them. 3. During the violent inspiratory efforts which attend cough, particles of secretion may be sucked into and infect still healthy portions of lung. Finally, repeated attacks of cough exhaust the patient's strength. They do so both by the fatigue attending such violent muscular exertion and by the attacks of vomiting which often accompany it. This is explained by the close association of the respiratory and gastric centres, an anatomical arrangement which also explains the fact that coughing is often produced by the ingestion of food. It is very common for patients to say that a cough which annoys them is nothing but a "stomach cough." In most cases they are mistaken in their diagnosis, but this does not disprove the fact that cough may be excited in a reflex manner by gastric irritation.

Having decided to relieve the cough, it is better to begin by trying to dispense with that remedy which one is compelled to resort to sooner or later in most cases, viz., opium and its alkaloids. One of the best sedatives for an abnormal irritability of the respiratory centre, is hydrocyanic acid, which may be combined with a tonic as in Begbie's mixture—a favorite English prescription :

R   Acid. hydrocyan. dil. . . . . . f ℥ i
    Acid. nitrici dil. . . . . . . f ℥ iii
    Glycerini . . . . f ℥ i
    Infus. quassiæ . . . . q. s. ad f ℥ vi
M. Sig. A tablespoonful in water, thrice daily, before food.

This, with the aid of the steam atomizer, by means of which a spray of compound tincture of benzoin and water is inhaled, may give great relief. The effect of these remedies may be aided by counter-irritants and cataplasms to the chest. If the cough continues unabated, or if, in the course of time, these measures seem to lose their effect, opium in some form will have to be resorted to. The following mixture, in which the dose of morphia is too large, has long been employed at the Episcopal Hospital :

R   Potass. cyanidi,
    Morphinæ acetat. . . . . . ãã gr. 1-10
    Acet. sanguinariæ . . . . . . ℳ v
    Syr. Tolutan . . . . f ℥ ss
    Aquæ . . . . q. s. ad f ℥ i
M. One drachm every six hours.

It is better to give a smaller dose, say one-twentieth grain of morphia, at shorter intervals. If morphia disagrees, codeine may be substituted for it. Spirit of chloroform is an excellent ingredient in an expectorant mixture. A mixture of equal parts of glycerine and whiskey is sometimes very soothing after the nocturnal attacks of cough, and it may enable the patient to sleep until the accumulation of secretions awakens him in the morning. With such measures as these and with others which will suggest themselves, the cough may be greatly relieved. When dependent upon laryngeal catarrh or ulceration, it will, of course, demand local treatment.

Pain.—Although, probably, no case of phthisis runs its course entirely without pain, the latter cannot be called a prominent symptom of the disease. Pleurisy, as is proved by the firm adhesions with which the two layers of the pleura are always bound together, is a constant accompaniment of phthisis. As a rule, the separate attacks of pleurisy by which these adhesions are effected, are subacute, but occasionally such an attack may give rise to severe pain and marked febrile movement. Such a case is now in the hospital, one in which the pain was so great that pneumothorax was suspected. Great relief may be afforded in such attacks by restraining the movements of the chest with straps of adhesive plaster.

Fever.—An attempt has been made to distinguish two types in the fever of phthisis, an inflammatory and a resorptive; the former depending upon the irritative and inflammatory processes going on in the lung, and the latter upon the absorption of products of inflammation and necrosis. The two types are generally combined in varying proportions, and it is held by some authorities that valuable prognostic and therapeutic data may be derived from a correct estimate of the degree in which one or the other preponderates. The inflammatory is characterized by a high temperature range, with slight fluctuations; the resorptive by marked fluctuations, shiverings, and sweatings. The former is to be treated by absolute rest in bed. Stimulants should be withheld, as a rule, and the drugs should be limited to an expectorant and a saline, such as the liquor ammoniæ acetatis. When the fever is indicative of resorption of inflammatory or caseous products, alcohol should be administered, as it not only tends to steady and lower the temperature but, at the same time, to check the profuse night sweats which so often accompany this type of fever. This brings us to the consideration of this latter symptom—night sweats—which are often so annoying and weakening to the patient.

Night Sweats.—It has been supposed by some that the perspirations are eliminative and, therefore, to some extent beneficial; but there is little ground for such an opinion. They are undoubtedly indicative of nervous exhaustion, and they accompany all sorts of enfeebled conditions in which there is no question whatever as to the elimination of any toxic or infectious material. If in any degree eliminative they are, like the cough, greatly in excess of such requirements. This is proved by the fact that the patient is rendered much more comfortable when they are checked. They may sometimes be controlled by the nocturnal administration of food, such as milk, soup, beef-tea, or an alcoholic stimulant; and such means should be employed before resorting to drugs. Sponging the surface with tepid water containing vinegar, or a little dilute mineral acid, will often prove of benefit. These measures failing, there are two drugs which exert a specific action in controlling night sweats, whether in phthisis or in any other disease, and I say this with great positiveness as the result of a large experience with them. The drugs to which I refer are picrotoxin and agaricin. They are both given in pill, the former in doses of one-eightieth of a grain; the latter in doses of one-tenth of a grain. I am accustomed to prescribe one grain of Dover's powder with each dose of agaricin. One of either of these pills given at bed time will prevent the sweating in many cases, but they may have to be given twice or thrice in twenty-four hours. Atropine, belladonna, and oxide of zinc are doubtless still largely employed in

the treatment of night sweats; but in my opinion are much less certain in their action than the two substances mentioned.

Pleuritic Adhesions.—The pleuritic adhesions to which reference has been made as being so constantly present in cases of phthisis, may be regarded to some extent as conservative. The adhesion of the wall of the cavity to the opposite costal pleura will prevent the rupture of that cavity into the pleural sac. Rupture gives rise to what is called pneumothorax. During a paroxysm of coughing, the patient feels a severe pain in the side, has the sensation of "something giving way," and immediately thereafter suffers from the severest form of orthopnœa. The other symptoms are those of collapse in general, such as a cold, clammy skin, and thready pulse. Death may be the almost immediate result of such an accident, or, on the other hand, the patient may survive its immediate effects and succumb to the pleurisy, generally purulent, which is sure to ensue. When death from dyspnœa seems imminent, the pleural cavity should be punctured and the air allowed to escape. The treatment of the ensuing pleurisy or empyema is partly medicinal and partly surgical and does not come within the scope of our subject.

Fistula in ano.—This is a complication of phthisis the frequency of which has been estimated by one authority to be about five per cent.; by others, between ten and fifteen per cent. The responsibility of deciding the question of an operation in such cases should be assumed by the physician, who is better acquainted with the recuperative powers of his patient than a surgeon who is called in consultation can be. If there are decided fever and severe paroxysms of cough, operation should not be undertaken; but if there is little or no febrile movement, slight cough and moderate expectoration, it may be advised, especially if the fistula gives rise to much discomfort and is attended with considerable discharge.

Lung Surgery.—The local treatment of pulmonary cavities is twofold. When seated near the apex, experience has proved that benefit may be derived by injecting into them various antiseptic solutions. The following are recommended: Lugol's solution, iodoform in ether, and solutions of carbolic acid, bichloride of mercury, creasote, and sulphocarbolate of sodium.

It is now a recognized surgical procedure to open certain tubercular cavities, insert drainage tubes, and, in short, treat them as abscesses are treated in other situations.

To be amenable to surgical treatment, a pulmonary cavity must fulfil certain conditions. It should be single, near the surface, and situated in the lower portions of the lung. The thoracic walls in the upper part of the chest are too rigid to permit of that contraction which is necessary to the cicatrization of a cavity. These operations should not be lightly undertaken, for the greatest skill in diagnosis is requisite to the proximate localization of a lung cavity.

There are many other symptoms and complications of phthisis to which want of time has prevented allusion. They are so numerous and varied that a case of chronic pulmonary phthisis may be regarded as an epitome of all other diseases It is an inflammation, a fever, and an infectious disease; and there is scarcely an organ or tissue of the body which may not be impaired, in structure or function, during the course of the disease. The study of pulmonary phthisis, therefore, although somewhat discouraging from a therapeutic, is instructive in the highest degree from every other point of view.

----◆◆◆----

COMMUNICATIONS.

GONORRHŒAL RHEUMATISM.[1]

BY CASPAR W. SHARPLES, M.D.,
RESIDENT PHYSICIAN, PHILADELPHIA HOSPITAL.

The following paper is based upon the study of eleven cases at the Philadelphia Hospital, chiefly in the wards of Professor Osler.

This subject we find treated of under the following synonyms, viz.: "Arthritie or Arthropathie Blennorrhagique," "Tripper-rheumatismus," "Urethral Rheumatism," and "Urethral Synovitis."

In 1784 the subject was first mentioned by Swediaur under the heading of "Arthrocele, Gonocele, or Blennorrhagic Swelling of the Knee." About the same time Selle recorded a similar note. Swediaur's account is unique, and for its historic interest worthy of repetition. It is as follows:

"A very considerable swelling of the knee (sometimes of both knees and the heel at once), attended by excruciating pains in the joints, sometimes occurs in men after blennorrhagia. These pains, accompanied by more or less symptomatic fever, continue for two or three weeks and gradually go off, leaving a stiffness in the joint, which lasts for many months. The disease particularly affects young men, who, after a debauch, have been infected with blennorrhagia, with which it seems to be intimately connected. It is surprising that no author has treated of this disease, as the consequence or symptom of blennorrhagia. It is not very uncommon, for in the course of my practice I have seen seven or eight cases, each of which came on about the sixth or eighth day of the blennorrhagia, and in every instance the discharge from the urethra was either sensibly diminished or totally suppressed. For want of sufficient observation, I have not been able to determine the character of the disease, but in all cases which have come within my knowledge this disease appeared to partake of the character of gout—with this exception, that all the persons were about the age of twenty-three or thirty, that the color of the skin was not changed, and that the swelling bore handling without exciting pain. The swelling gradually disappears by the free use of mild diluent drinks, and by frictions with the ammoniacal liniment; but above all, with a liniment made of gum ammoniac dissolved in the vinegar of "squills."

In this account we find the key note of many later descriptions of this disease. It is a very good account of that form of the trouble, chiefly affecting the knees, called chronic hydrarthrosis.

There has been, and is yet with certain physicians an idea that no such affection as gonorrhœal rheumatism exists. How we can avoid acknowledging its existence I do not know ; for in so many instances it has occurred in connection with gonorrhœa, and in the same cases there has been a return of rheumatism with each subsequent attack of gonorrhœa, without any extraneous rheumatic exciting causes. There is undoubtedly some connection, at least, with urethral conditions. As an example, Basset, of Fournier's clinic, reports a characteristic case, in which there were five attacks of gonorrhœa, and rheumatism with each attack. But a striking feature was that, after every introduction of an urethral instrument, fever immediately followed, and arthritic pains, with conjunctivitis throughout the attack. Rheumatism has existed resulting from irritation due to a stricture.

Petrone has found gonococci in the affected joints. In one case they were found on the fifth day and in another on the third day. Another observer found them the day after the fluid had collected in the

[1] Read before the Philadelphia County Medical Society, March 13, 1889.

joint, but on the fifteenth day they could not be found. Hall reported a case in which they were found to the Clinical Society of New York. These facts demonstrate more than a coincidence between gonorrhœa and rheumatism. Dr. Jameson attempted two cultures from cases, to which I shall refer later; one was a case of hydrarthrosis of the knee, one a case of general articular trouble. Only a negative result was obtained.

In new-born children there is sometimes seen a purulent ophthalmia, which is attributed to gonorrhœal infection during the passage of the head. Rheumatism has in a few instances been associated with this ophthalmia. Lucas reports a case with a good history. A mother obtained gonorrhœa three weeks before her confinement. Soon after delivery, the child had conjunctivitis, with a profuse discharge. Associated with this ophthalmia was swelling of the knee and later involvement of the wrist. Other cases of rheumatism soon after birth have been reported, without mention of gonorrhœal ophthalmia, and probably closer study would show such cases to be similar to Lucas's case.

From the resemblance of puerperal rheumatism to gonorrhœal rheumatism, many cases of the former are probably specific, though there exists a puerperal rheumatism quite distinct from gonorrhœal infection. It is proper to say that after the rheumatism has once appeared it runs a course independent of the urethral state, and does not cease when the gonorrhœa has ceased.

Gonorrhœal rheumatism holds no distinct time relation to the stage of the urethritis. It usually occurs from the third to the sixteenth day of the disease, but is quite common from the third to sixth week, and has been, in connection with gleet, delayed as long as the twelfth month. Dr. Pye Smith has tabulated the time of appearance of rheumatic symptoms in eleven of his twenty-nine cases: In 3 cases during the first week; in 1 case during the third; in 2.cases during the fourth; in 2 cases during the sixth; and in 3 cases during the ninth week.

To this list I would like to add the time of occurrence in nine of my eleven cases. In one case it occurred on the fourth day; in two on the sixth; in one on the twelfth; in one on the fourteenth; in one on the twenty-first; in one about the fiftieth; and in one on the sixty-third day.

Nothing remarkable is to noted as to the time of life at which this disease occurs. In my cases, the attack occurred in three before the age of twenty; in seven between twenty and thirty; and in one above the age of thirty years. The habits of people during the decade between twenty and thirty, and their exposure to infection then, account for the greater frequency of gonorrhœal rheumatism. The parts and the number of parts affected vary much. They do not seem to bear any relation in this respect to the severity or stage of the gonorrhœa. There may simply be an involvement of the synovial membrane, making a true but a specific synovitis. But there are said to be cases of gonorrhœal synovitis which have afterward become cases of arthritis, presenting a joint filled with pus and showing consequent destruction of bones and cartilages. The fibrous tissues around the joints are often first involved with affection, perhaps secondary, of the synoviæ and cartilages. Along with other fibrous tissues we may have involvement of the sclera, and accompanying iritis. The endocardium and pericardium are affected. Ligaments in all parts may be attacked, and it is not rare to have trouble in the fibrous tissues of the spinal column. A point of supposed involvement is the bursa under the os calcis. The sheaths of the tendons are affected, and there is an œdematous infiltration of the skin, which may become hard and brawny. The affection seems to have no predilection for certain joints, for almost every joint in the body has been involved, different parts suffering in different varieties.

In some instances we find a distinct gouty or rheumatic family history, and occasionally a history of a previous attack of ordinary rheumatism. Nolen's record of 88 cases gives six with ancestral rheumatic history, four with previous rheumatism, and twelve with gouty ancestors. Of my cases two had had previously acute rheumatism, and two had a family history in which rheumatism figured.

It affects men oftener than women. Of one hundred and eleven cases there were but seven in women (Nolen). Davies-Colley reports twelve cases of one form of this disease, nine of which were in women. Of the writer's group of cases only one was in a woman. It is stated that prostitutes possess an immunity from this disease, and of this fact I know of no explanation. Five out of nine cases of Davies-Colley's were in pregnant women, suggesting that perhaps a specific trouble in connection with pregnancy may render the person more susceptible to the rheumatic affection. It is usually found in women who are not prostitutes but who have had illicit intercourse, or in women who have been recently married.

In comparing the relative frequency of gonorrhœal rheumatism in men and in women, there may be an explanation found in the urethral and vaginal constituents. The female urethra consists of muscular, erectile, and mucous coats. The mucous coat has no special glandular communications except the few mucous follicles around the external orifice of the urethra. The male urethra also has the same coats. The mucous coat, however, is a part of the genito-urinary mucous membrane, and is prolonged into the ducts of the glands which open into it—viz., Cowper's, the prostatic, vesiculæ seminales through the ejaculatory duct, and the vasa deferentia. From this greater complexity and sensitiveness, as well as from the greater area of exposed mucous membrane, the attempt is made to explain the frequency of gonorrhœal rheumatism in men. Moreover, the vaginal wall is a tough, thick, and non-absorbent combination of tissues.

The immediate cause of gonorrhœal rheumatism is the specific urethritis. Often it comes without any apparent exciting causes, and at other times there is apparently a dependence on cold, fatigue, injuries, and exposure to wet, such as result in ordinary rheumatism.

Fournier has made three divisions of gonorrhœal rheumatism, which are : (1) Hydrarthrosis of Knee ; (2) Polyarticular, as in subacute rheumatism ; and (3) Ambulatory pains. But in Pepper's System of Medicine, Dr. Howard makes a division into five classes, viz : (1) Arthralgic ; (2) Rheumatic ; (3) Acute gonorrhœal arthritis ; (4) Chronic hydrarthrosis ; and (5) Bursitis and thecitis.

The arthralgic form may co-exist with the more acute forms, as ambulatory pains, shifting from joint to joint, without any swelling or tenderness on pressure, but a decided increase of pain on motion. There is no change in the color of the skin. Such a condition is found in a gonorrhœa of long standing, and without any apparent change in the urethral discharge. The patient is liable to exacerbations of pain. This form does not yield to treatment.

The rheumatic form may come with a premonitory chill, or may follow exertion, strain, exposure, etc. ; or it may occur without any of these apparent influences. Rheumatoid pains in the soles of the feet, ankles, loins, etc., lasting a day or so, may precede the

trouble. Then there is a sudden involvement of many joints, the attack perhaps coming on during the night. The joints are moderately swollen, are more or less changed in color, and are tender on pressure or on motion. This rheumatic form tends to involve all of the joints, and especially the smaller ones. Regarding the number of joints affected, it is interesting to note that in 120 cases, 212 joints were affected : the knees 83 times, the ankles 32 times, and the fingers and toes 75 times. In 25 cases collected by Pye Smith, the involvement is as follows: the wrist in 6, shoulder in 3, hip in 1, elbow in 1, and the knee in 14. In my 11 cases there were 60 joints affected, distributed as follows: the ankle in 10, wrist in 6, knee in 9, elbow in 4, temporomaxillary in 4, sterno-clavicular in 3, shoulder in 2, hips in 3, and the fingers and toes in seven cases. These eleven cases present twenty-two distinct attacks of gonorrhœal rheumatism. One patient had seven attacks and another three. Nevertheless, with all this general affection there is a tendency for the disease to settle in one joint, in which there may occur an effusion, consisting of leucocytes, flakes of lymph, and serum. Periarticular tissues are more commonly involved than in ordinary rheumatism. This is shown in the marked local œdema and the fusiform enlargements of the fingers. Pain, pseudo-anchylosis with deformity, are quite common, disappearing eventually, though the cartilages and bones may take such a part in the inflammatory process as to cause the affection to resemble rheumatoid arthritis. In this variety we see cardiac, pleural, cerebral, and ocular complications. The urine is often high colored, and contains transiently oxalates, urates and uric acid. Acid sweats are often present as a passing phenomenon. Local sweats are quite persistent. The temperature is not high, though at first it may rise to 103° F., but only to fall soon and remain down, in spite not only of a continuance of the arthritic trouble but also of an involvement of new joints.

Here I would like to submit the report of a few cases, some of which are of more than usual interest from the points they illustrate.

Case I.—H. H., 24 years old, admitted to the Philadelphia Hospital November 19, 1888. The patient's family history was good ; there was no history of rheumatism. He is a baker, and is exposed to sudden changes of temperature. Four years ago he had rheumatism in the feet and ankles.

Since then he has had a yearly attack. One attack was of nineteen weeks' duration. All this took place before he had gonorrhœa. On November 3, 1888, he became infected with gonorrhœa, and in eight days there was urethritis with much strangury. On the 17th he had pain in the joints following a wetting on the previous day. The pains were first in the metatarso-phalangeal joints of the great toe of the left foot, then in the great toe of the right foot. The morning before his admission, the fingers of the left hand, and on the 24th the right temporo-maxillary articulation, became involved. A urethral discharge was present on his admission, and continued to be thick and creamy. The joints were swollen and very tender. The pains required morphia to relieve them. The patient was given oil of gaultheria in twenty-five drop doses every two hours, with relief of the pain, and blisters were applied to the affected joints. The temperature was 103° on admission, but fell in two days and ran along about normal for nineteen days. Recovery was rapid, and on December 2, 1888, he was up, the trouble having almost gone from the joint. The urethral discharge had become very thin. On December 4, however, he injured the great toe, which became tender and swollen. On December 12, he complained of being cold, and had a chill followed by a rise in temperature to 101$\frac{4}{5}$°. The first phalangeal articulation of the left hand and the left knee became swollen, and there was at the same time pain in the back. The urethral discharge was also increased. On the 27th the patient was discharged, with some stiffness of the joints and some enlargement of the fingers. An examination of the heart, early in the attack, showed that the apex beat was in the fifth interspace, inside the nipple line ; there was no thrill. There was a distinct blowing systolic murmur at the apex and at the aortic cartilage. In May, 1888, the patient was in the hospital with rheumatism, and in a note made on his dismissal I find this statement: "Heart was carefully examined and no lesion found." His urine was acid and contained only pus cells.

Case II.—O. C., 31 years old, a paperhanger, was admitted to the Philadelphia Hospital November 4, 1888. There was no family rheumatic history. The patient has been a heavy drinker. When twelve years old he had inflammatory rheumatism. In 1876 he had his first attack of gonorrhœa, from which he recovered in three weeks. In July, 1884, he again had gonorrhœa, and in a few days gonorrhœal ophthalmia. The urethral discharge ceased in a few days, following four injections. His urine stopped for a few days. Soon he had soreness in the great toe of the left foot. The left ankle and knee, the right shoulder and right hip, the ball of the great toe, and left shoulder became affected in the order named. For this attack he was in bed six months, being unable to move or feed himself. For a year he was compelled to use crutches. During this attack the urethral discharge did not reappear. Preceding the joint trouble he had a thorough wetting, and convalescence was slow and gradual.

In September, 1886, he had a third attack of gonorrhœa, the discharge appearing four days after infection. During the progress of the gonorrhœa his ankle became swollen (the result of an injury as he thought), disabling him from September to January. At that time he was in bed five weeks. His present attack dates from October 13, 1888, when he became re-infected. Urethritis appeared in a few days and lasted a day or so after using injections. The urine was scanty and passed frequently. On the eighth day he first had pain in the back and about the heart ; he had never before experienced pain about the heart. The right hand and left foot were next affected, as was also the right wrist. The wrist and ankle were swollen, red, and tender ; it was impossible to move them. The patient said he had had a great deal of fever before his admission. Shortly after admission the left knee was affected ; then the right great toe and left foot, and then the sterno-clavicular articulation. The temporo-maxillary articulations on each side were much swollen and tender, so that he could not open his mouth. On October 26, his eyes became sore, with some discharge. There were intervals of days when the pains would be less, only to be followed by a recurrence, with painful and tender joints, for five or six days. The trouble was chiefly situated in the right knee and wrist. On December 21, 1888, he was discharged, with the right knee still somewhat swollen and stiff. The right hand could not be closed. On the patient's admission there was a distinct systolic murmur at the apex, which persisted during his stay, though its intensity became much less. The urine was strongly acid. His temperature, on admission, was 97°, but soon rose to 101$\frac{4}{5}$°, ranging between that and normal, rising sometimes, as a new joint was affected, and often with no apparent cause.

Treatment was with oil of gaultheria,

which seemed to lessen the pains and control the temperature; arseniate of iron was also used, but had no effect. The patient was given hot whiskey and pilocarpine, to produce sweats, and after the sweats he felt much better. Apart from these no sweats were noted in the course of the disease.

Case III.—W. L. C., 28 years old, was admitted to the Philadelphia Hospital December 12, 1888. There was no history of rheumatism in his family. The patient is a moderate drinker. Four years ago he had gonorrhœa, which followed three days after infection. In four days he had pain in his left foot, which continued for sometime before any swelling appeared. The left foot, the right knee, both hands, the fingers, elbows and temporo-maxillary, joints were affected. With this attack he was in bed three months; he did not have much fever, but had heavy night sweats. After getting up, the left ankle remained sore and stiff for a long time. The present attack began four days after the urethritis, and not after any unusual exposure. The secretion did not lessen when the joint trouble began. Pain appeared in the foot before the joints were involved, and affected the left toe, left ankle, right great toe and elbow, in the order named, with slight swelling. The elbows were extremely painful on exertion. On Dec. 27, 1888, he had an exacerbation of the pain in the elbow and right foot. He had conjunctivitis during the first attack and also in the exacerbation. The man had on admission a well-marked aortic regurgitation, which seemed to suffer no change during his stay. He had oil of gaultheria, local urethral treatment, and calcium sulphide in doses of ¼ to ½ grain, three times a day. He left the house with moderately good use of his joints, though they were stiffened. The Resident in charge of the case says that he thinks the calcium sulphide had some effect.

Case IV.—J. C., 28 years old, was admitted on October 9, 1888. The patient says that his father had rheumatism. He is a laborer and is much exposed to wet and cold, and has had gonorrhœa four or five times before the present attack, with the last of which, four years ago, he had a bubo. On July 28, 1888, he again had gonorrhœa, acutely for several days. On August 2, 1888, as a result of treatment, as he thought, the discharge ceased. Four days afterward he felt the first pain in the joint; the pain had been preceded for several days by constitutional disturbance and fever. On August 6, 1888, the pain appeared in the right ankle and on the 8th in the right knee, but without any swelling. He then entered the hospital. The left ankle and knee, right hand, and left wrist were involved in the order mentioned. Then followed the involvement of the right elbow and shoulder, and of the sterno-clavicular articulation. The temporo-maxillary joints and hips were also slightly affected. The most intense inflammation was in the left wrist and in the sheaths of the tendons along the dorsum of the hand. The affection here has been most acute and the swelling extreme, of a dense brawny character. The skin was dark and very firm in this region. On November 15 a fly-blister remained on for twenty-four hours without effect, as it did also on the 21st. Off and on, there was an orchitis of the left testis, and accompanying it a renewal of the urethral discharge, as a thin pus. In one attack, commencing Nov. 23, the testis swelled rapidly, with great pain extending up into the abdomen. The scrotum was much thickened. The urethral discharge persisted with the orchitis, and the two seemed to subside together gradually. About Dec. 11, there was a fresh outbreak of articular mischief, which appeared in the first phalangeal articulation of the right middle finger, and extended to the metacarpo-phalangeal joints. The thumb of this hand was also affected. The temperature rose to 103°. Dec. 16, there was well-marked lymphangitis of the right arm, red lines, ⅟₁₆ of an inch in width, extending from the seat of inflammation, with enlarged axillary glands and a temperature of 101° on the evening of the 17th, subsiding on the 18th. Dec. 20, there was again much swelling and pain in the left testis, with return of the urethral discharge, which had been absent for the preceding six weeks. Dec. 27, the right shoulder became very sore, and next day there was swelling of the right sterno-clavicular articulation, which was very red. Jan. 5, the left testis was again swollen, with return of the urethral discharge, burning micturition, and chordee. The testicle was not so large as upon former occasions. At each attack the swelling and urethral discharge were less, but this was the first occurrence of chordee. A few days before this attack of orchitis, there was pain in the shoulder. The right sterno-clavicular joint again became swollen and looked as if suppuration was going on, but no pus was found on opening it. Jan. 10, the patient was quite comfortable. The left wrist was stiff, the parts atrophied, the pain nearly gone, the legs and the sterno-clavicular articulation swollen. Since the last attack he has been in about the same condition.

The temperature in this case has presented the following features. On admission it registered 100°; the second evening 101⅖°, the next morning normal, and then it gradually rose until the 12th, when it was 100⅘°; on the 15th, when there was much pain, it was 101⅘°. From this time until the 28th it ranged from 99°–100°. Dec. 4, it rose to 102°, and since then it oscillated from normal to 101°. The highest record was 103°, which occurred during the trouble with the right hand. Quite early he had some sweats, which ceased; later he had night sweats and local sweats of his legs. After about six weeks some change was noted in the first sound of the heart, and subsequently a murmur became quite plain. In the treatment, means have been quite exhausted and without any result. Poultices and lead water and laudanum were used to no avail. The hand was put on a splint and bichloride towels were applied with marked relief. Oil of gaultheria had no effect. The patient was put on bichloride, iodide of potash, and arseniate of iron without effect. Morphia was administered to control pain. The parts were wrapped in cotton wool.

The above cases very well show, I think, that endocarditis does occur in connection with gonorrhœal rheumatism. In Case I there is a distinct note of absence of heart lesion, and of its subsequent appearance without any intermediate cause except gonorrhœal rheumatism; though it is possible that this may be a coincidence of gonorrhœa and rheumatism, and that the gonorrhœa acted as an exciting cause. In Case II there were noted the changes and symptoms of acute endocarditis and the gradually diminishing murmur. In Case III, though there is no positive evidence that the heart lesion was due to gonorrhœa, yet there is the history of a previous attack of gonorrhœal rheumatism and the absence of other rheumatic affections; and we know the proneness of the disease to affect the aortic leaflets. Case IV developed under observation as reported. Cases of gonorrhœa have been reported in which endocarditis occurred, without any rheumatic complications, though the endocarditis in these instances may have only been coincidences. One case, ulcerative endocarditis came on in the course of gonorrhœal rheumatism. Certainly endocarditis may appear in this disease, though proportionately much less frequently than in ordinary rheumatism.

(To be concluded.)

ARTHRECTOMY OF THE KNEE-JOINT AS A SUBSTITUTE FOR EXCISION.[1]

BY JOHN ASHHURST, Jr.; M.D.,

PHILADELPHIA.

PROFESSOR OF CLINICAL SURGERY IN THE UNIVERSITY OF PENNSYLVANIA.

The case brought before you to-night is of some interest, being illustrative of an operation which is attracting a good deal of attention among surgeons, especially those who have to do with diseases of childhood. This is a comparatively new operation, having been first suggested by Wright, of Manchester, some seven years ago. His first case was recorded in 1881. He has operated in a certain number of cases since then, but it has been within a very short time, hardly over a year, that the procedure has been taken up by other surgeons. It is now practised by Owen and Parker, of London, and by others. It has been adopted in Germany and in France. In France the sentiment is rather against the operation. The opinion of the majority of French surgeons who have employed this substitute for excision is, that it is equally as dangerous, and the result no better, and in some respects not as perfect. In Germany the sentiment is more favorable to arthrectomy, and in England it is still more so.

My experience with this operation is very limited, as I have employed it only twice. The second patient is still under treatment, and the case which I record to-night is, therefore, the only completed one which I have to report. I think that, as far as a single case can, it shows that the operation is a good one, and that it has a distinct field of usefulness in cases in which the surgeon hardly feels justified in resorting to excision. The history of this case is as follows:

The boy is twelve years of age, with a good family history. The father is living and healthy, the mother living and phthisical; but whether or not there is a tuberculous taint inherited from the mother is uncertain. The belief of the family is that the mother's health was broken down by nursing this boy, and that the phthisis was developed after his birth. The lad was under my care, in the Children's Hospital, more than seven years ago, when five years of age, for the same condition of the knee-joint. At that time I divided the hamstring ten-

[1] A verbal communication made at the meeting of the College of Physicians of Philadelphia, February 6, 1889.

dons and applied a splint, and he left the hospital. This is a practice that I have followed for a number of years in young children, for excision is not a very successful operation in the earliest years of life. In this way a serious operation can often be postponed for some time. The patient returned to the hospital this fall, having in the meantime been under the care of the surgeons in the out-department. His knee-joint, while not getting much worse, did not get better. It was one of those cases which seem too bad to be let alone, with no prospect of benefit from conservative measures, and, on the other hand, not bad enough to justify any very dangerous operation. This seemed to be a case in which it might be proper to do this comparatively new operation of arthrectomy.

The term arthrectomy might properly be applied to the operation of excision itself, but it is understood as applying to the removal of all of the diseased soft tissues, without disturbance of the bones. Some surgeons have employed a longitudinal incision on one or both sides, passing behind the patella and scraping away the soft tissues. Others make the incision across the patella, saw through that bone, clear out the joint, and bring the two segments of the patella together with stitches. The plan which I have adopted, and which is, I think, preferable, is to make the incision just as for excision, below the patella, through the ligament, turning up the patella and getting full exposure of the joint. Then with knife, scissors, and curette, I carefully remove all morbid tissues that can be dissected out, the synovial sac, semilunar cartilages, and any portions of the articular cartilages and bones that may be diseased. The greater portion of the synovial membrane can be dissected out with the knife, scissors, and forceps. The portion at the back of the joint cannot well be thus dealt with, but can be removed with the curette. The articular cartilages should be thoroughly scraped. If any patches of carious bone are found they should be removed. A drainage tube is then inserted, the wound closed, and the limb placed on a posterior splint just as after excision.

This boy was operated on October 3, 1888. Here is his temperature record, which was kept for two months. It shows that there was very little reaction from the operation. The highest point reached was 100.6°, and that upon only one occasion. On five occasions it reached 100°. The result of the operation is an almost perfectly straight leg,

with firm union between the articular cartilages. Some surgeons have attempted to obtain motion, but I think it better to be satisfied with fibrous anchylosis. This is simply imitating Nature's mode of effecting a cure in comparatively mild cases, where fibrous anchylosis takes place. In the same way, excision is an imitation of Nature's method of effecting a cure in bad cases, that is, by bony union.

The advantages of this operation over excision are, in the first place, that the length of the limb is not interfered with, and that there is no risk of consecutive shortening. One of the most serious prospective risks after excision is, that from implication of the epiphyseal cartilage, the growth of the limb may be prevented. Most surgeons are familiar with the case of Mr. Pemberton, of Birmingham, where the shortening amounted to eight or ten inches. This is, of course, unusual, but there is risk that the limb will not grow in proportion to the rest of the body. As this operation does not involve the epiphyseal cartilage, there is no risk of consecutive shortening. In the second place, the shape of the limb is preserved. This is, however, a point of minor importance. In the third place, there is no risk of that inward turning of the lower portion of the limb, so common after excision. Surgeons who have done many excisions are familiar with the fact that it is sometimes almost impossible to prevent a certain amount of axial deformity, the lower part of the limb turning in while the upper part rolls out. In arthrectomy the condyles are preserved and the head of the tibia fitting between them prevents the occurrence of this deformity.

An objection to the operation urged by French writers is, that there is apt to be consecutive flexion. This also occurs after excision, and can be avoided by maintaining a firm support as long as may be necessary. I think that in a case like the present it would be better to perform arthrectomy and then retain a plaster bandage or a leather support for even a long time, than it would be to perform excision.

I, of course, do not suppose that this operation will ever take the place of excision, for the majority of cases in which operative procedures are called for are so far advanced that excision is the only remedy; but there are cases in which the disease is limited to the soft parts, and here this operation has its legitimate field. In this case the boy had been under observation for eight years and the condition had finally become so bad that it seemed necessary that something should be done. There are then a certain number of cases in which this operation may properly be performed, coming in between the simple rectification of the deformity by tenotomy and the graver operation of excision.

It is about four months since this limb was operated on. It is now strong, and the boy can walk on level ground without crutches. He does not require a high shoe. Before the patient goes home, a plaster bandage will be applied, and he will wear this for a long while, reporting from time to time, so that the occurrence of consecutive flexion may be avoided.

CONTAGIOUSNESS OF ERYSIPELAS.

BY CHARLES P. WOODRING, M.D.,
MEADVILLE, PA.

I was called on March 13, to see Emma W., who was suffering with a sore throat. Upon inspection I observed the usual appearance seen in diphtheria, including a decidedly characteristic membrane. Belle W., 13 years old, and two years younger than her sister Emma, was also suffering from the same disease ; but hers was evidently a much milder attack and manifested itself three days earlier. When Emma's diphtheritic symptoms, both local and general, were at their height, she developed facial erysipelas, upon the appearance of which the patient referred *all* her pain and distress to the dusky-red, hard and swollen cheeks, to which the erysipelas was limited.

With the increase of the severity of the skin affection came a corresponding decrease in the severity of the local diphtheritic symptoms. This inverse ratio continued until the entire disappearance of any and all throat symptoms.

While the erysipelas was in full bloom, and just after Mrs. W. had applied one of the frequent dressings to it, Edward E., who was visiting the afflicted family, came into the room and asked Mrs. W. to dress a little cut upon the middle finger of the left hand, which he had a minute before inflicted upon himself. Mrs. W. immediately complied with his request, and nothing more was thought of the finger until twenty-four hours later, when Edward began to suffer the most excruciating pains in the injured finger. The pains, however, were not confined to the finger, but extended thence to the wrist, forearm, arm and axillary space.

My attention was then, for the first time, directed to this additional patient, whose finger then was only slightly swollen. The course of the lymphatics could, nevertheless, be distinctly traced all the way to the axilla. In a few days all of the worst symptoms of phlegmonous erysipelas had developed in the finger, which soon became the seat of extensive sloughing, and evident necrosis of the phalanges, while the swelling extended in alarming proportions and with the greatest rapidity to the elbow.

The treatment in all of the cases mentioned was supporting throughout : tincture of the chloride of iron, sulphate of quinine, whiskey, milk, and beef-tea internally, and for the diphtheria, turpentine locally. For the facial erysipelas a solution of sulphate of iron was used locally, and for the phlegmonous erysipelas of the finger hot water dressings were first used, and afterward deep and numerous incisions with charcoal poultices, followed by solutions of carbolic acid.

It is generally admitted that all forms of erysipelas must be preceded by a solution of continuity for the ready admittance of a blood poison. Possibly the facial erysipelas in the foregoing case owed its existence to the preceding diphtheria, but undoubtedly the digital erysipelas could claim the facial erysipelas for its parent. The case of phlegmonous erysipelas proves at least, if it proves nothing more, that we cannot be too careful in the handling of patients with facial erysipelas, both for our own safety and for that of other members of the household with whom we come in contact.

A SEDATIVE AND LAXATIVE MIXTURE FOR FUNCTIONAL NERVOUS DISORDERS.

BY J. B. JOHNSON, M.D.,
WASHINGTON CITY, D. C.

A young physician who is called to treat the various nervous affections of women, sometimes finds himself in doubt in selecting a suitable prescription, which will, in the larger number of such cases, meet the indications calling for prompt, pleasant and efficient relief. These disorders are known by the familiar name of functional nervous diseases, and all of them, to a greater or less extent, are attended with vitiated secretions of the alimentary canal, and constipation ; and these conditions always aggravate nervous disorders.

The usual causes of these functional nervous diseases are: chronic ovaritis, sub-involution of the womb, and painful menstruation. These derangements of the female organs of generation are foretold by mental depression, mental worry, nervous headache, sick stomach, sleeplessness, and those forms of menorrhagia that are often symptomatic of ovarian irritation or sub-involution of the uterus.

To allay the distress caused by these functional disorders, it is very important to have absolute rest in the recumbent posture, in order to give the organs involved time to regain and resume a healthy discharge of their functions. The next duty is to correct the vitiated secretions of the alimentary canal and to relieve constipation. For this purpose I know no better mixture than the following :

> R. Magnesiæ Sulph., ... ʒ j
> Aquæ Camphoræ, . . . f ʒ v
> Olei Menth. pip., . . gtt. ij
> Glycerini, ... f ʒ j
> Potassii Brom:di, ... ʒ ss
> Tinct. Hyoscyami, ... f ʒ iij

M. Sig. Shake well. Dose a tablespoonful every three hours

Should the tongue be much coated it will be necessary to give an alterative dose or two of calomel; and should it become advisable, a vegetable tonic may be added to the mixture with advantage. For this purpose the compound tincture of gentian, in half-drachm doses, will act well; and should menorrhagia or leucorrhœa be present, twenty drops of the fluid extract of ergot can also be added with beneficial results.

—Dr. Robert Abbey, of New York City, will address the Philadelphia County Medical Society, May 1, on Lateral Anastomosis of the Intestine.

—A Press dispatch from Mobile, Ala., to the daily papers states that all the condemned articles at the old Quarantine Station on Ship Island, opposite Biloxi, were destroyed by order April 12, and the Yellow Fever Hospital and fixtures and every particle of matter supposed to be capable of carrying infection were burned. There was a great mass of bedding, clothing, and refuse left there when quarantine was moved in March to Chandeleur Island, and as the mass was known to be infected with germs and visitors were not prevented from going on the island, there was a call through the press for its burning, with the result just mentioned.

SOCIETY REPORTS.

COLLEGE OF PHYSICIANS OF PHILA-DELPHIA.

Stated Meeting, February 6, 1889.

The President, D. HAYES AGNEW, M.D., in the Chair.

DR. WHARTON SINKLER communicated the following on

A Case of Pott's Disease from Injury, Followed by Complete Paraplegia. Treated Successfully by Suspension.

History of Patient.—John T., eighteen years old, native of Ohio, was admitted to the Orthopædic Hospital and Infirmary for Nervous Diseases, February 16, 1888. Father and mother both living and healthy. He is the eldest of three children; others are healthy; there is no history of consumption in the family; has never had any of the diseases of childhood; always healthy and strong.

In September, 1886, some of his schoolfellows "bumped" him against a tree. This was done by four boys, each taking a leg or arm and bringing the buttocks forcibly against the tree. Acute pain in the spine was produced by this at the time, and afterward, in either sitting or standing, pain was remarked; but when lying on his back he was comparatively easy and free from pain. The pain was first greatest in the epigastrium and radiated thence into the back, down into the legs, and up into the shoulders. About three weeks after the injury, he accidentally discovered a lump in the dorsal region of the spine. Soon after observing this, the lump became very painful and was sensitive to the touch. He continued to sit up and walk, but progressively became weaker, and after the second week in January, 1887, was unable to walk at all.

About three months after the injury, he began to lose sensation in the legs; the knees began to get stiff in the spring of 1887. He has been unable to sit up, but was comparatively comfortable in bed.

Condition on Admission.—A tall, slim boy; weight eighty-four pounds; angular curvature at seventh dorsal vertebra; can sit up with the aid of a leather corset which he has worn for some months. He is unable to move the legs at all; knees and ankles generally in a state of rigidity; knee-jerk grossly exaggerated; patella clonus present;

ankle clonus very marked on both sides; toe reflex present—(this is very striking on both sides). The condition known as *spinal epilepsy* readily induced; plantar reflex exaggerated; no cremasteric or abdominal reflex can be elicited; sensation is impaired, but is not lost. He can localize and distinguish touch anywhere on legs or feet; no interference with the functions of bladder or rectum. There is no pain in the spine.

There is a bed-sore the size of a ten-cent piece over the sacrum. The circulation in the legs is poor; the feet are constantly cold. His temperature is above normal, morning and evening; varying from 100° to 102° F. in the evening; in the morning, 99° to 100° F.

He was ordered massage, and the cautery was used on each side of the angular curvature. He was also ordered cod-liver oil and milk-punch. A plaster jacket was applied soon after his admission, but as he fainted before the plaster could set, it had to be removed, and in two days a second jacket was applied. This could be borne only for three or four days, on account of interference with respiration; and it was removed on the second day. A third jacket was applied at the end of another week, and in this he was comfortable. The bed-sore, however, continued to increase in size and depth.

On March 18, he was suspended by means of a padded leather chin and occipital piece from a bar of iron projecting over the head of his bed. This was placed high enough above the bed to allow him to sit upright upon the bed. He was able to bear the extension for nearly five minutes on the first day. On each subsequent day the time was extended, until he was able to bear the extension for half an hour twice a day.

On April 17, the plaster jacket having been removed on March 29, ice and hot water were applied to the spine over the region of the curvature, for ten minutes four times each day—the ice and hot water being applied alternately; first the cold, followed by the heat.

May 14, he was placed in a chair, and extension made from a rod attached to the back of the chair and bent over the head.

About this time he began to have slight power of motion of the toes; this was followed by power to flex the feet, and to flex the thighs.

June 25, fluid extract of ergot, twenty drops three times a day, was added to the treatment; and this was continued until July 31.

July 23, the following note was made: Condition much improved; complains of no pain; can move the legs, drawing up the knees lying on his back in bed; sensation is improved, but is not perfect; clonus is less, but still marked; knee-jerk still exaggerated; toe reflex still present.

The application of heat and cold to the spine was continued until October 18.

In August he was able to lift the feet from the floor as he sat on the chair. One of Kolbe's spinal apparatuses was applied on July 31, and he has continued to wear this when sitting up ever since; it is removed when he is in bed. In the middle of August he could walk a few steps in the wheel crutch.

In October he began to walk about with crutches. He has continued progressively gaining strength in the legs, and is now able to walk about at pleasure, but has not yet been allowed to dispense with his crutches, although quite strong enough to do so.

His weight is now ninety-seven pounds. There is no tenderness over the curvature, but there is no material change in its shape. The reflexes are all still exaggerated, but to a moderate extent; and the tremor of the legs is no longer excited by moving them vigorously.

REPORTS OF CLINICS.

UNIVERSITY HOSPITAL.

GYNECOLOGICAL CLINIC.—PROF. GOODELL.

Removal of an Ovarian Tumor.

While the gentlemen are assembling I shall make some remarks on the case before you. This girl is only sixteen years of age. Her health was good until one year ago, according to her statement; but her physician thinks that it was two years ago that she received the following accident. She and another girl were walking when she suddenly fell on her back, and her companion fell on her abdomen. The patient was menstruating at the time. The next day the pain ceased, but she "began to swell" and has never had but one menstruation since that time. She has lost much flesh, and is now merely skin and bones.

We ask ourselves the question: What is this tumor? It is clearly a cyst. Upon making an examination *per vaginam* I find that the uterus is small, and not connected with the tumor. Hence I am disposed to say that it is an ovarian growth. But if it is true that it has come in only one year, it is probably malignant.

In these large tumors I prefer the use of chloroform to ether for anæsthesia, because it does not tend like ether to congest the kidneys and suppress the secretion of urine. From this cause I have lost patients after laparotomy. My last thirty-four cases of oöphorectomy have been done mostly under chloroform, and they have all been successful. Then again chloroform does not tend to cause œdema of the lungs, which in the aged is liable to result from ether narcosis. In large tumors, such as this one is, the diaphragm cannot play while the patient lies on her back, and we are often compelled to give the anæsthetic and to empty the cyst while the patient lies on her side.

Now after thoroughly cleansing the abdominal walls with a 1 : 1000 bichloride of mercury solution, I begin my incision about four inches above the pubes, making it first down to the preperitoneal fat and then down to the tumor. I examine carefully for adhesions, and I find that I have mistaken the adherent peritoneum for the wall of the tumor. Fortunately I discovered my mistake before doing any mischief; but let this serve to impress upon you how very careful we have to be. Before going further now, all bleeding has to be stopped. In opening cysts the rule is to tap them high up, because the trochar will travel down as the fluid is removed, and otherwise the collapsed cyst may slip off from it. The fluid now ceases to flow, not because the whole cyst has been emptied, but because the cyst is multilocular and only one compartment has been emptied. There is another cyst and a solid body, which we must cut into. I leave these for a moment, while I examine higher up. I find that there are adhesions everywhere, though they are not very strong. I now extend the incision higher up in the median line, nearly to the navel. The catch forceps are more difficult than usual to apply, on account of the œdematous condition of the skin and underlying fascia. I now break up adhesions and incise the other cyst. It is smaller than the first one; but the fluid is thick, dark colored and probably irritating, so that I use every precaution to prevent its getting into the abdominal cavity, which I now enter after washing my hands. I have nearly detached the cyst from the front of the abdominal parietes. The omentum is also attached to the surface. To expedite matters, I catch it up in a pair of forceps and cut it away from the cyst. Within the cyst is a solid tumor, which I cannot reduce in size; and as the pedicle is quite broad and short I shall clamp it and cut off the tumor, so as to get more room.

Cleaning first the outside of the abdomen and packing the inside with sponges, I avoid the introduction of any septic matter, which might set up septicæmia. On the broad slender pedicle I introduce a sort of cobbler's stitch. That is to say, I transfix the pedicle three times before tying the ligature. As the pedicle is so short and broad I shall be on the safe side and put on another ligature, to prevent any possible hemorrhage. I now cut away the redundant portion of the pedicle-button, lest it might slough.

We now tie the omentum, which is held by the forceps *en masse*, and drop it. The removal of the omentum is a small affair. It is not a vital organ, and when necessary I have removed pieces as large as my hand. As such a procedure is not necessary now, I simply drop it back into the cavity.

As our patient is young, I wish to save the other ovary if it exhibits no symptoms of disease. It looks healthy, and as she has menstruated from it at least once since her illness began, I shall leave it.

I now put in one sponge in front of the bladder, another behind the womb, and a large flat sponge on both flanks, and one in the middle, over the intestines. Now, having protected the abdominal cavity, I search for any vessels that need ligating, first on the wall. There is very little bleeding anywhere here; but, if there were, the sponges would show it. Let me count the instruments while the sponges are in.

I now pass the sutures from within outward, because it is easier and safer. I include the peritoneum and the rectus muscle. The tumor does look like a malignant one, yet in apparently innocent cases I have seen growths develop on the pedicle and metastatic cancers riddle the liver. This is a case for drainage, because such a large raw surface as the pedicle and the denuded abdominal walls present will secrete a fluid very favorable for the development of septic germs. I put in four stitches to the inch, because there is less danger of hernia than with a smaller number, and I take in a good deal of all the tissues in every stitch. The largest tumor I ever removed weighed one hundred and twelve pounds. The patient recovered, but with a troublesome redundancy of abdominal skin. I have removed several weighing over eighty pounds, one of which was removed last Thanksgiving day. But the longest incision I ever made was in a successful case of hysterectomy, in which a fibroid weighing forty-four pounds was removed.

The operation to-day was not difficult, because the adhesions were easily broken down. Dr. Adler has weighed the tumor, and now tells me it tipped the beam at fifty-five pounds; but we must have lost several pounds of fluid on the floor, so that it comes very near the sixty pounds that I predicted it would weigh. We now flush out the cavity of the abdomen with several pitchers of water, although I do not think anything got in it from the tumor. I did not empty the bladder before the operation, because the presence of the urine serves to show where the bladder is, and saves it from injury.

I now paddle about and wash the intestines in the water. Such a procedure we would not have dared to do some years ago; but we now know that it is not the exposure and handling of the intestines that do mischief, but septic filth.

After this laundry of the peritoneal cavity, the sponges are removed and a drainage tube put in. I bring out the stitches close to the margin of the wound, so as to prevent doubling in of its edges. The wound being closed it is dressed antiseptically, with iodoform and iodoform gauze. The bowels will be opened on the fourth day, because otherwise the large pedicle may get fastened to an intestine and cause fatal obstruction.

The drainage tube will be pumped out every two hours for the first day, less frequently on the second day, and it will be removed as soon as the fluid withdrawn from it is straw-colored.

The patient will have no nourishment for twenty-four hours, and will have no opium. Then small doses of milk or of beef tea will be cautiously given. On the eighth day the stitches will be removed.

—*Public Opinion*, March 9, says: M. Mosso, of Turin, having carried out a series of experiments with the blood of eels, finds that it possesses marked poisonous properties. Even to the tongue it has an insupportable acridity, and a very small quantity of the serum is sufficient to kill a dog. Half a cubic centimeter (about ten minims) injected beneath the skin of a dog weighing 35 pounds killed it in four minutes. At this rate, an eel weighing five pounds would contain enough poison to kill ten men. The blood of the eel, however, is inert when taken into the stomach, and it loses its toxic properties when heated.

PERISCOPE.

Intubation of the Larynx in Diphtheritic Croup.

In a communication published in the *New York Medical Journal*, March 9, Dr. Dillon Brown gives an analysis of two hundred cases of diphtheritic croup in which intubation was performed. He states at the outset that in determining the value of any operation in the treatment of diphtheritic or membranous laryngitis it is necessary to give not only the number of operations and their result, but also the whole number of such cases seen, whether operated upon or not. Again, to compare the value of any two operations in the treatment of this disease, it is not sufficient to state simply the number of recoveries following each operation; it is essential to form some idea of the character of each case and compare the result only in similar cases. The physician must take into consideration the age, the duration, and the amount of laryngeal obstruction, the presence or absence of pharyngeal or post-nasal diphtheria and its duration, the condition of the kidneys, and the presence or absence of sepsis or other complications, as pneumonia, measles, scarlet fever, whooping-cough, etc.

As regards the character of the cases, he states that nearly one-half of the patients were either absolutely hopeless or under three years of age. He has not refused to operate in a single case of advanced laryngeal obstruction, however hopeless it seemed; and besides, he has never operated until the stenosis was extreme. Not a single patient died during the operation. On the primary introduction of the tube, membrane was pushed down in several instances, but every time it was either coughed out through the tube or it followed the tube on its withdrawal. In no case was membrane pushed down in sufficient quantity to produce fatal obstruction during the operation.

Regarding the value of intubation, he says: "If those physicians who oppose intubation in favor of tracheotomy, and who have operated sufficiently often to make their opinion of any value, will give us a *complete* report of their cases—including all the cases seen, whether operated upon or not—it would be of the greatest value in comparing these operations, and would quickly consign tracheotomy to the background, for use only in special cases."

Dr. Brown says he has operated upon two hundred patients with diphtheritic or membranous laryngitis, of which fifty-four, or twenty-seven per cent., recovered. The patients were divided as follows: males, 87; females, 113. The average age was 3 years 5 months; of those that died, 3 years 2 months; of those that recovered, 4 years 5 months. The urine contained albumin in 116 cases, no albumin in 15 cases, and was not examined in 69 cases. In fatal cases the average length of life after intubation was 2 days 23 hours; in cases of recovery the average time during which the tube remained in the larynx was 5 days 10 hours.

Dr. Brown then gives a tabular statement of his cases. With reference to internal medication, he says: "Since my last report in June, 1887, I have operated in one hundred and fifteen cases. Of these cases, fifty were treated without the use of bichloride of mercury, in most cases with some iron preparation; and twelve recovered, or 24 per cent. The other sixty-five cases were treated with bichloride of mercury in large doses (gr. $\frac{1}{40}$ to $\frac{1}{80}$ every hour), frequently with iron in addition to the mercury. Of these patients, twenty-four recovered, or 36.9 per cent. I am firmly convinced that the use of bichloride of mercury in the treatment of diphtheria and croup, as recommended by Professor A. Jacobi, of New York, offers us the best means of fighting this disease."

In concluding his paper Dr. Brown gives a summary of the cases of intubation hitherto reported. In this he says: "The foregoing list gives 2,368 cases, with 647 recoveries, or 27.3 per cent. It is the record of 166 operators, practising in Germany, France, England, Spain, Canada, and nearly every State in this country. The results of each operator, with twenty-six exceptions, were personally communicated to me since October 25, of this year [1888]."

Experiments with Creolin.

Some interesting experiments with creolin are mentioned in the *Wiener med. Presse*, Feb. 7, 1889. They were performed by Dr. Washbourn, of London, for the purpose of determining whether or not it is possible, without essential injury, so to saturate a living animal with creolin that the development of specific pathogenic microörganisms in it will be checked. He first proved the antiseptic and disinfecting action of the creolin in the case of microörganisms found in dead nutrients, and then, after inoculating mice and guinea pigs with virulent anthrax, he immediately injected a certain quantity of creolin in watery solution into their bellies and backs; the injection was made once or several times. The development of anthrax was checked or suppressed in this way, but only by the employment of such quantities of creolin as brought about the death of the animals of acute or chronic creolin poisoning These experiments establish irrefutably the fact that creolin acts as a strong poison upon the animal organism. The symptoms of acute creolin poisoning consist of clonic spasms of the muscles of the trunk and extremities, which are attended with or followed by a soporose condition. In guinea pigs there was also a great increase of the secretion of tears observed. The stronger the solution of creolin injected just so much more quickly the symptoms named developed and death occurred. The injection of fifteen minims of a ten per cent. solution in mice, and seventy-five minims of a ten per cent. solution into the peritoneums of guinea pigs, produced immediate symptoms of poisoning, and death resulted at latest in a few hours. These experiments do not prejudice the employment of creolin as a local antiseptic or disinfectant.

Mode of Transmission of Measles and of Diphtheria.

At the meeting of the Société Medicale des Hôpitaux, February 22, 1889, M. Sevestre said that for a long time it was thought that measles was contagious only during and after the eruption. It is now known that it is contagious during the period of invasion of the disease, and in M. Sevestre's opinion it is especially in this period that contagion occurs. But the disease is equally contagious during the period of eruption, at least in the first days of this period, for the contagious power becomes feeble soon. M. Sevestre thinks that the atmospheric air is the habitual vehicle of the germs of measles, which are expelled with the expired air to a certain distance, especially during the spells of coughing. The reason for this opinion is that the disease is contagious from the onset of the prodromic period, when as yet there is nothing upon the skin. Again, the microbe of measles very rapidly loses its harmful property; for if healthy children are brought into a room which a child with measles has left only two or three hours, contagion will practically never occur. From this brevity of duration of its virulence it necessarily follows that contagion is very rarely carried by persons or by objects.

In diphtheria, on the contrary, infection is most frequently mediate. Contagion is carried by some object, or by a sick person to a well one. Everybody is agreed upon this point. It seems also that contaminated objects preserve their virulence for a long time, even for several years.

The practical point to be learned from these facts is that patients with measles are to be isolated at once, as soon as the diagnosis is possible or even probable.

M. Graucher, however, does not think with M. Sevestre that contagion occurs from the expired air of a patient with measles, but holds that contagion is transmitted especially by soiled objects which, in turn, may infect the air. He does not deny the possibility of indirect contagion by the air, but regards its occurrence as much more rare than that by direct contact. And in accordance with his opinion as to the source of the contagion in most cases, he lays more stress upon the efficacy of disinfection. The microörganism of measles exists, according to him, in the nasal and bronchial mucus and in the tears. Contagion before the occurrence of the eruption is therefore quite natural. But he thinks that the vehicles of the contagion are linen, garments, etc., upon which the nasal and bronchial mucus, etc., have been deposited, and not the expired air of patients.— *Bulletin Médical*, February 24, 1889.

Case of Dyslexia.

L. Bruns (*Neurolog. Centralblatt*, No. 2, 1888) has observed a case of dyslexia, a condition first described by Berlin. The patient was a man 40 years old, who had had syphilis twenty years before and for seven years had repeatedly suffered with articular rheumatism. After frequent attacks of dizziness with headache and vomiting he was seized with an attack of apoplexy with subsequent left-sided hemiplegia. This improved, but soon there was a fresh apoplectic attack which was followed by a left-sided palsy; there were clonic convulsions of the right extremities. The patient died some days after the hemorrhage, and at the autopsy there was found pronounced atheroma of most of the larger cerebral arteries, as well as an area of softening in the right lens and right external capsule. Dyslexia had occurred after the first stroke: the patient was unable to proceed after reading

a few words; after a short pause he was able again to read, but very soon was again obliged to stop. As regards the writing itself, that which he did spontaneously showed no variation from the normal, while on the contrary, in writing performed at dictation the patient complained that his arm became stiff and the writing altered: it resembled that observed in the case of scrivener's palsy.

Whether the dyslexia is to be regarded as a pure functional disturbance or as a group-symptom can not be decided by present experiences.—*Centralblatt f. d. med. Wissenschaften*, Jan. 26, 1889.

Use of Antipyrin for Renal Calculus.

Huchard, says the *Wiener med. Presse*, Feb. 7, 1889, has recently discovered a new property of antipyrin, which leads him to recommend it in the treatment of renal calculus. He states in the *Revue gén. de clinique et de thérapeutique*, No. 4, 1889, that he gave fifteen grains of antipyrin daily to a man who was suffering with violent renal colic. The remedy acted so favorably against the pain that the patient without asking any questions continued to take thirty grains of antipyrin daily for the next two months. The effect of this self-medication was that the pain ceased entirely, the urine, which before contained constantly sand and small stones in pretty large amounts, became clear and contained, as shown by chemical analysis, only a normal amount of uric acid. In a second case, Dr. Schweig, of Carlsruhe, states that a man 70 years old had suffered since 1870 with kidney stones, and since 1887 had taken daily three doses of one and one-half grains of antipyrin; under this treatment the pains subsided and the excretion of urates and sand markedly diminished. Huchard believes that in this second case the dose of antipyrin was too small, and that fifteen to thirty grains a day are indicated. Although these two cases are not sufficient to prove that antipyrin has a lithotriptic action, Huchard thinks they are sufficient to warrant practitioners in further experimentation. He orders the antipyrin taken during meals and adds to it, to obviate disturbance of digestion, some bicarbonate of soda, as in the following formula:

R Antipyrin . . . . gr. cccxxv
   Bicarbonate of soda . . . . gr. lxxv
   M. Div. in pulv. No. xxx.
Sig. One or two powders at each meal.

THE

MEDICAL AND SURGICAL

REPORTER.

ISSUED EVERY SATURDAY.

CHARLES W. DULLES, M.D.,
EDITOR AND PUBLISHER.

The Terms of Subscription to the serial publications of this office are as follows, payable in advance:

Med. and Surg. Reporter (weekly), a year,	$5.00
Quarterly Compendium of Med. Science, -	2.50
Reporter and Compendium, - - - -	6.00
Physician's Daily Pocket Record, - - -	1.00
Reporter and Pocket Record, - - - -	6.00
Reporter, Compendium, and Pocket Record,	7.00

All checks and postal orders should be drawn to order of

CHARLES W. DULLES,
N. E. Cor. 13th and Walnut Streets,
P. O. Box 843.   Philadelphia, Pa.

☞SUGGESTIONS TO SUBSCRIBERS:
See that your address-label gives the date to which your subscription is paid.
In requesting a change of address, give the old address as well as the new one.
If your REPORTER does not reach you promptly and regularly, notify the publisher *at once*, so that the cause may be discovered and corrected.

☞SUGGESTIONS TO CONTRIBUTORS AND CORRESPONDENTS:
Write in ink.
Write on one side of paper only.
Write on paper of the size usually used for letters.
Make as few paragraphs as possible. Punctuate carefully. Do not abbreviate, or omit words like "the," and "a," or "an."
Make communications as short as possible.
NEVER ROLL A MANUSCRIPT! Try to get an envelope or wrapper which will fit it.
When it is desired to call our attention to something in a newspaper, mark the passage boldly with a colored pencil, and write on the wrapper "Marked copy." Unless this is done, newspapers are not looked at.
The Editor will be glad to get medical news, but it is important that brevity and actual interest shall characterize communications intended for publication.

THE FOUR YEARS' COURSE.

At a meeting of the Philadelphia County Homœopathic Medical Society, April 11, 1889, a resolution was passed which heartily endorsed any movement for elevating the standard of medical education. The sentiment was pretty general in favor of a four years' optional course, provided the hundred medical colleges of the country, which have a two-year course, will mend their ways or change their curriculums, so that this State may not be discriminated against.

If this resolution is correctly reported it is one which illustrates the importance of the word "if"; for there is no likelihood of the adoption of a four years' course—optional or obligatory—by any medical school which waits until all the other schools in the United States which have a two years' course mend their ways. The argument that a compulsory four years' course for men who wish to practise in Pennsylvania will discriminate against the State is one which shows that those who use it mean by "the State" the medical schools. How the State can be the worse for having in it only thoroughly educated physicians does not yet appear. The effect on some of the schools cannot be determined in advance. So far as men intending to practise here is concerned, the legal requirement of four years of study would compel them all to study in Pennsylvania or in the schools of other States for an equal length of time. The probability is that a law such as is proposed would for a time keep Pennsylvanians in Pennsylvania medical schools, and that this would more than make up for the loss of students who expect to practise in States where the law is less exacting. At the same time, there can be no doubt that it would bring a very strong pressure to bear upon all the Eastern schools to adopt a four years' course, and as little doubt, we think, that other States would follow the example of Pennsylvania in demanding more thorough preparation of those who wish to practise medicine within their borders.

So far as we understand it, the proposed requirement is one which ought to be heartily supported, unless it can be shown that a shorter term of study is sufficient to make good physicians and surgeons, and that the conditions of this country do not warrant a step which has so much in its favor. Most of the arguments against a four years' course of study have an air of being shaped in the interest of weak and inefficient medical schools, which care more for the number of their students than for their fitness to practise. This is a matter in regard to which the community may take a very different view, and those who expect to be practised upon may say that they will have none but well educated physicians in Pennsylvania—or any other State—and demand that the schools shall provide such physicians or go out of business.

DANGERS OF COCAINE INJECTIONS INTO THE URETHRA AND BLADDER.

The discovery of the local anæsthetic property of cocaine has proved of almost incalculable value in minor surgical operations. Perhaps no single remedy comes into play more frequently. Its use is now so common, and the evil effects from it usually so few, that there is risk of forgetting that it may act as a serious poison. It may be well, therefore, to call attention to several cases in which dangerous symptoms, and even death, have followed the employment of the remedy in what would seem at first thought to be a perfectly safe way, namely, by injection into the urethra and bladder.

One of the first recorded instances in which dangerous symptoms followed the injection of cocaine into the urethra is that mentioned by Dr. G. Frank Lydston, in the course of a clinical lecture published in the REPORTER, July 28, 1888. In this case the patient had been operated on for stricture by internal urethrotomy, and a four per cent. solution of cocaine was injected every second day subsequently to facilitate the passage of the sound. On the ninth day after the urethrotomy, however, the patient in a few minutes after receiving the injection complained of dizziness, and immediately fell back in convulsions, dying in less than five minutes. Nothing abnormal was found at a *post-mortem* examination except extremely congested kidneys. It is only fair to state that Dr. Lydston did not attribute the fatal result in this case to the action of cocaine, although otherwise no adequate cause of it seems to exist. Possibly sufficient cocaine had accumulated in the system from previous injections to explain the sudden result

following the last injection: the patient had received two fluid drachms of a four per cent. solution, or about five grains, at each injection.

In 1888, Dr. Simes reported, to the Philadelphia Academy of Surgery, a case in which a fatal result followed the injection into the urethra of one drachm of a twenty per cent. solution of cocaine. The patient was a man, 29 years old, and the injection was given to permit of painless internal urethrotomy. The nozzle of the syringe used in making the injection had scarcely been withdrawn from the urethra when the first symptoms appeared, and death occurred in twenty minutes from the first convulsion. It was preceded by symptoms of collapse, by convulsions, and cyanosis ; the respiration especially seemed to be affected.

Still another case is reported by Stewart, in the *Medical News*, August 18, 1888, in which the injection of one and a half fluid drachms of a four per cent. solution of cocaine into the urethra, preparatory to internal urethrotomy, was followed by the appearance of collapse and clonic convulsions. In this instance there was a previous history of *petit mal*. The patient was a man 32 years old. He recovered.

Dr. Alejandro Settier, of Madrid (*British Med. Journal*, February 16, 1889) has met with a case of poisoning from the injection of cocaine into the bladder of a patient suffering with painful cystitis and chronic prostatitis. The patient had himself been in the habit of injecting from five to eight fluid drachms of a four per cent. solution into his bladder daily for seven months. When he came under Dr. Settier's care the latter injected cocaine into the bladder and followed it, after twenty minutes, with a solution of nitrate of silver. The pain was so great that the patient again injected cocaine, so that in one day he received four injections of cocaine, and, notwithstanding the fact that he was well seasoned against the drug, alarming symptoms appeared. The patient, naturally taciturn, began to talk with great volubility. His sentences were unfinished, his speech indistinct, and his voice thick and quavering; he complained of giddiness and nausea, got up and sat down suddenly, and his gait was so unsteady that in walking he had to cling to the furniture. The tongue, mouth and fauces were quite dry, the mucous membrane blanched, the body covered with cold sweat; the pulse was small and thready, beating one hundred and five times in the minute; two or three times he vomited glairy matter. Eight hours after their onset all these symptoms disappeared, and the patient was quite well again.

At a recent meeting of the Neurological Society of Philadelphia (*Medical News,* April 6, 1889), Dr. J. Chalmers Da Costa reported four cases of poisoning from cocaine, in three of which the cocaine was injected into the urethra, and in one into the foreskin of the penis. The patients were all men; two of them were brothers, of nervous temperament and drinking habits; a third was also a drinking man, while the fourth was of nervous temperament but of unknown habits. The cases are interesting because in each the symptoms developed after a single injection, and in only one case did the quantity injected amount to as much as a grain and one-fifth (twenty minims of a six per cent. solution). In three of the cases collapse with unconsciousness soon developed, and was marked by embarrassed breathing, pale, clammy skin, dilated pupils, muscular relaxation, and general anæsthesia. This was followed by very pronounced delirium of an active type. In one case the delirium came on at once, not being preceded by collapse. The patients all recovered, and without any serious after-effects.

In attempting to estimate the part played by the cocaine in the production of the symptoms mentioned in the foregoing cases it should be recollected that operations about the genitalia give rise to shock more readily than operations in other regions; and also that in several of the cases, notably in those of Dr. Da Costa, the drinking habits of the patients and their nervous temperament predisposed them to shock. But the symptoms produced can not all be explained by the supposition that shock occurred. On the contrary, the symptoms were such as experiment has proved do actually result from the toxic effects of cocaine. The conclusion seems warranted, therefore, that while especial caution should be exercised in the employment of cocaine in urethral operations upon persons addicted to the use of alcohol or of a nervous temperament, yet its use is not to be regarded as free from danger in any persons. Moreover, the propriety of using a stronger solution than one of four or five per cent. is questionable, and so is the continued use of the remedy for local anæsthetic purposes.

RESECTION OF THE RECTUM.

In the REPORTER, February 18, 1888, we described the method of resection of the rectum proposed by Kraske, which has been carried out with marked success in a number of cases. At present we call attention to a method proposed by Dr. William Levy, of Berlin, which seems to be based on sound principles, although it has never been practised upon the living. Levy's method is as follows: A transverse incision about three inches long is made over the sacrum, about a finger's breadth above the horns of the coccyx, and going down to the bone. From each end of this incision another is carried of about the same length through the skin and the whole thickness of the gluteus maximus. In one of these latter incisions a retractor is placed and drawn strongly outward. The lateral border of the ischio-sacral ligament is exposed by pushing aside the fibres of the gluteus muscle, and the greater and lesser sacro-sciatic ligaments are divided close to the horizontal incision. This operation is then repeated on the other side. The periosteum is then pushed up from the sacrum above the transverse incision and the bone cut through with bone forceps. The flap of bone and soft parts between the three incisions is now drawn downward with a strong hook, carrying with it most of the sacro-sciatic ligaments on each side. This exposes a large part of the rectum, extending from about three-quarters of an inch above the anus to the sigmoid flexure. If necessary part of the alæ of the sacrum can now be removed, as in Kraske's method.

The remainder of Levy's method consists in removing so much of the rectum as may be necessary and any involved glands, uniting the divided ends of the rectum with a double row of sutures, replacing the flap and uniting the edges of the transverse incision with sutures of the bone and of the soft parts. The lateral incisions may be left open and tamponned with iodoform gauze, or they may be sutured except at the upper angles, leaving drainage tubes in the wound, going down to the rectum. As the patient is to lie upon his back, the drains will be in the best position for the purpose of drainage or irrigation.

The great advantage of Levy's method is that it does not interfere with the function of the outlet of the pelvis, which is robbed of its support in case part of the sacrum and the whole of the coccyx are sacrificed. About a year ago Heineke proposed (in the *Münchener med. Wochenschrift,* 1888, No. 37) a method embodying the principles of that suggested now, by Levy, but more complicated in its details, and, for this reason, less desirable. Both contemplate an improvement over any method we know of for removing morbid growths in the rectum out of reach of operations in which the bones do not have to be touched, and are deserving of the careful attention of American surgeons.

MICHIGAN STATE MEDICAL SOCIETY.— The Twenty-fourth Annual meeting of the Michigan State Medical Society will be held in Kalamazoo, Thursday and Friday, May 9 and 10, 1889, and preliminary arrangements for it are already completed.

The membership of this Society is rapidly growing, and added interest in its work is displayed from year to year, its members working together harmoniously to further the welfare of the Society. This is the first State Society to adopt the plan of division into Sections for the reading and discussion of papers, and this plan has greatly facilitated its work. Stenographers have been furnished each Section and verbatim reports of discussion are taken down. The recent volumes of Transactions shows the amount of work accomplished in this way. A similar plan will be carried out at the next meeting.

The morning sessions of the Society will be devoted to the general business meetings, the afternoons to work in the Sections.

———

STATE MEDICAL SOCIETY OF ARKANSAS.— A preliminary circular has been issued by Dr. L. P. Gibson, of Little Rock, Secretary of the State Medical Society of Arkansas, announcing that the fourteenth annual meeting of the Society will be held at Pine Bluff, beginning Tuesday, May 28, and lasting three days. All properly qualified physicians of the State are cordially invited to join the Society. The circular contains a list of the committees with the names of their members. A request is made that the secretaries of local societies shall send to Dr. Gibson a list of the delegates and others who will attend from their respective counties. A final circular, giving detailed information concerning railway rates, hotels, and titles of papers will be issued as soon as the necessary data can be obtained ; but in the meantime Dr. Gibson will give any further information.

———

—The Camden County Medical Society has resolved to recommend the establishment of a State Board of Medical Examiners in New Jersey.

BOOK REVIEWS.

[Any book reviewed in these columns may be obtained upon receipt of price, from the office of the REPORTER.]

THE DIAGNOSIS AND TREATMENT OF DISEASES OF THE RECTUM. By WM. ALLINGHAM, F R.C S., Senior Surgeon to St. Mark's Hospital, etc. Edited and revised, with much additional new matter and numerous diagrams, by HERBERT WM. ALLINGHAM, F.R.C S., Surgeon to the Great Northern Central Hospital, etc. Fifth edition, 8vo, pp. xvi, 366. London: J. & A. Churchill, 1888

Allingham's work on diseases of the rectum and anus is well known, and has an established position, and this edition is likely to meet with a cordial reception. Its greatest merit is that it represents the opinions of a man who has for years devoted himself to the treatment of the diseases discussed, and who has had a very large experience. For this it must be regarded as an important contribution to the literature of the subject.

It has however certain defects. One of these is that, in this edition, it is not always clear who speaks or who is referred to—the father or the son. Another is that the latter seems to have caught his father's unfortunate style of apparently magnifying himself and slighting the experience or opinions of others. In some cases the preferences of the authors seem to be due to prejudice; in others, to sheer ignorance. The former is illustrated, we think, in their expressions in regard to Mr. Henry Smith's and Mr. Whitehead's methods of treating hemorrhoids; and the latter is conspicuous in the chapter on excision of the rectum.

As in previous editions of the book, we note that it has a miserable index. It is remarkable that our British cousins, with the many examples of good indexing which this country has furnished them, should be so slow to learn how to make this very important part of a book.

In spite of all these drawbacks the book before us is a valuable one, and is likely—as it has always done—to continue to be regarded as one of the standard works in the English language.

THE PATHOLOGY AND TREATMENT OF DISPLACEMENTS OF THE UTERUS. By DR. B. S. SCHULTZE, Prof of Gynecology etc., in Jena. Translated from the German by Jameson J. Macan, M.A., M.R.C.S. Eng., etc., and Edited by Arthur V. Macan, M.B., M.Ch., etc., Master of the Rotunda Hospital, Dublin. 8vo pp. xx, 378, with 120 illustrations. New York: D. Appleton & Co., 1888.

All students of gynecology will welcome the appearance of an English translation of Schultze's work. No one man has done more than he to elucidate the subjects of the normal position, or positions of the uterus, and the etiology, nature and proper treatment of the various displacements of that organ. In this book is found a complete, philosophical exposition of the subject of the displacements of the uterus, and a record of years of faithful painstaking work, by which the author has arrived at the views here set forth.

The Editor states that this book has revolutionized the opinions formerly held as to displacements of the uterus, and he predicts that the views of Schultze will eventually receive universal acceptance. This is doubtless true in the main, but in several particulars we are not prepared to believe it. In view of the many diseased Fallopian tubes which surgeons are daily removing from women suffering with pelvic inflammation, of the frequency with which they find peritonitis, and of the rarity of parametritis, we are forced to believe that Schultze attaches far too great importance to parametritis, and too little to peritonitis in the causation of displacements of the uterus. Our space forbids a consideration of the difference between the views advocated by the author, and those generally held in this country, with reference to so-called congenital anteflexion and its relation to mechanical dysmenorrhœa. Many American and English gynecologists probably will not agree with Schultze that the only pessaries which should be used are his figure-of-eight and sledge-shaped pessaries.

The author's results in the treatment of retroflexion with adhesions command our admiration. It seems probable that by following his method of separating these adhesions by bi-manual manipulation, under anæsthesia, the number of cases requiring hysterorrhaphy may be lessened. At the same time too great care in diagnosis cannot be enjoined, or else a pyosalpinx—which may be rare in Jena, since Schultze does not mention the subject, but is certainly common in this country—will sometime be ruptured inadvertently.

Features of the book specially to be commended are the excellence of the diagrammatic illustrations; and the summaries which are appended to each chapter.

The translation is a most excellent one; and the publishers have issued the book in their usual good style.

HINTS FOR TEACHERS OF PHYSIOLOGY. GUIDES FOR SCIENCE-TEACHING, NO. XIV. By H. P. BOWDITCH, M.D., Professor of Physiology, Harvard Med. School. 16mo., pp. 58. Boston : D. C. Heath & Co., 1889. Price, 25 cents.

This little paper-covered book contains a large number of ingenious and valuable suggestions for teaching physiology in schools. The plan proposed is such as will lead scholars to learn for themselves—to observe and generalize, instead of accepting the mere dictum of their instructors The suggestions are made in simple and practical shape, and the main topics of physiology, appropriate to school-teaching, are well covered by the distinguished author. The book is one which may be heartily commended to the notice of teachers, who will find in it an excellent outline of instruction and illustration; and it would be a great help to parents who have some knowledge of physiology themselves and wish to give their children information in regard to this important branch of science

RECTAL AND ANAL SURGERY. By EDMUND ANDREWS, M.D., LL.D., Professor of Clinical Surgery in the Chicago Medical College, etc., and E. WYLLYS ANDREWS, A.M., M.D., Adjunct Professor of Surgery in the Chicago Medical College, etc. Illustrated. Second edition, revised and enlarged. Large 8vo, pp. xiv, 140. Chicago: W. T. Keener, 1889. Price, $1.50.

In noticing the first edition of this book, Nov. 26, 1887, we spoke of its admirable character and especially of its interesting protest against the folly and fraud of certain quacks who chiefly infest the Western States. The new edition has all the merits of its predecessor, and has been revised and enlarged so as to cover a little more ground than this did.

It is a book full of practical common sense, without being too elaborate, and will, we have no doubt, enjoy even a larger popularity than the first edition did.

PAMPHLET NOTICES.

[Any reader of the REPORTER who desires a copy of a pamphlet noticed in these columns will doubtless secure it by addressing the author with a request stating where the notice was seen and *enclosing a postage-stamp.*]

247. THE TECHNIQUE OF OVARIOTOMY, AS PRACTICED AT THE UNIVERSITY HOSPITAL BY PROF. GOODELL. BY LEWIS H. ADLER, JR., M.D., Philadelphia. From the *Medical News*, Dec. 29, 1888.

248. DIE VERBREITUNG DER TUBERKELBACILLEN AUSSERHALB DES KÖRPERS. VON DR. GEORG CORNET, prakt. Arzt in Berlin und Reichenhall. (From *Zeitschrift für Hygiene*, Vol. v, 1888.) 140 pages.

249. UEBER DAS VERHALTEN DER TUBERKELBACILLUS IN THIERISCHEN ORGANISMUS UNTER DEM EINFLUSS ENTWICKELUNGSHEMMENDER STOFFE. VON DR. GEORGE CORNET, prakt. Arzt in Berlin und Reichenhall (From *Zeitschrift für Hygiene*, Vol. v, 1888.) 33 pages.

247. This is a pamphlet which ought to be in the hands of all who have purchased Goodell's Lessons in Gynecology; because Dr. Goodell has modified his methods of preparatory and after treatment, as well as of operating, in very important ways since the last edition of his book was published. The article by Dr. Adler represents his present views and practice, and is both interesting and instructive.

248. This reprint treats of the distribution of the tubercle bacilli outside of the animal body, and is marked with a thoroughness which is a credit to its author. It assumes that the bacillus is the exclusive cause of tuberculosis, and then proceeds to prove by a large number of inoculation experiments that it is everywhere present in the surroundings of phthisical patients. But, if the bacillus is so ubiquitous, why should it be so difficult to infect animals by compelling them to inhale tubercular virus, or why should so infinitely few persons, who are exposed to it, contract tuberculosis? This incongruity is fully recognized by the author, but it is a question whether his theory of unequal distribution of the bacillus will account for it. His pamphlet will well reward careful perusal.

249. This is an effort to show the influence of germicides on the tubercle bacilli within the organism. The animals are infected, the medicament introduced, and with the usual result of the bacilli coming out of the contest with flying colors. The principal agents which were employed for this purpose were tannin, lead acetate, hydrogen sulphide, menthol, acid sublimate, and creasote. The mountain cure of Davos was also tested on six animals, with lamentable results. The pamphlet is valuable in showing to what desperate efforts those are driven who base their faith of curing tuberculosis on the hope that they may discover something which will annihilate the bacillus.

LITERARY NOTES.

—*The St. Louis Polyclinic* is the title of a new monthly magazine edited by L. A. Turnbull, M.D., in the interest of the St. Louis Post-Graduate School of Medicine. The first (April) number contains twenty-eight octavo pages of reading matter, and eight pages of advertisements and reading notices. Subscription price, one dollar a year.

NOTES AND COMMENTS.

Methods of Instruction in Medicine.

Dr. J. West Roosevelt speaks as follows in a paper on medical education, published in the *N. Y. Med. Journal*, March 16, 1889: Preliminary education is beginning to receive some of the attention it deserves. It is well to consider what is the best training for one who intends to study medicine. Let me avoid starting the old discussion of the relative value of classics or mathematics. It seems to me that, if it really be necessary to "train the mind" by the study of some language in the irritating and complicated way so long the fashion among teachers of Latin and Greek, German might be made quite as dull, quite as involved and complex as Latin. When the student finishes the "training process" he will end with a more or less confused notion of a language which he must use and can learn perhaps more easily because of the training. I am not speaking of the rational teaching of Latin and Greek, merely of the method of lifeless drill in grammar so long in vogue.

Let us suppose that a student has a fair general education; what does he need to prepare for medical studies? Surely the answer should be: Special training in some branch of science requiring observation, classification, and more or less delicate use of the hands and special senses. It does not make much difference what is selected— chemistry, botany, comparative anatomy, or any other. Whatever it be, let the student learn it not from a book alone, but let him do practical work. This does not preclude a good education in other matters; in fact, it presupposes such an education.

Perhaps the greatest need in medical education is some method for teaching medicine. It is almost unavoidable that medical instructors should go to work in an amateurish sort of way. Teaching to them is a small part of their aim in life. Most men really are practitioners first and teachers afterward. Many seek to teach merely because they can thereby advance their private practice. This is natural, as instructors are poorly paid. Unfortunately, many men teach without having the faintest idea of the difficulties of so doing.

It is not only necessary that a teacher should know his subject. He should also know precisely what he wishes to teach about it. He should appreciate the difficulties likely to trouble his pupils. He should cultivate the faculty of expressing himself clearly and concisely. Should be on the lookout for illustrations and similes. Above all, he should try to learn how to make his pupils think for themselves. As in all educational institutions, so in medical schools, the greatest object should be to show *how* work is done.

Schoolroom Space.

Mr. H. Courthope Bowen, whose opinions on all matters connected with the proper construction of schoolrooms are entitled to great weight, and are regarded as authori-tative by the leading medical journals of England, expresses somewhat as follows what, in his judgment, should be considered a good schoolroom. Taking the case of a room 14 feet high, fairly ventilated and always well aired in recess, he would assign two-thirds of the floor-space to the scholars and their desks, and keep the other third for the teacher, the blackboard, etc. With single desks, 22 inches should be allowed from side to side, and 3 feet from back to front, for each scholar. The passages need not be more than 18 inches for those running from back to front, and 1 foot for those running from side to side. In such arrangement, counting the passages, each scholar has (without reckoning the share of the space allotted to the teacher) a trifle more than 40 inches from side to side, and just 4 feet from back to front. In a room 25 feet by 20 feet the floor-space for scholars' desks will be 16 feet by 20 feet, with 4 feet from back to front per row, and accommodation is provided for 20 scholars. The whole floor-space is 500 square feet, and the cubic contents of the room 7,000 cubic feet, with 20 square feet and 280 cubic feet per person.—*Science*, April 12, 1889.

Amputation of the Penis.

The most unpleasant symptom following amputation of the penis is the funnel like retraction of the urethra, which causes the patient endless discomfort. Dr. Assaky, of Beucharest, says the *Centralblatt für Chirurgie*, March 30, 1889, overcomes this by dissecting the pars spongiosa of the urethra from the penis for about an inch beyond the superficial incision. Then the corpora cavernosa of the penis are cut through from below, leaving about a half inch of the urethra protruding beyond. The tunica albuginea and the skin are then brought over the stump of the pars cavernosa and stitched around the protruding urethra. This will retract to some extent leaving a very natural looking meatus.

A Doctor's Presence of Mind.

The Philadelphia *Ledger*, April 19, says that the superintendent of a private asylum in Russia (so the story runs) lately had complaints laid before him by one of the patients, who was considered convalescent, as to the poor quality of food which was given, especially the soup, which he stated was half water. The doctor, thinking it was not unlikely that the cooks took advantage of the weak intellects of the patients to tamper with the food, and acting upon the suggestion of the man who had laid his complaint in a very coherent manner, at once proceeded to the kitchen to inspect the soup which was boiling in a huge cauldron over the fire. He lifted the lid, and was about to take out a small quantity to test it, when he was startled by the patient, who had followed him into the kitchen, whispering in his ear, " Do you know. doctor, you are so nice and fat. you would make good strong broth." The man then seized him by the shoulders, preparatory to throwing him into the cauldron. The doctor knew that it would be useless to struggle with the lunatic, who was tall and powerful. With great presence of mind he said quietly, "I quite agree with you, it is an excellent idea, but I fear my clothes will spoil the flavor of the soup. Let me first go and take them off." The madman seemed to see the force of this reasonable request, and permitted the doctor to leave the kitchen. By this means the latter was able to call for assistance and have the man placed under arrest.

Hyperidrosis among Soldiers.

An official circular addressed to Prussian army surgeons, respecting excessive sweating of the feet and other parts in the soldiers as an affection demanding treatment, advises the use of chromic acid—of the strength of one part in ten of water—as an efficient and economical application. In cases of hyperidrosis of the feet, such a ten-per-cent. solution, applied at intervals of three, four, or six weeks, has proved sufficiently strong to remedy this source of disability. From the point of view of military hygiene, the prophylaxis of this affection is not merely a question of discomfort and inconvenience, but has its relations to the efficiency of the service, since all soldiers having hyperidrosis will be more or less prone to recurrent catarrhal troubles and to the evils attendant thereon. Hyperidrosis of the feet, moreover, impairs the marching capabilities of the men.—*New York Med. Journal*, April 20, 1889.

Sulphur Fumigation.

Fumigation by the burning of sulphur is the most common method employed by boards of health in the disinfection of apartments in which contagious disease has existed, and the clothing worn by the patients during their illness. In an address delivered by the distinguished chemist, Dr. E. R. Squibb, before the Kings County Medical Association, he called attention to the fact that there must always be an abundance of watery vapor in the room to be disinfected ; otherwise the sulphurous-acid gas generated by the burning of the sulphur is not an efficient disinfectant. The same is true of chlorine gas when used for disinfecting purposes.—*Science,* April 12, 1889.

Treatment of Variola with Cocaine.

Dr. E. Ory recommends (*Revue gén. de clin. et de thér.* No. 9) the treatment of variola and varioloid with cocaine. In a case of severe confluent varioloid (*sic*) immediate improvement occurred and the eruption quickly subsided after the patient had taken during the night more than one-third of a grain of cocaine. After some days ten drops of a four per cent. solution of hydrochlorate of cocaine were ordered four times daily, and in less than ten days the patient was cured. In a second case of variola recovery resulted under the cocaine treatment five days after the appearance of the pustules. A third patient with very severe hemorrhagic variola recovered without scarring in five days under the cocaine treatment. Two children likewise recovered from varioloid in five and six days respectively under the same treatment.

Ory gives to adults ten drops of a five per cent. solution of hydrochlorate of cocaine four times daily, to children he gives eight drops of a one per cent. solution four times a day. As in all cases the vesicles dried immediately after the employment of the cocaine, it cannot be positively declared that the disease was variola. Ory believes that as the cocaine so quickly neutralized the virus of variola in the infected organism it may check the development of it; and acting upon this belief he recommends its employment as a preventive remedy to be used by those persons about patients with variola.

The above account of Ory's employment of cocaine in variola and varioloid is taken from the *Wiener med. Presse,* March 17, 1889. If the results obtained by other clinicians are approximately as favorable as his, cocaine will prove to be an astonishingly valuable remedy. It should not be difficult, with small-pox widely distributed over this country as it has been during the past winter, to determine with certainty just how much credence is to be given to Ory's observations.

Oxychloride of Mercury as an Antiseptic.

At the meeting of the Ophthalmological Society, of Paris, Feb. 5, M. Chibret stated the following conclusions as the result of his bacteriological researches:

1. The micrococcus pyogenes aureus may be met in the normal human conjunctival sac. However rare, its presence may be expected.

2. Its presence at the time of an operation for cataract is, besides, compatible with a normal cicatrization.

3. Bathing the eyes with oxychloride of mercury 1 to 1500, for five or ten minutes during three days, seems to insure antisepsis better than irrigations.—*Bulletin Médical,* Feb. 10, 1889.

Bryonia Alba in Hemorrhage.

Petresca of Beucharest has been experimenting with the root of bryonia alba, and he finds, according to the *Berliner klin. Wochenschrift,* February 25, 1889, that it is an especially active hemostatic. He employs a decoction of twenty to twenty-five parts of bryonia root to three hundred parts water, reduced to 150 parts, then filtered. It is mixed with syrup, divided in four parts and taken every half-hour. He has also investigated the glucoside " brein," contained in bryonia. The watery and alcholic extracts, in doses of from fifteen to forty-five grains a day, have proved very useful in metrorrhagia, hematuria, hemoptysis and epistaxis.

Cystitis in Women.

Dr. Thomas Moore Madden, of Dublin, treats severe cystitis in women by dilatation of the urethra. This permits a continuous outflow of the secretions. In many cases this treatment, together with mild washing of the bladder, will effect a speedy cure. If not, the fundus and neck of the bladder should be wiped off with a tampon of cotton soaked in carbolized glycerine, and inserted through the dilated urethra. The use of cocaïne will relieve all pain caused by this operation.

Salol in the Treatment of Burns.

Two Italian physicians, Fato and Cabatelli highly recommend salol in the treatment of burns. They first wash the burned part carefully, then empty the blebs and apply small pieces of linen spread with the following ointment:

Lanolin	100 parts.
Salol	3 parts.

This dressing, renewed two or three times a day, rapidly allays the pain, the authors say, prevents inflammatory reaction, and allows rapid healing to take place without bad scars.—*Bulletin Médical*, Feb. 10, 1889.

Influence of Chronic Lead Poisoning on Pregnant Women.

The Paris correspondent of the *Therapeutic Gazette*, March, 1889, says that the influence of chronic lead poisoning on pregnant women and the fœtus was brought to light in 1860 and 1861 by Dr. Constantin Paul. A new instance, interesting on account of the thoroughness of the observation, has just been related to Drs. Hermann-Legrand and Winter of Paris. It occurred as follows: The patient, a woman, 27 years old, worked as a compositor in a printing establishment. She had six times been to the hospital before for lead colic. Five previous pregnancies resulted four times in abortion, and once in a full-term child, which died of convulsions seven months afterward. On the present occasion the patient entered Dr. Budin's service at the Charité Hospital, pregnant for the sixth time, and seven and a half months advanced. She recently suffered again from lead colic, and presented the usual symptoms of the poisoning. Three days after her reception she gave premature birth to a child, but recovered without accident. The husband, it should be added, is a compositor, also affected now and then with the lead-symptoms, but never to any serious extent; no syphilitic taint was observed in him, but a little alcoholism. The child, a boy, was puny, ashy-pale, weighed ten hundred and twenty grammes (about thirty-five ounces avoirdupois), and died after fifteen days. At the autopsy, besides the peculiar appearance and dwarfish size of the kidneys, and a cirrhosis of the liver, the remarkable point was the presence of considerable quantities of lead in the hepatic parenchyma. None was found in the kidneys; they had evidently been impeded in their development, but held no lead. This observation demonstrated that one of the most insoluble of poisons may be transmitted from mother to fœtus, and cause in the child's organs lesions sufficient to render them unfit to carry on life. This much so far may readily be taken for granted, as it is supported by clear evidence. But Drs. Hermann-Legrand and Winter go further, on ground scarcely solid enough. They think that besides hereditary saturnism, there exists quite a series of similar poisonings, not only mineral but also organic, and even bacteriological in their origin. For the present it seems safer to stop at lead, and, so far as other hereditary poisonings are concerned, to wait for further developments.

Adulterated Milk.

The Philadelphia *Ledger*, April 18, says that the Board of Health has adopted a report of its Sanitary Committee asking the City Councils of Philadelphia to pass an ordinance, framed under the provisions of the act of Assembly of April 20, 1869, "to prohibit the sale of adulterated or inpure milk in the city of Philadelphia." The ordinance comprises ten sections, the first of which prohibits the sale, under penalty, of milk which is offered as a pure article but has had any part of the cream removed, or which has been in any way adulterated. The second section permits the sale of skimmed milk, on condition that the vessels containing it are so marked in letters not less than two inches in length. The third section prohibits the sale of skimmed milk as such when it contains less than nine per cent. of the milk solids, exclusive of butter fat. In Section 4 it is made a punishable offence to sell impure or adulterated milk; to keep cows in a crowded or unhealthy condition, or feed them upon food of an unwholesome nature. Section 5 declares the addition of water to milk to be an adulteration; also, milk obtained from cows fed on distillery water or other unwholesome food; or from cows kept in a contaminated atmosphere, or from tuberculous cows. Section 6 provides that, for the purposes of prosecution under the ordinance, milk shown by analysis to contain more than 88 per cent. of watery fluids, or less than 12 per cent. of milk solids, or less than nine per cent. of milk solids exclusive of butter fat, shall be considered to be adulterated. Section 7 fixes a penalty of $50 for the first and $100 for the second and subsequent offences. The remaining sections of the ordinance provide for its proper enforcement.

Dried Potato.

In the *Voënno-Sanitarnoïë Dĕlo*, Dr. Jakov M. Shmulevitch emphatically draws attention to dried potato as an important food-article, possessing some very valuable advantages in comparison with the vegetable in a fresh state. The advantages claimed for the article are these : (1) while fresh potatoes easily rot, blacken, and sprout, dried potatoes, when kept duly protected from moisture, remain in the best condition for a very long time ; and (2), being by far lighter and less bulky than fresh potatoes, are by far more convenient for preservation and transportation, which point has a great practical importance, especially in time of war. To be fit for culinary use, the article requires a preliminary maceration in water for about ten or twelve hours.—*Science*, April 12, 1889.

The Suppression of Small-Pox.

An outbreak of small-pox is reported to have occurred recently in Minneapolis, and the health-officer of that city is credited with having summarily and successfully dealt with it. According to *The Journal of the American Medical Association*, as soon as a case was announced, a consultation was called to determine if the disease was small-pox. That being settled, the patient was removed to the quarantine hospital for treatment. The house where he lived was quarantined, and all the people directly exposed were confined in it. Dr. Kilvington's assistants then began to look up all people indirectly exposed, and vaccinated them. Quarantine houses had guards stationed about them, who allowed no one to go in or out during the season of quarantine. The quarantine people were vaccinated, and during the time until it could be determined whether the vaccination would take, they were supplied with food. When the vaccination took, the person under quarantine was bathed, given new clothing in the place of the old, which was burned, and he was then discharged. When a house had been emptied of people under quarantine, the bedding and curtains were burned, sulphur burned in all the rooms, and the walls sprayed with corrosive sublimate. None of the inspectors or guards were allowed to enter any of the houses under quarantine, when there was danger ; and *the doctors that did the vaccinating saturated their clothing with the corrosive sublimate before and after entering a house where there had been small-pox.* The clothing and bedding were either paid for at a reasonable price by the board of health, or were replaced by new articles. In one of the houses quarantined, *there were 31 laboring men who were inclined to object to the rules of quarantine.* One escaped, but he was taken back when found, *and a guard, with a rifle and instructions to shoot* should he attempt to escape, was put over him. Since Jan. 13, six thousand people have been vaccinated, and the schools, public and private, have been systematically visited, and unvaccinated children vaccinated.

The absurdity of saturating the clothing of the vaccinators before and after entering each house where there had been small-pox is self-evident. Nor do we believe that in this enlightened age any guard would be instructed by a health-officer to shoot a laboring man who, after being shut up forcibly in a house where a case of small-pox had been, should attempt to escape, especially when the house had been disinfected, and the man himself vaccinated. The account above given must, we think, have been obtained from some source outside the health-office of Minneapolis.—*Science*, April 12, 1889.

The Ritual of Circumcision.

Circumcision, says Dr. Messala Pogorelsky, in the *Centralblatt für Chirurgie*, March 30, 1889, is not only practiced by the Jews and Mohamedans, but also among many tribes and nations of America, Asia, Polynesia and especially in Africa, where, as in Abyssinia, for instance, the custom is also in vogue among the Christians. In Central and South Africa not only the men are circumcised but also the women, in whom the labia minora are cut away. Professional circumcisers go from town to town offering their services to the people.

The ritual of circumcision was originally practiced by the Jews for hygienic reasons. The Christians gradually dropped the practice ; those in Rome being the first to do so. Their reasons for abandoning the ritual were principally to make a distinction between themselves and the Jews, and also because they considered the right a hindrance to the spreading of Christianity.

From a surgical point of view, the operation is of great importance. Erichsen says, "all children born with phimosis should be circumcised, also those with an abnormally long prepuce, even if phimosis does not exist. The operation promotes health, cleanliness and propriety, and it would be well if we were to make its practice universal.'' Pogorelsky believes that many barren marriages are due solely to phimosis, and points out the dangers of paraphimosis, retention and the formation of stone, as the possible results of phimosis. Sayre speaks of its causing reflex paralysis and contractions of the lower extremities.

Erichsen quotes many spasmodic diseases as arising from infantile phimosis. Thomas cites 16 cases of trismus neonatorum which were cured by circumcision. Adams cured a case of nocturnal emission by the same operation. It has also proved itself of value in hypochondriac subjects and in cases of chorea minor, neuralgia, hysteria, hallucination and paresis.

Michigan State Medical Society.

Committees of the different sections of the Michigan State Medical Society urgently desire that members further the work of the Society by contributing brief papers. Those willing to do so are requested to fill out a blank, to be furnished by the Secretary, and return it by mail to the Secretary of the Section before which the paper is to appear. Papers should not exceed twenty minutes in length. Those presented must be fully completed, that the publication of the Transactions may not be retarded.

Applications for membership may be filled out by any regular physician desiring membership in the Society. They must be presented by the applicant in person at the annual meeting. Railroad certificates for reduced fare will be sent to all physicians, other than members, who desire them, on application to the Secretary.

The headquarters of the Society will be at the Burdick House, Kalamazoo. All Sessions of the Society will be held in the 1st Presbyterian Church, corner of Rose and South Streets. The Officers of the Society solicit the coöperation of all members, to the end that the next meeting at Kalamazoo may prove the largest and most successful in the history of the Society. The President of the Society is S. S. French, M.D., Battle Creek; and the Secretary is Geo. Duffield, M.D., 25 Washington Avenue, Detroit. The Secretaries of Sections are: Practice of Medicine, H. B. Hemenway, M.D., 524 South Park St., Kalamazoo; Surgery, F. W. Mann, M.D., 250 West Fort St., Detroit; Obstetrics and Gynecology, C. Henri Leonard, M.D., 18 John R. St., Detroit.

—It is stated that cholera is epidemic in the Philippine Islands, and that out of 1,500 cases, 1000 have proved fatal.

—Mr. Henry C. Gibson has given $2500 toward establishing a Chair in the Department of Hygiene of the University of Pennsylvania.

—The Shelby County (Indiana) Medical Society held an interesting meeting at Shelbyville April 9. The morning session was taken up with scientific discussions, and in the afternoon the members and invited guests sat down to a banquet.

—Dr. Sutton, of Pittsburgh, has just finished a series of 50 abdominal sections for diseased ovaries. In the 50 cases he has had 3 deaths. Of the last 36 cases, only 1 was fatal, and in the last 30 there were no deaths. Many of the cysts were very large and adherent.

—According to the *Berliner klinische Wochenblatt*, March 25, Berlin is becoming a healthier city. Although the increase of population was 3.68 per cent. greater last year than the year before, statistics show 32,086 deaths this year against 36,003 the year before. A notable feature is the great decrease in the mortality of children.

—The *Lancet*, March 23, states that the third obstetric clinic at the Vienna Hospital, the director of which is Dr. G. Braun, has had to be closed on account of the occurrence of an epidemic of puerperal fever. This is believed to be due, not to any want of antiseptic precautions, but to the unsatisfactory hygienic condition of the building, which is old, and in which there have been repeated epidemics of puerperal fever.

—The *Deutsche med. Wochenschrift*, Jan. 31, 1889, says that the number of physicians in Germany has so greatly increased in recent years as to have more than doubled since 1880–81. For the examination year 1887–88, according to the publication of the Chancellor, there were 1215 physicians, 562 of whom were in Prussia and the rest scattered throughout the other German States. The numbers of dentists, veterinarians and pharmacists have also increased.

—The Commission appointed by Commissioner Coleman to investigate the subject of hog cholera has nearly completed its work, but finds that additional time will be necessary to finish the report, which was expected April 1. Secretary Rusk has extended the time 30 days. The Commission consists of Dr. Shakespeare, of Philadelphia; Prof. Bolton, of Columbia, S. C., and Prof. Burrill, of Champaign, Ill. The Commissioners have been pursuing their investigations independently for the past five months, but have met from time to time for conference.

HUMOR.

MAN IS ABOUT the only animal who "draws in his horns" through his mouth.—*Danesville Breeze.*

TEACHER—"Now, children, I will give you three words: Boys, bees, and bears; and I want you to compose a sentence which will include all three words."

Small boy—"I have it."

Teacher—"Johnny McCarthy, you may give us your sentence."

Johnny McCarthy — "Boys bees bare whin they goes in swimmin'."—*Harper's Bazar.*

DOCTOR—"Well, there's only one thing for you to do—you must go yachting for nine months!"

Patient—"Oh, that costs so much money; besides I'm a bad sailor—is there no alternative?"

Doctor—"Well, yes—by no means an expensive one, nor one that will make you sick. Don't eat so much!" (Patient chooses the yacht.)—*London Punch.*

THE LAST THE WORST.—Dullard—"So old man Richly is dead at last."

Brightly—"I wonder he lived so long, with all the doctors. Why, Dr. Scalpel had a hack at him, Dr. Piller had a hack at him, and a dozen others."

Dullard—"And now the undertaker has him."

Brightly—"Yes, by gum! and he's the worst. He got seven hacks and a hearse at him."—*Lowell Citizen.*

DANGEROUS TITLES.—Pedestrian (to Washington Policeman)—"What is the meaning of this great crowd in the street, officer? Is anybody hurt?"

"No; there has been an accident and the street is blockaded, but things will soon be in shape again."

"But tell me what has happened."

"Why, you see, Vice President-elect Morton has just met First Assistant Postmaster General Stevenson, and their titles are too long to pass each other on the same thoroughfare. We are trying to induce the First Assistant Postmaster General to resign for half an hour while we get things in shape."—*Chicago News.*

A TRUE MORAL DISTINCTION.—"James," said the grocer, as he looked up from the morning paper, "they have begun to make maple sugar in Vermont already."

"Yes, sir," said the clerk, with ready comprehension. "Those maple sugar bricks left over from last year are down cellar. I'll have them sandpapered and put in the front window to-morrow morning."

"Have you the same sign you had last year to stick up in the box?"

"Yes. It reads 'Fresh from Vermont, strictly pure.'"

"You may use that sign again, James. I don't think it would be exactly right to paint a new one with that inscription."—*Chicago Tribune.*

AN ARTICLE which lately appeared in the *Lancet,* in relation to doctors who tried to appear very learned by using high-sounding technical words to their audiences, suggests to one of our readers an anecdote of the late Dr. Physick. Two doctors had a case of a rather obscure and obstinate character. Dr. Physick was requested to join them in consultation. On his arrival one of the doctors jumped up and began in high-toned and abstruse words to explain the case to Dr. Physick. In the course of his address he said : "Moreover we at last tried to act on the man's dermoid capillaries." This was more than Dr. Physick could stand, and he impatiently broke in and said : "Doctor, for mercy sake, as I have no medical dictionary with me, please explain. Do you mean to say that you tried to sweat the man?"

OBITUARY.

J. H. KIDDER, M.D.

Dr. J. H. Kidder, of the Smithsonian Institution, died in Washington, D. C., April 8, of pneumonia. Dr. Kidder served as a surgeon in the navy until about twelve years ago, when he resigned and became connected with the scientific branch of the Government service. Under Professor Baird he was connected with the Fish Commission, and during recent years was Director of the International Exchanges in the Smithsonian Institution. He leaves a wife and three children.

MEDICAL AND SURGICAL
REPORTER

No. 1679. PHILADELPHIA, MAY 4, 1889. VOL. LX.—No. 18.

CONTENTS:

CLINICAL LECTURE.

ABASIA FOLLOWING POISONING WITH CARBONIC OXIDE.

BY PROF. J. M. CHARCOT, M.D.,

PARIS, FRANCE.

Gentlemen: The case that I present to you to-day is one that is worthy of attention, as it is rare and of a kind but little known. The affection with which the patient is attacked came on after asphyxia from carbonic oxide.   The question arises here, does his trouble depend entirely upon the poisoning or on something else? You will remember that certain cases of poisoning have special relations with the nervous system ; and you know the effects that often follow lead poisoning, as well as that from alcohol. This morbid state appears sometimes not to merit the denomination of toxic hysteria, but simply tends to provoke certain disorders such as I think you will find in the case before us.

This man, as you see, seems to be vigorous, notwithstanding that he is a little pale and depressed. He has a nervous heredity and a history of acute nervous trouble in the past, which I will not speak of at present. He presents certain symptoms to which I wish to call your attention.   I have had him placed on a bed, although he can stand up, for I wish you to remark that, when lying down, he is in an absolutely normal state and does not present any signs of dynamic or organic affection.   His inferior members are supple and he can make all the movements that I ask him to do : he raises his legs, gives a kick, resists all efforts I make to bend the limbs or stretch them, so that coördination is perfect.   Sensibility is also good, and the patellar reflex is normal.   In a word, there is no paraplegia and no ataxia.   The general movements of the body are also normal, as he can turn easily on his back or front ; he can also make the motion of swimming— *he knows how to swim, and has not forgotten it ;* just notice that fact : when he is sitting it is the same, and when he rises we do not see anything abnormal ; for he can stand

531

still with his legs together, or when they are divided, or when in the position for fencing. But, you will ask, what is the matter with him then as he seems to coördinate all movements well? The moment I order him to walk the special incoördination of his case is shown; you will see a series of flexions and extensions of a rapid character which constitute a most singular method of walking. He can hardly turn and cannot walk backward to save him. Notice the way he starts, and this will allow us to analyze the trembling method of stamping or kicking about that he makes as he walks.

You know that in normal walking we commence by bending the knee, and then we raise the foot. Our patient tries to bend the knee also, but at that moment a contrary movement of extension seems to come over him, and he tremblingly lifts his foot from the ground and gives us the spasmodic trembling movement of paraplegia—which we know that he has not, however; we might define the movement by supposing a paraplegic patient who had at the same time a spinal trembling movement. This anomaly, which appears when he starts to walk, continues and increases if he continues to walk, and he goes on like an automaton, bent forward. There is a sort of rhythm in his incoördination which resembles rhythmical chorea, as Professor Grasset, of Montpellier, showed in a similar case; but this is only on appearance, as chorea of the rhythmic form comes not only while the patient is walking but also during repose; besides, it is involuntary, the patient has no power to stop the movements, while our patient has only to stop his movements when he likes.

This man then *does not know how to walk any more*, and does not present any incoördination except for that mode of progression and for that only. Certainly you can understand, *a priori*, that the different methods of progression, such as walking, jumping, dancing, swimming, etc., are quite independent of each other. And when I tell the patient to jump with his feet joined, he can do it. Well, this is explained by the fact that these movements are learned and can be unlearned. A child is born with the single predisposition to execute movements of walking, and to succeed in the regular production of this act he has to make a long apprenticeship. The memory of the movements needed to walk are represented in the cerebral shell by a cellular group that is quite distinct from that which corresponds to dancing and also from that

of swimming. I have shown you that the mechanism of swimming in our patient is intact, he has only interference with walking in a natural way.

I remember the case of a little boy, who could not walk but could jump about the garden of the establishment in which he was under treatment. This peculiarity is curious because it is unforeseen; but it is only a physiological demonstration of the fact that the mechanisms of the different methods of progression are isolated, and independent of each other. I compare the different cellular associations which in the medulla preside over the different modes of progression, to the rollers of an organ or of a music box. The combinations of little points on the rollers, you know, correspond to certain musical tunes or airs. The brain, in my comparison, plays the part of the strings that work the organ, to play or not, and to change the air or to stop it. In our patient the roller of walking is affected, so that there is a contrast between the movements of flexion and extension to the profit of the last; and apart from ordinary regular walking our patient can make any other movement. If he wishes to stride, as actors do in dramatic pieces, he can do so. And you can see him in the garden striding about like a tragedian. Another peculiarity is that he does not turn around like other people, but makes the "right about" of the soldiers. So that he can do almost anything except walk.

There is really nothing curious in nature, it is only our ignorance of these facts that makes things seem so. The first time I ever saw a phenomenon of this kind was in a little boy who was sent to me from Havre, and I was much surprised. He had developed his attack from fear at being charged to make a little speech to the superintendent of his school, who was visiting the house. The fact of having to speak before him, was enough to make this sensitive child ill, and two days afterward he could not walk. When I saw the little patient he was in his bed; he could make all the regular movements, and sensibility was intact, as well as the patellar reflex. On trying to make him stand up it was found that he could not do so, but fell to the ground, so that he could neither walk nor stand. When he got a little better he could jump up a tree and climb, but did not walk for some time. After a relapse he was cured finally.

I have known this affection only for a few years, and I think the first work that was published upon it was in 1883. With M. Richer, I called it a special form of motor impotency of the inferior members, owing to the want of relative coördination of standing and walking; but I wish to say that we found in a work of Dr. Jaccoud's, entitled "Paraplegia and Ataxia of Movement," a passage that briefly spoke of the defect of automatic movement. The author said: "The movements are normal when they are made in the sitting or lying posture, and become ataxic only when the patient stands or walks." M. Jaccoud thought that it was a reflex that came into action when the foot was put upon the ground; but this interpretation does not seem to be well founded. If his theory is not exact, the description of the affection was good. Besides this description, I found in a work by Weir Mitchell, published in 1885, a description which shows that this author has seen the disease also. Under the name of *hysteric ataxia* Dr. Mitchell gives two forms of it: one in which the trouble depends on anæsthesia, as Briquet and Lasègue also saw; and a second form that he describes thus: "The patient has the free use of his legs when he is lying down, but when standing or kneeling the incoördination is at once manifest," etc. The disease then is called now *Astasia-Abasia;* and you will find all that relates to it in a complete work by a former interne of mine, M. Blocq. I have seen several new cases since, and Professor Grasset is about to publish an account of one in the *Montpellier Médical.*

This then is the history of abasia. I have already told you that it attacks young people, but adults are not entirely exempt from it, as our present patient is 41 years of age. It gets well, unless it is complicated with organic trouble. In our case it is dynamic in nature, and I was even afraid the patient would be well before I could present him to the class.[1]

The description of abasia has another point that I must speak of. You must not imagine that it is always the same in its symptoms. There are different forms; for instance, my first patient could neither stand nor walk; the moment he was put on his feet, he fell. This form might be called paralytic. A second variety contains cases in which standing and walking of a kind are possible, but the walking is quite abnormal. One of my patients, whose history was published by Miliotti, was a type of this class. When lying down or sitting his

[1] Prof. Charcot presented this patient cured at the next lecture.

movements were normal, but on standing the contortions commenced; his thighs bent on his legs, and the trunk on the pelvis; then he straightened up only to fall again. In his case it was the reverse of the condition of our present patient, for flexion was increased instead of extension. In other abasic patients the contrary movements of extension will be most marked, so that we may divide them as follows:

Abasia | Paralytic |
       | Ataxic | Trembling form
       | | Choreiform

I must now detail the history of our patient. He is employed in Chaix's large printing office, and lives in a very small room. On November 15 last he desired to heat up a drink he had, and lighted an open fire to do so, and then laid down on his bed and fell asleep; when he woke up three days afterward he found himself in the Hôtel Dieu hospital. Was this loss of consciousness asphyxia-coma? I do not think so, as the latter never lasts three days—rarely over twelve or fifteen hours, when they either sleep or die. We know also that in his case on the second day, a child, who knows him, came to the hospital to see him, and the patient answered his questions without however seeming to recognize the child; and, moreover, he now does not remember this fact, so that he has amnesia, which you know often follows asphyxia from charcoal fumes.

We must ask now if all the phenomena seen in this case can be due to carbonic oxide poisoning? The nervous symptoms following such poisoning have been thoroughly studied by Bourdon, then by Leudet, Lancereau, and Rendu. They are of two classes: amnesia, of which I just spoke, and paraplegia, accompanied by anæsthesia; and trophic troubles—bullæ, scars, herpes, etc.—which get well sometimes, and are often attributed to peripheral neuritis. This paraplegia comes some twenty days afterward; during this time the patient comes out from his coma and returns to his usual occupations, although he is a little stupid; then hemiplegia comes on, which terminates quickly in death. Klebs and Gosetten at autopsies found symmetrical softening of the brain without any vascular obliteration; we do not know the pathogenisis of this trouble.

This is all the knowledge we have of this poisoning by carbonic oxide; what is wanting, and what should be shown, is hysteria. I say this with assurance, as I base my remark on analogy with the other poison-ings that occur from alcohol, lead, and sulphide of carbon, which all provoke neuroses. Nevertheless, if hysteria come after carbonic oxide asphyxia, it is not so important as the amnesia and other symp-toms; it is an hysteria of •a oxy-carbon nature. The toxic principle here is only the occasional cause that reveals the neurosis in a patient predisposed to it. The ante-cedent history of our patient is much in favor of my theory. He is predisposed to hysteria, and the asphyxic accident simply showed its manifestations. During his coma they applied mustard plasters to his legs, and on coming to he saw the scars. He staid at the Hôtel Dieu twelve days, and a short time afterward he found that he could not walk well; from this he became terribly frightened lest he would have serious diffi-culty from this infirmity; and in the mental situation he was then in, we can readily see that the phenomenon of auto-suggestion produced the actual disorder that came on then. However, he continued to walk for ten days when he struck against a person in walking, and from that moment commenced the trembling method of walking I show you. Just note the succession of events on his genealogical tree, which I placed on the black-board, which will give us an explana-tion of his actions:

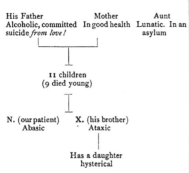

His Father	Mother	Aunt
Alcoholic, committed suicide *from love!*	In good health	Lunatic. In an asylum

11 children
(9 died young)

N. (our patient)	X. (his brother)
Abasic	Ataxic

Has a daughter
hysterical

The past of N. is also interesting. As a child he was tormented by a nightmare, which was always the same. This you are aware is a sign showing nervous origin. He constantly saw himself sleeping at the base of a high wall, on his left side; and he could see at the top of the wall the ends of a ladder, which was on the other side of the wall. On the ladder soon appeared an ugly, bloody figure of a man; the latter held an immense stone which he let fall on N, who awoke screaming. This dream came on almost every night up to the age of 14 or 15, and with such regularity that his mother watched his first sleep to wake him when he cried. His education was very good, and he read many books, among them Moliere, Lamartine and Moreau.

The patient tried the profession of lock-smith, but had to give it up owing to vertigo. Some three years ago a friend of his, in whom he had placed every confidence and affection, was arrested for theft, and since then the patient's existence has been broken; he cries for nothing, even the slightest cause brings on an emotional attack, so that we can readily conclude that he is suffering from hysteria.

We conclude then that we are in the presence of a very singular case, in which walking alone is affected. Where is the seat of the mechanism here? We are led to admit two centers. We know that there is one in the brain, where the mental acts hold their seats and give orders; the other is spinal, and receives the commands, while it also represents the mechanism of execu-tion of them. We have several reasons for believing this. It is told of the Emperor Commodus that he had ostrich's heads cut off, but they continued to walk; ducks also will flap their wings and walk a certain distance after decapitation; the same is true of serpents, which will coil themselves around a stick after losing their heads.

But does not man also walk automatically? I can cite an anatomico-pathological fact which is quite demonstrative of this. I have spoken to you before of spinal marrows, found in autopsies after Pott's disease, which were divided into two parts held together only by a few nerve fibres; and yet these patients walked. The mechanism of walk-ing is found then in the lumbar swelling, and you may readily figure to yourselves that there exists here, in the spinal axis, as many independent centers as there are modes of progression.

As to the prognosis of this case, I have already said that he can be cured quickly. What shall be the treatment? As he is depressed and anæmic, we shall use iron with hydrotherapy. We will also teach him how to walk in a certain way. Perhaps he is hypnotizable, and we can cure him by suggestion; but I admit that, in my service at least, I have not been spoiled by success in this method of cure, as most of the cases of hysterical manifestations in males have failed to be cured by suggestion.

COMMUNICATIONS.

REMARKS ON THE USE OF THE OBSTETRIC FORCEPS.[1]

BY CHARLES P. NOBLE, M.D.,
PHILADELPHIA.

It is by no means my intention to bring before you a formal disquisition upon the obstetric forceps; but rather to confine my remarks to the impressions or opinions concerning the forceps, their use and abuse, which have been impressed upon me by my observation and experience. I am the more inclined to bring the subject before you, because the subject of forceps delivery has occupied my attention to a considerable degree of late; for within a short time seven women have been under my care in private and consultation practice, who have required the aid of the forceps to enable them to complete their labors.

Forceps applications are naturally divided into high forceps and low forceps applications; that is, at or above the brim of the pelvis, and below the brim—in the cavity or at the outlet. This division has not only an anatomical, but also a very practical basis. For, as all the initiated know, a forceps application at the outlet, the indication being simple inertia, is one of the simplest of operative procedures; while the high forceps operation is apt to be exactly the reverse, and often requires the greatest skill and judgment to bring it to a successful termination.

My own experience with high forceps applications is small, being limited to three cases, but I have observed and have assisted at a number of others. The histories of the cases requiring high forceps application are as follows:

Mrs. E. C., 22 years old, a primipara. The patient fell in labor December 11, 1888. After eighteen hours the membranes ruptured; and sometime later, no progress being made, I was asked by her attendant to see her with him. I found her a healthy Englishwoman; but she was exhausted by her labor. The vagina was hot and dry; the cervix fully dilated, but prevented from slipping over the head by lack of descent of the head. The head was in the 3d position, R. O. P., semi-flexed, and impacted. It neither advanced nor receded with the pains, and the doctor informed me that it

occupied at the time I saw it the position it had originally assumed. My attention was arrested by a fleshy strip attached to the cervix, which, after it was drawn down, I found to be a strip of the cervix; and indeed, as examination some weeks after the labor showed, it was the entire anterior lip of the cervix. This strip of tissue was deeply congested, as was the vagina also. The indication was plain—the impacted head had to be brought down and the obstructed circulation relieved. The woman's general condition also demanded delivery.

The Wilson-Davis forceps were applied, twenty-three hours after labor began, and an hour was taken to complete delivery. There was so little room about the head that I thought the pelvis was rather small; but subsequent examination disproved this. The apparent lack of room was due partly to the large size of the child's head, partly to œdema of the soft parts, and partly to the absence of flexion. It was not possible to apply the forceps over the parietal eminences. One blade was applied over one frontal bos, the other over the opposite occipital bos. Very gentle traction efforts were made, due regard being paid to the already torn cervix, and to the œdematous tissues.

After the head was brought to the floor of the pelvis the forceps were removed and internal rotation assisted by manual efforts. The forceps were then reapplied and the head slowly delivered. Owing to the congestion of the tissues laceration of the perineum was anticipated, and it occurred. The child was born in the condition of asphyxia livida, but was easily resuscitated and afterward throve. There was some bruising and a slight laceration of the integument of the forehead, which healed in a few days. The torn strip of cervix was now pulled down, ligated, and removed. The perineum was sewed with much doubt as to the result; but excellent union was obtained. Full antisepsis with douching was employed. The puerperium was normal. Three weeks later I searched for the silk ligature in the cervix but did not find it. The patient was anæsthetized with chloroform.

Mrs. O., 26 years old, a primipara. The patient fell in labor January 27, 1889. She had had prodromal pains for some days. I saw her with her attendant twenty-one hours after he had been summoned. The pains at first had been distant, but later they became more frequent, and ultimately almost continuous. Her pulse was good

[1] Read before The Northern Medical Association of Philadelphia, March 8, 1889.

but she said she was very much exhausted, and was suffering severely. Palpation was unsatisfactory, owing to the rigidity of the uterus. The lower segment felt to me unusually thin. Auscultation detected the fœtal heart sounds. Touch showed that the occiput was presenting to the left iliac bone, and that the head was fixed in the brim. The cervix was half dilated and very flaccid. Incomplete dilatation was evidently due to non-descent of the head A bag of waters was present, although the attending physician told me the patient had been losing water. Through the membranes a well-marked caput succedaneum could be felt. The sacrum could easily be reached, and subsequent examination showed an indirect conjugate of four and a quarter inches. My opinion was that the patient could not deliver herself; so I ruptured the membranes. Chloroform was then ordered. About an hour elapsed from the time I saw her, until the forceps were applied; but in that time no progress was made. I applied Hodge's forceps with difficulty, and somewhat to my surprise I got them over the sides of the head. One hour was taken in extracting the head, and I was obliged to make more vigorous traction efforts than ever before. The brow slipped off the brim with a distinct shock, easily felt by the hands, and apparently with an audible sound. The child was born in the state of asphyxia pallida, the heart was pulsating about thirty times per minute. Efforts at resuscitation failed, and the heart ceased to beat twenty minutes after the birth of the child. A slight rent occurred in the perineum, started by backward pressure over the lock of the forceps. Two sutures were introduced, and partial union resulted. Full antisepsis was employed. The douche was used before and after the forceps. The puerperium was normal. The most striking feature in the case was the presence of a caput succedaneum, with a bag of waters.

Mrs. R., 30 years old. The patient had borne three children. She fell in labor February 3, 1889. Her two previous labors were lingering; one baby was still-born. I saw her in consultation with her physician about twenty-three hours after labor had begun. The brow could be made out by palpation to the right, and the fœtal dorsum to the left. The fœtal heart was plainly heard. Touch detected a cystocele; a dilated os, ready to slip over the head; and the head presenting in the first position—the occiput, however, was farther back than is usual in this position. The

attending physician stated that no progress had been made for some hours. On consultation we decided that labor could be completed spontaneously only after long delay; that probably the forceps would be necessary later for inertia; and that without early delivery the baby would likely be dead, as was the preceding baby.

We recommended the use of the forceps and I proceeded to apply the Hodge forceps, under ether anæsthesia. After the patient was etherized and a more careful examination became possible, the conjugate diameter was found shortened—the sacrum being within reach. No accurate measurements were taken ; the true conjugate was estimated at three and three-quarter inches. The application of the left blade was difficult, because the end of the blade impinged against the shoulder of the child. It was not possible to apply them to the sides of the child's head, so they were applied obliquely. Traction efforts easily brought down the head ; but unfortunately the bladder did not ascend, and it was not possible to push it above the head between the pains. Her attendant had no better success. After forty-five minutes—the head having meantime been brought into the cavity of the pelvis—it was thought best gently to pull the head by the bladder, which was accordingly done. The child was in the state of asphyxia pallida when born, and while it soon gasped occasionally, and later had shallow respirations, more than an hour elapsed before it was in a fairly satisfactory condition. Partial antisepsis was employed, and the douche used the following day. The woman was unable to pass her water for forty-eight hours, but afterward had no trouble. The puerperium was normal.

The problem as to how to manage the cystocele was a serious one. Had the labor been normal, I should have advised the knee-chest position. But under ether anæsthesia this was manifestly impossible. The bladder could not be pushed up because the head occupied all the space between the sacrum and pubes. The perineum was slightly rubbed by backward pressure with the forceps, but a suture was deemed unnecessary.

In these cases the forceps were applied according to the prescribed rules. The head was grasped as gently as possible, sufficient pressure being made to prevent slipping. Between the traction efforts the pressure was intermitted to allow of equalization of the cerebral circulation. When the head is grasped obliquely, unusual care is required to prevent the forceps from marking the child's head. This is especially true of the various modifications of the Davis forceps, and the Hodge forceps; it is less true of the heavier forceps with kite shaped fenestræ, such as the Simpson forceps. Traction efforts were made intermittently, as far as possible during the pains. The least traction was made that would cause the head to advance. To avoid undue traction the sitting posture was maintained, and the elbows allowed to rest on the knees, so that the traction was made principally by the forearms. By means of pressure over the lock in a downward-and-backward direction, in addition to the traction at the end of the handles, the head was drawn upon somewhat in the axis of the superior strait.

My experience with these cases is sufficient to convince me that the ordinary forceps is poorly adapted for use at the superior strait. The difference in the force which is necessary to bring the head through the superior strait as contrasted with that which will bring it through the inferior strait, is a sufficient demonstration that a very considerable part of the force employed when the ordinary forceps is used at the superior strait is wasted—worse than wasted, for it is lost in injurious pressure of the head against the soft parts covering the pubic bone. I have never employed Tarnier's forceps, but I fully accept the principles upon which that forceps is constructed; and from observation I have personal knowledge, that Tarnier's forceps will bring the head from the brim to the floor of the pelvis with far less effort on the part of the operator, than will the ordinary forceps. In the future I intend to use this instrument in high forceps applications.

I believe it best, with the head at the superior strait, to use forceps with a heavy, non-cutting blade, and with the kite-shaped fenestræ; and so to apply the forceps that the pelvic curve of the blades is approximately parallel with the curve of Carus. As already stated, I consider the axis-traction attachment of Tarnier a great advantage, as with its use less force is required to deliver in a given case, than without it.

I did not apply the forceps to the sides of the pelvis in the three cases reported, because I had with me either the modified Davis or the Hodge forceps, which, in my judgment, are not adapted to the application over the face and occiput of the child. The bevelled, sharp, almost cutting edges, of these forceps would almost certainly disfigure the face of the child; not to mention the danger of wounding the maternal soft parts with the projecting heel of the blade—especially of the Davis pattern—in which the heel is only out of harm's way when the blade is applied snugly to the side of the child's head.

The low forceps applications have been made because of inertia of the uterus. Sometimes their use has been hastened by recognizing weakness, extreme rapidity, or extreme slowness, of the fœtal heart beats. In general the forceps have been applied to the sides of the child's head. This is sometimes impossible when the occiput looks toward one ilium and the brow toward the other; no matter whether the position is primitive or the head undergoing internal rotation, the occiput having originally been posterior. Chloroform has generally been given to the "obstetrical degree."

Traction efforts have been made as nearly as possible in the axis of the birth-canal, and during the pains, when pains were present. Half an hour has usually been the time taken to deliver; the object being to secure relaxation and not rupture of the perineum. Delivery has been hastened several times when forceps were applied because of fœtal heart failure. Between the traction efforts the forceps have been allowed to lie loose in the birth-canal, compression being intermitted. The gentlest traction efforts have always succeeded; and vigorous traction has always been avoided. Great care has been taken to feel whether or not the heel of the forceps blade projects beneath the vertex, and to remedy this when it is found. Unless this is done it is extremely easy to cut the posterior wall of the vagina—especially before internal rotation has occurred. This is especially the case with the projecting heel of the modified Davis forceps. It is perhaps needless to say that such cases have come under my observation. When the occiput has crowned, the forceps usually have been removed, and the final delivery left to the patient, assisting her by manual efforts. In a few cases I have purposely left the forceps on; and a few times their removal has been difficult and they have been allowed to remain. When the forceps have remained on but little traction has been made, for as every one knows little force is required to effect the delivery of the head after the occiput has crowned.

The instruction of the books that the handles, while the head is delivering, should be very much elevated and finally lie almost parallel with the abdominal wall, has purposely not been followed. I am convinced that one of three accidents is often produced by this practice: 1. Extension is unduly hastened and exaggerated, and consequently the perineum is apt to be ruptured. 2. The extremity of the forceps blade is apt to cut the soft parts of the pelvic floor—especially when they are not snugly applied to the head. 3. The vascular tissues of the vestibule and lower anterior vaginal wall are apt to be cut by the anterior edge of the forceps blade. This is especially prone to occur with the comparatively straight blade of the Hodge forceps. I have known this accident to happen in good hands several times.

When the head is distending the perineum the reflex contractions of the abdominal wall and of the uterus are almost always sufficient to complete delivery. Hence traction efforts at this time are rarely necessary. It is sufficient to allow *gradual* extension of the head to occur, and at the same time to keep the sub-occipital region in close apposition to the pubic arch.

In occipito-posterior positions I have usually waited patiently for anterior rotation to occur, or I have assisted rotation manually by pressing the brow upward and backward during the pains, or by applying the thumb behind the occiput and two fingers in front of the brow, and impressing a rotary motion on the head. I have been surprised to see how easily rotation can be effected sometimes. When the natural powers have been unable to complete the delivery, the forceps have been applied. In the high forceps case already detailed the head was brought to the floor of the pelvis, rotation effected, and then the forceps reapplied.

The indications for the use of the forceps are various. In general, it may be stated that the forceps are indicated, after the head has engaged in the superior strait, whenever the natural forces are unable to effect delivery with safety to mother and child. This limitation excludes a discussion of the cases in which from contraction of the pelvis, large size of the head or other cause, the head remains movable above the superior strait. On the other hand, whenever the head engages in the superior strait, especially if the biparietal diameter is below the brim, there is reason to believe that the natural powers assisted by the forceps can effect delivery.

Of course the indication varies as to whether the head is at the brim, in the cavity, or at the outlet of the pelvis. A forceps application at the brim, even in skilled hands, has certain inherent dangers, and is an operation of gravity; whereas an application in the cavity or at the outlet is exceedingly simple, and of itself, in skilful hands, can hardly be considered in any case as adding to the danger of either mother or child. Perhaps an exception may be made when the occiput is posterior or toward one ilium. Under these circumstances there is some danger of injuring the child.

Labor may last for a long time when the membranes are unruptured, and the head not impacted in the brim, without serious consequences. Under such circumstances the only indication for instrumental interference would be exhaustion on the part of the mother or cardiac failure on the part of the child. When the cause of delay, or arrest of the head at the superior strait, is a slight disproportion between the size of the child's head and the pelvic inlet, instrumental interference should not be lightly undertaken. The head becomes moulded to correspond with the pelvis, and nature can often do better than art. In such cases the membranes should be preserved. When however the symptoms of exhaustion in the mother supervene, or the circulation of the child becomes embarrassed, delay is no longer permissible. As is well recognized, in order to apply the forceps at the brim, the cervix must be dilated or dilatable, and the membranes ruptured. If these conditions do not exist they must be induced. In case the membranes rupture, the conditions are quite similar to those in which delay occurs in the second stage of labor, with the head below the brim.

It is not my purpose to consider unusual indications for the use of the forceps either at or below the brim, such as heart disease in the mother, eclampsia, threatened rupture of the uterus, etc. The usual indication for the use of forceps in the cavity or at the outlet is a lack of relation between the expulsive force and the resistance to be overcome. Time elapses and little if any progress is made. More or less complete inertia of the uterus is present. The second stage of labor is normally completed in from thirty minutes to two hours; and the time may be somewhat extended without detriment to either mother or child. Still, when the second stage of labor is prolonged beyond two hours, this fact itself should be a cause of watchfulness—the condition of the soft parts of the mother and the life of the child being especially borne in mind. Since there is no fixed limit of time for the conclusion of the second stage of labor, it is evident that the length of the second stage cannot be a positive indication for the use of the forceps; at the same time it should ever be borne in mind that the danger to mother and child increases with the length of the labor, and especially with the length of the second stage of labor.

It is often stated that the forceps should be used whenever the head ceases to advance during the pains, or, what is the same thing, when the head ceases to recede in the intervals between the pains. This is unquestionably a sound general rule. Exhaustion on the part of the mother, which is not relieved by restoratives, is also a pressing indication for the use of forceps. A positive indication is extreme slowness or extreme rapidity of the fœtal heart beats. The fœtal heart should be listened to from time to time during every labor, and especially if the second stage is prolonged.

Finally, I think the question of the operator is a large factor in the indication for the forceps. The skilful man may apply them with relative frequency, and only good result; while the unskilful man may apply them seldom and only evil follow. In my own hands the forceps have been applied in fifteen per cent. of the cases; and yet I am an opponent of the too frequent use of the forceps. The apparent frequency is explained by the fact that most of the forceps applications were in consultation cases. Among my own private cases the forceps have been applied in seven per cent. of the cases. Probably this per cent. will increase in the future.

The dangers arising from the use of the forceps are seldom insisted on. Yet they are not the less real.

The forceps may injure both mother and child. The particular dangers differ with the peculiarities of the case. When the forceps are applied within the uterus, the head being at the superior strait, the uterus may be perforated, lacerated or contused. With proper care and gentleness it hardly seems possible to perforate or rupture the healthy uterus. The principal dangers to be apprehended are contusions of the lower segment of the uterus, and lacerations of the cervix. Contusions are to be avoided by making traction as nearly as possible in the axis of the superior strait, so that the tissues of the uterus may not be caught between the bony head and bony pelvis; and also by seeing that the edges of the forceps blades do not make injurious pressure on the tissues, more especially of the cervix. Laceration of the cervix is no doubt at times unavoidable. Laceration is to be avoided by securing full dilatation

before applying the forceps, if possible; and in every case by using gentle traction efforts, and by avoiding the hasty extraction of the head through the partly dilated os.

When the forceps are applied to the head, in the cavity of the pelvis, the danger of injuring the maternal tissues is not great. It is possible, however, in case the cervix has entirely drawn up over the head so as to be beyond reach, to catch the cervix between the end of the forceps blade and the child's head, and thus perforate the cervix or even tear loose more or less of it. This is especially apt to occur when the long blade of the Davis pattern is used, and it does not seem possible to prevent the accident when these forceps are used. I have known this accident to occur to experienced obstetricians, on two if not three occasions. Also, if the forceps are not applied over the parietal eminences, the projecting edge of one blade may cut the vagina and pelvic floor, unless great care is exercised. This is of course most apt to occur with forceps having wide blades. The nature of the injuries at the outlet which may be caused by the forceps and the methods of avoiding them have been sufficiently indicated already.

The possibility of introducing septic matter into the birth-canal with the forceps necessitates more than ordinary antiseptic precautions. In this connection the dangerous character of the ancient green flannel forceps-bag deserves attention.

The child, too, may suffer. I have seen the skull of the child fractured by the projecting sacrum in a case of labor in a woman having a rachitic, flat pelvis; and yet no undue force was applied with the forceps. Had inordinate traction been used what would have been the result? Undue compression of the forceps may lead to laceration of the integument of the head; depression of the skull; compression of the brain; rupture of blood vessels and hæmatoma, either within or without the skull; death of the child, or worse, paralysis or epilepsy. Such cases are not rare. A rarer accident is the compression of the umbilical cord by the blade of the forceps. These accidents in my judgment, are most liable to occur when a forceps with long, wide, closely approximated blades are used. These not remote possibilities should ever be borne in mind, and the greatest care exercised to avoid them.

It is commonly believed, and I think rightly, that the child is least liable to injury when the forceps are applied over the parietal eminences of its head, the blades being more or less parallel with the occipito-mental diameter; hence, except when the head is at the brim or high in the cavity, with the occiput directed toward one ilium, it is incumbent on the operator to endeavor to apply the forceps after this manner. Should it be impossible, however, the danger to the child is greatly increased. It is then necessary to apply the forceps over one frontal bos and opposite occipital bos, or directly over the brow and occiput. Under these circumstances the greatest gentleness is necessary to avoid injuring the child.

I purposely pass over a further discussion of the merits of various forceps in oblique applications when the head is in the cavity. Also I must omit mention of the use of forceps when the face or the breech presents.

I have not been able to make my remarks as systematic and concise as I wished, but I hope I have made clear the views I wished to elaborate and illustrate. It seems to me that the following are the requisites for the largest success in the use of the obstetric forceps:

1. A thorough knowledge of the anatomy of the organs concerned in parturition.

2. An intimate acquaintance with the mechanism of labor, both when it is normal and abnormal.

3. An equal knowledge of the accidents of labor, and of their prevention.

4. Knowledge of the principles upon which the forceps act; the differences between the action of the different varieties of forceps; and the advantages and disadvantages of each variety, in the varying conditions under which the use of the forceps becomes necessary.

5. The use of the least force, in compression and traction, that will complete delivery.

The object in using the forceps is not only to complete delivery, but also to complete it without injury to mother and child; or, when this is not possible, to complete it with the least injury to mother and child. It seems to me that this desirable end will be best secured when the forceps are used under the conditions named.

———————◆◆◆———————

—Drs. J. A. Watson, S. W. Battle, F. T. Merriweather and others give notice in the *North Carolina Medical Journal*, March, 1889, that an application will be made to the Legislature of North Carolina for a charter incorporating the Western North Carolina Medical College.

GONORRHŒAL RHEUMATISM.[1]

BY CASPAR W. SHARPLES, M.D.,
RESIDENT PHYSICIAN, PHILADELPHIA HOSPITAL.

(*Concluded from p.* 510.)

Case V.—Henry H., 27 years old, an iron-worker, with no family rheumatic history. The patient is a moderate drinker. Three years ago he had his first attack of gonorrhœa without complications. In May, 1887, he had a second attack, beginning six days after connection. During the acute stage he was working and using injections, and in three weeks articular trouble appeared, the urethral discharge having completely ceased two days before. The day before the joints became affected he was more exposed than usual. The next morning he could not get up on account of a sore and swollen left ankle. The sacro-iliac articulation and left knee next became involved. For six months he was disabled with the knee and ankle trouble. Fully eight months after the gonorrhœa, the right hip was affected and has so remained ever since. The right instep has also suffered. During all this period gleet persisted, but has now ceased. The ankles off and on have been so painful that he could not walk for a week or so. The heart has never been affected. Below the malleoli there is now an œdematous infiltration. There is swelling on the outer margin of the os calcis and about the tendo Achillis; the lateral movements of the joint are much impaired, though flexion and extension remain quite good. He has had the heel pain so often observed, and has had all forms of treatment except operative. He has had iodides, salicylates, bichloride, quinia, iron, and all with no effect. The cautery was applied to the hip, and repeated, with temporary results.

Case VI.—J. K., a man 18 years old, was admitted December 6, 1888. There was no history of rheumatism in his ancestors. One brother is rheumatic. The patient does not drink and he denies a venereal history. When he was admitted he had retention of urine for three days, with a small amount of pus at the meatus, which, on examination, showed gonococci. Far back in the urethra there was found a stricture. About the end of August he had an acute trouble in the left foot, the pain appearing before the swelling. There was no redness. The toes subsequently became involved; then the

[1] Read before the Philadelphia County Medical Society, March 13, 1889.

left knee and hip, with much pain and tenderness; the shoulders and lumbar region next became affected, after which pain appeared in the right ankle and foot without manifest change in their appearance. The sacro-iliac joints were last affected. The right elbow was repeatedly affected and remained sore for a month, and now there is partial false anchylosis. For the past six weeks, the left leg has been swollen, œdematous, not tender, but painful on motion. The patient's face presents a waxy dull appearance, a subjective heaviness, and a new fulness under his eyes, especially in the naso-malar fold. The mental region is also full. The patient is anæmic; he sweats a good deal in the feet and legs, and slightly over the rest of his body. He has had no fever while in the house. The disease has made no appreciable change. The heart has not been affected; the urine shows nothing. Treatment was with counter irritation, rest, and oil of gaultheria.

Case VII.—Robert H., 31 years old, was admitted August 27, 1888. No rheumatic history exists in the family. The patient is not a drinking man, but indulges freely in venery. He has had gonorrhœa four times; the first and second time without articular mischief, but at the third attack the joints were involved and have remained so ever since. November 4, 1884, he had an acute non-specific iritis, from which he recovered. In Jan., 1885, he had gonorrhœa, and a recurrence of iritis in the right eye, and soon after this pains came on in the joints, and within ten days after the onset of the gonorrhœa they were acutely inflamed, the inflammation being accompanied by a temperature of 106°. The knees, ankles, toes of the right foot, hip and the elbows were involved, and when the articular mischief appeared, the urethral discharge stopped, and did not reappear for six weeks. He was given twelve grammes of salicylic acid daily for forty days, with great relief from pain, though it caused much gastric distress. During this attack he had scleritis, tenderness of the right eye, and iritis. He was in bed till the middle of March, when his articular pains were relieved though not completely. In April, 1885, the joints were still sore. Three times daily he had rubber bandages applied for thirty minutes, and a daily hot bath, with temporary relief. In May, 1885, he had an iridectomy performed upon the right eye with some relief. Subsequently he took warm mud baths with great benefit. In June he had iritis of the left eye, during which he received iodide of potash and pilocarpine. Throughout the summer of 1885 he continued disabled. In Sept., 1885, he again had iritis. In Dec., 1885, he was quite free from joint trouble. At this time he again contracted gonorrhœa, and in eight days he had a recurrence of iritis in the right eye. The urethral discharge continued until March, 1886, when the left shoulder was involved, accompanied by double iritis lasting for six weeks. The joints of the feet were much affected. In the winter of 1886 and 1887 he was pretty well. In March he again had iritis in the right eye. In June he again had gonorrhœa, followed by involvement of the feet, toes and ankles. Since his admission he has had persistent gleet and attacks of iritis of long duration. The plantar arch is nearly gone. He walks with great difficulty and has a peculiar heavy appearance, with an enlarged naso-malar fold. He is anæmic and pale. The heart is normal. The urine contains oxalates. Treatment has been of no benefit.

Case VIII.—G. S., a man 52 years old, was admitted October 26, 1888. He had been in the house before with the same trouble. The family history is negative. At eighteen he had chancroids and buboes. At twenty-two he had his first attack of gonorrhœa, with gleet, lasting for a year. About three weeks after he seemed to be cured of the acute affection, the ankles and knees began to swell, confining him to bed for eight weeks. Four years after that he had a second attack of arthritic trouble, the ankles and knees becoming as when he had gleet. At this time he was laid up for eight weeks. Two years subsequently after gonorrhœa the rheumatic affection recurred. In two years he had a fourth attack, in which the joints were affected. In the first and second attacks he had ophthalmia, and with each subsequent attack the eyes became injected and their secretion increased. The present is his seventh attack, and began four months ago, following urethritis on the third day. The ankles, knees, phalangeal joints of the right index finger, the metacarpal joints and wrists were affected in the order of mention. The right sterno-clavicular joint has also been involved. The joints have always been red, with a moderate degree of swelling, which was more marked in the first than in subsequent attacks. For the first time the hands have been involved. The ankles and right carpus are stiff. Each subsequent attack seems milder. There has been no heart trouble and no sweats. Treatment of the urethra and joints was local, and sulphide of calcium was administered. The man left the house slightly relieved.

Case IX.—L. A., a colored man, 39 years old. No rheumatic family history exists. He has been much exposed to cold and wet, and especially for three years while in the army. He is not a drinking man. He has now advanced phthisis. In July, 1876, he had gonorrhœa, the discharge appearing in six days after infection. Two weeks later he had a severe wetting. The following morning he could not move. In three days the urethral discharge left, and the elbows and ankles became painful and swollen. The knees were stiff as well as the hips and shoulders. The temporo-maxillary joints were so swollen that he could not open his mouth. The left ankle was the part most affected. It was thirteen months before all the joint affection left. Up to the present he has had no further joint trouble. Early in Dec., 1888, he had pain and swelling in the left ankle, and extreme tenderness. With this again came some urethral disturbance, though he has not had gonorrhœa since the first attack. For the last attack he had iodine applied, massage employed, and salicylates administered with good effect. No murmur is found at the apex, but a distinct systolic murmur at the second left interspace.

Case X.—F. M., a woman 19 years old. The patient's mother had rheumatism. She herself has no previous venereal history, and never before had had rheumatism. She does not know the time of infection, but about nine weeks after she first saw the discharge, she had pain in the joints. The gonorrhœa was complicated by buboes. The swelling first began in the right wrist, which was only slightly red, and extended into the hand and fingers. There is now a peculiar induration and thickening of the dorsal surface of the hand. The skin is dark and over the fingers decidedly glossy. The temperature has not been above 100°. Improvement has been slow. The condition as above mentioned is at the end of the seventh week. The patient appears heavy in the face, with a large naso-malar fold, and she is anæmic and pale. The heart is normal. She has had iron and quinia and has made slow improvement.

The third class, or "acute gonorrhœal rheumatism," is much rarer than the former. The pains wander from joint to joint, and then suddenly, often at night, one joint suffers the severest pain, and soon periarticular œdema and fusiform enlargement appear, so that the affection has been described as

an enlargement of the bones. The pain is worse at the plane of articulation, from which point swelling extends, usually along the dorsal surfaces of the wrist or ankle. The joint has heat, but may be pale or red, and febrile disturbance is not marked. The trouble may undergo resolution, or may go on to suppuration, but most commonly ends by fibrous anchylosis. Such a class of cases may most readily be confounded with acute rheumatism, as it runs a less chronic course and comes on more rapidly. Though I have no case recorded here under this heading, yet I think that Case I properly belongs here; it was put with the others on account of the cardiac condition.

The fourth class, "chronic hydrarthrosis," may occur in connection with the polyarticular variety, or may be monarticular alone. It usually attacks the knee, and a few cases are recorded in which it attacked both knees at once. The effusion comes rapidly and insidiously into the joint, without any heat, change of color, tenderness, marked pain or fever. Pus formation following it, is rare. It is curious to note that in many books we find only this form described, and no mention made of other varieties of gonorrhœal rheumatism. From the case, which I have added as an example of this, an attempt was made to obtain cultures from the serum withdrawn from the joint, but with no success.

Case XI.—T. B., a man 23 years old, was admitted January 15, 1889. The patient is a temperate man. Fourteen months ago he had his first attack of gonorrhœa, during which he let a tub fall upon his foot, which became sore and swollen. Three weeks before his present admission, he again became affected with gonorrhœa. The discharge from the urethra became watery and thin. The right knee was swollen ten days after the discharge appeared. The swelling progressed rapidly, and within two days he could not get out of bed. He did not have much pain, but had a good deal of swelling. On admission there was marked distension and fluctuation in the affected joint. Cold bichloride towels were applied over it with apparent benefit and rapid disappearance of the effusion. On the 22d, the left wrist was swollen and the arm stiff and painful. On the 24th, the ankle became swollen, without pain. The urethral discharge has been slight and is now most abundant. Salicylate of soda internally and bichloride applications locally were ordered. The man is now better, with slight swelling and stiffness of the knee.

Dr. Osler has furnished me with notes of a case of "multiple arthritis" of gonorrhœal origin. A. B., 31 years old. In 1869 the patient had an attack of gonorrhœa, which was followed by inflammation for ten weeks. In 1876 he had a second attack, accompanied with swelling of both feet. The other joints gradually became affected and he had a prolonged illness, the attacks recurring alternately with periods of comparative comfort. He was incapacitated and had more or less joint trouble for eight years and eight months. He went about to various hot springs and sanitaria, at which he secured only temporary benefit. Dec., 1887, he had three attacks of gonorrhœal rheumatism, after nearly three years of fair health. Within a month of that time he was attacked in the ankles, knees, and hips. Jan. 12, 1888, it was noted that he had had pains with slight swelling in the metatarsal and phalangeal joints, and also in the right ankle, knees, hips, and shoulders. He was anæmic, thin and delicate looking, with slight fever and no heart affection. The ankles and toes were red and painful. At first he received gaultheria with benefit, but later Fowler's solution was substituted. He remained in the hospital but a few weeks and then went to the Hot Springs of Arkansas. This case, with some of the others, illustrates the extreme chronicity of this disease.

The fifth and last form needs no attention. It involves especially the sheaths of the tendons, the bursæ and, it is said, the periosteum. It often comes without any accompanying joint affection. There is great pain, tenderness and local swelling. The pain is more marked at night. Gonorrhœal bursitis is rare and for the most part occurs over the patella and around the olecranon. To this is due the peculiar pain, the small bursa beneath the os calcis being the one affected. Most of the above cases illustrate this class.

There is no constancy at all as regards the urethral discharge, and this does not need better proof than the fact that one author describes one period, and another another period, for the occurrence of rheumatic symptoms. Some say that the discharge stops with the appearance of gonorrhœal rheumatism, and others that it suffers no abatement. In some cases the discharge has stopped before the rheumatism appeared, and in others it persisted throughout, or to nearly the end of the attack. If the discharge stops before the attack, it may and usually does stop suddenly; and patients are apt to say that it stopped as the result of injections; or when the attack appears the discharge may suddenly be sensibly diminished and resemble gleet. The occurrence of an orchitis and an increase of the discharge, as took place in Case IV, I think quite anomalous. Otherwise the discharge presents no interest, unless it be for the purpose of diagnosis by staining it to discover gonococci. Many cases of rheumatism could be placed in this category if the genitals were carefully examined.

The theories as to the origin of this trouble are many, and are all alike in the fact that they cannot be proved. In former times it was said that the origin was by metastasis, and irritants were applied to increase the urethral discharge. There is a "reflex" theory, the physiology of which is simple. The irritation goes up through the sacral plexus into the spinal cord and to the trophic centers, and then we see the changes mentioned. Why any urethral irritant may not cause this is hard to explain, unless it be the fact that the specific element of gonorrhœa is more irritating. In some cases sciatica has been noted, due probably to the same cause.

At present the septic theory has the most supporters. In cases of septicæmia arising from gonorrhœa the prostatic plexus and urethra have been found full of pus. One line of treatment has been based on the septic view. The rheumatism is a general affection and the gonorrhœa a local one, and is so universally regarded; but in the light of the reported cases of endocarditis with gonorrhœa there may be something more in it. What the change is that occurs to make gonorrhœa a gonorrhœal rheumatism, I do not think we can yet say. In Van Buren and Keyes's article I find this statement, practically expressing nothing, but at the same time about all that we know: "It is then, an idiosyncrasy which causes a patient with gonorrhœa to develop rheumatism, and not any tendency to suffer with the latter complaint."

All measures of treatment have only little curative effect. If the urine should be too acid, use alkalies. Pain requires the application of leeches, the use of morphia and salicylates. Salicylates have the same effects as in ordinary rheumatism, viz.: to allay the pain and lower the temperature, but not to cure the affection; and they should be stopped when this end has been attained. Splints should be applied and the joints protected. Plaster has been applied even in the acute stage, with the result of relieving the pain and diminishing the swelling, but not hastening the cure. Small doses of mercury have been recommended, along with quinine and iron. The joints should be enveloped in cotton. The urethra should be treated. In later stages apply mercurial ointment, massage, pressure, and use passive motion. In the acuter stages perhaps the application of cold bichloride cloths may be deserving of more trial.

TRISMUS FOLLOWING DOG-BITE OF THE FINGER. RECOVERY AFTER AMPUTATION.

BY CHARLES B. PENROSE, PH.D., M.D.,
PHILADELPHIA.
OUT-PATIENT SURGEON TO THE PENNSYLVANIA HOSPITAL.

The following case occurred in the writer's service at the Pennsylvania Hospital.

J. M., a woman 40 years old, was bitten by a dog on the little finger of the right hand, in August 1888. The patient received on the palmar aspect of the finger a lacerated wound, two inches in length, which divided the tissues down to the periosteum. From the beginning she suffered intense pain, shooting from the finger along the arm, shoulder and neck to the right ear. This was followed in a few days by continual tinnitus and subsequent complete deafness in the right ear. The finger was never swollen or inflamed; the wound, however, showed no tendency to heal.

Six days after the injury the patient began to experience difficulty in swallowing and in opening her mouth; and she came under the charge of the writer on the seventh day after the injury. At this time the skin of the injured finger was dry, with several blebs on the palmar surface. The wound was unclosed, presented a gangrenous appearance, with no evidence of granulation. There was no swelling of the hand or of the finger. There was continual spasm of the muscles of mastication, which prevented her from opening the mouth except to a very slight extent. There was complete deafness in the right ear, and she complained of tinnitus in the left ear similar to that which had preceded the deafness in the right.

The wound was thoroughly washed, and frequently changed wet dressings of bichloride of mercury (1-2000) were applied; and large doses of bromide of potash were administered internally. This treatment was continued for ten days, with no marked effect either on the muscular spasm, the pain, deafness or tinnitus aurium.

The finger was consequently amputated at the metacarpo-phalangeal articulation. The next day the shooting pain and the trismus had disappeared. The amputation wound healed by first intention. The deafness and tinnitus aurium continued, and were still present two months after the amputation, though the general condition was in all other respects good.

SOCIETY REPORTS.

NORTHERN MEDICAL ASSOCIATION.

Stated Meetings, March 15 and 29, 1889.

The President, DR. JOSEPH S. GIBB, in the Chair.

DR. CHARLES P. NOBLE read a paper entitled

Remarks on the Use of the Obstetric Forceps.[1]

DR. HENRY LEAMAN, in opening the discussion, said: I am glad to have a subject of such practical importance brought before the Society. The essayist has covered the subject very well, and in most points I agree with him, especially in his summary of conclusions. I have gone over the last 950 labors occurring in my practice, of which I have notes, and find that the forceps have been used 137 times, about once in seven labors. The presentation in 91 of these cases was vertex to the front (left or right). In 40 it was posterior (right or left). The forceps were applied once with a presentation of the face, where the head had been impacted under the use of ergot (given by a midwife) for three hours; once, in an induced labor; once, during convulsions; and once to the after-coming head.

I have applied the forceps 10 times at the superior strait, the indication being a shortened conjugate diameter or obliquity of the pelvis. In the remaining cases they were applied when the head had more or less completely engaged in the pelvic cavity. The use of the low forceps was rendered necessary by weak abdominal muscles in two cases of obesity; once by mitral disease of the heart; but the usual indication was delay in the second stage of labor. This delay is invariably due to a want of sufficient flexion, owing to a lack of easy adjustment between the head and pelvic canal. The head is most frequently at fault either in size, irregularity of shape, or undue closure of the fontanelles. A resisting per-

[1] See REPORTER, p. 535.

ineum will occasionally call for the use of the forceps.

In all cases the os was either dilated or dilatable when the instruments were applied, except in the case of convulsions, when they were applied as soon as the os was dilated sufficiently to admit them.

The only injury done to the mother was a rupture of the fourchette in four cases, and of the perineum in four cases—making injury to the perineum once in sixteen labors. I have never seen any injury to the child except slight marking.

The instruments used were a long-handled forceps, known as Wallace's, and a short-handled forceps known as Davis's. These I have found sufficient for all purposes.

DR. H. W. RIHL said: How should the forceps be used? When we consider that the death of the child very often results from prolonged labor, if severe, it becomes a grave question as to how long we shall wait before interfering. My own experience has been that by far fewer children are born dead when instruments are used early. If the head has engaged for even one or two hours, the pains being frequent and severe without causing the head to advance, and if the position of the head can be accurately diagnosticated so that the forceps can be applied to the sides of the child's head, and if the os is well dilated or dilatable—I generally advise the application of the forceps. If the position is transverse, *i.e.*, if one ear is behind the symphysis pubis, I apply the blades to the sides of the head and rotate so as to bring the vertex under the symphysis. I would long hesitate before applying the forceps over the forehead and back of the head.

But the forceps are not only, as Dr. Meigs used to call them, "the child's instrument," they are also the mother's. Are we justified in allowing her to suffer hour after hour when we can easily and safely terminate her sufferings—under the plea that labor is a physiological process with which we must not meddle?

I use forceps also when convulsions occur or are impending, when labor is complicated by feebleness or disease of the heart, and when the mother is exhausted by the labor.

Many object to the forceps because the perineum is often lacerated when they are used. Do we give sufficient weight to the fact that the cases in which forceps are used are generally those in which the head is abnormally large? Would not the tear therefore be quite as likely to occur without them? Recently in a primiparous labor, after bringing down the head to the perineum, I removed the forceps, and made a careful examination of the perineum and found it intact. After the completion of the labor I found a laceration extending to the sphincter ani. Had the forceps not been removed, they would probably have been blamed for the tear.

The injuries which the forceps are supposed to entail upon the child are doubtful. Are epilepsy, idiocy, etc., due to the pressure of the forceps, or are they not rather the result of the prolonged pressure in the pelvis, before the forceps are applied? and would not an earlier use of the forceps prevent many of these unfortunate results of difficult labor?

Finally, I may remark that my opinions with reference to the forceps are drawn from an experience of more than 300 applications, in nearly 3000 obstetric cases. I almost always use the Bethel forceps, which I have had made with blades of about double the usual thickness. These thick blades are not so apt to mark the child as thinner blades. Of late years when the position of the child could not be determined with accuracy or when it was transverse, I have at times used Simpson's forceps.

DR. D. LONGAKER: If Dr. Noble's paper has been carefully followed you will have noticed, whenever injuries to mother or child have been mentioned, that he has stated that these injuries are most apt to happen when forceps are used having long, closely approximated blades, with wide fenestræ and projecting heels. My own experience and observation teach me that this is true. When I began practice I used the Hodge forceps. I gave these up, partly because of the dissatisfaction I felt with their action, but largely owing to the teaching of the late Dr. Albert H. Smith, my teacher, who was a strong advocate of the modified Davis instrument, which bears his name. Upon adopting this instrument I soon began to have accidents occurring in my hands. I pinched a hole in the anterior lip of the cervix by catching it between the end of the forceps blade and the side of the head. I have also known this accident to happen to others using this or a similar instrument. A moment's thought will show that this accident is unavoidable, when as in my case the head is in the pelvic cavity and the cervix retracted beyond reach. It is of course most likely to happen with a forceps such as this, the blades being long with the ends closely approximated and thin. I also found it extremely difficult to prevent scoring the vagina with the heel of the instrument. Nor did the child entirely escape. It was not uncommon to mark the scalp, especially when the forceps could not be applied over the parietal eminences. In one case in an oblique application one blade pinched the umbilical cord which was around the neck, and the other injured an eye. The child was born asphyxiated and subsequently died. With this experience I adopted the Simpson forceps, which I have used with the greatest satisfaction. Moreover, the modified Davis forceps is a powerful compresser, an action of the forceps which is least desirable to employ, as it can do only harm.

With reference to forceps for use at the superior strait, it seems to me that the verdict of obstetricians is in favor of Tarnier's instrument, especially when the indication is contraction of the pelvis. My own experience with the instrument has been most gratifying.

DR. LEAMAN: It by no means follows that all who use the modified Davis forceps, which is capable of producing marked compression of the head, bring into play this action of the forceps. I condemn undue compression with the forceps as strongly as any one. It is not my purpose to detail my method of employing the forceps this evening, as I am now engaged in writing a paper on the action of the forceps, but suffice it to say that I use them very differently than I was taught by the late Prof. Wallace.

DR. HORN exhibited a pair of Bethel forceps, which was owned by Dr. Bethel himself. The forceps had long narrow blades with a very marked pelvic curve. The blades were thin and springy, and were quite beveled. He said: I would not use this forceps owing to the exaggerated beveling of the blades. This would cause marking of the child's head, unless caught squarely. Such a forceps should only be applied to the head of a dead child.

DR. RIHL: I have used the Bethel forceps about 300 times on living children. I object, however, to the thin blades of the pair exhibited.

DR. G. W. VOGLER: I have a pair of Bethel's forceps which I occasionally use. When other forceps slip, Bethel's often will not slip. I think it is especially adapted for use within the uterus to make the head engage. When this has been accomplished this forceps should be removed and some other substituted, as owing to the great pelvic curve, the ends of the blades are apt to injure the anterior lip of the cervix.

I quite agree with those who advocate a moderately thick blade to the forceps. I think the forceps does not often cause injury, in good hands. I have not seen grave injury to the soft parts. I usually apply the forceps when the head has been stationary for one or two hours.

DR. JAMES COLLINS: But little has been said concerning the use of high forceps in the discussion. My rule is to apply high forceps when I think there is little prospect of being able to apply low forceps. I have seen the vagina scored and the perineum ruptured by the projecting heel of Wallace's forceps, as mentioned by the writer of the paper.

DR. STRITTMATTER: I agree in the main with the points which have been brought out in the paper and the discussion. I wish to emphasize that I am an advocate of the frequent use of forceps. I see no objection to applying the forceps in any case when the soft parts are relaxed. Palpation and auscultation are of great assistance in forming a diagnosis of the position of the head, especially when it is at the superior strait. I have seen some injured heads due to forceps delivery, but in these there was no subsequent idiocy or deformity.

With reference to axis-traction forceps, I do not think it is possible to draw exactly in the axis of the pelvis with any forceps. The chief merit of Tarnier's forceps is, that it interferes but little with the normal movements of the head—flexion, and internal rotation—during labor.

DR. ROBERT J. HESS: I have had a large experience among the insane, and considerable experience as an obstetrician, and have not been able to convince myself that the forceps are the cause of many cases of idiocy, epilepsy, or paralysis. I consider the forceps one of the most beneficent of instruments, and think that they can be used often with advantage. The only injury I have seen has been to the perineum.

DR. NOBLE: Dr. Leaman has found the Wallace and Davis forceps sufficient for all cases. It has not been my purpose to discuss particularly the many forceps in use. As I indicated in my paper, however, I do not believe that there is a "best" forceps. I still believe that we should use axis-traction forceps at the superior strait—either Tarnier or Poullet's. I have found the Hodge forceps a satisfactory instrument when applied to the sides of the child's head in the cavity or at the outlet. But it is not satisfactory when applied obliquely to the head or directly over the brow and face. Hence I am inclined to think that the best combination for the obstetrician to possess is a pair of Tarnier's and a pair of Simpson's forceps. With reference to applying the forceps for the sole object of relieving the mother's sufferings, as advocated by Dr. Rihl, I have not found this necessary. Chloral hydrate and morphia in the first and chloroform in the second stage, given when labor was unusually painful, have yielded good results.

REPORTS OF CLINICS.

HARLEM HOSPITAL.

SURGICAL CLINIC—DR. MANLEY.

Local Tuberculosis.

The first two patients presented by Dr. Manley at his clinic on April 8, 1889, were typical cases of what is at the present time described by pathologists as suppuration due to tubercular trouble, and what was formerly known as scrofula or struma. Indiscriminately classifying every kind of disease of bone or gland tissue as tubercular must lead to mischief, by tending to prevent what is rational and proper in such cases, namely, the removal by operative means of the source of ulceration.

This, however, is opening the way for the removal of an endless number of joints by resection, and to other needless mutilations, in order to eradicate the tubercle, under the false assumption that tubercle is always destructive when left alone. Dr. Manley observed that while the pathological or bacteriological elements found in the joints or gland tissues of a child are identical with those of pulmonary tubercle in the adult, still there exists—and this should be always borne in mind—a vast difference in the clinical peculiarities of each. In the one case, that of children, the disease is, as a rule, curable, and generally leaves the individual with no impaired vitality. It may leave an anchylosed joint, but it does not in any way interfere with the general health. Besides, repair is the rule in scrofula or early tubercular processes, not only of areolar tissue alone, but also of bone. On the other hand, with pulmonary tuberculosis in adults, death is the rule; recovery is seldom seen, and when it does occur, the cavities show none of the originally destroyed tissue reformed, but the void is filled with a shiny cicatricial tissue.

In the case of the first patient, no history of traumatism was elicited. The child,

three years old, complained of pain in the back, and weakness, which was diagnosticated as lumbar disease and treated by the plaster jacket. This having been worn three months, the pain disappeared, and the spinal lesion appeared to be arrested. A month later the mother noticed that the child could walk on the right limb only with difficulty, and that it complained of much pain at night. It was now evident, upon examination, that ulceration had commenced in or about the hip-joint, for a large accumulation of matter had formed over the great trochanter and was pressing toward the surface. This was opened, irrigated and drained, the part buried in moist antiseptic gauze, and the limb placed in an immovable dressing. No effort was made to search for the seat of bone disease, as it was decided to await results. It is well known that a small exfoliation of necrosed bone will work its own way out; besides, later, when the child has improved in strength, should a fistulous opening refusing to heal remain, the parts can be laid open and the sequestrum removed.

The second case, that of a boy nine years old, was one which was dependent largely on the same diathesis, but differed in not having originated or been hurried into action by an injury. Dr. Manley observed that while it was yet a disputed question in tubercular lesions in children, and especially those of bone, whether or not they were dependent upon injury or constitutional disturbance alone, he was decidedly of the opinion that a very large proportion was directly dependent on injury as an immediate cause. This boy injured his right forearm on its radial side by a fall some two months ago. It had been swollen and painful ever since, and was now evidently the seat of suppuration. A long incision was made, and the lower two-thirds of the radius found saturated in pus, but with a well-formed sheath of periosteal formation enclosing it. A large sequestrum of bone was then removed and the wound dressed with idoform gauze.

Knock-Knee.

The third case was one of knock-knee, due to a bowing outward of the femora. The lecturer was persuaded, from what he had seen of congenital and acquired deformities in the bones of children, that they were as often the result of weak ligaments and want of harmony in muscular action as of deficient inorganic matter. The modern method of treating these cases—which he thought decidedly unsurgical—was to break or to cut the bones—osteoclasis or osteotomy; but while these means readily remove the deformity, they do not remedy the defect. That they certainly remove the *visible* deformity—which both the patient and the parents are most anxious about— there can be no doubt; but it is a question if, as regards the strength and general usefulness of the limb, this practice does not leave more or less displacement of bone and consequently a defect in strength. In this instance a double osteotomy was performed, the parents refusing to allow the child to remain in the hospital a year.

Traumatic Gangrene of the Little Finger.

The fourth case was one of traumatic gangrene of the little finger, extending to the metacarpal bones. This case, according to Dr. Manley, was of more than ordinary interest for two reasons, first as to the cause and second as to the treatment. The patient gives the following particulars as to the origin of his complaint: two weeks ago he scratched the back part of the little finger of his left hand in handling some boards; he dressed the finger with adhesive plaster. A few days later the wound began to fester and commenced to give him great pain; the finger and hand then swelled to a great size. Here was mortification, or gangrene, of the hand coming from a mere scratch, a really typical case of wound infection with the germs of putrid wounds. Dr. Manley remarked that it was well to notice that wounds are usually more prone to take on erysipelatous action in the months of March and April. As regards the treatment, the part, he said, should be immediately opened when pus was suspected, and the wound treated on the most antiseptic principles. In this case he would cut down and remove all tainted tissue. This, he remarked, being a case of spreading gangrene, it could be arrested only by the prompt and free use of the knife.

The gangrenous process was found to extend into the metacarpo-phalangeal articulation, whereupon the little finger and the distal end of the fifth metacarpal bone were removed, the flaps loosely brought together, and the wound well drained.

———

—The child of Mr. C. J. Moore, a surgeon of West Middlesex, England, was attacked with diphtheria, and the father performed tracheotomy and sucked the tube clear. Both father and child died.

PERISCOPE.

Pathology of Chronic Alcoholism.

The Pathological Society of London has devoted much time recently to a consideration of the pathology of chronic alcoholism. The discussions have been prolonged and very interesting. The following brief review of them, taken from the *Quarterly Jour. of Inebriety*, April, 1889, will prove of interest to the readers of the REPORTER:

Dr. Payne, in his opening and closing of the debate, insisted clearly on stating his belief that the ordinary pathological conception of cirrhosis needs reconsideration. He demurred to regarding it as a mere inflammation of the interstitial stroma of the liver set up by alcohol introduced through the portal vein, and producing great quantities of new fibrous tissue, which by pressure destroys the hepatic cells. He insisted that the destruction of cells and the hyperplastic inflammation of connective tissue take place concurrently, and in this view he was supported by Dr. Lionel Beale, who held that the essence of cirrhosis is atrophy of cells, and not inflammation of connective tissue. Dr. Dickinson stoutly maintained that the overgrowth of fibrous tissue is the essence of cirrhosis; and Dr. Sharkey showed specimens of apparently healthy liver cells side by side with masses of newly-formed connective tissue even in advanced cases of cirrhosis. He suggests that the liver cells seen in such connection with newly-formed fibrous tissue may be newly-formed cells; his hopeful view of the formation of new cells and new bile ducts is especially noteworthy; in other words, there may be a restoration of tissue in a diseased liver, a possibility supported, as he says, by clinical experience of cases of recovery from grave degrees of hepatic disease.

Not the least interesting part of the debate was that having reference to alcoholic paralysis and other forms of nervous disease produced by alcohol. What is eminently worthy of the attention of practitioners in this connection is the frequency of tuberculous disease in cases of alcoholic paralysis. In fact, the association of chronic alcoholism in all forms, and tuberculosis, was brought out by almost every speaker, including Dr. Payne, who said truly that the inaccurate impression that habits of alcoholic excess are in any way antagonistic to tubercular diseases must be regarded as swept away. Dr. Dickinson's investigations into the comparatively much greater frequency of tuberculosis in publicans and others whose occupations and habits expose them to the evil of chronic alcoholism were the first to open the eyes of the profession to the fallacy that alcohol ·antagonizes tubercle. Many eminent medical men have felt with Dr. Dickinson that, as alcohol does so much harm, it surely must do some good. But, so far, the good that it does or the evil that it prevents has not been made very manifest. They need more definition. Dr. Izambard Owen says the statistics of the Collective Investigation Committee show that the consumption of alcoholic liquors appears to check malignant disease. This statement should now be tested very rigidly. Malignant disease is said to be on the increase. We have seen the demolition of the belief that alcohol is a preventive of tubercle; it would be some set-off against the mischief it works if it could be shown seriously to antagonize cancer.

The views and opinions of the many leading men who participated in this discussion were expressed in a scientific spirit, not as absolute or final, but as the most probable facts sustained by our present knowledge of the subject.

Relation Between Chlorosis and Menstruation.

At the meeting of the Obstetrical Society of London, March 6, Dr. W. Stephenson, Professor of Midwifery, University of Aberdeen, read a paper on the relation between chlorosis and menstruation; an analysis of 232 cases. The author observed that in the rapid progress of uterine specialism, chlorosis in its relation to menstruation had been too much neglected by the gynecologist. The 232 cases were divided into two groups: (1) where the illness was primary and occurred before the twenty-third year, comprising 183 cases; (2) where the attacks were of the nature of relapses after a period of good health (49 cases). Dr. Stephenson regards chlorosis as due to a constitutional state; but the diathesis. is not necessarily associated with an impairment of the development of the body, and is not, to any marked degree, connected with defective health previous to the onset of the disease. The influence of the chlorotic constitution on menstruation before chlorosis sets in was first discussed. Tables were given to show that the tendency of the chlorotic diathesis is to accelerate the age at which menstruation first appears, and that chlorosis by itself is not a cause of retarded appearance of the catamenia. At the same time, in one-half of the cases, the functional activity is defective, and is chiefly characterized by lengthening and irregularity of the intervals and scantiness in the amount of the flow. The author's statistics were against the opinion that there is a menorrhagic form of chlorosis. In 96.6 per cent. the effect was to diminish the activity of the function, the remaining fraction being complicated with ovarian irritation. In 58.7 per cent. menstruation became scanty and irregular, and in many cases painful, while in 37.8 per cent. there was amenorrhœa for various periods. A table was given to show that there are two marked chlorotic periods: the one, of primary attacks, from the age of fourteen to twenty-one; the other, of secondary attacks, from twenty-four to thirty-one. The number of cases of the disease presents a regular curve, beginning at the age of fourteen and rising steadily to a maximum between eighteen and nineteen, then rapidly falling, to disappear altogether at twenty-two. The tendency to secondary attacks manifests itself first at the age of twenty-four, rises to a maximum between twenty-six and twenty-eight, again to disappear at thirty-two. That there may be a third period is probable, as two cases were recorded at the ages of thirty-nine and forty-one. This law applies to attacks of the disease with distinct intervals of good health between, as distinguished from the simple relapses, after periods of imperfect convalescence, frequently met with after a primary attack. The curve of menstrual age, compared with the curve of the onset of chlorosis, does not bear out the opinion that "foremost in etiological importance is the period of the first appearance of the catamenia." The fact of a periodicity in the attacks is also against it. The cause of this periodicity was considered, and the general conclusion arrived at is that imperfect evolution of menstruation, as evidenced by scantiness of the flow and irregularity of the periods, is as regular a feature of chlorosis as the imperfect evolution of the red corpuscles of the blood. These constants are independent one of the other, though a close relationship exists between them whereby the reproduction and development of the red corpuscles of the blood are governed by, or form part of, the menstrual cycle; while both are influenced by a greater rhythmic action which determines the time and activity of development, growth, and reproduction.—*Lancet*, March 23, 1889.

Treatment of Chronic Cystitis in Women.

Dr. W. Symington Brown read a paper on chronic cystitis in women before the Gynecological Society of Boston, Dec. 13, 1888, in which he reported the case of a Mrs. B., whom he visited on Christmas-day, 1887. The patient is a married woman, 63 years of age, with a grown-up family, and had always enjoyed health until 1884, when she began to suffer pain in the bladder, accompanied with frequent calls to urinate, night and day. During the whole three years she has never been able to retain her urine for more than an hour at a time, and sometimes she has been obliged to use the urinal every half hour or so. Mrs. B. had been under the care of several physicians, regular and irregular. Although naturally of a placid, happy disposition, her face showed marks of suffering and anxiety. Her pulse was 85; the temperature 99.5°. Her urine, drawn with a soft catheter, contained pus, mucus, and crystals of the triple phosphates. There was no uterine or ovarian disease. A small caruncle, growing at the lower edge of the meatus urinarius, was removed by means of a wire snare. A similar but smaller growth was found at the neck of the bladder, and this was also removed. For a period of six weeks, she took a tablespoonful of the following solution every four hours during the day; and also used it as an injection into the bladder every night and morning:

R Benzoic acid, pure, ... ℥ ij
    Biborate of soda . . . . . . ℥ iv
    Distilled water . . . . f ℥ vj
Mix.

She took lithia water as a drink for several weeks, with apparent benefit. All kinds of fermented liquors were absolutely forbidden. Her diet was carefully regulated. Salt meat, salt fish, pork, lobster, beans, highly spiced soups, fried food, and pastry were prohibited. The usual directions to overcome constipation were given. Attention was paid to position in bed, by raising the pelvis with graded cushions, so as to avoid contact of the urine with the *trigonum vesicæ*, the most sensitive spot in the bladder. At the end of six weeks the urine was free from pus and triple phosphates, and it could be retained about two hours. Early in May, 1888, she considered herself cured. As the bladder had become much contracted, Dr. Brown made an attempt, toward the close of the treatment, to dilate it by means of tepid salt water from a fountain syringe. Dilatation should be effected, he says, very gradually; for there is some risk of paralysis from overdistention; and it seems possible, when the ureters are abnormally dilated, that the kidneys themselves may be injured. Reference was then made to the efficacy of hygienic, comfortable surroundings, admirable nursing and a contented coöperation on the part of the patient.—*Journal of the Amer. Med. Association*, March 16, 1889.

Unique Presentation of a Fœtus.

At the meeting of the Philadelphia County Medical Society April 10, 889, Dr. E. P. Bernardy described a case in which a fœtus had presented in a peculiar manner. The patient who gave birth to the child was a primipara, eighteen years old. Dr. Bernardy saw her for the first time at 8 o'clock on April 8, 1889; the membranes had been ruptured four hours, the fœtus was presenting in the right oblique diameter; the presenting part seemed to be the breech, the right side deeper in the pelvic cavity than the left; the fingers could be hooked in what appeared the groin, but did not have the full feeling one would expect in a breech presentation; a sort of sulcus or fissure was in the centre of the presenting part. Passing the fingers further upward, the bone of the skull was detected. Dr. Bernardy thought that he had to deal with a double pregnancy, the breech of one presenting and the head of the other imbedded in the chest of the first. External palpation showed the uterus divided in two by a deep dent in its fundus, a large body occupying the upper left portion, and a body occupying the lower portion of the right side. He did not introduce his hand into the vagina, for the maternal parts were rigid, and had not undergone any softening, and such examination would, he thinks, have undoubtedly caused a rupture of the perineum; the os was spasmodically contracted around the presenting part. The patient not having much pain, he left her for about two hours. On his return, the entire presenting portion was grasped by the vulva, and the child was delivered in this position. It was then found that both shoulders presented fair and square, the neck, somewhat stretched, thrown forward on the chest, and the head slightly twisted sideways, lying in a cavity in the chest; the arms laid on the top of the chest, right and left side, the head between. There was hardly any pain connected with the confinement.

Dr. Bernardy said he could not recall an instance of a similar presentation.

THE
MEDICAL AND SURGICAL
REPORTER.

ISSUED EVERY SATURDAY.

CHARLES W. DULLES, M.D.,
EDITOR AND PUBLISHER.

The Terms of Subscription to the publications of this office are as follows, payable in advance:
Med. and Surg. Reporter (weekly), a year, **$5.00**
Physician's Daily Pocket Record,   - -   1.00
Reporter and Pocket Record, - - -   6.00
All checks and postal orders should be drawn to order of
CHARLES W. DULLES,
N. E. Cor. 13th and Walnut Streets,
P. O. Box 843.   Philadelphia, Pa.

☞SUGGESTIONS TO SUBSCRIBERS:
See that your address-label gives the date to which your subscription is paid.
In requesting a change of address, give the old address as well as the new one.
If your REPORTER does not reach you promptly and regularly, notify the publisher *at once*, so that the cause may be discovered and corrected.
☞SUGGESTIONS TO CONTRIBUTORS AND CORRESPONDENTS:
Write in ink.
Write on one side of paper only.
Write on paper of the size usually used for letters.
Make as few paragraphs as possible. Punctuate carefully. Do not abbreviate, or omit Words like "the," and "a," or "an."
Make communications as short as possible.
NEVER ROLL A MANUSCRIPT! Try to get an envelope or wrapper which will fit it.
When it is desired to call our attention to something in a newspaper, mark the passage boldly with a colored pencil, and write on the wrapper "Marked copy." Unless this is done, newspapers are not looked at.
The Editor will be glad to get medical news, but it is important that brevity and actual interest shall characterize communications intended for publication.

WEIL'S DISEASE, OR INFECTIOUS JAUNDICE.

The tendency of modern pathological investigation has been toward reducing the number of separate diseases through a better understanding of the underlying processes at work in their production. As the result of this tendency, dropsy and jaundice, at one time regarded as diseases, are now universally looked upon as symptoms merely; and it is only a question of time when the whole group of symptomatic diseases will cease to exist except as symptoms. While this elimination is steadily going on, it is manifest that any new applicant to the rank of a disease will be very closely scrutinized, and will have to show very good grounds for the request. This is especially true when the disease bears a man's name—a kind of nomenclature always to be deprecated and discouraged.

Within the last few years a number of papers have appeared in Germany on "Weil's Disease," an abstract of one of the most important of these papers being published in the REPORTER, May 5, 1888. Weil described the affection as an acute infectious disease associated with swelling of the spleen, with jaundice and nephritis. All four of the patients originally studied by him were vigorous young men, who were taken sick, without special prodromes, with headache, dizziness, and fever, which in one case was introduced by a pronounced chill. In the first few days after the patients were admitted into the hospital the symptoms especially noteworthy were abnormal weakness and very marked cerebral symptoms—restless sleep, disposition to delirium, somnolence; in addition there was moderate jaundice of the skin and conjunctivæ, painful swelling of the liver and spleen, and albuminuria. Digestive disturbances were present and were manifested by coated tongue, loss of appetite, diarrhœa or constipation. These symptoms persisted unchanged, or they increased in intensity, for some days, and then abated rather quickly, so that from the fifth to the eighth day a change for the better occurred; and with subsidence of the jaundice and of the swelling of the liver and spleen, and lessening of the albuminuria, the temperature slowly and gradually fell to normal. But the disease was not over yet. After an afebrile period lasting from one to seven days the fever again rose in three cases, but ceased finally in five or six days. A striking feature of the affection was the protracted convalescence, due to great weakness resulting from very much lowered nutrition. This condition was so marked that the patients had to be kept in the hospital from four to ten weeks, before they could be dismissed cured.

Looking at the symptoms of the affection more in detail, we see that the whole duration of the first attack was from six to ten days. The highest temperature during this time was attained by a rapid rise, and reached 104°, or even 105° Fahr. Defervescence was by lysis, and was completed in four or five days In the relapse the fever did not rise so high, being on an average a degree lower than in the first attack. The pulse was moderately increased in frequency, rising to one hundred and four or one hundred and twelve. The jaundice present was not of a high grade, but was distinctly noticeable. The urine contained not only bile, but also bile acids. The stools in three cases corresponded with the moderate jaundice, while in a fourth they were clay-colored. Diarrhœa existed in three cases, and constipation in one. The urine was cloudy except in one case, and contained albumin, epithelial casts, red and white blood corpuscles—in a word, such products as are present in so-called infectious nephritis. One patient developed on the seventh day a marked roseola; another patient about the same time had red spots on the throat and face. During convalescence one patient was affected with irido-cyclitis. There was early and painful enlargement of the liver.

The diagnosis of an affection presenting such complex symptoms is unquestionably one of great difficulty. Weil regarded it as an infectious disease whose virus caused swelling of the abdominal organs, the point of entrance of the poison being probably the intestinal tract. Since his first paper, several observers have reported additional cases, and all have in the main accepted Weil's opinion. More recently, however, Professor A. Fraenkel has given a very careful study to the whole subject, and he communicates his results in a paper published in the *Deutsche med. Wochenschrift*, February 28, 1889. He rejects the opinion that "Weil's Disease" is an abortive form of acute atrophy of the liver; for the simultaneous involvement of the spleen, liver and kidneys, as well as the course of the fever, show that the process is a general infection, or—what is more prob-

able—that it is an intoxication. It is not a disease of the nature of recurrent fever or typhoid fever, although it resembles a special form of the former described by Griesinger; but Weil was unable to find in the blood of his patients the spirilla described by certain Russian physicians as occurring in relapsing fever. But for the relapses it would be extremely difficult to say that the affection is not typhoid fever with marked bilious symptoms. Weil himself left it an open question whether it is a disease *sui generis*, or a special form of typhus; yet he maintained that it was possibly a peculiar undescribed disease, depending upon a specific cause as yet unknown. He further states that the anatomical changes and functional disturbances of the different organs are to be considered as coordinate effects of the specific infection.

Fraenkel does not believe that all the cases reported as those of Weil's disease are identical in character. The only symptoms common to all are fever and jaundice. He asserts that the cases simply present a group of symptoms which to all appearances are produced by various agencies belonging to the category of septic infective material. Possibly the symptoms arise from intoxication with one or more chemical poisons acting after the manner of ptomaines. In his own case the point of entrance of the poison was a wound; as a rule it has been the intestinal tract. On account, therefore, of this diversity of symptoms and the probability that their cause is not single, Fraenkel recommends that the name "Weil's Disease" should be dropped, as it leads to false inferences.

Fraenkel is probably right in his conclusion that the affection is not a separate entity, but merely one of a group of possible intoxications. It should not be forgotten, however, that Weil's studies and those of others who followed him have made it possible to recognize the group, and that he has thus aided materially in the advancement of medical knowledge.

THE OBLIGATIONS OF HOMŒO-PATHIC PHYSICIANS.

In another part of this number of the REPORTER we publish a letter from Judge Barrett, of the Supreme Court of New York, to the *New York Medical Times,* in which he says that a physician designating himself an homœopathist, and called as such to a patient, has no legal or moral right to adopt other than homœopathic means in the treatment of the case.

This opinion is expressed without reserve and Judge Barrett gives his reasons for holding it. These reasons will meet the approval of all representatives of the regular school of medicine, for they are founded upon the belief that practitioners who assume a special designation, and are chosen as medical advisers on that account, ought not to violate the principles which that designation indicates that they hold.

At the present time it is well known that but a limited number of so-called homœopaths believe that the law of *similia similibus curantur* is one of universal applicability. The great majority practise on the same basis as do all intelligent physicians. Although their education gives them a leaning toward the use of certain medicinal preparations which are attenuated or diluted, yet in this they are guided by experience and observation and not by any such theories as Hahnemann promulgated. In fact they have no more right to call themselves homœopaths—though they cling to this title —than they have to call the members of the regular profession allopaths, as though they too followed an exclusive dogma.

The term homœopath, as Hahnemann understood it, does not fit the homœopaths of this day, and the community is deceived insofar as it believes that it does.

We know that there are men in the ranks of the homœopaths who feel the inconsistency of their professions with their practice, and who would be glad to escape from the awkwardness of their position. To such it must be trying to find a learned judge describing the lapses from homœopathy into which they fall as illegal, as well as immoral.

It is with no desire to give offense that we call attention to the way in which the attitude of the so-called homœopaths of our day impresses those who reject all exclusive dogmas, but rather in the hope that a plain statement of it may quicken the zeal of those among them who would be glad to abandon a designation which keeps them separated from the great mass of honest and intelligent medical men, and ties them to men who adopt the name solely as a trade distinction and carry it easily only because their intelligence or their moral sense is defective.

There is only one way in which the breach between the regular school of practice and the homœopaths—a breach which the homœopaths created and maintain—can be closed, and that is by the abandonment of the special name which the latter have assumed and the selection of that noble one which is borne by the members of the regular school.

THE SUPPRESSION OF SMALL-POX.

In the REPORTER, April 27, under "Notes and Comments," we published an account of the way the authorities of Minneapolis, Minn., are said to have dealt with a case of small-pox which was detected in that city, and the measures adopted to prevent the outbreak of an epidemic. As the Editor of *Science,* from which the account is taken, remarks, some of the proceedings reported were absurd, and some were brutal. The former criticism applies to the soaking with corrosive sublimate solution of the clothing of those who vaccinated the quarantined persons. As brutal, it is not unjust to characterize the wholesale quarantining, and the threat to shoot a laboring man if he attempted to escape from imprisonment in a suspected house in which he, with thirty others, was caught.

No doubt the authorities of Minneapolis would justify their conduct by the result; but we think the law in Minnesota must be peculiar if they could have justified themselves, had they carried out the threat to shoot. The day for shot-gun quarantines has gone by, and we believe that the most that can reasonably demanded of those who are suspected of having been exposed to infection from small-pox is that they shall be vaccinnated, washed thoroughly from head to heels, furnished with new clothing, and kept under *surveillance* for a moderate length of time.

This much we believe would be both feasible and prudent in any city, if a case of small-pox were discovered where none had existed before. We think that intelligent people would consent to the personal inconvenience without complaint, if the city met the expense—as it certainly should. Among the ignorant, resistance would have to be met by persuasion, and, if this failed, by the exercise of as much force as was necessary and legal; but persuasion would always be the best aid of sanitarians, because there is not much law in the United States to warrant such proceedings as are reported from Minneapolis.

HERNIA INGUINO-SUPERFICIALIS.

At the meeting of the Surgeons of Berlin, February 11, 1889, Prof. Küster presented four new cases of this form of hernia described by him under the name of hernia inguino-superficialis. Two of the patients had been operated upon with removal of the atrophied testicle. Two of the patients had double hernia, with atrophy and ectopia of the testicle. In these cases—if they are operated upon—Kuster proposes to save the testicle and to make an artificial tunica vaginalis—as he has already done in one case—although it is impossible now to bring the testicle down into the scrotum.

In the form of hernia described by Küster as hernia inguino-superficialis, the prolapsed bowel lies outside of the muscles of the abdominal wall and is covered only by skin and superficial fascia. This is a condition rarely recognized, and not a case of this sort has ever been reported by an American surgeon. It is closely allied to the inguino-properitoneal hernia which has been referred to in a pamphlet notice in the REPORTER, August 25, 1888, and which is better understood in this country.

Aside from the scientific advantage of accuracy in diagnosis, it is useful to be able to recognize these peculiar forms of hernia, because in some of them a correct diagnosis has a very important bearing upon the treatment to be adopted.

GENEROUS GIFT TO THE EPISCOPAL HOSPITAL OF PHILADELPHIA.—The family of the late George L. Harrison, of Philadelphia, has offered $200,000 to the board of trustees of the Protestant Episcopal Hospital to found and to endow a building for incurables in connection with that institution. Some years ago Bishop Stevens submitted to the Convention of the Diocese suggestions in reference to such an addition to the hospital. He wanted especially an endowment for a ward of such a character. The trustees of the hospital took the matter in hand, and some measures were adopted which brought a response, and a nucleus was formed by donations until the total, some of it given for building and some for an endowment, amounted to something less than $10,000. Now Mrs. Harrison has joined with the four sons of her late husband, Charles C., William W., Alfred C., and Mitchell Harrison, in making the gift to perpetuate the memory of George L. Harrison, one of the best and most generous friends the hospital ever had. It is almost unnecessary to add that the Board of Trustees has accepted the offer.

It is seldom that money is given so generously and so wisely as in the present instance; for instead of expending the whole sum in a building, one-half of the amount is to be reserved as an endowment, so that the building when erected will have ready to its hand the money necessary for accomplishing the good work for which it is intended.

BOOK REVIEWS.

[Any book reviewed in these columns may be obtained upon receipt of price, from the office of the REPORTER.]

THE OPERATIONS OF SURGERY. A SYSTEMATIC HANDBOOK FOR PRACTITIONERS, STUDENTS AND HOSPITAL SURGEONS. By W. H. A. JACOBSON, F.R C.S., Assistant Surgeon Guy's Hospital, etc. With 199 illustrations. 8vo, pp. 1006. Philadelphia: P. Blakiston, Son & Co., 1889. Price, $5.00.

This handsome book is one of the most admirable works on operative surgery which we have seen for a long time. The author has brought to its preparation a large observation and experience, and a very thorough acquaintance with the methods of other surgeons. His book is comprehensive, and its directions are clear and reliable. The most recent advances in surgery are represented in these pages, although we do not find any reference to operations for the removal of tumor within the canal of the spinal column, a few of which have been performed. It is gratifying to an American reader to find that full justice is done to the work of American surgeons by Mr. Jacobson, and that his book bears no marks of the distance which stretches between his land and ours. This is as it should be, and is no less an element in the excellence of the technical worth of his book, than it is an evidence of the cosmopolitan character of good scientific work.

The book is very well printed and bound, and we have no doubt will meet with general professional favor on both sides of the Atlantic.

PAMPHLET NOTICES.

[Any reader of the REPORTER who desires a copy of a pamphlet noticed in these columns will doubtless secure it by addressing the author with a request stating where the notice was seen and *enclosing a postage-stamp.*]

250. OUR INSANE. THE STATE HOSPITALS FOR THE INSANE POOR. BY HIRAM CORSON, M.D., Conshohocken, Pa., 13 pages.

251. CLINICAL STUDIES ON THE PULSE IN CHILDHOOD. BY JOHN M. KEATING, M.D., AND WILLIAM A. EDWARDS, M.D., Philadelphia. From the *Archives of Pediatrics,* December, 1888. 15 pages.

252. NOTES ON THE TREATMENT OF ACUTE CORYZA. BY FRANK HAMILTON POTTER, M.D., Buffalo, N. Y. From the *Buffalo Med. and Surg. Journal,* January, 1889. 5 pages.

253. FEMORAL OSTEOTOMY FOR THE CORRECTION OF DEFORMITY RESULTING FROM HIP-JOINT DISEASE. BY AP MORGAN VANCE, M.D., Louisville, Ky. From the *N. Y. Medical Journal,* December 1, 1888. 15 pages.

254. CASES IN ORTHOPÆDIC SURGERY. BY AP MORGAN VANCE, M.D., Louisville, Ky. From the *N. Y. Medical Journal,* November 7, 1885. 17 pages.

255. A CASE OF HODGKIN'S DISEASE ACCOMPANIED WITH A POSSIBLE RESULTING PARAPLEGIA. BY LEWIS H. ADLER, Jr., M.D., Philadelphia.

256. ZUR BEHANDLUNG GEWISSER FORMEN VON NEURASTHENIE UND HYSTERIE DURCH DIE WEIR-MITCHELL CUR. VON DR. JOSEF SCHREIBER, Aussee-Merau. From the *Berliner klin. Wochenschrift,* 1888, No. 52.

250. Dr. Corson's pamphlet bears on its cover the sub-title : "A plea to the Legislature for a reorganization of the Acts of Assembly regulating the State Hospitals." It contains an argument in favor of the government of hospitals for the insane by Trustees, as exemplified in the Hospital at Norristown, which is one of the best managed institutions of this sort in the world. Our readers are familiar with Dr. Corson's views, because they have been fully explained in the REPORTER during the past year; but his pamphlet will prove both interesting and instructive to those who wish to get light on the important subject which it discusses.

251. This pamphlet contains an instructive study of the pulse of infants and small children, in health and in certain organic affections of the heart. The frequency, rhythm, and force of the arterial impulse have been investigated by the writers, and the results of their investigations are recorded systematically, with mention of some rare peculiarities of the pulse which are seldom observed.

252. The readers of the REPORTER who have observed the stand it has taken in regard to ventilation of sleeping apartments will not wonder that Dr. Potter's pamphlet commends itself at the very outset to our approval ; and those who acquaint themselves with its contents will see, we think, the reasonableness of his suggestions as to best way to prevent and to treat coryza. His directions are simple and sensible, and can be heartily commended to the attention of our readers. An abstract of Dr. Potter's paper was published in the REPORTER, January 19.

253. This is a very interesting paper, containing an account of eight cases of deformity of the leg, due to chronic hip-joint disease, in which great relief was afforded by Dr. Vance, by an operation which consisted in partial division of the femur with a chisel, followed by breaking the bone—the whole being done subcutaneously—and placing the limb in a good position and retaining it so until bony union took place. The improvement in some of these cases was almost marvellous, and it is no wonder Dr. Vance has a high opinion of an operation which in his hands has yielded such good results.

254. This paper by Dr. Vance antedates the one noticed just before by three years, and contains accounts of five cases illustrating a variety of orthopædic difficulties and the way in which he treated them. One was a case of extreme valgus due to infantile paralysis, in which an artificial ankylosis of the ankle-joint was produced. Two more cases illustrate similar procedures at the knee and ankle respectively ; and in two he partly divided and partly broke the femur to correct deformities resulting from old hip-joint disease.

255. Dr. Adler's article contains a good report of a well-studied case of Hodgkin's disease, which was under the care of Prof. Horatio Wood at the Hospital of the University of Pennsylvania.

256. Dr. Schreiber's paper contains an admirable discussion of the value of Dr. Weir Mitchell's method for the treatment of neurasthenia, and of the modifications which should be made in it in certain cases. The discussion shows that Dr. Schreiber has not been a blind follower of the routine of this method, but has grasped its underlying principles, and recognized the fact that some of its details would be absolutely damaging to some patients to whom other parts of it would be very beneficial.

CORRESPONDENCE.

Formula for Boro-glyceride.

To THE EDITOR.

Sir: Will you be good enough to give me through the REPORTER the formula for the preparation of boro-glyceride, so much and so successfully used in middle-ear diseases and to which reference is so often made in The American System of Gynæcology? I desire the formula for the original boro-glyceride, and also the proportion of it in solution for use.

Yours truly,
S. H. BARHAM, M.D.

Lone Oak, Texas,
April 17, 1889.

[The preparation called Boro-Glyceride is regarded by some chemists as a mere chemical mixture, and by others as a true compound However this may be, its mode of preparation is as follows: 92 parts of glycerine are heated in a weighed porcelain capsule to a temperature not exceeding 302 degrees Fahrenheit, and 62 parts of boric acid are added in portions, constantly stirring. When all is added and dissolved, the heat is maintained at the same temperature and the stirring is continued, breaking up the film which forms on the surface. When the mixture has been reduced to a weight of 100 parts, it is poured on a flat surface, previously coated with a very small quantity of petrolinum and allowed to cool, when it is cut into pieces and transferred to bottles or jars.

Boro-Glyceride is a very hygroscopic and is best kept by being combined with, or dissolved in, an equal part or two parts of glycerine. This is the form in which it is usually employed in gynecological practice in tampons, etc. It is a sticky, tenacious liquid, which has to be kept in a very wide-mouthed bottle, or it is almost impossible to get it out.— EDITOR OF REPORTER.]

NOTES AND COMMENTS.

What a Patient May Demand of a Homœopath.

On March 11, 1889, the *N. Y. Medical Times* addressed a letter to the Hon. Geo. C. Barrett, Judge of the Supreme Court, asking him to answer the following question: "Has a physician designating himself an 'Homœopathist,' and called as such to a patient, any legal or moral right to adopt other than homœopathic means in the treatment of the case?"

To this Judge Barrett replied under date of March 13, 1889: "I have your note of the 11th inst., asking my opinion upon a question of professional ethics. In my judgment there can be but one answer to your question, and that is in the negative. If I call in a medical man who designates himself a 'Homœopathic physician,' it is because I do not wish to be treated allopathically, or eclectically, or otherwise than homœopathically. There is an implied understanding between myself and the homœopathist, that I shall receive the treatment which, by tradition and a general consensus of opinion, means small doses of a single drug administered upon the principle of 'similia similibus curantur.' If there is to be any variation from that method, I have a right to be informed of it and to be given an opportunity to decide. Common honesty demands that before a confiding patient is to be drugged with quinine, iron, morphine or other medicaments, either singly or in combination, he should be told that the 'Homœopathist' has failed, and that relief can only be afforded by a change of system. An honest 'Homœopath,' who has not succeeded, after doing his best with the appropriate homœopathic remedies administered on homœopathic principles, should undoubtedly try anything else which he believes may save or relieve his patient. But when he reaches that point, the duty of taking the patient into his confidence becomes imperative. The patient may refuse to submit to the other system, or he may agree but prefer a physician whose life has been specially devoted to practise under that other system. He may say to the 'Homœopathist,' you have failed, but I prefer to try another gentleman of your own school, before resorting to a system that I have long since turned my back upon. Or he may say, well, if homœopathy can not save me, I prefer to go to headquarters for allopathic treatment.

All this, gentlemen, is the logical sequence of the particular designation 'Homœopathist.' There may, of course, be gentlemen who in a general way favor the principle of small doses and 'similia similibus curantur,' to whom it would not apply. But such a physician would not stamp his school upon his work as a practitioner. If I call in such a man, I mean a physician pure and simple— calling himself neither homœopathist nor allopathist—the implied understanding is that I entrust myself to his best judgment in all respects. Such a man may be a graduate of the College of Physicians and Surgeons, and I will have no cause of complaint should he in an exigency deem it appropriate to administer the third potency of aconite. Or he may be a graduate of a college founded under homœopathic auspices, and yet I can not object if he thinks the occasion demands twenty grains of quinine. But if a physician calls himself allopathic and is summoned as such, it would be a fraud to resort to homœopathic treatment without full disclosure to the patient of what was proposed. If, however, we are to have a class of men who purpose, in the interest of humanity, to utilize the best that they can find in any and every school, 'pathist,' as a designation of fixed methods of practice, must be ignored, and the broad and noble title 'physician,' in its unreserved sense, be revived and substituted.

The patient will understand, when he sends for one of this class, that he is to have the physician's best judgment in the unprejudiced use of the ripest fruits of modern discovery in every field. I see that I have done more than simply answer your question. But I am sure you will pardon a layman for taking advantage of the occasion to intimate the need of greater clearness of professional attitude—both as a matter of justice to the patient and as due to the integrity of the physician."

Treatment of the Eczema of Dentition.

According to M. E. Besnier, eczema of dentition is a reflex eczema from the face, and at times from the back of the hand and wrist, with tenderness of the gums and salivation. There are three indications in its treatment: (1) to allay the itching of the gums; (2) to control insomnia; (3) to cure the local condition. To allay the irritation of the gums, he recommends frequent touchings and frictions of the gums with a finger dipped in the following solution:

> Hydrochlorate of cocaine . . . . . gr. ⅜
> Bromide of potassium . . . . . gr. viiss
> Distilled water,
> Glycerine . . . . of each ℳcl
> M.

To control insomnia, he employs teaspoonful doses in soup, every hour, of the following mixture:

> Bromide of sodium . . . . gr. ivss–viiss
> Syrup of orange flowers . . . . f℥iss

For the local condition he prescribes the following ointment:

> Oxide of zinc . . . . gr. cl
> Vaseline . . . . ℥iv

In addition, Besnier recommends to cover the affected regions with a mask of linen or muslin coated with gutta percha. In some affected parts a sheet of mackintosh may be used.—*Gazette Hebdomadaire*, March 29, 1889.

Ammonium Chloride in Fumes for Inhalation.

Dr. P. W. Maxwell says in the *Dublin Journal of Medical Science*, March, 1889, that his experience with ammonium chloride has been confined to catarrhal conditions of the nose and pharynx. He has found it most useful in cases in which the secretion is scanty or nearly absent, and also in those in which, though abundant, it is tenacious and difficult to dislodge. In such cases the greatest immediate benefit seems to be produced by a warm solution of the salt used as a nose wash; but he is inclined to think that, where repeated applications are necessary, the fumes produce in the long run the most good. For the production of the fumes he describes an apparatus which consists of a wide piece of glass tube, resembling the cylinder of an ordinary glass syringe; this tube is placed horizontally on two wooden supports. About fifteen grains of ammonium chloride are introduced by a spoon through the wide end of the tube, and are placed in a little heap in the centre. The base is then lightly stopped with cotton wool. A lighted spirit lamp placed beneath the tube volatilizes the salt. A piece of rubber tubing with a glass mouth-piece is attached to the narrow end of the tube, through which the fumes are inhaled. A current of cold air rushing in by the large end of the horizontal tube mixes with the fumes and reduces their temperature, so that they are not more than slightly warm. These fumes, he says, are neutral from first to last. When it is desired, they can be medicated with oleum pini sylvestris, eucalyptus, etc., by dropping about five minims of the oil upon the wool at the wide end of the tube.

Atropine in the Prevention of Shock.

At the meeting of the New York Surgical Society, Jan. 9, 1889, Dr. Lewis A. Stimson recommended the hypodermic injection of from $\frac{1}{75}$ to $\frac{1}{100}$ of a grain of atropine previous to giving ether for an operation, and instanced cases in which its good effects were shown. He has used atropine for this purpose for five or six years, having first observed its control of the inhibitory action on the heart in certain physiological experiments. How much influence it may exert it is not always easy to determine, but he believes it to be of great value.—*New York Medical Journal*, March 9, 1889.

Hysteria in Infants.

Prof. Grancher has recently stated that the diagnosis of hysteria in infants is often very difficult, as the disease presents anomalies not usually found in that affection in adults. The most distinctly marked symptoms are: very sudden convulsive crises, quick throwing back of the head, convulsive movements of the eyes, jerking strokes of the limbs, and pharyngeal spasm. The attacks usually last about half a minute; there does not appear to be a complete loss of consciousness. At first sight, such attacks would be regarded as epileptic. The general condition of the patient and the frequency of the accessions must decide the matter. Epilepsy soon involves the general health to a very marked degree, the crises increase in number and the patient becomes progressively dispirited. In infantile hysteria, on the contrary, these conditions do not exist, and we often find the child in high spirits very soon after the attack.— *New York Med. Abstract,* April, 1889.

Clinical Observations on Gonorrhœa.

Drs. John P. Bryson and Edwin C. Burnett communicate a very interesting paper to the *Journal of Cutaneous and Genito-Urinary Diseases,* April, 1889, based upon a study of a very large number of cases, 1394 of which were seen in dispensary practice; for the latter reason they regard their observations as not justifying definite conclusions regarding the average duration of gonorrhœa. They incline, however, to accept the generally expressed opinion of clinicians that, when treated according to the so-called "methodical" plan, the great majority of patients with gonorrhœa apparently get well in from six to eight weeks. This result they find to occur most frequently when all local treatment is abstained from in the increasing and stationary stages of the disease, and is reserved for the decreasing or subacute conditions, every effort being made to limit the inflamed areas to the anterior portion of the duct.

They conclude that gonorrhœa is a specific disease of which the gonococcus of Neisser is the essential etiological factor. The abortive treatment is held to be both inefficient and harmful. They recognize in the disease a marked tendency to persist in the chronic stage, and this tendency appears to them to be increased by the use of topical treatment in the first and second stages. In their opinion the internal administration of remedies (especially balsam of copaiba and oil of yellow sandal wood), combined with proper hygienic and dietetic regulations, does most to shorten the duration of the disease. In the third or declining stage mild vegetable and mineral astringents seem to be of service.

Treatment of Tetanus by Absolute Rest.

Prof. de Renzi, of Naples, has carried out the treatment of tetanus by absolute rest in four cases, and has obtained a successful result. He was led to try the treatment through noticing that a frog poisoned with one-twentieth milligramme of strychnia and exposed to the influence of light and sounds could not be saved; but if it were kept in absolute rest, it survived.

The following is the treatment adopted: the patient's ears are stopped with wax and cotton and he is brought into a very quiet and dark room, into which no noise is allowed to penetrate. It is impressed upon the patient that his recovery depends upon absolute quiet. The room is entered only every four hours, and with a dark lantern. Nourishment is fluid and is given by the mouth, so that chewing will be avoided. When there is marked pain some belladonna and ergot are given. Of five patients so treated four recovered.— *Wiener med. Presse,* March 17, 1889.

Digestion of Live Tapeworm.

As long ago as 1780, Dr. Masars de Cazelles described a tænia fenestrata. Drs. Notta and Marfan published notes of a suspected specimen two or three years ago. With regard to this specimen, Dr. Danysz gives, in the *Journal de l'Anatomie et de la Physiologie,* a series of observations by which he endeavors to show that the parasite was a tænia saginata, and that the perforations commence as little superficial erosions, which gradually extend through the entire thickness of the segment. Apparently the process begins by fatty degeneration of the cuticle of the tænia. The cuticular layer of the diseased segment breaks down at the points where the degeneration has taken place. The interior of the segment is then exposed to the digestive fluids of the host. In this way holes are soon made. Several segments may be reduced to the form of oblong frames. Dr. Danysz illustrates this singular change due to digestion of the live parasite.—*British Med. Journal,* Feb. 16, 1889.

A Dangerous Chlorate of Potassium Prescription.

A pharmacist writes to the *Bull. com.*, January, stating that he often gets a prescription as follows: Chlorate of potassium, 5 gm. (gr. 75); distilled water, 120 gm. (4 fl. oz.), simple syrup, 30 gm. (1 fl. oz.), a dessertspoonful every half-hour. "Children who take this," adds the pharmacist, "*always die.* M. Brouardel cites six cases of death in children after using a similar potion. Can I refuse to dispense this mixture?" The editor says the pharmacist cannot refuse; he can only state the facts to the doctor, "who will be likely to attribute the cause of death to the gravity of the disease." He adds: "Physicians, on account of the scant information we have as to the physiological action of chlorate of potassium, use this medicament with the same imprudence and the same indifference as they have formerly shown."—*American Journal of Pharmacy*, April, 1889.

Galvanism in Dysmenorrhœa and other Pelvic Pains.

Dr. Franklin H. Martin, Professor of Gynecology in the Post Graduate Medical School of Chicago, discusses in the *North American Practitioner*, April, 1889, the employment of galvanism in the treatment of dysmenorrhœa and other pelvic pains. He employs a current-strength of 100 milliampères. Externally he employs what he calls "a large animal membrane abdominal" electrode, large enough to cover the whole surface of the abdomen between the pubes and umbilicus. The vaginal electrode described consists of a metal exposure of 16 square cm., surrounded with wet absorbent cotton; it is crowded well up into the space between the uterus and the vaginal walls on one or the other side of the cervix, as may be indicated by the requirements of the case. With the electrodes held firmly in position, the current is gradually turned on until it reaches a strength of 100 milliampères. Here it is allowed to rest for five minutes, when it is gradually turned off, and the treatment finished.

Dr. Martin reports three cases in which this treatment was adapted to the relief of pain, and expresses the opinion that in certain conditions, in which pain is often the predominant symptom, galvanism will prove an infallible and prompt remedy. His propositions are:

1. Do not advise the removal of an ovary for persistent pain, until galvanism has been systematically and thoroughly applied, if any of the following conditions are suspected as a cause: (*a*) chronic ovaritis, either with or without hypertrophy; (*b*) where inflammatory deposits, either with or without adhesions, surround one or both organs; (*c*) ovarian neuralgia; (*d*) all pain coincident with menstruation; (*e*) in all cases of ovarian pain not known to be the result of active, acute inflammation; septic or specific inflammation; and cystic tumors.

2. Galvanism is a sure remedy for all pain resulting from tubular diseases, except when septic or specific inflammation is the cause, or the presence of pus is demonstrated.

3. Galvanism is positively indicated in dysmenorrhœa or other pelvic pain, when a result of chronic metritis; when a result of hyperplastic enlargement of the uterus; when a result of fibrous or other non-malignant growths of the uterus.

4. Galvanism is emphatically indicated in pelvic pain when a result of old pelvic exudates of all kinds, provided acute inflammatory action is absent and the presence of pus is not suspected or demonstrated.

5. Galvanism is indicated in pelvic pains, arising from reflex disturbances, or hystero-neuroses, the condition well defined by Engelmann as "a phenomenon which simulates a morbid condition in an organ that is anatomically in a healthy state."

6. Galvanism is indicated in dysmenorrhœa, when the result of cervical lacerations, with unyielding cicatrized plugs; when the result of cervical endometritis or uterine vegetation.

Commencement of the Medical and Dental Departments of the University of Pennsylvania.

The one hundred and fifteenth annual commencement of the Medical and Dental Departments of the University of Pennsylvania was held May 1, 1889, and the degree of Doctor of Medicine conferred on 124 graduates, and the degree of Doctor of Dentistry on 58 graduates. The valedictory address was delivered by Dr. Osler, the retiring Professor of Clinical Medicine. A portrait of Dr. Agnew, the retiring Professor of Surgery, was presented to the University by the three undergraduate classes of the Medical Department, and accepted on behalf of the Trustees by Dr. S. Weir Mitchell. In response to numerous calls, Dr. Agnew spoke a few earnest words to the graduating class, and was nearly overcome by his deep emotion.

NEWS.

—The Iowa State Medical Society will meet in Keokuk, May 15, 16 and 17.

—The Townsend Chapel of Bellevue Hospital, New York City, was dedicated April 22.

—Dr. James L. Manney, the son of Dr. James Manney, died in Wilmington, N. C., March 18.

—Dr. Lallement, Professor of Anatomy in the Medical Faculty of Nancy, recently died of apoplexy.

—The annual meeting of the Missouri State Medical Association will be held in Springfield, May 21.

—It is stated that the Roosevelt Hospital, New York City, will receive $350,000 from the estate of the late Mr. William J. Syms, to be used for building and maintaining a new operating theatre.

—The President of the Board of Heath of Sanford, Florida, stated April 23, that a case of yellow fever existed in that city. Every precaution has been taken to prevent a spread of the disease.

—Dr. W. F. Wilson is reported to have died in Denver, Colorado, April 19, from an overdose of morphine taken to induce sleep. He was only 29 years of age, but had been troubled with insomnia.

—The Kansas City Medical College held its twentieth annual commencement on March 11, and conferred the degree of Doctor of Medicine on 18, and the degree of Doctor of Dentistry on 11 graduates.

—Mr. John G. Borden, a winter resident of Florida, has, according to the *New York Medical Journal*, April 27, offered a prize of $1000 to the city within that State which shall be found in the most cleanly condition on July 1.

—Dr. R. C. Word, the managing editor of the *Southern Medical Record*, had his dwelling, furniture, library, instruments, his lecture notes, the manuscript of a work nearly ready for the press—all destroyed by fire on March 16.

—The Health Commissioner of Baltimore was notified, April 23, that at Santos and Rio, the ports from which the coffee importers of Baltimore receive nearly all their coffee, the yellow fever is raging more virulently than ever before. At the time of the last report from Rio there had been 186 deaths from yellow fever in four days.

HUMOR.

A GLASS EYE has one compensation— everybody else can see through the device if the wearer can't.—*Life.*

THE POOR OLD KING of Annam is dead. His is the most notable case of suspended Annamation on record.—*Philadelphia Press.*

A SMALL BOY sojourning on the coast of Maine sent the following clipping to his father in Boston:

Examiner—"What would you do in the case of a man with clammy sweats?"

Budding Sawbones—"Advise him to give up clams."

The boy appended the following:

" Dear papa, I thought you would appreciate the above, as you are having the sweats and I am having the clams." —*Western Medical Reporter.*

OBITUARY.

THOMAS S. SOZINSKEY, M.D.

Dr. Thomas S. Sozinskey died at his home in Philadelphia, April 19. He was born at Cabery, County Derry, Ireland, about 37 years ago. In 1869 he came to Philadelphia, where he has since resided. In 1872 he was admitted to the degree of M.D. by the University of Pennsylvania, which, the following year, also conferred upon him the complimentary title of Ph.D. He was for years a member of the Masonic Order. Three children survive him.

RESOLUTIONS ON THE DEATH OF DR. GROSS.

At a special meeting of the J. Aitken Meigs Medical Association, held April 22, 1889, the following minute was made: The ranks of the remaining few of the instructors of the members of this Association having been invaded by death, it is in grateful appreciation, Resolved, That we will cherish the memory of Dr. Samuel W. Gross, as a talented teacher, whose precepts then inculcated guide us in our daily pursuits; and that, together with the medical profession at large, we mourn the loss of a *savant* whose impressive teaching, erudite writing, and originality of thought and operative skill have made him a master in surgery.

J. MOORE CAMPBELL, *President*,
M. H. BOCHROCH, *Secretary*.

L. W. STEINBACH,
JOHN S. MILLER,
H. H. FREUND,
Committee.

MEDICAL AND SURGICAL REPORTER

No. 1680.   PHILADELPHIA, MAY 11, 1889.   VOL. LX.—No. 19.

CONTENTS:

CLINICAL LECTURE.

PYURIA. CONVALESCENCE FROM TYPHOID FEVER.[1]

BY JAMES B. WALKER, M.D.,
PHILADELPHIA.
PROFESSOR OF THEORY AND PRACTICE OF MEDICINE IN THE WOMAN'S MEDICAL COLLEGE OF PENNSYLVANIA.

Pyuria.

This patient is thirty-three years old and a glass-blower by occupation. He came into the house a few days ago with a fever, a cough and a pain in the right side rather low down, and in the back.

His history is as follows: Three weeks ago the pain began in the right side without apparent cause, and has continued off and on since. The past week it has become more severe, and cough has appeared. There is a little expectoration of a yellowish color, which occurs for the most part in the morning. The pain has remained on the right

[1] Delivered at the Philadelphia Hospital, April 24, 1889.

side, but it occasionally shoots to the left. The patient complains, at times, of pain in the cardiac region. He has been losing flesh for several months. He has no appetite; his bowels are regular. He has complained for two weeks of ringing noises in the ears. He has never been healthy; has had malaria almost every spring, and had typhoid fever two years ago. He was in the hospital six years ago with secondary syphilis, but he has had no symptoms of that disease since. His mother died at forty, and a sister at twenty—both with some heart trouble. One brother was living and well when last heard from.

The temperature on admission was 104.6°. It fell to 99.4°, then to 98.2°, and this morning it is 98.8°. His respirations have been in the neighborhood of 26, and his pulse about 92, the respiration being increased relatively to the pulse.

His urine is amber-colored, acid, with a dense sediment which consists chiefly of pus and epithelium. It contains one-eighth per cent. albumin, but no sugar. By pressing over the floating ribs near their spinal extremities, we find a tenderness which is exaggerated by counter-pressure from the back. This tenderness exists below the level of the ribs in the right lumbar region, but does not reach the umbilical region. There is slight tenderness on the left side also.

When he first came in, we supposed from his history of cough, his high temperature, and pain in the side that we would find pneumonic trouble, although the pain was low down; for the pain in pneumonia is very indefinite in location. Examination of the lung, however, showed that it was not involved.

Excluding, therefore, pneumonia and pleurisy, the urine was examined, with the result given. The pain and tenderness were in the region of the kidney. Generally the location of tenderness over a viscus is sufficient to refer the disease to that organ, but sometimes pain is radiated from its origin, and nerves at a distance are made sensitive. I have seen a case in which a renal calculus gave rise to such intense pain in the gluteal region that a diagnosis was made of lumbago and muscular rheumatism of the thigh. With, however, tenderness over the kidneys and the presence of acid urine containing pus, we have pretty clearly located the disease in the kidney itself. A chronic catarrh of the lining membrane of the bladder, when, as is usually the case, bacteria are present, will promote alkaline, ammoniacal changes in the urine; but if with pyuria the urine is persistently acid, it is almost pathognomonic of renal trouble.

What is the kidney trouble that can cause pyuria? It is a calculus more frequently than anything else, which gives rise to surgical kidney—but not always. We had at one time in this house a very interesting case, which taught us a lesson. The patient had a history somewhat similar to this man's. He would have high temperature, with severe pain in the region of the kidney. Then he would void a considerable amount of urine containing pus, and would experience relief from the fever for twelve to fifteen days; at the end of that time he would again have another attack lasting twenty-four or forty-eight hours, followed in turn by another remission. It was supposed, therefore, that there was a renal calculus blocking up the pelvis of the kidney and acting as a ball-valve.

It occurred to us, however, that there might be bladder trouble, and Dr. White, at my suggestion, examined the man and found strictures of the urethra from an old gonorrhœa. After having had the strictures dilated and after taking lithium borate and other antacids and diluents to keep the urine unirritating, the man recovered. Now, in that case, three of the visiting staff had agreed that it was wise to perform an exploratory operation and see if there was a stone in the pelvis of the kidney.

The case has impressed upon me the importance, in these cases, of always examining the bladder and urethra. I have asked, therefore, that it be done in the present case. In the meantime we must keep the urine in an unirritating condition. In most cases of the kind described, the urine is so acid that a small calculus of uric acid forms in the pelvis of the kidney and increases the irritation. The indication is, therefore, to prevent the further production of this form of calculus by rendering the urine alkaline. With this in view, that salt which is most solvent to uric acid should be used. It is probable that the uric acid calculus, once formed, is not soluble by the use of any known remedy which can be administered by the mouth and excreted by the kidney. But we can, at any rate, prevent the formation of new calculi. We must not, on the other hand, make the urine so strongly alkaline as to produce secondary alkaline deposits on the calculus. Therefore we should keep the urine in a very faintly alkaline or neutral condition.

Lithium salts are better than potassium salts for prolonged use; though, if you have a very severe case, I would recommend the occasional substitution of the potassium salts, because they act more rapidly, giving potassium bromide for nervous symptoms combined with potassium citrate or acetate for its action on the urine.

Lithium carbonate is given in three to five grain doses in pill form four times a day. If five grain doses are given, divide them into two pills each, for five grains in one pill would form a bolus too large to swallow. You may use in addition one of a number of alkaline waters, such as Waukesha, Buffalo Lithia, Londonderry or Lincoln Water. The increased amount of water taken by the mouth will in itself favor the washing out of the calculus, provided it be removable in this way. If not, surgical treatment alone will accomplish its removal.

The production of an offensive alkaline urine which undergoes ammoniacal changes, may be prevented by giving the patient boric acid, which tends to make the urine acid. The action of two grains of boric acid more than counteracts the alkaline tendency of three to five grains of lithium carbonate. It is not, however, the mere acidity of the urine that causes the deposition of calculi, but the presence of uric acid. Find out by experiment, therefore, how much alkali is necessary to make the urine slightly alkaline, and then administer in addition two to five grains of boric acid every day to prevent the decomposition of the urine, which otherwise would be likely to lead to extensive suppuration of the ureters and bladder. The sound revealed the presence of a decided stricture in this case, which may prove that the entire trouble is of gonorrhœal origin.

Convalescence from Typhoid Fever.

Case I.—This patient came before you three weeks ago with typhoid fever. His temperature was then running a pretty even rate, ranging from 102.3° in the morning to 103.2° in the evening. Since that time the temperature has showed very little variation until seven days ago, the twentieth day after admission, when it fell to 99°; and twenty-four days after admission, that is, day before yesterday, it fell below normal.

He had been sick for about two weeks before admission. He had not gone to bed until he was brought to the hospital. His pulse has rarely been above 100, and the temperature has not varied greatly between the above morning minimum and evening maximum. The case has gone on very nicely. When I showed the patient to you at first, he had quite marked diarrhœa—three or four movements a day—but since then he has had not more than two a day, and sometimes none at all. There has been no complication except bed-sores, which are fortunately rare in typhoid fever at present. All over the right trochanter major there is a puffy angry sore. There was also one over the sacrum, which has healed except a very small centre that is burrowing, with the formation of a little sanious pus. The sore should be syringed out with some antiseptic solution, and possibly it will need free incision.

Dujardin-Beaumetz, in his "Clinical Therapeutics," states that he accidentally used a one per cent. solution of chloral on a bed-sore, and with such good results that he has continued to use it since. As the bed-sore upon the hip did not yield very readily to chloral treatment, cinchona ointment (ʒi of the powdered bark to ʒi of simple ointment) was used.

In typhoid fever, especially in the nervous form, bed-sores are apt to occur in spite of the most careful treatment. To protect against bed-sores, we may make pads of elastic wool or cotton, or we may use a water-bed or cut a hole in the mattress so as to distribute the weight upon the thigh and the body above. If the threatened bed-sore is seen in time, we may prevent it not only by relieving pressure but by stimulating applications, such as alcohol, salt and whiskey, or alum solutions; but the removal of pressure is better than any washes that can be used. A doe-skin plaster, a quarter to half an inch thick, makes an excellent protective; but the trouble with this, as with most plasters, is that, unless carefully watched, a crease is formed which increases the irritation. It is better, therefore, to have the surface uncovered as long as it is unbroken.

This patient's tongue is now clearing off, though there is still some fur on it. His pulse is still dicrotic. We may not yet change the quality of his food, although his temperature is returning to normal. The use of vegetable foods in typhoid fever is very much to be deprecated. The starchy preparations should be especially avoided, because they are digested chiefly in the small bowel—which is the part of the intestine principally involved in typhoid fever—and also on account of their tendency to over-distend the bowels with gas, which embarrasses the heart and respiration and may even cause rupture of the intestine.

Rice is the starch first to be resorted to in these cases, as it does not produce much gas; but the solid animal foods, such as a soft boiled egg, a piece of tenderloin steak—nicely broiled and well masticated, and the pulp not swallowed at first—should be used early in convalescence.

During the disease, milk and meat broths—but *not* soups to which flour and other vegetable starchy matters have been added—should be employed. Beef and mutton are preferable to chicken and veal. Chicken broth is perhaps more laxative than any other meat broth.

Case II.—The next patient is a farmer, thirty-nine years old. Five weeks ago, without any apparent cause, he had a chill followed by pains all over his body, especially in the abdomen and head, which have continued and have grown worse. He went to bed and has remained in bed most of the time since. The bowels were sometimes constipated, sometimes loose, until a week ago, since which time he has had diarrhœa constantly, to the extent of having six or seven stools a day. There have been no hemorrhages of any kind.

On admission, his temperature was 101.6°, pulse 97, respiration 19. Since then his pulse has ranged from 76 to 84. His temperature ranged, for the first two days, between 101° and 102°, and then fell to normal—rising, however, to 100 in the evening—and since has risen and fallen, but has not been far from normal.

His tongue has improved quite decidedly since day before yesterday. It has now lost its dryness, but is somewhat coated and has a red tip and edge. His skin is normal to the touch. His pulse has a fair volume, is soft, very compressible, and slightly dicrotic. On whipping the deltoid muscle, contraction is evoked. This is rather a painful experiment, but it is said to be suggestive of typhoid fever. I have found it in all the cases of typhoid fever in which I have examined for it, but I have not tested to see whether it is present or not to the same degree in other weak conditions. There are the remains of a spot in the centre of the abdomen, which do not disappear on pressure. This is the case frequently with old typhoid spots. On Monday this spot disappeared on pressure, and was suggestive of a typhoid eruption. The tenderness over the abdomen is great, and is not confined to the right iliac region. There is no tympanites, but the abdomen is rather scaphoid.

He had been eating pretty much everything before he came into the house, so that his intestines are in a condition of widespread irritation.

The improvement in his condition just mentioned occurred under the administration of small doses of calomel and ipecac—one-twelfth of a grain each—repeated till the bowels moved. These remedies are indicated when the secretions are lacking and the skin and the tongue are dry, even if there is diarrhœa.

This spring there has been almost an epidemic of typhoid fever in Philadelphia, and many other cases have seemed to be on the verge of having typhoid fever. You know the general idea is that the typhoid fever germs, on entering the system and finding a lodgment, invariably develop and produce a well-marked attack of typhoid fever. The Germans believe that, although the system may not have the power to resist the entrance of germs, it may be able to prevent the full development of the disease. In a number of cases when head-

ache with dryness of the tongue and skin have manifested themselves, I have given calomel with ipecac or soda, not repeating this treatment unless the same symptoms recurred. This I have followed by quininæ sulph., gr. iss; caffeinæ, gr. ss, in pill form, every four hours. It is continued for about seven days, and additional doses of caffeine are given in the intervals, if they are necessary to control headache. Generally, under this treatment, the appearances of threatened typhoid have passed away, but I do not say that I have averted typhoid fever in any case.

I do not like to use antipyrin and antifebrin for the relief of headache in a case of threatened typhoid. They are depressing and have to be used in almost as large doses for headache as for their antipyretic effect. By avoiding them early in a threatened attack they may be reserved for their more important effect later, should the rise in temperature demand their use; although I am not in favor of their employment as antipyretics, unless the indications for them are urgent.

COMMUNICATIONS.

REMARKS UPON THE TREATMENT OF THE OPIUM HABIT AND KINDRED AFFECTIONS.[1]

BY J. C. WILSON, M.D.,

PHILADELPHIA.

PHYSICIAN TO THE HOSPITAL OF THE JEFFERSON COLLEGE, ETC., ETC.

There are clear indications that the habitual abuse of the more subtile and pernicious narcotics is a growing evil. Were the increase of the evil open to question, the manifest prevalence of these habits is wide enough to excite serious apprehension among those interested in social problems, and to render any apology for the discussion of the subject in this Society is unnecessary. Unlike alcohol, the addiction to which, however secret at first, sooner or later betrays itself by unequivocal signs, opium, chloral, and others of the group give rise to a vice essentially secret. The practitioner who is on the alert finds the consumption of some such drug, often in large amounts, to be the underlying cause of a noteworthy proportion of the cases of chronic invalidism that come under observation.

[1] Read before the Philadelphia Neurological Society, April 22, 1889.

The victims of these habits occupy a much higher social level than the victims of alcoholism. A large proportion of them are persons of intelligence and refinement. We find among them men of letters, professional men, especially physicians, in unfortunate preponderance, while the statistics of numerous observers point to even greater prevalence of the habit among women.

A certain proportion of the cases are incurable. A considerable number of them, although not permanently curable, may under proper management be freed from the vice for more or less prolonged periods. A third group comprises individuals who have fallen into vicious habits of this kind rather through unfortunate circumstances than through any defect of nervous organization, and who are, therefore, capable of permanent restoration to health. For these reasons the consideration of the subject of habitual narcotism merits the attention not only of those in the profession who have especially devoted themselves to the study and treatment of nervous diseases, but also of those engaged in general medical work.

The diagnosis of the opium habit is in many cases attended with considerable difficulty. Many *habitués*, it is true, do not hesitate to admit the real cause of their symptoms. Others, while seeking to conceal it, do so in such an indifferent manner that detection is not difficult. But the greater number for a long time sedulously conceal their passion not only from their friends, but also from the physician whom they select voluntarily or at the solicitations of those interested in them. If inquiries be made upon the subject, they deny the habit altogether, often with vehement protestations. If forced to admit it, they are very apt to mis-state the amount taken or the frequency of the dose.

As a rule, to which there are, however, not infrequent exceptions, emaciation is marked, the appetite is diminished and variable, the pulse is small, the circulation feeble, the respiration often sighing, the pupils occasionally strongly contracted, constipation is present, often alternating with diarrhœa. When to these conditions, for which no cause can be found upon careful examination, there are added marked change in disposition, periods of unaccountable dulness alternating with unusual vivacity and brightness, especially insomnia alternating with periods of prolonged and heavy sleep, the abuse of narcotics may be suspected. If the hypodermic syringe be used, the wounds made by the needle confirm the diagnosis. These punctures are usually found in groups upon the thighs, legs, arms, or abdomen. Close inquiry into the habits of the patient, who either goes himself, or sends at short intervals to some neighboring apothecary, for unusually large quantities of opium, morphia, or other narcotic drug, is sometimes necessary to confirm the diagnosis.

The diagnosis of the chloral habit is attended with much less difficulty than that of the morphine habit. In the first place, there is general and often serious derangement of health without adequate discoverable cause. The appetite is poor and capricious, the digestion imperfect and slowly performed; jaundice of variable intensity, often slight, sometimes severe, occurs in many cases; the bowels are not as a rule constipated. Dyspnœa upon slight exertion is, in the absence of pulmonary, cardiac, or renal trouble, of diagnostic importance. The circulation is as a rule feeble; disorders of the skin, persistent or easily provoked conjunctivitis, and a tendency to hemorrhages from mucous surfaces also occur. When with these •symptoms, irregularly grouped as they are apt to be, we find a tendency to recurring attacks of cerebral congestion, persistent or frequently recurring headaches, and the evidences of subacute peripheral neuritis, the abuse of chloral may be suspected. The pains of the limbs are almost characteristic; they are acute and persistent, neuralgic in character, but not localized to special nerve tracts; they are more common in the legs than in the arms and occupy by preference the calves of the legs and the flexor muscles between the elbows and wrists; they do not implicate the joints, are not aggravated to any great extent by movement, and are often temporarily relieved by gentle frictions. The pains of chloralism have deen described as though produced by encircling bands above the wrists and ankles. The suspicion of addiction to chloral becomes the more probable if there be a history of prolonged painful illness or prolonged insomnia in the past. This suspicion is confirmed when we encounter at the same time perversion of the moral nature, enfeeblement of the will and of the intellectual forces. It is rendered positive, notwithstanding the denials of the patient, by the discovery of the drug or the prescription by means of which it is procured.

The same diagnostic criteria are available in cases of vicious narcotism from cocaine and cannabis indica.

The treatment of these affections naturally ranges itself under two heads: (A) the prophylactic, and (B) the curative treatment.

A. Of these, broadly considered, the Prophylactic Treatment is the more important. This is, however, a complex subject, involving questions too far-reaching to admit of discussion in the present communication. I venture, however, to make the practical suggestions which follow. The therapeutic use of narcotic drugs when necessary, should be guarded with every possible precaution. 1. The patient should, when practicable, be kept in ignorance of the character of the anodyne used and of the dose. 2. The physician should personally control, as far as possible, the use of such drugs and the frequency of their administration, taking care that the minimum amount capable of producing the desired effect is employed. 3. The occasional alternation of anodyne medicaments is desirable. 4. Sedative doses of narcotic drugs, and especially hypodermic injections of morphia, should not be used except in acute cases or in chronic painful illnesses likely to terminate fatally. The prolonged habitual administration of hypodermic injections of morphia is inadmissable, where recovery is to be hoped for. 5. The danger of yielding to the temptation to allow a merely palliative treatment to assume too great importance in the management of painful affections must be shunned. 6. An effort, which is too often likely to be unsuccessful, should be made to prevent renewals of the prescription without the direct sanction, or indeed without the written order, of the physician himself.

Too often these precautions are neglected, and the patient, betrayed by a dangerous knowledge of the drug and of the dose, and tempted by the facility with which the coveted narcotic may be obtained, falls an easy victim to habitual excesses. The lowered moral tone of convalescence from severe illness and of habitual invalidism increases these dangers. The uniform and efficient regulation of the sale of narcotic drugs by law would constitute an important prophylactic measure against habitual narcotism. Unfortunately, the existing laws relating to this subject are a dead letter; they are neither adequate to control the evil, nor is their enforcement practicable.

B. The Curative Treatment of the opium and morphine habit consists in the isolation of the patient and the progressive diminution of the dose. The method of Levinstein, which consists in the abrupt discontinuance of the drug, is cruel and hazardous; and is, so far as I am aware, neither advocated nor practised in this country.

The substitution of other narcotics is neither desirable nor necessary, except to meet special indications, and forms no necessary part of the plan of the gradual withdrawal.

Whether the treatment may be most satisfactorily carried out in an institution devoted to the care of nervous and insane patients or in a private house, is a matter of opinion. Certain it is that no confirmed case of the opium habit can be successfully treated under ordinary circumstances at his own home or if he is permitted to go about. The cases in which the home-treatment proves successful in curing addiction to opium or morphine must be looked upon as exceptional. The reasons for this are obvious. They relate to a variety of circumstances which tend to weaken the mutual relations of control and dependence between the physician and his patient. The doubts, criticisms, remonstrances, even the active interference, of the patient's friends tend to weaken the authority of the physician and to hamper him in the management of the case; the discipline of the sick-room is maintained with greater difficulty; the absolute seclusion of the attendant with his patient is a practical impossibility. Affectionate but foolish friends come with sympathy at once disturbing and dangerous. Some devoted servant cunningly conveys from time to time new supplies of the coveted drug, or, if these accidents be averted, the very consciousness of a separation which amounts to only a few feet of hall-way is in itself a source of distress to the patient and his friends alike. Furthermore, the period of convalescence following the treatment is attended with the greatest danger of relapse— a danger which is much increased by the facility of procuring narcotics enjoyed by the patient in his own home as contrasted with the difficulties attending it away from home under the care of a watchful attendant.

The desirability of undertaking the treatment away from the patient's home can therefore scarcely be questioned. That this plan is more expensive, and that it involves a radical derangement of the ordinary relations of the patient's life, are apparent rather than real objections to it. The very expense of the cure within the limits of the patient's ability to pay, and the mortification and annoyance of temporary absence from usual occupations and seclusion from friends, are in themselves hardships that enhance the value of the cure when achieved, and constitute, to a certain extent, safeguards against relapse. Whether the treatment can be more advantageously carried out in an institution designed for the reception of several such cases, or in a private boarding house, is a question to be determined by circumstances. My own experience warrants the belief that these cases are best managed in suitably arranged apartments in private boarding houses, and by physicians, not necessarily specialists, but actively engaged in general clinical medicine. Under these circumstances the seclusion is more complete, and the patient is secured from even the chance contact of persons who may know him personally or by sight. It is not necessary that the proprietor of the house should know more than that he is a sufferer from some nervous ailment. Under this arrangement, many persons willingly leave home for treatment who could not under any circumstances be persuaded to enter a public or private institution for treatment; moreover, the control is more effectual and the personal relationship between the patient and his physician closer.

The symptoms which attend even the very gradual reduction of the dose are such as demand the most varied experience in clinical medicine and a wide range of therapeutic resources. They are familiar to you all; notwithstanding the utmost care in the management of the case, they are sometimes of dangerous severity.

The apartment occupied by the patient should be so arranged as to guard against attempts at suicide. The furniture should be of the simplest character; the heating and lighting arrangements must be such as to render any accident to the patient during paroxysms of sudden maniacal excitement quite impossible. From the beginning of the treatment the patient must under no circumstances be left alone. Two attendants are required, one for the day and one for the night. They should be not only skilful and experienced, but patient and firm, and as a considerable portion of the patients are persons of education and refinement, intelligence and good manners are desirable on the part of those who must be for a length of time not only the nurses, but also the companions of the sufferer. It is further desirable that the separation of the patient from his family and friends should be as complete as possible. During the continuance of the active treatment, no one should be admitted to the patient except his physician and regular attendants. So soon as the acute symptoms caused by the withdrawal of the drug subside and convalescence is fairly established, brief visits from judicious members of the family may be permitted in the presence of the nurse.

At the earliest possible moment open air exercise by walking or driving must be insisted upon, and change of scene, such as may be secured by short journeys or by visits to the sea-shore, is useful. These outings require the constant presence of a conscientious attendant.

Whatever may have been the form of self-administration of the drug, hypodermic injections of morphia should be chosen during the treatment by the physician. Three, sometimes four, doses should be administered in the course of each twenty-four hours. While the diminution should be in general terms progressive, it is desirable that the evening dose should be somewhat increased in amount in order to secure quietude during the night. The drug should in every instance be administered either by the physician himself or by a trustworthy medical assistant. This is a point of radical importance. It obviates all risk of excessive doses; it relieves the nurse from the importunities of the sufferer, which are always distressing and often intolerable; it keeps the patient in ignorance of the amount of the successive doses; and it establishes a degree of control and influence on the part of the physician which is of great advantage to all concerned. A large number of failures in treatment is due to the fact that the administration of the narcotic is entrusted to the care of the immediate attendants.

The rapidity with which the drug is withdrawn will be determined by the circumstances of the individual case. The time occupied is rarely less than a week, and not infrequently must be extended to a fortnight. If the administration of the morphia to correct urgent symptoms be at all required after this period, it will be at most on one or two occasions at intervals of twenty-four or forty-eight hours. When the process of reducing the dose is too gradually prolonged, the sufferings of the patient are unnecessarily aggravated. It is frequently desirable to continue the equivalent of the habitual dose for a few days after the isolation in order to investigate the peculiarities of the case and to establish the discipline of the sick-room. It is especially desirable during this period that the patient shall take large amounts of easily digested and nutritious food, and it is a cardinal rule that throughout the treatment suitable nourishment should be systematically administered at short intervals and in full amounts.

The diet should consist of milk and lime water or Vichy water, peptonized or sterilized milk, Koumiss, Kéfir, concentrated broths, the expressed juice of fresh, slightly broiled beef, and the various commercial foods used in the artificial feeding of infants. The commercial peptonoids and especially Reed and Carnrick's liquid peptonoids, have been found useful.

Efforts to control vomiting by medicines other than the administration of opium and morphine in some way are not usually attended by success. Diarrhœa is best managed by the administration from time to time of large doses of bismuth subnitrate (gr. xx–xxx) every second, third, or fourth hour. The sinking feeling at the pit of the stomach and the epigastric pain are to some extent relieved by external applications. Hot fomentations or hot, wet compresses with a few drops of chloroform or turpentine are useful. For the relief of symptoms due to flagging action of the heart, the recumbent posture, external warmth, friction of the extremities, the application of turpentine or mustard to the precordial and epigastric regions, the inhalation of ammonia, or the administration of preparations of ammonia, will be required. Digitalis, strophanthus, sparteine sulphate, and adonidine are all useful. It is frequently desirable to begin the systematic administration of agents of this kind early in the case. Alcohol will, however, prove in the greater number of cases an indispensable remedy. It may be given in the form of milk punch, hot toddy, champagne, etc. Failure of the circulation may, notwithstanding every effort to control it, reach such a degree as to jeopardize the patient's life. Under such circumstances, the progressive diminution of the dose must be interrupted by the immediate administration of efficient doses of morphine, which, if necessary, must be repeated. As the tendency to diarrhœa increases, the quantity of urine excreted rapidly diminishes. It is often reduced to six or eight fluid ounces in the course of twenty-four hours, and after a few days of treatment it frequently contains albumin and occasionally casts. The oliguria is largely due to the excessive loss of fluid by the bowel, and does not require treatment. Nor is active treatment demanded by the albuminuria, which usually spontaneously ceases in the course of a few days. In the rare instances where it persists for weeks or months, appropriate treatment must be instituted.

The nervous symptoms are favorably influenced by methodical alimentation and the free use of alcoholics. Care must be taken to reduce the amount of alcohol administered as convalescence progresses. The danger of replacing a vicious habit of morphine taking by the more brutalizing vice of chronic alcoholism must be ever held in view.

It is hardly necessary to describe in detail the treatment demanded for the relief of the varied disturbances of the nervous system. The occasional use of cannabis indica, either in the form of the tincture or the extract, exerts a favorable influence. Neither the nitrites alone, nor nitroglycerine in combination with sparteine, as first recommended by Jennings, have proved useful in my experience. The ethereal extract of lupulin exerts a favorable but not very powerful influence in tranquilizing the nervous system. For twenty-four or forty-eight hours after the final discontinuance of morphine, but little effect may be expected from other sleep inducing drugs. Chloral in single large doses, either alone or associated with correspondingly large doses of the bromides, administered on the second or third night after total suppression, is often followed by prolonged, tranquil, and refreshing sleep. Paraldehyde, although a less certain, is a less dangerous hypnotic under such circumstances. Sulphonal, in doses ranging from 15 to 20 grains, is often a serviceable hypnotic during convalescence. Hyoscine hydrobromate may be used with advantage when there is great motor excitement. Massage, hot baths, and the cold pack are all useful adjuvants to the treatment.

The abject mental state of the patient calls for much firmness, gentleness, and tact on the part of the physician and attendants. Every effort should be made to inspire courage and hope. Neither the importance of the symptoms nor the intensity of the sufferings of the patient should be underrated; nevertheless, the ordeal is a limited one. In the majority of instances, to get rid of the opium means to get well, because opium, unlike alcohol, does not leave permanent structural lesions of any organ. The expectation of a radical cure must therefore be confidently presented to the patient as a consolation in his sufferings.

Insomnia and muscular weakness usually persist into the convalescence for some weeks, and only gradually yield to careful regulation of the daily life of the patient, with abundant nutritious food, open-air exercise, and change of scene. The insomnia of this period constitutes a serious symptom, for the reason that it constantly subjects the patient to the temptation to return to indulgence in narcotics. In the course of time, however, the normal physical and mental condition is regained, and the patient may be permitted to return to his former pursuits and associations.

The time occupied in the withdrawal of the narcotic and in the convalescence, constitutes on the part of the nervous system a period of gradual readjustment to normal conditions. Efforts to unduly shorten this period must in the nature of things be unsuccessful. The patient must therefore understand that his complete restoration to health demands a certain length of time. Any attempt to abridge this period by the substitution of other narcotics, exercising a less intense, or at all events, a modified effect upon the nervous system, are less likely to be permanently useful than the systematic employment of measures tending to improve to the fullest extent the general nutrition of the body and to bring about a wholesome moral sense and reasonable exercise of the will.

The curative treatment of habitual addiction to chloral is attended by neither the difficulties nor the dangers which are encountered in the management of the opium habit. The symptoms attending the discontinuance of chloral are less severe and less persistent; in fact, individuals accustomed to the taking of large doses of chloral not infrequently voluntarily discontinue its use for considerable periods of time. As a rule, the treatment may be carried out at home, the patient, however, being isolated and cared for by a watchful attendant. The drug should be stopped at once. For the first few days alcoholic stimulants should be freely given. Systematic feeding, pepsin, full doses of quinine, followed after a time by strychnia, and, as soon as the condition of the digestive system will permit of it, by iron, fulfil the general indications. Cod-liver oil and malt extracts may be given with advantage. Cardiac failure, collapse, and delirium tremens are to be treated in the same manner as similar complications occurring in the treatment of the opium habit. Vomiting is much less likely to occur, and when present is less persistent and less difficult of management. Diarrhœa does not usually prove troublesome, the bowels, on the contrary, being constipated. The latter condition yields to mild laxatives or to simple enemata. Hemorrhages from the various mucous tracts may be controlled by fluid extract of ergot, the hypodermic injection of solution of ergotin, minute doses of wine of ipecac, or fluid extract of hamamelis.

Two serious cases only of addiction to cocaine have come under my observation. In both of these the drug was at once stopped, with immediate relief from the epigastric and cardiac distress and the extreme bodily and mental depression which the habit had induced.

In conclusion, the following propositions may be affirmed:

1. No confirmed case of the opium habit can be satisfactorily treated at home. Suitable rooms in a private boarding house are available for a large proportion of the patients, including those who cannot be induced to enter a public or private institution.

2. Hypodermic injections of morphine, administered by the physician or by a medical assistant, constitute the best means of administering the drug during its gradual withdrawal.

3. The substitution of other narcotics, while occasionally required for special symptoms, does not constitute any necessary part of the treatment.

4. Many of the more serious symptoms following the withdrawal of the drug are prevented by the systematic administration of suitable food at short intervals and the judicious use of alcoholic stimulants.

5. The insomnia and asthenia of convalescence are incidental to the re-adjustment of the nervous system to normal conditions. So long as these symptoms persist, there is danger of early relapse and the patient should be kept under observation.

6. The convalescent must be warned that in the future the first dose of opium or morphia, either by the mouth or hypodermically, is likely to lead to the formation of the habit anew.

1437 Walnut Street.

———————◆●◆———————

—Examinations in English schools go toward proving that color-blindness is frequently declared to be present when really no organic defect, but only poor training in the naming and distinction of colors, is found to be the trouble.

REPORT OF AMPUTATIONS PER-
FORMED AT THE HOSPITAL OF
THE UNIVERSITY OF PENNSYL-
VANIA FROM SEPTEMBER 30, 1874,
TO DECEMBER 31, 1888.

BY LEWIS H. ADLER, Jr., M.D.,

LATE RESIDENT PHYSICIAN, UNIVERSITY HOSPITAL.

The cases tabulated in the following paper comprise largely amputations done on account of railway accidents; which are always extremely dangerous, and are liable to be followed by bad results, even in subjects enjoying perfect health at the time of the accident, owing to the tendency to the development of mortification and pyemia.

Again, the results of the work of such men as Dr. D. Hayes Agnew, Dr. John Neill, and Dr. John Ashhurst, Jr., in a large institution such as the Hospital of the University of Pennsylvania, cannot but add somewhat to our knowledge of the mortality resulting from amputations.

The majority of these operations were done before the present strict antiseptic treatment came into vogue, and it is certain that the statistics of the future will make a better showing. But still, the care and personal attention of the Surgeon-in-chief, which have always characterized the treatment of such cases in this Hospital, both during the operation itself and during the period following it, are important factors in the reduction of the mortality from this operation.

I have followed in the arrangement of the statistics in this paper the plan adopted in similar papers, by both Dr. George W. Norris,[1] and Dr. Thomas G. Morton,[2] surgeons to the Pennsylvania Hospital, in their published reports of the statistics of amputation.

In the tables sub-joined, all amputations in which the operation was performed within twenty-four hours subsequent to the accident are included under the head of Primary. The other divisions—Secondary and Chronic—explain themselves.

Of 290 patients upon whom 320 amputations were performed during a period of a little over fourteen years—(extending from the opening of the hospital, in 1874, to 1889 inclusive) 73 died, or 25.1 per cent.

Of this number 21 were primary double amputations; 3 primary triple amputations; 1 secondary double amputation, and 2 were double amputations for chronic trouble.

Of the 21 primary double amputations 11 patients recovered; 10 died, or 47.6 per cent.

Of the three primary triple amputations 2 patients died, or 66⅔ per cent.

The case of secondary double amputation recovered.

Of the cases of secondary amputations for chronic trouble, all the patients recovered.

TABLES OF DOUBLE AND TRIPLE AMPUTA-
TIONS.

Double amputations:		Result.	Age.
Shoulder-joint and arm	Primary	Died	21
Arm and thigh	"	Rec.	28
" leg	"	D	21
" "	"	"	35
Forearm and leg . . .	"	R	48
" . " . . .	"	"	45
Hip-joint and leg . . .	"	"	15
Thigh and foot	"	D	25
Knee-joints (both) . .	"	R	28
" " . .	"	D	32
Knee-joint and leg . .	"	"	41
" " .	"	"	50
" " .	"	R	25
Legs (both)	"	"	22
"	"	"	21
"	Chronic	R	23
"	Primary	D	63
"	"	R	18
Leg and foot . . .	"	"	25
" . . .	"	"	19
" . . .	"	D	34
" . . .	"	R	21
Feet (both)	Secondary	"	29
"	Chronic	"	61

These cases number 24; 14 patients recovered; 10 died, or a percentage of 41.7.

Triple amputations:		Result.	Age.
Arms (both) and thigh .	Primary	D	15
Forearm, thigh and leg	"	R	26
Forearm and legs (both)	"	D	45

Of the 263 patients who had but one limb amputated, 202 recovered; 61 died, or 23.3 per cent.

180 cases were primary single amputations; of this number, 140 patients recovered; 40 died, or 22.2 per cent.

3 were cases of secondary single amputation; of this number all the patients died, or 100 per cent.

80 were cases of single amputation for diseases of a chronic nature; of this number 61 patients recovered; 19 died, or 23.75 per cent.

[1] *American Journal of the Medical Sciences*, vols. xxii, xxvi and xxviii. See also a similar account, dating from January 1, 1850, to January 1, 1860, with a general summary of the mortality following the operation in the Pennsylvania Hospital for 30 years. Contributions to Practical Surgery—Norris. Lindsay & Blakiston, 1873.

[2] *American Journal of the Medical Sciences*, 1870 and 1875.

TABLE SHOWING THE VARIOUS SINGLE AMPU-
TATIONS, WITH THE RESULTS.

			Result.
8 Shoulder-joint amputations . .	Primary	R
3 " " "	"	D
2 " " "	. . . Chronic	R
30 Arm amputations	Primary	R
5 " " . . . . . . "	"	D
4 " " . . . . . Chronic	R
20 Forearm ·-	Primary	R
2 " " . . . . . . "	D
5 " " . . . . Chronic	R
3 Wrist-joint amputations . . .	Primary	"
15 Hand amputations	"	"
3 " " . . . . Chronic	"
1 Hip-joint amputation	"	D
12 Thigh "	Primary	R
14 " "	"	D
11 " " . . . . Chronic	R
7 " " . . . . "	D
1 " " . . . . Secondary	"
11 Knee-joint "	Primary	R
3 " " . . . . "	D
3 " " . . Chronic	R
5 " " . . . . "	D
34 Leg amputations	Primary	R
12 " " .	"	D
26 " " . . . . Chronic	R
6 " " ·· . . . "	D
2 " " . . . . . Secondary	"
1 Ankle-joint amputation . . .	Primary	"
7 Foot amputations	··	R
7 " " . . . . . Chronic	"

upper extremity; of this number 10 patients.
died, or 10 per cent.

163 of the amputations were of the lower
extremity; of this number 52 patients died,
or 31.9 per cent.

In one of Dr. Geo. W. Norris's papers
upon amputations,[1] previously referred to,
mention is made of the mortality of such
operations in the following terms:—"In a
large hospital no operation is more frequently called for than that of amputation,
and even where the time for doing it is.
judiciously determined, and the operation
itself dexterously and well performed, the
dangers to which the patient is afterward
exposed, are so great as to render the subject worthy of all attention from the practical surgeon. Contrary to the opinion generally prevalent in this country, amputation,
even under favorable circumstances, is very
frequently followed by fatal results in civil
hospitals. In the practice of the Hôtel
Dieu, of Paris, it is said that not more than
half of the cases prove successful,[2] and I
have the authority of M. Hache, a former
interne of the hospital of St. Louis, of the
same city, for stating, that out of twenty

TABLE SHOWING THE INFLUENCE OF AGE UPON THE MORTALITY AFTER AMPUTATIONS.

AGE.	SINGLE AMPUTATIONS.						SYNCHRONOUS DOUBLE AMPUTATIONS.				SYNCHRONOUS. TRIPLE AMPU- TATIONS.	
	Primary.		Secondary.		Chronic.		Primary.		S'c'nd- ary.*	Chron- ic.*	Primary.	
	R	D	R	D	R	D	R	D	R	R	R	D
19 and under	39	5		1		1	9	0	3		1	
Between 20 and 30	55	9	1				12	5	6	4	1	1		1
" 30 and 40 . .	25	12	1		2		18	4	0	3			
40 and over , ...	21	14					22	10	2	3		1		1

*None died.

TABLE SHOWING THE PERCENTAGE OF MOR-
TALITY OF SINGLE AMPUTATIONS UPON
THE DIFFERENT PARTS OF THE BODY:

				Per cent.
13 shoulder-joint amputations, mortality 3			or	23
39 arm ·	"	5	"	13
27 forearm "	"	2	"	7.4
21 Wrist-joint & hand "	"	0	"	
1 hip-joint "	··	1	"	100
45 thigh ·	"	22	"	48.8
22 knee-joint "	"	8	"	36.4
80 leg "	"	20	"	25
15 ankle-joint & foot "	"	1	"	6⅔

100 of the above amputations were of the

successive amputations made in the year
1833, in that institution, twelve died, or 60
per cent. With one exception (that of a
toe) all these were capital amputations, and
at the time the statement was made some of
the patients were remaining still uncured."

When we recall the fact, which is often
overlooked in the comparisons of older statistics with those of the present day, that
anæsthetics have only been used to relieve

[1] *American Journal of Medical Sciences*, August,
1838.
[2] *Gazette des Hôpitaux*, 1834.

suffering in these capital operations for a little over 40 years, and that the additional suffering inflicted before their use added largely to the shock and consequent mortality of this operation—we must, in summing up our conclusions as to the more favorable results obtained now, give credit to anæsthetics as important factors.

Again, the facilities for handling cases requiring amputation are greater now; the perfection of the railway system permits of the early inspection of the patients by the surgeon; and the accommodations offered to patients recently injured in the numerous hospitals scattered over the land, where with careful nursing and the constant presence of the house-surgeon, dangers can be met and guarded against—all tend to lessen the mortality of amputations.

From this *résumé* of amputations performed in a little over 14 years at the University Hospital, it appears—

1. That amputations of the lower extremity are more liable to prove fatal than those of the upper extremity. (Norris.)

2. That the rate of mortality is greater in proportion to the proximity to the trunk of the part amputated.[1]

3. That, contrary to the statements usually made in other published statistics, the mortality of amputations for chronic disease is about the same as for recent injury—the former being 23.75 per cent., the latter 23.5 per cent. The explanation of this may be found in the fact that many of the cases were operated upon for chronic disease of a malignant character — sarcoma; etc.

4. That the danger increases with the age of the individual operated upon—a point previously brought forth in the investigations of Dr. Norris.[2]

5. That in double synchronous amputations the prognosis is very favorable when the patient is under 30. Above that age the mortality is at least 75 per cent.—one chance in four in favor of recovery.

41 North Twelfth Street.

————◆◆◆————

—The Charité, the largest medical institution in Berlin, is to be enlarged. In order to provide more space for beds, room for lecture halls will be provided in separate buildings, and the space thus gained will be used for patients. The same thing will be done with the out-patient rooms.

[1] Ashhurst, Principles and Practice of Surgery, 4th Ed. page 112.

[2] *American Journal of the Medical Sciences*, August, 1838.

ANCHYLOSIS OF LARYNGEAL ARTICULATIONS FROM CANCEROUS INFILTRATION. RELIEF BY INTUBATION.

BY JOHN J. REID, M.D.,
NEW YORK CITY.
SURGEON TO CHARITY HOSPITAL.

————

The following case is of interest in several respects. First, as to the cause of the dyspnœa; second, with regard to the impossibility of making a correct diagnosis, even if the operation of extirpation of the growth had been performed; and finally, because of the benefit derived from intubation whilst the case was under consideration.

The history is briefly as follows: The patient, a widow 70 years old, entered the Charity Hospital, giving a history of hemiplegia coming on six weeks previously. Subsequently a growth was noticed about the middle of the neck, and to the left of the median line. Hoarseness followed, which was succeeded by dyspnœa of a spasmodic character. This growth was soft and fluctuating, but when the needle was inserted, no fluid was obtained. The diagnosis rested between cancer of the thyroid gland and abscess. The rapid development and fluctuating character of the tumor favored the latter view, but the nodular feeling, together with its connection with the thyroid, strengthened the suspicion of carcinoma. The most important question was as to the connection of the growth with the dyspnœa, and the necessity of immediate operation inasmuch as the most rational supposition was that pressure of the mass from behind obstructed the calibre of the trachea.

While the case was under consideration an O'Dwyer tube was inserted. This relieved the breathing and lessened the urgency of operative interference. Within thirty-six hours the patient died of exhaustion.

Autopsy.—The mass proved to be a cancerous growth of the thyroid, which extended upward along the trachea, but did not obstruct its calibre. At its upper part it invaded the posterior wall of the larynx, but did not project into it. The vocal cords were perfectly rigid, and would permit only the tip of the little finger to enter the chink of the glottis.

It was evident from an examination of the specimen that the dyspnœa was not due to the mechanical effect of the growth, but to the infiltration of the larynx, which caused anchylosis of the articulations and resulting stenosis.

SOCIETY REPORTS.

MEDICAL SOCIETY OF THE COUNTY OF NEW YORK.

Stated Meeting, April 22, 1889.

The President, ALEXANDER S. HUNTER, M.D., in the Chair.

Dr. G. H. Fox read a paper on the

Treatment of Acne Without Arsenic, Sulphur Ointments, or Lotions,

and said that it was not to be inferred from the title that he objected to the use of arsenic, sulphur ointments, or lotions; he simply believes their field of usefulness to be limited. On the average, it is probable arsenic does more harm than good in these affections, because it is administered without discrimination.

He divided acne, for convenience in treatment, into two forms, the irritable and the indolent. In the irritable form the skin is usually fine and soft, quickly inflamed by applications, and admits of no other than the most soothing treatment. This form of the disease is largely of a reflex nature, due especially to disorders of digestion and of the sexual organs. It is chiefly benefited by diet and internal remedies. The indolent form shows usually a coarse, doughy, often greasy skin. In these cases the glands, which are the seat of comedones and pustules, should be evacuated; in other words, the skin should be kept clean; soap and water, ointments and lotions are not sufficient.

Most physicians place much reliance upon arsenic as an internal remedy in acne, but on the whole it is probable that patients would get along better if it were unknown. Sulphide of calcium has been recommended highly, but is likely to lead the physician to neglect more important measures. Ergot possesses greater value than is generally attributed to it, its chief benefit being achieved in the indolent form. In irritable acne Dr. Fox now seldom uses the many internal remedies with which he has formerly experimented. The chief principles of treatment to be followed in acne, are the regulation of the diet and the use of local massage. Massage can be applied by squeezing out the comedones, emptying the pustules, and scraping with the round curette, kneading with the fingers, etc. But no fixed plan of treatment can be laid down for all cases.

Dr. L. D. BULKLEY then read a paper on a

Clinical Study and Analysis of Cases of Psoriasis and their Treatment,

which was a review of twenty years' experience with the affection. The disease, being one of the most common and persistent of skin affections, deserves careful study. It rarely attacks the skin of the palms of the hands or soles of the feet. Dr. Bulkley has not seen it on the tongue. It formed over 4.3 per cent. of all the cases of skin disease which had come under his observation. According to statistics, it seems possible that changes in temperature with much moisture has something to do with its causation. He has treated 264 cases altogether. His statistics harmonize in most respects with those of general collections. He has found that between ten and fifteen years of age the female patients were double the number of male patients. While between fifteen and twenty-five years of age the males were double the females. Over forty per cent. of all cases appear before the second decade of life. The youngest patient seen by Dr. Bulkley was a little over a year old. Over one-third of all his cases had lasted over ten years, and some as long as forty or fifty years. Many patients ceased their visits long before the eruption disappeared. Over forty per cent. of this cases remained under observation less than six months; quite a proportion of these, however, yielded to treatment, and were apparently cured. As the disease advances in duration, a smaller proportion is benefited. But sometimes careful and continuous treatment will keep the eruption almost entirely in check even a great number of years.

The disease has scarcely any tendency to self-limitation. Although its virulence is largely due to the patient's carelessness, yet there are cases which prove intractable however carefully the treatment may be carried out. It is most curable in children. The cases in patients between the twentieth and twenty-fifth years of age are very rebellious. The treatment should include diet, general hygiene, medicinal measures, the bath, internal and external medication.

Psoriasis is not a local disease, but a constitutional one, more or less akin to rheumatism and gout. Excessive meat-eating increases its severity, and the use of stimulants precipitate an attack. Oils and fatty matter, if properly digested, favor a cure. Pure wool should be worn next the skin, and sudden changes of temperature avoided.

Patients get along better in a warm, equable climate. As regards internal medication, arsenic undoubtedly causes the eruption to disappear in some cases. He had one patient who had taken, it was estimated, a gallon of pure Fowler's solution within fourteen years. Alkalies are also beneficial. Local applications may prevent in a large degree development of the eruption, if they are applied early. He has about abandoned chrysophanic acid in private practice. He has used more of white precipitate ointment in various degrees of strength than of any other local application. Mineral waters seem to have little influence on the disease. Among them sulphur waters hold the best place.

The papers of Drs. Fox and Bulkley were discussed at considerable length by Drs. R. W. Taylor, H. G. Piffard, C. W. Allen, E. B. Bronson, Sherwell, William H. Thompson, Cranmer. In general they agreed with the authors. Drs. Piffard and Allen value sulphide of calcium in acne, and also chrysarobin in psoriasis, and so does Dr. Sherwell. Drs. Bronson, Sherwell, Piffard and Cranmer, laid stress on disturbance of the sexual system as a factor in the production or aggravation of acne, and all considered massage and evacuation of the pustules important. Dr. Taylor and some others referred to the probable influence of a microbe in some cases of acne. Dr. Fox in closing the discussion said that in writing his paper he had sought to present what was true rather than what was new.

<hr>

—The *Quarterly Jour. of Inebriety*, April, 1889, says that the Vienna School Board have for some time past made laudable but ineffectual efforts to prevent the sale of strong drinks to children. They have just passed a resolution to appeal for government intervention, and it is proposed to lay before Parliament during the present session a bill for prohibiting the sale of intoxicating liquors to boys and girls under fifteen years of age. As a matter of fact, inebriety among Austrian school children is not uncommon, and the little boy that appears in the class-room in a state of intoxication has ceased to be a phenomenon. During the winter months the children of the poor are often sent off to school on empty stomachs, and in many cases a glass of the very cheapest spirits is given to them to keep out the cold. Amongst the Slav portion of the population, urchins of five and six often take a liberal dose of alcoholic drink on their way to school, without apparently being the worse for it.

REPORTS OF CLINICS.

UNIVERSITY HOSPITAL.

SURGICAL CLINIC—PROF. AGNEW.

Commencing Arthritis.

Dr. Agnew showed to the class, on March 13, a boy about ten years old who had a commencing arthritis of the right ankle-joint. There was a slight amount of swelling on the internal side of the ankle, indicating the commencement of an arthritis. Dr. Agnew said it would be possible to abort this inflammation, by introducing around it a few turns of a roller bandage of plaster. This must be renewed in a few weeks, when, as the swelling went down, the first bandage would become loose. In the meantime the child should be kept in bed or on crutches, with the limb in an extended position, alterative tonics being administered and the general constitution carefully looked after.

Removal of a Cancerous Breast.

The next patient before the class was a woman, forty-five years old, who had a tumor of the left breast which began about eighteen months ago. It was now very painful and hard. The skin was adherent over the tumor and the nipple was decidedly retracted. Dr. Agnew regarded the growth as cancerous, and removed the breast, taking especial care, at the same time, to take out the neighboring glands, which had also become involved and which, when left after an operation, are either a cause of the return of the tumor or, at least, of its returning more quickly than it would otherwise do from the mere cancerous diathesis alone. Dr. White then closed the wound with an antiseptic iodoform dressing, having introduced a drainage tube. This dressing is allowed to remain on twenty-four hours. The tumor removed weighed two pounds, notwithstanding its small size, thus exhibiting the characteristics of this class of growths in having great weight in proportion to their size. It was already commencing to undergo degenerative change in the centre.

Multiple Exostoses.

The first patient showed to the class on March 20, was a woman twenty-one years old. Some time ago she had had removed an enormous exostosis from the posterior part of the thigh. She recovered satisfactorily from the effects of the operation ;

but the diathesis still continues, she having at present one hundred and twenty-seven bony prominences in different parts of the body. When these exostoses cause pain or spasm by pressing upon a nerve, or when by their mere position or size interfere with the action of muscles or tendons, they have to be removed. The one removed at this time was situated on the right leg, say an inch below the knee, and a little to the left of the median line, so that it slightly interfered with the action of the tendon of the quadriceps extensor. Upon cutting down to the bone the tumor was found to originate from three prominences, each of which had to be removed. The mallet and chisel were first used and then the forceps. The exostosis had also to be taken off where the tendon of the sartorius runs.

On the outside of the leg, but rather higher and farther back, another prominence had to be removed, because it interfered with the action of the insertion of the tendon of the biceps. Here more care had to be taken on account of the presence of the popliteal nerve. When the operations were completed, drainage tubes were introduced and the wounds closed with the usual antiseptic precautions, additional care being taken to have the joint bandaged in an extended position upon a splint covered with raw cotton, to guard against the possibility of healing taking place with the limb in a flexed position.

Removal of the Great Toe and its Metatarsal Bone for Necrosis.

It is always difficult on the foot to determine the extent of necrosis from the external appearances of the soft parts; because an apparently insignificant sinus may open down to many necrosed bones. This arises especially from the fact that the synovial membranes opened are large and open into one another, so that a large surface of synovial membrane may be brought in contact with the air; and, moreover, when the synovitis is once established, an arthritis is especially apt to follow, owing to the bones being so close together.

This man is forty years old, and his present trouble began three years ago without an injury. Let this fact serve to impress upon you the importance of early opening of abscesses on the foot, owing to the tendency of the pus to burrow and establish sinuses, because it is bound down by dense fasciæ. So, too, with an abscess in the ischio-rectal fossa, which, unless opened, will cause an incomplete internal fistula in ano.

After the patient had been etherized and the Esmarch bandage had been applied, the right foot over the internal metatarsal bone and even closer to the ankle was found riddled with sinuses, and upon cutting down along the internal metatarsal bone, it was found necessary to remove not only the latter, but also the cuneiform bone and the great toe. The bottom of the wound was then curetted by Dr. White, any exuberant granulation tissue being thus removed from the neighboring bones. Dr. White then introduced a drainage tube and dressed the wound antiseptically, leaving the foot in a very good condition for future usefulness.

PERISCOPE.

The Hughes Crematory.

The city of Savannah, Georgia, says *Science*, April 12, 1889, is soon to have a crematory for the destruction of garbage by fire. The model selected is that known as the Hughes Crematory, and is thus described by the *Savannah News*:

The crematory will be about 30 feet long, and from 15 to 20 feet wide. The main body of the kiln or furnace is a vertical shaft built of brick. At its base will be two hydrocarbon-burners. Upper and lower triangular flues extend across the middle of the shaft, and also an upper and lower set of baffles or side-wings, which are connected by means of wall passages or flues. Underneath these is a shelf, forming a retort in which air may mix with the flames from the burners. Flues are provided for the return of the gases arising from the incineration to a smoke-stack at the side of the shaft. A hydrocarbon-burner is placed at the bottom of the shaft conveying the gases to the chimney, which deodorizes them before they pass out into the air. Perforated steam-pipes are located over the top drop-shelf of the shaft, connecting the burner with the boiler, so that the fluids may be carried off.

The operation of the crematory is simple. When the furnace is brought to the required degree of heat, a load of the material to be burned is emptied into the top of the shaft. It falls on the first drop-shelf. After a suitable period this shelf is dropped, and the mass of material is allowed to fall on the second shelf, and a second is dumped into the kiln. After another interval the second drop-grate is allowed to fall, and the material is thrown upon the baffles and flues below, whence the residuum finally drops down into the ash-pit at the bottom of the shaft. The capacity of the crematory will be 50 tons of garbage per day, and the cost of the process is from 18 to 20 cents per ton.

In Montreal it costs just $43,000 to destroy by fire a year's miscellaneous refuse, and $8,000 additional for the burning of its night-soil. The destruction of the latter costs 75 cents per ton, and of the former 25 cents per ton. In Minneapolis it is estimated that 15 to 20 cents per ton of refuse pays for the labor employed and the fuel used. Within five days recently the refuse cremated consisted of 33 horses, 59 hogs, 103 barrels of hotel and commission-house refuse, 12 loads of market offal, and 70 loads of manure. The aggregate weight was 200 tons, but the ashes deposited in the course of consumption weighed considerably less than 1,000 pounds. The total cost of labor and fuel for this five days' period was $38.25.

On the Action of Antipyretics.

Aronsohm, Sachs, Richet and, later on, Girard in 1885, experimentally demonstrated the existence of a special thermic centre, situated in the striate body. Soon afterward, Zavadovsky and Vladimïr I. Podanovsky drew attention to the fact that the antipyretic effects of antipyrin and antifebrin are determined solely by their action on the cerebral thermic centre, any direct influence on tissues (their chemistry, blood-supply, etc.) being out of the question. Quite recently, Dr. Podanovsky and Professor Sergëi A. Popoff, of St. Petersburg, have carried out a long series of experiments on lower animals with the view of studying the mode of action of other antipyretics, such as quinine, resorcin, and thallin (*Proceedings of the Third General Meeting of Russian Medical Men at St. Petersburg,* No. 9, 1889, p. 283). In rough outlines, the authors made a division of the brain just behind the striate body, and then introduced into the animal this or that antipyretic drug. The main outcome of their important researches may be given as follows: 1. The division of the brain behind the striate body is immediately followed by a steadily increasing and permanent fall of the central systemic temperature. A subsequent introduction of even most powerful pyrogenic (septic) substances does not produce the slightest impression on the temperature, though it gives rise to other usual symptoms of septicæmia, such as initial fall and subsequent rise of the arterial tension, acceleration of breathing, cardiac action,

diarrhœa, etc. 2. The facts can be explained only by the admission, first, that there exists a special cerebral centre, capable of responding to a septic poisoning by an elevation of the systemic temperature; second, that the operation isolates the centre from the rest of the body; and third, that systemic tissues of themselves are powerless to bring about any rise of the body temperature. 3. In such animals, antipyretics—antipyrin, antifebrin, thallin, etc.—are similarly unable to cause any change in the central temperature. 4. Neither can they alter the peripheral (cutaneous) temperature, notwithstanding the fact that both irritability of the vasomotor centre in the medulla oblongata, and contractility of the cutaneous blood vessels remain quite normal. Meanwhile, in normal—*i. e.,* animals non-operated upon—the introduction of the antipyretics gives rise to a rapid and considerable increase of the peripheral temperature. 5. Generally, there does not exist any strict parallelism between the antipyretic action of the drugs and their property of elevating the cutaneous temperature. 6. All antipyretics act on the central and peripheral temperature in healthy animals by far less markedly than they do on that of febrile ones. 7. The antipyretic effects of the drugs are undoubtedly dependent upon their specific action on the cerebral thermic centre. 8. In the beginning, the action is exciting, but subsequently it is sedative. 9. The facts adduced under "4" point out that, beside a medullary vaso-motor centre, there exists a special higher one, situated in the anterior lobes of the brain. It appears to be designed for increasing the systemic heat-loss in cases in which there arises an excessive heat-formation.

Impotence Consequent on Varicocele.

Segoud reports on a case brought forward by M. Jamain in which the radical cure of a varicocele was followed by return of sexual power in a man 26 years old, in whom it had been in abeyance since puberty. This "frigidity" had resisted all methods of treatment, but ceased when the patient lay on his back. This position, or the use of a suspensory bandage, reducing the varicocele, caused an erection. Potency was readily brought about two months after resection of the spermatic veins. The author quotes various similar cases, especially one by Vidal de Cassis, in which the impotence and puerile voice peculiar to castrated persons disappeared after the operation.—*London Medical Recorder,* April, 1889.

Salicylic Acid in Chronic Tuberculous Joint Disease.

In the *Boston Med. and Surg. Journal*, April 11, 1889, Dr. Robert W. Lovett recommends salicylic acid in the treatment of chronic tuberculous joint disease, and cites cases illustrating its usefulness in subduing the pain, and especially in controlling the spasmodic pains so commonly manifested by "night cries." He states that in the cases coming under his observation no mishaps have occurred in the use of the drug, although in cases in which it was continued for a long time the kidneys were watched to see that no nephritis was set up; in hospital out-patients the drug was not ordered in cases in which the parents were not careful, and able to bring the child each week to the clinic. The salicylic acid was prescribed in the form of the salicylate of soda, made up in five-grain tablets; these were taken readily, without complaint. The experience in the use of the drug in this connection has led of late to its wider and earlier use in the hospital clinic, always, however, he is careful to say, as an adjunct to proper mechanical treatment.

His conclusions are: That salicylic acid in large doses is useful as an aid to the mechanical treatment of chronic tuberculous joint disease, not in routine conditions, but (1) when night cries are present; (2) when the diseased joint is very painful and sensitive to jar; (3) when vomiting and general discomfort are associated with an increase in the local disease.

Relief from pain and the diminished sensitiveness, he says, follow at once, as quickly as in acute articular rheumatism. He recommends that the drug should be given in as large doses as for articular rheumatism, until the pain is relieved or the physiological effect is produced.

Splenic Murmurs.

In a paper read before the Clinical Society of Paris (*La France Médicale*, No. 36) Prof. Bouchard drew attention to the existence of a bruit over the region of the spleen in cases of enlargement of this organ—a bruit not attributable to pressure upon vessels or to conduction from the heart, but apparently generated in the splenic artery or in the spleen itself. During the past three years he has constantly practised auscultation of the spleen, and on five occasions has detected such a bruit. Three times the splenic enlargement was due to cirrhosis of the liver; in one case the spleen was hypertrophied, as in leukæmia, but the blood was not altered; and in the other the swollen spleen was associated with a large liver in an obese subject. In several cases—notably in malarial spleen and in one marked case of leukæmia—no bruit was to be detected. He entered into details of his first case—one of cirrhosis of the liver,—in which the spleen was very large, measuring seventeen by eleven centimeters (about 6.3 by 3.9 inches) and was hard and smooth. Over its whole area there was audible a soft prolonged bruit synchronous with the pulse, but the bruit could not be traced beyond the splenic region. It was still audible when the patient was made to lie on the left side, to prevent the organ exercising any pressure upon the abdominal vessels. The bruit was audible whenever the patient was examined during the three years the patient was under observation. The case was otherwise interesting as an example of "cured cirrhosis," upon which the chief discussion took place. There had been considerable ascites, which required paracentesis on three occasions; but Prof. Bouchard attributed the arrest of the disease to the prolonged administration of calomel in small doses. The patient also had an attack of uræmia, which was successfully treated by naphthol, on the theory of intestinal antisepsis being needed to limit the operation of auto-intoxication in the production of the uræmia.—*Lancet*, April 6, 1889.

Infectiousness of Croupous Pneumonia.

Dr. N. I. Sokoloff lays down (*Transactions of the Third General Meeting of Russian Medical Men at St. Petersburg*, 1889, p. 384) the following propositions, based on researches of his own: 1. Croupous pneumonia is an infectious disease. 2. Typhoid fever patients are especially liable to be infected with the pneumonic virus. 3. The mortality amongst typhoid fever patients contracting pneumonia is truly enormous; in fact, it amounts, on an average, to 66 per cent. 4. In view of this fact, every hospital must be furnished with special wards for cases of pneumonia. 5. When pneumonia makes its appearance amongst hospital typhoid fever patients, the latter must be at once isolated, and the wards concerned must be disinfected most thoroughly. 6. The pneumonia wards must be similarly disinfected before they are used for patients suffering from other affections. 7. In view of a considerable general mortality from croupous pneumonia—which, even with the best possible management, proves to be as high as 12 per cent.—as well as in view of the intense infectiousness of the disease, the strictest sanitary precautions should be adopted as soon as a pneumonia epidemic breaks out at a given locality.

Tapping and Irrigation of the Ventricles.

At the meeting of the Philadelphia County Medical Society, Feb. 13, 1889, Dr. W. W. Keen read a preliminary report on a case of tapping and irrigation of the ventricles of the brain, and said : Last fall I made a proposition for tapping the lateral ventricles. At that time I was not aware that the procedure had ever before been suggested, but I have recently learned that, in 1881, Wernicke suggested it in a general way, and by the lateral route. I, however, first formulated definite rules, which have stood the test of actual trial. The operation, I believe, was never performed until I did it in a case of marked choked disc on both sides, with complete blindness dating from last Christmas, which I had the opportunity of seeing through the politeness of Dr. Strawbridge. I tapped the ventricle five weeks ago last Friday, reaching it by the lateral route, at a depth of one and three-fourths inches from the dura mater. A half-inch trephine opening was made, a crucial incision in the scalp and dura being employed, as I intended to keep up drainage. From two to four ounces of cerebrospinal fluid escape from this opening daily.

The case was examined from day to day to see the effect on the swelling of the optic discs. Before the operation this amounted in one eye to 2.3 mm., and in the other to 1.8 mm. After the operation, it eventually fell to 0.83 mm. on each side. At the end of a week the horse-hair drain, which was introduced at the time of the operation, was substituted by a rubber drainage tube passing into the ventricle. The discharge then became freer, amounting to four to eight ounces per diem.

In addition to this, I explored with a probe the occipital lobe on the left side, twice to a depth of three and a half inches, but found no tumor. I then made a small opening by a gouge under the cerebellum on the left side, and explored the left lobe, and then passed obliquely into the right side, but no tumor was found.

Last Friday I trephined the child on the opposite side, thinking that there might be a tumor in the posterior lobe on that side, but I found none, though I touched the tentorium and the falx. I then tapped the lateral ventricle on that side. Yesterday I washed out the lateral ventricles, passing about eight ounces of a solution of boracic acid (four grains to the ounce) from one side to the other. There was some little irritation resulting from the manipulations, but the moment the warm solution began to pass through the ventricles the child settled itself into a position of complete comfort.

I will pass around a bottle of the cerebrospinal fluid, which has been standing on my desk for a week. There are no signs of decomposition. The fluid contains both sugar and albumin. This with its continuous flow, proves it to be cerebro-spinal fluid.

The child did not suffer any notable rise of temperature after any of the operations, with the exception of the last one. Then there was a temporary sharp rise to 104°.

Acute Localized Œdema.

At the meeting of the Glasgow Pathological and Clinical Society, February 25, Dr. Napier described a case of acute localized œdema. The patient was not presented, as his eruption had in the meantime disappeared ; he was a strong, healthy-looking young man, 24 years old, whose illness had begun a year ago. In his early years he had masturbated frequently, but had suffered nothing apparently from the practice. About a year ago, he fell in with some quack literature of the ordinary kind, the study of which completely upset him mentally; he became "nervous," unable to keep his attention fixed on anything for any length of time, restless, and hypochondriac, and had to give up work for a considerable period. About three months ago, the swellings he complains of were first noticed. They are generally preceded by a sensation of irritation and heat, sometimes by no abnormal sensation at all; in an hour or two the part swells, forming elevations two to four inches long, and about two inches broad, tense, shining, hot, and tingling, and not pitting on pressure. In six or eight hours the swelling disappears, leaving no trace behind it. The affection has appeared in nearly every part of the body, chiefly on the face, limbs, and chest; several times it has occurred on the penis, tongue, and throat. Dr. Napier compared this case with a series of cases in which rapid swelling of face and hands had followed exposure to cold on emerging from a very warm atmosphere, the patients having been moulders and hammermen.—*Glasgow Medical Journal*, April, 1889.

THE
MEDICAL AND SURGICAL
REPORTER.

ISSUED EVERY SATURDAY.

CHARLES W. DULLES, M.D.,
EDITOR AND PUBLISHER.

The Terms of Subscription to the publications of this office are as follows, payable in advance :
Med. and Surg. Reporter (weekly), a year, $5.00
Physician's Daily Pocket Record,   -   -   -   1.00
Reporter and Pocket Record,   -   -   -   -   6.00
All checks and postal orders should be drawn to order of
CHARLES W. DULLES,
N. E. Cor. 13th and Walnut Streets,
P. O. Box 843.   Philadelphia, Pa.

☞SUGGESTIONS TO SUBSCRIBERS:
See that your address-label gives the date to which your subscription is paid.
In requesting a change of address, give the old address as well as the new one.
If your REPORTER does not reach you promptly and regularly, notify the publisher *at once*, so that the cause may be discovered and corrected.
☞SUGGESTIONS TO CONTRIBUTORS AND CORRESPONDENTS:
Write in ink.
Write on one side of paper only.
Write on paper of the size usually used for letters.
Make as few paragraphs as possible. Punctuate carefully. Do not abbreviate, or omit words like "the," and "a," or "an."
Make communications as short as possible.
NEVER ROLL A MANUSCRIPT! Try to get an envelope or wrapper which will fit it.
When it is desired to call our attention to something in a newspaper, mark the passage boldly with a colored pencil, and write on the wrapper "Marked copy." Unless this is done, newspapers are not looked at.
The Editor will be glad to get medical news, but it is important that brevity and actual interest shall characterize communications intended for publication.

THE PHILADELPHIA HOSPITAL AND THE MAYOR.

One of the positions held by the late Dr. Edward T. Bruen was that of Attending Physician to the Philadelphia Hospital. His death created a vacancy in the Medical Staff of that important institution, and this gave rise—as every vacancy there does—to an active canvass for the place. The usual effort was made by a number of worthy candidates to secure the endorsement of the surviving members of the Staff which, under the Civil Service Rules in force in this city, is the prerequisite of election by the Board of Charities and Correction.

While this was going on, another candidate, was put forward by the Mayor of the City, who first endeavored to have him appointed without reference to the wish of the Medical Staff, and, when told that its nomination was indispensable to an election, instructed the President of the Board of Charities and Correction—Dr. James W. White—to order the Staff to nominate him.

After expostulating in vain with the Mayor, Dr. White transmitted this order. The Medical Staff of the Hospital then met and nominated three candidates for the vacancy, but passed the Mayor's candidate by—he receiving only one vote out of seventy-eight cast by twenty-six voters, each voting for three candidates.

Thereupon the Mayor asked Dr. White, who has been a most faithful and efficient public officer, to resign ; and when this request was refused he issued an order that he be dismissed, and appointed a new member of the Board and a new President.

Our readers who have followed the story thus far will not be surprised to hear that this conduct of the Mayor has brought upon him scathing rebukes from almost every newspaper in Philadelphia, and that he stands before the citizens as a man set to enforce the law who has deliberately attempted to break one of its most salutory provisions. This is an aspect of the case which concerns every citizen, and the physicians of Philadelphia need not trouble themselves especially to condemn it, for the whole city has taken the matter up and will probably make its sentiment understood and, in time, respected.

But there is another aspect of the matter which concerns medical men more than others. This aspect relates, not to the Mayor but to the Medical Staff of the Hospital and to the candidate of the Mayor. The Medical Staff deserves the support and praise of all men who admire honor and courage. Its members were threatened with the hostility of the Mayor if they did not name a man to share their duties and responsibilities who was regarded as fit for the position—as the vote indicated—by only one out of twenty-six physicians, surgeons and accoucheurs who voted, and who can be assumed on general principles to know more about his character and ability than the Mayor, who says he has never seen him.

On the other hand the Mayor—censurable as he is—is not the only person to be censured. Those who persuaded him to his false step deserve censure also. The representatives of a medical school which has failed to secure the respect of the most intelligent and conscientious members of the medical profession in Philadelphia, and which has been so conducted that this last step is no surprise to those who have watched it carefully, have attempted, by posing as martyrs and by appealing to the autocratic part of the Mayor's nature, to secure what they could not get in the way open to those who have real merit.

In doing this they have forfeited any claim which they might think they had on the score of equal representation, and have justified the suspicion and disapproval which have heretofore stood between them and positions of honor in the medical profession of Philadelphia. They ought to know— and if they are not lost to reason they will yet learn—that integrity and ability are essential to gaining the approbation of their fellows in the medical profession, and that no success in persuading mere politicians is a desirable substitute for such approbation.

If this lesson is made prominent by the unhappy occurrence described above, it will not be without its uses, and good may yet come of what is in most respects a very shameful piece of business.

THE SACRO-COCCYGEAL ROUTE FOR INTRA-PELVIC OPERATIONS.

In the REPORTER of April 27 attention was called to the method of operation on the rectum which includes a temporary resection of the coccyx and a part of the sacrum, with division of the sacro-sciatic ligaments. It may be interesting, in connection with this, to advert to the fact that more than one surgeon has entertained the idea that the route to the cavity of the pelvis which can be made in this way might be utilized for the removal of various morbid products in the pelvis of women. Hochenegg and Herzfeld, last year, recommended this for total extirpation of the uterus, and tested the operation on the cadaver. The proposition has met, we believe, with approval from Hegar, and more recently— in the *Berliner klinische Wochenschrift*, March 11, 1889—by Dr. W. Wiedow, of Freiburg, who has discussed its value in regard to operating for pelvic abscesses, and diseases of the ovaries and Fallopian tubes, as well as for removal of the uterus.

In his paper Wiedow gives an account of three cases in which he adopted this method: once for a pelvic abscess; once for extirpation of a cancerous uterus; and once for the removal of diseased tubes. As a result of his experience and reflection, he concludes that the method referred to is of value in operations for pelvic abscess, and that it is preferable to vaginal hysterectomy. For operations on the Fallopian tubes he thinks it is not better than laparotomy.

These conclusions seem to be justified by what Wiedow reports of his cases, and they appear to be reasonable on general anatomical and pathological grounds. Certainly no one could ask a better method for operations upon the Fallopian tubes than that of Tait, which is practised so often and so successfully in this country, and especially in this city. We think the same may be said of the usual operation for what is called pelvic abscess; and that it is hardly likely that American surgeons will choose a route which involves a resection of the sacrum and division of the sacro-sciatic ligaments, when the route through the abdominal wall serves so well as it does nowadays.

But the case is different in regard to operations for removal of the uterus. Hysterectomy is, we believe, generally done through the vagina at present. It is often a very difficult and sometimes—as in two cases which the writer of this has witnessed—

a formidable operation. The greatest difficulty it presents depends upon the fact that its most delicate steps are conducted in the dark. The method of Kraske, or that of Levy, permits of bringing the field of operation into view, and eliminating the danger of wounding or ligating portions of the intestine. This is a theoretical advantage which will not be despised by those who have confronted the difficulties of vaginal hysterectomy.

Experience alone can determine whether, or not, the technical details of operation through the sacro-coccygeal region are so great as to outweigh the advantages it offers; but this method is certainly worthy of consideration. It may be that it will fulfil the expectations of those who propose it, and if so the field of its usefulness will doubtless widen in directions which have not yet been suggested. For example, it is among the possibilities that this method may, in some cases, supplant the Cæsarean section, and afford at the same time a means of radically curing defects which prevent normal parturition. This is a matter to which we invite the attention of our readers who practise largely in the field of operative obstetrics, in the hope that their judgment and experience may lead to a determination of the true value of this suggestion.

THE ADVANCE OF MEDICINE IN JAPAN.

History presents no parallel to the advance of the Japanese people during the past fifty years. Scarcely a half century ago anything foreign was looked upon with superstition and dread, and foreigners were distrusted and shunned. The country was in a barbaric state. Today Japan has schools rivalling those of Europe or America; a complete postal and telegraph system; a standing army, thoroughly drilled and armed with the most approved of modern weapons; a navy which ranks with those of European countries; a police force of strength and efficiency in every city and town; railroads traversing the country from end to end and fast increasing; reliable banks, thriving news-papers, a people's government, and lastly a University where the best talent of Europe and America is represented in the corps of instructors, and where degrees in law, science, physics, chemistry, philosophy, philology, civil engineering, medicine and dentistry may be obtained.

In the beginning of the sixteenth century Japan was fast becoming a Christian country. The Dutch traders were greatly liked by the *Shogun*, or ruling power, and foreign introductions were encouraged. More than this, Christianity was looked upon with favor, and the Jesuit missionaries found no opposition. This happy state of affairs continued for nearly a century. The Christians in the southern part of Japan numbered several hundreds of thousands; but at last the powers of the state began to realize that it was not only the doctrines of Christianity that the Jesuit fathers were teaching but also obedience to another earthly power, the Pope. An imperial edict was therefore issued, forbidding the continuance of the preaching of this faith. At this the priests only doubled their zeal and preached publicly in bold defiance to the Emperor's commands. They were then ordered to leave the country, but the order was taken no notice of. Then began their systematic persecution. All foreigners were forcibly driven out of the country, and those who insisted upon staying were put to death. The priests and hundreds of Japanese proselytes were crucified for their faith. An edict was issued condemning all those who professed Christianity to be crucified, and a fearful slaughter took place. This persecution lasted for nearly a century and ended in the complete expulsion of all foreigners. Medicine had been introduced by the Dutch physicians, and they had had many eager students, but now its practice, as taught by the Dutch, was a crime punishable by death.

From then, until the country was opened

again by our Admiral Perry, Japan remained free from foreign invasion.

After Perry's conquest the foreigners gradually returned and were left unmolested, excepting when they violated all laws of propriety. Medicine was again introduced, but its study strictly forbidden by the authorities. Nevertheless the foreign physicians found themselves overwhelmed by crowds of eager students, many of whom bought their knowledge with the penalty of death. Some were decapitated, others were allowed to commit suicide by disemboweling. Soon however the spirit of progress took hold of the government also, and with the beginning of the present reign, some twenty-three years ago, foreign arts and studies were not only allowed but earnestly encouraged. Schools and colleges sprang up all over the country and the University was founded. Education is now opened to every Japanese and there is a complete public school system.

The main feature of the Imperial University, which is now recognized by nearly all foreign colleges, is its magnificent Medical Department, which, as far as completeness and thoroughness of teaching go, ranks with any school in the world. The course extends over a period of five years; and a sixth, or post-graduate, year is strongly recommended. The first year is devoted exclusively to theory; the studies taken up are anatomy, inorganic chemistry, physics, medical botany, and histology. During the second and third years the student dissects, uses his microscope, does a good deal of work in practical physics, and has his place in the laboratories. Physiology and organic chemistry and a very complete course in embryology are also gone through with during these years. It is not until his third year that the student sees the inside of a Hospital and then he begins the didactic study of medicine and surgery and its branches. The most of the third-year student's time is however devoted to materia medica, therapeutics and pharmacy.

Practice is only taught during the fourth and fifth years, and during this time every student has his share of active work in the Hospital. The sixth year is more properly a "specialty year," during which the student is supposed to devote his time to some specialty. Strange to say a large proportion of the present students are taking up such specialties as medical jurisprudence, therapeutics, anatomy, etc., preferring to become teachers rather than practitioners. An able student in Japan will find no difficulty in the pursuance of his studies; for, if he has a certain average, the government will take charge of his education, remit his school fees and if necessary give him money for his board and finally send him to Germany or America to complete his studies under eminent specialists. Hospital positions are only obtainable by competitive examination. Wire-pulling is of little value.

The life of the medical student in Japan is of course totally different from what it is in America. A very military looking uniform is worn. Fencing and archery matches take the place of base ball and foot ball. Athletics are largely indulged in. The school fees amount to about $2.50 a month, and when four or five students club together they can live for less than three dollars a month. As a class they are usually refined and gentlemanly. At noon the student rests on soft white matting, in a picturesque teahouse, with a vista of minature waterfalls and bridges and fragrant plum and cherry-blossom trees in the distance, whilst a dainty little Japanese maiden in a gay gown serves him his lunch of beefsteak, rice, eggs and tea all for *six cents.*

There are Medical Societies in every large city of Japan, and Tokyo has about six or seven. The largest are the Tokyo Medical Society and the Sei-I-Kwai (Foreign Medicine Association). The latter holds an English meeting once a month, besides its regular meetings, and publishes transactions part of which are printed in English. These

Societies are very active, have large memberships and fine libraries.

Every city in Japan has its government hospital besides private institutions. Tokyo has about ten principal hospitals and a number of small ones. They include the City Hospital, the Naval Hospital, the University Hospital, the Children's Hospital, the Hospital for Diseases of the Lungs and Throat, the Maternity Hospital, the Eye and Ear Hospital, the Army Hospital, and the Insane Asylum. The Sanitary Bureau is most efficient and equipped with able officers. Quarantine Stations are located at every port and their regulations rigidly enforced.

Already Japanese physicians are being recognized abroad for their original investigations and untiring zeal. Dr. K. Miura, of Tokyo, has contributed valuably to therapeutics by his discovery of the new alkaloid, ephidrine, an extract from the *Ephedra vulgaris.* Professor Nagai of the Imperial University now ranks among the leading chemists of the day. Dr. Takaki, Surgeon General to the Navy, had two years ago performed thirty ovariotomies without losing a case—a record that no one need be ashamed of.

The latest experiments of European specialists are always carefully investigated in the laboratories of the University. Koch's and Pasteur's experiments were carried out in every detail. The latest medical and surgical works are translated into Japanese as fast as they are brought out; although every medical student is perfectly conversant with the German language, and very many with English besides.

In connection with these facts, it is interesting to learn, from the latest advices from Japan, that our country has agreed to revise the treaty with Japan on lines desired by the latter power. The *Mainichi Shimbun,* a leading newspaper in Tokyo, in speaking of the coming treaty revision says: "America is the first of all foreign powers to respond to our appeals, and with America rests the palm of giving effect to their liberality. America has helped Corea to achieve her independence, and America has interfered between powerful Germany and helpless Samoa, and it was America alone among all treaty powers, who returned her share of the Shimonoseki indemnity to Japan, and this last act is a worthy and fitting sequel to her consistently friendly proceedings in our country."

THE TIMES AND REGISTER.

There have come to this office the generous number of three copies of the first issue of a medical journal called the *Times and Register,* which is the successor of the *Philadelphia Medical Times,* the *Medical Register,* and the *Dietetic Gazette.* It has the general appearance of the *Register,* and the general character of the *Times.*

Those who admired the latter journals will probably regard this as praise; those who did not, will perhaps be disappointed that we cannot say more.

The number before us contains nothing above the standard of the latest issues of the *Philadelphia Medical Times,* which was once an admirable journal, but which fell into sad decrepitude before it entered upon the process of metempsychosis. If its editor improves his new opportunity, to show that he can produce a journal which will tend to elevate the standard of medical journalism, and not to debase it, his venture will have our best wishes, and, we have no doubt, will meet with success.

Ohio State Medical Society.—The forty-fourth annual meeting of the Ohio State Medical Society will be held at Youngstown, Ohio, May 22, 23 and 24, 1889. The President is Dr. P. S. Conner, of Cincinnati. The sessions of the Society will be held in Wick Hall, No. 134 West Federal Street, and the first session will begin at 2.00 P. M., Wednesday, May 22.

Reduced rates may be obtained on all railroads running to Youngstown, on certain conditions. Further information may be obtained from the Secretary, G. A. Collamore, M.D., of Toledo.

BOOK REVIEWS.

[Any book reviewed in these columns may be obtained upon receipt of price, from the office of the REPORTER.]

LECTURES ON THE ERRORS OF REFRAC-
TION AND THEIR CORRECTION WITH
GLASSES. By FRANCIS VALK, M.D., Lecturer
on disease of the eye, New York Post-graduate
Medical School, etc. Large 8vo, pp. 241. New
York and London: G. P. Putnam's Sons, 1889.
Price, $3.00.

The preface of this book asserts that it is offered
to the general profession "as a simple and at the
same time complete method for the diagnosis and
correction of all the errors of refraction." As such,
it seems to us a complete failure. Error begins in the
first lecture upon Anatomy, to end only with the
termination of the volume. Faulty construction, bad
grammar, and incorrect spelling of proper names,
meet us upon every page; whilst the sketches—with
the exception of the cuts borrowed from the instrument makers—prominent amongst which is the
author's self-styled "Valk's Improvement on Loring's Ophthalmoscope"—are frightfully and wonderfully made.

A book so full of faults as this one requires treatment at the hands of the reviewer which is far from
pleasant to him; but the consideration which would
spare the feelings of an author and thereby mislead
the readers of a review would be an injustice to the
latter. To tell the truth is the critic's duty, and the
truth about Dr. Valk's book is that it is unworthy to be
as a scientific or practical guide, and likely to lead
astray those who may put their trust in it.

MATERIA MEDICA AND THERAPEUTICS,
FOR PHYSICIANS AND STUDENTS. By
JOHN B. BIDDLE, M.D., late Professor of Materia
Medica and Therapeutics in the Jefferson Medical
College, etc. Eleventh edition, revised and
enlarged, by Clement Biddle, M.D., U. S. Navy,
and Henry Morris, M.D., Fellow of the College of
Physicians, Phila., etc., with numerous illustrations.
Large 8vo, pp. 607. Philadelphia: P. Blakiston,
Son & Co., 1889. Price, $4.25.

Biddle's Materia Medica is about as familiar to
students of medicine in this country as is Gray's
Anatomy, and it has always been popular because it
combined sufficient scientific detail with an easy and
pleasant style. These two characteristics marked the
earlier editions of this text book, and they mark the
latest, which appears long after the death of the
original author. His successors have kept his book
in step with the progress of the age without changing
the features which made it so popular at first. The
book has grown much beyond its first proportions:
but symmetrically and harmoniously. It is still one
of the best works on materia medica and therapeutics
with which we are familiar, and may safely be commended as a text book to both students and physicians.

PHOTOGRAPHIC ILLUSTRATIONS OF SKIN
DISEASES. AN ATLAS AND TEXT-BOOK
COMBINED. By GEORGE HENRY FOX, A.M.,
M.D., Clinical Professor of Diseases of the Skin,
College of Physicians and Surgeons, New York,
etc. Parts 1–6. New York: E. B. Treat.

This is the second series of a well known work by
one of the best dermatologists in this country. The
six parts before us contain over one hundred pages of
text, and twenty-four photographs, colored by hand.
The plates are exceedingly graphic, and life-like, and
are especially interesting as being exact reproductions
of the conditions represented. They have not the
brilliancy of lithographs, but they are more true to
nature.

The whole work is sold, by subscription only, at
two dollars for each part, and it is to be completed
in twelve parts.

PAMPHLET NOTICES.

[Any reader of the REPORTER who desires a copy of a
pamphlet noticed in these columns will doubtless secure
it by addressing the author with a request stating where
the notice was seen and *enclosing a postage-stamp*.]

257. THE BRAIN AND NERVOUS SYSTEM. By E.
W. RUSH, M.D., Paris, Texas. 18 pages.

258. SCIENCE IN MEDICINE. By HORACE N.
MATEER, M.D., Ph.D., Wooster, Ohio. From the
Post-Graduate and Wooster Quarterly, April, 1888.
15 pages.

259. THE CORTICAL LOCATION OF THE CUTANEOUS
SENSATIONS. By CHARLES L. DANA, M.D., New
York. From the *Journal of Nervous and Mental
Diseases*, October, 1888. 31 pages.

257. This pamphlet contains a lecture delivered by
Dr. Rush before the Teacher's State Normal School,
at Aikin Institute, last July. It is stated to be a
lecture on "Temperaments, or Temperamental Physiology, which embraces the Brain and Nervous System." In concluding it the author says he "has
had to deal with truths and facts, elicited from subjective and objective clinical history of diseases, and
he has long since learned to make the greatest allowance in human testimony, both in clientele, as well as
in social statements."

258. Dr. Mateer's pamphlet contains his thesis
for the degree of Doctor of Philosophy in the Post-
graduate course of the University of Wooster. It is
an interesting essay upon the claim of Medicine to
be called a Science. It touches on the history of
medicine, and the theories which have ruled in its
development, and discusses the proper method for
studying disease and the principles which should
govern its treatment.

259. Dr. Dana's paper, which was read before the
American Neurological Association, at Washington,
last September, contains a learned and thorough discussion of the question whether, or not, the cortical
areas in the brain for touch, pain and heat-sensation
are identical with the motor areas for similar parts of
the body. This question the author answers in the
affirmative. The reasons for his opinion are founded
chiefly upon a careful and exhaustive analysis of the
histories of 142 cases, in which the symptoms were
noted during life, and an autopsy was made after
death. Four of the cases were under Dr. Dana's
personal observation. The symptoms and the location of the brain lesion are noted upon charts of the
brain published in his pamphlet, and the correspondence of the latter to the motor areas is very conclusively shown.

As a whole, this study is one not only of great
interest, but also of great value to students of cerebral pathology and physiology, and is an admirable
example of thorough and painstaking investigation
in a very important and difficult field.

NOTES AND COMMENTS.

Criminal Abortionists Punished.

The Paris correspondent of the *Lancet*, March 2, 1889, says that a rather curious case of a series of criminal abortions was recently tried at the Court of Assizes of the Eure, and caused a great sensation. This trial has brought to light one of the probable causes of the increasing depopulation of France in general, and of Normandy · in particular. The accused, a man named Martin, was denounced by some of his own accomplices. He was a clockmaker by trade, and fifty-one years old. Seeing that it was impossible to deny the charge against him, he decided upon making a confession, and at the same time denounced his accomplices, as well as those who had submitted to the operation, which he performed with a reed. The list was a long one, but there were nineteen persons directly implicated. Martin, the principal, showed during the trial an imperturbable assurance, as if he failed to realize the gravity of the charges against him. "I wished simply," he said, "to render service to those who addressed themselves to me. As to the fees which I received, they were the just remuneration for my trouble." He added, with incredible cynicism: "Moreover, medical men, pharmacists, and herbalists have rendered justice to my ability in sending me patients." Martin was condemned to eight years and his accomplices to shorter periods of imprisonment.

Creasote in the Lung Affections of Children.

Soltmann says in the *Wiener med. Blätter* that with a few exceptions almost all observers speak well of the value of creasote in tuberculosis, and agree in saying that, even if recovery is not to be hoped for, marked improvement of the chief symptoms follows its employment. All the communications hitherto published relate to adults, and Professor Soltmann, of Breslau, is the first to record his experience of the remedy in children. He has, he says, given creasote in chronic lung diseases with little or advanced destruction, without considering the presence or absence of bacilli. After all due allowance is made for care in hospital, suitable nourishment, baths, good air, etc., considerable advantage is evidently derived from the administration of creasote, since cases which were not doing well began to improve unmistakably under increasing doses of creasote. He gives from two to seven drops of creasote a day. Soltmann's prescription is this:

R Creasoti . . . . gtt. iv–xiv
  Spir. æther. . . . . . . gtt. vj–xij
  Aq. destil. . . . . . . f ℥ iss
  Sacch. albi . . . . . ℥ iiss

A teaspoonful every two hours.

It merits especial mention that the creasote was well borne by all the children. Stomachache, nausea, vomiting, diarrhœa—inconveniences which often render treatment by creasote impossible in adults—never occurred. Even in high fever, which by all authors is spoken of as a contraindication, the creasote was taken without disadvantage. That the large doses helped to give the good results is probable from Guttmann's experiments on the antiseptic power of creasote over many microörganisms. Very remarkable in many cases was the increase of appetite and gain in body-weight, the diminution of cough and expectoration, and the gradual disappearance of pathological lung-symptoms. Soltmann concludes that creasote exerts in chronic lung-disease in which there is a suspicion of tuberculosis a markedly favorable influence, especially where there is not much destruction .of lung or other severe complication, and where there is not too high fever, the general strength being relatively good.—*London Medical Recorder*, March, 1889.

Damages for Death from Inebriety.

A man in New York drank to intoxication in a saloon and was drowned on his way home in a small stream. His widow sued the saloon-keeper for damages. The jury brought in a verdict for the widow and the case was appealed. In the Supreme Court the judgment was confirmed. The judge said the evidence was clear that the death of the plaintiff's husband was caused by his intoxication, arising in whole or in part by the liquor furnished by the defendant. The law in this case was the Civil Damage Act of 1873, of New York State, which provides as follows: "Every husband, wife, child, parent, guardian, employer, or other person who shall be injured in person, property, or means of support by an intoxicated person, or in consequence of the intoxication, habitual or otherwise, of any person, shall have a right of action against any person or persons who shall by selling or giving away intoxicating liquor have caused the intoxication in whole or in part." —*Quarterly Jour. of Inebriety*, April, 1889.

For Chronic Chills.

Daniel's Texas Medical Journal, April, 1889, says that for chronic chills, and that peculiar but very common condition of chronic malarial blood poisoning seen in swampy and other malarial sections, in which there is a "fever cake" or enlarged spleen, and a general dropsical tendency, there is no remedy, or combination of remedies, which has a better effect than that known throughout the South as Gadberry's Spleen Mixture. It is a solution of the oxy-sulphate of iron and potassa, and is made as follows:

   R Pulv. ferri sulph. . . . . ℥ i
      Acidi nitrici . . . . f ℥ i

Mix, and when reaction has ceased, add one ounce of some aromatic water, mint or cinnamon; to this add quinine ℥ i, little by little, stirring constantly.

   R Potas. citratis *vel* nitratis . . . ℥ i.
      Aquæ menth. pip. *vel* cinnam. . f ℥ vii

Mix and dissolve and add slowly to the above, stirring constantly. Filter and wrap in blue or other dark paper, to exclude the light.

When properly made the mixture should be a perfectly clear, green fluid. The dose for an adult is a tablespoonful, three times a day, and in cases of long standing, it should be given every day for a month. On the days on which the chill is expected, the mixture should be given in anticipation, the same as quinine is given, and for children the dose should be proportioned to the age.

If old, dried sulphate of iron is used, the mixture is apt to be brown, and to deposit a sediment. If the sulphate is used in the natural state as found in the shops, and it is preferable, the mixture will be a bright green, and clear.

Care is necessary in adding the quinine to the acid solution of iron, to prevent its lumping; if added gradually and stirred with a grass rod it will dissolve like snow.

Pilocarpine in the Itching of Jaundice.

Dr. Goodhart states in the *British Med. Journal*, January 19, 1889, that he has found pilocarpine very effective in controlling the itching which is such an annoying symptom in many cases of jaundice. One patient had one-third of a grain injected subcutaneously many times, and always with the result that for the first twenty-four hours he was quite free, the second he was fairly free, and the third day he was getting bad again, and the dose had to be repeated. He has had six cases in all, and in none has it failed.

The Immisch Patent Metal Thermometer.

One of the most important aids to a correct diagnosis is a knowledge of the temperature of the patient. With our present means it takes fully ten minutes to ascertain this with our clinical thermometers. Further than this, the instrument is extremely delicate, easily broken, and often inaccurate. Immisch claims to have invented an instrument that does away with all these difficulties. His metal thermometer is supposed to register correct temperatures inside of five minutes or less, and it is claimed that it never varies. The instrument, however, has failed to stand practical tests. According to a report in the *Berliner klin. Wochenschrift*, March 25, 1889, Dr. F. Huebner has carefully compared it with other thermometers and has found that it is very inaccurate and not to be depended upon, and also that it takes fully ten minutes to reach the correct temperature. The instrument is very compact and well made, but in Dr. Huebner's opinion its good points are entirely overbalanced by its inaccuracy.

Febriline, a so-called "Tasteless Quinine."

Dr. R. G. Eccles declares in the *Druggists Circular*, May, 1889, that he has investigated a preparation sold under the name "Febriline or Tasteless Syrup of Amorphous Quinine (Lyons)," by the Paris Medicine Company, of Paris, Tenn., and finds that it contains no quinine at all. Instead of quinine quinidine is used, another alkaloid of cinchona bark, which is described as follows in the National Dispensatory, edition of 1879, page 1181: "Quinidia is not officinal. Being very slightly soluble, it should be administered in mucilage or syrup. Its lack of bitterness renders it convenient for administration to children, and its imperfect solubility is not disadvantageous when a slow or tonic action is alone required."

Chair of Surgery at Burlington, Vermont.

The Chair of Surgery at the University of Vermont has been filled by the election of Dr. A. M. Phelps, of New York City, who will begin his instructions on May 15. Dr. Phelps has already done service in the Medical Department of the University as Lecturer upon Orthopædic Surgery.

Treatment of Buboes.

In the Polish weekly *Gazeta Lekarska,* Nos. 15, 16, 17 and 18, 1888, Dr. Karol Szadek (pron. "Shadek"), house surgeon to the Kïëv Military Hospital, communicates an account of 274 cases of chancroidal buboes treated by him during 1881–86, the whole number of chancroid patients during the same period being 1084. The buboes, therefore, occurred in 25 per cent. of patients with soft chancres. The treatment consisted in absolute rest and the application of warming carbolic compresses on the appearance of cutaneous redness. As soon as fluctuation became distinct, he made a free incision, extirpated the affected lymphatic glands, scraped out carefully the whole abscess cavity with a sharp spoon, washed it out with a corrosive sublimate lotion, dusted on iodoform, and finally applied a tight bandage. The dressing was changed every four or five days. The wound healed in from ten to forty-five days, the average duration being about thirty days. In 5 cases, erysipelas, and in 12 eczema, occurred about the wound. Dr. Szadek never saw any toxic symptoms following the use of iodoform. He also treated, after the same method, 26 cases of buboes in syphilitic patients, and 12 of tuberculosis of the inguinal glands. The results were similarly very satisfactory, though here sometimes, especially in very exhausted tuberculous patients, recovery was rather slow.

A Disagreeable Summons.

A lawsuit interesting to medical men in obstetric practice has recently been tried in London. Dr. A. was engaged to attend Mrs. B. in her approaching confinement. In the dead of night Mr. B. summoned the doctor through the speaking tube at the side of the hall door. There was no undue delay, but still the anxious husband kept up such a din that the accoucheur declined to answer the summons, and refused to have anything to do with such an unpleasant patient. Another medical man attended the patient, who appears to have been delivered most satisfactorily; but not satisfied with the course of events, the discontented husband sought Dr. A. in his consulting-room, and attacked him both with tongue and fist. The magistrate, who presided at the subsequent action for assault held that a medical man was quite justified in declining an obstetric engagement under such circumstances, and fined the defendant accordingly.

NEWS.

—Southern California is to have a hospital for the insane.

—Dr. Craik succeeds the late Dr. Howard as Dean of the McGill Medical College, Montreal.

—The American Surgical Association will be held in Washington, D. C., May 14, 15 and 16, 1889.

—The American Climatological Association will hold its next annual meeting in Boston, June 24 and 25, 1889.

—Dr. F. E. Stewart has been appointed Demonstrator of Therapeutics in the Jefferson Medical College of Philadelphia.

—The next meeting of the American Association of Genito-Urinary Surgeons will be held in Newport, May 21 to 23, 1889.

—It is stated that Duke Karl Theodor, of Bavaria, who is an ophthalmologist, is about to establish an eye hospital at Meran, in the Tyrol.

—Dr. H. J. Harriman, of Revere, died at East Peacham, Vt., April 14, after a long illness. He was graduated from Dartmouth Medical College.

—The commencement of the Southern Medical College was held at Atlanta March 2, and degrees conferred 34 graduates in medicine and 17 graduates in dentistry.

—The municipal authorities of St. Louis have passed an ordinance to pay $500 to Dr. A. C. Bernays, to reward him for performing a successful laparotomy upon a policeman who was shot.

—Mr. Thomas Downs died in Philadelphia April 23, 1889, at the great age of ninety-four years. He was the father of Dr. R. N. Downs, of Germantown, and of Dr. Thomas A. Downs, of West Philadelphia. Mr. Downs was also the father-in-law of Dr. R. A. Martin, of Albion, Mich., the grandfather of Dr. Norton Downs and Dr. J. W. Mecaskey of Philadelphia, and the uncle of Dr. M. J. Grier, also of Philadelphia.

—The fourth session of the French Congress of Surgery will be held at Paris from October 7 to 13, 1889, under the presidency of Baron Larrey. The following questions have been set for discussion: 1. Immediate and remote results of operations done for local tuberculosis. 2. Surgical treatment of peritonitis. 3. Treatment of aneurisms in the limbs. All communications should be addressed to Dr. S. Pozzi, General Secretary, 10 Place Vendôme, Paris.

HUMOR.

To Young Physicians.—There is said to be a barber's sign near the Palais Royal, Paris, bearing the following legend in the vernacular: "Callileucocapillaire water which colors the hair white. For the use of young physicians and magistrates.—*Sanitarian.*

Mr. Rambo (at dime museum), in great alarm—"Nancy, do you see anything in that cage next to the monkeys?" Mrs. Rambo—"Yes, there's a lot of snakes." Mr. Rambo—(with recovered self-possession)—"So they are. Fine specimens too, aren't they?"

Pleasant for Uncle Jack.—(Uncle Jack returns from a long walk, and, being somewhat thirsty, drinks from a tumbler he finds on the table. Enter his little niece Allie, who instantly sets up a yell of despair.) Uncle Jack: "What's the matter, Allie?" Allie (weeping): "You've drinked up my aquarium and swallowed my free 'ittle polly-wogs."—*Daniel's Texas Medical Journal.*

OBITUARY.

RESOLUTIONS ON THE DEATH OF DR. GROSS.

At a meeting of the Philadelphia County Medical Society, April 24, 1889, the following minute was unanimously adopted:

By the death of Dr. Samuel W. Gross this Society has lost an industrious co-laborer, a wise counsellor, and the profession one of its most brilliant ornaments. As a student, practitioner and teacher he possessed, with remarkable surgical acumen, unusual power of analysis and deduction, and his lectures, like his mental workings, were conspicuously clear, concise, logical and vigorous. He was an earnest student of the progress of surgery in all countries, with more respect for the experience of the present than the traditions of the past; never satisfied to stand still, and ever advancing with the progress of science, he kept his teaching always apace with the rapid strides of surgical knowledge. As an operator he was bold, conscientious and successful. Possessed of broad views, he was quick to recognize merit and to welcome truth by whomsoever presented. He took an active interest in all that pertained to the welfare of the profession and was ever ready to work for its promotion. He possessed positive convictions and was frank in their expression. As a companion he was genial and entertaining; as a friend generous and true.

HARVEY LINDSLY, M.D.

Dr. Harvey Lindsly, the oldest physician in Washington, D. C., died there April 28. Dr. Lindsly was born in Morris County, N. J., January 11, 1804. He was descended through both parents from English ancestry, the representatives of which came to this country two hundred years ago, and settled in New Jersey. He was prepared for college at the classical academy in Somerset County, N. J., and was subsequently graduated from Princeton College, which later conferred upon him the honorary degree of LL.D. At the time of his death he was one of the oldest living graduates of the college. He studied medicine in New York, and before completing his studies there he came to Washington, D. C., in 1827. He entered the National Medical College and took his degree in the year 1828. He became associated with Dr. Sewall, then the leading physician of the city, first as a medical student and then as a partner. Upon the death of Dr. Sewall, Dr. Lindsly succeeded to his practice. Sixty-one years ago he married Emeline C. Webster, a niece of Dr. Sewall, who survives him. Last year this aged couple celebrated the sixtieth anniversary of their marriage. He continued in active practice from the year 1828 until the year 1872, when he retired. Dr. Lindsly had a large practice, and in his day was associated with Drs. J. C. Hall, Thomas Miller, W. P. Johnson, Noble Young, J. F. May, Joseph Burrows, and other leading members of the profession. The two latter are still alive.

Dr. Lindsly was a member of the Medical society of Washington and of the American Medical Association. In 1858 he had the honor of being made President of the latter body. He was an honorary member of the Rhode Island Medical Society, of the Historical Society of New Jersey, and a number of other organizations. He was a contributor to a number of medical periodicals. For several years he was Professor of Obstetrics, and subsequently of the Principles and Practice of Medicine in the National Medical College of Washington. He was President of the Washington Board of Health for many years, beginning in 1833. For over thirty years he was a member of the American Colonization Society, and for a number of years he was President of the Princeton Alumni Association of the District of Columbia, holding that office at the time of his death.

Dr. Lindsly leaves a wife and four daughters.

MEDICAL AND SURGICAL
REPORTER

No. 1681.   PHILADELPHIA, MAY 18, 1889.   Vol. LX.—No. 20.

CONTENTS:

COMMUNICATIONS.

OBSTRUCTION OF THE NASAL PASSAGES: ITS EFFECTS AND ITS TREATMENT.

BY C. A. BUCKLIN, M.D.,

NEW YORK.

Extensive obstruction to nasal respiration causes an individual to become an habitual mouth breather. When the obstruction is less complete, it causes a partial vacuum to be formed beyond the point of obstruction with each respiratory act through the nose. Mucous membranes become chronically congested when subjected to constantly varying atmospheric pressures which fall below the normal atmospheric pressure with each inspiration. It is self evident that mouth breathing or constant changes in the atmospheric pressure gives a rational cause for the production of catarrhal diseases.

During the stage of congestion we have acute catarrh. The stage of hypertrophy which follows chronic congestion is called hypertrophic catarrh. The atrophy which finally results from the increase of connective tissue in the mucous membrane occasions dry or atrophic catarrh.

Structural changes in the mucous membrane produce a change in the character of the mucus secreted. It is much thicker and produces the sensation of a foreign body on the mucous membrane. The constant attempt to dislodge this thick mucus, causes one to believe that there is a great increase in the amount of mucus secreted, when the quantity is in reality diminished. In health there is more mucus secreted, but its quality being normal, its presence is not appreciated and there is no desire to expectorate.

I am convinced as a result of clinical observation, that with the exception of persons one or two generations removed from tubercular ancestors and those affected with some infectious disease, nasal catarrh is developed as a result of obstruction in the nose and usually of obstruction due to some mechanical deformity in the bony walls of the nostrils.

589

Nasal obstruction also causes, indirectly, most of the incurable ear and annoying throat diseases of this latitude. It is also a cause of chronic bronchitis and catarrhal diseases of the eyelids.

Further, chronic congestion of the mucous membrane of the entire nasal cavities and of the connecting sinuses has a most decided influence in producing functional disturbances of the brain. Individuals so affected appear drowsy and stupid and complain of feeling so.

It may be said that these ideas are illogical, unfounded, and they may be received with incredulity by the profession.

For this reason all reference to obscure reflex nervous symptoms said to occur with nasal obstructions, will be avoided in this paper and only those easily demonstrated consequences, which arise from imperfect nasal respiration, will be considered. These my readers may be induced to accept, because frequent opportunity will offer in practice to verify the conclusions advanced. These conclusions have been forced upon me as a result of twelve years of careful thought and experimental investigation, combined with an extensive experience and extended observation of the methods employed and results obtained by Austrian, German, American and English specialists, in their daily hospital work.

I do not take the liberty of advancing a single idea which has not—as I believe—been fully confirmed by clinical observation, and which will not stand thorough investigation by others. The most convincing testimony in favor of the conclusions which the profession are asked to accept, is the history of intelligent persons, who have been operated upon. When the nasal obstruction has been properly relieved, these patients state, unsolicited, that they have been greatly relieved of annoying symptoms.

Nature of Nasal Obstructions.—These differ widely in their nature, their extent, and the amount of trouble they produce. The same amount of nasal obstruction does not produce anything like the same degree of annoyance with one individual, that it produces in another; while in a third person, possibly no annoyance would be experienced from a like defect.

Three per cent. of the children in the schools of New York have adenoid growths from the vault of the pharynx. These are a common cause of nasal obstruction, when they attain sufficient size. The other form of nasal obstruction most commonly found in children is hypertrophy of the mucous membrane covering the turbinated bones. Occasionally, a congenital mal-position of a turbinated bone is the underlying cause of the trouble. Deviations of the septum are very rarely seen until after the tenth year of age.

Children having the adenoid form of obstruction are invariably strumous. When the examination is made among half orphans, the percentage will run higher, than it will among public school children. If made among full orphans, the percentage will be found higher than in either of the other cases; which simply points more strongly to the strumous origin of the adenoid growth. This form of trouble is also very frequently complicated with enlarged tonsils.

Excessive hypertrophy very frequently develops in strumous children on the turbinated bones, as a result of frequent colds, nasal diphtheria, scarlatina, measles and other acute infectious diseases. This hypertrophy frequently produces a permanent nasal obstruction.

In adult life, in addition to the diseased condition of childhood, we have all possible deformities of the nasal septum, and polypoid degeneration of the mucous membrane of the nose, as causes of obstruction.

We have various neurotic conditions of the nose, which cause the mucous membrane to react so violently under the slightest irritation, such as a change of temperature, that its almost constant swollen condition produces a hypertrophy as a further cause of nasal obstruction.

We also have that strikingly peculiar so-called neurotic condition known as "hayfever," which produces complete closure of the nose during the attack. In these patients, there is a peculiar susceptibility to poisoning by "rag weed," which blooms all along the Atlantic coast from Florida to the St. Lawrence River between the 1st and 14th days of August. I am told by my most intelligent patients, that this weed produces their attack of hay fever during its blooming period; that they can decide by examining the vegetation of a vicinity whether they will be able to avoid an attack of hay fever in that locality or not. They also tell me that at certain altitudes they are entirely free from hay fever. I think that most hay fever patients have the attack between the 1st and 14th of August. These troubles at this time, are certainly due to rag weed. Those patients who have hay fever severely commencing during June or July, are evidently poisoned by other forms of vegetation. I have not observed such cases in my own practice.

In adult life there are three prominent factors which enter into the etiology of nasal obstruction. The first and most common factor is an abnormal relation between the bony walls of the nostrils, which so encroach on their caliber that there is not room for the normal swelling of the mucous membrane incidental to sudden changes of temperature.

All individuals in the same latitude are exposed to about the same changes in temperature. In some persons these changes always produce most annoying symptoms, which with each successive cold in the head are of longer duration, until at last the trouble becomes chronic. In other individuals, there is plenty of room for the normal swelling of the mucous membrane incidental to sudden changes in the temperature, without its producing decided nasal obstruction or more than temporary annoyances.

Individuals of the first class are constantly catching cold in their heads, while individuals of the second class are rarely troubled in this way.

The normal relations between the bony walls of the nostrils are disturbed by all deformities in the nasal septum, either bony or cartilaginous. The abnormal development of position of the turbinated bone, occasionally produces the trouble where there is not any deformity of the septum.

These bony deformities are the most common cause of nasal obstruction in adult life. They are frequently of sufficient magnitude to produce direct obstruction in the nose, but they most frequently produce obstruction indirectly by the unequal atmospheric pressures they cause the mucous membrane to be subjected to, during respiration. It is exactly in this special field, where the greatest success should be obtained, that the greatest failures have been made in treating nasal catarrh resulting from nasal obstructions.

These difficulties being mainly mechanical promise much better results from treatment, than difficulties which are largely due to constitutional diseases.

The second factor in producing nasal obstruction in adult life, is the nature of the mucous membrane which covers a bony or cartilaginous deformity in the nostrils. Cachexy and neurotic disturbances, produce conditions in the mucous membrane which cause it to swell excessively as the result of the slightest irritation. This explains why two individuals with the same bony deformity, suffer, under like circumstances, in such widely differing degrees.

The third factor in producing nasal obstruction is the climate in which the individual resides. In the tropics, but little room is necessary to accommodate the swelling of the mucous membrane, which in our latitude is necessarily so great, because of the sudden falls of the temperature. Consequently, individuals suffering intensely from nasal catarrh in our climate—which trouble has been the result of a bony deformity obstructing the nostril—will immediately improve upon change of residence to a milder climate.

Another form of nasal obstruction which very frequently escapes observation, is enchondrosis of the septum very low down. With a nasal speculum introduced and distended, the difficulty is not readily detected unless it is carefully searched for, because it becomes displaced by the speculum. The slight fall of the alæ of the nose with each inspiratory act, brings them in close contact with the thickened septum, making a valve-like obstruction which closes the nose to a greater or less extent with each inspiration.

Nasal obstruction from polypoid degeneration of the mucous membrane, is usually complete and very annoying. Relief is easily obtained by removing the polypoid growth which obstructs respiration. When the growths are very extensive, it will be found very difficult to prevent their frequent return.

Having considered the various forms of nasal obstruction, and how it brings about catarrhal diseases by producing in the air tract unequal atmospheric pressures with each inspiratory act, we will consider the effects of nasal obstruction on diseases of the eyelid, the ear, the brain, the throat and the lungs. We will also consider its special effect on the throat and lungs of tubercular patients.

I am thoroughly aware that the majority of my readers, may regard my attempt to show the relations between diseases of the eyelid, the ear, the brain, the throat, the lungs, the fatal termination in tubercular patients and nasal obstruction as groundless. I, however, state what I honestly believe my clinical experience has taught me, and having read the suggestions, I only ask my readers to accept such parts of these views as their clinical experience will confirm.

Effect of Nasal Obstruction on the Eyelid.— Ophthalmologists as a class acknowledge that one of the most frequent causes of chronic conjunctival disease is nasal catarrh.

It communicates, through the lachrymal passages, most annoying catarrhal disease to the conjunctival sac. The following four cases have been selected as samples of the evidence which has convinced me of the relations between nasal catarrh and conjunctival disease.

Case I.—Mr. L. came to me in 1880. He had been treated for some months by prominent specialists for trachoma. They had tried sulphate of copper and also nitrate of silver. The eyes had been growing steadily worse during the treatment. I tried the same treatment for two weeks, and must confess the eye-lids, which were one mass of granulations, grew steadily worse. The patient told me he had a badly obstructed nose and every time he caught an additional cold in his head, his eyes were decidedly worse. Acting upon this suggestion, without the slightest expectation of success, I thoroughly cleared his nose of all obstructions. In three weeks his granular eye-lids did not annoy him; and I heard within a month that he never has had any return of the trouble.

Case II.—Miss C., a case referred to me by Dr. Fields of this City, had been treated by skilled specialists every second day for about four years by the usual means of copper and silver. The opacity of the cornea continued to grow worse. She told the same story about the nose being obstructed and the eyes much worse every time she caught cold in her head. At the time I first saw her, she could not count fingers at a greater distance than four feet. The opacity of the cornea rapidly disappeared, and after four weeks she refused to come to the office any more because she considered herself well.

Cases III and *IV*—were two children treated for three months with sulphate of copper. I found they were not benefitted, and removed the nasal obstructions which existed in both children. They improved more in ten days than during the previous three months' treatment. The change for the better was so marked, that it attracted the attention of every one who came in contact with the children.

Effect of Nasal Obstruction on the Ear.— The ear is probably affected in two ways. The first is by direct extension of the inflammation to the middle ear. The second and more probable way is that the swollen condition of the mucous membrane of the pharynx causes the opening of the Eustachian tube to become obstructed in such a manner that the swollen end of the tube acts like a check valve. When we swallow, the air from the middle ear is partially exhausted, and the swollen mouth of the tube is so closed that a partial vacuum is constantly maintained within the middle ear. It is easy to understand what will happen in the blood vessels of the membrane lining this cavity if they are under a continuous partial vacuum. They will become chronically congested, the lining membrane of the tympanic cavity will hypertrophy or thicken, and we very soon have an incurable catarrhal disease in the middle ear. This condition has a tendency to keep up an annoying and unmusical buzz in the ear.

The fact that a large number of persons affected with catarrhal disease of the middle ear can hear distinctly when in a noisy railway carriage, or during the existence of any similar noise, is interesting and astonishing to the persons afflicted as well as to their friends. This phenomenon is especially prominent in proportion as the inflammatory disease has stiffened the joints of the little chain of bones which transmits the vibrations of the drum to the inner ear, which contains the nerve terminations necessary for appreciating sounds. When the stiffened joints of these little bones are set in vibration by a rumbling sound, any additional sound waves emanating from the human voice are easily appreciated. The moment the louder noise ceases, the sound waves from the voice are not of sufficient force to move these stiffened joints. With these individuals the stopping of a train interrupts entirely an animated conversation which was in progress while the train was running. This peculiarity is present in the most hopeless of incurable ear diseases.

I do not pretend by treating the nose to cure an ear which has been destroyed by catarrhal disease; but I do propose to arrest this horrible disease by proper treatment of the nose, if the treatment is undertaken before the ear is ruined. The slightest uneasiness or buzz in the ear should seriously attract immediate attention. You have only to look at the text books on otology and to observe cuts of Eustachian catheters made to inflate an ear, the Eustachian tube of which must be reached from the nostril of the opposite side, owing to a bony obstruction on the affected side, and no other testimony is required in support of the statement that cases of incipient catarrhal congestion of the middle ear have not received proper treatment. Treatment for catarrhal disease of the middle ear is usually commenced too late to be successful; when it is commenced in time the recognized treatment is of such a nature as greatly to annoy the sufferer without giving him any chance of permanent benefit. The examination of the nasal cavities of school children is of more importance in averting future ear disease than the examination of the eyes is in averting future eye diseases.

Persons without nasal obstruction, having ventilation through the nasal passages sufficiently free to prevent the rarefaction of air during respiration, never develop catarrhal disease of the middle ear. The disease of the middle ear which comes on with the early secondary manifestations of syphilis must not, however, be confounded with catarrhal diseases of the middle ear by those who wish to criticize the above sweeping statement. The confusion which exists between these two forms of ear disease is very general among specialists.

Effect of Nasal Obstruction on the Throat and Lungs.—The throat and lungs become affected when the nose is obstructed, in three ways, viz.: by direct extension of the inflammation to these parts; by the rarefaction of the air within the parts during each respiratory act; and by the irritating influence of breathing directly into the air passages atmosphere which is cold, and laden with particles of foreign matter. When respiration is carried on through the nose this atmosphere is warmed, and the particles of foreign matter are removed by adhering to the moist mucous surface of the nose, which is especially adapted to receive such foreign bodies without injurious effects.

Persons frequently have a distressing cough for years, from continual irritation of the throat, caused by mouth breathing. Such a cough is greatly improved or entirely disappears upon the restoration of perfect nasal respiration.

Special Effects of Nasal Obstruction on Consumptive Individuals.—A consumptive person has a very irritable condition of the mucous membranes of the nose, throat and lungs, which for this reason are much more susceptible to the injurious effects of mouth breathing than the same organs of those who are not consumptive. The nasal obstruction in such cases should be relieved with the greatest possible rapidity.

Forced feeding, with intelligent use of pepsine, should be resorted to for the purpose of increasing the weight of the individual. The results should be carefully watched and if the weight increases steadily though very slowly, the prospects are encouraging. The individual need not be

hastened away for climatic influences under these circumstances, for having changed one from a mouth breather to a nose breather, you have most materially changed the climate he lives in. Tubercle being a neoplastic or new cell growth without blood vessels, the general sloughing or breaking down of which is a result of its loss of nutrition, our object should be to avoid these consequences which lead so rapidly to a fatal termination. This can only be done by increasing the general nutrition of the body by forced feeding, and this cannot always be carried on without artificial assistance to digestion by pepsine. The increase or loss of weight decides quite accurately whether our efforts are meeting with success or not. Should the weight continue to decrease the individual should not be detained for the medical treatment of his nasal or throat trouble, but should be urged at once to avail himself of the only possible chance of averting the fatal tendencies of his disease by a speedy removal to a more favorable climate. The restoring of nasal respiration as a means of treating throat and lung diseases in consumptive persons will be successful in proportion as it is resorted to very early.

Effect of Nasal Obstruction on the Voice.—Singers, both professional and amateur, lose their voice as the result of nasal obstruction. Many have the most serious difficulty in attaining a given note. "E" being the note with which the difficulty is most frequently experienced. I have seen such a difficulty, which had annoyed a professional singer for twenty years, disappear one week after the removal from the nostrils of a bony obstruction which had disturbed the normal relations existing between those parts of the sound waves which are emitted through the mouth and nose. Any singer may observe the pure mechanical effects upon the resonance of a head tone by closing both nostrils when producing the tone. Those having the obstruction in the nostril suffer from more than its immediate mechanical effects—they also suffer from the chronic congestion of the mucous surfaces lining the entire respiratory tract. This congestion is directly due to the nasal obstruction, and as a secondary cause, most seriously damages the quality of any musical tone produced by the vocal organs.

Headache produced by Nasal Obstruction.—Persons having chronic congestion of the mucous membrane of the entire pharyngeal and nasal cavities complain of "full feelings" in the head. They are drowsy and find it difficult to remain awake at public meetings or amusements. They suffer from mental depression and some with each cold in the head have intense frontal headaches due to obstruction of the frontal sinus.

The fact that the above described symptoms, existing in this class of individuals, are frequently relieved by restoring perfect ventilation through the nose is convincing of the relations existing between the nasal obstruction and the cerebral symptoms complained of.

Having considered how nasal obstruction produces such a variety of annoying diseases, we will consider the treatment of nasal obstruction.

Treatment of Nasal Obstruction.—The nature of the obstruction which is to be overcome must be thoroughly investigated before the means for its treatment can be chosen. Inspection frequently shows the anterior end of an obstruction which is so complete that we cannot see anything beyond it. The trouble may be due to chronic congestion of the mucous membrane alone. This can be decided only by using cocaine thoroughly, which will, in a few minutes, cause the temporary disappearance of the hyperæmia. We then have an opportunity to examine for further causes of obstruction, such as deformities of the nasal septum, or the turbinated bones, adenoid growths from the vault of the pharynx and true hypertrophies.

A carefully manipulated probe is of great additional assistance in determining the length, extent, and best manner of removing the bony deformity in the nose.

In obstructions due to simple congestion of the mucous membrane constitutional treatment with iron and quinine is sufficient to relieve the trouble.

It has been tried for years to reduce the thickening which occurs in the diseases of the mucous membrane of the nose by the use of all kinds of astringent sprays. The word failure is a mild expression for the negative results gained by this method of treatment. The only spray which should be used in the nose is an alkaline spray which is non-irritating deodorizing and antiseptic. I find a spray of the following description very valuable in cleaning the nostrils and neutralizing the irritating and decomposing nasal secretions both before and after operations. It is also valuable in the treatment of acute inflammation of the nasal mucous membrane.

This solution has been recommended by Carl Seiler of Philadelphia. It contains the following ingredients and is superior to any other alkaline spray I have used :

Sodii bicarb.	. . . .	ʒ viij
Sodii bibor.	. . . .	ʒ viij
Sodii benzoat,		
Sodii salicylat,	. . . . . .	āā gr. xx
Eucalyptol,		
Thymol,	. . . .	āā gr. xx
Menthol,	. . . .	gr. v
Ol. gaultheriæ,	. . . .	gtt. vj
Glycerini,	. . . .	ʒ viiiss
Alcoholis,	. . . .	ʒ ij
Aquæ,	. . . .	q. s. ad Oxvi

This formula gives a solution which is sufficiently alkaline to dissolve the thickened secretion adhering to the nasal mucous membrane, and as it is of the proper density, it is bland and unirritating, leaving a pleasant feeling in the nose. At the same time it is antiseptic and acts as a deodorizer, being in this respect far superior to Dobell's solution or any other non-irritating deodorizer and antiseptic. As it is, however, inconvenient for many patients to have so large a quantity of solution on hand, a Philadelphia drug-house (Wm. R. Warner & Co.) has made the solid ingredients into a compressed tablet, so that one, when dissolved in two ounces of water, will make a solution identical in its effects with the solution made after the above formula.

When there is no bony deformity in the nostril and the obstruction is due to a chronic thickening of the mucous membrane, good results may be obtained by making use of the contracting tendencies of a scar produced by the removal of a portion of the mucous membrane covering the turbinated bone, or by the application of caustics or galvano-cautery at the point where the contracting effects of the scar is desired.

I, however, discovered as early as 1880, that in the majority of cases the true cause of the difficulty was not a thickening of the mucous membrane alone, but a bony deformity which left too narrow an opening between the bony walls of the nostrils. In such cases the septum by its deflections or exostoses usually so encroaches on the caliber of the nostril as to make it impossible by the destruction of the soft tissues with cautery or caustics to obtain satisfactory nasal respiration, because the room gained by the destruction of soft tissue is lost as soon as collateral circulation is fully established.

Occasionally an enlargement or malposition of a turbinated bone, is also the cause of serious nasal obstruction.

My first attempts to remedy these bony

deformities were made nine years ago and they were the first thoroughly satisfactory ones ever made.

The instrument used was a No. 10 jeweller's saw, clamped in a sheet of metal to give the saw the requisite stiffness. One and one-half inches of the saw were left free to cut. The metal sheath was firmly clasped in a pin vice, which was driven into an ebony file handle. Seventy-five cents furnished the instrument complete, with a dozen blades. Although cocaine was not then in use, I obtained some most satisfactory results with this instrument in treating bony obstructions in the anterior parts of the nostril, owing to exostoses or deflections of the septum. I regard this instrument with such classic reverence that I give a cut of it in its original simplicity.

I was not long in discovering bony obstructions in the nostril, which were rather heavy for this little saw, some of them protruding at least one-fourth of an inch into the nostril and having a length of one inch. These difficulties led to the construction of a heavier and longer nasal saw, manufactured by Tiemann & Co., and kown as Bucklin's reversible nasal saw. It has two blades which are reversible in the handle.

Fig. 1.

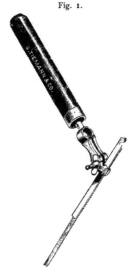

Figure 2 represents this saw as it is in use at present. With it I can remove from the nose any bony obstruction which is detrimental to perfect nasal respiration.

I am satisfied that from native timidity in a field where there was no precedent to follow I have erred in the past by failing to avail myself of all the room possible to

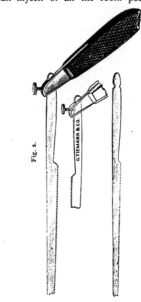

Fig. 2.

obtain a thorough removal of the deformity of the septum. I have tried to make good what I failed to do on the septum by the use of the cautery on the turbinated bones.

Exceptional cases are encountered where the displacement of the septum is so great that the difficulty cannot be relieved by its removal. In these cases the complete removal of one turbinated bone, although in its normal position, will usually give satisfactory breathing room. The rapidity with which the saw does this work is illustrated by the fact that the entire lower turbinated bone can be removed in less than one minute.

The complaints of intelligent patients plainly teach me that the mere opening of a hole through the nose gives little or no relief. The necessary requirement is a hole of sufficient size to admit sufficient air to prevent its rarefaction during the inspiratory act, and if the removal of the turbinated bone is necessary to secure this, it must be removed.

Dr. Bosworth of New York City has constructed a saw since I invented mine, but as far as I know he did so without any previous knowledge of my instrument. He has done much to demonstrate that satisfactory results can be obtained by this method, and to expose the erroneous conception of that class of specialists who introduce an electric cautery into every nose they treat.

For the removal of excessive hypertrophies from the posterior extremity of the inferior turbinated bones and adenoid growth from the vault of the pharynx I can usually obtain better results with the steel wire snare introduced through the nose, the loop being carefully adjusted by means of a rhinoscopic mirror held in the other hand.

Special cases of this description may require the use of various forceps or the curette.

Conclusion.—The restoration of the normal relations between the bony walls of the nostrils by removing bony deformities is one of the most successful means of treating catarrhal diseases of the eye-lids, the ear, the throat, the lungs, and frontal headaches caused by catarrhal disease in the nasal passages.

The operations necessary to restore these normal relations are free from pain or danger when cocaine and carefully disinfected instruments are used.

The relief to the sufferer in nearly all instances has been simply magical. The changed nature of the mucous secreted by mucous membranes which have in old cases undergo extensive connective tissue changes, cannot always be remedied, consequently abnormal expectoration does not entirely disappear, in all cases.

206 West Forty-second Street.

REPORT OF A CASE OF SPINAL HEMORRHAGE.[1]

BY FREDERICK A. PACKARD, M.D.,

PHILADELPHIA.

The following case is of interest as one of hemorrhage into and possible partial rupture of the spinal cord in its upper portion, the patient having recovered in spite of the great extent of the consequent paralysis. .

The patient applied for treatment at the Medical Dispensary of the Episcopal Hospital in March, 1889, giving the following history:

[1] Read at the meeting of the Philadelphia County Medical Society, April 24, 1889.

F. R., white, thirty-eight years old; was born in New Jersey; lives in Philadelphia; spar-maker by occupation. He has been married for fifteen years, and has had three healthy children. His family history is purely negative, except for the fact that one sister died in childhood from "some brain trouble." He has always been a very strong, healthy man, having had no previous illness, except malarial fever, of which he had attacks at various times until three or four years ago. He has been a *very* moderate drinker. Has had no venereal trouble of any kind.

He felt in his usual condition of health, and did a full day's work at his trade on September 22, 1888. In the evening he drank some old ale, not enough actually to intoxicate, but enough to make him a little uncertain in his gait. He went up stairs at 11 P.M., and when near the top of the first flight of fourteen steps lost his balance and fell to the landing on the first floor. He is positive that he fell from lack of balancing power and vertigo, and *not* from loss of power. The back of his head and neck struck the washboard at the foot of the staircase, while his back was bent over the edge of the lowest step. He endeavored to move, but found that he had no power in the extremities or trunk. He thinks also that common sensibility was lost from below the shoulders. His breathing, he remembers, was rapid, and there was a sensation as of a heavy weight pressing upon the chest. When found he was able to talk, see, and hear perfectly well, but was unable to use any muscles below the shoulder-girdle. There was no loss of consciousness, nor had he any convulsive movements. He felt as though the hands and feet were cold, and his impression is that they were soon found actually to be so by his family.

A physician was summoned and administered a powder that produced sleep. On the day after his fall he was undressed and put to bed. Hot irons were applied to his feet, and he was catheterized. He lay in bed perfectly powerless, except for head and neck, for two weeks, at the end of which time. he became able to move his right shoulder. At about this time (*i.e.*, at the end of two weeks) there was noticed a linear series of blisters on the soles running from the ball of the foot to the heel. Nothing could be elicited to throw any light upon the question as to whether the blisters were traumatic, due to accidental contact with the hot irons, or trophic, although the former origin is much the more likely.

Soon after regaining some power in the right shoulder he became able to accomplish coarse movements with the arms. At the end of three weeks he regained some power over the right leg. The left leg remained powerless for two months. At the end of six weeks he was able to grasp an apple or other large object. At that time he tried to get out of bed with assistance, but was merely able to sit on the side of the bed, and that for not more than five minutes, owing to a feeling of being crushed from above. At this time (six weeks after his fall) he also first regained sensation, beginning in the thumb and index finger of the right hand and gradually extending to other parts.

During this time he had but little, if any, fever until the fifth week of his illness, when he had a pronounced chill followed by fever, and in four days another chill. After his second chill his "temperature reached 106°" on one occasion, at which time he was for a while delirious. He had no bed-sores at any time (careful attention having been directed to the condition of his skin). His bowels were extremely constipated, and catheterization was necessary for two months. He ate well. Sleep was broken by a feeling of intense soreness across the back. He had no very severe pain, but felt as though a tight belt were being drawn about the chest and abdomen. He first noticed twitching of the muscles and extremities about three or four weeks after his fall.

Shortly after turning his sixth week he was propped up in a chair, after which time he gradually became able to walk with a great amount of assistance. He could not trust himself alone until two months ago (four months after his injury). At that time he thinks that he had regained as much sensibility as he now possesses.

His condition at the time of presenting himself at the Dispensary was as follows: General health seems good; he eats and sleeps well; the bowels are constipated, being unmoved for a week at a time unless aided; his urinary apparatus is apparently in good working order; he has no symptoms referable to the heart; he gets short of breath easily and, in addition to a sensation of weight upon the thorax, has a pronounced "girdle-pain;" he has not, nor has he had any vomiting or hiccough; his hearing is excellent, but his vision seems to him to be impaired; he has almost constant pain in the back of his neck, at times shooting over the occiput in straight lines on either side; his greatest complaint is of weakness in arms and legs, most marked on left side, and of coarse tremor occurring in all but a few positions that he assumes; he is able to walk about one block with the aid of a cane, but having accomplished that distance his right knee gets stiff and he is unable to lift the toe from the ground; he has both sexual desire and power.

Examination of the patient revealed the following conditions: Intelligent man, well nourished; speech natural; face and neck appeared entirely normal except for slight myosis. Examination of the pupils showed that they were equally contracted when shaded, but reacted feebly to light. There was no accommodative change in the size of the pupil. Heart and lungs normal. The urinary examination was negative, except for a slight excess of mucus, as revealed by the microscope. He stands with the knees in slight over-extension, the feet apart and the body inclined forward from the hips. On walking with the aid of a cane there is seen to be a marked spastic gait with some flinging of the feet in addition. On throwing the weight of the body from the hinder to the advanced foot there is seen to be a marked clonus in each, more marked in the advanced foot, and while produced in the forward foot by the weight of the body upon the ball of the dragged toes, it is, a little later, produced in the hinder foot by the effort of pushing the body forward by the ball. On closing the eyes there is marked oscillation, but apparently in great part from weakness, as the same symptom, to a very slightly less extent, occurs with the eyes open when he is deprived of his cane.

The spine is straight and regular. At the fourth and eighth dorsal spines are points tender on percussion. The muscles of the back are markedly wasted. Breathing is entirely abdominal at rest. Forced inspiration is accomplished practically entirely by means of the diaphragm and the muscles of the neck, including the platysma myoides. The intercostal spaces are plainly marked and not obliterated by the respiratory acts. On the occurrence of a deep inspiration there is marked bulging in the left lumbar and iliac regions as compared to the right, showing probably more powerful diaphragmatic contraction on the right side, or possibly more powerful action of the right parietal abdominal muscles. The grasp is weakened, especially and markedly on the left side. The nails show no transverse markings.

The sterno-cleido-mastoid, platysma, trapezius, and levator anguli scapulæ of both sides are well preserved, as are also the supra- and infra-spinati. The serratus and latissimus dorsi are on each side wasted and feeble. Both arms appear wasted, the right slightly, the left markedly. On the right side the deltoid is of a size disproportionately large as compared with the arm; on the left side it is more equally wasted. Both arms can be abducted, the left with but small force. The right biceps is small but firm, the left is much wasted and flabby. The triceps on each side shows the same relative conditions. On each side the upper (clavicular) portions of the pectoralis major are in good condition, whereas the lower (sternal) portions are only seen on exertion and even then only with moderate distinctness.

Supination is very feeble in the left arm; in the right arm it is more forcible. The fingers are kept in a position more marked than semi-flexion, as is more markedly seen on the left side. Power of extension of the right wrist and fingers is feeble; on the left side extension beyond a right angle is impossible. The intrinsic muscles of the hands are wasted; on the left there is almost complete absence of thenar and hypothenar eminences.

Both thighs and legs on each side are wasted, the left much more than the right. The left thigh and leg, when the patient is seated, cannot be elevated even by great effort on his part. The right can be only slightly raised from the chair seat. There is very marked "clasp-knife" rigidity of the knees. There is no marked alteration in tactile sensibility. Of the superficial reflexes none could be elicited except the abdominal and cremasteric, and these were but poorly marked.

All of the "muscle phenomena" were marked, there being present: Knee-jerk in great excess, ankle clonus, paradoxical muscular contraction of the flexors of the ankle, great toe reflex, wrist and triceps reflexes. The phenomena excited by forcible flexion of the great toe existed only to the extent of contraction of the inner hamstring muscles.

In regard to the action of electricity, there was found to be diminution in Faradic excitability to a slight but noticeable extent, while to the constant current the excitability was much diminished.

Time did not permit of a detailed examination of all of even the principal muscles for qualitative changes. Those tested were the deltoids, biceps, quadriceps femoris, and the muscles of the calf. In all the formula presented was uniformly: 1. KClC; 2. KOC; 3. AnClC; 4. AnOC. The strength of current required to obtain KOC was five cells of a Fleming galvanic battery, more than were required to develop KClC; that for AnClC one or two cells more than were necessary to develop KOC, while many cells had to be added to obtain AnOC.

Examination of the eyes, kindly made by Dr. Randall, showed no abnormality except for hypermetropia, the fields of vision showing no change.

Taking the history and conditions present in this case, there would seem to have been hemorrhage into and around the cord with probably also partial rupture. That the lesion was hemorrhage or in the nature of partial rupture is made certain by the sudden onset in a previously healthy man of paralysis of motion and loss of sensation. That it was high up, in the cervical segment, is shown not only by the history of complete motor and sensory paralysis below the shoulder-girdle, but also by the signs presented at the present time.

The conditions no doubt have been a hemorrhage into and around the cord at about the sixth cervical segment, with probably partial rupture of the cord on the left side of the median line. This primary effect was followed by shrinking of the clot and restoration to some extent of the abolished functions. Secondary myelitis probably then occurred with, later, the descending degeneration of the lateral columns giving the greatly increased myotatic irritability below the parts supplied by nerves from the injured area. A secondary meningitis also probably occurred about the site of the lesion giving rise to the pain in the nape, and possibly also to the "girdle-pain" of which he now complains. There are present no signs to indicate any posterior ascending degeneration, but the lesion is so high up in the cord that they would be difficult of recognition.

Concerning the reactions obtained with the galvanic current, I do not know what significance the formula 1. KClC; 2. KOC; 3. AnClC; 4. AnOC may possess. It is rather hard to see how it can indicate degeneration from polar-cell disease, since it is so widely distributed beyond the site of the lesion as to preclude the idea of direct damage to the multipolar cells in the dorsal and lumbar regions.

—The Governor of Pennsylvania has signed the bill prohibiting the sale of cigarettes to children.

CASE OF CHYLURIA, WITH EXHIBITION OF PATIENT AND SPECIMENS.[1]

BY SOLOMON SOLIS-COHEN, M.D.,

PROFESSOR OF CLINICAL MEDICINE AND APPLIED THERAPEUTICS IN THE PHILADELPHIA POLYCLINIC AND COLLEGE FOR GRADUATES IN MEDICINE.

This patient and these specimens are exhibited at this time to give members an opportunity to see what is a rarity in this climate, and to make a record of the case. I trust to be able to present a more elaborate study of the condition at some future meeting.

The first specimen of urine exhibited was passed four days ago, and shows the characteristics of chylous urine to a marked degree. It looks like so much milk. The second specimen, passed two days ago, is not so marked; and the third specimen, passed this morning, is perfectly clear.

The patient is a colored boy, sixteen years of age, who was brought to Philadelphia from the island of St. Thomas nine years ago. I can obtain from his grandmother, who is an intelligent woman, no history of disease prior to four years ago, at this season of the year, when she noticed for the first time that he passed white urine. He was given a prescription by a physician, and in two weeks the urine resumed its normal appearance. There was no further trouble until about April 8, of the present year, when he again began to pass this milky urine. A week ago he applied at the medical department of the Philadelphia Polyclinic. After obtaining the history narrated, and having the patient urinate in my presence, a prescription was given which, to the mind of the patient, has exhibited startling virtues. It consisted of six drops, thrice daily, of aqua mentha piperita. The urine has become perfectly clear, as shown in this morning's specimen.

I have failed to discover in the urine either embryos or ova of the filaria sanguinis hominis. It has been kindly examined at my request by Professor Angelo Heilprin and Professor Joseph Leidy; but neither has found evidence of this parasite. I have also failed to discover it in the blood, either by day or night. The blood has also been examined (on one occasion, two nights ago, in this hall) by Dr. Griffith and Dr. Tyson, with the same negative result.

Now as to what we do find. The urine is acid in reaction and has a specific gravity of 1,010. On agitation with ether this milky appearance gives place to a slight cloudiness; showing it to be largely due to fat. On chemical examination of the urine, after the removal of the fatty matter, a notable quantity of albumin is found, but no sugar. A promised accurate chemical analysis has been prevented by the activity of our therapeutics—or the perversity of the disease. Under the microscope the milkiness, as stated in the report of Dr. Leidy, "appears to be due to an exceedingly fine and scarcely perceptible molecular basis, as well as to the presence of lymph corpuscles."

On three occasions I have found fragments of finely granular tube casts, and twice a few red blood-corpuscles. After solution in ether, the presence of oil globules is very plainly shown. Bacteria of various kinds were numerous in all specimens examined, even the one freshly passed. No unusual form was recognized as such. The long, slender rod described by Sir William Roberts was invariably absent.

When first noticed, the urine all day long presented more or less the chylous appearance. That passed before me, at about twelve o'clock, noon, a week ago, was of about the color that would be produced by mixing two specimens, one clear, one chylous. Later, the milkiness was present only in the morning urine, and now it is not present, even in the morning. The clear specimen of urine shows neither oil, corpuscles, albumin, nor sugar.

The boy, although not fatty or fleshy, and probably much under weight, is not wasted. He is active, extremely intelligent, and possesses much physical endurance. Heart and breath sounds are normal. No disturbance in any other function has been observed and no lesion of any kind has been detected. Liver and spleen give normal percussion; there is no œdema or swelling anywhere. No enlarged glands, except a few shot-like enlargements back of the sterno-mastoid muscle, can be discovered. The chyluria has evidently run the same course as before, spontaneously intermitting; and I have thus been prevented from making extended observations as to the effect of diet, exercise, etc. The case seems to be non-parasitic, but I am not prepared to explain its origin with present data. I shall try to keep the patient under observation.

[1] Read at the meeting of the Philadelphia County Medical Society, April 24, 1889.

MUMPS IN AN AGED PERSON.

BY CHARLES W. MUSGROVE, M.D.,
AUSTINVILLE, PA.

April 20, 1889, I was summoned to see Mrs. Wolf, 84 years old, and found her afflicted with catarrhal fever. The catarrhal inflammation did not extend beyond the bronchial tubes, and by the tenth day the patient was convalescing very nicely. However, this day my attention was directed to a pain complained of by the patient during deglutition, occurring in the region of the angle of the jaw. On examination, I found the lower part of the left parotid gland slightly swollen, and tender to the touch, and the next day the entire gland was inflamed, and the right one slightly so, and tender to the touch. I now concluded that my patient simply had the mumps, regardless of her extreme old age. There were no symptoms except such as might be expected in this disease, and by the fifth day the inflammation appeared to be subsiding, and the patient doing extremely well.

On the morning of the sixth day I was sent for in a hurry, the messenger informing me that the patient was supposed to be much worse. On my arrival I found her with the following symptoms: Stupor, stertorous respiration, and jactitation. She could swallow liquids, when aroused from the stupor; but in spite of our efforts to save her life she died at 4 o'clock the next morning.

Deeming this a case of mumps with metastasis to the brain, occurring in an extremely aged person, I thought it might prove interesting to the readers of the REPORTER.

—The *Chemist and Druggist*, April 20, 1889, says that Dr. Lamal, of Anvers, has arrived at the conclusion that watery solutions of salts of morphine become turbid, colored, and of an acid reaction when kept for some time. This turbidity is due to two causes—the formation of mycelia, and the deposition of crystals. The coloration and the acidity have also in part a common cause, the formation of acid morphetine; more or less oxymorphine is also generated, which sets free a part of the acid in combination with the morphine. Oxymorphine has no therapeutic properties, so that these old solutions do decrease in narcotic strength. It would have been important for Dr. Lamal to have told us how much.

SOCIETY REPORTS.

INDIANA STATE MEDICAL SOCIETY.

FORTIETH ANNUAL MEETING, AT INDIANAPOLIS, MAY 1 AND 2, 1889.

President's Address.

The President's Address was delivered by Dr. W. H. WISHARD, of Indianapolis, and was an interesting review of the practice of medicine during the past fifty years. He asked the question, have we as medical men kept abreast of the times? His answer was a masterly effort to prove that we had. The primitive Indiana doctors, he said, had not advantages of medical education. The Transylvania University, at Lexington, Kentucky, opened a medical department in 1817, which soon grew to be the second medical school of the United States. In 1819 the Medical College of Ohio, at Cincinnati, and in 1837 the Medical department of the University of Louisville were formed. Only twenty to twenty-five of the physicians of Indiana had taken one course of lectures in medicine in 1825. Ephraim McDowell was not a graduate in medicine, but after he had practised thirty years the University of Maryland gave him the honorary degree of doctor of medicine. The *Medical Repository*, of Philadelphia, was the only medical journal in the United States at the beginning of the early part of this century. Dr. Lunsford P. Yandell, of Louisville, first instituted the treatment of fevers more in accordance with modern ideas.

Dr. Wishard well remembers when quinine first came into use. He was given a prescription consisting of thirty grains of quinine, ten drops of diluted sulphuric acid and six ounces of water: dose, teaspoonful to be taken three times a day, with great care. He has known an old thumb lancet to descend as an heirloom in families for several generations, and it had drawn more blood than some regiments in the civil war. An old theory of mighty weight was, that if you drew blood from the right arm when pain was in the left the pain would be drawn across the heart and the patient would be killed. Obstetric business was of necessity in the hands of women in the early days. Physicians were scarce, women were robust, hardy nature required but little assistance. Early settlers were almost exempt from tuberculosis, diphtheria and cerebro-spinal meningitis; in winter, pleurisy and pneumonia raged. Four-fifths of the cases were treated by the old women until hopeless, then the doctor was called. The doctor was looked upon with suspicion in obstetric cases, and was not summoned until there was dire necessity; then the news spread like wildfire and the neighborhood turned out as to a wedding or a funeral. The good dame of fifty years ago would show with pride her ten or twelve sons and daughters. To-day we are shown one son or daughter and a poodle dog, sometimes only the poodle dog, as the hope of the family.

The doctor then made some scathing remarks on criminal abortion, and after some statements relative to the fortieth anniversary of the Indiana State Medical Society,—which was organized June 6, 1849, with twenty-eight physicians, of whom only five are now living—his interesting address was closed amidst applause.

The report of the Secretary showed a gain of six county societies and seventy members over last year. No doctor can be a member of the State Society unless he belongs to the County Association, and being a member of the latter makes him a member of the State Society. The whole number of members is twelve hundred. The Treasurer's report exhibited a prosperous condition of the financial affairs of the Society.

Dr. Kate Corey, a graduate of Michigan University and Superintendent of the Methodist Hospital at Foochow, China, was introduced to the society, and made a brief speech. The motion to make her an honorary member was passed without a dissenting voice.

The following officers were elected: *President*, Dr. J. D. Gatch, Lawrenceburg; *Vice-President*, Dr. S. Y. Yonte, Lafayette; *Secretary*, Dr. E. S. Elder, Indianapolis; *Assistant Secretary*, Dr. T. C. Kennedy, Shelbyville; *Treasurer*, Dr. F. C. Ferguson, Indianapolis.

Dr. G. W. Vernon, of Indianapolis, read a paper on

Broncho-Pneumonia in Children.

He thought the use of natural gas had become an important factor in this and other catarrhal diseases. In treating measles, whooping cough, etc., he said we should bear in mind the possibility of this disease: it may commence in the tubes and extend into the alveoli, or it may begin in the interstitial tissue.

Dr. Johnson, of Indianapolis, thought there were more recoveries from acute lobar pneumonia than from broncho-pneumonia. He considers catarrhal diseases essentially belonging to childhood.

Dr. G. W. Smythe, of Greencastle, read a paper on

The Hydro-Therapeutic Treatment of Typhoid Fever,

which was followed by a paper on

Atypical Typhoid Fever,

by Dr. H. McCullough, of Fort Wayne.

Dr. M. F. Porter thought there were more cases of the atypical than of typical typhoid fever. He opposed the routine treatment by cold baths.

Dr. Mendenhall said: there are 300,000 cases of typhoid fever in the United States each year, and 30,000 of these prove fatal. We should be interested in the disease.

The discussion on the subject grew quite strong, and the conclusion reached was that the whole question is simply one of diagnosis.

Dr. W. N. Wishard, of Indianapolis, discussed

Urethral Stricture in the Male.

Otis's operation is the only method by which he feels confident of success, as he is still dissatisfied with electrolysis.

Dr. A. C. Porter, of Lebanon, read a paper on

Nervous Sick Headache.

He said little was written and little known about this disease, though it is so frequent. He thinks a large majority of cases is due to a deficient supply of blood in the brain or some part of it. When due to stomach trouble, bismuth and fluid extract of quassia are good.

Dr. R. F. Stone, of Indianapolis, read a paper on the

Nature and Etiology of Tuberculosis.

He opposed bacteriology and all the theories of Koch. He disbelieves in contagion, thinks the germ theory a fallacious one, and antiseptics useful only so far as they induce cleanliness. This paper produced considerable discussion among the disciples of Koch.

Dr. James F. Hibberd, of Richmond, read an interesting paper on

Myxœdema,

and gave a report of a case under his care, and went extensively into the literature of this recently described and rare disease.

He pronounces it a distinct disease, with well-marked symptoms, not amenable to treatment, and says that, though persons may live for years, they never recover normal health.

Dr. G. W. KEMPER, of Muncie, Ind., read a paper on

Antiseptics in Normal Labor,

and said that his experience in 900 cases of labor had taught him that antiseptics are uncalled for in cases in which the patient is surrounded by healthy environments, and he regards the complicated details of antiseptic midwifery in such cases as tiresome, expensive, and unnecessary.

TENNESSEE STATE MEDICAL SOCIETY.

ANNUAL SESSION, AT NASHVILLE, APRIL 30, MAY 1 AND 2, 1889.

The President, DR. T. J. HAPPEL, of Trenton, in the Chair.

The Treasurer's report showed a balance of $169.68 in the treasury. A report was made showing that after forty years of solicitation the legislature of Tennessee had at last passed a law regulating the practice of medicine. Though far from perfect, it was a great gain and should receive the hearty support of all. The Society recommended the following for appointment as a Board of Medical Examiners: Drs. C. Deadrick, Nashville; J. B. Murfree, Murfreesboro; D. D. Saunders, Memphis. A resolution requesting the legislature to pass the bill now pending requiring the registration of births and marriages was carried.

The following officers were elected: *President*, Dr. Duncan Eve, Nashville; *Vice-Presidents*, Drs. Henry Berlin, Chattanooga, J. B. Neil, Marshall, and J. P. C. Walker, Dyersburg; *Secretary*, Dr. E. D. Nelson, Chattanooga; *Treasurer*, Richard Cheatham, Nashville. The next meeting will be held at Memphis, the second Tuesday in April, 1890.

—Hypnotism, says the *Boston Journal*, has become very conspicuous in Europe of late. It has been used in the place of chloroform in some surgical operations at Paris, and when, in a recent murder case there, it was charged that the murderer had hypnotized the victim and forced her to kill herself, public opinion accepted the possibility of the fact in a way quite remarkable.

MEDICAL AND CHIRURGICAL FACULTY OF MARYLAND.

NINETY-FIRST ANNUAL SESSION, AT BALTIMORE, MD., APRIL 23–25, 1889.

DR. JOHN MORRIS, President, in the chair. On Tuesday, April 23, after greeting the members, the President made his address on

The Physiology and Pathogenesis of Crime.

To prevent a man from becoming a criminal, he said, we must begin with him as a child. Every one cries out against immorality, but no steps are taken to create morality, to make morality a public sentiment; to make it a subject of national pride. Yet these are the prominent, the prevailing influences in Japan. There, crimes of violence and outrage are scarcely known.

Where the law of heredity is recognized, it is the duty of the medical man to forewarn parents and to suggest the proper education and surroundings, to render innocuous this taint of blood. The law of heredity obtains even more in moral than in physical traits. The family doctor has disappeared, but he must be brought back to occupy a higher and a wider field. We are born with unalterable tendencies which are not always evil. The Jew and the gypsy are examples of unalterable types. Ordinarily the physician treats the body alone irrespective of the mental organization. He is but half a physician. The body yields to the mind, the mind to the body rarely. The weakness or total absence of certain powers of mind is rarely noticed in children, and yet this observation is of the highest importance in shaping their future lives. The physician should be consulted in regard to the education of a family of children, and to do this he must have been trained by a long course of mental observation.

Marriage should be regulated by law. Paupers and criminals should be prevented from marrying. It is as harmful to bring insane children into the world as it is to drive them insane by bad usage. The habitual criminal, man or woman, should be deprived of the power to procreate.

On Wednesday, April 24, the Annual Oration was delivered by PROF. WILLIAM OSLER, the Physician recently elected professor of theory and practice of medicine in Johns Hopkins University,

On the License to Practise.

He spoke principally of the need of state boards of examiners to decide on the fitness of medical graduates to practise. In this country, he said, a man can follow the vocation he pleases, subject only to such restrictions as may be necessary for the public welfare. The right to regulate the practice of medicine rests with the state. At present this power is variously exercised in different states. In many no regulations whatever exist. In a majority of states, however, there are restrictions which demand evidence on the part of the practitioner that he has studied for a longer or a shorter period at an incorporated school. Practically the rule prevails that, with a diploma from a chartered school, he can begin at once, without any hindrance other than that relating to registration. The educational duties of the state do not here extend beyond the system of common and normal schools, though in a few higher university works are also undertaken. Special education does not receive support from the public revenues. Schools of law, medicine, engineering, theology, all the special branches of study, are private enterprises chartered by the state, and maintained by fees from pupils, or by the munificence of private friends. Certain privileges are granted to these institutions by the state, the most important of which, in the medical school, is the recognition of the diploma as a qualification for practice. So unsatisfactory, however, has this system proved, that there is, on the part of the public and the profession, a growing sense of the necessity for a radical change, as shown by the number of states in which bills have either been already passed or have been before the legislatures dealing with the problem, and if we wish legislation for the protection of the public, we have got to get it together, not singly. I know that this is gall and wormwood to many, but it is a question which has to be met fairly and squarely. When we think of the nine or ten subjects we have in common, we may surely, in the interest of the public, bury animosities and agree to differ on the question of therapeutics. In connection with license to practise there are, it seems to me, three courses open:

"First. A continuance in the plan at present prevailing, which makes the college the judge of the fitness of the candidate, and state supervision is only so far exercised that the diplomas are registered if from legally incorporated schools.

"Second. The appointment by the state or by parties so deputized of a board of examiners which shall, irrespective of diplomas, examine all candidates for the license.

"Third. The organization of the entire profession in each state into an electorate, which shall send representatives to a central parliament, having full control of all questions relating to medical education, examination and registration. These various plans are at present in operation in different parts of the continent. Colleges have practically had a monopoly for years, as the diploma has carried with it the privileges of registration. To all intents and purposes, the medical schools of the country are private organizations, and have direct pecuniary interests in the size of the classes. These chartered corporations are wholly irresponsible, without supervision by the state, the profession or the public. It would not be difficult, without fear of just rebuke, to bring a railing accusation against them for persistently acting in their own interest, and not in the interest of the public, but the time has passed for this. Yet it is surprising to think that so many men, distinguished in every way in their profession, cultured and liberal, still cling to and even advocate the advantages of an irresponsibility which has made the American system of medical education a by-word among the nations."

In the Section on Surgery, DR. RANDOLPH WINSLOW, Chairman, called attention to the subject of

Surgery of the Central Nervous System,

dwelling first on the importance of understanding thoroughly the general and topical anatomy of the brain, and then referring to the important results obtained by experiments on animals, by clinical observations, post-mortem examinations and by electrical stimulation of the exposed human brain during the performance of surgical operations. The cortex and base are most accessible and amenable to surgical procedure. Tumors of the brain are of more frequent occurrence than general practitioners think. W. Hale White and Victor Horsley have done the best work here. Cranio-cerebral topography is a new and very important study and has been mainly used in the surgical treatment of epilepsy, brain abscesses, etc. The study of surgery of the spinal cord is of more recent date. Few cases have been reported.

In the same section, DR. OSCAR J. COSKERY reported a case of

Trephining for Cerebral Abscess,

with the result of removing the pus and giving motion to a paralyzed arm and leg, but the patient eventually died.

Dr. John G. Jay then reported a case of

Exsection of the Entire Ulna with Resection of the Humerus and Radius,

in a woman 49 years old. Complete anchylosis did not occur and the elbow remained movable to the extent of several inches, and the thumb and two fingers could be used. The operation was fully justified by the excellent results.

In the Section on Practice of Medicine, Dr. William B. Canfield, Chairman, spoke of

The Relation of Dusty Occupations to Pulmonary Phthisis.

He began by saying that the pulmonary diseases caused by the different kinds of dust had received a variety of names according to the character of the dust inhaled, but collectively they were all covered by the name pneumonkoniosis. Ever since Koch's discovery of the tubercle bacillus, and the gradually improved classification of lung diseases, there seemed to be doubt whether these dust diseases were tuberculous or not. The particles inhaled by miners in badly ventilated mines gradually overcame the action of the ciliated epithelium and penetrated to the alveoli of the lung, whence they found their way into the subepithelial layer where, unless rendered harmless or devoured by the greedy phagocytes, they set up a fibroid condition of the lung. Most writers agree that the fibroid condition is a barrier to the growth and multiplication of the bacillus.

Pneumonia, he said, results from something more than "catching cold." Sailors lead an exposed life and rarely have it. A large number of investigators have been looking for the specific organism. Salamon did some excellent work; Friedländer's pneumococcus was accepted for a time, but the investigations of Fränkel and Weichselbaum have shown Friedländer's organism to be only an accidental accompaniment of pneumonia. Good work has also been done by Gamaleia, Sternberg, Lipari and others. He referred to the theory of phagocytosis in connection with this subject and related his own experience in the bacteriological study of the organism.

Dr. W. S. Forwood of Darlington, Md., said that what was called "flint disease"

by the workmen was very common and fatal in the quarries of Harford County. It begins insidiously with cough but not like consumption. It is generally fatal and ends like consumption. In answer to Drs. R. Winslow and A. K. Bond, he said that at the end of one year the lungs were permanently affected.

Dr. J. T. Wrightson, of Newark, N. J., said that lung trouble was very common and fatal among the hat makers of his city, but it was attributed more to drinking than to the dust.

On Thursday, April 25, in the section on Obstetrics and Gynecology, Dr. T. A. Ashby, the Chairman, spoke of the growing tendency to abandon empirical methods in gynecological work and the position of exploratory laparotomy. He then discussed the various diseases for which electricity had been used and then showed how much had been accomplished by it in a short time.

Dr. L. E. Neale then exhibited A New Obstetrical Forceps, which was a modification of Howard's modification of Tarnier's. He called it "Neale's Forceps." He claims superiority on the ground that it is all hard metal and can be made thoroughly aseptic, has Simpson's lock; the blades are narrowing, preventing rupture of the perineum.

In the section on Materia Medica and Chemistry Dr. T. Barton Brune, Chairman, read a paper on

Sugar Testing with Special Reference to "Alkaptonuria,"

in which he reviewed the various substances giving a sugar reaction, and spoke of the danger of trusting too much to one test alone.

In the same section Dr. W. B. Platt took up the subject of

Surgical Therapeutics,

in which he considered the curative, non-mechanical agencies employed in surgical cases, whether after accident, operation, or for surgical diseases. These he classified as Anæsthetics, Antisyphilitic and Antiseptics. In the first class he discussed protoxide of nitrogen, chloride of methyl, and cocaine.

Under antisyphilitics were mentioned mercury by inunction, hypodermic injections, and gray oil. The antiseptics were carbolic acid, creolin and iodoform.

Dr. Whitfield Winsey read a paper on

Hypnotics and Antipyretics.

In the former class he reviewed what is now

known of sulphonal, of which he spoke very highly.

Dr. H. Salzer read a very exhaustive paper on

Lavage,

and gave the indication for its use in adults and children, and his experience with it.

In the section on Anatomy, Physiology and Pathology, Dr. William H. Welch, Chairman, read an elaborate paper on Hydrophobia, in which he supported the opinions of Pasteur in regard to its nature and cited with approbation the statistics which Pasteur's supporters bring forward to show its efficiency.

Dr. F. T. Miles then read a paper describing a Case of Dilatation of the Stomach dependent upon Contraction of the Pylorus, in which tetany of a typical character occurred, and was speedily followed by death. He could find nothing in the vomited matter to account for it.

Dr. George I. Preston reported a case of Tumor of the Cerebellum pressing on the middle lobe.

Dr. I. W. Chambers submitted a paper on Cystic Tumor of the Lower Jaw, which was read by title.

Dr. J. D. Blake, in referring to Dr. Welch's paper, asked how the poison could be transmitted by the nerves alone. If injection into the blood does not kill, but makes the animal proof against future attacks, why not inject the substance directly into the blood of man to prevent hydrophobia?

Dr. W. C. Van Bibber said if the temperature stated would kill the organism of rabies, this should give a valuable idea in the treatment.

Dr. W. H. Welch remarked in conclusion that many facts about rabies were known which could not be explained. It was not understood how the virus was transmitted along the nerves, but the fact remains, and still further this did not seem to disturb the function of the nerve. It might extend along the lymph vessels of the nerves; we know little of the composition of the lymph. He did not mean to be understood as saying that the virus did not extend through the blood, lymphatics, etc., but that we have no evidence of this. In reply to Dr. Van Bibber, he said that the method of cauterization is a good one, but it does not prevent rabies. The virus must penetrate into the nerve to be transmitted by it and the chance of piercing a nerve in the skin by puncture is very small.

On Saturday, April 27, in the section on Psychology and Medical Jurisprudence, Dr. Richard Gundry, Chairman, read a paper on The Relation of the Physician to the Insane, and spoke particularly of the frequency of monomania and of the difficulties of recognizing true insanity by the unskilled, for a person may be entirely sane on many subjects and insane only on a few. A person totally insane has no recollection of a deed committed, while a person partly insane may remember the past partly.

PERISCOPE.

Simultaneous Amputation of Both Arms: Recovery.

At the meeting of the Philadelphia County Medical Society, April 10, 1889, Dr. W. W. Keen read the notes of the following case, which he puts upon record as a contribution to the statistics of multiple amputations.

Paul K., fifteen years old, was run over by a street car, at 5 o'clock P.M., on November 13, 1887. He was admitted to St. Mary's Hospital two hours later. The right hand, forearm, and elbow, as well as the left hand and lower part of the forearm, were crushed; both clavicles, also, were fractured. The boy had lost a great deal of blood before his admission, and was in profound shock when admitted; so grave was his condition that it was doubtful if he would live through the night. Dr. J. B. Roberts saw him late in the evening, and ordered whiskey and digitalis. At 10.45 o'clock P.M. his temperature was 97°; his pulse 120.

The next morning the temperature was 102.5°; pulse 142. At 1 o'clock P.M. his condition was very grave, but, as he had rallied from the shock, Dr. Keen decided to give him the only chance of his life, by amputating both arms. The right arm was amputated below the insertion of the deltoid; the left forearm at its middle. The moment that the first amputation was done, during the dressing of that arm by his assistants, Dr. Keen proceeded with the second, so as to lose as little time as possible. The patient bore the ether badly, and his pulse at times was almost imperceptible. Almost no blood was lost during the operations, the Esmarch bandage being applied above, but not including, the crushed parts. Of course, the most careful antisepsis was carried out. There was no need for hot bottles, etc., as his temperature was well maintained. From the time of the opera-tions his recovery was a perfectly steady one. For the first three days the morning and evening temperatures were about 100° and 102° respectively. From that time on the temperature fluctuated between 99° and 100°, reaching the normal by the tenth day.

On the third day after the operation the anterior flap on the left forearm began to slough; by the end of a week a piece two inches transversely by half an inch in the axis of the limb was completely separated. The gaping wound now exposed the end of the radius covered with granulations spring-ing from both the periosteum and the medulla. In order to promote adhesion of the flaps extension was applied to them by means of adhesive strips, on which traction was made by a rubber band. This band extended to the end of a straight splint applied to the forearm, counter-extension being maintained also by adhesive plaster which was tacked to the upper end of the splint. At the end of two weeks the lips of the wound were united, and the splint was taken off. The right stump healed kindly, all the sutures being removed by the twelfth day. The boy was up ten days after the operations, and was sent home six days later to come to the hospital as an out-patient until he was entirely well. He was finally discharged at the end of January. Two small circular sequestra separated from the ulna and the radius of the left stump, and were removed January 9 and 24. The recumbent posture was the only treatment used for the fractured clavicles. They united very well, and with but little deform-ity.

Furunculus of the Ear.

In an interesting work by Dr. Löwenberg, a well-known aurist, entitled "Therapeutical and Bacteriological Studies on Furunculus of the Ear," the author gives as the results of his investigations the following summary of his conclusions: 1. Furunculus is caused by a microbic infection proceeding from external media, the invasion taking place by the excretory ducts of the cutaneous follicles. 2. The successive appearance of furunculi in the same individual proceeds from auto-contagion, which is effected by the transportation of cocci to the level of the cutaneous surface. 3. The same process may propagate the affection from one person to another or to several persons; furunculus is therefore contagious. 4. The entrance of microbes into the blood produces internal complications (metastatic abscesses) in cer-tain cases of carbuncle, and even of furun-culi, and often terminates in death. The author affirms that the micro-organism most frequently present in this affection is the staphylococcus albus, which was absent in one case only. The staphylococcus aureus and citreus were found equally often. In only one case were all three forms of staphy-lococci present together, and they were found in a certain number of unopened furunculi. Taking his stand on these researches, Dr. Löwenberg completely rejects the emollient treatment of this affection, which has hitherto been the clas-sical one. He proposed, as long ago as 1881, to replace this treatment by another method which is antiseptic or antibacteric, destined not only to abort the affection at its commencement but also to prevent its recurrence. This he effects by the use of saturated solutions of boric acid and alcohol, which he drops into the ear in cases of otorrhœa, and in cases of unbroken furun-culi he employs a supersaturated solution of boric acid in alcohol, from which the author has never experienced any bad effects. Milder solutions, he says, are of little or no use in these cases.—*Lancet,* April 6, 1889.

The Prevention of Conception.

At the Third General Meeting of Russian Medical Men at St. Petersburg, Dr. Petr N. Seidler read an interesting paper on the truly burning subject of the prevention of conception. While condemn-ing an indiscriminate employment of any preventive means, the author believes that the practitioner is fully justified in interfer-ing with conception in the following three categories of cases: 1. In women suffering with a more or less advanced pulmonary phthisis. 2. In women with organic car-diac disease. 3. In women suffering from profound anæmia, or failure of the general systemic nutrition with a hereditary tend-ency to pulmonary tuberculosis.

During a discussion following Dr. Seid-ler's communication, Dr. Nil I. Voblyi sug-gested that prevention is indicated, further, in such women as have once or oftener passed through extra-uterine pregnancy.

—The Connecticut Legislature has passed a bill prohibiting the manufacture or sale of oleomargarine colored in imitation of butter, and also prohibiting the sale of imitation cheese.

THE
MEDICAL AND SURGICAL
REPORTER.

ISSUED EVERY SATURDAY.

CHARLES W. DULLES, M.D.,
EDITOR AND PUBLISHER.

The Terms of Subscription to the publications of this office are as follows, payable in advance:

Med. and Surg. Reporter (weekly), a year, **$5.00**
Physician's Daily Pocket Record, - - - 1.00
Reporter and Pocket Record, - - - - 6.00
    All checks and postal orders should be drawn to order of
            CHARLES W. DULLES,
    N. E. Cor. 13th and Walnut Streets,
P. O. Box 843.   Philadelphia, Pa.

☞SUGGESTIONS TO SUBSCRIBERS:
    See that your address-label gives the date to which your subscription is paid.
    In requesting a change of address, give the old address as well as the new one.
    If your REPORTER does not reach you promptly and regularly, notify the publisher *at once*, so that the cause may be discovered and corrected.
☞SUGGESTIONS TO CONTRIBUTORS AND CORRESPONDENTS:
    Write in ink.
    Write on one side of paper only.
    Write on paper of the size usually used for letters.
    Make as few paragraphs as possible. Punctuate carefully. Do not abbreviate, or omit words like "the," and "a," or "an."
    Make communications as short as possible.
    NEVER ROLL A MANUSCRIPT! Try to get an envelope or wrapper which will fit it.
    When it is desired to call our attention to something in a newspaper, mark the passage boldly with a colored pencil, and write on the wrapper "Marked copy." Unless this is done, newspapers are not looked at.
    The Editor will be glad to get medical news, but it is important that brevity and actual interest shall characterize communications intended for publication.

SECONDARY OCCLUSION OF THE BOWELS FOLLOWING LAPAROTOMY.

With the aid of antisepsis and the technique of modern surgery we are now enabled to cope with the two greatest dangers of abdominal surgery, viz., septic infection, what for a long time was known by the name of "shock," and secondary hemorrhage. Of late years laparotomy has become an almost common operation, and although there are but few surgeons who can boast of having done it one thousand times like Sir Spencer Wells and Lawson Tait, yet the records of many hospitals show that the operation is becoming a more frequent one.

But now another great enemy to the success of laparotomies is agitating the minds of surgeons, viz., secondary occlusion of the bowels, which is caused almost exclusively by adhesions to the peritoneum. Dr. Alfred Obalinski, in the *Berliner klinische Wochenschrift*, March 25, 1889, speaks of three cases of occlusion of the bowels out of eighty-six laparotomies performed by him. Two of the cases were operated upon and recovered, the third came too late for treatment, and died. The causes for such adhesions are, according to the statements of various surgeons, first, the presence of foreign bodies, such as catgut, silk ligatures and the like; second, the presence of irritating fluids, such as solution of bichloride of mercury or carbolic acid, and third, overlooked wounds or lacerations of the peritoneum.

Dr. Th. v. Dembowski states that, after experimenting largely upon animals, he has found that adhesions can be produced with certainty only through the presence of foreign bodies or as a result of cauterization; also that the presence of iodoform, blood-clots, irritative antiseptic solutions, or even wounds of the peritoneum, never give rise to any adhesions. The experiences of Obalinski agree with the conclusions of Dembowski. In the three cases mentioned above, the adhesions were not in the vicinity of the sutures or ligatures nor near any lacerations of the peritoneum. He explains their cause as follows: Those portions of the bowels which are exposed to the atmosphere during the operation gradually assume a reddish color and then become covered with a fibrinous deposit. The same parts are necessarily handled both by the operator and his assistant, and it was at these portions of the bowels that Obalinski invariably found the occlusions.

The adhesions are not caused by septic peritonitis; for if such were the case, death would invariably follow. Early diagnosis of such occlusions is of the greatest importance. The principal and most infallible symptom is the anti-peristaltic movement of the bowels above the obstruction. The symptoms of occlusion should not be confounded with those of peritonitis; for, although fever may accompany it and there may be distension of the abdomen, yet the latter will always remain soft and will not be sensitive. That this mistake has been made, however, has been frequently proved by autopsies where the peritoneum has been found to be smooth and shining and the occlusion to be merely a mechanical one.

Secondary occlusions of the bowel are far more easy to diagnosticate than primary occlusion, for, as they occur after laparotomy, they are watched for by the surgeon, and they may be treated before delay has precluded the possibility of recovery. Sibileau (*Annales de Gynécologie*, February, 1889) and many other authorities are against the immediate use of the knife, as soon as the existence of occlusion has been proved, and they state that in many cases such symptoms as vomiting and stoppage of the bowels, distention of the abdomen, collicky pain and the presence of albumin in the urine, may be overcome by large doses of belladonna. Obalinski, on the contrary, considers such symptoms a direct indication for speedy operation.

The prognosis of such cases is not so gloomy as is generally supposed. Sir Spencer Wells tells of eleven deaths from occlusion out of one thousand laparotomies. The prophylaxis of occlusion after laparotomy has been much discussed in gynecological societies, both here and abroad, and many theories in regard to it have been advanced. Muller (*Archiv. für Gynäkologie*, vol. xxiv, p. 1) suggests the injection of a sterilized solution of salt and water (seven per cent.) into the peritoneal cavity, in order to prevent the irritated surfaces from coming in contact with each other. A similar use of olive oil has also been suggested. Dembowski, by a large number of experiments upon animals, has proved the untrustworthiness of both of the above proceedings. The salt and water solution

is absorbed too quickly to be of any value, and the oil causes suppuration and peritonitis. The same experimenter also proved that the use of iodoform, bichloride and carbolic acid, could not cause any adhesions.

In conclusion, it seems that reducing the exposure and manipulation of the bowels and peritoneum to the lowest limit possible would greatly lessen the chances of adhesions; while the occurrence of secondary occlusion should not cause the surgeon to despair, as the condition is easily recognized and in many cases not difficult to overcome.

CAPILLARY PULSATION IN AORTIC REGURGITATION.

General practitioners and life-insurance examiners are sometimes puzzled to decide whether or not obscure first and second sounds of the heart, heard over the aortic area, are due to a lesion of the aortic valves. It is well known that the distinctness or volume of a heart murmur bears no relation to the gravity of the lesion of the valves causing it; and the importance of determining with precision the existence or non-existence of the lesion must therefore be as great as far as prognosis is concerned in the case of a very faint murmur as it is in the case of a very loud one.

In such instances as we refer to, in which the diagnosis is otherwise doubtful, assistance may sometimes be obtained from the detection of capillary pulsation, according to the method suggested by Mr. W. S. Lazarus-Barlow, in the *Practitioner*, March, 1889. Capillary pulsation, it will be recollected, is a manifestation in the capillaries of the intermittent action of the heart. It is too slight to be detected by the sense of touch, but its existence may be inferred when the capillaries can be observed to grow alternately redder and paler with each systole and diastole of the heart. Of course, to be seen at all it must be looked for in a tissue richly supplied with blood and with but a thin covering over the capillaries. Mr. Barlow's studies have led him to regard the mucous membrane of the lower lip as the best point at which to study capillary pulsation for practical purposes.

In examining for capillary pulsation he everts the mucous membrane of the lower lip and presses against it a microscopic slide. What is then seen in a typical case is a central patch into which no blood comes, owing to the pressure of the slide; but at some varying distance from the centre is a narrow zone in which the color intermittently becomes deeper red and then paler over the whole patch, while the edge seems to be in continuous movement, now encroaching upon, now receding from the area of greater anemia which lies next it. It is important in manipulating the slide to heed the caution insisted upon by Mr. Barlow, namely, that trembling of the observer's hands, or powerful pulsation of his arteries may lead to error in diagnosis by producing a varying anemia of the area under inspection, due to unsteady pressure of the slide against the mucous membrane. To constitute capillary pulsation, therefore, the flushings observed must correspond with the frequency of the heart beats.

Now as to the application of this phenomenon to the detection of disease. Mr. Barlow believes that capillary pulsation practically never occurs in health. In thirty-nine out of forty-six cases in which it occurred, the patients had some greater or less degree of affection of the aortic semilunar valves, as estimated by the condition of the second sound. Eighty-three per cent., therefore, of the cases in which it was found presented aortic valvular affection. The practical outcome of Mr. Barlow's observations is that capillary pulsation seems to be diagnostic of aortic disease, or—to be more exact—of aortic regurgitation, since twenty-eight of the thirty-nine patients had double aortic murmurs.

Mr. Barlow's paper is an interesting and valuable contribution to the value of capillary pulsation in the diagnosis of heart disease. But it is only just to say that the question cannot yet be regarded as settled in the affirmative; for while Fagge cites capillary pulsation seen under the finger nail as one of the symptoms of aortic regurgitation, Balfour, one of the most careful and accurate students of heart disease, declares that it has neither pathological significance nor diagnostic value, but is a "physiological curiosity" only. It is remarkable that such decided differences of opinion, as these statements of Barlow and Balfour indicate, should be held regarding the significance of a phenomenon so accessible to observation as capillary pulsation. This much can be said, it undoubtedly exists, and just how helpful its presence is in the diagnosis of aortic disease the readers of the REPORTER are as competent to decide as any other persons. Moreover, as intimated in the first part of this editorial, to determine the matter is of great clinical importance; for if, as seems probable, capillary pulsation is of diagnostic value in aortic regurgitation, then it may be possible to recognize this grave valvular lesion at an earlier period than is possible at present by other physical signs, and as a consequence the person affected may be placed in the best circumstances for the prolongation of his life.

SULPHATE OF SPARTEINE.

Sparteine, the alkaloid of Cytisus Scoparius, or the common broom plant, is a colorless liquid alkaloid, of a penetrating odor and extremely bitter taste, and soluble in alcohol, in ether, and in chloroform. It has been very little used in this country but is in common use in France and Germany, if we may judge by the number of papers which have been written upon it. In the *Deutsches Archiv für klinische Medicin*, March 14, 1889, Dr. L. Anton Gluzinski, of the University of Cracow, has a communication on the physiological and clinical action of sparteine. He finds that it exerts a pronounced influence upon the circulation. This influence is more marked in cold-blooded animals than in mammals, and in the former its effect is more marked when sparteine is applied directly to the heart muscle than when it is injected into a vein or under the skin. The principal symptom of its action, according to Gluzinski, is retardation of the heart's action, and in a less degree also rise in the blood pressure—results which appear to be brought about by the action of the drug on the pneumogastric nerves and on the muscles. In toxic doses the inhibitory center of the heart is paralyzed; and death results from asphyxia.

The rapidity with which the effects of sparteine manifest themselves leads Gluzinski to recommend its employment when threatening or very severe symptoms develop in non-compensated heart lesions, and when the slower effects induced by digitalis cannot be awaited. It is, therefore, in his opinion, an adjuvant to digitalis and to be prescribed simultaneously with it. Moreover, it may be prescribed when digitalis produces no effect, or when its administration is for any reason contra-indicated.

It will be seen from the foregoing that Gluzinski does not regard sparteine as a remedy with a very wide range of application. . It is, apparently, a heart stimulant less rapid and fleeting in its action than the ammonia preparations, and more rapid than digitalis. It has, therefore, a distinct though limited field of usefulness. The sulphate of sparteine, the salt most used, is freely soluble in water, and the smallness of its dose—one-twentieth of a grain at the beginning—fits it especially for hypodermic medication.

We may remind our readers, in conclusion, that Gluzinski's opinion as to the value of sparteine in the therapeutics of heart disease is substantially that previously stated by Jacobi, in his paper on the treatment of diphtheria, which was published in the REPORTER June 30, 1888. Jacobi, however, uses it in much larger dose than that recommended in this editorial as the one proper to begin with. Since, therefore, experimental. therapeutics and clinical experience seem to be in accord with regard to the utility of sparteine, it may be fairly assumed that they represent its actual value.

A REPORTER IN AN HOSPITAL FOR THE INSANE.

A good deal of interest has been aroused within a few days in Philadelphia, in consequence of an adventure of a newspaper reporter, who feigned insanity in order to investigate the workings of the Insane Department of the Philadelphia Hospital. This is not a new device, but it is a one which has opportunities of usefulness. In the present case the reporter learned by experience that it is possible to feign insanity so as to deceive for a time even those who have had much experience in diagnosticating the condition. This, however, is a fact which he could have learned with much less risk to his health and comfort by consulting any authority on the subject. He also learned the way in which hospital attendants sometimes treat the inmates when not restrained by the eye of the physicians: a thing he could hardly have learned without some such enterprise as he undertook. In doing this he has rendered a service to the authorities of the hospital in question, and a service also to his fellow men.

It seems as if there were no way in which occasional acts of cruelty to helpless insane persons can be prevented, and the greatest vigilance of humane physicians and superintendents is not sufficient to insure invariably kind treatment of these unfortunates. As this is the case, they may well be thankful to any person who is willing to become an inmate of an institution for the care of the insane in order to ascertain how keepers behave when they think there is no responsible person watching them.

Those who read the story of the reporter

of the *Philadelphia Inquirer* may well bear in mind that reporters who undertake enterprises of this sort do not usually spoil their descriptions by making them too tame, and there may be some exaggeration in the interesting account which this one gives of what he saw in the·Philadelphia Hospital. But the story is published by a respectable and responsible paper, it is signed with the name of the reporter, and if it receives careful and wise attention, it may be turned to profit by the management of the institution.

STATE MEDICAL SOCIETY OF WISCONSIN.— A preliminary announcement of the meeting of the State Medical Society of Wisconsin has been issued. The next meeting of the Society will be held in Milwaukee, commencing Tuesday, June 4. All members of Committees especially, and all others·who have voluntary papers to present, are requested to forward at once the titles and probable length of such papers, that they may be properly stated in the official announcement and programme of the meeting. As the President is absent from the State, all correspondence should be directed to the Secretary, Dr. J. T. Reeve, Appleton, Wis., who will also be glad to receive the names and addresses of any physicians deemed worthy of membership in the Society.

CHAIR OF SURGERY AT THE JEFFERSON MEDICAL COLLEGE.—The Trustees of the Jefferson Medical College have elected Dr. William W. Keen to the chair of Principles and Practice of Surgery and of Clinical Surgery, made vacant by the death of Dr. Samuel W. Gross. Dr. Keen was graduated from Brown University in 1859, and from the Jefferson Medical College in 1862. For two years he was a surgeon in the United States Army, and subsequently studied in Europe for two years. Later he taught, for nine years, pathological anatomy in the Jefferson College, and also conducted the Philadelphia School of Anatomy. Since

1884 he has held the chair of Surgery in the Woman's Medical College of Pennsylvania, and he also is Professor of Artistic Anatomy in the Pennsylvania Academy of the Fine Arts. Dr. Keen is well known as an accomplished anatomist, a skilful surgeon, an admirable teacher and a man of high personal character. Those who have had the pleasure of attending his lectures in the Philadelphia School of Anatomy will feel that the teaching force of the Jefferson College has received in him a very important addition.

PENNSYLVANIA STATE MEDICAL SOCIETY. —The Thirty-seventh annual session of the Pennsylvania State Medical Society will be held in Pittsburgh, June 4 to 7, instead of on May 21 to 23, as at first intended. It is to be hoped that there will be a full attendance of all the members.

PAMPHLET NOTICES.

[Any reader of the REPORTER who desires a copy of a pamphlet noticed in these columns will doubtless secure it by addressing the author with a request stating where the notice was seen and *enclosing a postage-stamp*.]

260. FIFTY-SIXTH ANNUAL REPORT OF THE MANAGERS OF THE PENNSYLVANIA INSTITUTION FOR THE INSTRUCTION OF THE BLIND, PHILADELPHIA. December, 1888. 33 pages.

261. THE CAUSES AND MODES OF DEATH FROM ECLAMPSIA, AND THEIR PREVENTION. BY A S. V. MANSFELDE, M.D., Quality Hill, Nebraska. From the *Proceedings of the Nebraska State Med. Society*, for 1888. 6 pages.

262. THE COMPARATIVE DANGER TO LIFE OF THE ALTERNATING AND CONTINUOUS CURRENTS. BY HAROLD P. BROWN, Electrical Engineer, New York. 61 pages.

263. SUCCESS AND FAILURE OF ELECTROLYSIS IN URETHRAL STRICTURES, ESPECIALLY DR. KEYES' METHOD REVIEWED. BY ROBERT NEWMAN, M.D., New York. From the *Philadelphia Medical Times*, December 15, 1888. 36 pages.

264. BIENNIAL MESSAGE OF RICHARD J. OGELSBY, Governor of Illinois. January 9, 1889. Springfield, Ill., 23 pages.

260. This Report of one of the best and most celebrated institutions for the blind in the world contains matter of interest in regard to its general management; but its most interesting feature for most readers will be the report of the Principal, Mr. Frank Battles This gives an outline of the methods of instruction pursued in the Institution, and valuable suggestions in regard to the way in which the blind, as a class, should be regarded and treated. It can be warmly commended to the attention of all who

haVe an interest in any blind person or persons, and will abundantly reWard any humanitarian for its careful perusal.

261. Dr. von Mansfelde gives his vieWs in regard to the factors Which most frequently contribute to bring about eclampsia, and the method best calculated to preVent its deVelopment or to cure it if it appears. For the former he recommends rational habits and dress, With examination for the occurrence of albuminuria and treatment of it—especially With a milk-diet ; and for the latter morphia, chloroform, clysters, speedy deliVery, and ergot. Bleeding he adVises only in a limited number of cases.

262. The question as to the comparatiVe danger to life of alternating and continuous electrical currents has been someWhat complicated of late by the arguments of persons interested in shoWing the comparatiVe safety of one or the other method of lighting. After all, howeVer, we believe that Mr. BroWn demonstrates beyond reasonable doubt that alternating currents are far more dangerous than continuous currents of equal electric poWer. His pamphlet contains an imposing statement of facts and description of experiments, and leaVes little room to doubt the justice of his conclusions.

263. Dr. NeWman, in this paper, continues the defense of his method of treating strictures. It is principally occupied With a denial of the conclusions arrived at by Dr. Keyes from the results obtained in the case of one of his patients Whom he turned oVer to Dr. NeWman for treatment. The discussion is not altogether pleasant, and cannot counteract the impression that must be made by the fact that this method has so far failed to secure the approVal of a single well-knoWn specialist in genito-urinary diseases.

264. The part of GoVernor Ogelsby's report which is of most immediate interest for medical men refers to the Working of the State Board of Health, which has done so much to eleVate the standard of medical practice in that State, and to benefit the Whole community. The praise accorded to this Board, and to its efficient Secretary, Dr. Rauch, is abundantly deserVed, and other States might well study and folloW the example they haVe set.

LITERARY NOTES.

—The *Kansas Medical Journal* is the title of a new medical magazine, published monthly in Topeka, Kansas. The first (May) number contains 31 octaVo pages of reading matter, and 9 pages of adVertisements, including the coVer. The subscription price is two dollars a year; single copies, tWenty-five cents.

—The *Annals of Surgery* for May, 1889, has as its leading article a report by Dr. George R. Fowler, of Brooklyn, of a unique case of an air tumor of the neck caused by a hernia of the pleura in a case of pneumothorax. It is well illustrated by a lithographic plate and by a photo-engraving. The editorial articles take up the topics of Injuries of the Heart, The Treatment of Cerebral Abscess, Cancer of the Larynx, and the Treatment of Enlarged Prostate by Electrolysis. The Department of Index of Surgical Progress contains an unusually copious and exhaustive series of classified abstracts of articles from foreign and domestic sources, under about 40 different titles. The usual number of book reVieWs conclude the number. The *Annals* continues to maintain its position as a publication of high scientific merit.

CORRESPONDENCE.

Euphorbia Pilulifera.

To the Editor.

Sir : So many physicians from all over the country have written to me desiring to know where Euphorbia Pilulifera may be obtained, owing to their attention having been directed to it by my article in the REPORTER of March 16, 1889, that you will confer a great favor by publishing this note. It is prepared in the form of a Fluid Extract, by Parke, Davis & Co., of Detroit, Mich. They give the dose as fʒi, but I have used gtt. xxx in a wineglassful of water, three or four times daily, *pro re nata.*

Yours truly,
M. GRAHAM TULL, M.D.

4807 Woodland Avenue,
Philadelphia,
May 9, 1889.

NOTES AND COMMENTS.

Cæsarean Section.

On May 10, 1889, Dr. Howard A. Kelly, of Philadelphia, performed the Cæsarean section for the third time, delivering a well-developed male child. The obstruction to normal labor consisted in an osteo-sarcoma of the sacrum and coccyx which blocked up the superior strait of the pelvis and reduced the conjugate diameter to about one-third of an inch.

Treatment of Seminal Emissions.

Dr. J. K. Mitchell remarks in the *University Medical Magazine,* May, 1889, that the treatment of cases of nervousness from masturbation, or more properly nervousness *about* former masturbation, is commonly not satisfactory. He has, however, found one measure which has proved very useful in several cases under his care. He thinks it was originally suggested by Dr. John H. Brinton, some years since. It consists in the application of a blister over the sacrum. This measure he admits, is a somewhat severe one, but the patients are apt to have suffered many things of doctors, from advertising quacks up, and various treatments, mostly of a depressing or a merely palliative sort, with small results, and he finds that they offer little objection. What is more, the improvement is usually lasting. Of course, the use of the blister need not preclude other and additional treatment, hygienic and medicinal.

The cases are, roughly speaking, divisible into two classes. In the first, the patient has emissions, usually during sleep, without an erection or with only an attempt at an erection; in the other the semen is only voided during erection or upon some irritation, mental or physical. In the former, the treatment should be tonic. Dr. Mitchell likes a mixture of dilute phosphoric acid and strychnia, as in the following formula:

R Strychniæ, ... gr. j
Acidi phosphorici dil., . . . f℥ ij
M. Sig. 25 drops in water after each meal.

In the latter, bromides, or better, a mixture of hydrobromic acid and bromide of soda or of lithium, have done good service. The usual precautions of course must be taken that no old stricture be left to keep up an irritation, and hygienic directions given—a hard bed, not too heavy coverings, light suppers, little meat, a sponge bath in the mornings, the bowels kept free, and all causes of sexual excitement avoided.

Dr. Mitchell then gives the following brief notes of three cases:

"A. B., æt. twenty-four, dyer, self-abuse from the age of twelve until fifteen, very frequently. After about one year began to have emissions involuntarily during the night, three or four times weekly. For some years now they occur every second night. Despondent, suffers with headache, weak back, general nervousness and costiveness. Heart and lungs sound, nothing wrong with urine. Pulse weak and seventy-four to the minute. Always has an erection before emission. Ordered phosphoric acid mixture, and a blister, four by four inches, over sacrum. Returned in five weeks to say had had emissions not oftener than once a week since blister. This patient reported himself as continuing well after several months.

"C. D., æt. twenty. Butcher. Masturbated until nineteen from childhood. Suffers little except from bad sleep and frequent emissions, with erection, several times a week. Eats much meat. Ordered hydrobromic acid, minims xv, with bromide of soda, gr. x, at night and four by four blister.

"Reported in a week that he had had no emissions, and at the end of a month that he had had only two.

"E. F., æt. twenty-nine. Weaver. Masturbated from the age of fourteen until twenty-one, once or twice daily. Has had emissions three or more times a week for 'some years,' sometimes without, but more usually with erection. Has pain in the chest and is languid, and nervous. Heart and lungs perfect. No urethral trouble and general health fairly good.

"Ordered hydrobromic acid mixture, and after two weeks' trial, with very slight improvement, blistered the sacrum. The resulting improvement has been permanent, and he has now emissions very rarely."

Analysis of Butter.

It is reported from Washington, under date of May 4, that the Agricultural Department has been making an analysis of butter from cows fed on cotton seed meal, which produces unlooked for results. The analysis showed remarkable points:

1. A low percentage of volatile acids.
2. A phenomenally high melting point.
3. A strong persistence of the reducing agent.

The first point is of importance as showing that mixing cotton seed with the feed of cows in the South will tend to raise the melting point of butter, thus rendering it more suitable for consumption in hot climates.

According to Professor Wiley the results are of great importance from an analytical point of view, since they show that a butter derived from a cow fed on cotton seed meal might be condemned as adulterated, when judged by the amount of volatile solids present. Since cottonseed-meal is destined to be a cattle food of great importance, especially in the southern part of the United States, this is a fact of the greatest interest to analysts and to dealers.

Voice Lozenge.

Dr. Hinkle, according to the *Chemist and Druggist*, March 30, 1889, recommends the following formula as the best for a "voice lozenge" in the ordinary hoarseness of singers and speakers. A small piece should be allowed to dissolve in the mouth just before using the voice:

Cubebs . . . . ½ grain
Benzoic acid . . . . ⅓ "
Hydrochlorate of cocaine . . . 1/15 "
Powdered tragacanth . . . . . ¼ "
Extract of liquorice . . . . . . 5 grains
Sugar . . . . 13 "
Eucalyptol . . . . ¼ minim
Oil of anise . . . . 1/16 "
Black currant paste, enough to make 20 grains.

Treatment of Hæmaturia.

Professor Ultzmann, according to the *Deutsche med. Wochenschrift,* Feb. 28, 1889, suggests the following formulæ for use in hæmaturia:

R   Ext. Ergotæ . . . . gr. xv
    Sacchari albi . . . . gr. xxx
M. Div. in pulv. No. vi.
Sig. One powder every 3 hours.

R   Aluminis,
    Sacchari albi . . . . aa gr. xlv
M. Div. in pulv. No. vi.
Sig. One powder every hour.

R   Ext. Ergotæ . . . . gr. xlv
    Ol. Theobrom. . . . . gr. clxxx
M. Ft. suppos. No. vi.
Sig. Four suppositories a day.

R   Argenti nitrat. fus. . . . . . gr. xv
    Aquæ destill. . . . . fℨ xvi
M. Sig. To be put in equal or double the quantity of cold water and used for injection into the bladder.

In the same way the following is to be employed:

R   Ferri sesquichloridi . . gr. xvii ss *vel* xv
    Aquæ destill. . . . . . fℨ vi
M.

The Potter Railroad Hospital.

A memorial hospital, for the benefit of railroad men, of the Chicago, Burlington and Quincy line chiefly, is proposed. About a year ago, a railway king, Mr. Thomas J. Potter, died and it was agreed to honor his memory by a fine statue. Later his friends abandoned this plan and substituted for it the foundation of a hospital, to be called the Potter Hospital. The estimated first cost of this construction is stated at $25,000; the city in Iowa which contributes most generously will be the one chosen for the site of the hospital.

Sodium Bromide to Counteract Quinine Idiosyncrasy.

Dr. Krastilevsky has met with the case of a young girl, nine years old, affected with intermittent fever, in whom even small doses of quinine always provoked an erythema accompanied with intense itching. He succeeded in stopping this idiosyncrasy by the use of the bromides. By giving the patient every two hours a teaspoonful to a dessert-spoonful of a solution of bromide of sodium, one part to forty, he could administer the quinine with impunity, that is to say, without provoking in the patient either an erythema or itching.—*Bulletin Médical,* April 7, 1889.

Specialists for Asylums for the Insane.

At the meeting of the Alumni of Niagara Medical College, Buffalo, an address was delivered by Dr. C. A. L. Reed, of Cincinnati, on the great number of unrelieved cases of insanity among women, in the asylums of this country, by reason of inability on the part of the attendants to diagnosticate and treat uterine diseases. Some States have recognized this as a fact, and have ordered the appointment of one or more women physicians upon each asylum staff; but this does not, in Dr. Reed's opinion, reach the root of the trouble, for the number of these appointments is not proportionate to the numbers of the cases. He advises the abandonment of the present system of superintendents and assistants and the substitution of a visiting staff of specialists, made up from every branch of practice.

Dr. W. S. Tremaine, U. S. A., is reported to have endorsed the propositions of Dr. Reed, and added his conviction that rapidly made specialists are not desirable. No physician, he said, should assume to practice a specialty until he had passed ten years as a general practitioner.

"Take Your Medicine."

Dr. C. R. Illingworth says in the *British Med. Journal,* Feb. 9, 1889: As is only too well known, children and infants frequently refuse to take medicines, however palatable they may have been made. A great deal of trouble may be saved, I find, by fixing the cheeks firmly with the finger and thumb of the left hand, whilst the spoon is inserted with the right. By this method, which I first observed practised by a young married lady recently, the first essential in the act of deglutition is provided for, namely, a fixed point for the pharyngeal muscles. Ordinarily this provision is effected by closing the mouth, and there cannot, I think, be any doubt that the prevention of the natural process by the presence of the spoon leads in great part to the struggle to avoid taking medicine. When the approximation of the lips is prevented by the firm forward pressure of the finger and thumb, medicine may be poured into the pharynx without fear of its being spat out, and the most refractory child will, as a rule, discreetly swallow it. The practice of nipping the nose should, I am sure, be strongly condemned because of the risk incurred of forcing the medicine along the Eustachian tube.

Phenacetin and Antipyrin.

Professor Masius of Liege has communicated to the Belgian Academy of Medicine the results of a somewhat extended trial of phenacetin, which he has been making in his wards during several months past. In fevers of all sorts a reduction of temperature could generally be obtained by suitable doses; usually a dose of from fifty to seventy-five centigrammes ($\frac{3}{4}$–1$\frac{1}{4}$ grains) was sufficient for this purpose; it was found that the same effect could not be produced by smaller quantities, even when given repeatedly. Two grammes (30 grs.) during the twenty-four hours sufficed to keep the temperature down. The patients said that they felt a great deal better as the temperature fell; the pulse, too, became slower and stronger, and appetite and sleep returned under the influence of the drug. M. Masius also employed phenacetin as an analgesic not only in rheumatic, but in various other cases, with considerable effect. He did not, however, find that in this respect it was equal to antipyrin. It has been claimed for phenacetin that it has several advantages over antipyrin, such as more rapid action and an absence of disagreeable secondary effects, but according to the experience of M. Masius, though it is true that the lowering of temperature is more rapid than with antipyrin, it is of much shorter duration, besides which there is a liability to the occurrence of rigors and cyanosis, and neither its antithermic nor its analgesic action is so well marked as that of antipyrin. It has certainly the advantages of not disordering the digestion and of being cheap.—*Lancet*, March 9, 1889.

Diseases of the Antrum of Highmore.

Dr. Moritz Schmidt (*Brit. Jour. of Dental Science*, March 1, 1889) diagnosticates empyema of the antrum by making a small puncture below the inferior turbinated body with a fine canula, rather thicker and less pointed than a hypodermic needle, and curved like a Eustachian catheter. A pledget, soaked with 20 per cent. cocaine, is first inserted. He has diagnosticated in this manner an empyema in sixteen cases, and once a collection of colloid fluid. In twelve cases the exploratory puncture was made with a negative result, but without causing any injury. If pus is found he recommends free drainage through an alveolus. A silver tube is to be kept in.—*London Med. Recorder*, April, 1889.

NEWS.

—The Hospital of the Johns Hopkins University, at Baltimore, was opened with appropriate ceremonies May 7.

—The *Western Medical Reporter*, April, 1889, says that the Illinois Legislature has cut off the financial supplies of the Illinois State Board of Health.

—The Legislature of Massachusetts has appropriated $55,000 for the purchase of land and the erection of buildings for an epileptic hospital at Baldwinsville.

—Dr. Edward H. Williams has given $10,000 for the establishment of a separate department for convalescents in the new building for the Western Temporary Home, in West Philadelphia.

—Dr. Harrison Allen will deliver the next Toner Lecture at the National Museum, in Washington, on the evening of May 29. His subject is "The Clinical Study of the Skull, especially undertaken in Connection with the Morbid Conditions of the Jaws and Nasal Chambers."

—The authorities of the University of Pennsylvania have submitted a proposition to the Academy of Natural Sciences to remove the Academy collections and library to new buildings to be erected on grounds adjacent to the University, with a view to the mutual advantage of both institutions. The matter has been referred to the Council of the Academy for consideration.

—The *British Med. Journal*, April 27, 1889, says the Italian Ministry of Agriculture has, in compliance with requests from each of the localities, granted subventions to the Veterinary Schools at Turin, Bologna and Pisa, to promote the practice of vaccination against charbon (splenic fever) in the province of Sassari, and at Foligno and Civitavecchia, where the disease is causing great loss of cattle.

—Dr. Elliott Coues, of Washington, and formerly Surgeon, U. S. A., it is announced, is about to go abroad as a representative of the Theosophical Society, of which he is President. He intends to visit France, Egypt and India, with his gospel of mysticism. While in New York City, April 24, before taking the steamer, he lectured on modern miracles and ancient ghosts, before an audience composed chiefly, as one of the papers states, of women whose hair was short, with a few men whose hair was long. Dr. Coues is well known as a naturalist and as a contributor to the Smithsonian Institute publications.

—The Michigan House of Representatives has passed by a majority of six votes a Liquor Tax bill, which requires retailers to pay $600 a year; distillers, $1000; brewers, $200; wholesale liquor dealers, $800; wholesale beer and wine dealers, $500, and prevents druggists selling liquor except upon written application, which must be recorded in a public book. Under no circumstances can druggists sell by the drink or mix liquors with soda water or any other beverage to be drunk on the premises. The law will not go into effect this year.

—The daily papers state that contracts were signed May 7 by which the State of New York purchased for the electrical execution of condemned criminals three Westinghouse alternating current electric light dynamos. The State prisons at Sing Sing, Auburn and Clinton are each to have one of these deadly machines, which will be driven by the engines already in place. The current will be applied to the unfortunates at the same pressure used by the system for electric lighting, and the State's experiments have shown that death will ensue in less than 30 seconds.

—The *British Med. Journal,* April 20, 1889, announces that the three-hundredth anniversary of the invention of the microscope will be celebrated by the Executive Committee of the International Exhibition of Geographical, Commercial, and Industrial Botany, at Antwerp, in 1890. A retrospective exhibition will be got together from all available quarters, illustrating the history of the microscope, as well as an exhibition of the modern instruments of existing makers. A variety of conferences relating to technical and scientific questions connected with the microscope will be arranged. Already great interest is being expressed in the proposed exhibition.

HUMOR.

NOTHING will trip the light fantastic toe with more ease than a loose brick in the sidewalk.—*Merchant Traveller.*

IT MUST HAVE MADE the former Dandy Mayor green with jealousy to see the present one put on Waugh-paint and turn out White.—*Philadelphia Ledger.*

MISS MINERVA.—"If it is a proper question, please tell me, Mr. Longlocks, if the magazines ever return any of your poems? I have such ill luck myself." "No; never." Grumps (inaudibly).—"He never sends stamps."—*To-day.*

ANXIOUS MOTHER.—"I wish, Susan, that when you give baby a bath you would be careful to ascertain whether the water is at the proper temperature." Susan.—"Oh, don't you worry about that, ma'am. I don't need no 'mometers. If the little one turns red the water is too hot; if it turns blue it's too cold, and that's all there is about it!"—*Boston Commonwealth.*

OBITUARY.

F. S. McMAHON, M.D.

Dr. F. S. McMahon, of Courtland, Alabama, died April 12, 1889. He had been in poor health for two years. Dr. McMahon was born in Courtland July 10, 1836, and was graduated from the University of Pennsylvania in 1857. He practised his profession successfully until the breaking out of the war, when he enlisted, was appointed Assistant Surgeon, 16th Alabama Volunteers, rose step by step until at the close of the war he was Brigade Surgeon.

Dr. McMahon was a courteous gentleman, true, brave to a fault, and faithful in his dealings with all men. He died beloved by all, and deeply loved and lamented by his professional brethren.

MORTIMER O'CONNOR, M.D.

A cablegram received in Harrisburg May 3, announced the death of Dr. Mortimer O'Connor, in Paris, of pneumonia. Dr. O'Connor was born about sixty years ago in Ireland, and studied medicine at Glasgow. Immediately after graduating he was appointed surgeon in an English regiment of the line, and went to India, where he served during the Sepoy mutiny. On his return to England he was made surgeon in the Cunard steamship service between Liverpool and New York. In 1864 he was married, in Paris, to Miss Susan B. Haldeman, of Harrisburg, whom he first met on the steamer, and since that year he has resided in Harrisburg. His wife and son, Haldeman Mortimer, survive him.

About ten months ago a cancer, similar to that which afflicted General Grant, developed in Dr. O'Connor's throat, and his general health became bad. In company with his wife and son he spent the past winter in Algeria, but the climate did not agree with him and he went to Nice, and subsequently to Paris, where he died. Dr. O'Connor was a gentleman of liberal mind and culture, with very many friends.

MEDICAL AND SURGICAL
REPORTER

No. 1682.   PHILADELPHIA, MAY 25, 1889.   VOL. LX.—No. 21.

CONTENTS:

LECTURE.

PRACTICAL VALUE OF THE KNOWLEDGE OF PATHOGENY.[1]

BY PROFESSOR BOUCHARD,

PARIS, FRANCE.

PROFESSOR OF GENERAL PATHOLOGY AND THERAPEUTICS IN THE PARIS MEDICAL SCHOOL.

Gentlemen: To know why we do a certain thing, and what we do, is very rare knowledge, and for the physician it is a new thing. Medicine, as the other sciences which are practically applied, necessitates directing ideas for its intervention. Before the laws of resistance had been established by the science of mechanics, architects studied the old and most ancient monuments, which had resisted the trying influence of time, and then applied to new buildings the methods of construction which had preserved from destruction the works of the past, the excellence of which was in that manner empirically demonstrated.

Medicine has not overlooked empiricism; formulas have been compiled and adopted without knowing how the remedies act, but only on account of the observations of past centuries which have recommended them for the cure of certain diseases. This empirical therapeutics, however, did not prevent the physician from acquainting himself, following the example of Hippocrates, with the processes of Nature's medication; he ignored, however, the real cause of the cures, knowing only by external manifestations, which usually preceded the cure, that this naturalistic medication would relieve and help the symptoms. The particular indications were also not neglected, and the physician fought against the dangerous symptoms—pain, fever, and even insomnia. This is the therapeutics of symptoms and accidents; this is the palliative therapeutics which, some forty years ago, took up the name of physiological therapeutics and is still to-day in great favor.

I have always spoken in a respectful way

---

[1] Delivered at the Paris Medical School.

of palliative or physiological therapeutics, which I use to-day, when I cannot do better; but I should like those who use this method exclusively to speak of it with modesty. I admit that this method of therapeutics oftentimes relieves and even sometimes prevents death; this happens when, in a case of cardiac asystoly, the heart is stimulated to more energetic and regular contractions; and when, in a case of left pleurisy, the dangerous pressure upon the heart is suppressed by aspiration; but while to evacuate what is found in the pleura might sometimes prevent a man from dying, yet it will not cure his pleurisy.

Using the physiological method a high elevation of temperature might be prevented from becoming dangerous or the pain from becoming unbearable; intervention may be useful, may be satisfying to the suffering man, but it will not cure him; and the morbid process will continue its work, overlooking your intervention, and according to its natural laws proceed toward cure or toward death. If the patient recovers, he owes it to himself; nature has furnished the material for his cure.

Oftentimes the physician has very much contributed to the cure; he has attacked the cause of the disease, has interfered with the pathogenic process; he has very often done it unconsciously, the means having been furnished by empiricism. To the latter we owe the knowledge of administering quinine in intermittent fever, mercury in syphilis, the salicylates in acute rheumatism; these are precious acquisitions, which must not be overlooked to show that empiricism has done good. We are beginning to find out their mode of action, of some of them, and gradually they will be classified in the pathogenic therapeutics, of which method I said, ten years ago, that to it belonged the future.

In diseases the pathogeny of which is partly known pathogenic therapeutics pursues its researches in a logical direction, finding out what is better than drugs, the methods of treatment. Empiricism had given to it mercury, while pathogenic therapeutics has discovered its antiseptic property, and at once, more than a hundred antiseptic drugs. My excellent master, M. Charcot, said twenty-three years ago: "it is necessary for the physician to think anatomically"; one of his students said, some twelve years ago: "the physician must learn to think physiologically." These two precepts are excellent and one can say that Laennec, Cruveilhier, and Claude Ber-

nard had prepared physicians to accept those precepts.

It is certainly useful that the physician should accustom himself to have, so to say, an internal view of the state of the parts in which the pathological process is going on. It is also necessary that he should be able to comprehend what interferes with the natural function of the part, and of the physiological disturbances produced by it in the other organs. But it is much more useful for the clinician and for the pathologist that they should accustom their minds to search the reasons why and how these lesions arise, why and how they persist or increase, and how they disappear. For the past ten years, I have always recommended that the physician should think pathogenically. What distinguishes scientifically medicine from natural history is this pathogenic point of view.

It is this which practically can enable one to apply curative therapeutics with some appearance of logic. This is a new view in medicine, and I shall surprise nobody when I say that a number of our professional brethren have never been embarrassed or preoccupied by it, having never employed it. This is because pathogeny is a new science. I must say, however, that in all the past life of medicine, physicians have always tried to find out the mode of action of causes and deduce from this knowledge a rational therapeutics; but they had false conceptions and made wrong deductions.

Only some thirty years ago has medicine slowly engaged itself in this pathogenic path, and pathogeny begins to-day to become beneficial to therapeutics by its discoveries. If we consider that Hippocrates was the heir of what he himself called "Ancient medicine," and that since his time more than two thousand years have been necessary to establish the nosology, to know what diseases are, by what lesions they are characterized, what symptoms reveal them, one is entitled to think that ever so many years will be necessary to know how diseases are produced, to penetrate into their intimate nature, to establish their pathogeny; and we might fear that thousands of years still separate us from the moment when we shall be able rationally to institute a pathogenic therapeutics. This would be true if each disease had a special pathogeny; but if the morbid causes are not numerous, then the number of pathogenic processes is limited. For the past ten years I have repeated and demonstrated that there are only four pathogenic processes. Certain diseases are the result of a previous interference in the nutrition. Life can vary in quality and in intensity without stepping out of the physiological state. There are certain men in whom the cells elaborating the organic matter push this function to its extremest degree of destruction or oxidation, transforming the organic matter into water, carbonic acid, urea, etc. This perfection is however the exception, and is nearer to disease than to health. There are other men, and these constitute the majority, who, besides those perfect products, elaborate in a variable quantity incompletely transformed materials—such as uric acid, oxalic acid, the other organic acids and, in particular, the volatile fatty acids, etc. ; this does not constitute and does not necessarily originate a disease. This imperfection of nutrition, which is the rule, brings on disease only when it is carried beyond certain limits. The quantity of transformed organic matter varies just as much as the different degrees of metamorphosis, even in a state of health.

One kilogramme of living human material can in twenty-four hours furnish one gramme (fifteen grains) of urea in the child ; about forty centigrammes (six grains) in the adolescent ; thirty centigrammes (four and a half grains) in the adult man ; and twenty centigrammes (three grains) in the old man. In the same individual, not considering the age or the kind of feeding, many different conditions can influence the production of urea beyond or below the average daily quantity, without there being any cause or consequences capable of altering the state of health.

When we consider the intensity of nutrition only by the variations in quantity of one of the products of disassimilation, we observe that the physiological state is not allied to an invariable percentage of organic matter metamorphosis, but that it can exist when this matter is more or less completely transformed, or when this matter is more or less abundantly transformed. But there are certain limits of intensity and duration beyond which this deviation from the average nutritive type can bring about only a pathological state. I have demonstrated to you a type of these durable interferences with nutrition ; they bring on diseases—such as biliary calculi, obesity, diabetes, gout, etc.—which are apparently different but the parentage of which has been established by clinical observations.

The physical, mechanical or chemical-morbid causes can involve, in a direct manner, the cells of a circumscribed part or the cells of the whole organism, and produce in them—without there having been previously an interference in the nutrition (a disturbance of life) of their functions that group of diseases of which the traumatisms and intoxications are the principal types, and which belong to a pathogenic process which I have designated under the name of "primitive cellular dystrophy." This is the simplest pathogenic process, but it is the least known and the most difficult one to study.

The morbid causes can also disturb the nutrition and the cellular function in an organ, in an apparatus, in the whole body, by an indirect action, using the intervention of the nervous system, and producing those diseases of nervous reaction to which I have devoted one year of my teaching.

Finally, infection constitutes the fourth pathogenic process, the knowledge of which is the most recent. · This classification of the different ways in which diseases are produced you hear me refer to every year ; I repeat it again to-day, for I am convinced that it is the expression of a just and prolific idea, which is not enough recognized. There is not a single disease the genesis of which does not recognize one of these processes, either isolated or in combination ; the physician is therefore enabled to-day to think pathogenically.

Those who have a knowledge of pathogeny profit by it as well as their patients ; this knowledge ought to be useful to others, but the generation of to-day does not familiarize itself with these notions ; does not follow the oral lectures, but remains at home and makes their education by reading books which are still all built on an anatomical basis. Practitioners, although admitting the reality of the new doctrines, do not use them to direct their conduct.

Do the learned men of our profession derive all the benefit which is found in a knowledge of the pathogenic notions? I fear not, most of them only see one side of pathogeny, namely, infection. How many are they who take into consideration a morbid predisposition, diathesis or the premonitory interferences with nutrition? This enables us to see the most eminent masters in our profession use lithium for gout, or treat diabetes with the bromides. They do not comprehend that a remedy, which has a passing action, cannot, even if it has a momentary effect, overcome a chronic disease, which is chronic owing to a permanent vicious mode of life and which can only be suppressed if life, that is, nutrition, is modified in a more durable form.

The surgeons of to-day protect wounds against *all* the microörganisms, to be more sure to prevent the influence of the pathogenic ones. If you treat in this manner, a wound in a diabetic patient, this wound will be cured by first intention; but at the same time, at some other part of the surface of the skin where no abrasion of the skin is to be found, will suddenly develop some formidable carbuncle. This is the result of the invasion at some portion of the subcutaneous system of the staphylococcus aureus, which, if it had only reached the surface of the wound, might only have produced a very slight suppuration. Many practitioners do not reflect on this point, others who think over it are discouraged; they do not see that in an infection, the infectious agent is not everything and that for its realization the interference of the organism is necessary; they overlook or forget that if the state of health is a safeguard against infection, certain deteriorations of health are favorable to the development of infectious agents and that there are nutritive changes which produce these deteriorations. They do not seem to know that the staphylococcus, which would not even produce the slightest reaction in a healthy man, will bring on pustules, boils and carbuncles in the diabetic patient. In the example I have just given, the wound has been carefully protected against the influence of the staphylococcus; and has united without suppuration; but the skin has not been protected everywhere, and the infectious agent, which resides everywhere around us, has penetrated into one of the follicles in which it has developed, having found a very favorable field for his development.

It is not the doctrine which is at fault in this case, but the physician who has failed to recognize the association between the two pathogenic processes, the premonitory disturbances of nutrition and then the infection; others are astonished when, during the convalescence of an acute abscess, they meet, owing to an exposure of the patient to cold, to fatigue, to a moral impression, with an unexpected complication, such as erysipelas. They know that it is not a new infection, but that the primitive infection extends itself beyond the at first circumscribed limit of organic reaction. They do not know, however, that the nervous action has modified the nutrition and rendered the organism favorable to the microbe, which

before the nervous shock had not been able to penetrate it deep enough. They accuse the doctrine of not explaining the clinical facts, because they have failed to associate the two pathogenic processes—the nervous reaction and the infection. To have a knowledge of infection constitutes progress; to see infection alone will prevent one from understanding many morbid processes. This scientific fault is detrimental not only to preventive or curative therapeutic, but also to prognosis and diagnosis.

If a fracture or a contusion have produced a large effusion of blood, and the skin is not injured so as to prevent the introduction of the infectious agent, a favorable prognosis will be given. But there are microbes in the intestines and you must not think that the epithelial layer is a great protection against them; they continually try to invade the organism, but the phagacytes prevent and destroy them after a short time. If, however, the life of the cells is suspended by the traumatic shock, the inhibitory action of which on nutrition has been demonstrated by the able experiments of M. Brown-Séquard, then phagocytism[1] is interfered with for some time, and as a result the microörganisms pass into the blood and

---

[[1] Phagocytism is a theory advanced by Professor Metschnikoff, of Odessa, which explains the fight between the organic cell and the microörganism. He asserts that there are certain cells in the organism, whose function it is to envelope, to digest, to eat up any bacteria which penetrate into the organism. This can be very well studied in the most simple form of organic matter, the amœba; but while this living matter employs this process of absorption and digestion of bacteria for its nutrition, in the higher organism, this same function of certain cells exists, with the object, however, of protecting the organism against the invasion of pathogenic microbes.

Metschnikoff has given the name *Phagocytes* to the cells which have the property of digesting microbes. He has divided them into two classes: first, the microphagous phagocytes, which are the migrating cells or leucocytes, found in all the tissues, but especially in lymphatics and blood organs. Second, the macrophagous phag· cytes, which are the fixed cells of connective tissue, the endothelial cells of the lung, the cells of the spleen, of the marrow of bones, and all the cells which have a large nucleus.

Whenever a foreign body, living or dead, penetrates into the organism, there is an assembly, a meeting of phagocytes, of leucocytes. If the foreign body is small enough to be enveloped by the isolated cells, it will be found in the interior of the phagocytes, such as is seen in malarial fever. If, however, the foreign body is large, the phagocytes will surround it and will form gradually an isolating envelope of connective tissue, which is what we observe in what is called eliminating inflammation; the hypertrophy of lymphoid organs in infection can also thus be explained, for those organs are really an agglomeration of leucocytes.]

reach the favorable spot. The surgeon astonished notices the development of a gaseous crepitation, fever appears, and infection is produced when he thought it impossible. Infection has taken place by a door which he thought carefully closed and which opened itself by a process which he did not suspect.

Phthisis is infectious, the tubercule bacillus is eliminated with the pus and fragments of pulmonary tissue, its presence is discovered in the sputa, which is a certain sign. What is the value besides these facts of the minutiæ of diagnosis? A bacteriological research gives you in ten minutes an absolute certainty, which the strictest and most careful clinical exploration will never give you. But the bacilli may not be present in the expectoration, even after a number of examinations, and precisely in cases in which the signs of auscultation are the more delicate. Are we not to fear lest a too exclusive notion of infection may lead the physician to neglect the education of his organs of sense and to diminish his skill in the difficult art of diagnosis? I could multiply examples to demonstrate how dangerous for the intelligence or practice of medicine it would be to overlook pathogenic processes and to attach ourselves exclusively to one of these processes. The notion of infection, when applied too exclusively, becomes excessive in its applications; the most difficult operations, owing to this knowledge of infection, have become much less dangerous. Still I am afraid it will become a too great stimulant to operative skill. The operation which was to be a curative one has already become exploratory. As I said a few minutes ago, for clinical medicine, the surgeon will become more careless and will neglect all the delicate and difficult means of clinical exploration; and, like the physician, he will allow himself to search for the absolute certainty in a more easy way but in a more dangerous one. Still, I cannot say that I am opposed to the exploratory operation, for I consider it a good procedure when necessity requires it. The exploratory operation becomes indispensable only when it is to be the first step in a probably curative intervention and when all other methods of diagnosis have failed. When diplomacy is powerless, there is some good in using a cannon; the same applies to exploratory operations.

The knowledge of infection has been very beneficial to the practice of medicine; but its practical application is such an easy one that if one allows himself to apply it too freely, some mischief may arise from it, were it only the delicacy of diagnostic means which is liable to be neglected or even the operative intervention which is liable to become temporary in character.

The therapeutic applications of our knowledge of infection have been very beneficial to both surgery and obstetrics; this knowledge has been extended to operations in all the serous cavities and to the greater part of the mucous surfaces. As to intestinal antisepsis in particular, I can say that it can render in certain cases the same services as external antisepsis in surgery. Interstitial antiseptic therapeutics has also given good results, but general antisepsis barring a few exceptions, is more theoretical than practical. A few years ago it was considered sufficient for therapeutical application to a disease to know its infectious nature; we cannot have to-day this same certainty, for we have gone deeper into the knowledge of virulence and infection. We understand that the infectious agent acts in different ways, that a virulent disease is not, as was believed, a battle between the microbes and the animal cells, but that the real action is more often directed by the cells toward the microbes, than from the microbes toward the cells; and that it is more a process of defence of the organism than attack on the part of the pathogenic element.

We have found, also, that the microörganisms are really dangerous through the poison they secrete. This was first asserted without any experimental proofs by M. Toussaint, then indicated by M. Chauveau as explaining more readily certain results of inoculation; from M. Pasteur it received the beginning of an experimental demonstration. It has finally been definitively asserted by M. Charrin, for the pyocyanic disease; by MM. Roux and Chamberland for gaseous gangrene; by MM. Chantemesse and Widal for typhoid fever; and by MM. Roux and Yersin for diphtheria. If the virulence of a certain disease is due to the toxicity of the matter secreted by the microbes, our therapeutical intervention must change, for poisons are not neutralized by antiseptics; yet, during the active period of the disease, when the infectious agent is multiplying rapidly, it is quite necessary that we should prevent its development, although we must not forget the poison which alone produces morbid accidents.

If this poison be secreted on an accessible surface, it can be evacuated or precipitated, to prevent it from being absorbed; if the absorption has already taken place, or if the poison has been primarily formed in the middle of tissues, it can still be reached, burnt, by calling into action the process of combustion, or eliminated by the excreting organs. We can also combat its physiological effects by administering antagonistic substances. Amongst all these different processes, the elimination of the morbid poison is the one that is really established or demonstrated. I have demonstrated that in infectious diseases the urine carries out of the organism the greatest part of the soluble toxic substances which have been secreted in the body by the microbes during the course of the disease; that one can, in injecting the previously sterilized urine of an animal which died of the pyocyanic disease, produce in a healthy animal the principal and special symptoms encountered in this disease. MM. Charrin and Ruffier, after having injected into an animal the sterilized culture of the pyocyanic bacillus and having collected the urine, by injecting it into a healthy animal produced the characteristic paralysis met with in the pyocyanic disease.

The morbid poisons, and especially those of microbian origin, are then eliminated by the kidneys as the natural poisons are. If antiseptics can be used with advantage in the period of development of the general infectious disease, why should they be used in the later stages of the disease when the microbe ceases to be reproduced? But then, the virulent accidents have not disappeared, for they are slowly eliminated, this elimination seeming not to be complete before twelve or fourteen days. This better knowledge of infection which we possess to-day makes it possible to comprehend that in the treatment of infectious diseases antiseptics are useful sometimes but in some cases are absolutely irrational, especially when microbes or poisons no longer exist; and this is what occurs when, a long time after an infectious disease, accidents present themselves. These accidents are not infectious, they are not even toxic; but the poison has previously weakened the cells and injured their nutrition in a lasting manner. It is not with antiseptics that you will be able to repair the lasting injuries due to the infectious disease; it is only by agents which will generally modify the nutrition. There are many practitioners who, according to the modern doctrines, will treat a diphtheritic paralysis with iodine, oxygen, or carbolic acid; if better instructed in the contemporary pathogenic discoveries, they would return to the older practice and use the neutral salts, the alkalies, iodides, sulphides, and resort especially to nervous stimulation, to frictions, to hydrotherapy, to balneo-therapy, etc. This shows that the better we come to understand pathogeny, the better we are able to place by the side of new acquisitions the remedies obtained from empiricism, and the better we can explain the success which occurred in the old medical practice. It is said that to each specific infectious disease there corresponds a special microörganism; this is not so. A pathogenic microörganism of a determined species may produce nothing, or it may start a local lesion, or again it may bring on death without a lesion. The local lesion, if it develops, may be unique, circumscribed, diffused or multiple. The disease, when it occurs, may be trifling or temporary in character, or bring on death or become chronic. The streptococcus pyogenes can produce a phlegmonous inflammation, phlebitis, angioleucitis, erysipelas, meningitis, pyæmia, puerperal fever, etc.; this puerperal fever may be accompanied by a diphtheritic exudation into the uterus, infiltration of this organ, peritonitis, venous coagulations, metastatic abscesses, suppuration of the serous membranes; or again the puerperal fever may be without any lesions. As to the local lesions, suppuration is not necessary. Such a variability of action of one single kind of microörganism was thought impossible a few years ago. To-day, the fact being recognized, it is explained by the influence of the "*terrain*" (general state of the organism) which is variable with each individual. I certainly do not contest the influence of the *terrain;* I have sustained its influence and have tried to establish it as a factor at a time when it was regarded with suspicion. The influence of the *terrain* does not explain every thing, while the microbe can account for the differences existing.

Virulence is very variable.; it has degrees, it may be weaker or may be stronger. A great many circumstances influence it; the field of development, especially, the composition of the nutritive substance; the presence of air or of too much oxygen can reduce or suppress it; too little oxygen stimulates it; it becomes weakened in a medium previously poor or in a medium which has been impoverished by the growth of the microörganism; it increases when it is animalized in a nutritive medium, such as has been lately shown by M. Chauveau, who restored the lost virulence of the bacillus of malignant carbuncle by cultivating it in broth to which blood has been added. It is rendered much stronger when it passes from an inert medium into a series of living organisms; this increase in virulence varies according to the animal species, so that it can be reduced by transplanting the microbe from a more favorable animal species to a more refractory kind.

Some of these conditions are encountered in human pathology. When the streptococcus, moderately virulent, multiplies itself in an irregular wound, in fetid cloaca in the uterine cavity, its virulence increases and can produce dangerous symptoms, which are much rarer when the streptococci are found on a wound exposed to the air. Meeting so many varieties of action, we may ask ourselves, Which is the type of the normal virulence? and we are forced to conclude that this normal does not exist.

Among the chemical functions of the pathogenic microbes, there is one which produces the toxic substance; this function is more or less active, feeble or strong. According to the case, the same microbe has a negative virulence, a feeble, a moderate, an intense or an excessive one. In this manner we explain the variability of action of the same virus, which misled the adepts of the new doctrine and made them doubt the validity of their belief.

Virulence can extinguish itself; the microbe can even cease to develop. It is not dead, however, but remains asleep in the organism, and one day awakens as a result of a local traumatism or of some disturbance of the general health; it has recovered its virulence. The return of a disease succeeds upon a short sleep. The return of the disease at the same place or at some distant point from the one primarily infected is the effect of the awakening which follows a very long sleep, and is a clinical justification of what M. Verneuil has expressed in one word, the *latent microbism.*

All this, however, appeared in contradiction to the doctrine: one could not understand why, in certain women, the regular appearance of the menses would bring on periodically an erysipelas without a new infection. The resurrection of a microbe is sometimes due to the invasion of the organism by another pathogenic agent; it is known that wherever two different microbes are in conflict in the same organism, one will overcome the other, and the result will be for this last one a neutralized effect, an attenuation. For the bacteria of malignant carbuncle, Emerich has established that its development is interfered with by the presence of the streptococcus of erysipelas, and Pawlowsky has shown that the pneumococcus prevents its development. I have myself brought about the recovery of a rabbit inoculated with a culture of malignant carbuncle bacilli, by inoculating it afterward with the pyocyanic bacillus.

But if on the same field or medium two microbes can interfere with each other, they can also assist each other. Has not M. Roger lately demonstrated that the inoculation of the bacillus prodigiosus renders possible in the rabbit the development of a special species of gaseous gangrene to which this animal is refractory when the two microbes are not associated?

Every day, science clears away apparent contradictions. It has pursued the microbe where it lies hidden, not only in the spleen, in the marrow of bones, in the lymphatic organs but also in the lungs, in the liver, in the kidneys and in the vascular endothelium. If its presence does not produce in those parts an appreciable pathological change, it has impressed the nutritive type; and later, when it has disappeared, chronic lesions are liable to appear,—cirrhosis, nephritis, endarteritis, valvular alteration having infection for its cause, but as a distant cause. These are all diseases of infectious origin, to combat which antiseptics are of no avail. These late localizations of infectious diseases do not proceed directly from infection, they are the result of a permanent interference with the nutrition of the cells of certain organs, which have been impressed previously by an infectious agent. They have the greatest resemblance, as regards anatomical lesions or pathogenic processes to similar alterations of these same organs which occur in general diseases of nutrition or in certain intoxications. It is for this reason that in my lectures of this year, when I am to study the localizations in general diseases, I shall consider in parallel line those proceeding from infection, those derived from a diathesis, and those which are produced by an intoxication.

To-day, before separating, I should like to leave in your mind this thought: that pathogenic notions are useful; that to possess one single pathogenic notion alone condemns one to powerlessness; that the contradictions, of which so much has been said, between clinical facts and pathogenic doctrines are only apparent, and that the scientific work of every day contributes to dissipate them in giving to the facts their real interpretation.

COMMUNICATIONS.

EARLY DIAGNOSIS OF LATERAL CURVATURE OF THE SPINE.[1]

BY JOHN RIDLON, M.D.
NEW YORK CITY.

Upon the early diagnosis and the rational treatment of the conditions presenting in lateral curvature of the spine will depend the successful or unsuccessful termination of the case. When the distortion has advanced so far that the diagnosis is made by the dress-maker or some lay-friend, it may fairly be said to have passed the time for an early diagnosis, and generally passed the time for a complete eradication of the deformity.

It is not easy to say how early a case of lateral curvature can be diagnosticated. I am inclined to think that it will depend upon the cause of the curvature; for upon the cause will depend the first symptoms. A curvature following and depending upon one of the fevers, as scarlatina or typhoid, will present early symptoms differing greatly from those of a curvature following a pleurisy and depending upon the contraction of the pleuritic exudation, although, when well advanced, the distortion is in no way different. So also, a case depending upon a shortening of one lower extremity, congenital or acquired, will, in its early symptoms, differ from one due to poliomyelitis anterior, although both may progress to the same characteristic deformity. In a word, a case may begin with curvature and rotation, or without curvature, or without rotation, or without either curvature or rotation, and still present diagnostic symptoms.

An early diagnosis may be characterized as such when there is as yet no deformity of the spine, or only such deformity as can by posture or manipulation be temporarily eradicated. A deformity which, at the first examination, cannot be made to disappear, will pretty generally resist treatment, at least so far as the primary curve is concerned; although some do remarkably well, as will be seen in the case which I shall present to demonstrate the exercises.

In a case in which there is actual bony anchylosis of the vertebræ on the concave side, we can not hope in any measure to change the primary curve, although much can be done to render the deformity apparently less by reducing the prominent hip and the compensatory curves above and below the area of anchylosis. '

A successful termination may mean an eradication of the deformity and an erect and graceful carriage, or only an arrest of the primary and a reduction of the secondary curvatures with increase of health and strength; or it may mean any degree between these extremes; a termination is not considered successful which leaves the patient encumbered with a brace or jacket, and with muscles so weak and flabby that the supported position can not be maintained when the support is removed; neither do we consider as successful, cases that present a greater deformity at the end than at the beginning of treatment.

By rational treatment is understood the attempt to meet indications, as presented by causation and symptoms, in each individual case, with the end constantly in view to restore the figure so far as possible to the normal contour, and so to strengthen the muscles that this normal contour may be easily and instinctively maintained. Routine treatment of any kind is to be deprecated, but the routine treatment of every case of lateral curvature, no matter what its cause or how varied its symptoms, by any one kind of brace or any one exercise is opposed to our idea of rational treatment.

Rotation of the vertebral bodies, causing the convexity and concavity—the bulging and the falling in—is the characteristic symptom of this deformity, and in a very large number of cases it appears very early. This bulging can be best seen by causing the patient, stripped to the hips, to bend forward, the arms hanging and the knees straight and rigid. But even before this rotation can be detected there are, in some cases, characteristic symptoms: as the patient walks, if unconscious of observation, the head is carried somewhat to one side, the shoulder of that side is slightly advanced, and the foot of the same side is rotated out.

If the patient is asked to lie down upon some plane surface, as a table or the floor, and is simply told to "lie straight," this carrying of the head to one side and outward rotation of the foot will become more easily apparent. If then, with the arms straight and the elbows and wrists rigid, the patient is made to grasp a stick lying across the thighs, with the hands so far apart that the arms are parallel, and is directed to carry the stick forward and upward over the head, it will be seen that the plane through which either arm passes is not parallel with the antero-posterior plane of the body, but that, as the arms pass upward, they will swerve to one side—the side toward which the head leans and the foot points. If the surgeon now grasps the stick between the patient's hands when it is resting on the thighs and forcibly makes the arms follow planes parallel to the antero-posterior plane of the patient's body he will distinctly see and feel the stick twist in his hand. At starting, one end of the stick will be lower than the other, that is, farther down the thigh and that arm appear the longer arm; when it has passed through ninety degrees and is opposite the face, the other arm will appear the longer; and when it has been carried ninety degrees more, the first arm will again appear the longer.[1] This phenomenon appears to depend upon the advancing of one shoulder beyond the other, and, together with the deviation of the head and the rotation of the lower extremity, can doubtless be traced to the same central lesion that causes the subsequent vertebral rotation.

In cases in which these symptoms have been noted, distinct rotation has been observed for a very considerable time before any lateral deviation of the line of spinous processes began to appear. On the other hand, when the lateral deviation appears before rotation, as in curvature depending upon one short lower extremity, I have not found the neck and shoulder symptoms and the outward rotation of the foot.

. It may be asked if *true* scoliosis can be caused by a short leg or a contracted pleural cavity, and I should answer, in the present uncertainty as to the etiology of true scoliosis, that lateral deviation of the spine with rotation of the vertebræ, and all the characteristic forms in the late stage do follow, and may undoubtedly be caused by, a short leg or a contracted pleural cavity, and that such a curvature is to all intents and purposes as true a scoliosis as one that comes without known causation.

For the sake of greater clearness in arranging symptoms I shall divide our cases into two classes: (1) those that present rotation before curvature, and (2) those that present curvature before rotation.

In the first class, in which rotation appears before the curvature, the symptoms generally appear in the following order: Outward rotation of the foot on the side toward which the convexity is to look—this is more marked when the patient lies supine than when he is standing; the head is carried somewhat toward the same side; the

shoulder is carried forward, separating the scapula from the line of the vertebral spines farther than on the opposite side. If the patient be a woman with mammæ developed, there will be found on palpation atrophy of the gland on the side of the advanced shoulder. Then comes bulging of the ribs on this side and sinking in of those on the other side—this is best seen when the patient bends forward. About this time comes the lateral deviation of the line of the spinous processes. I shall not venture an explanation why this is more frequently seen in the dorsal than in the lumbar spine, and more frequently to the right than to the left. As the curve increases the shoulder of the concave side drops lower than that of the convex side, and either a compensatory curve appears in the lumbar region, or the hip of that side becomes elevated and prominent. When there is a compensatory curve in the lumbar region it is the hip on the side of the convexity of the primary curve that becomes prominent. As the bulging of the ribs increases, the shoulder on that side is carried further forward, and the lower angle of the scapula is tilted out in marked contrast to the one on the opposite side, which lies abnormally flat against the sunken chest wall. If the deformity is far advanced this scapula, on the convex side, can not be carried back into place by any effort of the patient; while if the deformity is not far advanced it can be pretty nearly replaced. After a time the compensatory curve, which at first was simply a lateral deviation, undergoes rotation, and it may even become rigid. Lordosis, also, is of not infrequent occurrence. In some few cases there is found to be some degree of shortening of the muscles of the calf of one or both legs, and even a slight degree of talipes equinus.

The symptoms above enumerated may go progressively on to almost any degree of deformity, or they may cease to progress at any time, either with or without treatment. One patient, for instance, wore a brace for some two years, and grew gradually worse. She was then treated for some months by electricity and certain passive manipulative exercises, with little or no gain. During the following two years she had no treatment, yet the progress of the distortion stopped and she became somewhat straighter. Another patient wore the same brace and had passive manipulative exercises for about ten months, during which time she grew gradually worse; but with the brace removed and under active manipulative exercises and

[1] This latter condition is reversed when the deformity has progressed so far that one shoulder is higher than the other.

gymnastics she has become rapidly straighter. The progress of the distortion is sometimes very slow, going on for upward of ten years; in other instances the same degree of deformity may be reached in a few months.

In the second class of cases, in which the curvature precedes the rotation, the first symptom appearing is the lateral deviation of the line of the spinous processes. This, however, is not usually noted, since the curve, not being rigid, is not permanent; and the symptom which is usually first noted is the prominent hip. Not infrequently, however, we can obtain a history of an uneven gait and a faulty habit of standing or sitting in a flabby and rapidly growing child. The relation of the prominent hip to the curvature, that is, to the convexity or concavity, will depend upon the location of the curve. If it is lumbar, the prominent hip will be on the side of the concavity; and so it will be if there is only one curve occupying most of the dorsal and lumbar spine; whereas, if there is a double curve, to the right in the dorsal and the left in the lumbar spine, the prominent hip will be that on the side of the dorsal convexity. After a curvature of this kind has existed for a certain time, usually many months or some years, rotation supervenes and with it all the consequent symptoms: bulging of the ribs on one side in the back and of the other side in the front; flattening of the ribs of the first side in front and of the opposite side in the back; tilting out of the lower angle of the scapula and elevation of shoulder on the side of the convexity, and flattening of the scapula and lowering of the shoulder on the side of the concavity. In this class we have not found outward rotation of the foot, and the peculiar advanced shoulder during locomotion, which is so often seen in the cases of the first class; but the lateral deviation of the head appears subsequent to the lateral deviation of the line of the spinous processes. It is very doubtful if true mammary atrophy occurs in the cases of this second class, but I have observed a smaller but not a flabby gland on the side of the convexity. A considerable number of patients also present a condition of flat-foot.

The spinal rigidity comes slowly as compared with the cases of the other class, and these are, therefore, by so much, more amenable to treatment. In the cases in which there is a short lower extremity it is an advantage to have the length equalized by a high shoe, but this is not absolutely necessary for a good result. In cases in which the deformity is due to, or associated with, the contraction of a pleuritic exudation great care should be exercised in the use of active manipulation, lest the inflammatory process be renewed again.

Treatment should consist in the reduction of the deformity, and the development of the muscular strength to maintain the acquired position. This is gained by posture, manipulation, massage, and gymnastics with assistance and with resistance. In many cases electricity is of use, and the proper arrangement of the clothing is of no small importance; but of more importance than any other one thing I believe to be the constant maintenance, *by voluntary effort,* both during the exercises, and in the intervals between the exercises, of the *best possible position*—the "keynote position" of Roth. As to the use of braces, supports, jackets, and corsets, it is difficult to lay down any uniform rule. In some cases they are unnecessary, in some even harmful, while in some they are of great comfort to the patient; but it should not be lost sight of that their use is prejudicial to muscular development, and delays the ultimate favorable result.

THE PATHOLOGY AND SURGICAL TREATMENT OF SEBACEOUS TUMORS.[1]

BY CHARLES. B. WILLIAMS, M.D.,

PHILADELPHIA.

Sebaceous tumors, or as they have been variously called by different authors, *encysted tumors; atheromatous cysts*—and *wens,* are classified pathologically among the sebaceous cysts. The pathology of the sebaceous tumor makes quite an interesting study, and, in fact, a certain knowledge of this pathology is essential before we can intelligently perform the radical operation. Sebaceous tumors, or as they are more generally called, wens, are quite frequent among hairy persons.

Their favorite seats are in the sub-cutaneous connective tissue, especially of the scalp and scrotum. In the interior of the body they are more rare. These tumors consist of accumulated masses of epidermis and sebaceous matter in the hair follicles, and are a result of the distension of the sebaceous gland and its duct, with hypertrophy of the walls, which forms a thick, tough sac or cyst. They vary in size from that of

---

[1] Read before the D. Hayes Agnew Surgical Society, Feb. 14, 1889.

a pea to that of a walnut or a pigeon's egg, or are even larger, and may occur singly or in numbers.

In shape they are habitually flattened and lenticular. According as their contents are fluid or solid they are termed *mélicerous* or *steatomatous* wens.

The *melicerous* wens (μελι—honey; χηρος —wax) contain a substance semi-fluid in consistency like honey, comprising a large quantity of free fat and isolated epidermal cells.

The *steatomatous* wens (στεαρ, στεατος— solid fat) have more solid contents, consisting of the same elements as the melicerous wens, only there are more epidermal cells and less free fat. In both forms the fat undergoes a metamorphosis, and as it is no longer subjected to nutritive changes it gives rise to crystals of stearic acid, margarin and cholesterin. The cyst is located in the sub-cutaneous tissue. The skin covering it is thinned at the surface, and its papillæ are flattened or they have disappeared entirely—while the surface is smooth, more or less devoid of hair, and with atrophy of the sebaceous glands.

As regards the microscopical structure of the cyst itself we have to consider first its fibrous wall, which consists of connective tissue with flattened spindle shaped cells, a tissue identical with that of the inner coat of arteries and that of fibroma. This disposition, we are told, is caused by pressure exerted upon the walls by the incessant accumulation of the elements contained within the cyst. Fatty, atheromatous, and calcareous degenerations may take place in this connective tissue wall, and this still further increases the analogy of this membrane with the internal coat of arteries. Hence also the name *atheromatous* cyst. Next to the fibrous membrane we have layers of stratified pavement epithelium which undergo evolution similar to that found in sebaceous glands.

The cells nearest to the spindle cells have large nuclei surrounded by a small quantity of protoplasm; and it is probably here that new cells are constantly being formed. Next we have a layer of horn-like cells which are devoid of nuclei. And lastly an innermost layer containing sebaceous globules. Often the horn-like layer of cells detaches itself from the wall of the cyst and forms a shell-like membrane, slightly translucent and almost cartilaginous in texture. It is within this membrane that we find the melicerous or steatomatous contents. Hence the necessity, in operating, of removing this membrane along with the contents of the sac. For if one should leave the membrane behind and merely evacuate the contents of the cyst, new cells would be engendered and cast off, together with the formation of more sebaceous globules which would in turn be cast off, and from this increase of new material we would have, in a short time, a recurrence of the sebaceous tumor.

The diagnosis of sebaceous tumors is an easy one, and probably the only tumor with which it may be confounded is the lipoma. In the lipoma or fatty tumor we have the fatty mass invested by a capsule. From this capsule septa pass inwardly, dividing the tumor into lobes of various sizes. Making the skin tense and passing the fingers over the lipoma, then, we get the dimpling which is characteristic of this tumor. And besides we may feel its lobular structure by careful manipulation. Another final proof we derive from our knowledge that all fatty matters become hardened by the application of cold; hence if a spray of ether be directed upon a lipoma, its contents will be rendered hard and firm. The treatment, however, would be the same in both tumors, i.e., excision; and a slight error in diagnosis would, therefore, not be accompanied by any serious results.

In an operation for sebaceous tumors, at which I assisted last autumn, three wens were removed from the head of the patient, without the use of ether. A sharp bistoury was, by a rapid thrust, carried through the longest diameter of each tumor, slitting up the cyst and disclosing its contents, which were of a greenish yellow color and *melicerous*, or semi-fluid in consistency, containing flakes of sebaceous matter and broken down cells. The contents were evacuated and with the aid of a pair of forceps the membranous wall of the cyst was carefully dissected away from the scalp. The hemorrhage was very slight and was easily controlled by pressure with sponges. The operation was conducted with antiseptic precautions, and afterward the parts were washed with bichloride solution, the edges of the wound were brought together and held by a single suture, an antiseptic dressing was applied and held in place by a few turns of a roller bandage.

As regards the use of an anæsthetic in these operations, I may say, that it depends entirely on the patient:—Should he happen to be as great a stoic as the patient referred to above was, he will require no anæsthetic; but if he be timid and afraid of a little pain then ether had better be administered.

SOCIETY REPORTS.

SIXTH CONGRESS OF THE ITALIAN SOCIETY OF SURGERY.

AT BOLOGNA, APRIL 16, 17 AND 18, 1889.

(Specially reported for the MEDICAL AND SURGICAL REPORTER)

The meeting of the Italian Society of Medicine took place at the University of Bologna, which celebrated last year its eighth centennial anniversary. The meeting was presided over by DR. LORETA, Professor of Clinical Surgery at the Faculty of Medicine of Bologna.

PROF. CECCHERELLI, of Parma, read the first scientific paper on

Surgical Intervention in Cases of Tubercular Peritonitis.

Sometimes after the diagnosis of abdominal tumor has been admitted in a certain case, we find, after opening the abdomen, that we are in the presence of a tubercular peritonitis; this mistake of diagnosis, however, can become, in certain cases, of some utility to the patient. In view of the fact just mentioned, I have tried to consider in which cases of tubercular peritonitis we are enabled, by the aid of surgery, to be of some use to the patient, and what are the reasons of the utility of our intervention.

I have had the opportunity of studying this question on four patients, who presented themselves at my clinic. The first case was that of a woman, 32 years old, who had had five children; after her fifth child she suddenly lost her appetite, and her abdomen became enormously enlarged, due to the collection of a great quantity of liquid in the peritoneal cavity. On opening the abdominal cavity, tubercles were discovered; and after the withdrawal of several pints of liquid, and washing out the serous membrane with a solution of thymol, and the dusting of the parts with iodoform, all the symptoms disappeared and the patient was cured. In a second case, in a young boy of eleven, who was suffering from a progressive ascites, the same treatment as in the preceding case—thymol and iodoform over the involved tubercular part—was employed. Several weeks later, however, the ascites reproduced itself, and I had to resort to a second laparotomy, which exposed numerous adhesions between the coils of the small intestine and between the parietal and visceral layers of the peritoneum; cultures made from these new formations gave neg-

ative results. The boy is very much improved as regards his abdominal condition, but for some time past he has shown signs of involvement of the apex of one lung.

My last two laparotomies were performed on children; one 6 years the other 8 years old; the ascites was very pronounced, and encysted in separate pockets, which I was able to empty and disinfect very easily. A microscopical examination showed the specific tubercle bacillus. Both these patients were cured and in both the diagnosis of tubercular peritonitis was well proven by physical test.

Up to date, 86 cases of tubercular peritonitis have been recorded as having been treated by laparotomy; out of which 52 have been cured, six improved, in five cases the result was unknown, the patients having been lost sight of; and, finally, twenty-five died.

I divide tubercular peritonitis into two forms: first, dry tubercular peritonitis; second, ascitic tubercular peritonitis. In the first form, surgical interference is of no avail and would be impossible or useless on account of the numerous adhesions that exist, which it would be very difficult and very dangerous to remove. In the ascitic form, however, surgical intervention is to be recommended, especially if the liquid is encapsulated; if the liquid is free in the abdominal cavity, simple puncture, accompanied by washing out of the serous cavity, is all that we can do.

The cure in cases of laparotomy is produced by an adhesive peritonitis subsequent to the operation; this leads to the formation of connective tissue bands which surround and strangulate the tubercles; when these adhesions already exist, as in the dry form of peritonitis, operative interference would be much more harmful than useful.

PROF. DURANTE, of Rome, does not believe that tubercular peritonitis can be absolutely cured; he thinks that these so-called cures are only of a temporary character, as we all know that tubercular peritonitis can remain localized for over ten years. Moreover, tubercular peritonitis is also liable to be diagnosticated when we have to deal with a pseudo-tubercular state of this serous membrane.

PROF. BASSINI, of Padua, mentions the fact of two of his patients with tubercular peritonitis, who died from pulmonary tuberculosis, one eighteen months and the other two years after the laparotomy.

DR. FERRARI also accepts the operation as a palliative against serous peritonitis which complicates tubercular abdominal affections; but he does not believe in the final cure of the disease.

PROF. RUGGI, of Bologna, read a paper on the

Use of Corrosive Sublimate in Laparotomies.

I present to you to-day, a statistical account of a series of 115 cases of laparotomies, which I performed last year in my hospital, as well as in my private practice, and in which bichloride of mercury solutions have been used. My cases are divided into:

Single oöphorectomies, 21; cured, 21. Oöphorectomies and salpingectomies, 10; cured 10. Castration for several causes, 14; cured 14. Extirpation of sub-peritoneal fibroids, 4; cured 4. Salpingectomies, 15; cured 4. Supra-vaginal amputations of the uterus for fibroid tumors, 24; cured 19; deaths 5. Laparo-hysterotomy for sarcoma, 1; death 1. Hysterotomies by Antona's method, 3; cured 3. Extirpation of cysts of the parametrium, 2; cured 1; death 1. Intra-abdominal straightening of the uterus by my method, 19; cured 19. Laparotomies for tuberculosis of the peritoneum, 3; cured 3. Echinococcus cysts of the peritoneum and liver, 2; cured, 2. Exploratory laparotomies 5; cured 5. Ascites, 1; cured 1. Laparotomy for foreign body, 1; cured 1.

I have had in all 107 cures and eight deaths, two of which I attribute to poisoning by corrosive sublimate. These two patients I operated upon for fibroid tumors of the uterus; death occurred in less than twenty-four hours and was preceded by a rapid collapse. On *post-mortem* examination, we found a degeneration of the renal and hepatic cells of toxic origin. The poisoning must have taken place as follows: the napkins to be used for the dressing of the peritoneum had been dipped in and kept for too long a time in a solution of corrosive sublimate, which had probably caused the deposition of the salt on the napkins themselves. Hereafter I intend to use exclusively boiled water, instead of the sublimate solution.

PROF. BASSINI has observed two cases of death as a result of poisoning with corrosive sublimate; he now uses salicylic acid instead.

PROF. DURANTE, of Rome, asserts that peritoneal absorption readily takes place only when we have to deal with a normal serous membrane; but he thinks that when there exists an irritated condition of the peritoneum, we can safely wash this serous membrane even with a 1 to 1000 solution.

PROF. D'ANTONA, of Naples, has made a series of thirty-two ovariotomies, with not one death, which he attributes to the use of corrosive sublimate employed with all due care. Among his cases he mentions two of adeno-carcinoma, cured by extirpation, without a recurrence of the disease.

PROF. D'ANTONA, of Naples, reported a case of

Cure of Hystero-Epilepsy by the Extirpation of the Uterine Appendages.

I have operated on a young woman, who, after having suffered from metrorrhagia due to a uterine retroflexion, presented all the classical symptoms of hysteria, namely: ovarian pain; anæsthesia, shortening of the visual field, hystero-epileptic attacks which could be brought on by compression of the ovaries. The reposition of the uterus brought about a temporary amelioration, but soon afterward the metrorrhagia occurred again, and I was compelled to remove the appendages. The tubes were found in a state of congestion, and the left ovary was undergoing cystic degeneration, while the right one was in a much advanced stage; still the patient recovered perfectly.

DR. M. FRANGELINI, of Frosinone, reported a case of

Extirpation of an Ovarian Cyst in a Pregnant Woman.

I have extirpated a very large ovarian cyst from a woman who was in her sixth month of pregnancy, the pregnant condition being recognized only at the time of the operation. The incision started at the symphysis pubis and extended to about four inches above the umbilicus. The patient was walking fourteen days after the operation. The pregnancy did not come to full term. The patient did some hard household work, besides indulging in too frequent sexual connection; these brought on labor, which was uncomplicated. This observation demonstrates that we can extirpate ovarian tumors during pregnancy without bringing on abortion.

DR. BOGGI, of Bologna, read a paper on

Dilatation of Strictures of the Cardia and Pylorus.

In presenting to you the statistics of the laparotomies which have been performed at the clinic of Bologna, I shall call your attention especially to those which have been made for diseases of the stomach, to produce a digital dilatation of the pyloric strictures and an instrumental dilatation of the cardia. I shall not attempt to give you the *modus operandi* of the process, but shall confine myself to recording observations made upon my two last patients.

Case I.—A man 56 years old, had been sick for eight years past, vomiting every two or three days, about seven hours after the meal, a quantity of badly digested food. The hypogastric region was in a tumefied condition, while the inferior portion of the abdomen was quite retracted. He evacuated his bowels only every eight or nine days. As a result of my examination I concluded that I had to deal with a fibroid stenosis of the pylorus. After having opened the abdomen and then the stomach, the pylorus was hardly large enough to allow the passage of the little finger; but gradually dilatation occurred and I first could introduce one index finger, then the other one, and then was able to make a forcible stretching. The patient is to-day cured, eats well, has no more vomiting, and his digestive functions are in a perfect state.

Case II.—My second patient was a man, 48 years old, who had been suffering for several years. On examination we found a cicatricial stricture of the cardia, with dilatation of the œsophagus immediately above it; the stomach was very much retracted.

After opening the abdomen and stomach, the latter organ was very difficult to find or recognize, on account of its small retracted form. The closed extremity of Dupuytren's *revulseur* was introduced into the cardia, and dilatation was made, after which a large œsophageal sound was introduced into the stomach. Fourteen days later, the patient left the hospital completely cured. This man had been suffering for twenty years, and since the operation he has been feeling perfectly well, having no more any rejection of food after his meals

DR. BENDANDI, of Bologna, cannot admit that a temporary dilatation, such as is made with the fingers, can really bring about a permanent cure. He admits the persistency of the dilatation of the cardia, as this dilatation can be maintained by the œsophageal tube; but he cannot understand how dilatation of the pylorus can remain permanent.

DR. PUTLI, of Bologna, like the preceding gentlemen, cannot admit the persistency of the dilatation of the pylorus, considering that for stricture of the urethra we are obliged, after the stricture has been cut, to maintain the dilatation by the occasional passage of a sound.

DR. D'ANTONA says that strictures of the pylorus cannot be compared with strictures of the urethra; they are more analogous to strictures of the anus, which when once forcibly dilated remain pervious.

DR. POGGI : I have studied the effects of forcible divulsion on healthy sphincters and on cicatricial tissues, and as a result of my researches, I think I can affirm that if divulsion does not succeed in certain very rare cases where the pyloric ring is completely transformed into a cicatricial tissue, there exists on the other hand a very large series of retractions caused by partial and superficial cicatrices, which are easily dilatable. I have made on the normal pylorus of several dogs, a dilatation which was still recognizable one year and a half after the operation.

DR. POSTEMPSKI, of Rome, read a paper on the

Reduction of Diaphragmatic Hernia.

At the Hospital of Consolation, in Rome, I observed, some four months ago, a patient who had been wounded in 'the left seventh intercostal space, and who, while he was lifting a heavy weight, was suddenly seized with pulmonary, cardiac and intestinal symptoms, and presented in addition the symptoms of intestinal obstruction with displacement of the heart.

The diagnosis of diaphragmatic hernia was confirmed by the *post-mortem;* the hernial part was not adherent to the diaphragmatic opening, it was only compressed and strangulated. I then thought that we might bring about a radical cure of such hernias, by penetrating through the thorax instead of through the abdomen ; several experiments on the cadaver convinced me that it was a feasible operation, which six weeks later I had the opportunity to perform on the living subject. The patient was a young man who had received a wound in the eleventh intercostal space, of three and a half inches in length; after having enlarged the opening three-fourths of an inch more, I made two perpendicular incisions, as if I was going to make a thoracoplastic operation ; the opening being more dilated, I had all the light and space desired. I had to deal with a hernia of the omentum. I freed it from its strangulation and then brought the lips of the diaphragmatic wounds together by the aid of forceps. I then sutured with a very long needle-holder. Next the external wound was sutured. After the operation, a very large pneumothorax made its appearance, but it progressively diminished until the twelfth day, when it had entirely disappeared. Eighteen days later, my patient was presented before the Academy of Medicine of Rome, completely cured.

PROF. DURANTE reported a case of

Extirpation of the Cæcum,

which he had performed on a woman, 52 years old, who for four or five years past had suffered very much in the right iliac fossa, when she evacuated her bowels. In this region, a resistant tumor could be felt extending down as far as the superior strait of the pelvis; the diagnosis was atrophic or fibrous cancer of the cæcum and adjoining parts.

The operation was a very tedious one, on account of the numerous adhesions which existed between the small intestine and peritoneum and the tumor, and for the additional reason that it was difficult to differentiate the small from the large intestine, on account of the unusual displacement of the parts. I succeeded, however, in cutting the cæcum, and I united the intestinal stumps by means of sutures in three rows. The patient was rapidly cured.

Seven days after the operation, the patient had her first fæcal passage, on the tenth she left her bed. An examination of the extirpated parts showed that we had to deal not with a cancer, but with a case of chronic, indurated typhlitis or perityphlitis of tuberculous origin.

DR. TROMBETTA has also extirpated the cæcum with the ascending colon, thinking he had to deal with a case of cancer, while it was one of chronic typhlitis and perityphlitis accompanied by numerous small abscesses. He formed an external fistula, but the patient died on the fourteenth day from peritonitis due to rupture of the intestine.

PROF. TIZZONI, of Bologna, read a paper on the

Etiology of Tetanus.

A case of tetanus, which has lately taken place at the surgical clinic of Bologna, has given me the opportunity to make, in collaboration with Miss Cattani, *privat-docent* of our Faculty of Medicine, bacteriological researches on this very dangerous affection. The patient was a workman, who fell and sustained a complicated fracture of the arm; the fractured bone had gone through the skin, and had implanted itself in the earth.

The blood of the wounded person appeared normal on microscopical examination; perhaps it coagulated too rapidly. Cultures on serum, made with this blood, remained negative, and inoculation of rabbits gave no pathogenic effect. We next made cultures with the liquid obtained on the surface of the fracture, and with liquid obtained at some distance from the immediate wound, but still in the inflamed region. Of all these cultures, the only ones which have given positive results are those which have been made with liquids obtained from the surface of the wound. After the death of the patient, I tried to ascertain in what organs the virus had propagated itself, from the seat of fracture. For this purpose, I made cultures from the nervous system and spleen; but all have given negative results; the liquid alone which was derived from the wound itself produced positive cultures and killed the animals which were inoculated with them. The cultures obtained on the gelatinized blood-serum are mixed cultures; they liquefy the serum, which is transformed into a yellow liquid, having tetanizing qualities highly developed; injected into animals, it kills them in twenty-four hours, with well defined tetanic symptoms.

We have cultivated this liquid, and we have assisted the development of mixed colonies, in which we have been able to isolate three species of microörganisms: (1) a streptococcus in globular colonies, which do not liquefy the gelatine; (2) a diplococcus, exactly similar to the one of Fraenkel, and having all its biological characters; (3) a bacillus, identical in every way with the tetanic bacillus of Nicolaier and Rosenbach.

We have been able to isolate these bacilli, the culture of which is rapidly weakened when on serum, but which will keep much longer on agar-agar. We have been able to bring them up to the ninth generation. The injection of such cultures invariably produces tetanus.

PROF. LAMPIASI, of Trapani, said: The microbe of tetanus which I have discovered has well defined characters, and has always produced a typical case of tetanus in the numerous animals in which it has been inoculated. I have a culture of this microbe which has kept its virulence for the past two years. As my results differ from other experimenters I am led to believe that traumatic tetanus differs from the rheumatic form, and that each can be developed by a different microbe.

DR. Lampiasi also mentioned the fact

that cultures made with Rosenbach's bacillus produce no tetanic phenomena.

DR. TIZZONI: I admit that the pure cultures of the bacillus of Rosenbach have no pathological action, it is only by the entire liquid and its contained bacilli that the tetanic symptoms are produced. My researches are different from those of Dr. Lampiasi, for I have started from a case of traumatic tetanus while the one which has been studied by Dr. Lampiasi was a case of spontaneous tetanus. In the inoculated rabbits signs of infection were found only in the spleen.

(*To be continued.*)

KENTUCKY STATE MEDICAL SOCIETY.

THIRTY-FOURTH ANNUAL MEETING, AT RICHMOND, MAY 8-10, 1889.

The Kentucky State Medical Society held its thirty-fourth annual meeting at Richmond, Ky., May 8, 9 and 10, 1889. The reports of the various officers and committees showed the society to be in a prosperous condition.

The address of the President, DR. L. S. McMURTRY, was a history of the society. It was brief and to the point. Much satisfaction was expressed by the various members at the new medical practice law which has just gone into effect, and on motion of Dr. J. N. McCormac, of Bowling Green, the President was instructed to appoint a committee, consisting of three in each county, to look after the enforcement of the new law. The surplus funds in the treasury at the close of this meeting are to go toward the prosecution of violators of the law.

A banquet was given at the Garnet house, and was a very pleasant affair. Toasts were responded to by the President, Dr. McMurtry; Ex-Governor McCreary, of Richmond; Dr. W. H. Wathen, of Louisville; Dr. D. S. Reynolds, of Louisville; Dr. J. M. Mathews, of Louisville; and Dr. O. D. Todd, of Eminence. A hop was also given the Society at the rooms of the Madison Club.

The officers elected for the ensuing year are as follows : *President*, Dr. John A. Ouchterlony, of Louisville; *Senior Vice-President*, Dr. William Jennings, of Richmond; *Junior Vice-President*, Dr. R. L. Willis, of Lexington; *Permanent Secretary*, Dr. Steele Bailey, of Stanford; *Assistant*

Secretary, Dr. John Young Brown, of Henderson; *Treasurer*, Dr. J. B. Kinnaird, of Lancaster; Chairman of the *Committee of Arrangements*, Dr. James H. Letcher, of Henderson.

A good feature of the scientific part of the programme was the reports on progress in the different departments. That on Surgery was made by Dr. W. L. Rodman, of Louisville; that on Medicine by Dr. J. W. Gilbert, of Lawrenceburg; on Hygiene, by Dr. J. N. McCormac, of Bowling Green; on Gynecology, by Dr. W. H. Wathen, of Louisville; that on Obstetrics by Dr. J. G. Cecil, of Louisville; on Laparotomy for Penetrating Shot Wound of the Abdomen, by Dr. David Barrow, of Lexington; on Medical Ethics, by Dr. Dudley S. Reynolds, of Louisville; on Diseases of the Rectum, by Dr. J. M. Mathews, of Louisville; on Ophthalmology, by Dr. S. G. Dabney, of Louisville; on Otology, by Dr. J. M. Ray, of Louisville; on Progress and Treatment of Pulmonary Tuberculosis, by Dr. F. C. Wilson, of Louisville; on Vital Statistics, by Dr. T. B. Greenley, of West Point.

Cincinnati was represented at the meeting by Drs. T. P. White, A. B. Thrasher and E. S. McKee. Drs. Thrasher and McKee read papers ; the latter was a delegate from the Ohio State Medical Society.

DR. J. A. OUCHTERLONY, of Louisville, read a paper on the Transmissibility of Tuberculosis, which was of much interest. The theory of inheritance he thought had been thoroughly shaken. Tuberculosis is rarely if ever congenital. The object of the paper was to show that tuberculosis can be transmitted from the lower animals to man. There can be no security from tuberculosis as long as tuberculous meat and milk are used. He insisted that the medical profession should bring this matter before the public and instruct them thereon. On motion, such a committee was appointed for such a purpose.

Several reports of cases and papers on the subject of extra-uterine pregnancy were furnished. The general opinion was in favor of operation, and not much faith was placed in the treatment by electricity, as it was thought practically impossible to diagnosticate this condition before the twelfth week; and what to do with the tumor when the child was killed by electricity was a question of difficulty.

DR. JOSEPH M. MATHEWS, of Louisville, read a paper on the Importance of Rectal Examinations to Life Insurance Companies. No company, to his knowledge, demands rectal examinations. He reported several cases in which applicants were received who had serious rectal trouble, which soon proved fatal and the insurance companies were heavy losers.

The discussion of acute traumatic tetanus was one of considerable interest, and drew out a number of case reports and treatment. The general opinion was that bromide of potassium is the best remedy. The only fear is that it may not be given in doses of sufficient quantity. Dr. j. C. Brooks, of Paducah, had given five grains of morphia hypodermically to a man once who was given over to die of traumatic tetanus, and the man recovered and remained well.

REPORTS OF CLINICS.

PHILADELPHIA HOSPITAL.

SURGICAL CLINIC—DR. STEINBACH.

Syphilitic Disease of the Tibia.

The patient before you, a girl twenty-two years old, is suffering from some severe bone lesion. The region of the tibia near the knee is riddled by several sinuses. The knee itself is anchylosed. Whenever there is severe disease near a joint, the joint itself will necessarily be fixed to avoid pain and, from the inflammation in the neighborhood, the joint structures will be bound together, not in a bony union but in a false anchylosis.

I do not know what I shall do here. I shall examine first and, if the joint is involved at all, will resect it and give the patient a fixed limb to walk on. Still, the bony tissue left may be too little to allow a resection at present and, in that case, there is danger that an amputation may have to be done at no distant time.

Bone diseases may be caused by traumatism, occasionally by struma, but, I believe, in this case it is due to a specific disease, which I need not name. The indications of knee-joint trouble are not very apparent here; still, the patella is hardly movable and the joint is fixed at an obtuse angle. It is supposed that an obtuse angle in the leg is better than a straight limb, but I do not find it so.

A long incision will be made over the tibia, and the dead bone found and removed. The probe entering a sinus goes straight up to the cartilage of the joint. The head of the tibia is the usual seat of necrosis and here the cancellous tissue immediately beneath the articular surface is so badly involved that my finger sinks into the bone. I have already invaded the knee-joint in following up the diseased structures. The bone is a mere shell, so that resection can not be thought of, there being no structure underneath to build on. The probability is that we shall have to amputate this limb, and it would be proper to amputate at once; but we have not the consent of the patient.

A large portion of the head of the tibia was curetted away, so that only a layer of cartilage was between the finger and the knee joint, which was distinctly involved. An Esmarch bandage had to be applied to control hemorrhage. Continuing, Dr. Steinbach said: In young subjects it is possible to remove large masses of bone and still have the cavity fill up. Care must be taken to leave no dead bone behind, otherwise the operation will be a failure. It is the same work as a dentist's, only on a larger scale. In removing the dead bone, I have left only a thin shell posteriorly, but the popliteal and the posterior tibial are so well covered with soft tissues that there is hardly any risk of injuring them.

It will be necessary to take even greater care of the limb than if it had been amputated, for the bone will break readily, so that a splint will be used. I curette thoroughly all the sinuses which led to the dead bone, and, although it is to be treated as an open wound. We desire to approximate the soft parts to some extent, and I will insert a few sutures and then the cavity will be packed with iodoform gauze.

Vertebral Abscess.

Abscess in the lumbar region almost always indicates caries of the vertebræ. It would be proper to speak of abscesses commonly called lumbar or psoas as vertebral abscesses, since it is entirely accidental whether they present below or above Poupart's ligament or in the region of the lumbar muscles. There is a villous membrane, apparently pyogenic, but the pus is really secreted from the vertebræ or intervertebral cartilages. We cannot, as in the last case, go down and remove the carious bone, but must be content with palliative treatment, and, as the internal organs are generally infiltrated with tubercles, palliative treatment is all that is really indicated. Before the days of antisepsis it was considered fatal to open these abscesses, but now we open them with impunity.

This patient has had other abscesses of this kind opened at different times during the last few years, so that she evidently has considerable vitality.

This abscess presents in the hollow between the lower lumbar vertebræ and the crest of the ilium, and near the median line. This is by no means an indication that the subjacent parts are affected. It may come down from the dorsal region, but more probably from the lumbar vertebræ. Since the parts have no large blood vessels, special care in making the incision is not necessary. Possibly this abscess communicates with the track of an old psoas abscess, which has been opened in front. Incising the abscess and introducing the finger, I find that this is the case, the abscess is only a compartment of a regular psoas abscess which has found its way around the crest of the ilium. I shall have the abscess washed out, a drainage-tube introduced, and the wound dressed antiseptically.

New York Correspondence.

Operations for Multilocular Ovarian Cyst, Pyolsalpinx and Pelvic Abscess, Lacerated Perineum, Spina Bifida and Necrosis of the Tibia.—The Hot Air Treatment of Phthisis.—Some Favorite Bellevue Prescriptions.

New York, May 6, 1889.

Dr. W. E. Bullard, of the Post-Graduate School and Hospital, removed a multilocular ovarian cyst, March 30, which was interesting from its size and contents. The patient was Catherine D., 45 years old, and a seamstress by occupation. Her history was rheumatic. She began to menstruate at 17, and was fairly regular until seven years ago, when her flow began to diminish. A year later it stopped entirely, and has not since returned. About this time, a tumor was felt in her abdomen. It grew gradually until when she entered the Post-Graduate Hospital last month it had attained an enormous size. The diagnosis of an ovarian cyst was easily made, and operation was necessitated by the dangerous symptoms of pressure, etc. Dr. Bullard cut down on the tumor and drew off the contents. There were in all 67 pounds of it, chiefly albuminous. One sac connected with the cyst contained a quart of colloid matter and several small ones contained dark grumous fluid. The solid part of the tumor weighed seven and a half pounds. Both ovaries were diseased and it was necessary to remove all the uterine appendages. The stump was secured to the incision in the abdominal walls, not with pins, but with silver sutures. By this means the abdominal cavity is closed and the stump left open for treatment. Dr. Bullard is a brilliant surgeon, rapid and sure, and the operation was not a long one considering its gravity. The patient rallied well, with little fever. A week later, when the wound was dressed, a mural abscess of considerable size was found, connecting with the sloughing pedicle. Treated with thorough antisepsis, however, it rapidly improved and the patient is now recovering.

March 31, Dr. A. P. Dudley, of the Post-Graduate and Women's Hospitals, operated at the former place for left pyosalpinx and pelvic abscess. The patient was a domestic, 31 years old, a widow with no children, having had one miscarriage two years ago. The latter was followed by an illness lasting six months, during which pus flowed from the rectum. There was a history of repeated pelvic abscess, from which the woman was also suffering on her entrance into the Hospital. Dr. Dudley performed laparotomy, removing both tubes and ovaries, which were diseased, curetting the walls of the abscess, breaking up the numerous adhesions, and stitching the rectum to the abscess walls. The result was a rapid and complete recovery. Dr. Dudley has his own way of closing the abdominal incision, using, instead of silver wire, three rows of catgut stitches. First he unites the peritoneum and lets it drop; next the fascia, the seam of which he includes in the next sutures which take in the abdominal muscles and integument.

Dr. A. F. Currier, of the Post-Graduate Hospital and School, performed an operation for lacerated perineum and rectocele, a few weeks ago, under cocaine. The patient was an American, 36 years old. She menstruated at 13, married at 14, her husband dying two years later. At her first menstruation she had a severe cold, which was followed by amenorrhœa for four months. At 15 she aborted with twins, and at 16 gave birth to a child weighing sixteen pounds. The labor was instrumental, long and difficult, and was followed by an illness lasting five months. She was remarried two years ago, and has since aborted twice. Three weeks before operation she was troubled with incontinence. Physical examination revealed extensive laceration of the cervix anteriorly and posteriorly, cystocele, recto-cele and lacerated perineum. Dr. Currier first operated for the lacerated cervix and cystocele, suturing the former with silver wire and the latter with catgut. The patient bore ether badly, and at the second operation for lacerated perineum and rectocele she had severe bronchitis, which contra-indicated ether. Accordingly the double operation was done under cocaine, and very successfully, the patient experiencing little pain.

Dr. L. A. Stimson, at a Bellevue clinic, operated on a case of spina bifida. The patient was a year and a half old, the son of Italian parents. He was born with a tumor the size of a walnut over the sacral region. It gradually increased in size until, at the time of the operation, it was as large as a double fist and had a broad base. The diagnosis lay between a cystic tumor and spina bifida, with indications favoring the former. It was aspirated and then a depression could be felt communicating with the spinal canal, which settled the question. At the aspiration ten ounces of clear fluid were withdrawn. The sac immediately refilled and the child grew weaker. It was decided to dissect out the sac and ligate it, hoping to save the child's life. He was given ether and an attempt made at dissection. The sac was so adherent, however, and the child took ether so badly that the operation had to be abandoned for the time. April 22, Dr. Stimson, by operating very rapidly, succeeded in getting rid of the tumor and bringing the child safely out from under the influence of the ether. An incision was made directly down through the sac wall and the sac emptied. The membranes of the cord and the cord itself in part protruded through the opening in the spinal canal, and numerous filaments were attached to the walls of the sac. These, with the terminal end of the cord, were all ligated, the inner part of the sac was cut away, the hæmorrhage was stopped, an elliptical piece of skin was removed, and by these means the sides of the collapsed tumor were nicely brought together and sutured with silk. A drainage tube was inserted at the lower angle and an ordinary antiseptic bandage applied. The child suffered from shock, but stimulation brought him around and left him in fair condition. The wound did nicely, primary union being obtained throughout. Meningitis, however, was developed; there was a temperature of 104°, projectile vomiting, rigidity of the neck, etc. At latest accounts he was doing well under bichloride of mercury internally and cold tubes to the spine externally.

At his clinic, April 15, Dr. Stimson exhibited a case of extensive necrosis of the tibia, upon which Dr. Gwyer operated for him. The patient, a boy thirteen years of age, had slipped on an orange peel nine months before, striking his right leg on the pavement. This accident was followed by fever, swelling, and a discharge. Since then he has been unable to walk upon it. There was enlargement throughout, a sequestrum involving a large part if not all of the tibia being evidently present. There were congestion and chronic inflammation, and the whole leg was literally honeycombed with sinuses. An incision was made over the whole length of the shaft of the tibia, and the periosteum raised, leaving the involucrum bare. This was chiselled away in front and several large and many small sequestra removed. These were easily loosened, being enclosed in pulpy granulation tissue and *débris* with some newly formed bone. The whole of the shaft was necrotic, and below extended to the epiphyseal line, and perhaps involving the epiphysis itself. However, it was thought best not to interfere with it. The involucrum extended entirely around the bone, and with the exception of what was chiselled away in front, it was left undisturbed. The pulpy tissues of the sinuses were scraped out and the cavity packed with bunches of cat-gut, drainage being obtained from the sinuses near the lower angle. Silk sutures were put in at each end and supporting sutures in the centre. Over this a dressing of curled hair soaked in bichloride of mercury was applied.

The operation was a long one but the boy recovered from the ether well and is doing nicely. This hair dressing is a new thing that promises well. It is aseptic, light, comfortable, and furnishes perfect absorption and drainage; and, where pressure is wanted, as in fractures, it is exceptionally good as it equalizes the pressure.

The treatment of phthisis by the inhalation of hot air apparently is not a success in Bellevue. It is being quite extensively tried, air at a temperature of 450° being used. Although the visiting physician is not ready to make a report of his experience it is understood that the patients have not yet shown much if any improvement.

The operation of grafting a rabbit's cornea on to the eye of a man was successfully performed here last week. The details will appear in the REPORTER very soon.

The following is the prescription for an expectorant mixture much used in Bellevue Hospital:

R Ammonii Carbonatis . . . . . gr. xxxij
   Extr. Senegæ Fluidi,
   Extr. Scillæ Fluidi   . . aa f ℥ j
   Tr. Opii Camph. . . . . f ℥ vj
   Aquæ . . . . f ℥ iv
   Syr. Tolutan. . . . . . q. s. ad f ℥ iv
Dissolve and mix. Dose, a teaspoonful.

As a gargle for inflammatory troubles, Dr. Abraham Jacobi's "Special" is used:

R Potassi Chloratis . . . . gr. lxxx
   Tr. Ferri Chloridi . . . . . . ♏ clx
   Glycerini . . . . f ℥ ij
   Aquæ . . . . q. s. ad f ℥ viij
Dissolve and mix. Used as a gargle and internally in doses of half ounce.

PERISCOPE.

Hysterical Monoplegia in a Man.

At the meeting of the New York Academy of Medicine, March 11, 1889, Dr. Robert Abbe presented a young man, about twenty-five years old, in whom hysterial mono-plegia was developed, the mild clonic spasm and its occurrence in a male patient making the case an uncommon one. This patient had fallen and struck on his back on a slip-pery pavement, had felt a sharp pain, and had at once lost full power to use the right leg. From this time on the right limb had been affected with anæsthesia, the gait had been irregular, and if the patient lay down and moved the limb about, a clonic spasm appearing like an exaggerated tremor was at once produced. Any general effort pro-duced violent trembling due to clonic spasm in the muscles of the neck and abdomen, and partial stoppage of respiration. Exqui-site sensitiveness was complained of when a portion of the spinal column opposite the first dorsal vertebra was pressed with a piece of ice. However, the anæsthesia was dimin-ishing, and when ether had been given, though the affected limb had remained weak while the patient was going under its influence, as he was coming out it had been used with the utmost vigor. It had become quite evident that the case was largely hys-terical in its nature, when it was also found that by suggestion the patient could be made to complain of the same pain in any other portion of the spinal column touched with the ice. On being forced to run along the wards quite rapidly, he had used the affected limb freely and had not stumbled. Mild clonus, said Dr. Abbe, is a rare affection, and has not been classified among any of the diseases of the nervous system. The monoplegia does not suggest a spinal paral-ysis. The condition present is probably an hysterical neurosis, perhaps due to shock, and existing without the patient's being conscious that his own ideas are so largely the cause of it.—*New York Med. Journal*, April 20, 1889.

Treatment of Certain Cases of Chronic Uræmia.

At the meeting of the Medical Society of London, April 8, 1889, Dr. Stephen Mackenzie read a paper on the treatment of certain cases of chronic uræmia. He regards uræmia as a poisoning of the nervous system—a toxæmia; and as the poison is developed within the body of the patient, it is an autotoxæmia. References were made to the writings of Grainger Stewart, Dick-inson, and Carter, and more especially to the researches of Bouchard, who had described seven toxic elements in the blood in uræmia. The principles of the treatment of uræmia he declared to be three: (1) the elimination of the poisons; (2) the counter-action of the poisons; (3) the prevention of the retention of further poisons. After discussing the first and last principles of treatment, which should always be employed, he proceeded to point out that the value of morphine is to fulfil the second indication. The author next discussed the nature of uræmic dyspnœa, headache, and convul-sions, and attributed the beneficial effects of morphine to its freeing the blood-vessels from the spasm induced by the poison in the blood. He referred to the writings of Loomis and his followers, and to cases recently recorded by Mr. Alfred Grace, in which morphine had been administered in as large quantities as from one-half to one whole grain for a dose, by hypodermic injections, with the best results. He con-cluded by saying he thought enough evi-dence had been brought forward to show that morphine deserves further trial in uræmia. He does not recommend its indis-criminate use, and in the light of the asserted susceptibility of patients with disease of the kidneys to the toxic effects of opium, it should be given with eyes open to its possible danger. There can, however, be no doubt as to its immediate good in suitable cases, and it is probable more lasting good will result in cases of a cura-ble kind.—*British Med. Journal*, April 13, 1889.

THE
MEDICAL AND SURGICAL
REPORTER.

ISSUED EVERY SATURDAY.

CHARLES W. DULLES, M.D.,
EDITOR AND PUBLISHER.

The Terms of Subscription to the publications of this office are as follows, payable in advance:

Med. and Surg. Reporter (weekly), a year, **$5.00**
Physician's Daily Pocket Record, -   -   - 1.00
Reporter and Pocket Record, -   -   -   - 6.00
All checks and postal orders should be drawn to order of

CHARLES W. DULLES,
N. E. Cor. 13th and Walnut Streets,
P. O. Box 843. Philadelphia, Pa.

☞SUGGESTIONS TO SUBSCRIBERS:
See that your address-label gives the date to which your subscription is paid.
In requesting a change of address, give the old address as well as the new one.
If your REPORTER does not reach you promptly and regularly, notify the publisher *at once,* so that the cause may be discovered and corrected.
☞SUGGESTIONS TO CONTRIBUTORS AND CORRESPONDENTS:
Write in ink.
Write on one side of paper only.
Write on paper of the size usually used for letters.
Make as few paragraphs as possible. Punctuate carefully. Do not abbreviate, or omit words like "the," and "a," or "an."
Make communications as short as possible.
NEVER ROLL A MANUSCRIPT! Try to get an envelope or wrapper which will fit it.
When it is desired to call our attention to something in a newspaper, mark the passage boldly with a colored pencil, and write on the Wrapper "Marked copy." Unless this is done, newspapers are not looked at.
The Editor will be glad to get medical news, but it is important that brevity and actual interest shall characterize communications intended for publication.

THE CHARGE AGAINST THE PHILADELPHIA HOSPITAL.

The last issue of the REPORTER contained an editorial describing the charges brought against certain nurses, or helpers, in the Insane Department of the Philadelphia Hospital, by a newspaper reporter, who had feigned insanity in order to investigate the management of the institution. These charges have been met in a manner highly creditable to the Board of Charities and Correction, which governs the hospital. The President of the Board acting for it, at once addressed an official communication to the District Attorney, reciting the published accusation and asking him to make such an investigation as shall discover in how far they may be true, and to take steps to bring to justice any person who may be shown to have been guilty of cruelty to the inmates. He has also taken steps to have the charges formulated in such a way as to bring them formally before the District Attorney for official notice.

In doing this the Board of Charities and Correction has taken the best step possible to strengthen the confidence reposed in it by the community. It is rather a new thing, in the history of institutions like the Philadelphia Hospital, to invite a thorough judicial investigation of charges made against them. The usual course is to deny the charges and to endeavor to screen those individuals who are directly implicated by them. In deviating from this course the authorities of the hospital have disarmed captious criticism, and shown that they know how to concede what is proper to an excited public sentiment, while awaiting with patience a vindication which shall be without favor or a correction which shall be without prejudice. Whatever the issue may be, as to the details of the charges of cruelty on the part of a few subordinates, the community will be sure to approve the wise and just attitude assumed by those who are indirectly involved in them; and the reputation for humane and skilful management, which the Philadelphia Hospital has of late years come to enjoy, will, we have no doubt, be enhanced by the manner in which the present exigency has been met.

A CASE OF HYSTERO-EPILEPSY IN A MAN.

On account of the comparative rarity of hysteria in men and especially of its severer forms much interest attaches to the history of a case reported by Drs. Andrée and Knoblauch in the *Berliner klin. Wochenschrift,* March 11, 1889. The case was observed at the garrison hospital at Karlsruhe. Instantaneous photographs were made during the several periods of the spasms and from them engravings which illustrate the paper. The following is an outline of the history of the case. A grenadier, twenty-three years of age, never having had any nervous disease or hereditary tendency of this sort, after great mental agitation, combined with great bodily exertion, was suddenly taken ill with violent spasms, and was brought to the hospital in a state of unconsciousness, on March 4, 1888. On examination in the hospital he was found to be a strongly built, very muscular and well nourished man; all the organs were normal, the pulse was full, bounding and regular, with about ninety-six beats per minute. The respirations were quiet and deep, and somewhat accelerated. There was no contraction of the muscles or wounding of the tongue or lips. A short time after being placed in a bed, the man had an attack of spasms lasting four minutes, succeeded during the same day by similar attacks. From the fifth to the seventh of March the patient had from six to nine attacks of spasms daily, of varying duration and intensity. From this time on, the attacks diminished in frequency, but increased in duration and in intensity, until finally there was developed the typical attack of *"grande hystérie,"* or hystero-epilepsy, with the three well marked stages described by Charcot, Richer and others. Always before an attack began, the patient had sensations on the breast, neck and the head, similar to the *aura epileptica.* A most remarkable feature of the case was the fact that the lightest touch upon the right nipple produced the hysterical aura, and this was followed by a typical attack when the nipple was pressed somewhat more firmly or when the skin was rubbed with the finger in a direction from the nipple upward toward the right side of the neck. On the other hand it was possible to suppress the attack in all its periods, and to put the patient in a state of a profound sleep, by rubbing the skin in the opposite direction—from the neck to the right nipple. An attack could not be produced by acting on the testicle, but it was possible to suppress one for a short time by strong pressure on one or both testicles, and also, in like manner, by strong pressure on the abdominal regions on both sides which corresponded with the position of the ovaries in women.

After the fifth day of the patient's stay at the hospital the frequency of the attacks diminished rapidly, and when they had failed to appear for six weeks, he was discharged. After two weeks he had a new attack lasting fifteen minutes. A final attack, lasting five minutes occurred five weeks afterward. During the last five months he had not had any more attacks, but was very well and able to work; and of late he had not had any evidence of having had a nervous disease.

This remarkable case is of great interest, as it illustrates the strange character of grave hysteria, to which the name is etymologically as inappropriate in women as in men. The possibility of developing an attack by pressing the nipple of one side or rubbing the skin of the breast in one direction, and of curtailing the attacks by rubbing the same skin in an opposite direction or pressing upon the testicles is as curious as any of the phenomena observed in hysteria in women. More curious still is the fact that pressure upon the abdomen, over the region corresponding to that of the ovaries in women, should have produced an effect similar to that observed when the ovaries themselves are pressed in hysterical women. This may be partly accounted for upon the theory that the pressure caused a sensation in the spermatic cord which was referred to the testicles, but the fact is none the less interesting.

MILK AND THE PUBLIC HEALTH.

The relation of adulterated, fermented, putrified or infected milk to the public health is a question which has assumed greater importance with the increase of knowledge of the etiology of disease. Adulteration of so necessary a food product as milk needs only to be mentioned to be condemned. It is now generally admitted that milk which has undergone fermentative and putrifactive changes, is a very frequent cause of diarrhœa in artificially-fed infants. The causative relation between certain products of the putrefaction of milk and other albumenoid substances and choleraic attacks in those ingesting them—known as picnic ice-cream poisoning, stale cream-puff poisoning, etc.—has been demonstrated, and largely through the investigations of Prof. Vaughan. The occasional dependence of epidemics, especially of scarlet fever, and other contagious diseases, upon infected milk is an accepted fact. That milk from tuberculous animals may prove a source of infection has long been a prevalent belief in the profession. This belief finds expression in the axiom that a tuberculous mother should not nurse her offspring. At the French Congress for the Study of Tuberculosis, held in 1888, the opinion was strongly supported that milk from tuberculous cows is a frequent source of infection. A case in point is that of Demme, of Berne, which was mentioned in the REPORTER, August 18, 1888. In this case an infant artificially-fed, and not hereditarily disposed to phthisis, died of tuberculosis of the mesenteric glands, as shown by the autopsy. The cow from which milk for the infant was obtained was killed and tubercle and bacilli were found in abundance in the left lung and pleura. Bacilli were also found in milk expressed from the deepest parts of the mammary gland. The statement that the relation between bad milk and the public health is an important one is seen to rest upon a solid basis. Unquestionably, however, the question of bad milk as a cause of disease and death among infants is relatively so great as to overtop the other evil influences arising from this cause.

The methods of milk supply in general use in Philadelphia and other cities do not protect the consumer against bad milk ; in fact, the incentive to the honest producer and dealer is to adulterate the milk, because he is in close competition with dishonest dealers who do. A number of methods have been suggested and tried to protect the consumer and the honest dealer. Systematic inspection has done much to improve the milk supply of New York, among other cities. It is conceded that proper inspection of milk to detect adulteration, together with stringent laws for the punishment of the adulterators, are powerful factors in ensuring pure milk to the consumer. But, however much the accomplishment of this end is to be desired, it really solves but a part of the problem. Milk which has undergone putrefactive changes, or which contains the contagium of scarlatina or the bacillus of tuberculosis is far more to be dreaded than milk which contains an undue percentage of water.

The method of delivering milk in sealed bottles or glass cans is advocated and practised quite extensively. In Philadelphia the method has been employed by Dr. J. Cheston Morris and others. In 1884, Dr. Morris read a paper before the Social Science Association of Philadelphia, in which he advocated the general adoption of this method of milk delivery. It is claimed for the method that since the seal is placed upon the bottle at the dairy, the consumer is protected against the dishonest retailer ; and since the producer's name appears upon each bottle, the demand for his brand depends solely upon its quality. Hence the producer has a constant incentive to furnish a good quality of milk. On the other hand, it is urged that the multiplicity of milk vessels increases the probability of the use of unclean vessels ; and that the liability of milk to be a means of propagating the infectious diseases is increased by the method, since the vessels are left at houses indiscriminately, whether their inmates are suffering from contagious diseases or not ; also that no protection is afforded against tuberculosis.

Prof. Vaughan, so well known for his researches in connection with the putrefaction of milk, has formulated certain rules which, if followed, would ensure a supply of good milk; though the spread of the contagious diseases and tuberculosis by means of milk might not be prevented. These rules comprise the exclusion of diseased cattle from dairies, provision for the sanitary condition of stables, exclusion of improper food, and cleanliness of the cattle. In this way good milk is secured. In order that it may be good when delivered to the consumer, it is to be strained in perfectly sweet and clean cans, and chilled by being placed in running water or ice water until its temperature is at or below 65° F. During this time the milk must be exposed to the air; only refrigerator cars must be used in its transshipment; and its temperature must never be above 65° F. when received by the consumer. To ensure the results sought by this method necessitates a large force of inspectors.

With a supply of whole, unfermented milk ensured the consumer, the problem of preventing putrefactive changes, and of destroying the germs of tuberculosis or the contagium of the exanthemata is probably solved by sterilization with heat. The usual method of boiling milk in open vessels probably destroys any germs it contains—the germs of disease as well as those of fermentation; but the method is open to objections. It is necessary to pour the milk into other vessels, thus it is freely exposed to the air and fermentation is favored. Practically, Caillé has found that "store-milk," after being boiled in an open vessel, when placed in an open dish in an ice-box "turned" after eighteen hours; and that good "bottle-milk" treated in the same way "turned" in twenty-six hours; and that the same milk when left standing in an open room with a temperature of 75° F., had a distinct sour taste and smell after from eight to fifteen hours. Milk boiled under pressure in small bottles for thirty minutes and left in the bottles remained good eighteen days. The very superior results obtained by boiling the milk under pressure would indicate this as the most desirable method.

The method followed and the apparatus used by Caillé were those of Soxhlet. The method is intended more especially for the sterilization of milk for infant feeding in private families. The apparatus is very simple and inexpensive. Practically the method consists in putting milk into five or six ounce bottles, into which a perforated rubber cork is inserted. The bottles are put in a water bath and the water raised to the boiling point. Glass stoppers are then inserted in the perforated rubber corks and the boiling process is continued for twenty minutes. This method and apparatus are largely used in Munich and Southern Germany, and to a certain extent in this country.

It appears that the principle involved in this method is so simple that it could easily be applied to the milk supply of a city. In discussing the method of supplying milk in sealed bottles, it was found that the two objections to the method were the greater probability of milk contamination from unclean vessels, and the danger of spreading contagious diseases from house to house. These objections would be overcome by boiling the bottles after cleaning them; and sterilizing the milk in the bottles before sealing them. Milk so prepared could not cause diarrhœa or cholera infantum, or be the means of spreading tuberculosis or any one of the infectious diseases.

A COUNTY SOCIETY SUSTAINED IN COURT.

It is interesting to note that judgment has lately been entered on a final order of Judge Ingraham of the Supreme Court of New York, sustaining the Medical Society of the County of New York in expelling from membership Dr. James O'Reilly, who advertises a so-called "Woman's Infirmary and Maternity Home," in which the special object seems to be to care for unmarried pregnant women.

In the circulars issued when this institution was first started there were intimations which might easily be construed into a willingness to relieve mothers of illegitimate children of all the responsibilities of their motherhood, as well as to furnish them a place of concealment during the latter part of their pregnancy and their lying-in period. These intimations, and the general methods of Dr. O'Reilly were calculated to arouse suspicion in regard to the motives and intentions of his institution, which posed as a charity, and the New York County Society expelled him, for a violation of the code of ethics—as we understand the case.

As the members of the profession in the city in which Dr. O'Reilly lives and has his "Infirmary" are best fitted to judge of the propriety of conduct which at this distance seems open to suspicion, we have no doubt that he got but his deserts in being expelled from the County Society, and are glad to find that the Society's action is now fully sustained by a judicial decision.

ANOTHER MURDER BY AN INSANE MAN.— A dispatch from Chicago to the daily papers states that a young man, twenty-six years of age, became suddenly insane while in bed, on May 5. After a desperate struggle with his wife, he took their babe from its crib and dashed its brains out against the wall. He then got a butcher knife and tried to kill his wife, but she escaped to the street. The man then cut his own throat with the knife, but did not kill himself. He was secured and taken to the hospital.

It is possible that the man in question had been insane for some time, but had been kept at home by his affectionate but misguided family. The case points to the importance of putting persons with certain forms of mental derangement under proper supervision and, if necessary, restraint at the earliest possible period. This is best as regards the patient's recovery, and is the only way to prevent such horrible acts as are illustrated in the present instance.

BOOK REVIEWS.

[Any book reviewed in these columns may be obtained upon receipt of price, from the office of the REPORTER.]

ELECTRICITY IN THE DISEASES OF WOMEN, WITH SPECIAL REFERENCE TO THE APPLICATION OF STRONG CURRENTS. By G. BETTON MASSEY, M.D., Physician to the Nervous Dept. of Howard Hospital, etc. Small 8vo, pp. viii, 210. Philadelphia and London: F. A. Davis, 1888. Price, $1.50.

The appearance of Dr. Massey's book at this time is opportune, and, unlike many books, we believe it will fill a "want," felt by the profession, which has been produced by the publication of the researches and results of Apostoli, Engelmann and others.

The introductory part of the work consists of a concise presentation of the laws of electricity, together with a description of the electrical apparatus necessary for the application of this agent to the treatment of certain diseases peculiar to women. Then follows a systematic consideration of the uses of electricity in gynecology. The author's claims are in general moderate, and fully justified by the present status of the subject. His moderation in statement is less apparent when he strays slightly from the domain of electricity into that of surgery proper. This is perhaps to be expected from one who has studied the subject from the standpoint of the neurologist and electrician rather than from that of the gynecologist.

It is especially pleasing to note that the author regards the presence of pus in the pelvis as a positive contra-indication to the use of electricity.

As already stated we believe the book will fill a "want," and owing to its scientific character and moderate claims it can be recommended to all who treat the diseases of women.

PAMPHLET NOTICES.

[Any reader of the REPORTER who desires a copy of a pamphlet noticed in these columns will doubtless secure it by addressing the author with a request stating where the notice was seen and *enclosing a postage-stamp.*]

265. REPRESSION OF MENSTRUATION AS A CURATIVE AGENT IN GYNECOLOGY. By EUGENE C. GEHRUNG, M.D., St. Louis, Mo. From the *American Journal of Obstetrics*, November, 1888. 12 pages.

266. FOOD VERSUS BACILLI IN CONSUMPTION. By EPHRAIM CUTTER, M.D., New York. From the *Virginia Medical Monthly*, December, 1888. 24 pages.

265. Dr. Gehrung, after a short consideration of the functions of menstruation in general, advances and defends the rather startling view that it may be advantageously interrupted by artificial means—vaginal tampons—whenever the flow seems to be greater than a woman can afford to lose. He believes that a flow of from two to four ounces of blood should be regarded as the maximum, and that the loss of quantities in excess of this is injurious to health.

266. It is not pleasant to criticise persons whose motives may be excellent; but how anybody can read patiently the stuff published by Dr. Cutter, we cannot see. The pamphlet before us is like all the rest of his productions which we have seen, and commends itself as little to our approval.

CORRESPONDENCE.

Catarrh of the Middle Ear.

To the Editor.

Sir: For the past two years we have had numerous cases of acute inflammation of the middle ear, of a catarrhal nature. So frequently have they appeared that they may justly be considered epidemic. Some cases are mild and are relieved after only two or three days of "ear ache," while others are very severe, having a destruction of the tympanum; the chain of bones, and deeper structures, with loss of hearing, leaving an offensive discharge from the ear which continues for months. When there is extensive inflammation in the tympanic cavity there are excruciating pains. In one case of four days standing, symptoms of compression of the brain appeared, after which the patient survived only twenty-four hours. In another case an opening was made above the mastoid process, from which there was a discharge of fœtid pus for several months.

In some of these cases the inflammation seemed to start in the ear, and in others it travelled up the Eustachian tube developing into intense severity after reaching the tympanic cavity Those attacked were of various ages, from one year to middle life. I have not seen one above fifty years of age. The most severe cases were in adult males.

Catarrhs have not been more prevalent during this period of time than in former years, but this particular form seems to be more prevalent.

Diphtheria has prevailed to some extent, but in not one of these cases of diphtheria has there been an extension into the tympanic cavity. I am a firm believer in the germ origin of diphtheria—but am not quite ready to attribute this epidemic to any form of micro-organisms. I believe the cause to be exposure to extreme cold winds; but I cannot explain why we should have such an epidemic, for one does not always follow such severe cold winds when

These cases are seemingly cut short by vigorous and persistent use of anodynes and sedatives—remedies which in diphtheria would be extremely pernicious. Opium alone does not control the pain; I usually combine it with gelsemium, and bromide of potass.

Yours truly,
John M. Currier, M.D.

Newport, Vermont,
May 6, 1889.

NOTES AND COMMENTS.

Useful Formulæ in Skin Diseases.

Dr. M. J. Epstein gives the following formulæ as in use in the service of Dr. W. A. Hardaway, at the skin clinic of the St. Louis Post-Graduate School of Medicine (*St. Louis Polyclinic*, May, 1889):

R Unguenti vaselini plumbici . . ℥ iv
S. Spread on cotton cloth.

One of the most universally applicable and valuable ointments in eczema is the diachylon ointment of Hebra; but owing to the difficulty of preparing it after the original formula, it is now generally made by melting together equal parts of vaseline and lead plaster. It should be neatly and evenly spread on strips of cotton cloth, and fastened to the parts with a roller bandage.

R Ung. picis liquidæ . . . . . . ℥ ss
   Ung. aquæ rosæ . . . . ℥ iss
   Zinci oxidi . . . . ℥ i
M. S Spread on lint.

This is of especial value in the eczema (chronic?) of children.

R Ol. rusci . . . . f℥ i-ii
   Ung. aquæ rosæ . . . . ℥ i
M. S. Rub in thoroughly.

Useful in sqamous eczema and also sometimes in psoriasis.

R Hydrargyri ammoniati . . . . ℥ ss
   Liq. picis alkalin . . . . . . f℥ i
   Ung. aq. rosæ . . . . ℥ i
M. S. Local use.

Employed in infiltrated eczema and in psoriasis of the scalp. It must not be used, over too large a surface.

R Acidi salicylici . . . . . . ℈ i
   Sulphuris præcipitati . . . ℥ i
   Vaselini . . . . ℥ i
   Ol. rosæ . . . . q. s.
M. S. Rub in thoroughly.

The range of application of this preparation is very wide, viz: seborrhœa and scaly eczema of scalp, tinea versicolor, keratosis senilis, and lupus erythematosus.

R Emplastri plumbi . . . . . . ℥ xxv
   Pulv. saponis . . . . . . ℈ iv
   Aquæ . . . . q. s.
   Vaselini . . . . ℥ v
   Camphoræ . . . . gr. xx
   Acidi salicylici . . . . ℈ v
M. S. Spread on lint.

This is a modification of Pick's compound salicylated soap plaster. It is much prescribed in the clinic for infiltrated eczema, especially of the hands and feet, and is now largely used in place of the more expensive Hamburg plasters of a certain kind. The amount of salicylic acid may be varied to suit the case.

R   Chrysarobini . . . . gr. xl
    Acidi salicylici . . . . gr. xl
    Traumaticini . . . . f ℥ i
M. S. Apply with a camel's hair pencil.

This combination affords the best results in psoriasis. After thorough removal of the scales, it should be painted directly on the patches, being careful not to put it on the face, or about the genitals. As is well known, chrysarobin occasions considerable dermatitis, and its effects must be watched.

R   Quininæ sulphatis . . . . . . gr. x
    Spir. myrciæ . . . . f ℥ iii
    Glycerinæ . . . . f ℥ i
    Sodii chloridi . . . . ℥ ii
    Aquæ . . . . . . q. s. ad f ℥ viii
M. S. Local use.

There are hundreds of so-called hair tonics, containing more or less of these ingredients, but the one here given is one of the most satisfactory of its kind.

R   Acidi salicylici . . . . ℥ ss
    Zinci oxidi,
    Amyli . . . . aa ℥ ii
    Vaselini . . . . ℥ ii
M.

The formula above constitutes the well-known Lassar's paste. It may be applied on strips of cloth, or in chronic scaly patches directly rubbed in with the finger. It is of value in many varieties of eczema and intertrigo.

R   Zinci oxidi . . . . ℥ i
    Glycerini,
    Mucilag. acaciæ . . . . . aa f ℥ ii
M. Apply with a brush.

In extensive patches of eczema this paste is very agreeable. If itching is severe, one per cent. of carbolic acid may be added.

The Death of Father Damien.

Father Damien, the heroic Belgian priest who devoted his life to the service of the leper colony in the Sandwich Islands, fell a victim to the disease on April 10. The readers of the REPORTER will recollect that mention was made of his desperate condition in the issue of January 26, and a brief statement of his self-denying labors in the issue of February 16, of this year. Father Damien had resided among the lepers for sixteen years when death came to his relief, and he had seen the population of Molokai renew itself three times, as the average duration of a leper's life is about seven years. Years ago, he became afflicted with leprosy himself, and for a long time before his death was a painful sufferer from the scourge.

The latest letters from the leper colony stated that his health was so broken that his death was likely to occur at any time. Father Damien had for assistants two men as heroic as himself. One of these was an Irishman named Walsh. He was a mason by trade, and had been a soldier in the English army. Walsh reached Honolulu in broken health and reduced circumstances just at the time a superintendent was needed to keep the colony in order. He accepted the position, with the result that he is a leper himself to-day and pining for relief in death. Father Damien's other helper was the Rev. M. Conrardy, a Catholic priest formerly connected with the Archdiocese of Oregon, who voluntarily went to Molokai about two years ago to become Father Damien's assistant.

Dr. W. W. Keen and the Woman's Medical College.

At a stated meeting of the Faculty of the Woman's Medical College of Pennsylvania, held May 18, 1889, the following resolution was adopted :

"*Resolved*, that the Faculty of the Woman's Medical College of Pennsylvania have learned with deep regret of the resignation by Prof. W. W. Keen, of the Chair of Surgery in this College. Dr. Keen's enthusiasm as a teacher in a department for which he is eminently qualified, and his unhesitating surrender of time in doing a generous share of Faculty work, have made his connection with the College conspicuously valuable and helpful.

The Faculty also desire to express their sense of personal loss in this severance of relations which have ever been most harmonious and agreeable, and to proffer their congratulations to Dr. Keen in view of his new appointment, with warmest wishes for success and happiness in his future work.''

CLARA MARSHALL,
Dean of the Faculty.

—Roger and Gaume have made a report to the Biological Society of Paris upon experiments concerning the toxicity of the urine of pneumonia patients. During the febrile period they state that the urine is two or three times less poisonous than otherwise ; with the crisis it reaches its least degree of toxicity, while after the crisis for two or three days it is considerably increased. They think the cause of the toxicity is an unknown poison, perhaps a substance produced by bacteria.

NEWS.

—The Legislature of Tennessee has passed a bill to regulate the practice of medicine in that State.

—The German Ophthalmological Society will meet at Heidelberg from September 13 to 15, 1889.

—An International Congress of Otology and Laryngology will be held in Paris from September 16 to 21, 1889.

—The annual meeting of the American Surgical Association was held in Washington, D. C., May 15, 16 and 17, 1889.

—Dr. William A. Douglass, Emeritus Professor of Anatomy in the Cooper Medical College, died in San Francisco, Cal., March 26.

—The *Nashville Journal of Medicine and Surgery*, April, 1889, announces that the plans for the new city hospital have been submitted, and that bids for the erection of the building will be opened at an early day.

—Dr. Duane B. Simmons, who has done so much for medical education in Japan, died there recently. The *Sei-I-Kwai* Medical Journal, April, 1889, contains a number of appreciative notices of his life and services.

—The Eleventh Annual Congress of the American Laryngological Association will meet at the Arlington House, Washington, D. C., May 30, 31 and June 1. A cordial invitation to attend the meeting is given to members of the medical profession.

—Under date of April 27, 1889, it is reported from Japan that a terrible disease, resembling malignant typhus, has broken out in Anagawa Ken. Of 64 cases, 40 ended fatally within 24 hours. The doctors attribute the disease to the use of bad rice.

—Dr. Charles E. West, of Brooklyn, who began teaching when only 18 years old, is now about to retire at the age of 80 years. For the last fifty years he has been connected with three schools, of one of which, the Brooklyn Heights Seminary, he is now President.

—Willard Perkins, a restaurateur, of Waterbury, Connecticut, died there on April 27, from congestion of the lungs and heart failure, attributed to excessive fat. He was born in Philadelphia, and at the age of 12 years weighed 250 pounds. At one time he weighed 452 pounds. Until he was 20 years of age he was exhibited throughout the country as "Billy Bates, the Philadelphia giant."

—A law to punish drunkenness went into effect in Minnesota on May 16. It provides that "whoever becomes intoxicated by voluntary drinking intoxicating liquors shall be deemed guilty of the crime of drunkenness, and, upon conviction thereof, shall be punished as follows: For the first offense, by a fine of not less than $10, nor more than $40, or by imprisonment for not less than ten, nor more than forty, days; for the second offense, by imprisonment for not less than thirty nor more than sixty days, or by a fine of not less than $20 nor more than $50; for the third and all subsequent offenses, by imprisonment of not less than sixty days nor more than ninety days."

HUMOR.

OUR NATIONAL NAVY should be rapidly doubled up with the Cramps working so persistently at it.—*Washington Critic.*

IF YOU FEEL mad when some rude person runs into you in the street, how must you feel when a locomotor ataxia?—*N. Y. Commercial Advertiser.*

JINGS.—"Chops is all broke up. The Sheriff has just seized his meat market." Jangs.—"Is that so? I saw him this morning, and I thought he looked as if he'd lost flesh."—*Lowell Citizen.*

A SUCCESSFUL AFFAIR.—Wife (to her husband, a physician)—"Did you stop at the Vancouver ball to-night, William?" Physician—For a few minutes, my dear." Wife—"Did it seem to be a successful affair?" Physician—"Oh, yes; while I was there a young lady fell in a faint, and I prescribed for her. Here is her father's card."

WALT WHITMAN, it is related, was called upon the other day by a young man with a large manuscript, which the visitor exhibited, remarking "Mr. Whitman, I should like to read you my drama and get your opinion of its merits." "No; I thank you," responded the good gray poet, "I've been paralyzed once." So was the young man forthwith.—*Ledger.*

SYMPATHIZED WITH NATURE.—Granger.— "Doc, thar mus' be suthin' left whar ye pulled thet tooth for me, last week. It's ached ever sence." Dentist (examining the mouth).—"Nothing there, sir, but a vacuum." "How big?" "Why, about the size of a tooth, of course." "Wal' yank 'er out, Doc. I knowed suthin' was wrong. I've heerd that nacher obhors a vackeyum, an' dinged if I blame 'er, 'f she ever got one stuck inter her jaw."

MEDICAL AND SURGICAL REPORTER

No. 1683. PHILADELPHIA, JUNE 1, 1889. VOL. LX.—No. 22.

CONTENTS:

COMMUNICATIONS.

THE SUBCUTANEOUS USE OF MERCURY IN SYPHILITIC AFFECTIONS.

BY E. BALDWIN GLEASON, M.D.,

PHILADELPHIA.

The treatment of syphilis by the injection of various salts of mercury, both soluble and insoluble, either into the subcutaneous cellular tissue or deep into the muscular tissue, has lately attracted considerable attention. In France the favorite method seems to be the deep injection of calomel suspended in fluid cosmoline; while in Germany a formula consisting of calomel, common salt and distilled water has been extensively used. It is claimed for these methods that abscesses seldom occur, and that the calomel, being slowly changed by the chlorides of the blood into the soluble bichloride, is more slowly absorbed, and thus a more constant and prolonged influence of the drug is obtained than is possible by other methods. It is also asserted that the injections need not be repeated at frequent intervals, as some days must elapse before all the calomel has been converted into a soluble salt and absorbed.

My own experience in the use of subcutaneous injections of mercury has been wholly in the treatment of severe syphilitic disease of the nose and throat, where the prompt action of an antisyphilitic remedy seemed essential to save my patient from disaster. I have always employed corrosive sublimate dissolved in distilled water, and used it in the manner taught me by Dr. Carl Seiler. When a solution of corrosive sublimate is injected into the tissues, an insoluble albuminate of mercury is formed, which is somewhat slowly changed into a more soluble compound and absorbed. Undoubtedly subcutaneous injections of bichloride of mercury are more quickly absorbed than those of calomel; yet I am persuaded that if they are repeated not oftener than once in twenty-four hours, a constant and unvarying mercurial action may be obtained as readily as by the injec-

645

tion of the mild chloride, and with less danger of producing an abscess.

If three grains of corrosive sublimate are dissolved in an ounce of distilled water, a solution is obtained which remains apparently unchanged for months, and is very convenient for use hypodermically. Ten minims of this solution contain one-sixteenth of a grain of corrosive sublimate, which is perhaps the average dose employed by the subcutaneous method in the treatment of syphilis, although it is well to begin with a somewhat smaller quantity and not increase the dose until the susceptibility of the patient to the effects of the drug have been ascertained. The injection may be safely made in the following manner: The syringe having been filled with the quantity of the solution to be used, and the patient's back exposed, he is made to kneel before a chair, and bend somewhat forward. The point of the needle of the syringe is then introduced deeply into the cellular tissue just below the scapula, and moved about in a quarter-circle to be certain that the point is entirely free. The injection is thrown into the tissues somewhat slowly. Placing a finger over the small wound made by the needle, the operator should thoroughly knead and rub the injected fluid into the tissues. Upon the thoroughness with which this is done depends the subsequent freedom on the part of the patient both from pain and also from the danger of an abscess. This is a matter of the greatest importance and should not be overlooked. No immediate pain is caused by the injection. Within half an hour, however, some pain and soreness are experienced by the patient, the degree seeming to vary inversely with the depth of the injection into the cellular tissues and the thoroughness with which the irritating solution is distributed and, as it were, diluted by being rubbed into a large area of cellular tissue. If the injection is simply thrown beneath the skin and allowed to remain there without being distributed, great pain will be experienced by the patient, and, although I have not seen it result, I think an abscess would not be unlikely to occur.

It is hardly necessary to remark that an special syringe should be reserved for this kind of work, to avoid any possible danger of contagion. Corrosive sublimate rusts the needles and, unless especial pains are taken to prevent it, in a short time renders them unfit for use. A good rule is always to wash out both syringe and needle after each injection with clean water, and then draw into the needle a few drops of fluid cosmoline before inserting the wire and putting the instrument away in its case. Even with these precautions the point of the needle soon becomes rough and dull and should be frequently sharpened to avoid inflicting needless pain. The following cases now under treatment will illustrate what may be accomplished by the subcutaneous injection of bichloride of mercury.

Case I.—The patient was a nursing mother, 26 years old, with a puny infant three months old. She had had three miscarriages and had, when she applied for treatment, pains in the bones; her hair had also become much thinner than it had formerly been. The woman was fat and appeared to be in robust, blooming health; but she complained that her throat was sore and that it hurt her to swallow food. Upon examination, the fauces presented the characteristic red lines of syphilitic erythema, running up each of the anterior pillars of the fauces and ending abruptly at the root of the uvula. These red lines are to be seen in every case of syphilitic disease of the nose and throat, although they are not pathognomonic of syphilis, as a similar appearance is presented in other conditions. At the first view, nothing further abnormal was presented; but, upon lifting the uvula and soft palate, upon the pharynx was seen what was probably the lower border of a large ulcerating gumma. Realizing the danger, as stated by Bumstead and Taylor, that a lesion so situated might "even invade the vertebræ and produce necrosis, or even inflammation of the contents of the vertebral canal," the woman was immediately ordered large doses (f℥iii) three times a day of the following mixture:

R Hydrarg. bichlor. . . . . . . gr. i
   Potass. iodidi . . . . . . ℥ ii
   Aquæ . . . . f℥iii

The nose and throat were thoroughly cleansed by means of a spray of Dobell's solution, and the surface of the ulcer carefully dried with absorbent cotton. The soft palate being now drawn forward out of harm's way, acid nitrate of mercury, one part to five of water, was thoroughly applied to the surface of the ulcer, and the patient requested to present herself each day that these applications might be continued.

In spite of this local and constitutional treatment, however, the ulcer continued to increase in size. Within a few days the posterior aspect of the palate and upper part of the posterior pillars became involved.

Knowing that if vigorous measures were not at once adopted to stop the progress of the ulcer, adhesions would form during the healing process which would glue the soft palate irremediably to the pharynx, subcutaneous injections of mercury were resorted to; one-sixteenth of a grain of the bichloride of mercury being at first used daily and afterward every other day; the former treatment in the meanwhile was continued. Within forty-eight hours after the first injection, the ulcer presented a more healthy appearance. In about two weeks it had entirely healed, leaving the fauces entirely normal in appearance, except for the red lines previously noted, which still extended along the anterior pillars and ended abruptly at the base of the uvula.

I was the more anxious as to the prognosis in this case from the fact that I had at the same time under treatment a young woman, who, as the result of a similar affection in a worse degree, had the posterior aspect of the vomer, vault of the pharynx, and remains of the soft palate glued together. Only a small opening from the mouth into the nose, which was just large enough to admit a small knitting needle existed at the junction of the hard and the soft palates. It having been found impossible, even after tracheotomy had been performed and the patient etherized, to dissect through the hard cicatricial tissues with a knife, the small opening already existing in the palate was gradually enlarged by means of the galvano-cautery, until nasal respiration was secured. The voice also was somewhat improved by securing some degree of nasal resonance; but in spite of her improved state the young woman's condition still remains deplorable. In the literature of the subject I find no surgeon claiming very brilliant results in such cases; every operation undertaken has resulted in a partial or complete failure. It would seem then, that the timely use of the subcutaneous injections saved the first patient from great and irremediable damage.

Case II.—The patient was an Irish servant girl, 24 years old. No history of syphilis could be obtained from the patient, but it was subsequently ascertained that she had been treated the year before for a gumma of the septum. She came to me suffering from obstructive nasal catarrh; and a small shelf-like exostosis was accordingly chiseled from the septum. For some days the wound made by the operation apparently did well, but suddenly the nostril operated upon became occluded, while mucous patches in the mouth and upon the pillars of the fauces showed plainly enough what was going on in the nose. Antisyphilitic treatment was at once instituted, subcutaneous injections of one sixteenth of a grain of mercuric chloride being given once a day. In about ten days the nose and throat presented a normal appearance. It is probable that only the prompt effects of the mercury used subcutaneously prevented permanent and complete occlusion of the affected nostril from cicatricial contraction. This case also illustrates the danger of performing any operation about the nose on a syphilitic, until the patient has been mercurialized. Yet after the exhibition of mercury for some days I have seen an obstinate gumma curetted from the nose and a speedy and brilliant result obtained.

Case III.—The patient was an unmarried woman, thirty years old. She had had three miscarriages, and was suffering from a painful swelling upon the left tibia. She presented herself for treatment for a catarrhal affection of the nose and throat, which was, however, of a mild type; but the characteristic red lines upon the fauces, previously referred to, were well marked. She was at once placed upon antisyphilitic treatment, but for some weeks no progress was made. The periosteal pain indeed became almost unendurable, especially at night. Subcutaneous injections of the bichloride had been proposed and rejected by the patient. They were finally, however, resorted to, one sixteenth of a grain of corrosive sublimate being used twice a week. After four of these injections had been used, the periosteal pain ceased at night and the swelling upon the tibia grew less. The injections were now discontinued, the patient continuing to improve upon the treatment which before had had little effect.

Case IV.—This patient was a respectable married woman, who some years ago contracted syphilis from her husband. Large ulcerating gummata existed upon the upper part of each tonsil and extended upon the palate. The patient was extremely emaciated and debilitated. She was ordered cod-liver oil and the mixture given the first patient. One-sixteenth of a grain of mercuric chloride was also injected subcutaneously every other day; and the lesions in the throat, after careful cleansing by the spray of an atomizer, were touched with acid nitrate of mercury, one part to five of water. Under this treatment the patient's health rapidly improved and she gained in weight. At the end of four weeks the gummata in the throat had left scarcely a trace of their former presence. Unfortunately the woman was obliged to leave for New York City, where she placed herself under the care of another physician. After the lapse of three or four months, she returned in about the same condition as when first seen. Injections again brought about as good a result as in the first instance.

These four cases illustrate fairly well what can be accomplished by the use of corrosive sublimate subcutaneously. It will perhaps be claimed that an equally good result might have been obtained from using mercury either by inunction or by fumigation. If this be so, the filthiness of inunctions or the bother and inconvenience of giving mercurial fumigations render either method much more objectionable than that by hypodermic injection.

Many physicians have doubtless been deterred from using mercury subcutaneously from the fear of giving their patients pain or producing an abscess. The third patient, in the cases cited above, was the only one who complained of the pain caused by an injection. The injection complained of in this instance was the first, which is always the most painful; and in this instance also the injection was not given deeply enough beneath the skin and was not sufficiently well rubbed into the cellular tissue. In other words, the injection was "given in a hurry." The danger of an abscess must be very slight when the method that I have advised is carefully followed. The nearest approach to an abscess that I have observed was a redness and soreness of the skin, which persisted one or two days.

Since writing the above my friend, Dr. Lawrence Wolff, has kindly placed at my disposal an unpublished paper read by him before the James Arthur Meigs Medical Society, at their January meeting. After giving the history of the "hypodermatic use," as he prefers to call it, of mercurials in the treatment of syphilis, both in this country and abroad, and the various preparations of mercury that have been used in this manner, the Doctor states his own experience. Commencing to use mercurials hypodermically in the year 1876, he is among the first, if not the very first, so to employ them in this country. During 1876, Dr. Wolff and his friend Dr. Rosentral gave seventy-seven hypodermic injections, each containing the average daily dose of from one-eighth to one-half grain of corrosive sublimate. In none of the cases thus treated in that year did an abscess occur. Since that time he has given over one thousand hypodermic injections, of never less than one-eighth of a grain and frequently as much as one-third of a grain of the bichloride, without producing an abscess. He employs a half per cent. solution of the bichloride of mercury in distilled water, and injects daily from twenty-five to fifty minims into the cellular tissue of the back and sides of the chest. In none of his cases were more than twenty-five injections given; and, as a rule, a total disappearance of the syphilides resulted after the tenth injection. Even late secondary and commencing tertiary syphilis yielded rapidly under this treatment, when inunctions had failed. No other antisyphilitic remedies were administered during the time that the injections were employed; but an after treatment of five grain doses of iodide of potassium or Blanchards pill was kept up for three months. Only a small percentage of Dr. Wolff's cases showed any relapse and required subsequent injections of the sublimate; while only one case had a second relapse and required the use of the injections for the third time.

1346 Spruce Street.

WESTERN NORTH CAROLINA AS A HEALTH RESORT.

BY JAMES GRAHAM, M.D.,
PHILADELPHIA.

The frightful mortality from the different forms of phthisis in the northern section of our country proves only too conclusively the inefficiency of the medical treatment of the disease. Each winter has witnessed a larger migration to our southern States of sufferers from this and other diseases which our rigorous climate affects injuriously; and as, with our progressive people, supply follows close upon the heels of demand and frequently runs far ahead of it, winter resorts have become so numerous that the physician is now able to show as much judgment in selecting a place as he is in choosing a remedy for his patient.

Western North Carolina has a climate peculiarly adapted to some classes of cases and unfitted for others. Its location makes it easily accessible to our largest centres of population, as good lines of railroad enter it, both from the northeast and also from the northwest, and traverse it, so that almost any part can be reached by a day's journey by stage. The extreme western portion of

North Carolina is about three hundred and fifty miles west of the Atlantic Ocean, and contains a plateau between the Blue Ridge and Allegheny mountains. This is crossed by seven ranges, and extends from southwest to northeast for two hundred miles from the thirty-fifth degree of north latitude. Its northern and southern portions are narrowed by the nearer approach of the mountains which border it. It varies in width from fifteen to sixty-five miles, and includes some six thousand square miles of territory. Most of this territory is occupied by immense forests of almost every variety of tree, with valleys varying in altitude from fifteen hundred to four thousand feet above sea-level. It contains the highest peaks in the United States east of the Rocky mountains, more than fifty of them being more than six thousand feet high. The Blue Ridge is the water-shed of the country, and the plateau is traversed by many rivers.

The temperature of this region varies considerably in different years and is liable at all seasons to sudden changes. The late evenings, the nights and the early mornings are cool in summer and cold in winter, while the middle of the day is hot in the former and warm in the latter season. Frequently a bright sunny day will be followed by a cold damp one.

The sensory nerves of a sick man are a better, though less scientific, indicator of the weather than the thermometer and barometer; and if, as he certainly should, he leads an out-door life, the matter of clothing will be a perplexing one to him. Flannel or silk underwear, heavy or light according to the season of year, is the most suitable, as it will tend to prevent a sudden chilling of the surface of the body; and as at these altitudes one perspires easily on taking active exercise, it will also be found the most comfortable on account of its absorbent qualities. A patient should also be provided with convenient outside wraps, to be worn as required.

/The soil in many parts of Western North Carolina contains a red clay, which makes the roads sticky and muddy for days after a heavy rain or snow. These drawbacks are largely overbalanced by the invigorating character of the atmosphere. It affects him like a stimulating draught; it revives his courage, tempts him to exercise, lessens the feeling of fatigue that follows, and, provided he has followed the dictates of his feelings and taken out-door exercise, he is astonished at the keen appetite he enjoys and his freedom from dyspepsia.

We may infer from the foregoing that this mountainous country is no place for persons with cavities in their lungs, or for patients with low vitality from any incurable disease, or for those afflicted with laziness. In the early stages of phthisis, on the other hand, when the patient has still considerable bodily vigor, in convalescence from acute diseases, and for those who are worn down by over-work or worry, this elevated peninsula of the North projecting into the South offers a temperate, bracing climate during the autumn, winter and spring, which is much superior to the enervating climate of the warmer lowlands of the South. When, however, the patient cannot or will not take out-door exercise, then he should go further South, where he can remain at rest in the open air for a large part of the day without suffering from the cold.

While this country has only enjoyed for the last few years a reputation as a Winter resort for Northern invalids, it has been a Summer resort for sixty years for the families of the wealthy planters and merchants of the South. For most of our patients requiring an elevated location in the summer months, the Adirondacks or the Alleghenies in Pennsylvania are preferable to the mountains of North Carolina; but the latter might offer a pleasant change, or even be more suitable for special cases. Here the Summer temperature will frequently run up to 90° in the middle of the day, but the nights are always cool enough to make a blanket comfortable, and there is almost entire exemption from those hot weather plagues—mosquitoes and flies.

Climate is not the only requisite in a health resort, pure water is a good second; and here it can be found in abundance and of the best quality, and where—as is frequently the case—it is brought direct from the spring, the epicure and the critic are both satisfied. When we come to speak of the food, our praise has to be changed to condemnation, as it is bad, even for the South. In the first-class hotels it is probably equal to that supplied in hotels of the same class in the North; but everywhere else the Northern palate will fail to be satisfied, excepting in those houses—which are now numerous—that are kept by Northern men.

Scenery and objects of interest are also important factors in assisting convalescence of patients, and in these respects Western North Carolina is difficult to excel. From many of the mountains there are magnificent and extensive views, but from most of them, the outlook is disappointing; for there is such an innumerable number of surrounding peaks that when one ascends to the summit he sees nothing but a succession of mountain tops, like billows of the ocean. Frequently, however, one side of the mountain will be so precipitous that the view from its brink will be grand and imposing. But, if the views from the mountains are not all that could be desired, the rivers and streams must ever be the delight of the lovers of the beautiful. The Little Tennessee, the Tuckaseigee, the Nantahalah, the Ocona Lufty, the French Broad, north of Asheville and especially at the Tennessee border line,—these, with their noisy, rapid currents, dashing over rocky beds, through narrow valleys with precipitous sides many hundreds of feet high, afford a never ending delight to the poor invalid. Then the primitive inhabitants one meets, their peculiar dialect, their strange customs and their miserable log-huts, make a progressive Northern man feel as if he had been wafted into a foreign land.

Asheville, the metropolis of Western North Carolina and its railroad centre, is as progressive as a Western town. It has a population of about ten thousand, with electric street-cars, electric lights, underground drainage, banks, telegraph offices, large stores, abundant hotel, boarding and lodging house accommodations and an unfailing supply of pure spring-water, flowing through the town from a huge tank situated high up on the mountain. Its principal hotel, "The Battery Park," is charmingly located above the level of the rest of the town, and is without a rival in the State or a superior in the whole South. But Asheville was not built as a health resort. It is situated on a large open space at an altitude of 2250 feet above sea-level, and is altogether unprotected on the north and west; whereas, on the southeast, where it should be open to the cool breezes of summer, it is hid behind a mountain range; consequently the cold northwest winds sweep it in the winter, and in the summer it is often oppressively warm.

Hot Springs, thirty-seven miles north of Asheville, is beautifully located in the valley of the French Broad, at an altitude of 1326 feet. It has an excellent, large hotel, attached to which are the warm springs; these have a temperature of from 90° to 100°. They are enclosed in two frame buildings; one of these contains a swimming-tank, where ladies, gentlemen and children bathe together; in the other are separate, marble-lined pools, with all the accessories to a most luxurious bath.

Waynesville, on the Western North Carolina Railroad, thirty miles west of Asheville, is a thriving town at an elevation of 2756 feet, and is admirably located for a summer resort. A few miles to the west of it is the majestic Balsam Range of mountains, the tops of which are black from the thick foliage of the trees.

Forty-five miles further west, on the same railroad, is Bryson City, the county seat of Swain. It is a town of 300 or 400 inhabitants, lying in a beautiful valley on the banks of the Tuckaseigee. It has a good hotel, kept by a Michigan family, and numerous boarding houses. There are abundant and easily accessible springs on the adjacent mountains, but it gets its water supply from wells. Its elevation is 1747 feet above sea-level, and with a pure water supply it would be a desirable winter resort. Ten miles away, on the Ocona Lufty river, is an Indian settlement and training school.

Franklin, on the Little Tennessee, is twenty miles south of the railroad, has 300 or 400 inhabitants, is in a rich agricultural country, and is at an altitude of 2141 feet. The scenery is uninteresting and the water supply objectionable.

The Highlands, a new resort settled by Northern people, is on the main stem of the Blue Ridge, at an elevation of 3817 feet. It has an admirably-kept hotel. Satulah and Whiteside mountains are easily accessible and, being isolated peaks, afford extensive views. Highlands and Oweacaluco Falls are within short distances. The Highlands are a delightfully cool and popular resort in the summer, but the water is obtained from wells; as it is situated on the top of the Blue Ridge, showers of rain are of frequent occurrence.

Twenty miles south of Asheville by rail is Hendersonville, a prosperous town of 1200 inhabitants, built at an elevation of 2167 feet. Three miles away and charmingly located is Flat Rock, the oldest of these summer resorts.

Thirteen miles east of Asheville the railroad crosses the Blue Ridge, and half-way down its eastern slope passes "The Round Knob Hotel," 2000 feet above sea-level. It is in the neighborhood of the highest peaks, is a summer hotel, and has an abundant supply of the best water, and also a more than abundant rainfall.

These are only a few of the resorts of Western North Carolina; "the woods are full of them," and each one claims to be the best—not of the State, but of the United States.

A pleasant and beneficial way of changing one's banishment into a vacation is to take a tramping or riding tour. Saddle horses can be hired at five dollars a week. A plentiful supply of pockets will carry all the essential luggage, and, if desired, a trunk can be forwarded by express from town to town. It would be advisable to spend the first week at, say, Asheville, taking a walk each morning and afternoon. After this preliminary training, with a map and compass in the pocket—but no firearms, as only honest, innocent and hospitable people will be met—you start forth, being careful not to attempt too long walks at first. Any house you stop at will provide you with dinner, and also put you up for the night. A request (not a hint) for chickens, eggs, butter and milk may supply you with a palatable meal; but if not, your appetite will show its quality and edge by feasting on fried pork, saur kraut, hot corn-bread with molasses, and black coffee; the stomach will digest it as easily as it would a meal at home that had been ordered by the doctor and prepared by the nurse. As there will probably be only one room in the house, the guest will occupy it as a bedroom in common with the host and his family. On account of the difficulty of getting an abundance of nourishing food, and as such a supply is so important for an invalid, it would be advisable, when possible, for the patient who is taking this tramp to stop overnight at a town where reasonably good fare can be obtained.

The most important fact in regard to this country is that, owing to the cheapness of living, the thousands of the working classes who are excluded by the expense from a prolonged stay at most health resorts, can here live more cheaply than they could at home. Boarding at farm-houses, off the line of the railroad, can be obtained at from five to seven dollars a month. To a Northern man it would be wretchedly poor living, but if he were willing to pay ten dollars a month, the fare would probably be found satisfying. For many consumptives nothing but a permanent change of climate is of any avail, and frequently such a change is required by the entire family. If their financial resources are limited, Western North Carolina offers them peculiar advantages. Building material is plentiful and cheap, eligible locations are innumerable, land can be bought for a trifle, and with, in the winter months, chickens selling at eight cents a piece, eggs at eight cents a dozen, and in season an abundance of delicious fruit worth so little that it is almost given away, a family could be provided with every comfort, be surrounded by the grandest scenery, breathe the most invigorating air, and be exposed to no extremes of temperature at any season of the year. These advantages are so numerous that the probable result will be, in the course of years, that this section of country will be inhabited mainly by Northern invalids and by those who follow in their train.

COLOR-SENSE, AND COLOR-BLINDNESS AMONG THE CHINESE, BASED ON AN EXAMINATION OF TWELVE HUNDRED PERSONS.

BY ADELE M. FIELDE, M.D.,

SWATOW, CHINA.

A love of vivid colors is manifested in all branches of Chinese decorative art. The walls of public buildings are commonly adorned with paintings—historical, dramatic or conventional. Porcelain dishes, paper scrolls, and gauze fans are made to glow with tints that are at once delicate and brilliant. The shoes of all bound-footed women and the costumes of all actors are covered with variegated embroidery. Countless hues are shown in the silken fabrics which are made into gala-dresses for both men and women. Children, on festive occasions, are always gorgeously attired. Not only little Joseph, but also all his brethren appear in coats of divers colors; and no one thinks it amiss to put on a cap of scarlet, a tunic of buff, trousers of green and shoes of pink. Whether in garb or in pictures, there is nothing in Chinese taste that forbids the juxtaposition of purple and green, of rose and orange, or of any other known tints. Like nature herself, they boldly array themselves in all colors, and the experienced eye is no more offended by their tegument than by that of a mandarin duck or a macaw.

A few colors—black, white, red, yellow, light blue, dark blue, bright green, dull green, and flesh color—have each a name of one independent syllable, while their shades are indicated by prefixed adjectives. Many other colors are designated by reference to familiar objects, as "peach-blossom" for pink; "pig's liver" for brown; "coir-palm" for russet; "ashes" for drab; and "grapes" for purple. Dye-stuffs furnish terms for several colors, and "ink-water," thus used, becomes a comprehensive appellation for pale gray; but it is not easy to see why the effects of logwood dyeing should be termed "celestial green" when manifested in satin, though "red night" has a poetic sound for the same shade in cotton goods.

The fact that the cloudless sky is always called green by the Chinese, and their lack of precision generally in regard to colors, led me long ago to consider them deficient in color-sense. As I could find no account of their ever having been scientifically tested for this defect, I read last· year the books of Prof. Holmgren and Dr. Jeffries, procured Dr. Thomson's stick of Berlin wool-tests, and thought myself equipped for preliminary investigations. I have now tested twelve hundred persons, and have found among them twenty who are either red- or green-blind. The two sexes were equally represented in the number tested. Among the six hundred Chinese women, I found only one who was color-blind by Thomson's tests. This woman was completely green-blind; and all her four sons were color-blind—the eldest three completely green-blind and the youngest completely red-blind.

Among the six hundred men tested, nineteen were found to be color-blind. This number includes the four sons of the color-blind woman just mentioned. Of these nineteen men, thirteen were completely green-blind, five were completely red-blind, and one was incompletely red-blind. The last was a brother of one who was completely red-blind. The nineteen color-blind men included eleven farmers, two teachers, two students, one hospital-assistant, one clergyman, one mason, and one boatman.

By taking the forty skeins of yarn, which are suspended upon Thomson's stick, and piling them in confusion upon a white cloth, I was able to observe, as recommended by Holmgren, the action of the hands in the selection of colors; while the brass tags upon the skeins helped me in making quick record, for future reference and comparison, of the selections made by each individual. I did not, in testing, use the names of the colors; but I first held up the green sample skein, and said: "I am going to pick out, from the pile of yarns, all that are of the same color as this one, whether light shades or dark. Then I shall mix all the yarns together again, and ask you to pick out the same ones that I picked out." When I had taken out all the green yarns, I asked all to look sharply at them, so that they might easily recognize them again. By first showing what I wished them to pick out of the pile, I saved much time in testing the normal-eyed, while I gave no undue assistance to the color-blind.

Upon those found to be color-blind, the tests were repeated, often many times. One color-blind man was very desirous of learning how to distinguish the colors, and as he was at leisure, he remained by my side and gave close attention while a hundred other persons were tested; and yet, after having been repeatedly allowed to "try again," he made precisely the same mistakes as in his first examination. To green he not only added the usual "colors of confusion," but also pale pinks; while with pink he invariably matched bright blues, without adding any of the greens. This young man, like many others, made marked effort to discover differences in the fibres of the wools, or to find some means of distinguishing the skeins otherwise than by their color. Nine other of the twenty color-blinds in the first test also matched green with pink; but of these nine, eight were proven by the second test to be green-blind, matching pink with green.

In all cases where there was doubt of the patient's clearness of vision, tests for form were applied before the tests for color.

I have, following Young and Helmholtz, set down as red-blind all those who, in the second test, matched pink with blues only; and have set down as green-blind those who in the same test matched pink with greens alone, or with both greens and blues. Nine among the thirteen set down as green-blind matched pink with both blue and green.

The persistence with which more than half of the twelve hundred persons tested matched green with blue is remarkable. Even the brightest blues were added to the selected greens after repeated injunctions against so doing. While the tests established the fact that a much smaller percentage of· Chinese women than of Chinese men are color-blind, yet those men who by their out of door lives had gained a greater degree of mental training than is possessed by their secluded women-folk chose the correct colors as rapidly as did the women, and no oftener added blues to greens. While there was an almost universal lack of discrimination between green and· blue, two colors distinctly named in their own language, the tests afforded by Thomson's skeins, prepared expressly for testing railroad employés for red and green blindness only, were insufficient to prove, what I now suspect, that many Chinese are violet-blind.

The number examined, twelve hundred, is too small to rely upon for a percentage of red- and green-blindness among the Chinese. Further tests would add nothing to its value, unless subjection to the examination were made compulsory, for many of the color-blind would avoid being tested through fear of appearing stupid before their neighbors. Moreover, the dislike of the Chinese to everything which is not evidently profitable, and their dread of evils that may come to them through occult influences, make it difficult to test any large number. Those examined by me were mostly members of the mission schools and patients in the mission hospital, together with the dwellers in some hamlets, where I endeavored to omit no one from the test.

The proofs of color-blindness must always appear startling to normal vision. It gives one qualms to realize how little one knows of the consciousness of one's neighbor, and how difficult it is to think how the world must look to one who sees the same hue in a tea-rose and a pea-pod, in a rosy cheek and an azure eye, or in a bay horse and a peacock's tail. Even the stolid Chinese appear to be deeply impressed by the exposition of color-blindness.

REPORT OF A DEATH UNDER ETHER.

BY. A. W. RANSLEY, M.D.,
VISITING SURGEON TO THE PHILADELPHIA HOSPITAL.

Death under ether is a comparatively rare accident; but it occurs often enough to make it desirable that every case should be placed on record to assist medical men in forming their judgment of the relative value and safety of different agents used for anæsthesia. For this reason, I give here a brief account of a death which recently took place during an operation undertaken by me in the clinic of the Philadelphia Hospital.

The patient, D. A., 36 years old, was admitted into the Surgical wards of the Philadelphia Hospital about three months ago. The diagnosis was: Coxalgia. On taking charge of the wards on the 1st day of April, 1889, I found the patient suffering extreme pain. He was anæsthetized and examined, and extension was applied. The suffering was considerably ameliorated, the relief continuing for about one week, when his suffering returned and it was found expedient to take off the extension. It was now found on examination that pus had commenced to be formed, and an operation was advised for its speedy evacuation. Accordingly, I had the man brought before the class on May 18, and etherized. The condition of the patient did not contraindicate the use of ether or the performance of the operation. In fact it was imperatively necessary that free vent should be given to the pus.

The patient acted well under the ether (the pulse being moderately strong and regular) until the joint had been opened, when an enormous quantity of pus was evacuated. It was not until the abscess had been opened that any evidences of the terrible calamity that was to follow, showed themselves. Now, however, the patient's countenance suddenly changed; his face became cyanosed; his respirations became shallow and gasping; his heart fluttered, and death speedily ensued. Although everything that could be done for the patient was resorted to, the man died almost as if struck by lightning. It took fully twenty-five minutes to get the patient under the influence of the ether, but the operation was performed in a very short space of time,—fifteen minutes, so that the death occurred about forty minutes after the etherization was begun. Ten fluid ounces of Squibb's ether had been administered, by means of a cone formed with a towel, an opening being left at its apex, by one of the Residents of the Hospital.

In accordance with the law, an autopsy was held by the Coroner's physician; and no direct cause of death was discovered. To my mind it appears that the cause was the effect of the comparatively sudden evacuation of an enormous quantity of pus from a subject already weakened by disease and under the influence of an anæsthetic which—however rarely—certainly *sometimes* acts as a dangerous depressant.

The previous etherisation was without alarming symptoms, and the last gave rise to no anxiety until immediately before the fatal termination.

Whatever may be the correct theory as to the manner in which death was produced in this case, I think it proper to state the facts of it for the information of my professional brethren.

—Professor Billroth, of Vienna, celebrated his sixtieth birthday April 26.

SOCIETY REPORTS.

SIXTH CONGRESS OF THE ITALIAN SOCIETY OF SURGERY.

AT BOLOGNA, APRIL 16, 17 AND 18, 1889.

(Specially reported for the MEDICAL AND SURGICAL REPORTER)

(Concluded from p. 632.)

PROF. CASELLI, of Genoa, read a paper on the

Extirpation of Goitre,

in which he said: Up to date, I have done seventy-eight extirpations of goitre, with but one case in which complications occurred. Out of this number, I think I have extirpated the thyroid gland entirely in fourteen cases; I say I think I have done so, for during the operation, amidst the blood and numerous ligatures, one cannot positively state that some of the degenerated gland might not have been left in the wound. The latter accident is sometimes a happy occurrence for the patient, for the function of the part left preserves the patient from the grave general accidents which are often consecutive to a complete extirpation.

In one case, I operated upon a woman who presented an enormous tri-lobed goitre; ·I first extirpated the right and median lobes of the tumor. One year later, I extirpated the remnant of the goitre, the left lobe; seven days later the patient presented already very severe symptoms of the goitre cachexia; the urine was albuminous, and the number of blood globules had fallen to 2,900,000 in a cubic millimeter. These symptoms, however, became less marked; seventeen days later the number of blood globules had risen to 3,600,000, and this favorable change was explained when simultaneously a small tumor appeared in the crico-thyroid space, formed by a fragment of the gland which had escaped extirpation, and the consecutive development of this saved the patient from a fatal cachexia.

As regards the consecutive general phenomena, I think that a total extirpation of the thyroid body is much more serious if it is practised on young persons. It seems that the importance of the thyroid body in reference to the functions of the organism diminishes with increase of years. The nature of the tumor must also be taken into consideration. The tumors which have brought about a complete abolition of the physiological function of the thyroid body, can be extirpated without any fear of subsequent bad results; but if one has to deal with young persons, to whom the thyroid body is necessary, it would be useful to leave in place a certain portion of the gland.

Bruns and Kocher attribute the alterations of the tracheal and laryngeal cartilages, which are met with in goitre, to a fault of nutrition, due to a compression of the inferior thyroid artery. I myself think that these alterations are due to the direct compression of the tumor, for these alterations disappear when the goitre is extirpated.

DR. BASSINI, of Padua, said: In 1884, I extirpated a large goitre in the case of a young woman, who, after the operation was seized with symptoms of the cachexia strumipriva; but these symptoms soon disappeared. At the same time, there appeared on the sides of the neck, in the supra-clavicular fossæ, little tumors, which brought about the complete cure of the patient. Three of these nodules I extirpated for microscopical examination; they were thyroid adenomas, which convinces me that the tumor which developed in the neck of our patient was of thyroid origin.

DR. TRICOMI, of Rome, read a paper on the

Absorbent Power of the Bladder.

I have studied the power of absorption of the bladder with the healthy and pathological epithelium, in rabbits, dogs and guinea-pigs. I have used mechanical irritation, such as the introduction of a foreign body into the bladder, to produce the epithelial alterations. The following are my results, taking as a comparison the absorption of the same substances by the hypodermic method of administration.

In a bladder, having a healthy epithelium, the absorption is equal to that which takes place from hypodermic injection, with the following substances: sulphate of strychnine, medicinal prussic acid, chloroform, sulphuretted hydrogen. The absorption is less rapid for cantharidine, carbolic acid, corrosive sublimate, morphine, and especially for cocaine; for, to obtain in rabbits the same toxic effect as with one-half grain injected hypodermically, we must inject into the bladder from two to two and a half grains of cocaine. Again, if we inject putrefied liquids into a healthy bladder, we get no results.

In cases in which the vesical epithelium is in a pathological state, absorption of substances of the first series—strychnia, hydrocyanic acid, and chloroform—is the same as by the hypodermic method. The absorption of substances of the second series is less rapid than in cases in which the bladder is normal. Injections of micro-örganisms has always been followed by positive signs of intoxication in a bladder the epithelium of which has been mechanically and chemically altered. In a bladder undergoing a suppurative process, the absorption of gaseous substances is as rapid as after hypodermic injection; the absorption of bacilli is also very rapid.

DR. D'ANTONA read a paper on

Splenectomy following a new Febrile Infection due to a Special Bacillus.

The following case occurred in a patient who presented himself at my clinic, and it constitutes what I think to be a new disease. A child, two years and a half old, son of a physician, was attacked with a left pleurisy with effusion; he recovered, the exudation being absorbed. Two weeks after the disappearance of the effusion, a gastro-intestinal catarrh accompanied by jaundice set in. The child recovered; but from this moment began a sub-febrile state, with a temperature that has gradually increased from 100.2°, 102.1° up to 104° Fahr. in the evening, the thermometer marking 100.2° in the morning. An examination of the abdomen gave evidence of a tumor of the spleen. The child was then taken to the country and for several days he became worse; the thermometer in the evening went as far up as 105.4°; but on the thirteenth day the fever disappeared.

During these stages of aggravation, the spleen was excessively hypertrophied; later the splenic tumor persisted, notwithstanding the general amelioration in the state of the patient, who was treated with quinine, arsenic, and the mercurial preparations. When he was brought back to town in a splendid house and in a most healthy locality, far from any malarial influence, he was again seized with fever, and one month after his return, he still had a temperature of 101° in the axilla. His general state, however, remained good; he had a very good appetite, ate a great deal, was on his feet, and walked even with a temperature of 104° Fahr. The fever was of the continuous type; it never was intermittent and was never accompanied by chills or sweats. The spleen, however, always increased in volume. An antimalarial treatment was then recommended, but it proved useless. The pulse was small and gaseous. The intellectual faculties were well preserved. All belief in a malarial influence had to be put aside; we had to deal with a special infection of the spleen, as this organ increased in size with the fever.

I proposed the extirpation of the spleen, which was so much hypertrophied and indurated that it reached down to the right iliac fossa. The operation was permitted, and on the same day on which splenectomy was performed there was a reduction of temperature to 99°; then a slight fever, reaching in the evening to 100.2° and even 102° developed. The child ate well. Then supervened a gastro-intestinal catarrh, the temperature went up to 104°; then came a purulent otitis, with a temperature of 105.5°; the liver increased in volume, until it extended beyond the umbilical line, but decreased in size afterward and returned to its normal size. The child was at this time in good health for about five months, when he died of tubercular meningitis, which might have been transmitted to him by his father, who was then treating two patients suffering with the same disease.

The extirpated spleen weighed as much as one-tenth the total weight of the body. An examination of the blood before the operation gave a negative result. The blood obtained from the spleen, gave rise, eight days after the operation, to colonies of bacilli exactly similar to typhoid bacilli. Bacilli developed very rapidly on gelatin and water at the temperature of 64.4°; but on potatoes this bacillus proved absolutely sterile, which is an important point in the differential diagnosis from the typhoid bacillus. Inoculation of animals with this bacillus gave negative results. From these studies I infer that we had to deal with an infectious disease, not yet described.

DR. CECI draws attention to the unexplainable relation which seems to exist between tumors of the thyroid body, spleen and tonsils, and menstruation. The following observations he made on a young woman from whom he removed the spleen, three years ago. Twenty days after the operation an hypertrophy of the thyroid gland developed; four months later, the tonsils became very much enlarged and one had to be removed. Ten days after this last operation the goitre had disappeared.

DR. SALVATI, of Naples, read a note on

Cerebral Grafting,

and said : I have made the following experiment on two dogs; I have exposed a part of the cerebral cortex, with an oculist's lancet, and removed a small portion, about the size of a pea, from a convolution, and placed it in sterilized water at 77° Fahr. To obtain complete checking of bleeding, I used electricity; one of the electrodes was placed on the back of the dog, the other, which terminated in a platinum wire, in the convolution which had been cut; the hemorrhage was checked completely in ten seconds. The divided part was then reapplied as a grafting; the adhesion and result were perfect, as shown by the specimen before you. It is therefore possible to rely upon the uniting of two fragments of cerebral tissue.

DR. RUGGI, of Bologna, reported a case of

Resection of the Liver.

A woman came to me with a bi-lobed tumor in the right hypochondriac region, which by percussion appeared to be covered with intestine. An hydatid cyst of the kidney was suspected; but this hypothesis was soon given up, for we found no blood and no albumin in the urine. I performed laparotomy, and found two enormous echinococcus cysts in the liver, one anterior and superficial, the other posterior and deep. I enucleated them and then tried to unite the sides of the large opening which I had made in the liver; but I could not succeed. I then resected three inches of liver tissue so as to make the cut regular, and fixed the surface of the liver to the border of the abdominal parietes. In the first few days, I was obliged to change the dressing very often, on account of the persistent flow of bile which escaped from the cut section of the liver; but gradually this secretion diminished, and the patient recovered.

A microscopical examination of the resected portion of the liver showed me that the orifices of the biliary channels remained open on account of a new formation of connective tissue. I do not think that we must follow Loreta's process, which consists in letting the liver remain free in the abdominal cavity, after having excised a portion from it; although this practice succeeds in lower animals. I shall always recommend, in operations on man, to suture the margins of the hepatic wound to the sides of the wound in the abdominal parietes.

DR. CECCHERELLI says that he uses Paquelin's thermo-cautery as a hemostatic. He wishes to know how Dr. Ruggi stops the hemorrhage, which is ordinarily very severe and which has often been the cause of death of the animals on which he has experimented. He also thinks that the animal dies if a quantity of the organ greater than one-third of the total volume of this organ is extirpated.

DR. CECI: Can not the biliary channels, which remain gaping on the cut surface, be tied, and how is the bile carried out when the section has been made with the knife or the thermo-cautery?

DR. BOTTINI: How is it that Dr. Ruggi, in his experiments, cuts portions of the liver and then allows the organ to return into the abdomen, without concerning himself about the hemorrhage; and yet the animals live, while those of Dr. Ceccherelli all die of hemorrhage?

DR. DURANTE explains this difference by the fact that Ruggi's animals were rabbits and guinea-pigs, and those of Ceccherelli were dogs, in which the liver bleeds very readily. With a good control of the bleeding, one-half of the liver of an animal can be removed without killing it. As to ligaturing the opened biliary ducts on the surface of the cut, this is impossible. To prevent the external flowing out of the bile, we must, before we operate on the liver, excite a localized adhesive peritonitis between the parietal and visceral layers, and then cut the liver with the thermo-cautery.

DR. LORETA does not think that the effusion of bile into the peritoneum can have any bad consequences. He thinks that the bile of the biliary vesicles has toxic properties which the bile of the liver does not possess.

DR. POSTEMPSKI has made experiments on dogs to study the resistance of the peritoneum to the action of the bile; he has found that the peritoneum of dogs supports very well a certain quantity of bile, if it is effused at once; but it does not resist a continual flowing out. He has found biliary pigments in the urine. He thinks that the cause of death is peritonitis, but a non-septic peritonitis. He has seen that in dogs limited resections of the border of the liver occasion a very slight hemorrhage, while incisions on the concave or convex surfaces of this organ are followed by death.

DR. CECCHINI says that, in his numerous experiments, he never had any hemorrhage either in rabbits or in dogs.

DR. TANSINI asks what are the symptoms presented in case of bile effusion into the peritoneum?

PROF. CLEMENTI read a paper on

Battey's Operation,

and said: This method deserves to be seriously considered as it is a certain method of curing rebellious metrorrhagias. In the case of a woman 40 years old operated on by me three years ago, the patient had suffered with very severe metrorrhagia for eight years previous. The trouble was probably multiple fibro-myoma of the uterus. As every means employed had failed, I did a salpingo-oöphorectomy, in preference to a supra-vaginal hysterectomy, the first operation being much less serious than the second one. The cure was complete in nineteen days, and has persisted up to date, which makes three years.

The bottom of the uterus, which before the operation, was three inches above the symphysis pubis, is now on a level with it. The general state is very much better. The only things of which the patient complains are headache and congestion of the face which occur at periods corresponding to menstruation. Is Battey's operation to be performed in all cases of metrorrhagia or tumors of the uterus? Yes, for all the cases in which other treatment has failed.

DR. BOTTINI: After the publication of Meyer's statistics the operation of Battey has lost ground, and it seems to-day that the intervention is justified only in cases of grave hysteria. It is true, that after the extirpation of the ovaries the uterine tumors diminish in volume and cease to grow, but when the abdomen is open why should we restrict ourselves to the extirpation of the ovaries and leave the uterus in position?

DR. BASSINI: Although I am very much in favor of the extirpation of the uterus, I nevertheless meet with cases in which I am obliged to employ Battey's operation; that is, in cases in which the tumor is interstitial and deeply situated in the posterior wall of the uterus. The results obtained have been good—cessation of metrorrhagia and sometimes a considerable diminution in the size of the tumor.

DR. DURANTE: By the electric treatment, much better results are obtained than by oöphorectomies. With this method I have had but one failure. I think that before having recourse to the operation, the surgeon must first try the electric treatment; a few seatings will be sufficient to tell whether or not electrolysis will do any good.

DR. BENDANTI read a paper on

Trephining in Epilepsy.

I have applied the trephine in the case of a man, 37 years old, for extremely severe convulsive phenomena; he was suffering at the same time from an intercurrent hemiparesis. No neoplasms could be discovered, although the cerebral cortex was incised. Still recovery from the operation was obtained, and the epileptic phenomena have not reappeared; this I attribute to the strong effect of the operation on the œdema of the centers of this region; and I think the treatment of epilepsy by trephining is justifiable.

DR. CLEMENTI does not think that the brain should be too often exposed, as the results of intervention, except in cases of abscess, are often negative.

DR. BASSINI: As it is always difficult to arrive at a certain diagnosis in lesions of the cortex, I think it is allowable to interfere, if only for exploratory reasons; especially if we meet with incurable epilepsy. I remember one case in which there was very severe excitement, and a depression of the left parietal region; the condition was very much ameliorated by an operation; hence, I think that our colleague is too absolute in his proscription.

DR. BENDANDI: I do not think that trephining has been abused in the treatment of epilepsy, and if in tumors of the cerebrum surgery has not always been the high trump, yet we must recognize that it is our only chance of cure.

DR. MARACEO, of Naples, reported two cases of

Oöphoro-salpingectomy for Severe Nervous Troubles.

A young woman suffered from the age of 15 with convulsive attacks, especially severe during her menstruation; she tried to commit suicide on three different occasions. She had complete retroflexion of the uterus, with lesions of the appendages. As she attempted a fourth time to commit suicide, I had recourse to the following operation: I removed the two ovaries, which had undergone cystic degeneration, and the two tubes, which were chronically inflamed; I destroyed the numerous adhesions which existed between the intestinal coils and the anterior surface of the uterus, and having straightened this organ, I fixed it to the abdominal wall. The painful attacks disappeared, and the patient is perfectly well.

I also performed oöphoro-salpingectomy on a woman, suffering with very severe nervous trouble. For several years after, she suffered with periodical hematemesis, but without any bad effect on her general health.

Drs. Cizzoni and Poggi, of Bologna, read a note on

Reconstruction of a Bladder,

and presented a dog from which they had removed the bladder completely. This organ was then reconstructed with a portion of the intestine, to which the operators sutured the urethra and both the ureters. The animal is perfectly well and his urinary functions are perfect.

Dr. Babacci, of Macerat, read a note on

Elastic Suture of the Liver.

To obtain a complete checking of bleeding, after an incision has been made into the liver, it is necessary to suture this organ, in such a way as to establish perfect adhesion to the affected surfaces. For this purpose elastic sutures are best. Not one single animal on which I have tried this method of suture has suffered from peritonitis or other infectious disease. These sutures with the elastic thread, allow a certain increase in size of the organ, without tearing the tissues. The extremities of the elastic thread are connected with the sutures by a silk ligature.

REPORTS OF CLINICS.

PHILADELPHIA HOSPITAL.

CLINIC ON DISEASES OF CHILDREN—
DR. STRYKER.

Jaundice and Ophthalmia Neonatorum.

I am able to illustrate this morning, in the same patient, two affections of very early childhood which you will be called upon to treat. This child is hardly six days old. It has an intense yellow staining affecting the whole face and body. As a general rule, the affection is much less marked than in this case. The coloration comes on upon the fourth or fifth day after birth, and remains from five or six days to two weeks, and then gradually shades off in color as the biliary pigment is taken up. It is a species of jaundice, and is called icterus neonatorum. The exact cause is unknown, but it is supposed to be due to the alteration of the circulation through the liver at birth. In most cases it calls for no treatment, but in other cases a gentle purge, such as sweet oil or castor-oil, is indicated.

Another interesting feature of this patient is an irritation about the eyes, which has been quite severe. It was first noticed on the second evening after its birth. Although the eyes have been carefully treated and great improvement has occurred, you can see the redness of the conjunctivæ and the yellowish matter that seems to be smeared over them. This is purulent ophthalmia, ophthalmia neonatorum, and it demands prompt attention. An ordinary catarrhal conjunctivitis, in which only a little dry mucus is found in the corner of the eye in the morning, will usually require little attention except bathing with warm water. Breast-milk is used for it by the mothers. In ophthalmia, however, the conjunctiva becomes red and swollen, and inside of twenty-four hours, it begins to pour out a secretion, at first thin as in all such inflammations, but soon becoming viscid and gluing together the edges of the lids and filling up the chamber between the eye-ball and the glued lids. It soon, also, presses so much on the eye-ball as to jeopardize it, to say nothing of the danger of the extension of the inflammation to the corneal conjunctiva.

What is supposed to be the cause of this disease? In an ordinary mild case, possibly the effect of cold or of dust getting into the eye, or an irritation of the eye from washing may be sufficient explanation. But in an attack such as this, the source of the infection is either in an irritating leucorrhœa or in a gonorrhœa. In the great majority of cases, the eye is destroyed or there is such a deposition of inflammatory products as to leave trouble for life.

Rapidity is of all importance in the treatment of such cases. First cleanse the eye thoroughly, and repeat the cleansing as often as necessary—even to the extent of fifty times a day. In addition, use a solution of silver nitrate (5 or 10 grains to the fluid ounce). Make the applications yourself. Take your seat opposite the nurse who holds the child, and place the child's head between your knees so as to hold it securely. Raise the upper eye-lid with the fingers of your left-hand while the nurse pulls down the lower lid with the fingers of her right hand. When the lids are swollen, as in this case, it is difficult to evert them; and it may be absolutely impossible to see the eye-ball. Examine it if possible, as it is important to keep track of the case. When the lids have been opened, briskly paint over the eye, with a camel's hair brush, your solution of silver nitrate. After a minute or two, neutralize it with a solution of common salt.

For cleansing the eye between the applications, use plain warm water, or mercuric chloride, 1–4000, and keep light cloths, soaked in a cold solution of the same strength of corrosive sublimate, constantly over the eyes.

It will not be necessary to continue this vigorous treatment more than twenty-four hours. You may continue to use silver nitrate (gr. ss to f ℥ j), but I prefer to change to zinc sulphate (gr. ss–i to f ℥ j) and put three or four drops in the eye, three times a day. Other methods are suggested, such as syringing out the eye, which may be useful at times when the lids can not be opened so as to expose the eye-ball; but I think you can do just as well with the brush or with absorbent cotton as with anything else.

FOREIGN CORRESPONDENCE.

LETTER FROM BERLIN.

(FROM OUR SPECIAL CORRESPONDENT.)

Prof. Leyden.—Trichinosis of Twenty-seven Years Standing.—Disorders of School-Children.—Maximum Dose of Sulphonal. —A Young Poisoner.—The Bacillus of Musk.—A Monstrous Whale.—Congress of Internal Medicine at Wiesbaden.— Good Specialists must first be General Practitioners.—German Laws to Prevent Deception by Quacks.—Dettweiler on Tuberculosis.—Fibrinous Rhinitis.—Chronic Prostatitis.—Electric Massage.

BERLIN, April 13, 1889.

Prof. Ernst Leyden, of the University of Berlin, celebrated this week his twenty-fifth anniversary as a teacher of clinical medicine. The *curriculum vitæ* of Leyden, Germany's greatest living clinician, is full of interest. He started in Berlin, as all Professors *in spe* do, as a *privat-docent*, but was very soon called to Königsberg, then to Strassburg, and returned to Berlin after an absence of nine years. In Königsberg he worked in conjunction with Recklinghausen and Spiegelberg, and in Strassburg with Waldeyer and Gusserow, who are now both his colleagues at the Berlin University. After Frerichs's death he took charge of what is called the first medical clinic of the Charité. Leyden was the pupil and *protégé* of Traube, the great clinician, and has followed closely in his footsteps. Traube and Leyden can claim the credit of having introduced into Germany experiments on animals in the study of morbid conditions. Leyden studied at the Berlin Military Medical Institute, and counted among his fellow-students such men as Virchow, Helmholtz, Nothnagel, Fräntzel, Schmidt-Rimpler, Reichert and other now famous medical men. Among Leyden's prominent works, the following deserve particular mention: "Observations on poisoning with sulphuric acid" (his doctorate thesis, 1853); "Researches on the sensibility of healthy and sick individuals"; "The gray degeneration of the posterior columns of the spinal cord"; "Acute poisoning with phosphorus"; "The pathology of icterus." His most eminent work was 'the clinic of spinal affections.' Leyden can be regarded as a worthy successor to Frerichs, though many declare that no living physician equals Frerichs even approximately, while others regard Prof. Senator as Germany's most eminent clinician.

Speaking of Prof. Senator, a singular case, coming recently under the observation of this physician, is recalled to my mind. A patient, who had been treated for œsophageal cancer, had died and an autopsy was instituted. The examination showed the entire body crowded with trichinæ. There was not a single fibre of a tissue in which hundreds of the spiral parasite could not be detected; in a single muscular flap, weighing one and two-thirds grains, 280 trichinæ were counted. The clinical history showed that the patient had been a night-watchman, and that in an epidemic of trichinosis which had visited his native place in 1862 he had also become infected, but had recovered again. He attended to his duties uninterruptedly, but complained occasionally of rheumatic pains. The man, therefore, had a case of chronic trichinosis of twenty-seven years standing, which probably has no equal in the literature of this disease.

The German Imperial Government has ordered a special investigation of certain disorders occurring among school-children, believing that there is an etiological relation between the disorders and the modern school methods. First came the investigations in regard to myopia, which had become of alarming frequency, especially in the higher schools of Germany. Prof. H. Cohn, the famous Breslau oculist, was in charge of these examinations, which have not been wholly without success, as henceforth such examinations are to be made at regular intervals throughout the Empire.

Of greater interest were the observations

made on school-children by Dr. Bresgen, of Frankfort-on-the-Main. He found that in many children, who were notoriously inattentive and slow in making head-way, neglected disorders of the ear or nose, such as catarrhs or slight inflammations, could be detected. Dr. Bresgen pointed out that an impeded nasal inspiration caused a pressure in the frontal region, which could readily produce a bad effect on mental development. Such children complain of headaches, ringing in the ears and similar conditions, grow more and more inattentive and lazy. Dr. Bresgen's pertinent reports to the Secretary of Instruction were not heeded until the observations of Prof. Guye, of Amsterdam, confirmed the experience of the German observer. Guye found in adults that nasal catarrhs of long standing and of a neglected character exert a most deleterious influence over the entire mental condition of the patient. He found as results of the conditions mentioned morbid headaches, vertigo, progressive decrease of the perceptive faculties, disinclination and even inability to work. All of these symptoms disappeared after the cure of the nasal affection. Other observers have also confirmed the views and assertions of Bresgen and Guye. As after measles and scarlet fever disorders of the nose and ear are of especially frequent occurrence, it seems the duty of the teachers or rather, of a special school physician, to attend immediately to these conditions. Great mental disturbances can in this way be prevented by a timely and trivial attention.

It has been left to a workingman to answer satisfactorily the question of the maximum dose of sulphonal, regarding which therapeutists have hitherto not agreed altogether. Hans Knickebein, a workingman engaged with Riedel and Co., the Berlin manufacturers of sulphonal, decided to exhibit this hypnotic to his spouse, in order to alleviate her insomnia which, of course, is rather troublesome to a husband accustomed to coming home late, as was the practice of Hans. He consequently took home a good quantity of the drug, but, as a conscientious physician, he decided to determine previously the proper dose on himself. He took two tablespoonfuls of the salt. The effect of the drug was good ; the man slept *ninety hours*, awoke and slept again for *twenty-four* more hours. He had taken *eight drachms* of sulphonal, which had produced a sleep of one hundred and fourteen hours' duration, but, fortunately, no other ill effects.

A half-grown girl, 14 years old, was recently tried before the Berlin Courts for three attempts to poison children with oxalic acid. In two instances the girl had mixed the poison with the milk intended for the children on whom she waited, and in the third instance she had poured the acid into Hungarian wine which she sent to the parents of her intended victims by mail, as if coming from their family physician, after previous notification by a postal card. The special interest attaching to the case is the fact that no reason whatever could be assigned to the criminal attempts of the young poisoner. Possibly we have to deal here with a new type of mental aberration, which could be properly termed toxomania.

There are about twenty-five Japanese students attending the medical schools of Berlin, and it has been noted with satisfaction by the University authorities that nearly all of them have shown special inclination and aptitude for original work and researches. Dr. Ritasato has just published an interesting report on a new bacillus, belonging to the class of *fuxisporium*, which has the peculiarity of producing the smell of musk. Hitherto we knew only of bacteria which produced special colors or poisons or of such as were luminous, while a smell-producing bacterium was never heard of. The musk-bacillus was first discovered in an infusion of hay, and can be cultivated on various culture-soils, especially on rice and potatoes. Its cultures are at first reddish, then brick-red, and always give out the distinct and characteristic odor of musk. Dr. Ritasato's name is already known in medical literature through his contributions on the cholera-bacillus.

The sensation of the day in Berlin is a monstrous whale, which however has not been caught in the Spree, but has been transported to Berlin from a Danish island, where it had stranded and perished of hunger. The whale on exhibition belongs to the order known as *mysticetes*, which has barbs on the upper jaw instead of teeth, and to the family of *balænoptera musculus*. The stupendous business of embalming the monster has been undertaken by Dr. Wickersheimer, of Berlin, in connection with a Danish chemist. The height of the animal is sixteen feet, its length sixty-four feet. The number of barbs is about three hundred and seventy-five. This variety of whale, in spite of its gigantic proportions, swims with ease and a rapidity, it is said, fifty miles an hour, so that for a trip around the world about twenty-five days would be sufficient. The animal's intestines, which were taken out in Copenhagen, weighed about twelve thousand pounds. It is hoped to preserve the animal for a long time, and possibly ultimately to mummify it. From Berlin the whale is to be taken to Vienna.

The annual Congress of Internal Medicine, at Wiesbaden, is always regarded as an important event by the German profession, and is sure to attract many clinicians and teachers of fame and a multitude of practitioners from all parts of the Empire. Among the host of notable medical men present at the Congress this year, were Liebermeister, of Tübingen; Leube, of Würzburg; Vieror, of Leipzig; Jürgensen, of Tübingen; Curschmann, of Leipzig; Rosenthal, of Breslau; Bäumler, of Freiburg; Ebstein, of Göttingen; Fürbringer, of Berlin; Immermann, of Basle; and Petersen, of Copenhagen.

The Congress was opened on April 15 by an address by Liebermeister, who spoke of the aims and purposes of the annual discussions on internal medicine, as originally planned by Frerichs and Leyden, the founders of the Congress. The expanse of specialties, Prof. Liebermeister said, has of late been enormous, and, while it testifies to the ever progressing development of medical science and practice and as such is to be welcomed, it is not devoid of serious danger. The young physician selects, possibly already during his collegiate career, frequently a specialty and devotes his time and attention to the great neglect of internal medicine and general practice. No physician can ever become a specialist of note, unless he is a good general practitioner, and to be a good general practitioner means to have devoted many years of studious care and hard work to general practice. Internal medicine is the trunk of all medical practice, and to its furthering and fostering German practitioners have decided to meet annually in beautiful Wiesbaden, to exchange their views and to discuss the recent advances of their art.

Liebermeister, in the course of his felicitous address, complimented the German Government on its constant endeavors to protect both the public and the regular practitioners from the unscrupulous devices of patent medicine men and quacks. The public, Liebermeister said, can expect from the Government the same protection regarding their bodies which their purses receive with respect to the lottery and confidence men. For the sake of a better understand-

ing of the protection German citizens receive in regard to medicine and treatment, your correspondent begs to explain that no patent medicine whatever, which consists of more than one constituent, is allowed to be advertised by a paper or by any other means. The Government, besides, publishes in all daily papers a precise analysis, including medicinal worth and actual cost, of all remedies sold by patent medicine venders. The following advertisement, for example, can be found in all papers: "Attention! Druggist H. H. Darner, of Rochsburg, formerly a carpenter, sells a remedy, under the name of 'H. H. Darner's Safe Dyspepsia Cure,' at the price of three marks (75 cts.). The alleged remedy consists of (here follows an analysis of the ordinarily very simple composition). Medicinal value, none; but it may under certain conditions be injurious. Actual cost, three pfennigs (four-fifths of a cent). The public is warned against buying the above article. V. Richthofer, President of Police, Berlin. No physician, besides,—and this refers to every other sign—is allowed to hang out a sign unless the police have given, after careful investigation, their sanction. (How would it do to treat similarly all pretenders in the medical line in America?)

The most interesting paper of the Congress, and one which elicited most valuable discussions, was that of Dr. Dettweiler on Tuberculosis. The researches made some time ago by Dr. Cornet, of Reichenhall, in the Hygienic Institute of Berlin, under the directions of Prof. Koch, have thrown a new light on the mode of propagation of tuberculosis. A consumptive person, Dr. Dettweiler said, *per se* is quite harmless as far as contagion is concerned, provided his sputa are at once thoroughly disinfected. Tuberculosis can, in his opinion, based on numerous and careful bacteriological and clinical observations, be propagated only through the sputum of the patient. A tubercular patient who uses either a handkerchief, or an ordinary spittoon, or spits on the floor, can communicate the disease to his neighbors, and the atmosphere surrounding such a patient is impregnated with the pathogenic bacilli. After the sputa, which have been thrown into an ordinary spittoon, on the floor, or into a handkerchief, have become dried, the bacilli reach the atmosphere, mingle with the fine atmospheric dust and are disseminated at large. They may settle on walls or pieces of furniture, and may for a long period retain their vitality. The question arises, what can we do to check the propagation of the disease under this new etiological light? The answer would be: very little without direct legislation on the subject and strict enforcement of the ordinances to be passed eventually. The point to be reached is evidently a compulsory disinfection of either all sputa —which of course is impossible—or, at least, of the expectorations of tubercular persons, which is also a matter of great difficulty. In countries with a powerful and well-concentrated police apparatus the prospects of success or, at least, of improvement in the direction indicated are somewhat more hopeful than in a free country such as America. Legislation should, according to Dr. Dettweiler, enforce the placing of spittoons filled with an antiseptic solution in all public places, hospitals, schools, etc., and see to the instruction of the school and public at large on the subject. Tubercular subjects, besides, should be compelled immediately to render their sputa antiseptic. To facilitate this desideratum, Dr. Dettweiler has constructed an ingenious little antiseptic pocket-spittoon for the permanent use of consumptives. The little instrument in question has two openings; the upper one serves for emptying the sputum, and has a screw lid which, as in pocket ink-stands, prevents the flowing out; and the lower one serves for the antisepsis and elimination of the sputum. In this manner both the hygienic and æsthetic requisites could be fulfilled.

The remarks of Dr. Seifert, of Würzburg, on fibrinous rhinitis proved also of considerable interest. The speaker illustrated the subject by microscopic specimens. The affection occurs, Seifert said, both in a primary and in a secondary form; the former is principally found in children, and the latter is extremely rare. To call the affection *rhinitis crouposa* Seifert regards as little commendable, all the more as the line of demarcation between croup and diphtheria is not yet accurately fixed.

Dr. Posner, of Berlin, read a valuable paper on the diagnosis and therapeutics of chronic prostatitis. This affection, Posner maintained, is very often overlooked and mostly difficult to diagnosticate because of its symptoms, which are chiefly internal ones, and because a local examination is frequently neglected. It is not a rare occurrence to have a patient treated for years for sexual disease, until its prostatic character is revealed. Within a rather recent period, the speaker said, the diagnosis of chronic prostatitis has been materially facilitated. Seifert referred then to his own researches on the nature of the prostatic secretion, which allowed of a ready determination of the disease.

The paper of Dr. Nordhorst, of Wiesbaden, on electric massage, was of special interest. In order to utilize in chronic affections of a traumatic and rheumatic type simultaneously, the beneficial action of massage and of the constant current, Nordhorst has constructed a massage-electrode (in the form of a little roller) which not only conducts the current, but also as an instrument of massage is far superior to the hand. The electrical massage is performed in exactly the same manner as an ordinary massage. The advantages of an electrical massage are not merely of a theoretical nature but have also been practically confirmed. Of 208 cases treated with this form of massage all could be discharged as either completely cured or materially improved. Precisely the same disorders as are eligible for ordinary massage are suitable for electric massage. It is, however, especially indicated in all rheumatic affections of joints, muscles, nerves and tendons. In migraine this treatment is also of value. The results obtained with the electric massage in the Wilhelms Heilanstalt, of Wiesbaden, harmonize with the speaker's experience: Of 33 grave and inveterate cases, treated for months with massage and electricity without success, 23 were cured by the combined treatment. Nordhorst then referred to a pamphlet entitled "Therapeutic Success of Electrical Massage," in which he had embodied all pertinent information.

Prof. Liebermeister closed the Congress, which he regarded as the most successful one of all Wiesbaden meetings, both as regards scientific value and also as regards general attendance. The Congress had been visited by 300 physicians.

———————◆◆◆———————

—Dr. Pinel, of Paris, according to the *Electrical World,* has succeeded in hypnotizing several subjects by means of the phonograph. All the commands given through this channel were as readily obeyed as those uttered directly, and "suggestions" of every possible sort were as effectually communicated through the medium of the machine as if made *vivâ voce.* The conclusion deduced by Dr. Pinel is that the theory of a magnetic current passing from the operator to the subject is entirely baseless, and that the real cause of the phenomena of hypnotism is nervous derangement on the part of those subject to them.

THE
MEDICAL AND SURGICAL
REPORTER.

ISSUED EVERY SATURDAY.

CHARLES W. DULLES, M.D.,
EDITOR AND PUBLISHER.

The Terms of Subscription to the publications of this office are as follows, payable in advance :

Med. and Surg. Reporter (weekly), a year, **$5.00**
Physician's Daily Pocket Record,　-　-　- 1.00
Reporter and Pocket Record, - - - - 6.00
All checks and postal orders should be drawn to order of
CHARLES W. DULLES,
N. E. Cor. 13th and Walnut Streets,
P. O. Box 843.　　　　Philadelphia, Pa.

☞SUGGESTIONS TO SUBSCRIBERS:
See that your address-label gives the date to which your subscription is paid.
In requesting a change of address, give the old address as well as the new one.
If your REPORTER does not reach you promptly and regularly, notify the publisher *at once*, so that the cause may be discovered and corrected.
☞SUGGESTIONS TO CONTRIBUTORS AND CORRESPONDENTS:
Write in ink.
Write on one side of paper only.
Write on paper of the size usually used for letters.
Make as few paragraphs as possible. Punctuate carefully. Do not abbreviate, or omit words like "the," and "a," or "an."
Make communications as short as possible.
NEVER ROLL A MANUSCRIPT! Try to get an envelope or wrapper which will fit it.
When it is desired to call our attention to something in a newspaper, mark the passage boldly with a colored pencil, and write on the wrapper "Marked copy." Unless this is done, newspapers are not looked at.
The Editor will be glad to get medical news, but it is important that brevity and actual interest shall characterize communications intended for publication.

THE AUTOPSY ON MR. BISHOP.

The daily papers all over the United States have during the past week contained a great deal about the autopsy made upon Washington Irving Bishop, who was widely known as "the mind-reader." Mr. Bishop died suddenly in New York, with no relatives at hand. Within six hours an autopsy was conducted by a pathologist who was called in for that purpose by the attending physician, and soon after the story was started that, when this was done, the subject was not dead, but merely in a trance.

Nothing could be more calculated to excite widespread notice,—and it is not surprising that a judicial investigation has been begun by the Coroner of the city of New York to get at the facts in regard to the case.

Medical men will be slow to believe that any pathologist of experience could commit the horrible blunder of opening the body of a living person. It is not to be disguised however that there would be some risk in making an autopsy within six hours after the apparent death of a person of an intense neurotic nature—like Mr. Bishop—who had been in vigorous life but a few hours before, and who was subject to cataleptic attacks, unless more precautions were taken, to be sure of the fact of death, than are needed in ordinary cases. It is not impossible that the condition of so-called trance should deceive those who are unfamiliar with its manifestations, or not on their guard against the possibility of its occurrence.

But in the case of Mr. Bishop, the physician who had the autopsy made was one who had known him for years and who was aware of the fact that he was said to have had periods of trance during the past; and he, as well as the pathologist, may be presumed to have been acquainted with the phenomena of this condition.

Besides this, if they had made the mistake with which a grief-stricken mother has charged them, they could not have been in doubt in regard to the matter as soon as they opened the thorax and abdomen of the subject. In the thorax they would have found the heart beating, and in the abdomen the intestines would probably have manifested vermiform contractions under the stimulus of the air or the mechanical conditions of the operation.

But, with these and other means of knowing what they did the physicians who conducted the autopsy declare that there were no signs of life in the body; and they do this with the manner of men conscious of being right, and not of men endeavoring to hide an appalling blunder.

For these reasons, we think no medical man will hesitate to accept their statement, or fail to sympathize with them as they protest against the clamor excited by the horrible suspicion which has been raised in the minds of the general public.

There is another phase of this occurrence which is not so easy to see the end of just now. This concerns the right of the medical men to make an autopsy without the consent of a near relative. At present they have been placed under heavy bonds to answer at court, and their rights—or error—will soon be decided according to the law of the State of New York. The law in regard to autopsies is not uniform or clear in this country, and the physicians who made one on the body of Mr. Bishop may have committed a technical breach of the law in doing so. The attorney employed by Mr. Bishop's mother asserts that they have committed a misdemeanor; but they can no doubt get plenty of lawyers to assert that they have not, and it will be interesting to see what the Court will say. Meanwhile other medical men may take warning from the annoying predicament in which these medical men are now placed, and make sure, before they undertake any autopsy, that the subject is certainly dead and that they have legal authority to act.

VACCINATION AND SMALL-POX AT SHEFFIELD.

The opponents of vaccination for small-pox will not receive much comfort from reading the report of Dr. Barry to the Local Government Board on the recent outbreak of small-pox at Sheffield, England. The London correspondent of the *New York Medical Journal*, May 11, refers to the anti-vaccination agitation which is in progress in England, and to the jubilation over the fact that the English Government has granted the request made by these agitators for a Royal Commission to investigate the working of the vaccination acts. It is noticeable, however, that they have made no use in the debate of the facts contained in Dr. Barry's report. The latter dealt with

6,088 cases, of which 590 were fatal. Dr. Barry investigated the circumstances of every fatal case, of every case alleged to have occurred in children under ten who had been vaccinated, and of every case alleged to have taken place after previous small-pox or re-vaccination. He found that the attack-rate of the vaccinated children under ten was 5 in a thousand, and that that of the unvaccinated children of the same age was 101; the death-rate of the vaccinated children under ten was 0.09, and that of the unvaccinated 44. The experience in reference to those over ten was similar. For every 100,000 of those twice vaccinated, there were 8 deaths; of those once vaccinated, 100 deaths; and of the unvaccinated, 5,100 deaths. The outcome of the report was that, if the vaccinated children had been attacked at the same rate as the unvaccinated, there would have been 7,000 attacks in place of 353 and 3,000 deaths in place of 6; or, up to the conclusion of the epidemic, there would have been 4,400 deaths in place of 9.

These statistics furnish evidence of a sort which it would not be easy to gainsay; and they seem to justify the practice of vaccination, in spite of the theoretical objections which are sometimes raised against it.

THE HYMEN AS AN EVIDENCE OF VIRGINITY.

The presence of an intact hymen has long been regarded by mankind in general as a proof of virginity, and its significance has been said, by certain writers, to have led to the adoption of the crescent as the symbol of Diana, by the Romans, who were supposed thereby to suggest, in a figure, her unapproachable chastity. This belief is more interesting as a sign of the disposition some men have to discover obscure allusions to sexual matters in the pictures and statues of the ancients, than valuable as a mark of real erudition; and it is not generally held by mythologists. But the belief that an unruptured hymen is good evidence that its possessor has never indulged in sexual intercourse is almost universal among the laity, and is apparently held by many medical men of reputation. Meymott Tidy, in his work on Forensic Medicine, says that of late years Barnes, Oldham and Tyler Smith have sworn to the fact of females being *virgines intactæ*, chiefly on the ground of the integrity of the hymen ; and he himself thinks a physician who finds a hymen absolutely unruptured, and no signs of pregnancy, is justified in giving a positive opinion as to the existence of virginity.

Notwithstanding the apparent absence of qualification in these statements, they can hardly be supposed to have been intended to mean exactly what appears on their face ; for men so well informed must have known that they are subject to exception. Medical literature contains many illustrations of the fact that sexual intercourse may, in some cases, be indulged in repeatedly without laceration of the hymen, and that labor may be obstructed by the presence of the very condition which has been presumed to be a mark of virginity.

Very recently, in the *Transactions of the Royal Academy of Medicine in Ireland,* Dr. R. J. Kinkead, of Galway, reports a case in which he found labor obstructed by an unruptured hymen, the opening of which was no larger than the diameter of a crow's quill, and two other cases coming under his own observation, in which intercourse had taken place without laceration of this membrane, one of the subjects being a young woman who had been seduced when seventeen years old and who had led the life of a prostitute for about seven years afterward.

These cases indicate that the presence of an unruptured hymen can by no means be regarded as a proof of virginity. It may be so regarded in most cases, but not in all ; and a medical witness called upon to testify as to the significance of this condition would make a serious mistake if he asserted that it furnished anything more than presumptive evidence of the chastity of the subject.

REPLACING THE BONE AFTER TREPHINING.

The custom of dividing the button of bone removed by the trephine and placing the fragments in the opening is now more or less general, and seems to be of use in securing a bony closure of the defect in the skull instead of a membranous one. It has been proposed, also, to replace the entire button, and the *Deutsche med. Wochenschrift*, March 28, 1889, contains a report of a case to the Freie Vereinigung der Chirurgen Berlins, in which Prof. Küster adopted this method with apparent success. The operation was an exploratory one. The patient had months before had a severe wound of the scalp caused by a blow and followed by symptoms of brain disorder. Splintering of the inner table of the skull was suspected, and the skull was trephined. No splintering was found, so Küster did not open the dura mater. He replaced the button of bone entire, and it grew fast to the skull.

Whether the union will persist or not, and whether the piece of bone will remain without necrosis or absorption after months or years have elapsed, cannot be certainly predicted ; but at the time when Küster exhibited his patient the result was all that could be desired. So far the replacing of the bone may be approved, although it is by no means clear that the a bony covering to an opening made with a trephine is so superior to the usual membranous covering as to make it worth while to take the trouble and incur the risks to primary union which are inseparable from the method of replacing the button entire or after its division into small pieces.

THE CHICAGO INSANE ASYLUM.

Just now, when the Department for the Insane of the Philadelphia Hospital is under fire in regard to the treatment of its inmates, it is interesting to note that the authorities of the Cook County Insane Asylum, Chicago, are in a somewhat similar position before the public. They have been put in a very unpleasant position by recent statements of Dr. Clevenger, who was formerly a member of the medical staff of the Hospital. According to these statements the patients are not only shamefully neglected and allowed to become very unclean, but they are also cruelly treated. This disgraceful state of affairs is attributed by Dr. Clevenger to political jobbery.

Whether the charges made against the Chicago Insane Asylum are true or not, they indicate that such practices as he alleges occur there, are likely to develop in any charitable institution which has been allowed to fall into the hands of persons who manage it for political purposes or from mercenary motives.

MEDICAL SOCIETY OF NEW JERSEY.—The one hundred and twenty-third annual meeting of the Medical Society of New Jersey will be held at the Coleman House, Asbury Park, N. J., on Tuesday and Wednesday, June 18 and 19, 1889. An interesting and instructive programme has been provided. A reception will be given to the members of the Society on Tuesday evening.

—The Philadelphia *Ledger*, May 2, 1889, says that the French Council of State has concluded the examination of a series of public administrative rules applicable to the various modes of burial and cremation. With regard to the burning of the bodies of the dead, no apparatus for cremation is to be made use of without authority from the Prefect, who will grant it after consultation with the Hygienic Council. Every burning of a body is to be authorized by the Registrar on an application from the family, and the production of a certificate from the doctor who attended the deceased that death was due to a natural cause, or, in the absence of this, a report of the inquiry conducted by the municipal doctor. A report will be drawn up recording the reception of the body and its incineration, which will be transmitted to the municipal authority. The ashes will not be allowed to be deposited, even provisionally, anywhere except in places of burial regularly established, or to be removed without consent of the municipal authorities.

BOOK REVIEWS.

[Any book reviewed in these columns may be obtained upon receipt of price, from the office of the REPORTER.]

THE INSANE IN FOREIGN COUNTRIES. AN EXAMINATION OF EUROPEAN METHODS OF CARING FOR THE INSANE. By THE HON. WM. P. LETCHWORTH, President of the New York State Board of Charities. 8vo, cloth, pp. xii, 374. New York and London: G. P. Putnam's Sons, 1889. Price, $3.00.

This magnificently illustrated and handsomely printed book is one which is calculated to be of great interest and value not only to all persons connected with institutions for the care of the insane, but equally, we believe, to all humanitarians and persons interested in the history of medicine.

The introductory chapter contains a brief historical sketch of the treatment of the insane in various countries from the earliest times to the present day. Then follow chapters devoted to the lunacy systems of England, Scotland, and Ireland, and to representative institutions of these and Continental countries, and a chapter each is given to the remarkable insane colony of Gheel and to the noted asylum at Alt-Scherbitz, near Leipzig, which latter illustrates the combined excellencies of a colony and a hospital.

The final chapter presents a *résumé* of the author's observations and his conclusions drawn from them. Based upon the results of his inspections of foreign and American asylums and of his own ripe experience in the supervision of the defective classes of New York State, Mr. Letchworth offers his views as regards the selection of sites and locations of asylums, the kind of buildings to be provided, the questions of sewage disposal, water supply, protection against fire, the laying out of the grounds, the furnishing and decoration of wards and rooms, the difficult problem of the disposition of the acute, the chronic, and the criminal insane, the practice of restraint and the amount of liberty that may be granted, the character of the attendants to be chosen, the religious exercises, amusements, employments, dress and clothing, visitation and correspondence of patients, *post-mortem* examinations, the question of voluntary admission, the methods of admission and discharge, and the value of summer resorts. All of these subjects are treated clearly and explicitly. Besides these, the author gives his personal views respecting the insane in poorhouses, local or district care of the insane, state care, the boarding-out system, state supervision, and kindred topics.

The book is beautifully printed and richly illustrated with engravings and heliotype reproductions of plans of buildings and asylum interiors and pictures of historical interest, and is as creditable to the publishers as to the author.

THE ILLUSTRATED OPTICAL MANUAL OR HANDBOOK OF INSTRUCTIONS FOR THE GUIDANCE OF SURGEONS, ETC. By SURGEON-GENERAL SIR T. LONGMORE, C.B., F.R C.S., Professor of Military Surgery at the Army Medical School, etc. Fourth edition, enlarged and illustrated by 74 figures from drawings and diagrams by Inspector General Dr. Macdonald, R.N., F.R.S., etc. London and New York: Longmans, Green & Co., 1888. Large 8vo, pp. xx, 239. Price, $4.50.

There is such a marked contrast between the general appearance of the present edition of this manual and the first, which appeared nearly twenty-three years ago, that we are tempted to read the new work—which practically it is—most thoroughly and carefully.

As we reach the closing pages, we feel convinced that our labor has been both pleasant and instructive. Physiological optics have been brought to date; methods for the determination of refractive and accommodative error are accurately described in detail; and excellent wood-cuts have been discriminately distributed throughout the text. The errors, as for instance, the designation of Retinal Shadow Test by the incorrect term Keratoscopy; and the coinage and use of curious and meaningless technicalities, may all be excused. The author is to be congratulated upon his endeavors, as the contents are both valuable and instructive, not only to the Military and Naval Surgeon, for whom the volume is especially intended, but also to the general and special surgeon whose duty it may be from time to time to obtain adequate knowledge upon such subjects. It is to be regretted that our English friends will persist in giving their American cousins a binding that is only adapted for their own climate, and which breaks and splits upon the slightest usage.

LA MORT PAR LA DÉCAPITATION. Par le Dr. Paul Loye, Preparateur du Laboratoire de Physiologie de la Sorbonne, Paris, etc 8vo, pp. xii, 285. Paris: Bureau du Progrès médical, 1888.

In this curious volume, Dr. Loye discusses the question whether or not consciousness lasts after decapitation. By a number of careful observations and ingenious experiments, he has been led to the conclusion—in which we think the reader will certainly follow him—that in man consciousness is immediately terminated by decapitation, although in dogs manifestations of reflex excitation, due probably to deprivation of oxygen in the brain, last for some time, unless the knife has been made to pass through the medulla oblongata.

Dr. Loye's book contains very much that is of interest to the physiologist, as well as to those who may discuss the question of the best mode of executing criminals. In France decapitation is regarded as the best method of execution, and the conclusions of this book support this opinion.

In this country, the attempt to make the death penalty as free from horrors as possible has led one state to adopt the method of execution by electricity. It is not to be expected that Guillotining will ever be adopted here; but we think it would be a more rational and decidedly more merciful method than hanging, or even the mode now legal in New York.

LITERARY NOTES.

—The *Annales Médico Chirurgicales* with its May issue assumes the title of *Annales de thérapeutique Médico-Chirurgicales*. It will be published monthly under the direction of Dr. Constantin Paul, Dr. L. Duchastelet still continuing in the position of Editor in Chief.

—Dr. Desesquelles has recommended as a topical antiseptic a mixture of one part of powdered β naphthol with two of powdered camphor. The two are triturated together, dry, until they unite to form a colorless or creamy liquid.

NOTES AND COMMENTS.

Dr. Macewen on Aneurism and Epilepsy.

At a recent meeting of the Glasgow branch of the British Medical Association one of the most interesting demonstrations was that by Dr. Macewen. He showed, first, a man who had been subject to epileptic seizures for many years. A year ago Dr. Macewen removed a tumor from the cerebrum, with the result that the seizures have entirely ceased. The second subject demonstrated was a new method for the cure of aneurism, in which the object of the surgeon is to produce in the cavity, not blood-clot, but a "white thrombus" of connective tissue. This is accomplished by passing needles into the aneurism in such a way as to pass through one wall of the sac and just to touch the lining of the opposite wall; the current of blood causes an oscillation of the needle and a number of fine scratches on the inner surface of the endothelium, irritating it slightly and leading to the proliferation of leucocytes. From these connective tissue is formed, and a white fibrous mass develops on the inner surface of the sac. The irritation is repeated at intervals of days, the needle being introduced at different spots. The result is the formation of a strong layer of connective tissue, which is firmer than red clot, and involves no danger from embolism.—*Lancet*, March 2, 1889.

Yellow Fever in Brazil.

The extent of the yellow-fever scourge in South America has been only partly known to us. In Rio de Janeiro the mortality has been severe, but recent despatches show that it has declined. At Santos there has been no abatement; in that city of 14,000 inhabitants there have been more than five hundred deaths in a single month—which is equivalent to an annual death-rate of 420 per 1000, from that one cause. At Campinas the streets are almost deserted, and the poor are making appeals for aid and succor. The corps of nurses at Santos has done admirable work, and several members of the Italian White Cross Volunteers have died at the post of duty. The mercantile community at Santos has suffered greatly and it is stated that there is not a business house there that has not lost some of its employés. There is a government Committee of Relief with considerable means at its disposal.

Hemorrhagic Malarial Fever.

Dr. W. C. C. Stirling, of Weaver, Texas, says in the *Atlanta Med. and Surg. Journal,* April, 1889, that hemorrhagic malarial fever is quite common in Texas on the creeks and rivers. Its distinguishing feature is hæmaturia. It has been called hæmaturic malarial fever, and is known in the malarial localities as "black jaundice" and "swamp fever." A great many practitioners, he says, give it the name black jaundice, on account of the dark, black urine and yellowness of the skin and eye-balls. Dr. Stirling prefers the term hemorrhagic, as the hæmaturia is accompanied by hemorrhage in other situations. Malaria is not a poison inducing hemorrhage. The most experienced and accurate observers of malarial affections concur in the opinion that malaria establishes the hemorrhagic diathesis only through changes effected in the human economy by its prolonged influence.

The late Prof. S. M. Bemiss, of New Orleans, classes the morbid conditions of malarial fever with its tendency to hemorrhage as follows: First, the blood-changes of chronic malarial toxæmia so alter the consistency of that fluid as to favor the occurrence of hemorrhage. Second, the long persistent states of malnutrition in chronic malarial cachexias produce textural weakening of the vascular walls and increased liability to their rupture. Third, the increased blood-pressure put upon the vascular walls by passive congestion during a malarial paroxysm. The hemorrhage generally takes place in the kidneys, but also takes place in other situations, viz., stomach, bowels, nose, gums, and blistered surfaces. Sometimes the hemorrhage is into closed cavities.

After detailing several of his own cases, Dr. Stirling states that all forms of the disease are dangerous, and should be treated promptly. The first important thing is to administer cinchona as early as possible. Drs. Louis and Lynch, of Carroll's Prairie, Texas, assert that quinine sometimes produces the hemorrhage. While admitting that they are old physicians, and have treated a great many cases, the author does not agree with them. He has never seen hemorrhage follow the administration of quinine. He thinks in their cases the hemorrhage would have occurred if the quinine had not been given. Prof. S. M. Bemiss, who practised in a malarial locality for almost a half century, says that he has never witnessed any symptoms following the administration of chincona salts which justified a belief that they increased the hemorrhage.

After administering cinchona in some form, the next thing is to arrest the extravasation of blood, and to sustain the patient's strength. The best hemostatic is chloride of iron. The tincture should be given every two hours in ten-drop doses. Ergot, and gallic and sulphuric acids are valuable remedies to prevent hemorrhage into the stroma of the kidneys and Malpighian tufts. Bitartrate of potassium, he says, acts as a hemostatic by keeping up the flow of urine through the kidneys. For the jaundice there is no better remedy than calomel. It should be given at suitable intervals, until catharsis has been produced. Milk, eggs, and milk-punch, should be given when they are necessary. Enfeebled action of the heart always calls for stimulants. In many cases the danger of the disease is manifested chiefly by the enfeebled action of the heart. Coldness of the surface is an indication for the external application of heat, by means of warm blankets, hot mustard foot bath, etc. Morphine and atropine should be given hypodermically for restlessness, delirium and convulsions. After the interruption of the paroxysm, quinine should be given in tonic doses, and tincture of the chloride of iron in twenty-drop doses after each meal, together with a nutritious diet.

A slow, imperfect convalescence not unfrequently follows a violent attack, and is attended with feeble digestion and muscular and nervous debility. Good tonics that contain quinine, and something to act on the liver, are about all that is needed.

Anatomical Basis of the Phthisical Habit.

Rudolph Frels, of Munich, in his inaugural dissertation, 1888, states that he has studied one hundred bodies in Bollinger's Pathological Institute with reference to the origin of the phthisical habit. He believes that the following anatomical changes should be considered as the basis of the disease: 1. Narrowing of the upper section of the thorax, especially with shortening of the upper sagittal diameter. 2. Smallness of the heart and narrowing of the great arterial trunks, and especially of the pulmonary artery. 3. Disproportion between the volume of the heart and that of the lungs.

Frels makes no attempt to answer the important question as to the cause of these anatomical changes.—*Deutsche Medizinal-Zeitung,* April 4, 1889.

Chloroform as An Internal Remedy.

Dr. Stepp, of Nürnberg, noting the observations of Salkowski on the disinfecting power of chloroform water, determined to make trial of chloroform internally in a considerable number of diseases. It may here be remarked that the use of chloroform in aqueous or alcoholic solution is less common in Germany than in England, where the familiar so-called "æther chlor." forms a portion of a very large number of prescriptions. In gastric ulcer Dr. Stepp gave chloroform (fifteen grains in a five-ounce bismuth mixture) with great effect, and believes this to be due to its disinfecting, astringent, and stimulating properties. In various affections of the mouth and throat—as follicular pharyngitis, catarrh of the pharynx, gingivitis, and diphtheria—washes and gargles containing chloroform proved very beneficial. In one case of severe psoriasis of the mucous membrane of the mouth, which had been unsuccessfully treated by several medical men, chloroform water effected a complete cure. Two cases of pneumonia treated with chloroform did so well that Dr. Stepp means to make a further trial of it in this disease. Perhaps the most encouraging results were obtained in cases of typhoid fever, though only six of these were thus treated. The value of chloroform in some cases of fever was shown some twenty-five years ago in the Dublin hospitals, but it has never come into general use even in Ireland as an antipyretic.—*Lancet*, March 9, 1889.

Voluntary Co-operation of Micro-Organisms.

Binet states in his Psychic Life of Micro-örganisms that there exist organisms which lead a life of habitual isolation, but which understand how to unite for the purpose of attacking prey at the desired time, thus profiting by the superiority which numbers give. The *Bodo caudatus* is a voracious Flagellate possessed of extraordinary audacity; it combines into troops to attack animacula one hundred times as large as itself, as the Colpods, for instance, which are veritable giants when placed alongside the *Bodo*. Like a horse attacked by a pack of wolves, the Colpod is soon rendered powerless, twenty, thirty, forty *Bodos* throw themselves upon him, eviscerate and devour him completely. All these facts are of primary importance and interest, but it is plain that their interpretation presents difficulties. It may be asked whether the *Bodos* combine designedly in groups of ten or twenty, understanding that they are more powerful when united than when divided. But it is more probable that voluntary combinations for purposes of attack do not take place among these organisms; that would be to grant them a high mental capacity. We may more readily admit that the meeting of a number of *Bodos* happens by chance. When one of them begins an attack upon a Colpod, the other animacula lurking in the vicinity, dash into the combat to profit by a favorable opportunity.

Labor in Occipito-Posterior Positions.

Dr. T. G. Comstock, in a paper published in the *Clinical Reporter*, March, 1889, states his opinions in the following propositions, in which he will be seen to differ from the opinion of the better teachers of to-day:

1. When the occiput does not rotate normally, and it is driven down into the cavity of the pelvis, it has to travel at least three times as far as when it is anteriorly situated.

2. In this vicious position, the whole body of the child is jammed down into the cavity of the pelvis, and this is necessary before the occiput can escape over the perineum.

3. In this position, the occiput is at first forced a downward grade, into the hollow of the sacrum, and then to advance further, it must take an up-grade in order to glide over the perineum.

4. In posterior rotation, as I have stated, the occiput has to travel at least ten inches before reaching the outlet whereby it can escape into the world, and the whole fœtal ellipse (which only measures eleven inches) becomes jammed down into the cavity of the pelvis, and then the uterine power for expulsion is lost, although the pains still continue, and exhaust the mother.

5. One of the most frequent accidents of delivery when the occiput rotates posteriorly is, if the head is delivered in this position, that the perineum is ruptured.

6. When such cases occur, and we cannot deliver with the forceps, I would propose that lateral section of the perineum be made (episiotomy), and then the delivery can be accomplished. After such a proceeding, I should advise that the lateral cuts be closed at once by catgut sutures. Experience has proved that such wounds made by the knife will heal much easier than jagged wounds made in the central line by long pressure of the head producing traumatism.

Bromide of Ethyl as an Anæsthetic.

Dr. Charles E. Diehl, a dentist of Pittsburgh, in the *Pittsburgh Med. Review*, April, 1889, recommends the bromide of ethyl as an anæsthetic in minor but painful surgical operations, such as the opening of abscesses, the dressing of injuries, etc. His own experience with it, however, is limited to dental surgery. Our readers may recall the fact that Dr. Simpson recommended its use in labor, in the REPORTER, September 8, 1888. The advantages Dr. Diehl claims for it are :

1. Its rapid action ; two or three minutes will produce complete insensibility to pain. 2. The extreme fugaciousness of its effect ; the patient will regain complete sensibility within a few minutes after the inhalations are stopped. 3. Very often there is utter insensibility to pain, yet with full control of the mental faculties. 4. The absence of all irritating properties in the vapor, and the consequent ease with which it is taken. 5. The absence of after-effects, nausea, giddiness, etc., which usually follow ether and chloroform. 6. The harmlessness of the *pure* drug. The author reports ten cases in which he has used it, and says that since July, 1888, he has employed the bromide of ethyl in one hundred cases.

Mercury-Lanolin in Certain Affections of the Cornea.

At the meeting of the Paris Ophthalmological Society March 12, 1889, Darier recommended the émployment of mercurylanolin in certain affections of the cornea. Local inunctions of this ointment, he says, do very good service in diffuse infiltrations of the cornea unaccompanied with symptoms of acute irritation. Certain slight forms of interstitial keratitis, superficial keratitis, and spreading leucoma may be completely cured by this treatment. Hypodermic injections of corrosive sublimate are the only effective remedy in intense parenchymatous keratitis; but if the disease process relapses inunctions of mercury-lanolin are a valuable remedy to make the cornea translucent. These inunctions have both a mechanical action through the massage and also an antiseptic and solvent action. They are employed as follows: A piece of the ointment half the size of a grain of corn is introduced into the lower conjunctival sac upon a pencil, and then moderate massage of the cornea and eye-ball is practised by the thumb applied to the upper lid. The inunctions referred to are employed morning and evening, and are well borne even by children. The mercury-lanolin is composed of equal parts mercury and lanolin ; one-fourth part vaseline may be added to make it so that it will keep longer. Darier states that the cornea absorbs the ointment so rapidly that stomatitis has occurred in several patients after using it some time.

In the discussion upon Darier's paper, Abadie stated that in chronic inflammations of the lachrymal sac, with fungosities and fistulæ—a condition frequently present in scrofulous children—local inunctions of iodoform in lanolin in the neighborhood of the lachrymal sack, in addition to general treatment, effected surprisingly favorable results.—*Wiener med. Presse*, April 7, 1889.

Formulæ for the Use of Naphthol as a Local Antiseptic.

Naphthol is much used abroad as an antiseptic. Dr. Charles Éloy suggests the following convenient formulæ for its employment in the *Gazette Hebdomadaire*, April 19, 1889.

The following is for a weak solution :

Naphthol β . . . . gr. xv
Alcohol (60°). . . . . . . f ℥ xxx

It may be used upon hairy regions which it is desired to render aseptic.

A strong solution may be made as follows :

Naphthol . . . . gr. cl–ccxxv
Alcohol (60°) . . . . f ℥ xxx

It serves to disinfect denuded cutaneous surfaces.

For injections, the solution should be prepared warm, and subjected to a mild temperature. Before injecting it into serous cavities, therefore, and into abscesses it will be prudent to heat the syringe previously. The following is a formula :

Naphthol β . . . . . gr. cl
Alcohol (90°) . . . . . . f ℥ iiss
Water . . . . f ℥ iii ℥ v

As a mouth wash, some drops of the following solution may be used in a glass of water :

Botot Water . . . . f ℥ ii
Naphthol β . . . . gr. ix

For purposes of friction, camphorated naphthol may be used. This last is obtained by triturating to liquefaction the following :

Pulverized camphor . . . . . parts 2
Pulverized beta naphthol . . part 1

Influence of Saccharin upon Digestion.

Although saccharin was discovered in 1879, it was not until 1886 that it was introduced into the practice of medicine. It was highly recommended and extensively used in diabetes, until Worms, of the "Académie de Médecine" of Paris, and Dujardin-Beaumetz cautioned against its use and asserted that it materially retarded and injured the digestion. Of late however the subject has been brought up again, and a number of experimenters have been testing the drug. The majority of the results do not coincide with the opinions of Dujardin-Beaumetz.

Dr. Edgar Gans, of Carlsbad, gives the result of a very complete series of experiments and comes to the conclusion that saccharin does not injure the digestion in any way. Saccharin in powder form seems to retard slightly the digestion of albumen, but in solution it—if anything—aids it. A valuable property of saccharin is its ability to retard fermenting processes in the bowels and to prevent rapid decomposition. In one of his experiments, Dr. Ganz partly filled two test-tubes with intestinal fluid, and closed them with a wad of cotton. To the one a small quantity of saccharin had been added. The contents of the test tube without saccharin became highly decomposed and discolored in two days, while that containing it remained the same for over four weeks.—*Berliner klinische Wochenschrift*, April 1, 1889.

Useful Formulæ in Chronic Rheumatism.

Dr. Daniel R. Brower, in a clinical lecture on a patient suffering with chronic rheumatism, fatty heart and fatty liver, published in the *North American Practitioner*, May, 1889, suggests the following formulæ to aid in the removal of uric acid from the system, and to sustain and improve the action of the heart and of the liver:

R Lithiæ citrat. . . . . ℥ ii
   Strychnniæ . . . . gr. i
   Tinct. Strophanthi . . . . . . f ℥ iss
   Aquæ Menth. pip. . . . . q. s. ad f ℥ iv
M. Sig. Teaspoonful before each meal in water.

R Aloes . . . . gr. ii
   Pulv. Ipecac. . . . . gr. i
   Pulv. Rhei,
   Ferri sulph. exsiccat.,
   Ext. Hyoscyami . . . . . . aa gr. x
M. Div. in capsules No. X.
Sig. One at bed-time.

Uralium, a New Hypnotic.

Gustavo Poppi, of Bologna, very recently made a communication to the Medico-Chirurgical Society of Bologna, upon a new hypnotic, uralium. This is a combination of chloral with urethan. Poppi concludes, as the result of experiments upon animals and men, that the uralium induces sleep more quickly and surely than all the known hypnotics. It occasions, according to him, no change in blood pressure, and has no untoward secondary effects. It is said to have been given with success to patients with heart disease, mental disorders, hysteria, etc., and always with the best results, even in cases in which other hypnotics had failed.—*Wiener med. Presse*, April 7, 1889.

Orthopædic Shop at the University of Pennsylvania.

The shop for the manufacture of Orthopædic apparatus at the University Hospital has been reopened, and a plan has been adopted for permitting it to be used by any of the gentlemen connected with the University, for their charity cases, or for patients in moderate circumstances, upon application to the Clinical Professor, Dr. De Forest Willard, or to either of the Attending Surgeons in the Orthopædic Department. One of these will be in attendance every day from 12 to 1.00 P. M at the Dispensary.

Unless desired by the attending physician, no control will be exercised over the patient or over the apparatus, except a mere countersign in order to regulate properly the administration of the shop, which will be under personal management. The charge for charity cases will be regulated so as simply to cover the cost of material and labor. For higher class work, nickel plating, etc., a slight advance in price will be made.

Druggists Violating the Law.

The New Jersey Pharmaceutical Association began its annual session in Bridgeton May 22. According to a newspaper report, Chairman Rennells said that he had been advised by Cortland Parker that there was no law prohibiting druggists from selling liquor as a medicine. He further said that Senator Werts advised them to go on selling as heretofore, provided they were selling honestly. A prominent druggist is said to have stated at the meeting that he violated this law every day, and that every other druggist in the State did openly violate it, and that they would continue to do so.

NEWS.

—Dr. Frank Baker has been appointed Assistant General Superintendent of the Life-saving Service.

—The annual meeting of the Association of Medical Superintendents of American Institutions for the Insane will be held in Newport, R. I., June 18.

—It is reported that Dr. William G. Eggleston, who has for several years been a member of the editorial staff of the *Journal of the American Medical Association*, has retired from that position.

—The Iowa State Board of Health, it is reported, has decided that Iowa medical colleges should, after 1891, be required to give a four years' course to secure their graduates admission to practise in that State.

—Dr. Howard A. Kelly, Associate Professor of Obstetrics and Diseases of Women and Children in the University of Pennsylvania, has been elected Professor of Obstetrics and Gynecology in the Johns Hopkins University, at Baltimore.

—Doctors Beecher, Bell and Horwitz, Demonstrators of Anatomy at Jefferson Medical College, have resigned, and Dr. A. Hewson, Jr., has been appointed Demonstrator-in-Charge. Dr. Hewson was Dr. Forbes's assistant for seven years.

—The number of deaths in Philadelphia for the week ending May 25 was 339, which is 81 less than during the preceding week and 31 less than during the corresponding period of last year. There were 5 deaths from scarlet fever, 5 from measles, and 15 from typhoid fever.

—In experiments recently made in France on the elasticity of cork, it was found that disks of that substance, when submitted to a pressure of sixty-six tons to the square inch, were compressed to one-fifth their thickness, and recovered their original dimensions in exactly ten minutes after the pressure was removed.

—Dr. L. G. Hardman states in the *Atlanta Medical and Surgical Journal,* April, 1889, that he has successfully employed hypodermic injections of cocaine in operations upon the horse. The use of cocaine obviates the necessity of throwing the horse, or securing him in other ways which may do him damage.

—The *Medical Age*, May 10, publishes letters from a number of physicians bearing upon the question of the propriety of removing the Medical Department of the University of Michigan from Ann Arbor to Detroit. Many favor the change because there are greater clinical advantages at Detroit than at Ann Arbor.

—The Governor of Michigan has issued a proclamation prohibiting the importation of Texas cattle, or any other cattle raised south of the 36th parallel of North latitude, until the first day of November 1889, except such as are in transit across the State. The latter may be unloaded only at yards designated for the purpose and which are placarded: "For the feeding of Texas cattle only."

—Dr. Hobart A. Hare has been appointed Editor of the *Medical News*, to succeed Dr. I. Minis Hays, who will have charge in future of the *Amer. Journal of the Medical Sciences.* Dr. Hare has been one of the Editors of the *University Medical Magazine.* He is well known throughout the country as an author, and will no doubt maintain the present standard of the *Medical News.* The new arrangement in regard to the *Medical News* goes into operation on October 1.

—The annual meeting of the Maryland State Board of Health was held in Baltimore, May 14. It was resolved to coöperate with other State Boards of Health to secure the passage of a law absolutely prohibiting the transportation of bodies of persons who have died from small-pox, Asiatic cholera, leprosy, typhus or yellow fever, and to compel those forwarding the bodies of those who have died from diphtheria, scarlet fever or any other infectious disease, to prepare and encase them properly, in order that passengers should not be exposed to the dangers arising from the proximity of their baggage to the bodies when the latter are transported in baggage cars.

HUMOR.

Mrs. A.—"Isn't that an awful smelling cigar that man's smoking?" Mrs. B.— "Yes; but I can bear the smell of it when I think how much worse it must be to smoke it. Poor man! He deserves our pity rather than our blame."—*Boston Transcript.*

Pat Cole, the Irishman who killed Coombs in a fight some years since in Brunswick, on being arrested by the Sheriff, said: "It was a fair fight, Mr. Officer; if Coombs had killed me I wouldn't have said a word about it."—*Lewiston (Me.) Gazette.*

MEDICAL AND SURGICAL
REPORTER

No. 1684.   PHILADELPHIA, JUNE 8, 1889.   VOL. LX.—No. 23.

CONTENTS:

COMMUNICATIONS.

TAIT'S OPERATION FOR PARTIAL RUPTURE OF THE PERINEUM.

BY THEOPHILUS PARVIN, M.D.,

PHILADELPHIA.

PROFESSOR OF OBSTETRICS AND OF THE DISEASES OF WOMEN AND CHILDREN IN THE JEFFERSON MEDICAL COLLEGE.

The operation devised and done by Lawson Tait in an incomplete tear of the perineum, is probably not as well known by the profession in this country as it should be. Mr. Tait's method rests upon a rational basis, and its results have been pronounced by him, after a large experience, most satisfactory. Having had the opportunity of seeing him operate, and having repeated his operation in twenty-two cases,[1] it has seemed

[1] In addition to these twenty-two, I operated last winter on two patients for complete rupture of the perineum, using the method advised by Mr. Tait in such injury. Possibly a description of the operation may be given in another paper.

to me that a detailed description of the method, aided by suitable illustrations, might be useful to at least some of the readers of the REPORTER. A remark just made must be qualified—that relating to the repetition of Mr. Tait's operation; for in one particular, as will be explained hereafter, I have deviated from his method, though really the deviation is not great. Further, in referring to my own operations I shall frankly mention the mistakes that I have made, so that others may be guarded against their repetition.

Mr. Tait's method of operating will first be given in his own words, and his illustrations presented. Then will follow my description of the operations, the description being made clearer by illustrations, some of them drawn from actual cases during or after operation, by Mr. Burt W. Swayze, a student of Jefferson Medical College; and it is believed that by these means as good an understanding of the operation will be given as can possibly be obtained without actually seeing it.

673

Mr. Tait[1] says that when the marginal folds of the buttocks are fully drawn asunder in a case of torn perineum, the old tear is displayed by a thin line of cicatrix extending transversely to the axis of the rent, which of course was at right angles to the plane of the perineum. "The healing of the tear has taken another direction altogether, and we have the cicatrix at right angles to the wound. This is, so far as I can think out the question or know the facts, wholly unique in its occurrence. It forms the basis of the principles of the operation which I perform, and that is absolutely the opposite, as I have already said in a correspondence on this subject with Dr. Percy Boulton, of the principle of all denuding operations. The scheme of my operation is to restore the old rent and unite it at right angles to its representative cicatrix; that is, at right angles to the plane of the perineum. In this way, and in this way only, can the perineum be truly restored, and from this operation only can it be hoped that the restoration will stand the attacks of subsequent labors, as a large number of my restorations have done. I do not know of one having been torn a second time. ·

"Having the folds of the buttocks pulled firmly apart, so that the cicatrix is put on the stretch, I enter the scissors at its extreme end on one side, and keeping strictly to its line, I run through to its other extremity. The incision is about three eighths of an inch deep, and it forms two flaps, a rectal and a vaginal. From each end of the incision it is carried forward into the tissue of each labium for about an inch, and again backward for about a third of an inch, making a wound like this—

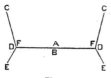

Fig. 1.

The vaginal flap A is held upward, the patient being on her back, and the rectal flap B being turned downward, the angles A F C being pulled by forceps diagonally upward and inward toward the middle line, and the angles B D E being pulled down-

[1] This description. given by Mr. Tait, is found in the third edition of H. Macnaughton Jones's Practical Manual of Diseases of Women London, 1888. The author of the Manual, by the way, strongly endorses the method.

ward and inward. The lines C E thus become straight, and the wound takes this form—

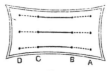

Fig. 2.

"By means of a stout-handled and well-curved needle the silkworm-gut sutures are entered on one side about an eighth of an inch within the margin of the wound, so as not to include the skin, at the dots A. They are buried deeply in the tissue as far as B, and then the needle is made to emerge so as to miss the angle of the wound. The needle again enters at the large dots C, and emerges at the dots B. By thus missing the upper or deep angle of the wound between B and C, the two great and divided masses of the old perineum, which lie in the parallelograms respectively bounded by the lines of large dots A—B and C—D, are respectively adapted. The rectal and vaginal flaps respectively point into the rectum and vagina, and like an old-fashioned flap-valve prevent noxious material entering the wound. The resulting mass of perineum is amazingly large; union is almost inevitable, for I have failed only twice in many hundreds of cases, and then because there had been previous denuding operations, the resulting cicatrix is absolutely linear, and so resembles the natural *raphé*, that in three or four months after the operation it is quite impossible to determine, from the appearance of the parts, that the perineum has ever been injured, for there are no stitch-holes left to tell the story. The pain after the operation is trifling compared to the old method of quilled or shotted sutures. I leave the stitches in for three or four weeks, and take great care that the rectum and vagina are washed out twice daily."

Obviously, as pointed out by Mr. Tait, this operation will prove useful in many cases of rectocele; for, by splitting the recto-vaginal wall to a greater height, we can fill in the triangular space made apparent when the free margins of the rectal and of the vaginal flaps are separated, with the tissues drawn by the sutures from each side, and thus present a barrier to further descent, while at the same time we have lessened the projecting mass; furthermore, by making a horse-shoe separation at the sides of the vulvar entrance we can throw the vaginal flap further forward, and thus greatly lessen that entrance. Mr. Taịt informed me that he was trying a somewhat similar operation for cystocele, but had not yet brought it to such perfection of method that he was willing to describe it.

Mr. Tait, in his operation, employs for stitches, as has been mentioned, silkworm gut, and the statement made in Vulliet's and Lutaud's recent [1] volume, that silver wire is used, is an error.

The next illustration, Figure 3, shows the operation as begun ; the patient is lying upon her back, two assistants, one on each side, while supporting the lower limbs well-flexed upon the body, press with the thumb

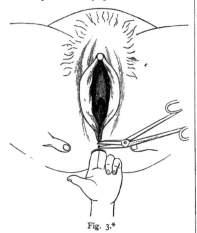

Fig. 3.*

or index finger so as to make the perineum tense ; the operator has two fingers of the left hand in the rectum, and enters the scissors about midway in the transverse line to be incised. This beginning at the middle, instead of upon one side as advised by Mr. Tait, is of course not an essential, but it has seemed to me somewhat easier. Next, one-half of the transverse line, as shown in Figure 1 is made, then the other half ; the two oblique lines toward the anus are next cut, then those at the vulvar margin, the extent of the latter being longer, as greater lessening of the outlet is required. Finally, the two flaps are by quick clips of the scis-

sors separated to a uniform distance on each side, and to such height as may be necessary.

Figure 4 represents the appearance of the fresh surfaces made by splitting the recto-vaginal wall, the vaginal flap being drawn up with tenacula.

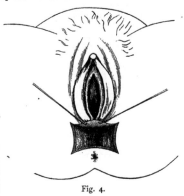

Fig. 4.

The next step is the introduction of the stitches ; and the following illustration

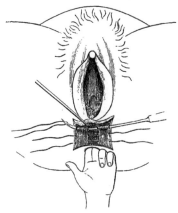

Fig. 5.

shows this process, according to Mr. Tait's method. The operator, still keeping the index and medius of the left hand in the rectum, passes the needle, as has been described, entering on the one side below the skin margin, and first emerging before reaching the apex of the wound, then after

---

[1] Leçons de Gynécologie Opératoire, Paris, 1889.

* The figure represents the flat of the scissors as parallel to the skin, whereas it should be perpendicular to it, so that a transverse incision will be made.

crossing, thus exposed in the sulcus, reenters the tissues, and comes out upon the opposite side of the raw surface, but does not include the skin; as soon as the eye of the instrument is exposed the assistant upon that side threads the needle with silkworm gut, the operator withdraws the needle, and the suture is in place; then the second and the third sutures are similarly introduced; in most cases these three are sufficient. The wound is now cleansed, and the operator ties the sutures beginning at the one nearest the anus.

In most of my operations, however, I have deviated from Mr. Tait's method in that the stitches have been passed through the skin; for I was not successful in bringing the margins of the skin wound in such close apposition as seemed to me necessary without this inclusion. Nevertheless I mean to try again until the method pursued by me shall be completely that of Mr. Tait, though I confess that I cannot see any harm of at least serious character if the stitches do include the skin in most cases, provided the last stitch be not drawn too tight, the consequence of which will be referred to hereafter.

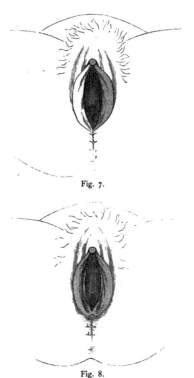

Fig. 7.

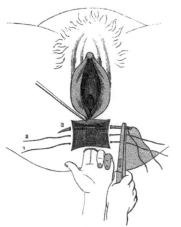

Fig. 6.

Figure 6 represents the introduction of the sutures, a strongly-curved needle and forceps being used, the method which I have generally used.

Fig. 8.

Figures 7 and 8 represent the appearance presented after the stitches have been tied, the first when the sutures do not include the skin.

The following illustrations show a strongly curved needle, and the forceps which I have generally used in my operations.

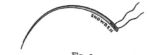

Fig. 9.

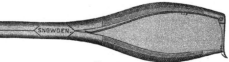

Fig. 10.

In regard to the after-treatment, I believe that washing out the vagina once a day with warm carbolized water, and evacuating the bowels daily by a warm water injection, the patient remaining in bed for the first ten days, are the most important parts. Of course the bladder must be catheterized, if spontaneous evacuation does not occur, and in some cases the bowels not being sufficiently moved by an enema, the use of a mild laxative is indicated. The removal of the stitches I have tried at different periods varying from ten days to three weeks; and my impression is decidedly in favor of late rather than early removal. The newly-united tissues are certainly in no condition to bear any severe strain under three weeks; for in one instance in which I had operated for cystocele,—by denuding an oval surface upon the anterior vaginal wall, and stitching the margins together with silkworm gut, following this operation by a perineal operation, materially lessening the vulvar opening,— three weeks after, in removing the stitches used for the cystocele, I introduced a Sims speculum for the purpose of retracting the perineum so as to expose the stitches, and found that although no great force was used in the retraction, it caused part of the perineal wound to give way. Two stitches were at once introduced, and the result was entirely satisfactory; but I had learned a practical lesson of some value. Nevertheless, if the stitches in the perineum are left much longer than ten days, they are liable to cause some external ulceration, and, more especially if the sutures have been tied too tight, partial cutting through the tissues occurs, with resulting transverse depressions marking the places of the stitches, and elevations in their intervals. From the latter statement a practical lesson is to be drawn: in tying the silkworm gut threads, see that the parts are brought only in apposition, with no wrinkling of the skin, and no strain upon the tissues.

The results in the cases upon which I have operated, have, as a rule, been most satisfactory; and one complete failure and some partial successes have been the result of the error of the operator. The failure occurred in a case operated upon at the Philadelphia Hospital; but the operation was done too soon after the woman's delivery, union did not take place, and the vaginal flap disappeared. In cases of partial success, the cause of the unfavorable result was in drawing the final stitch—that is, the one nearest the vulvar opening—too strongly, so that the lower portion of the vaginal flap projected, form-ing a tongue-like process; in one instance a week after the operation I found this projection so great, swollen and threatening to slough, that I cut it off, and in two other instances after the removal of the stitches there was an unnatural prominence made by it just at the vulvar entrance.

In some instances, too, immediate union of the entire surfaces brought in apposition did not take place. Possibly the failure may have occurred from the sutures not having been properly introduced or tied, or it may have been from not thoroughly cleansing the surfaces before the sutures were fastened.

The operation that has been described commends itself by its simplicity, by the readiness of its performance, by no tissue being sacrificed, and by its usually immediately satisfactory results. As to the remote results, of course, I can say nothing from personal knowledge, for my first operation was done in October, but I am quite willing to fully accept Mr. Tait's statement as to those results. Vulliet in describing Tait's operation, as he saw it done by Fancourt Barnes, states that it was completed in five minutes; it may be done in less than four minutes if one has assistants who are familiar with their duties. The operation will be found useful not only in uncomplicated partial rupture of the perineum, but also in many cases in which the injury is complicated with rectocele, and may also often be done with advantage after the usual operation for cystocele, supplementing that operation and contributing to prevent recurrence of the accident.

It certainly seems probable that a perineum restored by Tait's method would be much more likely to bear without injury the strain of childbirth than a perineum restored by the common method. Quite recently there was at the Dispensary for Diseases of Women and Children of Jefferson Medical College Hospital a woman who, after having her perineum badly torn in labor, had the usual denuding operation done, but childbirth again had caused as bad a tear as the original one. It is probable such examples are not infrequent. Again, I have been called to a case of labor, in consultation, where the unyielding cicatricial tissue of a restored perineum compelled episiotomy.

In conclusion, and without entering into comparison with other perineoplastic operations, some of which remind one in their diagrams of the many and various curves made by expert skaters upon the fresh ice— an American reviewer of a well-known work upon diseases of women, some years ago compared one of these marvellous diagrams to a Chinese puzzle—I will only say that it seems to me Mr. Tait's operation has very much to commend it to the profession.

THE INFECTIOUSNESS OF TUBER-CULOSIS: A STATISTICAL STUDY.

BY LAWRENCE F. FLICK, M.D.,

PHILADELPHIA.

Because of the confusing and indefinite nomenclature of tubercular diseases, and because also of the incompetence to make a diagnosis of some physicians who practise medicine, the deductions drawn from Board of Health reports cannot be accepted with any great degree of confidence. Nevertheless, with a disease from which there are as many deaths as there are from tuberculosis, we ought at least to arrive at general truths by careful topographical studies of such reports; and it is with the object of throwing some further light upon the question of the contagiousness of tuberculosis that I present this brief paper.

The Fifth Ward of the city of Philadelphia has an area of .321 of a square mile, has a population of about 16,000, and contains in the neighborhood of 3,500 houses. The population consists mostly of poor people, about twenty per cent. being colored, and has in its make up foreigners of every description and nationality; but in no part of the ward can there be said to be great overcrowding.

During the twenty-five years preceding 1888, about 1,500 deaths were returned from the ward under the various terms for consumption of the lungs and bowels, and such other terms as have the word "tubercular" attached or have that word for their basis; and they occurred in about 950 houses, or about thirty per cent. of the houses of the ward. Deaths returned under the heading of "marasmus" and other erroneous names, and which were really due to tuberculosis, are not included in the 1,500; hence thirty per cent. may be looked upon as too low a representation of the number of infected houses. But, inasmuch as deaths from such diseases occur largely in the same houses as deaths from tuberculosis of the lungs—as will be seen from the report for 1888—their exclusion in determining the number of infected houses cannot materially alter the result, and 30 per cent. may be accepted as approximately correct. I have selected twenty-five years as the most remote period by which to determine the infection of a house, for two reasons: First, because a house may retain its infection for a long time by intercurrent cases, which may get well, may move away and die somewhere else, or may die and be returned under some false name; and second, because the more remote the period, the stronger the emphasis on the non-infectedness of those houses which are set down as such.

During the year 1888 there occurred in the Fifth Ward of the city of Philadelphia 103 deaths which may be plausibly ascribed to some form of tuberculosis. Of these, 60 were returned under the various names for consumption; 17 under the heading of marasmus; 7 under that of meningitis, three having the word "tubercular" attached; 5 under that of hæmoptysis; 4 under inanition; 2 each under the names tabes mesenterica and consumption of the bowels; and one each under the name tuberculosis, general tuberculosis, chronic bronchitis, empyema, scrofula, and asthma.

Of the 103, 15 were returned from the residences of undertakers; 3 from the Consumptives' Home, on Spruce Street; one from a lodging room; and one from the Almshouse. Of the cases returned from the residence of undertakers, 11 were cases of phthisis, 2 of marasmus, and one each of scrofula and general tuberculosis. The cases from the Consumptives Home, the case from the lodging room, and the case from the Almshouse, were all cases of phthisis. Four of the cases returned from the residences of undertakers died at the Almshouse, 2 at the Pennsylvania Hospital, one at St. Mary's Hospital, one at St. Joseph's Hospital, one at the Consumptive's Home at Chestnut Hill, and one at Moyamensing prison. Inquiries as to the dwelling-places of these patients before their entry into the hospitals were attended with unsatisfactory results; but some of them at least lived outside of the ward.

Deducting the cases returned from the residence of undertakers, the Consumptives Home, etc.—20 in number, we find that of 103—the number returned from the ward—we have 83 cases which were reported from the residences in which they presumably died. Of these, 44 were cases of tuberculosis of the lung, returned under its various names, 15 were returned as marasmus, 7 as meningitis, 5 as hæmoptysis, 4 as inanition, 2 each as consumption of the bowels and tabes mesenterica, and one each as tuberculosis, asthma, empyema, and chronic bronchitis.

Of these 83 cases, I find that 48 were returned as having died in infected houses—that is, houses in which a death from some form of phthisis, or some disease with the word tubercular attached, had occurred sometime within 25 years; and 35 in non-infected houses—that is, houses in which no such death had occurred within 25 years. Of the patients which died in infected houses, 23 were returned as dying of phthisis under its various names; 10 as of marasmus; 5 as of meningitis; 2 each as of tabes mesenterica, inanition, and hæmoptysis; and one each as dying of tuberculosis, asthma, empyema, and consumption of the bowels. Of the persons who died in non-infected houses, 21 were returned as dying under the names for phthisis, 5 under that of marasmus, 3 under hæmoptysis, 2 each under those of meningitis and inanition, and one each under names consumption of the bowels and chronic bronchitis.

Of the 23 infected houses from which a death from tuberculosis of the lungs was reported, 18 had had a death from tuber-·culosis in them within 10 years, 14 within 7 years, 12 within 4 years, and 8 within 2 years. Of the 10 infected houses from which a death from marasmus was reported, 9 had had a death from tuberculosis in them within 10 years, 8 within 7 years, 7 within 5 years, 4 within one year. Of the 5 infected houses from which a death from meningitis was reported, 2 had had a death from tuberculosis in them within 10 years, and one within 3 years. Of the 2 infected houses from which a death from inanition was reported, one had had a death from tuberculosis in it within 5 years. Of the 2 infected houses from which a death from tabes mesenterica was reported, one had had a death from tuberculosis in it within one year. The infected house from which a death from consumption of the bowels was reported had had a death from tuberculosis in it within 3 years. Thus it will be seen that out of the 48 infected houses in which deaths from tuberculosis occurred during the year 1888, 32 had had deaths from tuberculosis in them within 10 years prior to 1888.

In only 5 of the 48 cases which were returned from infected houses during the year 1888 was the name the same as that of the person who had died in the house before, and of these, 2 probably bore the relation of husband and wife to the person who had died in the house first.

About the 23 cases of tuberculosis of the lungs which were returned from infected houses, I was given the following information at the houses from which they were reported: First, that 4 of the persons did not die in the house from which they were returned as having died. Upon inquiry, I was able to locate the place of death of two of these, one having died at a hospital and the other having lived and died in an infected house. Second, that 8 of them had consumption before they moved into the houses in which they died. Of 3 of these I was able to discover the former dwelling place, and all three of them contracted the disease whilst living in recently infected houses.

About the 21 cases of tuberculosis of the lung which were returned from non-infected houses, I was given the following information at the houses from which they were reported and by neighbors and friends of the deceased: First, that one of them did not die of consumption, but was reported to have died of that disease from motives of delicacy. Second, that 2 of them did not die in the houses from which they were returned. In both of these I was able to locate the place of death, and in one of them I found that the house was an infected one, that the person had lived there a year, but that he probably had the disease when he moved there. Third, that 7 of them had had consumption when they moved into the houses in which they died. Of 2 of these I was able to discover the previous residence, and in both instances I found it to be in an infected house. Fourth, that 2 of them had been associated with consumptives in their business. In neither of these cases was there any family history of consumption. Fifth, that 5 of them lived in lodging houses, where there was a constantly changing population, and that 3 of these were drinking persons.

This information, I am sorry to say, even meagre as it is, is not very reliable. The fears, suspicions, and prejudices of many of the people from whom I sought it, prevented them from telling the entire truth, and even led them to misstate facts. I give it, however, as I got it, so that every one with the entire picture before him may draw his own conclusions.

Even the data which I took from the Board of Health records I cannot endorse as entirely trustworthy. The custom of returning deaths from the place of burial instead of the place of death, the carelessness of undertakers in giving the numbers of houses and wards, and the indefiniteness of the nomenclature used by physicians, I am sure engendered mistakes which· I have not in every instance been able to correct.

The moving about from place to place of persons suffering from tuberculosis ought likewise to be taken into consideration in drawing conclusions, when the infection of houses, as determined upon mortality statistics alone, forms part of the premises of the argument. To what extent such change of residence alters the actual percentage of infected houses, and consequently invalidates the conclusions based upon the facts and figures I have given, must of course remain an unknown quantity, and must be approximately measured by every one for himself.

In spite, however, of all these sources of inaccuracy, which I have just mentioned, the figures which I have given, bearing upon tuberculosis in the Fifth Ward of this city for the year 1888, point unmistakably to the fact that tuberculosis is not only contagious in the broad sense of that word, but that a house in which that disease has existed remains a centre of infection for an indefinite time. Upon no other theory than this can a rational explanation be given of the fact that, whilst less than one-third of the houses of the ward became infected with tuberculosis during the 25 years prior to 1888, considerably more than one-half of the deaths from tuberculosis during the year 1888 occurred in those infected houses. Inasmuch as there were more than twice as many non-infected houses in the ward, as there were infected houses, we would naturally expect a preponderance of deaths in non-infected houses. Why this great preponderance of deaths in infected houses?

The conclusion that houses once infected by tuberculosis retain that infection for some time, is even more strongly borne out by individual cases than by the aggregate number of cases during the year. A death from tuberculosis occurred in a house on Gaskill street, in 1880. The family moved out and R. H. moved in. He was quite well when he moved there. He was a travelling salesman, and was away from home a good deal, but had his home there. In time he developed consumption, and he died in 1888. L. M. lived in the house in which she died for many years. A person who was no relative of hers died from consumption in the house in 1887. She took the disease in a very acute form, and died in 1888. H. M. suffered from chronic tuberculous diarrhœa, and died from it during the year 1888. During that same year there occurred a death from marasmus in the same

house. A death from consumption of the bowels was returned during January, of 1888, from a certain house on Hurst street; a woman who died from phthisis during September of the same year on Lombard street probably contracted the disease in that same house, as she lived there about that same time. During the latter part of 1887, a person died of phthisis in a certain house in the ward; during July, of 1888, a child 9 months old, not of the same family, died in the same house from tabes mesenterica. During the month of September, 1888, there occurred 2 deaths in an infected house in the ward—one from marasmus, in a child one year old, and one from meningitis, in a child 2 years old. The house had had 3 deaths from tuberculosis within recent years, the last one reported being in 1885. In a house on St. Mary street a death occurred from consumption during the latter part of 1887; during July, 1888, a child 17 months old died in the same house from marasmus. A woman is reported to have died from phthisis in a house on Union street during the year 1888, from which no cases of tuberculosis had ever been returned before. The house is a lodging house, and she is said to have taken the disease whilst living there. A man who died in a non-infected house on Spruce street, during the same year, was found to have contracted the disease in that same house about the same time. A death from tuberculosis is returned from a house on Dock street, in 1882. J. C. moved into the house sometime in 1884. He contracted consumption and died in 1888.

These cases are all taken from among those who died from tuberculosis in the Fifth Ward during the year 1888. By going back of that year I could cite from my notes hundreds of equally striking cases, illustrating the infectious etiology of tuberculosis.

Perhaps one of the most interesting lessons to be learned from this inquiry into the relation which the deaths from tuberculosis in the Fifth Ward during the year 1888 bore to those from the same disease during the 25 years prior thereto, is that bearing upon marasmus and meningitis in children. It will be remembered that out of 22 deaths from these two diseases, 17 occurred in houses which had been infected by tuberculosis of the lungs and bowels in adults. It would appear from this that marasmus and tubercular meningitis in children are apt to be concurrent with tuberculosis of the lungs and bowels in adults; that is to say, where an adult is suffering from phthisis or consumption of the bowels in any house, the children of that house are prone to develop marasmus or tubercular meningitis, and that these diseases are not apt to become centres of infection themselves.

It is somewhat surprising that only 7 deaths were returned from the ward under the heading of meningitis for the entire year, and that really only 3 of those had the word tubercular attached. The number of cases of tubercular meningitis which I meet with in my own practice would lead me to believe that these figures do not correctly represent the relative frequency of the disease, and that in all probability many deaths which are ascribed to convulsions are really due to tubercular meningitis. I have within the last year seen four deaths from tubercular meningitis in children, three of which occurred in houses in which there was a case of phthisis in an adult.

It is greatly to be regretted that our nomenclature of tubercular diseases is not more definite and more uniform than it is; for until it becomes so, statistical and clinical study of the disease will necessarily remain difficult. We cannot hope, however, to make much progress in this direction until the etiology of tuberculosis is settled, and until precise knowledge upon the subject shall be dispensed from every seat of medical learning. It is with the desire of hastening that day that I present this statistical analysis, if I may so call it, hoping thereby to stimulate others to enter this promising field of study.

Many interesting deductions, besides the few which I have made, might be drawn from the figures which I present, and many criticisms made upon the practical operation of our sanitary laws, as a legitimate part of this paper; but it would lead to subjects which in themselves furnish material for extensive papers. I will therefore, for the present, rest content with stating the facts and calling attention to a few of the most striking conclusions which grow out of those facts.

—The question of the origin of the dog has recently been discussed by Prof. Nehing, who believes that it has descended from various still surviving species of wolves and jackals. The latter animals can be tamed, and many attempts to domesticate wolves have been successfully made in recent times. Herr Ronge has so completely tamed a young wolf that it follows him exactly as a dog might do.

HYSTERECTOMY FOR LARGE FIBRO-MYOMA.

BY D. BENJAMIN, M.D.,
CAMDEN, N. J.
SURGEON TO THE COOPER HOSPITAL.

H. M., 30 years old, living in the southern part of New Jersey, came to me on March 24, 1888, suffering from a large abdominal tumor, which physicians had called an ovarian tumor. I obtained the following history: Her mother died of erysipelas, one sister died with cerebro-spinal meningitis. The patient's past condition was stated to have been moderately healthy until last summer, when she commenced to lose flesh; at this time there was noticed a slight enlargement of the abdomen, which was attributed to dropsy.

In October, 1887, the patient was examined by a physician, who stated that there was a tumor in the left ovarian region, then about the size of a fist. Two months afterward she was subjected to another examination, and the tumor was found to have increased in size to that of a child's head. No history of any injury to this region could be obtained. Her menstrual flow had been regular, sometimes profuse; it had skipped one month, which she attributed to a cold.

The patient began to suffer from vomiting and constipation, and occasional abdominal pains; these symptoms steadily grew worse, until almost every meal was vomited, and constipation became more and more obstinate, so that powerful purgatives had to be administered, but were losing their effect; symptoms of obstruction were becoming marked. She had lost fifty pounds in weight within a few months, but as she had been previously inclined to be stout, her emaciation was not extreme. The tumor appeared symmetrical and mobile, did not feel so hard as is common with fibroid tumors, nor so soft as a cyst, was not nodular, felt very much like a pregnant womb in the early part of the ninth month. Fluctuation could not be positively demonstrated. The percussion note was dull, except over a small area in each flank. Vaginal examination indicated that the cervix was drawn up; there was an enlargement in Douglas's pouch about the size of a retroverted womb. Examination of the rectum gave no additional information. A flexible urethral sound passed into the os uteri about two inches, taking a forward direction. Before using the sound pregnancy was eliminated by examination. A diagnosis of solid or semi-solid tumor involving the womb could be made, but the exact relation of the ovaries to this tumor was not clear. Exploratory incision was advised, with a view of ascertaining the exact relation of the tumor to the pelvic organs, and the possibility of its removal, with the understanding that any beneficial operation that would seem feasible should be proceeded with.

Accordingly, on March 29, the patient was etherized, the usual incision was made in the median line, and the surface of the tumor exposed. The tumor was quite elastic, and of a dark flesh color, and wedged so tightly in the superior straight of the pelvis that only one ovary, the left, which was enlarged, could be reached. As adhesions were slight, the incision was extended upward with scissors—sufficiently to enable the upper part of the tumor to be reached ; this part was free, but was in contact with the stomach and liver. The incision was then extended upward and downward sufficiently to enable the tumor to be delivered forward through the abdominal incision.

Both ovaries and Fallopian tubes could then be easily reached, while the large tumor was held upward, out of the abdominal cavity, by an assistant. The pedicle could not be thoroughly examined at this stage. The right ovary was enlarged, was found crowded down into Douglas's pouch, and was enlarged to about the size of a hen's egg, and roughened on the surface. The right Fallopian tube was also much enlarged ; the left tube was about double the normal size, and adherent. Both ovaries, and both Fallopian tubes were carefully ligated and cut away. The exact relation of the base of the tumor to the womb could now be clearly made out, and it was apparent that room enough could be obtained above the insertion of the vaginal wall into the cervix to remove the tumor and body of the womb—which was thoroughly and uniformally fused together—without necessarily wounding the ureters, bladder, or other pelvic organ. I then determined to remove the entire tumor and womb, since to return it to the abdominal cavity would have been equivalent to leaving her in almost as bad a condition as before the operation, with respect to the obstruction, and other difficulties which the tumor caused ; and at the same time the operation would then be little less dangerous to the patient's life than complete hysterectomy. I then carried the incision downward as close to the pubic bone as the bladder would permit, ligated each of the round ligaments in two places and cut between, applied Koeberle's clamp and cut away the tumor. The stump was at least three inches in diameter. The tumor was about thirty inches in circumference. After all bleeding points had been properly secured, and all clots removed from the abdominal cavity, the bowels and peritoneum was thoroughly washed off by pouring three or four gallons of warm water into the abdominal cavity.

The omentum, which had been lying on a towel, was returned and arranged over the bowels. The pedicle was fixed in the lower angle of the womb, and the incision closed with silk sutures at intervals of less than half an inch. The wound was dressed antiseptically, and the patient placed in bed.

The temperature, which had been normal before the operation, was taken three quarters of an hour afterward, and found to be 97.2° ; at 4 P. M., 100.8°. The second day, at 7 P. M., it reached 100.4°, pulse 128, respiration 28. Third day, 7 A. M., temperature 101° ; 7 P. M., temperature 101.4°, pulse 116, breathing 24. Fourth day, 7 A. M., temperature 99.4° ; 7 P. M., 100.6°. Fifth day, 7 A. M., temperature 99° ; catherization was stopped on account of irritation of the bladder. The patient constantly improved without any untoward symptoms, and was discharged in six weeks after the operation. The clamp came off on the twenty-third day. She has not vomited since the operation, has had no pain, and all her functions are normal. The patient states that it is the first time she has felt well for four or five years. She has returned to her home in the country, with rosy cheeks, full of life, and at this date, May, 1889, is in perfect health. She has not been sick a day since the operation, and is glad that she parted with her womb and ovaries.

In determining the value to humanity of the operation of hysterectomy, it is important that all cases should be reported, as I found the literature on the subject so meagre at the time of the operation just described that reliable data could not be obtained in this country. The operation had never, so far as I can learn, been performed' in New Jersey ; but as hysterectomies are becoming more frequent and successful, ample statistics will soon be forthcoming.

—Dr. W. D. Johnson, who is delivering a series of scientific lectures in San Francisco on the lower forms of animal life, says the oyster is capable of being educated in a limited way.

REPORTS OF CLINICS.

HARLEM HOSPITAL, N. Y.

SURGICAL CLINIC—DR. MANLEY.

Necrosis of Lower Jaw.

The first case for operation was one of resection of the lower jaw on the right side, for necrosis. The patient, a young woman, 25 years old, stated that she had suffered more or less pain along the whole line of the bone for more than three years; that she was never injured in the locality of the disease, and could give no cause for it; that abscesses of large size had formed at different times, between the ramus and ear, and had been evacuated by various physicians. At the time of operation, the patient presented a care-worn, cachectic, and very anæmic appearance, which was no doubt largely due to inability to masticate food, as well as to the want of sleep and the effect of pain and worry.

Dr. Manley, in his opening remarks, said that if he found exfoliation or limited caries, the case could be easily dealt with, as far as operative procedure went; but from what he had learned of the history alone, without examination of the patient, he strongly suspected a necrosis of the whole shaft, and its removal might, in spite of all precaution and care, entail considerable loss of blood.

On opening the larger pus accumulation, the bare and denuded bone could be seen stripped of its periosteum, from the symphysis to above the insertion of the masseter muscle. All the teeth formerly inserted into the true bone had long since decayed or dropped out, except the right central incisor, which was easily lifted up with the finger and thumb.

"In the removal of the inferior maxilla for disease," Dr. Manley remarked, "there are a few points which should be constantly borne in mind, and the neglect of which might not only place our patient's life in great jeopardy, but also leave her in a condition more lamentable than that which we are attempting to relieve. The first is, in a young person, to use every care in preserving the periosteum for the future reproduction of the bone; the second, carefully to avoid wounding Steno's duct, an accident which may leave a fistula difficult or even impossible to close. As this duct passes directly across the ramus of the upper jaw over the masseter muscle, this is no imaginary danger; the third,—and perhaps the most important of all—is to provide against excessive hemorrhage. The numerous great vessels which pass close to the angle—the internal maxillary, facial, transverse facial, and the internal carotid arteries, besides the internal jugular vein and its large tributaries, which drain all the tissues anterior to the ear—are to be avoided as far as possible, though some of them under certain circumstances are necessarily divided. If the bone readily shells out of the periosteum, throughout its whole length, its removal will be a simple matter."

Dr. Manley began his operation by passing a temporary transfixion stitch under the distal and proximal ends of the facial artery, which step cut off one important source of bleeding. An incision was then made in the usual way along the body of the jaw to the outer border of the masseter muscle, when a severe hemorrhage took place, apparently from every direction, but largely from the trunks of some large vessel. The wound was immediately filled and packed with sponges, but yet the blood welled up through and beside them. They were now quickly removed and the common carotid compressed against the cervical vertebræ. This at once checked the arterial admixture, but the hemorrhage still continued with a frightful rush. Clamp after clamp was applied in rapid succession, and the ligature used wherever a visible point of bleeding was observed; but the tissues seemed so soft and friable that the ligatures were of little avail. Dr. Manley now passed the index and middle finger within the mouth of the bleeding patient, along the right side of the buccal cavity, and rapidly pushed the tissues outward. This procedure, while firm pressure was continued, diminished the torrents of blood, which threatened quickly to end fatally if not arrested. The temporary transfixion stitch was again applied above and below, and it immediately arrested all bleeding. The termination of the operation was then completed leisurely.

Double Genu-Varum.

Among other instructive operations at the clinic was one of some interest for the manner in which it was done. It occurred in a case of double genu-varum, in a child two years old. Dr. Manley remarked that, in all cases in young children, when it is deemed advisable to remove the deformity, there is no method yet devised which will take the place of the hand in fracturing the bone, providing this was not too strong.

There is no osteoclast like it, and it should always be preferred to osteotomy, when practicable, as we do not make a slit-wound or create a compound fracture. Besides, he observed, with the osteotome and mallet, owing not only to the different consistency of bone which sometimes exists in the two limbs of the same child, there is danger of applying too much force on the mallet; as what would readily divide one bone would make very little impression on the other. He believes the iron osteoclast to be a dangerous apparatus, as he knows from experience; he says that when the hand will not break a bone, the osteotome should always be used in preference to any other means. In the present case, both bones were readily snapped with the hands; after which the limbs were put in plaster dressings, and the child sent home.

NEW YORK CORRESPONDENCE.

Locomotor Ataxia Treated by Extension— A Rabbit's Cornea Grafted on a Human Eye—How to Treat Chronic Ulcers— Tubercular Ostitis of the Ankle-joint.

NEW YORK, May 19, 1889.

Prof. Charles L. Dana, of the Post-Graduate School and Women's College, is using the new treatment of extension for locomotor ataxia on a patient in the Post-Graduate Hospital, and is having marked success. The patient is an expressman from Vermont, 44 years of age. He is married, the father of two children, and his personal history is excellent. His father died of rheumatism. His case is a typical one. Two years ago, he had wandering pains in his legs and feet, with a burning sensation. They also felt as if swollen and large. Then followed difficulty in walking, especially in the dark and when his eyes were closed. He has the feeling of a constriction around the thighs and chest, his patellar reflex is gone, there is incontinence of urine, no sexual desire, diarrhœa usually, and the characteristic ataxic gait. He was treated by a noted Boston specialist, but was given only iodide of potassium, with galvanism to his spine and Faradism to the muscles of the leg. Not improving, he placed himself under the care of Dr. Dana, who is using extension. To obtain it, he uses the ordinary tripod and harness which orthopœdists employ in applying plaster jackets. As is well known, this consists of a strap under each arm, and one under the chin and the back of his head. On the latter strap falls most of the weight. By means of pulleys the man is lifted entirely off his feet. The extension at first lasted only thirty seconds, but the time has been slowly increased until now, after three weeks, it lasts five minutes. In the meantime, the patient is getting nitrate of silver and chloride of gold and potassium, with foot-baths, rest in bed and a highly nutritious diet. Already the man is improving. He has less pain, the sensation in his feet has improved, and he holds his urine better. Dr. Dana is also using the extension treatment on a patient in Bellevue Hospital, to which he is a visiting physician.

Writing of locomotor ataxia brings to mind an instructive incident which occurred in Bellevue Hospital last week. One of the visiting physicians was making the ordinary tests for tabes dorsalis, and told the patient to walk with his eyes closed. He tried to do so, but fell so heavily that he broke his arm. This was in the presence of fifteen physicians, but none was near enough to catch the patient.

Dr. Francis Valk, Professor of Diseases of the Eye and Ear at the Post-Graduate School, has succeeded in grafting the cornea of a rabbit upon the eye of a woman, his being, as the writer understands, only the second successful case. The patient was 44 years old, born in Ireland, the mother of three healthy children, and the possessor of an unusually good personal and family history. Three years ago she had a gonorrhœal ophthalmia which left her totally blind, so that she could not distinguish light from darkness, the cause of the blindness being opacity of the cornea. On April 26, Dr. Valk operated on the left eye. With a trephine, specially constructed for the purpose, a piece of cornea as large as the end of a lead pencil was removed from the woman's eye. Then a rabbit was chloroformed and a similar piece removed from its cornea. This was immediately carried over to the woman's eye on a spatula and nicely fitted in. The eye was washed out with boracic acid, the lid lifted into place, a piece of cotton placed on it and a circular head-bandage applied. Nothing else was done. The operation was short and simple and, though the rabbit died under the chloroform before the piece of cornea was removed, the graft lived and united by first intention. There was no fever and at the first dressing, a week later, the union was perfect. The grafted cornea was at first totally opaque, but it is gradually clearing up, until now the woman appreciates not only light but also color, and a perfectly clear cornea is the anticipated result. The right eye was operated on May 11, with a similarly successful result. The second rabbit, however, was not chloroformed, cocaine being used instead. The trephine used is an ingenious little instrument. It has a sharp cutting edge and works with a spring. It is wound up, and then, when in place, a lever is touched and the spring causes the cylinder to whirl around, the cylinder being gauged to go to a certain depth and no deeper. As the membrane covering the aqueous humor is not ruptured, this fluid is not lost. In one eye this membrane was also opaque, hence the sight can not be regained in that eye. The patient, however, will have one good eye and the doctor has succeeded in demonstrating that the operation can be successfully done. The antiseptic precautions used were surprisingly few. The eye was not washed and the instruments were not placed in any solution. The operator did not even wash his hands. In short, the only antisepsis used was a slight wash with a solution of boracic acid after the graft was in place. The graft, after being taken from the rabbit's eye, was not dipped in an antiseptic solution but was carried immediately to the patient's eye on a spatula, which was previously wiped clean on the operator's coat sleeve. Notwithstanding all this, there was primary union throughout in both operations.

Dr. Valk has also made another step forward in eye surgery, by devising a means of removing a cataract without iridectomy. He makes the ordinary incision in front of the iris and then, by means of a retractor which he has invented, he dilates the pupil so that the opaque lens can be scooped out. This leaves the iris intact. It is a neat operation and will doubtless be popular.

For chronic indolent ulcers, Dr. S. J. White, Jr., House Surgeon of Bellevue Hospital, uses a paste of balsam of Peru and iodoform, over which is placed an antiseptic dressing of bichloride of mercury gauze. It works admirably, and the ulcers close up rapidly. There are no fixed proportions of the ingredients, the iodoform being stirred into the balsam until the desired thickness of paste is obtained.

Dr. V. P. McGibney being detained by the sickness of his son, his clinic on orthopœdic surgery at the New York Polyclinic last week was held by Dr. J. B. Bissell of Bellevue and Forty-second Street Hospitals. The subject was tubercular ostitis of the ankle, a child with this disease, commonly known as white swelling, being presented. The disease is comparatively rarely found at the ankle. Out of 321 cases treated at the Forty-second Street Hospital last year, the ankle was affected only eleven times. Most frequently it is found at the hip, then in the knee, shoulder, and lastly in the ankle. Its symptoms are : swelling—uniform and not localized ; stiffness—little, perhaps no, motion ; atrophy of the muscles—the patient's leg showed a marked diminution in size ; flabby muscles ; heat ; lameness and pain not proportioned to the amount of disease, as extensive disease may not be accompanied by much lameness or pain, or the contrary. Lastly is the cry of ostitis, chiefly heard at night. The lameness is characteristic and once seen is always a valuable sign. The nature of the disease is acknowledged to be tubercular. The New York Clinical Society last year appointed a committee to investigate the matter. It thoroughly analyzed forty cases, and found an hereditary taint in all. If traumatism occurs it acts only as an exciting cause. Though the treatment may not much vary, the affection is to be differentiated from acute arthritis, acute epiphysitis, bursitis, sprains, contusions, etc. The patient had been ill for a year, and hence all affections except bursitis were excluded. In the latter, the swelling is localized over one point, usually externally and anteriorly, where are located the bursæ of the tibialis anticus, extensor proprius pollicis, extensor longus digitorum and peronei muscles. In acute synovitis, the swelling is across the anterior portion of the joint where the capsule is thinnest. Acute arthritis is marked by an exceedingly rapid progress and great infiltration of pus ; abscesses form, the bones are affected, and there are marked pyæmic symptoms. The treatment is very generally conceded to be complete rest. Some use felt or leather splints, but more preferable are plaster-of-Paris splints, with the foot placed at a right angle to the leg so that, if anchylosis does occur, the limb is in the best possible position. In children able to walk, a Thomas splint is used. It is simply two bars of iron surmounted by a ring through which the leg goes, and hence the child walks with all his weight caught on the perineum. The sole of the other shoe is enlarged. Cases last from six months to six years. Some go on quietly, with the patient in good health ; but as a rule abscesses develop, sinuses form, there is hectic, etc. The question arises, shall the abscess be opened ? It is a mooted question, but the best men are in agreement that if it is very large and acute, and pyæmic symptoms develop, the abscess should be opened ; otherwise that it be let alone. If it is opened, as little bone as possible should be removed, as excision gives bad results, and if too much is removed, no union results and there is a worse than useless joint. The best plan of treatment is the expectant, giving cod-liver oil, iron, good air, etc., and treating symptoms as they arise.

FOREIGN CORRESPONDENCE.

LETTER FROM BERLIN.

(FROM OUR SPECIAL CORRESPONDENT.)

BERLIN, April 27, 1889.

The Eighteenth Congress of Surgery.—Esmarch on Carcinoma.—Horsley on Injuries of the Cortical motor Region.—Heidenhain on the Causes of Relapse in Cancer.—Schuchardt on Ozæna.—Bramann on Symmetrical Gangrene.—Schinzinger on the Prevention of Relapse of Mammary Cancer.—Thiersch on Extraction of Nerves.—Angerer on Diagnosis of and Operation for Stenosis of the Pylorus.—Schmidt on Extirpation of the Larynx.—Oppenheim on Traumatic Neurosis.—Lauenstein on Complete Extirpation of the Knee joint.—Gerstein on artificial Closure of Cranial Defects.—Mikulicz on the Operative Treatment of Perforating Peritonitis.—Leser on Actinomycosis.—Hanau on Inoculation of Carcinoma.—Mosler on Myxœdema.—Hoffa on newly discovered Ptomaïnes.—Ritasato on pure Cultures of the Tetanus Microbes.—Credé on Surgery of the Gall-bladder.—Waitz on Congenital Elephantiasis.

The Eighteenth Annual Congress of Surgery was opened in the great hall of the University by an address by Prof. Bergmann, in which he bade the numerous and distinguished guests welcome. After a brief reference to the case of Emperor Frederick, he called for three cheers for Emperor William II, the protector of art and science. Among the notable foreign guests were Horsley, of London and Billroth, of Vienna, whose sixtieth birthday just happened to be on the opening day of the Congress. The following are the essential features of the most interesting papers read :

In speaking of carcinoma, Prof. Esmarch said : "Every surgeon is familiar with a type of ulcerating neoplasms, occurring on any portion of the body but preferably on the tongue and lips, which in appearance and course are sometimes scarcely distinguishable from cancer. The differential diagnosis in such cases is, however, of great importance, as these pseudo-cancers often yield to medicinal treatment and trifling operations, while true cancers call for an early and thorough removal by the knife. In all doubtful cases a careful microscopical examination is an absolute necessity, even if, to obtain a particle of the tumor for examination, repeated and deep incisions are required. The greatest resemblance to cancer is presented by the syphilomata, especially if they appear many years after the infection or late in life as the result of hereditary transmission. Often the diagnosis is to be made by exclusion; and syphiloma can be diagnosticated if, after microscopical examination, cancer, tuberculosis, and actinomycosis have been excluded. A syphiloma readily assumes a malignant nature if not extirpated in time. The question as to the origin of malignant tumors is of vital interest, though, unfortunately, it is not yet definitely settled. An irritation, especially a continued one, appears to be the principal etiological factor, taken in connection with a certain predisposition—mostly inherited—and a lowered power of resistance. Besides, it is unquestioned that papillomata, atheromata, syphilomata, and condylomata *can assume a malignant character.* All other theories of the pathogenesis of cancer—such as Scheurlen's (microbic origin) or Cohnheim's (from embryonic cells), or those advanced by Thiersch and Waldeyer—are no longer tenable. The formation of sarcomata on a syphilitic base gives us a general idea of the origin of malignant neoplasms. A syphilitic affection apparently extinct leaves behind it a tendency toward proliferation of the connective tissue which, if removed by the knife, returns obstinately and, like the most malignant cancer, may lead to a general metastasis. The hereditary predisposition to syphiloma may have been transmitted from remote ancestors, several intervening generations being exempt."

In speaking of the recognition of injuries of the cortical motor region, Mr. Victor Horsley said that his researches proved a connection between certain points of the motor centre of the brain and various extremities. Thus, he had determined the central points presiding over the motility of the single fingers, the wrist-joint, the arm, the hip-joint, the knee-joint, and the toes. *Vice versâ* he was enabled to judge of the condition of those central points by the phenomena presented by the corresponding extremities. He has succeeded in this way in ascertaining and localizing various injuries of the motor region.

Heidenhain said that relapses in cases of cancer are invariably caused by cancerous portions left behind, and as his observations have shown this is especially the case after operations for cancer of the breast. It is, consequently, important to remove not only the cancerous portion of the breast, but also the pectoral fascia and a part or the whole of the pectoral muscle, according to the extent of its implication. This operation, which in addition has the advantage of removing the ordinarily suspected Mohrenheim's cavity, is not a bloodier one than the usual operation, and does not induce greater functional disturbances. It is very desirable to trace the migration of the cancer cells in order to get the proper limits for the operation.

Schuchardt remarked that the investigations on ozæna of Volkmann and himself have revealed, as the cause of ozæna, a transformation of the nasal ciliary epithelium into pavement epithelium, accompanied by putrid decomposition.

Bramann presented three boys, brothers, ranging in age from seven to thirteen years, suffering from gangrenous lesions on the fingers and toes. A close inspection demonstrate the symmetrical nature of the lesions. As there is not the slightest traceable cause for the affection, a nervous predisposition or, possibly, disease of the spinal cord must be regarded as an etiological factor. In the discussion on the subject several similar cases, for the most part of a traumatic character, were reported.

Schinzinger, in speaking of the prevention of relapse of mammary cancer, made a bold and original proposal. To prevent the return of cancer of the breast he advocated, if the woman had not yet reached her change of life, the removal of the ovaries. Cancer of the breast is the more malignant the younger the patient is, and the removal of the ovaries, the author said, would cause the woman rapidly and prematurely to grow old and the breasts to wither. The results of Schinzinger's heroic treatment will be looked for with great interest.

Thiersch said that many cases of neuralgia have been successfully treated by extraction of nerves. The great obstacle in this operation is the difficulty of getting well up near the origin of the nerve, which is of course very desirable. To facilitate this aim Thiersch has constructed a number of forceps which have proven very valuable, especially in extraction of branches of the trifacial nerve. In this connection he referred to a smith living near Leipzig, who enjoyed quite a reputation for instantly removing even the most violent toothache by a puncture of the face. He evidently punctured the auriculotemporal nerve. Such an operation, however, is to be condemned, as the destruction of so important a nerve causes serious injury to the muscles supplied by it. There is, besides, considerable danger of injuring the facial nerve, which runs near the auriculotemporal nerve.

Angerer said the diagnosis of pyloric stenosis is made by inflating the stomach with carbonic acid gas—generated by the administration of bicarbonate of sodium and tartaric acid—or by pumping air into the stomach. These measures serve to show whether the suspected swelling is in the stomach or in some neighboring organ. In the former case, resection affords fair prospects of success, and in the latter instance, a gastro-intestinal fistula will at least bring alleviation. The results of such operations are the better the sooner they are performed. As an anæsthetic for these operations, Thiersch recommended Rocher's plan, viz., giving chloroform in the beginning and ether later. Lauenstein called attention to the diuresis produced by the preparatory washing out of the stomach, one patient voiding fifty-five ounces of urine on the day following the washing out of the stomach. The cause of this diuresis appears to be the sucking up of the water by the tissues, though physiologists have doubted this capacity when there is so serious an affection of the stomach.

Schmidt presented a patient from whom about two years ago the entire larynx had been removed on account of cancer. The patient enjoyed good health, and his speech was all that could be desired; he had no artificial larynx and breathed through a canula.

Oppenheim's paper on traumatic neurosis created universal interest, all the more as it was illustrated by five patients suffering with the affection. The first patient was thrown and fell upon his left shoulder; the second was bruised by a car; the third was caught by an engine and injured in the back; the fourth fell from a locomotive; and the fifth was injured on the head by a falling wall. The nervous phenomena presenting themselves after disappearance of the immediate consequences of the injuries—such as swelling, etc.—consisted in various nervous disturbances, such as paralysis, anæsthesia, loss of mental activity, and difficulties of speaking and hearing. In the first and second patients the lesions remained limited to the injured half of the body; the third patient presented a singular and sad appearance; all the muscles of the trunk were in a state of violent and permanent convulsion. The pulse ranged in all the cases from 100 to 140, and great mental depression and insomnia were also universally present. Formerly such affections were frequently interpreted as simulations, as the existence of such nervous phenomena was regarded as impossible without a palpable spinal lesion. The present light of neurological science has dispersed this erroneous view.

Lauenstein's paper on complete exsection of the knee-joint gave rise to an interesting discussion regarding the significance of the ligamenta cruciata, the preservation of which he regarded as essential to functional integrity of the joint. König, on the other hand, said these ligaments served merely as an inhibitory apparatus for rotation, and could be cut without any scruples, all the more as they were sure to reunite again.

Gerstein described his method of reinserting portions of the skull which, by some traumatic cause, have been blown off. If strict antiseptic precautions are taken, bony reunion will result in the majority of cases. Horsley emphasized the importance of immediate replacement.

Mikulicz dwelt especially on the difference between the acute, diffuse, septic form of peritonitis and the progressive purulent, fibrinous, perforating form. In the former, laparotomy is a useless measure, while in the latter this operation is a necessity. The operator has to find out the several foci of suppuration and to empty them; but has to be careful not to disturb the natural connection of the intestinal loops which form a very desirable obstacle to the extension of suppuration. Antisepsis is of little importance here, a mechanical elimination of the pus being solely required. Nor is it necessary to hunt anxiously for the perforation, which heals spontaneously in a short time. To prevent the coming forward of intestines on coughing and vomiting, loose sutures are to be inserted, and a careful after-treatment (diet, opium, etc.) is to be instituted.

Leser said that actinomycosis, which has been hitherto believed to exist only in the cavities of the mouth, throat and abdomen, has by him been observed also in the skin in three cases. The affection is a rather frequent one in the vicinity of Graz, Austria, where it attacks especially mowers who have injured their fingers. Rotter also denies the rare occurrence of actinomycosis of the skin, as he has himself observed six cases.

Hanau stated that nearly all attempts to produce carcinoma artificially in animals through inoculation with carcinomatous matter, have hitherto proved futile. He, however, has succeeded in this inoculation in dogs and rabbits, and in a single instance in a man, whose case was an absolutely hopeless one.

Mossler presented a case of myxœdema of unusual interest. The patient, a lady in the prime of life, was suddenly attacked by the disease without any apparent cause. The affection was ushered in with a swelling of the skin beginning on the thumb of the left hand, and soon spread over the entire body, causing a dreadful disfiguration of the once handsome woman. The expression of the face is dull and stupid, and the swollen eyelids render the eyes exceedingly small in appearance. Speech and hearing are perceptibly defective as the result of the extensive swelling of the mucous membranes. The use of her limbs is likewise greatly impeded. Both the etiology and the therapeutics of the disease are absolutely blanks as yet. As usual, nervous conditions are said to be the causative agencies. Some observers have pointed to the thyroid gland as the possible cause of the disease, as this organ is usually found greatly diminished in size in this and in similar affections. In the patient presented, the thyroid gland is so small that it can scarcely be felt, and the entire affection recalls strikingly the phenomena of cachexia strumipriva, which is observed after total extirpation of goitre. Horsley, who has studied this disease in particular, presented various sections taken from patients with myxœdema, and also called attention to the peculiar contraction of the pupil always observed in this affection.

Hoffa said that the researches of numerous bacteriologists have established the doctrine that all intoxications of the septicæmic type are caused by certain ptomaines, which are regarded as the products of tissue changes or of secretions of specific microörganisms in the blood. Hitherto the exact nature and the chemical composition of these ptomaines have eluded all investigation. The author claims the credit of having first ascertained the exact chemical constituents of this poison. Experimenting on rabbits which had died of septicæmia, he succeeded in isolating the pathogenic ptomaine and in ascertaining its chemical nature. The composition of the ptomaine of septicæmia is that of methylic guanidin, and is represented by the formula of $C_2 H_7 N_3$. This chemical, injected into the lymphatic glands of healthy rabbits, causes the exact phenomena of septicæmia, which the author proved before the Congress. Hoffa has also discovered the specific ptomaine of anthrax, the formula of which he found to be $C_3 H_6 N_2$.

Ritasato, who was mentioned in the last Berlin letter as the discoverer of the musk bacillus, is the first bacteriologist who has succeeded in preparing a pure culture of the specific microbe of tetanus. It is a bristle-bacillus, which occurs in the superficial strata of the earth, and, when injected into animals, causes tetanus. Rosenbach has detected this bacillus also in the oral secretions of men affected with tetanus. Ritasato's method of obtaining a pure culture of the bristle-bacillus is as follows: The mixture containing this bacillus, in conjunction with other microörganisms, was placed in an incubating stove at a temperature of 97°-100.2° F., where a prolific multiplication could take place. He found that at a temperature of 176° F.—provided it was not kept up too long—all germ life perished with the exception of the spores of the bristle-bacillus, which could thus be obtained in a pure culture. Ritasato presented a pure culture and tried its action on mice, with the anticipated result, before the Congress. The tetanus bacillus is able to resist both heat and chemical agents to a considerable degree; it perishes when exposed to steam at the temperature of 212° F. in five minutes, and in five hours if exposed to the action of a five per cent. solution of carbolic acid. Its toxic effects are not attenuated through inoculation, but are destroyed by the action of dilute muriatic acid.

Credé, in speaking of the surgery of the gall-bladder, said that dogs in which the gall-bladder has been removed show great voracity for some time, but soon decrease in weight; later their weight increases again. Credé has observed the very same condition in two patients in whom he had removed the gall-bladder. The explanation is, that at first the fatty matters cannot well be digested in the intestines, owing to the absence of a sufficient quantity of bile, which after removal of the gall-bladder enters the intes-

tines constantly in a small quantity instead of the physiological plentiful supply at the needed time. Nature, however, forms—as the autopsy of animals and men has shown—an artificial reservoir in the common bile duct, and thus re-establishes the lost physiological conditions, which result in the subsequent increase of weight.

Waitz presented a child with congenital elephantiasis. The legs of the otherwise well-formed child, which was one year and a half old, showed an enormous hypertrophy both in length and thickness, especially marked in the left leg. The clinical history was very unsatisfactory. The mother knew of no possible cause except a great excitement experienced by her during a visit to a circus, shortly before her confinement.

In conclusion, I may mention that a magnificent exhibition of surgical instruments and of bacteriological specimens was prepared in connection with this Congress, which, as all agree, was a perfect success.

PERISCOPE.

Treatment of Aneurisms of the Aorta.

In a communication to the Berlin Medical Society, April 3, Dr. Litten said that there were some aneurisms of the aorta with which the patients can live from ten to twenty years; but the average duration of life is from fifteen to eighteen months. Death may arise from marasmus, from compression of the trachea or of a bronchus, through an intercurrent disease, or even by rupture of the aneurism into the pleura, pericardium, trachea or bronchus. Danger to life resides chiefly in the tendency of aneurisms to increase progressively in volume.

Treatment is essentially symptomatic. Hypodermic injections of antipyrin are excellent for the pain. For the insomnia, sulphonal should be tried before having recourse to morphine. In England and France iodide of potash is considered a specific for aneurism. This opinion is the result of the belief in the syphilitic origin of the great majority of aneurisms; however that may be, the iodide acts favorably, especially when used along with digitalis. In the paralyses of the recurrent laryngeal nerve electricity renders real service. Although the vocal cord that is paralyzed does not recover its mobility, yet the other one is benefited by the electricity. In the case of perforation of bony walls—as of the sternum, etc.—it will be necessary to protect the aneurism by means of appropriate bandages. Radical treatment of aneurisms, by galvano-puncture, by injection of coagulating liquids, or by the introduction of foreign bodies, etc., always fails and often even accelerates death.

Dr. Senator said that he could not accept Dr. Litten's opinion, which he called nihilistic. In aneurisms of the abdominal aorta, he says he has often succeeded in arresting the affection by putting the patient on his back for several months, by methodical compression, and by the use of iodide of potassium. Of eight cases of this kind three have been, so to speak, cured. Prognosis is naturally much worse for aneurisms of the thoracic aorta. Iodide of potash may be considered as a curative remedy.

Dr. B. Fraenkel declared that in his experience electricity was of no service whatever in paralysis of the recurrent laryngeal nerve in aneurism.

Dr. Ewald said his own experience was analogous to that of Dr. Senator. In addition, he stated that even in persons who present no visible manifestation of syphilis, an autopsy frequently establishes the syphilitic aspect, and atrophy of the base of the tongue, which is characteristic of syphilis.—*Bulletin Médical*, April 10, 1889.

Eczema of the Nails.

Dr. de la Harpe, *privat-docent* in the University of Geneva, mentions in the *Revue Médicale de la Suisse Romande* a somewhat rare case of eczema of the nails which came under his notice while he was acting as medical officer at the well-known baths of Louèche, or Leuk. The patient was a man of sixty, who had been sent to Louèche by Professor Hardy. There was no history of gout or other hereditary disease, and up to two years previously the nails had been in excellent condition. The first sign of anything wrong that was noticed was a slight redness about the ungual furrow of the ring finger of the right hand, which was at first supposed to be panaris, but instead of going on to suppuration it was followed by morbid changes in the nail itself, which soon became thickened and friable, with a roughened surface. The nails of the other fingers on both hands subsequently became affected, as shown in figures appended to the paper. When seen by Dr. de la Harpe, the affected nails were swollen, bent transversely, and marked with longitudinal striæ or grooves. Two apparently healthy nails showed fine depressed points. Regarding the cause of these appearances, which are the first signs of the commencement of the affection in otherwise normal nails, Dr. de la Harpe remarks that he has seen a case of chronic eczema of the hand in which there were a number of longitudinal grooves on the nails, some of them interrupted—that is to say, in sections. The punctate marks on the nails in the case in question may possibly be analogous to the interruptions noticed in this latter case. As to the treatment by means of the Louèche waters, it appears to have effected marked improvement.—*Lancet*, March 23, 1889.

New Cocaines by Synthesis.

The endless activity of synthetical chemistry has lately been markedly demonstrated in connection with cocaine. It is not so long since cocaine became of such great surgical importance, in spite of the difficulty of separating it from the leaves, and already it has been prepared artificially from benzoyl-ecgonine by introducing the methyl group into it. Recently Einhorn has announced and described three further substitution compounds in which the place of methyl is taken by other groups. One of these is the lower homologue of true cocaine, while the others are metameric or higher homologues. Two of these could not be obtained in a crystalline form, but only in the form of oil. The third, however, and the salts of all three, are crystallizable. So far, it has not been stated whether any of these new "cocaines" possess any special therapeutic properties. Judging from experience with other artificial drugs, it seems probable that they may in course of time be substituted for the true vegetable alkaloid, but that, until they can be prepared absolutely free from impurities, we shall be likely to hear further of untoward results from the use of cocaine. On the other hand, the importance of this discovery can scarcely be over-estimated if it can be worked with sufficient precision to provide for an increased supply of cocaine of certain composition and good quality. Any increase in the quantity of cocaine in the market will reduce the price and favor its more extensive employment. It remains to be seen whether the new cocaines possess similar therapeutic properties, and whether they can be prepared artificially more economically than the natural alkaloid, or will exist only as chemical curiosities.—*Lancet*, April 6, 1889.

THE
MEDICAL AND SURGICAL
REPORTER.

ISSUED EVERY SATURDAY.

CHARLES W. DULLES, M.D.,
EDITOR AND PUBLISHER.

The Terms of Subscription to the publications of this office are as follows, payable in advance:

Med. and Surg. Reporter (weekly), a year, **$5.00**
Physician's Daily Pocket Record, - - 1.00
Reporter and Pocket Record, - - - - 6.00

All checks and postal orders should be drawn to order of

CHARLES W. DULLES,
N. E. Cor. 13th and Walnut Streets,
P. O. Box 843.   Philadelphia, Pa.

☞ SUGGESTIONS TO SUBSCRIBERS:
See that your address-label gives the date to which your subscription is paid.
In requesting a change of address, give the old address as well as the new one.
If your REPORTER does not reach you promptly and regularly, notify the publisher *at once*, so that the cause may be discovered and corrected.

☞ SUGGESTIONS TO CONTRIBUTORS AND CORRESPONDENTS:
Write in ink.
Write on one side of paper only.
Write on paper of the size usually used for letters.
Make as few paragraphs as possible. Punctuate carefully. Do not abbreviate, or omit words like "the," and "a," or "an."
Make communications as short as possible.
NEVER ROLL A MANUSCRIPT! Try to get an envelope or wrapper which will fit it.
When it is desired to call our attention to something in a newspaper, mark the passage boldly with a colored pencil, and write on the wrapper "Marked copy." Unless this is done, newspapers are not looked at.
The Editor will be glad to get medical news, but it is important that brevity and actual interest shall characterize communications intended for publication.

THE DISASTER AT JOHNSTOWN, PA.

In the accounts of the terrible disaster which suddenly overwhelmed the town of Johnstown, in Pennsylvania, on Friday, May 31, it is not surprising to read of the heroism of the physicians of the ill-fated valley of the Conemaugh; nor is it surprising to find that, as soon as the news reached their professional brethren in all parts of the State, they hastened to the assistance of those involved in ruin or distress. This is just what the common life of physicians prepares them for; and such a response is precisely what would be expected. None the less is it gratifying and inspiriting to find the action of the physicians of Pennsylvania so quick and so spontaneous. Their willingness to run to the help of the distressed contributes to illuminate a cloud of disaster which, even with this relief, is appalling to contemplate.

The present needs of the sufferers is—it is to be feared—but a portion of the whole; and the physicians of this State may be—and probably will be, called upon for further aid. Men may be needed to go to the help of those who are on the spot, in caring for the sick and injured, and in warding off the effects of the pestilence which may follow the flood and fire. No doubt, also, money will be needed there, and the benevolence of our fellow citizens may be insufficient for the needs of our professional brethren. If this shall prove to be the case, we must be ready to add to what has been done already, and to fill up the measure of our fraternal aid to those whose misfortunes we have been spared.

At this writing there is no indication as to the best channel in which to direct even the best intentions; but this will come soon, and then the REPORTER will be happy to be the medium of communication between the members of the profession as to what shall be done in the emergency which has arisen.

PROGNOSIS OF HEART DISEASE.

The invention and improvement of the stethoscope and of the sphygmograph have led to a closer study of diseases of the heart, as the result of which our ability to recognize them early has been materially increased. In more recent years, also, the treatment of heart diseases has improved, especially by the judicious use of Oertel's method, a good description of which was published in the REPORTER, May 26, 1888. These two factors—greater power in diagnosis and improved methods of treatment—have naturally tended to make the prognosis of affections of the heart more hopeful.

Prof. Leyden recently drew attention to this circumstance in a communication published in the *Deutsche med. Wochenschrift,*

April 11, 1889. This distinguished clinician says that sudden death is liable to occur in aortic insufficiency, both in grave cases associated with considerable dilatation and hypertrophy, and also in cases in which the lesion is slighter and better compensated. He admits that it may also occur in true angina pectoris—that is to say, in the form which is dependent upon sclerosis of the coronary arteries; but he declares that in all other varieties of heart disease sudden death is a relatively rare occurrence. In mitral affections, for example, it occurs in only about two per cent. of the cases, and is therefore so rare that the physician may neglect it in prognosis. In fatty degeneration of the heart sudden death occasionally occurs, it is true, as it does in the later stages of acute diseases and in the beginning of convalescence from them. It may also occur under the influence of overexertion or strong emotions; but, as Leyden points out, these are rather general conditions which lead to heart weakness than affections of the heart themselves. And, after all, they result in sudden death so rarely that they need not be reckoned in prognosis.

In addition to the information gained by an examination of the heart and the condition of the circulation, it should be borne in mind, in making a prognosis, that the age, sex and circumstances of the patient, as well as the apparent effect of treatment, have each to be considered in estimating the probable result of the disease. For instance, little children do not bear heart affections well, while older children and young persons, on the contrary, do bear them well. In the aged the prognosis is grave, because heart affections are, at this period, very commonly the consequence of arterio-sclerosis—a disease which progresses steadily and is never arrested.

As regards sex, the prognosis of heart disease in general may be said to be more favorable in women than in men, as would naturally be supposed from the fact that women are less exposed to the influences which determine arterio-sclerosis and grave cardiac affections, namely, physical overwork, venereal excesses, and alcoholism. Moreover, aortic insufficiency—the most unfavorable form of heart disease—predominates in men, whereas women are more subject to mitral stenosis. The latter lesion, Leyden states, is relatively benign; but he should have made an exception in the cases in which pregnancy complicates it, for then it is very fatal.

The patient's manner of life and his ability to take proper care of himself are important elements in the prognosis of heart disease; and it is for this reason that better results are obtained in the treatment of heart disease in private than in hospital practice. Furthermore, the readiness with which the heart is found to respond to cardiac tonics and stimulants is of importance. If such remedies fail, the outlook is of course more gloomy, as a lack of recuperative power on the part of the heart is indicated. Digitalis is the best remedy for use in judging of the power of the heart to respond to stimulation. But failure with it does not leave us entirely powerless, in spite of the fact that the effect of analogous remedies and methods of treatment is more uncertain.

Medical men, and the more intelligent of laymen, have long known that the existence of heart disease, in which compensation is good, is compatible with long life and comparative comfort, if the patient's circumstances permit him to live on a comparatively even plane of life, and with the best treatment of his heart trouble. They have also known that, when death results from heart disease, it is the exception, and not the rule, for it to come suddenly. Nevertheless, the average layman still regards the diagnosis of heart disease as equivalent to a sentence of death at no very distant period, and is continually in dread of sudden death.

This false conception will continue to influence the public mind until general practitioners, and especially family physicians, succeed in establishing a correct view of the matter in the minds of their patients.

It is to be hoped, therefore, that the views which we have just cited may be carefully considered in order that as hopeful a conception as is proper may be formed of the prognosis of heart disease in general.

WOMEN TEACHERS OF PHYSIOLOGY TO GIRLS.

It is reported that the principal of a school in a New Jersey village has recently been charged with using the opportunity afforded him when teaching physiology to the school girls to make remarks which they thought to be immoral. The charge has been denied, and on investigation it has fallen to the ground. The teacher, however, has expressed the opinion that its mere discussion would probably compel him to give up his position and to leave the village.

This is an unfortunate outcome of what was doubtless meant to be an instructive exercise, and it illustrates the dangers that beset men who discuss before young women topics which are not usually broached under these circumstances. The study of physiology by girls cannot well be directed by a man, unless it is kept within restricted limits. There are matters connected with physiology which no man can discuss with girls without impropriety, but which it would be well for them to know about. For this reason it would be better if physiology should be taught them by a woman. There are now so many intelligent women physicians in this country that few places of any consequence are without them, and it ought not to be hard to find enough to teach all the physiology that is needed in the education of girls.

This work offers a field of usefulness to women physicians which is of great importance, and if it were occupied rightly by them the result could not fail to be of advantage to girls, many of whom grow up ignorant of physiological facts, a knowledge of which might save them from much unhappiness and some misfortunes.

THE PENNSYLVANIA STATE SOCIETY.

The members of the Pennsylvania State Society present at Pittsburgh have adjourned to September 3 the meeting which was to have been held in that city during the current week, in view of the fact that the disaster at Johnstown, and the floods which visited almost the whole of the State at the same time, have so disorganized the railroad service, that it has been impossible for the members of the Society, in any numbers, to attend the meeting.

The arrangements of the REPORTER have been interfered with by this postponement; for we had prepared to publish a number of the most valuable papers of the Society immediately after its adjournment. Regard for the rights of the Society and the wishes of the authors has, however, necessitated our withholding them from the press until the matter can be adjusted satisfactorily to all concerned. These circumstances have led to a delay in the appearance of this issue of the REPORTER which our readers will understand.

NEW HAMPSHIRE STATE MEDICAL SOCIETY.—The Ninety-eighth Annual Meeting of the New Hampshire State Medical Society will be held in Concord, Monday and Tuesday, June 17 and 18, 1889. All applications for membership in the Society must be made to the Secretary, Dr. Granville P. Conn, of Concord, before the meeting of the Councillors, on Monday evening, June 17. The programme issued by the Committee of Arrangements promises to be interesting; it contains, in addition to other useful information, a list of the stations at which it will be necessary to purchase tickets in order to obtain them at reduced rates.

BOOK REVIEWS.

[Any book reviewed in these columns may be obtained upon receipt of price, from the office of the REPORTER.]

A COMPENDIUM OF DENTISTRY FOR THE USE OF STUDENTS AND PRACTITIONERS. By JUL. PAREIDT, Dental Surgeon to the Surgical Polyclinic at the Institute of the University of Leipsig, etc. Authorized translation, by LOUIS OTTOFY, D.D.S., Lecturer on Physiology, Chicago College of Dental Surgery, with notes and additions by G. V. BLACK, M.D., D.D.S., Professor of Pathology, Chicago College of Dental Surgery, with numerous illustrations. Large 8vo, pp. xii, 229. Chicago: W. T. Keener, 1889. Price, $2.50.

This book contains an able discussion of the disease processes which attack the teeth, the maxillary bones and the mucous membrane of the mouth, as well as of the anomalies to which the teeth are liable. This, and the treatment of these conditions is considered in a most thorough and scholarly manner, as might be expected of the competent hands through which the work has passed. The part of the book devoted to mechanical dentistry is brief, but good. In the preface, the author calls attention to the importance of a knowledge of the diseases of the teeth to the general practitioner, and recommends a study of this subject to those who usually do not care to give it much attention. In this we think he is quite right, and can second his recommendation with the firm conviction that at least an elementary knowledge of the principles of dentistry would be of the greatest service to most physicians.

PAMPHLET NOTICES.

[Any reader of the REPORTER who desires a copy of a pamphlet noticed in these columns will doubtless secure it by addressing the author with a request stating where the notice was seen and *enclosing a postage-stamp*.]

267. SHOULD THE STATE TAKE CARE OF ITS INEBRIATES? By E. J. KEMPF, M.D., Jasper, Indiana. 24 pages. Price, 10 cents.

268. GRAVES' DISEASE. By WILLIAM C. BAILEY, M.D., Albion, N. Y. From the *Buffalo Med. and Surg. Journal*, August, 1886. 21 pages.

269. THE ELECTROLYTIC DECOMPOSITION OF ORGANIC TISSUES. By GEORGE H. ROHÉ, M.D., Baltimore, Md. From the *New York Med. Journal*, December 1, 1888. 15 pages.

270. POISONING BY CHROME YELLOW USED AS A CAKE DYE. By DAVID DENISON STEWART, M.D., Philadelphia. From the *Medical News*, January 26, 1889. 24 pages.

271. ANGINA AND PNEUMONIA BEFORE 1857 AND SINCE, WITH THE PATHOLOGY OF DIPHTHERIA IN ITS VARIOUS PHASES. By WILLIAM HENRY THAYER, M.D., Brooklyn, N. Y. From the *New York Medical Journal*, January 26, 1889. 22 pages.

272. A DEFENCE OF ELECTROLYSIS IN URETHRAL STRICTURES, WITH DOCUMENTARY EVIDENCE. By ROBERT NEWMAN, M.D., New York. From the *Medical Register*, January 5, 1889. 20 pages.

273. THE IMMEDIATE APPLICATION OF THE FORCEPS TO THE AFTER-COMING HEAD IN CASES OF VERSION WITH PARTIAL DILATATION OF THE CERVIX. By H. C. COE, M.D., New York. From the *Medical Record*, January 19, 1889. 7 pages.

274. DREAMS, SLEEP, CONSCIOUSNESS. A PSYCHOLOGICAL STUDY. By GEORGE M. GOULD, M.D., Philadelphia. From *The Open Court*, January 24 and 31, 1889. 24 pages.

275. REPORT OF THE COMMITTEE ON OPHTHALMOLOGY AND OTOLOGY. By SETH M. BISHOP, M.D., Chicago. From the *Transactions of the Illinois State Med. Soc.*, May 17, 1888. 11 pages.

276. ON CORPULENCE, ESPECIALLY ITS TREATMENT BY A PURE MILK DIET. By GEORGE H. ROHÉ, M.D., Baltimore. From the *Maryland Med. Journal*, Feb. 9, 1889. 4 pages.

277. ON THE MICROSCOPICAL EXAMINATION OF URINARY SEDIMENT. By WILLIAM B. CANFIELD, M.D., Baltimore. From the *Transactions of the Medico-Chirurgical Faculty of Maryland*, 1888. 4 pages.

278. THE GONOCOCCUS. By WILLIAM B. CANFIELD, M.D., Baltimore. From *The Microscope*, July, 1888. 3 pages.

279. REPORT ON A CASE OF PREGNANCY IN THE RIGHT HORN OF A UTERUS BICORNIS, ETC. By B. F. BAER, M.D., Philadelphia. From the *Transactions of the Amer. Gynecological Society*, 1888. 16 pages.

267. Dr. Kempf opens his pamphlet with the statement that he is not presenting a temperance tract, but a more interesting temperance tract, or a more entertaining arraignment of the system of licensing the liquor traffic we have never seen. The keynote of the argument is found in the sentence: "The State considers 'becoming a drunkard' a personal right, and 'being a drunkard' a crime. Science holds 'becoming a drunkard' to be a sin, and 'being a drunkard' a disease." The question in the title he answers in the affirmative, asserting that the State should erect and maintain homes for inebriates, using for this purpose the money collected for licenses to sell alcoholic beverages, and the fines levied upon those who break the law in consequence of drinking.

As a whole this pamphlet is calculated to do a great deal of good, and as its style is exceedingly interesting, none of our readers will regret it if they follow our recommendation and apply to the author for a copy of it.

268. Dr. Bailey's paper contains an instructive study of Graves' Disease, to which he was led by the experience gained in treating successfully a case of this disorder. The history of his own case is very well described, and the whole subject is gone over in a way which makes his pamphlet a valuable contribution to its literature.

269. After a preliminary discussion of the general principles of electrolysis, Dr. Rohé considers its applicability to the decomposition of morbid organic tissues, and warmly advocates its employment. Without going much into detail, he defends its use in the treatment of fibroids and strictures of the urethra. In regard to both of these he speaks with scorn of those who reject electrolysis, and intimates that a fair trial would convince them of its utility.

270. In this pamphlet Dr. Stewart follows up the history of a number of cases of poisoning with chrome yellow, used by bakers as a coloring agent in cakes, which came under his observation in 1887. He has studied these cases with praiseworthy industry and persistence, and the results of his study are both interesting and instructive. His work furnishes a needed lesson in regard to the danger which may follow the use of artificial dyes in articles of food,

and deserves the attention of all hygienists and toxi-ologists.

271. Contrary to the opinion of many recent writers, Dr. Thayer holds that diphtheria is essentially a constitutional disease " often with little manifestation in the fauces, and sometimes an entire absence there of the exudation - membrane from which its name is derived." His pamphlet is so full of interesting matter that it would be impossible to summarize it in our limited space, but it will abundantly repay perusal.

272. This is another controversial paper by Dr. Newman, in which he defends his method of treating strictures against the attack of Dr. F. Tilden Brown. Like all of his recent papers this one of Dr. Newman is interesting, and will arouse sympathy. As we have said before, he maintains a struggle against the prevalent opinion of genito-urinary surgeons. But it is evident from this and other of his writings that there is a considerable number of men who share his views and approve of his method. The principle of hearing both sides is peculiarly appropriate to this case, and it is to be regretted that the argument has developed so much acerbity.

273. Dr. Coe makes a warm argument for the immediate use of the forceps to deliver the head after version by the feet, and supports it by reference to a number of cases in which delay proved fatal to the child. He defends the procedure as easy of execution, and as involving no risk except that of lacerating the cervix, which he thinks is not to be compared with the risk of life to the child in case delivery of the head is delayed.

274. This pamphlet is what might be expected from its title. It is a study of the phenomena of dreaming and sleep and consciousness, with a section on " Character, the Soul, and Consciousness." It is vague and unsatisfying, and leads to nothing in particular. It is interesting and furnishes food for reflection, but is too much founded upon the writer's personal experience to admit of general application to the subject discussed.

275. In this paper Dr. Bishop is principally occupied with a description of three instruments of his invention: a pneumatic otoscope, an improved tonsillotome and a nasal speculum. The instruments are ingenious in principle, and calculated to be useful in practice.

276. The title of Dr. Rohé's paper indicates its contents. He discusses the physiological phenomena of corpulence and advocates treating the condition by means of an exclusive diet of skimmed milk, citing two observations which strengthen his conviction of its value.

277. This is a most instructive pamphlet, and every medical man who attempts to examine the sediment of urine microscopically would do well to learn and to follow Dr. Canfield's admirable and practical suggestions.

278. After a short review of the literature of the gonococcus, Dr. Canfield describes the method of searching for it in suspected pus.

279. Dr. Baer reports an exceedingly interesting case of a woman who missed her labor, and came under his care with a diagnosis of extra uterine pregnancy a year afterward. He operated, removed the dead fetus by a modified Cæsarean section, but had to leave the cyst-wall behind. The patient made a good recovery. The case is well described, and interesting remarks are added on the subject of pregnancy in a bicornate uterus in general.

CORRESPONDENCE.

Effects of Sulphonal.

To the Editor.

Sir: The much talked of sulfonal has lately revealed to me some weak points and ugly traits. For instance—

(1) Mr. G., aged forty-nine, married, has periodical attacks of dipsomania, about once a month, after which he cannot sleep. For several years morphia and bromide of potassium would quiet him pretty fairly. In December, 1888, I began giving him from twenty to thirty, and even forty-five grains of sulfonal, dissolved in hot water, at bed-time or an hour before. The drug invariably keeps him awake and comfortable during the night, and sleep follows, as a rule, sometime the next day. He says it intoxicates him.

(2) W. P., aged thirty-five, married, farmer; had gastro-enteritis during April last. During convalescence he could not sleep day or night. I gave sulfonal, in twenty grain doses an hour before bedtime. He did not " sleep a wink," and was a little delirious.

(3) Miss Mamie W., aged twenty-three, single; is on a visit East from Colorado, where she resides, on account of tendency to consumption. Both parents died of phthisis. After living here from two to four weeks, she always has loss of appetite, rapid and feeble pulse, great debility, a little cough and wonderful sleeplessness, but no fever. This (May) is her fourth visit East in the last four years, and her fourth attack of sickness, with above mentioned symptoms. The evening of the 18th inst. I gave her fifteen grains of sulfonal in very weak hot coffee, at nine P.M., and repeated the dose at half past ten. She scratched all night; was slightly delirious, and did not sleep. The next night I gave her thirty grains, in hot water, at 9 P.M. The same symptoms followed, with nausea and vomiting and marked debility.

Yours truly,
C. H. Shivers, M.D.

Haddonfield, N. J.,
May 21, 1889.

—The total number of students at all the Austrian Universities during the winter semester of 1888–1889 was 13,801, 1,388 of which were in the Universities of Lemberg and Czernowitz, which have no medical faculties.

NOTES AND COMMENTS.

No Yellow Fever in Florida.

Dr. Jerome Cochran, State Health Officer of Alabama, returned May 30 from a trip to South Florida and Havana, made for the purpose of investigating the yellow fever situation. He says that there has been no yellow fever in Florida since January, except one case *reported* in April, at Sanford. In Havana he found little fever, only a dozen to twenty cases a week. The general health of the people is exceptionally good, and Dr. Cochran gives it as his opinion that there will be no fresh outbreak of yellow fever in Florida this summer, unless there is a fresh importation of the disease.

The Disaster at Johnstown.

As our readers have already learned from the daily papers, about five o'clock on the afternoon of May 31 a most disastrous flood, caused by the bursting of an artificial lake, near Johnstown, Pennsylvania, overwhelmed that town and the valley in which it lies. The sympathy of physicians all over the State was at once aroused, and those who could offered their services at once. On receiving a telegram from Dr. Lowman, of Johnstown, asking for medical aid, Dr. William S. Forbes, of Philadelphia, organized a relief party of physicians and promptly started to aid the sufferers, in spite of great difficulties and of the uncertainty of reaching the afflicted city. He took with him as large a stock of provisions, clothing and medical supplies as could be gathered in the short space of time at his disposal.

Other physicians were not idle. At a meeting of the Faculty of Jefferson Medical College it was resolved that an additional relief corps from the staff of the surgical clinic of the hospital should be sent by the earliest train to report to Professor Forbes.

A largely attended meeting of physicians was held at the office of Dr. Harrison Allen, 1933 Chestnut Street, with the view to arrange for the furnishing of medical aid to the sufferers. Dr. John Ashhurst, Jr., presided and Dr. Allen acted as secretary. A committee was appointed to complete arrangements. At a meeting of this committee, held immediately, it was agreed to report to the Mayor and the Citizens' Relief Association, of Philadelphia, and to the Red Cross Society the names of physicians willing at a moment's notice to go to Johnstown in aid of the sufferers. Twenty-five physicians volunteered their services. .

The response from Pittsburgh was equally prompt, and accomplished more because access to Johnstown was not cut off from the West, while it was from the East for some days. The details of the work done by medical men from points other than Philadelphia are not as yet fully reported, and due credit can be given to them only in a general way. Further reports will only enhance their credit.

Relations of Scientific Experts to the Administration of the Law.

Willard Bartlett, Justice of the Supreme Court of New York, in a paper read before the Society of Medical Jurisprudence and published in the *Brooklyn Medical Journal*, May, 1889, gives some good advice to physicians called as medical experts in any case. He says:

"Upon the trial, except in the comparatively rare instances in which there is no dispute as to the nature, extent, and consequences of the plaintiff's injuries, the respective parties are assisted by physicians or surgeons, or both, who testify in reference to these matters, and often advise counsel as to the conduct of the medical or surgical part of the case.

"The wise doctor, as it seems to me, will take care not to act in both capacities. If he is to testify in the case, he will not act as assistant counsel; if he acts as assistant counsel, he will keep off the witness stand. There is no good reason why the most distinguished physician should not place his professional knowledge and experience at the service of one of the parties to a litigation which involves questions of medical science. To do so cannot justly subject him to reproach; but it does lessen his fitness and his usefulness as a witness in that litigation. In assisting counsel, he will inevitably come to share the sentiments of counsel as to the result. Just as counsel will seek to bring out every fact that may prove beneficial to the cause of his client, and will endeavor to destroy, as far as may be, the effect of any proof which is injurious to him, so the medical man thus employed will suggest questions for the examination of witnesses on the other side, which will call out answers favorable to the party at whose instance he has been brought into the case. All this goes on before the jury, who fully comprehend where the medical questions really come from. If, afterward, they see the doctor take the witness stand, it is impossible that they should regard him as otherwise than prejudiced. However truthful his testimony may be, and however correct his opinions, his evidence is the evidence of a partisan, and this fact invariably detracts from its force and effect."

Sulphonal in Night Sweats.

In addition to the hypnotic properties enjoyed by sulphonal, this drug is capable, according to Dr. Böttrich of Hagen, Westphalia, of exercising a most beneficial influence in night sweats. It acts, he thinks, very similarly to atropine, but, unlike it, is quite free from any undesirable effects. He found this property out by accident, having prescribed a quarter of a gramme (nearly four grains) for an old woman of eighty as a sleeping powder. The patient had been suffering from the most profuse night sweats, obliging her to change her things twice during the same night. After the first dose she asked the doctor whether he had not put something into the powder to prevent the sweats. On making further observations, Dr. Böttrich convinced himself that as a rule half a gramme (seven grains and a half) of sulphonal will stop night sweats. Its effects seem fortunately to be somewhat permanent, as even after the drug has been stopped the night sweats are found to be much less severe than they were previously to taking it.—*Lancet*, April 27, 1889.

State Board of Medical Examiners in Tennessee.

The *Southern Practitioner*, May, 1889, contains the full text of the act to regulate the practice of medicine in Tennessee, which was passed very recently by the legislature of that State and signed by the governor. Graduates of medical colleges must appear before the Board of Examiners, present their diplomas, and pass an examination before they can be allowed to practise in Tennessee. The act provides that regular physicians, homœopaths and eclectics, shall be represented on the Board, and that each candidate shall be examined by the representative on the Board of the school to which he belongs. A majority of votes are necessary for a rejection. Quacks are to be fined in any sum not less than $100 nor more than $400 for each offense. Any person practising without the certificate issued by the Board is to be fined $25 for the first offense and $200 for each subsequent offense. The Board is also granted power to revoke licenses for cause.

Death due to Somnambulism.

The *British Med. Journal*, May 11, 1889, states that a Dr. Davidson retired to rest about eleven o'clock one night, and about two hours afterward the attention of the servants was attracted by the noise of some heavy object falling. Dr. Davidson was found lying in his nightdress outside the house, having apparently fallen from his bedroom, which was situated on the third floor. Medical aid was obtained, but he succumbed to the injuries he had received. Dr. Davidson had been for several years subject to attacks of somnambulism, and there can be no doubt that the accident took place while he was in an unconscious condition.

Diagnosis and Treatment of Tubercular Peritonitis.

Dr. Samuel Fenwick, in the course of his lectures on cases of difficult diagnosis, writes as follows upon the diagnosis of tubercular peritonitis in the adult (*Lancet*, March 9, 1889): The diseases with which we are most apt to confound acute tubercular peritonitis are typhoid fever and acute non-tubercular peritonitis, and in some instances the resemblance is so close that it is only by great care and watchfulness that we can avoid falling into error.

As a general rule, tubercular peritonitis of this kind begins suddenly, whilst typhoid is usually preceded by a period in which the patient has been weak, feeble, and feverish. In the former, pain in the abdomen is more marked, and there is tenderness over different parts; whilst pain in the latter is rarely severe, and any tenderness that may be present is confined to the iliac region. In tubercular peritonitis the temperature rises at once, and not regularly, as in enteric fever, and the pulse is usually more rapid. As the case proceeds the temperature varies more in peritonitis, spots are rarely observed, and the stools have not generally the typical appearance of those passed in typhoid; whilst at a later period the persistence or frequent returns of abdominal pain and tenderness and of vomiting, the variations of the temperature, the alternations of constipation with diarrhœa, and the increasing prostration, will in most instances enable you to distinguish between these diseases. In addition to these differences, you will in many cases be able to render your diagnosis more certain by the discovery of fluid in the peritoneum, or by the detection of a tumor in the abdomen; or you may find the signs of effusion in the pleura or of a consolidation in the apex of one or both lungs.

Still more difficult is it to distinguish between acute tubercular peritonitis and ordinary peritonitis when the former does not assume from the first the typhoid form. In many cases I believe it is impossible to arrive at a certain conclusion in the early stage, for both may attack persons previously healthy, both may be ushered in by similar abdominal symptoms, and it is only by watching the progress of the disease that you can form an accurate opinion. As a general rule, the pain, tenderness, and vomiting are less distressing in the tubercular form, the temperature is lower, and there is more usually diarrhœa than constipation. As the disease progresses, the abdominal symptoms recur from time to time instead of slowly subsiding, the temperature remains high, emaciation becomes more marked, the effusion into the peritoneum is very slowly absorbed, and you may discover signs indicating effusion into the pleuræ or pulmonary consolidation.

As regards the treatment of acute tubercular peritonitis in the adult, he says: In the typhoid form I have usually treated the case as if it were one of enteric fever ; that is, the patient has been kept at rest, the food has been restricted to liquids, and cold sponging has been employed whenever the temperature has been unduly high. Quinine in moderate doses in combination with opium has been prescribed to relieve pain and to check diarrhœa. In the cases in which the symptoms were chiefly abdominal the treatment has been directed as in ordinary peritonitis ; poultices and hot fomentations have been applied to the abdomen, and small doses of opium have been given to relieve pain and diarrhœa. You must, however, be careful not to induce constipation, for it is usually followed by attacks of vomiting that quickly reduce the strength of the patient.

You may ask whether the washing out of the peritoneum, which is so successful in some cases of suppurative peritonitis, is likely to prove beneficial in this kind of case. I have never seen it tried, chiefly because the real nature of the disease has more frequently been suspected than actually diagnosticated during life; but I do not think it would be of much value, as I have found the fluid serous, not purulent, and the patients have seemed to me to sink from the general acute tuberculosis, and not from the effects of the inflammation of the peritoneum.

Expert Testimony as to Death by Poison.

The Supreme Court of Wisconsin has recently formulated a rule of testimony according to which, when a trial for murder by poisoning is on, any physician whose only knowledge of poisons is that which has come to him from books and college training is not competent to give an opinion relative to the symptoms of the final illness of the deceased with regard to their probable causation by poisoning. This is probably the first time that any court has prescribed such a regulation, but it has so much in its favor that we count upon its gradual extension from court to court as questions arise in regard to poisoning cases. No person may justly be put in jeopardy of his life on the quasi-expert testimony of a witness who has gleaned all that he knows of the subject from the printed page or half-remembered lecture.—*New York Med. Journal*, April 20, 1889.

Ichthyol.

Despite its disagreeable odor, ichthyol has been gradually establishing itself as a remedy of no mean properties. Unna says: "In my opinion we have not up to the present time possessed so effectual a remedy [as ichthyol] for rheumatism." According to Nussbaum—and his opinion is the same as that of Unna, Blittersdorf, and Lorenz—ichthyol is of special service in all diseases associated with hyperæmia and distended capillaries. Though very disagreeable at first to take, the palate and stomach soon become used to it, and it is said to improve the appetite in those cases in which it is indicated internally, as in intestinal, renal, cystic, or urethral catarrh. It is quite compatible with lanolin and other unguent bases, is miscible with mercury, zinc ointment, etc., and dissolves completely in water. A mild ointment (5 per cent.) is pronounced regenerative, a strong one (50 per cent.) resolvent. — *London Medical Recorder*, February, 1889.

Formula for "Lemonade Iron."

The following is the formula for "lemonade iron," a favorite combination with Dr. Goodell :

℞ Strychninæ sulph.	. . . .	gr. ss
Tinct. Ferri chlor.	. . . .	f℥ iv
Acidi Phosph. dil.	. . . .	f℥ vi
Syr. Limonis	. . . . .	q. s. ad f℥ vi

M. Sig. Dose, two teaspoonfuls three times a day.

Mr. Bishop was Dead.

After all the fuss made over the death of Mr. Bishop, and the assertion that an autopsy had been made on him while he was still alive, the Coroner's jury found the following verdict on May 29: "We, the jury in the case of Washington Irving Bishop, find: First, that he died at the Lambs' Club on May 13, 1889; second, cause of death was coma; third, we further find that while Drs. Irwin, Ferguson and Hance acted in good faith in performing the autopsy upon the body of the deceased, we would state that Dr. Irwin, through overzeal, acted in some haste respecting the direction of the performance of the autopsy." Coroner Levy thereupon discharged the three physicians, who had been held in $2,500 bail each.

Formula for Use in Nervous Anæmic Women.

Dr. Goodell thinks highly of the following combination for use in the case of nervous anæmic women, perhaps with dysmenorrhœa:

    Ext. Sumbuli,
    Ferri sulph. exsiccat. . . . . aa gr. i
    Asafetidæ . . . . gr. ii
    Acidi arseniosi . . . . gr. $\frac{1}{40}$
    M. et ft. pil. No. I.
    Sig. One pill after meals, to be increased to six pills a day.

Saccharin for Thrush.

Since it has been known that saccharin possesses the property of checking fermentative processes in the intestine it has been frequently employed as an antiseptic. Maurice Fourcier has used saccharin for some time in cases of thrush, and with very good result. In the *Revue gén. de clin. et de Thér.*, No. 11, he speaks of his experience with ten cases, which he treated with applications of a solution of saccharin; in eight cases the thrush disappeared within twenty-four to thirty-six hours, and lasted twice only as long as three days until complete healing occurred. In these cases the applications were badly made. Fourcier employs the following solution:

    R Saccharin . . . . gr. xv
    Alcohol . . . . f$\mathring{3}$iss

A coffee-spoonful of this solution is added to a half-glass of water, and the affected parts painted with the resulting mixture five times a day. A concentrated solution should not be employed, as it can be injurious. An apothecary who prepared the above solution tasted it by frequently putting his finger, which had been dipped in it, into his mouth. The same evening he was seized with a burning sensation in the mouth and on the day following had an aphthous eruption in the mouth, which however disappeared spontaneously in five days. In the way in which Fourcier employs the remedy it is entirely harmless and very effective.—*Wiener med. Presse*, April 14, 1889.

Proposed Tribute to Dr. Levis.

A Committee, including a number of physicians of Philadelphia, has invited subscriptions for the purpose of endowing a free bed in the Philadelphia Polyclinic, in recognition of the eminent professional services of Dr. Richard J. Levis, who was one of the founders of the Polyclinic, its first Professor of Clinical and Operative Surgery, and from its organization has been President of the Board of Trustees. The sum of five thousand dollars is needed for this purpose, and the Committee which has charge of raising the money requests that subscriptions be sent as soon as possible to the Treasurer, Dr. H. Augustus Wilson, 1611 Spruce Street, Philadelphia.

The Sanitarium at Red Bank.

The Sanitarium Association of Philadelphia, designed to furnish a day's outing to young children, infants and their caretakers, had its thirteenth annual opening at Red Bank, New Jersey, on Thursday, June 6. This excellent institution is the means of giving happiness and health during the summer season to hundreds of infants and young children which otherwise would have little opportunity to obtain much-needed fresh air and recreation. Those contributing to its fund have the right to send children to spend the day at the Sanitarium. Persons affected with any contagious or infectious disease are, of course, excluded.

The Howard Hospital.

The new building of the Howard Hospital, in Philadelphia, which has heretofore been conducted as a Dispensary, was opened May 23. The building will accommodate ten hospital patients besides the necessary rooms for matron, nurses, etc. Accident cases will be admitted at all hours, and clinical instruction will be given by members of the staff. A peculiar feature of the new service will be the sick-diet kitchen, which is intended to benefit invalids unable to get suitable food at their homes.

NEWS.

—Yellow fever is reported to be "very bad" in Vera Cruz, Mexico.

—Dr. G. E. de Schweinitz, of Philadelphia, has removed to 1401 Locust street.

—Prof. H. A. Bardeleben, of Berlin, celebrated his seventieth birthday on March 1.

—Up to Feb. 20 Dr. Waxham had had 188 cases of intubation of the larynx with 60 recoveries, or 31.36 per cent.

—Dr. R. J. Levis, who is summering with the Duke of Sutherland, instead of at Cedarcroft, has lately bought a winter home in Florida.

—A case of leprosy is said to have been discovered at Spring Lake, Wisconsin. The victim is a woman. The character of the disease is well marked.

—Dr. Roswell Park, of Buffalo, has been using powdered sulphate of cinchonidia in surgical dressings. He says it is both better and cheaper than iodoform.

—It is announced that Dr. Robert W. Taylor has been appointed Professor of Diseases of the Skin in the New York Post-graduate Medical School and Hospital.

—Dr. S. P. Moore, who was Surgeon-General of the Confederate States, died suddenly at his residence in Richmond, Va., May 31, of congestion of the lungs.

—The American Society for Psychical Research announces that, unless its income is increased by its members, it will be necessary to close its work by the end of June next.

—Dr. Erasmus M. Pond, a distinguished physician of Vermont, died at Rutland May 31, aged 61 years. He had invented Pond's Sphymograph, and several other important instruments. He was graduated from the Medical Department of Harvard University in 1853.

—Governor Bulkley, of Connecticut, on May 24, vetoed the bill to prevent deception in the manufacture and sale of butter and cheese. This is the bill which was designed to prohibit the coloring of oleomargarine to resemble genuine butter and cheese. The Governor's reasons for the veto are said to be that oleomargarine has been pronounced a wholesome article of food; that the present law sufficiently guards against its sale under false pretenses; and that to prohibit its manufacture entirely would be detrimental to the interests of the people.

HUMOR.

IT WAS A SCOTCH GRAVE-DIGGER who said, "Trade's very dull noo. I have na buried a leevin' cretur for a fortnight."—*San Francisco Alta.*

VERY SHOPPY.—Miss Reeder—"You should read Dr. Weir Mitchell's last story; the scene is laid in the lumber regions." Dr. Schmerz—"Oh, I see; in the small-of-the-back-woods you mean."—*Puck.*

HEALTH JOURNALS insist upon reposing on the right side only, and claim that it is injurious to lie on both sides, but we don't know where they will find a healthier-looking set of men than lawyers.—*Salem (Ore.) Statesman.*

THE CERTAINTY OF THE DOCTORS.—"But, doctor, you said last week that the patient would certainly die, and now he is perfectly well." "Madam, the confirmation of my prognosis is only a question of time."—*Fliegende Blätter.*

A CIGARETTE PREMIUM.—Cigarette smokers will be interested in the report, not yet confirmed, however, that a certain manufacturer of cigarettes offers a nice cemetery lot to every one who smokes twelve dozen packages of his cigarettes. Probably he wants to make the punishment fit the crime.

A YOUNG LADY'S PET PUG recently swallowed a threaded needle, and instead of administering a needle cushion, she had the animal etherized and the needle extracted by surgical means. She went to a great deal of trouble and expense to recover a needle that couldn't have cost any more than a cent.—*Norristown Herald.*

A REFINING PROCESS.—"I am somewhat astonished, Carper," remarked Bigbee, as he looked around the room, "to find that so great a book-worm as you are should possess so small a library."

"Ah, my boy," returned the other, "it takes a great deal of reading to find out what isn't worth keeping."—*Boston Saturday Gazette.*

DELICATE ATTENTION TO THE AUTHOR.— Daughter (*to mother*).—"Young Mr. Lightsome has just written a book, and has presented me with a copy." Mother.—"That is very nice, Laura." Daughter.—"Yes; and as Mr. Lightsome said something about making a call this evening, and I am very busy, I wish you would sit down and cut the leaves for me, and place it in a conspicuous place on the parlor table."— *Harper's Magazine.*

MEDICAL AND SURGICAL
REPORTER

No. 1685.   PHILADELPHIA, JUNE 15, 1889.   VOL. LX.—No. 24.

CONTENTS:

COMMUNICATIONS.

A PLEA FOR PROMPT INTERFERENCE IN ABDOMINAL DISEASES.[1]

BY J. M. BALDY, M.D.,

PHILADELPHIA, PA.

"Surgery becomes conservative when it tends to alleviate suffering without resorting to operative interference." "An element weakened by disease works viciously, it is true, or perhaps not at all; but if we seek to restore it to normal, we should not eliminate it altogether, but endeavor to heal the trouble, and thus restore the element to at least a measure of healthy action." "Carried into effect without exact diagnosis, and before the merits of a more conservative plan have been tried . . . it becomes a dangerous procedure, if not absolutely criminal." Such expressions are not of unfrequent occurrence in our medical literature.

[1] Intended to be read before the Medical Society of the State of Pennsylvania, June 6, 1889.

By the side of this, and in contrast to it, allow me to place with equal clearness, my own convictions. When an element weakened by disease, works viciously or not at all, and by so doing renders a patient's life miserable or eventually threatens that life itself, the man who stays his hand from eliminating that element, provided it can be done with reasonable safety, and rests satisfied merely with "a measure of healthy action," is, to say the least, not doing his whole duty to his patient. There are many cases of disease, calling for surgical interference, which threaten life, in which an attempt at an exact diagnosis or a trial of the merits of a more conservative plan of treatment becomes, with our present surgical knowledge, not only dangerous but almost, if not entirely, unjustifiable. Statements as strong as these must needs be qualified, that they may not be misunderstood; but it is equally necessary also to qualify such statements as those made in the interests of so-called conservative surgery. No one can appreciate the need of true conservative surgery more than myself, nor the importance of men being thoroughly instructed and trained in the rudiments of our science; but this cry of conservative surgery is too often set up as a mere cloak of ignorance and cowardice. Our sins of omission are oftener greater than our sins of commission.

M. M.; æt. 17; single; family history good; had been in perfect health until present attack. Without any apparent cause she was seized with a pain in the abdomen, which increased rapidly in violence. She was seen the second day of the attack; belly tympanitic and swollen; much colicky pain in abdomen; pulse rapid; and some slight elevation of temperature; anxious expression of face; constipation for several days. Rectal enemata and other appropriate treatment were ordered. From unavoidable delay, the nurse did not give enema until next day. At noon a large solid passage followed the enema, and all the abdominal symptoms became better. Toward night vomiting, which had a suspicious smell, occurred. The patient was now made to drink large quantities of hot water and then vomit it. This gave great relief, and all the symptoms subsided, so much so, that for a second time operative interference was postponed. In the meanwhile the bowels could not be made to act again. Operation was decided on if the bowels did not again move, or if vomiting returned. During the next day the patient was remarkably bright, and in the afternoon ate largely and very greedily of corn-starch, enjoying it very much and retaining it all. Later she rose from her bed and emptied a pint vessel of the same food, retaining and enjoying it. She was apparently better in every way, and an operation was now thought to be unnecessary. Although the bowels had not been opened she said she felt as if they would be at any moment. It was presumed that, by the next day, she would be well over her troubles. At six o'clock in the morning she vomited two or three times, and then suddenly died. The autopsy disclosed a strangulation of the small intestine near the cæcum, by a band. A single snip of the scissors would have relieved it, and the patient would have been saved.

Here we have a picture which all of us have seen only too many times, and in the vast majority of cases we have seen it end in death. A case of intestinal obstruction is one of such a character that there is little room for hesitation. The disease is caused by such a variety of factors, and is so fatal in its ending, that to waste valuable time attempting an exact diagnosis or going

beyond certain limits in the trial of the merits of a so-called conservative plan of treatment, is folly. Lusk never spoke truer words than when he said : "The resources of surgery are rarely successful when practiced on the dying." Why, with our past experience in these diseases, we should continue in the old beaten track of hoping against hope, only to see one valuable life after another slip through our fingers, without an effort to save them, I cannot comprehend. Mr. Treves states that in England, from this disease alone, over two thousand individuals die every year; and I think we are all agreed that in the United States we are equally unfortunate. Surely with such a frightful mortality as this staring us in the face, there can be little use for so-called conservatism. Here, at least, if this tremendous death rate is to be stopped, our only hope lies in bold, aggressive surgery. If a loop of intestine be caught under an adhesive band and strangulated, where one case may be relieved by purely medicinal treatment, ninety-nine will succumb. Of course, all cases of intestinal obstruction are not due to bands, intussusceptions and such causes; some are simply the result of fecal impaction, a slight temporary paralysis of the gut or some other cause amenable to medicinal treatment. If we knew that these were the causes, then it would be eminently right to persist for a considerable time in proper medical treatment. But this is just the point—we never know, or are never sure of the cause. The organic causes are so vastly in the majority, and the symptoms of all varieties are so much alike, that it is only safe to act always on the assumption that all are serious. Should a mistake be made, and an abdomen be opened for a case of obstruction due, for instance, to a fecal impaction, it would be a cause of regret that an unnecessary step had been taken. But our compensation would be even greater in such a case as this, than would be our chagrin. The diagnosis of an obscure and apparently dangerous case would be cleared up, and we could then proceed with confidence and certainty in our treatment, to a final cure. The harm done would be absolutely nothing. Such a mistake would however seldom be made and the number of curable cases, otherwise necessarily fatal, which would be reached and saved would over and over again triumphantly justify such procedures.

In the case cited above, the indications should have induced an early operation. The symptom of suspicious vomiting alone should have been sufficient to have settled the question ; and so it would have done, had not a passage of the bowels been obtained. From this point on, everything was in a position of uncertainty, and the old adage: "He who hesitates is lost," was again exemplified. The feces obtained were, of course, what was impacted below the seat of the obstruction, and that having come away, there was no more to follow. Fecal vomiting should always and invariably be taken as the limit of waiting in these cases. This having occurred once, opportunity should not be given for it to happen a second time, no difference what the other symptoms may be. It will be the rarest exception in the world that a mistake will be found to have been made. If relief has not been obtained within twenty-four hours by means of persistent and gently applied rectal enemata, the abdomen should always be laid open and explored, and whatever is found properly treated.

Two cases have recently come under my notice. Both were operated on after considerable delay, and, when the operation was finally done, a single stroke of the knife ended the strangulation and freed the bowel. In both cases several good passages occurred *per rectum* before the death of the patients. Both died from simple exhaustion. Here are three cases within a very short while, in all of which the subjects should be alive to-day, all young women and holding valuable places in the community. I could go back through the past three or four years of my experience and recall a dozen or more such examples, all of whom died for want of an early operation. The mortality of laparotomy for these diseases has been and is large—most frightfully so. Treves has collected 122 cases, with a mortality of over 63 per cent. According to Schramm the mortality in 193 collected laparotomies for intestinal obstruction is over 65 per cent. "Some of the patients were almost moribund at the time the laparotomy was performed, others were in a condition of profound exhaustion. In some there was general acute peritonitis, in others fecal extravasation had already taken place. Laparotomy has, indeed, been looked upon as a last resource instead of as a primary measure. This table shows in a graphic manner how serious is the delay, even of twenty-four hours" (Treves). An examination of the records shows very clearly that in cases in which the operation has been undertaken early enough, it is not a very dangerous one. In fact to those familiar with the present status of abdominal surgery, a simple incision into the abdominal cavity is a comparatively trifling measure. The great and only danger comes from delaying until the individual is past recovery.

These remarks as in regard to intestinal obstruction are equally true when applied to any other disease occurring in the peritoneal cavity. In a list of laparotomies collected by myself more than a year ago, there were 93 operations done for non-malignant diseases. Of these, eleven were followed by death. Of the eleven deaths—all after simple exploratory incisions—seven occurred for no other reason than that the operation was undertaken too late and the patient was in a dying condition. All the patients could have been saved had they been taken in hand in time. This element of time is being more generally recognized as of the utmost importance. We now accept it as one of the primary requisites in the Cæsarean section, and it is undoubtedly the one element which has chiefly contributed to raise that operation to its present successful status. If this be of such vital importance in the Cæsarean section, it is none the less so in cases of intra-peritoneal diseases. We daily see cases die shortly after an operation which should almost certainly have recovered.

Mrs. P., after an operation for an ovarian cyst, developed a purulent peritonitis. The case was temporized with day after day, because she became at times better and seemed on the way to recovery, in spite of the fact that the presence of pus was strongly suspected. She struggled on for three or four weeks, or more, and was finally given the benefit of an operation. Pus was found in large quantities. She made a brave fight for six days, and then died of exhaustion and sepsis. An operation one week earlier would undoubtedly have saved her.

X., medical student, was suddenly attacked with pain in his stomach and retired to bed. From the first there was well marked and exaggerated symptoms of peritoneal inflammation in the region of the cæcum. He was temporized with for four days, and was fed on morphia to ease his pain, with other so-called conservative treatment. He was told that there was not much the matter with him, and that he would get well. The attendant had seen many worse cases recover. A surgeon saw the patient the next day, and immediately operated. An ileo-cæcal abscess, with a badly diseased appendix vermiformis, was found. The patient died the same night.

Mrs. R. suffered for seven or eight years

with pelvic trouble, being treated conservatively (?) all the time. Suddenly she developed acute symptoms of intestinal obstruction. So-called conservative treatment was renewed. The patient went into collapse and an operation was advised. The consultant physician objected. The patient recovered from her collapsed condition, and in twenty-four hours had a similar attack. An operation was even yet opposed. The patient made a partial recovery from this second collapse, only to fall into the same condition for a third time. At this late hour an operation was agreed upon, and disclosed large pus tubes, with intestines so tightly bound upon them as to strangulate them. Death followed in twenty-four hours.

Miss L., suffering plainly referable to calculus, and a large stone, immovably fixed in one of the ureters, plainly felt by vaginal examination. Whole cause of trouble clearly recognized and the impossibility of spontaneous delivery realized. Patient in good condition and willing for anything' to gain relief. Allowed to drift on under hopeless conservatism until operation was impossible.

Mrs. C., clear history and diagnosis of extra-uterine pregnancy, with rupture of the gestation sac. Condition of patient fully realized and yet temporized with. Operation after two days delay, and, naturally enough, death followed from exhaustion.

But why should I cite more illustrations? You have all seen them and fully realize the truth of the statement that where one individual is killed by an unnecessary operation, hundreds die for want of one. An exploratory operation, with the patient in good condition, is a very harmless thing ; and those of us in future, who allow patients to die from well marked intra-abdominal disease and stand in the way of an operation, can no longer hide our want of skill and knowledge under this false cry of conservatism. Bantock and Price have both entered strong pleas for early interference, especially in ovarian tumors. It is folly to wait "until the heart and lungs, digestive organs, kidneys, bladder and rectum, no longer discharge their functions without disturbance," or "until the general health has become impaired," or "until all other means of relief have failed, and the patient's health is giving way under the extension of the disease," or "until the patient is failing in strength and becoming emaciated, depressed and nervous," as advised by many prominent men and teachers. In the words of Bantock, I am not aware that there is any operation in the whole range of surgery, in any other part of the body, *that must be a matter of necessity sooner or later,* if the patient's life is to be saved, in which it is considered advisable to await this contingency. Many cases are being refused for operation by operators, because of their having been left so late and handled by a more conservative plan of treatment until it is too late for surgery to have even a half chance of success.

I have in my practice at the present time half a dozen women, all of whom have run the gauntlet of the dangers of peritonitis two or more times and have come out of each attack in a much worse condition than they were before. They all refuse operative interference because they know, or have been told of, some friend who has died after an operation. Of these deaths, two to my personal knowledge were hopeless cases and should never have been touched with the knife. The consequence of the conservative treatment which had encouraged them on to death, with pus tubes in their abdomens, is that a dozen or more women are gradually dying for want of proper treatment. When a patient is dying it is simply a blow to good surgery to attempt any operation whatever.

In the words of one of Philadelphia's most brilliant gynæcologists : "The day is coming when Abdominal Surgeons will be the most arbitrary of men and will refuse to interfere, when called in only at the eleventh hour, merely as a last resource." If surgery has any place in intra-abdominal diseases it most emphatically is not as a last resource, but as a primary measure. As a last resource, abdominal surgery, the world over, has proven a dismal failure ; as an early and primary procedure, there is no branch of our art which has achieved such brilliant and lasting results.

We have only to look at the records of the prominent gynecologists, to see who have, and who have not, accepted this principle of early and timely interference. It is unnecessary to go beyond this city to find such a man, one whose work has made him an ornament to our profession ; and Dr. R. S. Sutton can rest well content that, in his last thirty abdominal sections, for various diseases, he has saved every one of his patients.

As an end of this short and imperfect plea for the necessity of prompt and intelligent work in abdominal diseases, I cannot do better than quote the words of Dr. John B. Roberts, in his address to the Philadelphia

Academy of Surgery, 1888: "Above all, the successful surgeon is a man of action. Experience and knowledge must be there, but they are of little value without action. Inexperience and ignorance are the parents of timidity and recklessness. To avoid these dangers he must have experience and knowledge, which though power, are mere possibilities until used as a source of deeds. The victory of battle is to the leader who does most, not to him who knows most. The true surgeon often takes the offensive, which is for the intrepid alone ; but the weak surgeon falters and lets death come because of his offensive hesitancy."

PHYSICAL EDUCATION.

BY C. F. McGUIRE, M.D.,
BROOKLYN, N. Y.

At present the subject of Physical Education is engaging the attention of educators to an extent that is surprising. When we consider its importance, however, we are more surprised at its almost universal neglect hitherto. The ancients paid great attention to this department of education, and, moreover, did not consider physical strength incompatible with intellectual vigor; on the contrary, their idea of the subject was aptly expressed by the axiom: "a sound mind in a sound body."

It is strange that this important fact was lost sight of by modern educators, and that we should only now be attempting what was an accomplished fact hundreds of years ago. We have had physical training, but usually mercenary in intent, and not in connection with a regular course of study. Yet people have always admired the trained athlete, and no doubt would have taken up the subject, if they but knew how to go about the matter. The trouble has arisen, in a great measure, from the fact that the men who were accepted as the exponents of this art, were not as a rule men whom fathers of families would care to have their children associated with.

Comparatively a short time ago, a body of educated men took the matter up, and, as a consequence, we are beginning now to see in our schools and colleges the fruits of their laudable efforts. It is for this reason that Dr. Anderson, of the Brooklyn Normal Training School for Physical Culture, has been trying for some time past to get the medical profession interested in this matter, especially the younger members, who have more time at their disposal, and to whom it offers a lucrative business. Dr. Anderson reasons that this department of education rightly belongs to the medical profession, as its members are the only ones that are qualified, both by training and education, to fulfil properly the functions of a teacher of this art.

I would suggest that doctors before engaging in this profession should master some one of the various systems now practised, as by so doing they will have a foundation to start from and also save themselves much trouble and anxiety. After they have acquired the necessary ground-work, they can then begin originating, improving, or correcting, as they may find necessary.

There is a great deal to be accomplished in this department—many household gods to be destroyed, many errors to be corrected. This has been well illustrated in the case of Dr. Leuf, of Philadelphia, whose articles in the MEDICAL AND SURGICAL REPORTER have been quite a revelation to many. The doctor has ably shown that many popular works on this subject are, to say the least, fallacious in their teachings and erroneous in their deductions. As an example of erroneous teaching, we have only to take up the subject of so-called abdominal breathing. This method is claimed by many excellent teachers of music to be the only true one, and that any other will surely lead the victim into consumption or else destroy the voice in time. If any one will take the trouble to investigate for himself or to read his works on anatomy, he will be quickly convinced that forcible expansion of the abdominal walls must lead, in the end, to injury. What should be aimed at, in the art of breathing, is a flexible condition of the thorax ; and the muscle which will bring about this flexibility, principally, is the serratus magnus. The diaphragm will take care of itself; for if the ribs are well drawn out by the serrati muscles, it will quickly descend, without any effort on the part of the subject.

Another point, which has been overlooked, is what we will term: individualizing the person—a method always adopted by the successful physician when engaged in diagnosticating disease. By this method the strong points of the person in question can be ascertained and the weak points developed. Most men are weak in the abdominal region, and for that reason this should be the part first attended to. And, moreover, in my opinion, it is the most important part of the body to be developed, for various reasons, best known to physicians. The muscles of this part of the body, together with the serrati muscles, should be plainly visible to the naked eye; and when a man is thus developed, the developing of the rest of the body is accomplished with comparative ease. The main object should be the uniform development of the whole body, never exercising one or two parts at the expense of the others. This point can be readily proven by a visit to one of the German "Turn-Schools," or—as we call them—gymnasiums. There one can see pupils who are experts in certain feats, but whose general make up is not flattering to the system.

When a man is once properly developed, he will remain so, provided, he practises a correct carriage of body and a proper method of breathing. This is well illustrated in the person of a certain Mr. Checkly, of Brooklyn, who is at present engaged in teaching physical culture. This man claims to have taken no special exercise previous to last January, for the space of ten years; yet at the end of that time he was able to handle his body with far greater ease than many men who were engaged constantly in gymnasiums.

What we need in this country are institutions devoted to rational gymnastics, also to the study of physiology, anatomy, hygiene and instruction in the art of cooking; for it must be remembered that the ordinary trainer knows what kind of food is necessary for his pupil. This instruction is vital; for without the proper fuel, no matter how good the machinery, we cannot get the same results. If a man, or woman, could show a diploma from an institution, conducted on these principles, then we might expect to see men and women who would not only be a credit to themselves but a great gain to the state. As a result of such teachings men would have more regard for their bodies and be less likely to abuse them by vile practices; and society in general would put on a different aspect. Instead of crowding rum-shops and other places of evil resort, they would flock to the gymnasiums or the open fields, there to exercise their new found powers, which, instead of making them feel wearied or exhausted, would, on the contrary, better prepare them for the successful prosecution of their business.

It remains with the medical profession especially, to bring about this grand result, and also to interest philanthropists in a scheme that will be far more beneficial to humanity than the erection of a thousand hospitals.

TUBERCULOSIS OF THE TESTICLE IN A CHILD NINE MONTHS OF AGE.

BY CHARLES B. PENROSE, Ph.D., M.D.,
PHILADELPHIA.
SURGEON TO OUT-PATIENT DEPARTMENT, PENNSYLVANIA HOSPITAL.

The following case is of interest on account of the very young age of the patient, and the complete recovery after excision of the diseased testicle.

A. B., black, nine months old, was brought to the Out-Patient Surgical Clinic of the Pennsylvania Hospital, during the writer's service in January, 1889. The patient's right testicle had begun to swell five months before, and an abscess had formed three months later and ruptured through the scrotum. When the child was first brought for treatment, there was a fungous outgrowth about one inch in diameter on the right side of the scrotum, attached to the right testicle, which was enlarged to the size of a pigeon's egg. There was a profuse purulent discharge, which had produced many superficial ulcers on the buttocks and inner aspects of the thighs.

The spermatic cord was knotty and about one-third of an inch in diameter. The left testicle was healthy. There were scars on the neck caused by previous suppuration of the submaxillary lymphatics. With the exception of the diseased testicle there was no sign of active tubercular disease. The mother was healthy and had had nine healthy children; the father had had a cough for several years.

The fungous outgrowth, the right testicle and the thickened portion of the spermatic cord were cut away; the indurated and thickened edges of the scrotal opening were removed; the cavity was thoroughly dusted with iodoform, a rubber drain was introduced, and the wound closed. The attempt to obtain primary union, however, was not successful, and the wound healed by granulation.

Examination of the removed gland showed that there was complete destruction of the epididymis by tubercular abscess, and that miliary tubercles were scattered throughout the body of the testicle. When the child was last seen, in April, 1889, there was no sign of tubercular disease in the right cord or in the remaining testicle, and the general health was fair.

In well-recognized general tubercular disease of the testicle, the gland should always be removed if the disease has not extended beyond the reach of the knife. If rectal examination shows that there is involvement of the seminal vesicles, the prostate or the bladder, removal of the testicle will not delay the course of the disease. The danger of such extension, and of extension to the other testicle, when operation for tubercular disease of the testicle is delayed, should always be remembered; and also the danger of general tuberculosis originating from this focus. Dr. E. H. Monks, in the *British Med. Journal*, Dec. 27, 1884, reports a case of tuberculosis of the testicle in a child five months of age, in which the removal of the gland was refused by the parents, and the child died soon afterward of general tuberculosis. And Laennec (*Gazette Méd. de Nantes*, 1886–1887, V, 117) reports a case of general tuberculosis which followed the late removal of a tubercular testicle. In localized tuberculosis of the testicle, even when an abscess has formed and a sinus exists through the scrotum, recovery occasionally takes place, either without surgical interference, or after destruction of the tubercular focus with the curette or cautery. But when the disease is generalized, the gland becomes functionally useless, and the dangers of extension and of general tuberculosis demand its removal.

1331 Spruce St.

TWO MONTHS IN THE HOSPITALS OF PHILADELPHIA.

BY GEORGE R. DEAN, M.D.,

SPARTANSBURG, S. C.

A busy practitioner, especially if located in the country, has but little time, and often less means available, to leave his labor and visit the great medical centres of our country. There are always a few old cases on hand, and a few new ones expected which will deter him from appointing a day to start, so that his trip North, South, or East, as the case may be, is delayed from time to time, until he finally gives up and plods on in the same old rut. Occasionally, however, one is found who in sheer desperation breaks over all difficulties, as did your correspondent, and drinks afresh at the fountain's source, so pleasant to one who is isolated from medical societies and opportunities and all sources of information save from his own limited and often sad experiences. The reports of those who have returned from Philadelphia have not always been the most encouraging or reassuring to those who wish to return to the city of their Alma Mater. What they want and need most, is clinical work, with short lectures descriptive of the various diseases and treatments, and opportunity to assist personally where it is possible. This, and this alone, can give them the information they most need.

It has been said that physicians and surgeons occupying positions in the hospitals and dispensaries of Philadelphia, which would enable them to do much in this direction, have not been as generous with their courtesies to the profession as those occupying similar positions in other cities. For this reason many of our Southern physicians have gone elsewhere to refresh their minds in medical knowledge when their inclinations were otherwise in favor of Philadelphia. Be this as it may, my own experience in this respect has been altogether different. I visited many hospitals and dispensaries, and received the most genuine hospitality and courtesy from both chiefs and assistants, in each and every instance. I therefore gladly record my evidence on the other side of the question, for a more generous, kindly interest could not have been shown to friend or stranger than was extended to me by those with whom I came in contact, during my two months stay in that city.

A man who expects to receive courtesies must himself be courteous, and when men complain of mistreatment at the hands of others, it is but just to inquire if they have been without blame themselves.

Some of the best clinics in Europe have been closed to visitors by the indiscretion of a few men who forgot themselves and the obligations due those whose courtesies they were enjoying. I saw in Philadelphia much of advanced surgery and gynecology, and it is my belief that our countrymen can find all they want and need here in the way of knowledge and skill in every department of the healing art, and men with nerve and brain to demonstrate them satisfactorily. A long trip to Europe, therefore, with a possibility of snubs from those whose skill is equalled if not exceeded in our own country, is not necessary to those who wish to keep abreast with the advance of the profession. I believe if a physician will go to Philadelphia with the earnest desire to see and learn, and will deport himself as is becoming a true gentleman, he will find physicians who are ready, willing and capable to give him just what he wants.

The improvement in the treatment of the diseases of women has been greatly advanced in the last few years. Antiseptics truly revolutionized this field of the physician's work, and now asepsis, in the hands of some of the most expert and advanced operators, has superseded this. Operative treatment of tubal and ovarian diseases is now a well-established procedure, and as now performed by a few of the profession gives results almost beyond belief, as witness the records of Dr. Goodell, Dr. Charles B. Penrose, Dr. Joseph Hoffman, Dr. John B. Deaver, Dr. M. Price, and Dr. Joseph Price with his 63 consecutive cases without a death. Through the kindness of Dr. Goodell, I was permitted to witness and assist in several ovariotomies in his private hospital. Through the kindness of Drs. M. Price and Hoffman, I saw many cases in their private practice—the former showing me several cases of great interest and permitting me to assist him in several of them. To Dr. Joseph Price I am indebted for the many advantages afforded by my visits to the Philadelphia Dispensary and the Gynecean Hospital. This hospital, in charge of Dr. J. Price and Dr. Charles Penrose, is a model in its way. It is new and small and lacks many conveniences of some other hospitals, but the lack of these is more than counterbalanced by the skill and enthusiasm of its chiefs, and their determination to achieve a success for it second to none in the world. It already stands at the head of such institutions in the United States. Their success is very gratifying, both to themselves and to the friends of the institution. I witnessed many operations while there—abdominal sections, and plastic operations upon womb and perineum—success in every case followed. I have seen pus tubes as large as small intestines, adhesions so great that the bowel would tear before the adhesions would break, and all anatomical relations obliterated in the pelvis; and yet these patients made an uninterrupted recovery. As to the results following ovariotomy for tubal and ovarian disease, I made many inquiries of the patients themselves, through the kindness of Dr. Price at the Philadelphia Dispensary. The verdict in every case was the same: the patients had either been cured entirely or were passing through the phases of a premature menopause. Not one single woman did I see, who did not express herself as being greatly benefited by the operation. So, from being a skeptic, I became a believer in surgical interference in these troubles, which unfit a woman for performing the ordinary duties of life; and I shall devote the balance of my life to this special

department for the relief of suffering womankind. In the Gynecean Hospital there are no antiseptics used in abdominal operations, but the asepsis is perfect, as far as human efforts and skill can make it so. The whole staff, from nurse to chiefs, is in full sympathy with its chief design; and success crowns their labors.

My experience in other dispensaries was very pleasant. To the physicians who extended me so many courtesies and so much kind consideration, I am under lasting gratitude; and I assure them that I will not soon forget their pleasant faces. Indeed, Philadelphia has hosts of good and true men in the profession, who are ready and willing to assist those who are truly and honestly trying to gain information.

HEMORRHAGE FROM THE UMBILICUS.[1]

BY H. F. WILLIS, M.D.,

PRESTON, MD.

The recent occurrence in my practice of a case of fatal hemorrhage from the umbilicus, being an event so rare, led me to give some attention to the literature of umbilical hemorrhage. I was surprised to find all of the old authors, whose writings I had an opportunity to consult, were silent upon the subject. A gentleman, to whose paper I am indebted for most of the information upon which this paper has been based, says that Cazeaux, Ramsbotham, Leischman and Lusk say nothing on the subject.

Dr. Joseph S. Gibb, of Philadelphia, in a paper read before the Philadelphia Clinical Society, March 28, 1884, and published in the *Medical Times*, of that city, May 17, 1884, has tabulated all the cases upon record up to that time. Various authors had reported, up to 1881, 236 cases. Between 1881 and 1884, Dr. Gibb found 5 more cases reported in the medical journals, all of which was seen by himself. This record proves the rarity of umbilical hemorrhage; yet it is liable to happen at almost any time.

Following the classification of Dr. Gibb, umbilical hemorrhage may be divided into three classes: First, hemorrhage from improper ligation of the cord; second, hemorrhage from traumatism; third, hemorrhage of spontaneous origin.

The first variety, or hemorrhage from improper ligation of the cord, is liable to

---

[1] Read before the Caroline County Medical Association.

occur at any time from carelessness on the part of the attending physician or the nurse. It is especially liable to occur when the cord is large and full of gelatinous matter; for, as it becomes smaller, the ligature is loosened, even when it has been properly applied in the first place. It is important to examine the ligature around the cord after the child has been dressed, to be sure that such a disagreeable accident may not occur. If you, Mr. President and gentlemen, have always been so fortunate as to escape being roused from a delightful sleep by the announcement that the baby was bleeding from the navel, you are more fortunate than the speaker, who remembers regretfully one such incident in his professional career. No life was lost, but it was an occurrence certainly not to be proud of. I think this form of hemorrhage is rarely fatal. Proper tying of the cord is the remedy.

The second variety of hemorrhage is occasioned by unnecessary handling of the infant. I have seen some poor little babies pretty roughly treated, and it is possible that after the dressing has been completed that undue pulling of the clothing and bandage might produce hemorrhage before the cord has had time to dry sufficiently; and any tearing of the cord near the umbilical surface might set up an alarming bleeding. If the part of the cord torn is too near the surface of the abdomen to be tied, the dependence for treatment would be upon styptics and compression.

The third variety—hemorrhage from spontaneous origin—is the variety which most concerns us. The hemorrhage may occur at almost any time. It generally sets in, I believe, about the time the cord begins to come away. You have all watched the drying up of the cord—undoubtedly a physiological process in ninety-nine cases out of every hundred. It begins at the outer end of the cord and extends toward the umbilicus; and, unless nature has been interrupted in her work by meddlesomeness or disease, a few days suffice to bring the cord away as a foreign substance, leaving a clean healthy surface to heal as rapidly as possible with the mildest and simplest dressings. It occasionally happens that the babe will bleed two or three days after birth. Examination will then reveal the fact that the outer extremity of the severed cord has undergone the true process of drying, but that the cord next the umbilicus has undergone softening, and you witness a sphacelated or gangrenous condition, with blood oozing from the edges of the umbilical depression. Fetor and softening warn you that the usual physiological process has been converted into a pathological disturbance of a serious character. The oozing may have begun slowly; styptics and pressure may control it for a time. Let it not be forgotten that it is very liable to recur in a short time. The blood is generally thin, watery, and lacking in the power to coagulate firmly enough to satisfy you that the danger is over.

As to the causation of this form of umbilical hemorrhage, it is evident that there is generally something at fault in the constitutional condition of the child, either hereditary or congenital. Jaundice is frequently found associated with this form of hemorrhage, and hence it is sometimes set down as the cause. Is it not more than probable that both symptoms—hemorrhage and jaundice—depend upon some blood dyscrasia? Dr. Gibb believes this to be the case, and argues forcibly in favor of his belief. I am led to believe with him that hemophilia is generally *the* disease of such infants, and that the jaundice is only "an indication that the liver is not receiving its proper healthy pabulum, and hence refuses to carry on its functions properly."

In my own practice, I now remember only two cases. The first occurred in January, 1884. The second day after the birth of the infant, I was hastily summoned to arrest the bleeding. The blood was oozing from the outer surface of the umbilical depression quite freely. The cord was nearly completely separated close to the belly. It was soft and fetid. The child was jaundiced. In this case the mother was young, strong and healthy at that time. I think she still remains so, although some of her relatives on the mother's side—her mother also—had died of phthisis. The child recovered, finally, but I think the hemorrhage returned two or three times.

The second and last case occurred in March last. On March 7, I was called, in the absence of the family physician, to attend Mrs. A., who was in labor. Upon my arrival, I found that the child had been born and dressed an hour before. As I approached the bedside of the mother, I was struck with her anæmic look. The placenta not being delivered I feared hemorrhage, but it was only the ordinary appearance of the woman. Inquiry elicited the statement that before her pregnancy she had had two profuse hemorrhages from the lungs. I saw her on the 8th; both mother and child were apparently doing well. On the morning of the 10th, I was hastily summoned to see the child. When I reached the house I found it almost in a dying condition, the clothing saturated with blood. I lowered its head and shoulders, and proceeded to remove the bandages and clothing. The cord was ready to come away; the end farthest from the umbilicus had dried in the physiological manner; the portion nearest the abdomen was soft and fetid—in a condition we might properly call soft gangrene. The child was thoroughly bloodless. With the anæmic color the icteric hue was marked. The child continued to moan for several hours, but never rallied. A styptic and compress prevented any further hemorrhage. Was this a true hemophilia, or only a manifestation of the hereditary hemorrhagic diathesis?

How shall we treat such cases? The result in my first case is in favor of the use of styptics and compression. Whether I gave calomel to the child or not I do not now remember. The styptic used was Monsel's solution. The second case was necessarily fatal at the time I saw it. I do not know that it should discourage us from attempting internal treatment, if the case is seen in time.

In this paper I claim little of originality. To Dr. Gibb, of whom I have frequently made mention, belongs the credit of bringing the subject prominently before the profession. If to you, Mr. President and gentlemen of the Society, I have succeeded in investing the subject with some degree of the interest which I have experienced while devoting some hours to the preparation of this paper, I shall be abundantly repaid for the time and labor.

—It would be an excellent idea, says the *Manchester Union*, if physicians of the present day would invent some other reason for about all of the deaths which occur nowadays than the cheap fraud, "heart failure." This might not be of serious moment were it not for the fact that hundreds of people are being nearly frightened to death by the constant use of the cause for sudden deaths, and many people who are sick and necessarily have some heart symptoms are kept in constant terror by reading or hearing in other ways of death after death by heart failure. There are probably no more deaths from heart failure in these times than heretofore, but a new cause for death has been coined and the nervous and timid are being severely injured by it.

REPORTS OF CLINICS.

PHILADELPHIA HOSPITAL.

CLINIC FOR DISEASES OF CHILDREN—
DR. STRYKER.

Hare-Lip and Cleft-Palate.

Here is a case that tells you the whole story. You will see at once that it is hare-lip, and that it came very near being double. In addition, there is a deficiency in the palate on each side, leaving quite a prominent intermaxillary bone in the middle. The union is complete behind. These cases, of course, call for operation. The hare-lip should be operated upon first, because the bringing together of the lip has some controlling action over the gap in the roof of the mouth, so that when the staphylorrhaphy is performed when the child is five or six years old, there will then be a much smaller chink in the palate to close up. The time for operation is a question about which surgeons are a little unsettled; but the best time is when the child is two or three months old, unless there is some pressing need of operating earlier.

The operation consists simply in freshening the edges, bringing them together, and liberating the lip from its attachment to the mucous membrane covering the jaw. Some surgeons recommend an elliptical, others an angular incision in the lip, the object being to avoid a little depression that is likely to occur just at the point of union at the free border of the lip. In this case the left intermaxillary bone projects forward, and by pressing against the lip may prevent its uniting. Sometimes the prominent portion of the bone has to be removed so as to allow the cut surfaces to be brought together.

Non-Inflammatory Diarrhœa.

I have three or four little patients whom I wish to bring before you this morning, to introduce the subject of affections of the alimentary canal, which, as the season advances, will become more common. Irritations of the alimentary tract in the spring season are due generally either to cold, to some fault of digestion or to some similar cause, and are certainly not due to heat, as they are apt to be during the summer season. We will consider this morning only the mild diarrhœas of children, and it might be well to call them the non-inflammatory diarrhœas, they are so evanescent.

The attack occurs so suddenly that there are no marked premonitory symptoms. At the time of the attack there may be a slight increase of temperature and an acceleration of the pulse, a certain amount of thirst, indisposition to eat, and there may be also a furred tongue or a patchy tongue—red in spots and white-furred in other spots. Such a tongue always indicates some disturbance of digestion. The attack is usually of short duration, although it may run into a more marked enteric irritation. If the child should die, there would be found very little to account for it except a slight engorgement of the blood-vessels of the intestine.

In institutions like the Philadelphia Hospital, we are liable to have cases of this sort at all seasons of the year, because the large majority of children in our nurseries and foundling wards are artificially fed. But even with nursing babies the milk may be irritating, and it will then give rise to just the same conditions as are found in babies artificially fed. If the breast-milk is persistently irritating, resort to artificial feeding, or, if the family can afford it, get a wet-nurse.

Here are two diapers containing the stools. You see a certain amount of lumpy matter, consisting of curds. Here in spots is a greenish-color, due to acidity. This is the result, possibly, of feeble stomach digestion in these children, and the consequent passing into the intestine of undigested particles, which give rise to intestinal indigestion and produce a diarrhœa. The number of passages varies from three or four to eight or ten in the twenty-four hours.

The best treatment consists in getting rid of the exciting cause, and, for this purpose, a mild purgative is indicated. The *Mistura Olei* of the old Dispensatory, consisting of a little castor oil, a few drops of oil of peppermint, and mucilage of acacia, is a good combination. Small repeated doses of castor oil will do better than a single large dose. Spiced syrup of rhubarb is a remedy that is in every household, and is used for just such a condition. Avoid over-feeding. A little chalk mixture may be necessary as an astringent later. The important part of the general treatment is so to regulate the child's diet as to prevent a continuance of the condition. A little bismuth or pepsin, or a drop of brandy with the meal, will stimulate digestion and allow the child to become properly nourished. As a rule, the child suffers very little pain, so that anodynes are seldom necessary.

SPECIAL CORRESPONDENCE.

LETTER FROM CHINA.

As Canton City is on the great highway around the world, and is what we might term the New York of China, there are naturally a great many tourists and travelers who visit us. The large medical Missionary Hospital for the Chinese is nearly always visited by those who come to Canton. I have thought it might prove interesting to answer, through the pages of the REPORTER, a few of the many questions asked by medical men and those interested in medical work in China.

Are there any native schools in China where medicine or surgery is taught? There are none. Native doctors there are in abundance—self-made doctors, they might be called; for they have never been under any system of medical education. No license of any kind is required of those who practise medicine. With the exception of a few native drugs, they are ignorant of the action of the many (supposed) remedies that they use. One wishing to qualify himself for the practice of medicine must be at least forty years of age, and generally a period of four or five years is spent with a native doctor, or perhaps part of the time in a native drug shop. It is indeed strange that, while much of their knowledge is derived from practical experience, yet their views on the whole subject are most erroneous.

Do the Chinese practise surgery? Not in any way. They stand aloof from the surgeon's knife, and do not attempt the simplest operations. Even those who have studied our western science of medicine and surgery find a great barrier to their practice of the same; for, should any accident whatever happen to a patient under their care, they would most likely have to pay heavy damages; and, should the case terminate fatally, the doctor would probably lose his head.

Do native physicians attend obstetrical cases? They do not. They may write prescriptions for certain cases, but are never in direct attendance. As a rule, a midwife is employed. If not, the ever-present mother-in-law assumes charge of affairs. The Chinese have no mechanical appliances to use where complications arise, and they have no knowledge of the mechanism of labor. There is a wide field here for the gynecologist and obstetrician. The foreign doctors from the hospital are very frequently called where complications arise in confinements, and little attention is paid to sex. The male physician is generally as readily admitted to the homes in such cases as the female physician is.

Do the Chinese readily submit to operations and are their powers of endurance good? As a rule, the Chinaman has implicit faith in the foreign surgeon, and is about as ready to go on the operating table as to lie down on his bed. So far as their nervous system is concerned, they are far less liable to suffer from shock than the European is, and their powers of endurance in severe operations seem to be much greater.

Are the diseases and surgical affections met with of much the same nature as those met with in America? So far as Southern China is concerned they are, generally speaking, the same. The eruptive fevers, except small-pox, are seldom met with. Pneumonia and diphtheria are rarely seen or heard of. Leprosy and elephantiasis are common, and Asiatic cholera is present every summer. The field of surgery is wide and almost any variety of surgical affection may be met with. Tumors, both malignant and non-malignant, of all varieties, are met with very frequently. Two wards of the Canton Hospital are set apart for patients who have urinary calculus, and there are from three to fifteen cases constantly present the year round. Calculus is found at any age, from that of the child one year old to that of the old man of eighty. This affection, however, is confined to a few districts near Canton City, and is very seldom met with in other places.

Much more might be said on these various points than can be included in a letter.

The first of the year 1887 there was organized "*The Medical Missionary Association of China.*" It has for its object—*First.*—The promotion of the Science of Medicine and Surgery among the Chinese, and mutual assistance derived from the varied experiences of medical missionaries. *Second.*—The cultivation and advancement of mission work and the science of medicine in general. *Third.*—The promotion of the character, interest and honor of the fraternity by maintaining union and harmony of the regular profession. All members are graduates of recognized regular medical colleges, and persons of every nationality are eligible for membership. The representative organ of this association is "*The China Medical Missionary Journal,*" which is published quarterly by Kelly and Walsh, Shanghai; price, two dollars per year. Those interested

in the progress of western medical science in the east will find a store of information in this journal.

One can scarcely imagine the untold value of Western medicine and surgery to the Chinese. They may hate the foreigner and all that belongs to him *except* the healing art—that they always welcome. It has been the entering wedge for Christianity and has done more to open up China to our western civilization than all the cannon of Europe.

J. M. SWAN, M.D.

Canton Hospital,
  Canton, China.
April 20, 1889.

PERISCOPE.

Mumps and Double Orchitis.

In June, 1887, Dr. Manbrac noted an interesting case which occurred at Bizerte during an epidemic of mumps. A man, 45 years old, was suddenly seized with painful swelling of the left parotid gland. For four days there was much tumefaction, and the patient was feverish. On the sixth day the swelling had slightly diminished, but orchitis of the left testicle set in. The complication lasted five days; during that time the parotid swelling became smaller. The patient then appeared to be convalescent. On the sixteenth day, however, the patient complained of much pain in the right testicle. The entire gland appeared to be involved in very acute inflammation. By the twenty-fourth day the patient was nearly well; the buccal mucous membrane remained somewhat œdematous, but the patient could open his mouth and masticate food without pain. Both testicles seemed to have returned to a perfectly healthy condition. Dr. Manbrac, writing in the *Gazette Médicale de Paris,* notes that the epidemic occurred amidst a population of 7,000; nearly ninety children were attacked, yet the above patient was the only one older than 20 who suffered from mumps. He lived in a house where a child aged 6 was laid up with mumps. His teeth were remarkably sound, and his health when attacked was good. He had no trace of syphilitic, gonorrhœal, or malarial taint. The case is of distinct interest, as the undoubted occasional association of mumps and orchitis is as interesting as the singular association occasionally observed between parotitis and injuries of the abdomen or abdominal section.—*British Med. Journal,* Feb. 16, 1889.

Influence of Carlsbad Water on the Secretion of Uric Acid.

At the meeting of the New York Academy of Medicine, January 15, 1889, Dr. S. LeClercq, of Carlsbad, Germany, said he had made careful experiments on himself to determine whether, as had been supposed, the secretion of uric acid is lessened by drinking freely of Carlsbad water. With a uniform diet and taking increasing doses of the water, he found the amount of uric acid unaltered, as compared with the amount noted in the five weeks previous to taking the water. He has found that on a fixed diet the daily amount of uric acid, nevertheless, varies. Niemeyer has stated that this variation depends on unknown changes of action in the internal economy. He believed that in the future the influence of any drug on the production of uric acid would be found to have no special relation to its value in the treatment of gout. Our theories as to the nature of gout and the action of Carlsbad salts must both change. He has found Carlsbad water acting in several ways, some of which are : 1. The condition of the patient is improved through its causing the production of better blood (without any solution or dissipation of the tophi). The taking of warm water of itself acts favorably by diluting the fluids and washing out the channels of the body. 2. In certain cases the gouty diathesis is not perceptibly modified. 3. In other cases the water seems to lessen the synthetic formation of uric acid. 4. It often acts on other anomalies of function, and improves the general health. The digestion is in some cases improved, or deleterious by-products are taken up and excreted more rapidly. Perhaps the topical effect of the water on the stomach explains much of the benefit obtained. The exercise, bathing, pure air, and change of surroundings also must exert considerable influence on the peristalsis and circulation, and thus increase the general tone of the body.

Dr. F. N. Otis spoke from his own impressions derived from a recent prolonged stay at Carlsbad, and from the results obtained by sending patients there. He had gone to Carlsbad himself to obtain relief from what was either a gouty or a nervous dyspepsia, with mental depression and inaptitude for work. His diet while there had contained little sugar or starch, but an abundance of meat, with a little bread and claret. Although he had taken but little exercise, he had lost a pound in weight every day for a month. A feeling of debility had been noticeable during his stay at the Springs, and had continued for about a month after his departure. It had then slowly disappeared; he had regained flesh, and had had no return of digestive troubles. He thinks the patients who can anticipate benefit at Carlsbad are those whose sickness is due to free living and too little exercise. When a patient can not be sent to Carlsbad, he recommends the giving of remedies which act on the skin and liver; also abundant exercise. Mercury he regards as a most valuable remedy ; it has relieved the condition when a visit to Carlsbad has failed to do so. He gives one, two, or even three grains of calomel a day, and does not find the system deteriorated by it. He has found that when there is Bright's disease, with abundant albumin, the Carlsbad waters depress the vitality, and are the reverse of beneficial.—*N. Y. Med. Journal*, March 9, 1889.

Hegar's Sign of Pregnancy.

The most conclusive signs of pregnancy in the first three months are to be found in the changes which take place in the size, shape, and consistence of the body of the uterus. These changes are the natural result of the lodgment and growth of the globular ovum in the uterine cavity. The body of the uterus bulges out as the ovum develops, its lateral borders become rounded, and there is a distinctly marked bellying of the anterior wall. After from four to six weeks' development this segment of the uterus presents in a very perceptible degree the characteristic elasticity of the fluid cyst which it contains. To the well-trained touch the bellying of the lower segment of the uterus, especially its anterior wall, and its fluid elasticity, are sufficient for the diagnosis of pregnancy in a large number of cases from the fourth to sixth week. These signs are obtained by the "bimanual" touch, as practised in ordinary gynæcological examinations.

To the signs above mentioned, Hegar has added another. This consists in the marked softening and thinning of that portion of the corpus uteri immediately above the cervix, especially as obtained by Hegar's method. His method of examination is as follows :

A preliminary distention of the rectum with water may be necessary to facilitate the manipulation. Chloroform may be used if required. Depressing the uterus with one hand over the abdomen, pass the index finger of the other hand into the rectum, up through the third sphincter, and press the finger tip

against the posterior wall of the uterus immediately above the utero-sacral ligaments.
Pass the thumb of the same hand into the
vagina and bring it in contact with the
anterior wall of the uterus just above the
cervix. The intervening tissues may in
most cases, during the last half of the second
month, be compressed by the grip of the
thumb and finger almost to the thinness of
a visiting card. This compressibility of the
lower uterine segment thus obtained is
Hegar's sign. It has been confounded by
writers with the before-mentioned changes
in the uterus, from which, as a sign of pregnancy, it is entirely separate and distinct.—
Brooklyn Med. Journal, March, 1889.

Fecal Fistula.

In a short note on fecal fistula, in the
Canadian Practitioner, March 1, 1889,
Dr. James F. W. Ross, Surgeon to the
Woman's Hospital in Toronto, says that
within the last three months he has seen
some curious occurrences in connection
with operations inside the abdomen, which
if not well authenticated by those engaged
in this work all over the world, would be
regarded as fabrications.

The idea of the terrible consequences of
injuring the bowel during an operation now
belongs to a bygone age. This accident
was regarded as a very untoward one, but
to his mind it has been proved that it is less
dangerous to injure the bowel than to leave
the source of illness behind. Unfinished
operations in experienced hands have shown
a large mortality. Operations a few years
ago left unfinished from want of pluck, are
to-day completed and the patient cured.
He had seen, during the short space of three
weeks, three cases of fecal fistula following
abdominal section. In one case the ovaries
and tubes were matted down after fourteen
years of the old fashioned expectant treatment. It was hoped to relieve symptoms
due to diseased ovaries, which were riddled
with abscesses, by other means than those of
operation. At last when the patient could
not endure life longer in such a miserable
condition, an operation was performed,
before the difficulties of which hysterectomy
pales into insignificance. A drainage tube
was inserted, as there was much hemorrhage,
and it was feared that during the separation
of adhesions some damage might have been
done to the bowel. The operation was
brilliantly performed, and there are few
men who could have carried it through to
completion.

In twenty-four hours the patient was passing feces through the drainage tube, without
the slightest inconvenience. In a few days
the tube was taken out and the fistula began
to contract. Enemata that were given washed
out through the abdominal opening.

In the second case the patient was operated
on for pyosalpinx, following a severe labor.
The enucleation of the large adherent suppurating mass was very difficult and accompanied by severe hemorrhage. This patient
also passed feces through the drainage tube,
and made an excellent though rather tedious
recovery. Her enemata also washed through
the fistula.

The third case was one of supposed malignant disease, matting the small intestine
and colon together in the left lower half of
the abdomen. Nothing was done except
to explore the mass. It was soft, felt as if
malignant, and certainly could not be
removed. The finger tore into it during
examination. In this case a drainage tube
was not used, but a fecal fistula resulted.
Death was regarded as only a matter of time.
The patient made a good recovery from the
operation and the fecal fistula soon healed.
The sequel shows the danger of giving an
absolute opinion in such cases. The thickening disappeared and the operator concluded that the growth was not malignant.
The moral from these cases is that fecal matter
is not poisonous to the peritoneum, if it can
readily escape. The old idea of the poisonous microbes in intestinal contents can
hardly be worth consideration in the face of
such clinical facts. No carbolic acid or
any other disinfectant was used in any of
these cases. Only cotton wool was used for
a dressing. A glass tube, taken out of a
card-board box, was inserted for a drainage
tube. No turpentine and corrosive sublimate scrubbing of the abdominal walls was
performed. Yet the instruments were clean,
cleansed with soap and water; hands were
clean, cleansed with soap and water; towels
were clean, fresh from the laundry.

Any one who has passed his finger down
the twenty-four hour old track of a glass
drainage tube will have recognized its tube-
like character. It is just like putting one's
finger into a rubber tube. It is wonderful
how nature effects such a channeling down
to the pouch of Douglas, or any spot on
which the drainage tube has rested. It is
easy to understand how fæcal matter can
readily be discharged into such a channel,
while the rest of the peritoneum remains
shut off by inflammatory, or at any rate by
an adhesive, process.

Pathological Anatomy in Cases of Death after Extensive Burns.

In the *Deutsche med. Wochenschrift*, xv, 2, 1889, Dr. Eugen Fränkel asks how rapid death after extensive burns is to be explained? Ponfick has answered that death is the result of extensive disintegration of blood corpuscles and certain parenchymatous changes of the internal organs, which are the result of heat. Sonnenburg has cast doubt upon this opinion, but Fränkel is in a position to support it by investigations of the pathological anatomy. He found not only a large quantity of *débris* of blood corpuscles, but he could also demonstrate parenchymatous degenerations, especially in the liver and kidneys; and he thinks that the combination of degeneration of the secreting epithelium of the kidney with extensive obstruction of the uriniferous tubules by masses of hæmoglobin especially fatal. In one point Fränkel differs from Ponfick. He considers the parenchymatous degenerations not the result of disintegration of the blood corpuscles, but thinks that both the disintegration and the degeneration are effects of a poisonous product to be sought in the burns of the skin. How extraordinarily rapidly this poison acts may be judged from a case of Fränkel's, in which death occurred fifteen hours after the burn, and yet the autopsy showed marked conditions.—*Schmidt's Jahrbücher*, April, 1889.

Operation for Depressed Nipple.

Dr. W. L. Axford, of Chicago, says in the *Annals of Surgery*, April, 1889, that Mrs. H., a young German woman about three months advanced in her third pregnancy, was referred to him by Dr. F. B. Norcom, who wished to see if anything could be done for her badly retracted nipples. In her two preceding lactations she had not been able to nurse her children, though all known mechanical devices had been resorted to. The only relief for the woman was to suppress the milk as soon as possible. She was very anxious to nurse the expected child. Dr. Norcom said that some ten years ago he had succeeded in improving a depressed nipple by excising an elliptical piece of skin and drawing the edges of the wound together, and that, although the present case was much more unfavorable, he believed an operation feasible. The idea was entirely new to Dr. Axford.

On examination it was found that where there should have been a projecting nipple there was actually a depression into which the end of the little finger could be inserted. The breasts were perfectly healthy and otherwise well formed. The woman was a brunette, and the depressed nipple in its dark areola presented much the appearance of the invaginated finger of a dark brown kid glove. The right breast was deeper than the other.

Seizing the ends of the ducts with toothed forceps, the nipple could be easily drawn out to any reasonable extent. There were no adhesions or bands holding it down. An operation was proposed and accepted, and with the assistance of Drs. Norcom and Parsons, was done as follows: The right nipple was seized with the volsellum and drawn out till the skin was well on the stretch; beginning about one-third of an inch from the apex two curved incisions enclosing a crescent-shaped piece of skin were extended out in the breast for two and a half inches, and the skin and fat down to the fascia removed.

This area of denudation, Dr. Axford says, should have its greatest breadth at the base of the newly formed nipple. Three such excisions, radiating from the nipple were made. A catgut suture was now passed in and out, purse-string fashion, through the fascia, encircling the base of the nipple, and snugly tied at the point of entrance. This served to pucker up the fascia so that when the volsellum was removed the nipple showed no tendency to return to its inverted condition. This suture, he says, becomes completely buried when the denuded areas are closed. These areas were then closed with the continuous silk suture.

The result in the right and more depressed nipple was so satisfactory that it was decided to attempt an operation on the other. A similar operation was done, the lunes a little broader and the buried sutures a little deeper, with a much more satisfactory result. An antiseptic dressing was applied and the patient put to bed. The sutures were removed at the end of the seventh day, and the immediate result found to be excellent.

The anatomical construction of the breast, he states, furnishes the key to the operation. The fascia everywhere covering the surface of the gland protects the lactiferous ducts from injury, and when puckered up around the base of the well-drawn-out nipple forms a support for the soft yielding tissues of which it is composed, holding it out in its proper place. In both cases after tying the buried suture the nipples stood out without the aid of the forceps. The closure of the lune-shaped areas in turn furnishes an additional support to that given by the puckered fascia, and adds to the projection of the nipple.

In conclusion, he calls attention to the fact that the field for this operation is limited, and states that it should be done only after the failure of mechanical devices fairly tried.

Iodol in Diseases of the Respiratory Organs.

In the *Canadian Practitioner*, March 1, 1889, there is a translation of an article by Dr. Dante Cervisato, of Padua, in which he says that the utility of iodine preparations in diseases of the respiratory organs has been disputed because it is feared that by their direct influence on the air passages, their bad influence on the digestive system, and their power of accelerating tissue change, instead of preventing the advance of the disease and promoting a cure, they may only hasten the course of the disease. In consideration of the many recently published successes in the treatment of diseases of the bronchi and lungs, particularly tuberculosis, by iodoform, he has, owing to the similarity of iodol to iodoform, used the former in the treatment of similar cases. The iodol was given internally in doses of 15 to 45 grains daily, and besides was applied locally in the form of inhalation, or insufflation to the larynx.

For inhalation, a watery alcoholic glycerine solution was used, in which very finely divided iodol was suspended.

In far advanced tuberculosis of the lung, with extensive cavities, no perceptible influence on the fever, cough, expectoration and general condition, could be observed. Cases of primary laryngeal tuberculosis were much improved both as to local condition and general symptoms. Sometimes apparently complete arrest of the process, and in many cases the transplanting of the disease in the lung, so long as the patient was under observation, prevented. Still he is not yet in the happy position of being able to publish cases of complete cure.

Great success attended the treatment of acute and chronic catarrh of the larynx by means of insufflation; especially in the acute and subacute forms rapid improvement was immediately noticeable. Iodol was very well borne even in cases where other kinds of treatment could not be carried on. In a case of extensive catarrh of the small bronchi (dry catarrh) with recurring fits of asthma, which occurred every ten to fifteen days, treated by iodol, internally and by inhalation, the catarrhal condition was much improved, cough much more seldom and easier, and the asthma did not recur during the two months the patient was under observation.

In two cases of dry bronchitis in children, one three, the other five, the internal administration of iodol caused increase of bronchial secretion and general improvement.

In three cases of stationary pleuritic exudation in children, pretty rapid resorption and final disappearance of the exudation was the result.

In some cases of chronic bronchial catarrh in children, in which the bronchial glands were supposed to be implicated, the general result was good, and particularly in two of the cases there was positive improvement of the general condition and bronchial symptoms, and disappearance of those symptoms supposed to be caused by the diseased glands.

Excessive Sensory Cortical Discharges and their Effects.

Dr. A. Hughes Bennett has a communication on this subject in the *Lancet*, March 30, and April 6, 1889. He uses the expression "cortical discharge" to mean a sudden liberation of the functional activity of any portion of the cortex cerebri. Excessive cortical discharge, he says, is consequent upon a state of hyper-excitability of the cellular elements of the brain caused by their irritation, which irritation may be induced either by mechanical, chemical, electrical, and other artificial agents, or by diseases of various kinds. This internal central change generates a corresponding series of external manifestations which take the form of explosions or sudden exaggerated paroxysms of that special function which is represented by the affected central gray matter. For example, if the motor area of the cortex be involved, a convulsion results; if the sensory region, a violent subjective storm of one or more senses. A "discharging lesion," therefore, is the state of instability of cortical cells, which in its turn may be due to a variety of pathological causes. The "discharge" itself is the sudden, excessive, concentrated liberation of their function, which as a consequence follows. The "symptoms of the discharge" are the paroxysmal exhibitions of excess of action of different kinds in different regions by those elements throughout the body whose functions are represented in the centres which are involved by the disease.

Dr. Bennett has undertaken an investigation with a view to the localization of the special senses—sight, hearing, smell, taste, touch—using for this purpose the sensory symptoms which often precede and accompany an epileptic seizure. His experience is derived from a careful analysis of 500 consecutive cases of epilepsy and epileptiform attacks under his own care and investigated by himself. In few of these there was a *post-mortem* examination, but the symptoms observed speak for themselves. No exact statistical method, he says, is attempted, as those who deal with epilepsy will recognize the difficulty and uselessness attendant on such a method of investigation. In most instances the physician has to rely upon the statements of the patient or his friends, having rarely himself the opportunity of actually witnessing the seizure; but he states that in this inquiry every effort has been made, by the strictest cross-examination, to elucidate the facts. He was fortunate enough in a few but important exceptions to have actually been present at some of the attacks, and to have personally tested and confirmed the previous statements of the patient. As a matter of convenience he takes the consideration of the five special senses in the order of the frequency with which they are affected, namely: (1) touch; (2) sight; (3) hearing; (4) taste; and (5) smell.

The general conclusions which he derives from his investigation may be summarized as follows: 1. In a given series of cases of epilepsy or of epileptiform attacks there is a certain percentage in which a pronounced feature consists of an aura of one of the special senses. In 500 cases there was in round numbers an aura of the sense of touch in 10 per cent., of sight in 3 per cent., of hearing in 1.5 per cent., of smell in 0.75 per cent., and of taste in 0.75 per cent. 2. These auræ take the form of the development of crude subjective sensations of one of the special senses, and consist of a sudden attack of exaggerated sensation of pain, light, noise, smell, or taste. 3. These exaggerated sensations of sense are immediately succeeded by the opposite condition—namely, by a temporary abolition or diminution of the special sense previously affected, which results in anæsthesia, amblyopia, deafness, loss of taste, and anosmia. 4. These facts seem to indicate that each of the special senses is separately represented in the cerebral cortex, and that each of them is liable to disease. When by irritation they are in a hyper-physiological condition, they discharge their respective functions, the result being a crude subjective sensation of the corresponding sense. When destroyed or exhausted, the function is abolished or temporarily depressed. 5. The sensory cortical centres thus obey the same general laws, in their relations to disease, as do the motor cortical centres.

Sulphur in Chronic Diseases of the Alimentary Canal, Liver, Skin and Joints.

Sir Alfred B. Garrod, Consulting Physician to King's College Hospital, London, who is well known for his studies upon gout, communicates to the *Lancet*, April 6, 1889, an interesting paper on some chronic diseases of the alimentary canal, liver, skin and articulations, and their treatment by long-continued small doses of sulphur. Dr. Garrod states that sulphur influences the alimentary canal partly by a direct action upon its mucous membrane, partly by the circulation of sulphuretted hydrogen through the intestinal capillary system, and partly by the altered and increased flow of bile from the liver. A single lozenge taken at bedtime is sufficient to obviate the necessity for ordinary aperients. The lozenges he uses contain five grains of precipitated sulphur and one grain of cream of tartar. He finds them of great value in many morbid states of the alimentary canal and liver, as in cases of sluggishness of the liver and in piles; the bleeding in the latter condition is often completely stopped, and great relief of all the symptoms, especially of the accompanying pruritus, is obtained. The continued use of the lozenges is often quite effectual in overcoming habitual constipation without producing the unpleasant action often pertaining to ordinary aperient medicine.

In acne, psoriasis, and prurigo it is useful, either given alone or as an adjunct to other treatment. It is also useful in some of the localized forms of eczema, especially those connected with a gouty diathesis, as pruritus ani. Under the influence of small doses of sulphur when long continued, the complexion of the patient often improves to a marked degree.

Some arthritic diseases, especially chronic forms of rheumatoid arthritis and gout, and also many cases of muscular rheumatism, are much benefited by the treatment in question. The more chronic the disease the more likely is sulphur to prove beneficial. In true gouty states of the joints, when the disease is both chronic and asthenic, sulphur is often a valuable adjunct to other remedies.

It will be seen from the foregoing that Dr. Garrod lays great stress upon the continued administration of the remedy, and the small dose. He is in the habit of giving one lozenge at bedtime for weeks, months, and in some cases years.

Recent Advances in the Treatment of Obstruction of the Nose.

At the recent meeting of the Harveian Society of London, Jan. 31, 1889, Dr. Scanes Spicer, after expressing his conviction that the importance of the nose in the economy is not yet sufficiently appreciated, made some preliminary remarks as to the recent proofs which have been afforded by physiologists that almost the whole of the warming, moistening, and filtering of the inspired air is done in the nose ; and on the dangers and troubles which arise from the pernicious habit of mouth-breathing, a necessary consequent of chronic obstruction of the nose. He also referred to the frequently observed clinical association between abnormal conditions of the nasal fossæ and walls and many chronic functional derangements of the nervous system, such as depression, hypochondriasis, drowsiness, lassitude, inability to keep the attention fixed, as well as neuralgia, headache, paroxysmal sneezing, and asthma. He then passed critically in review the chief modern methods advocated for dealing with the various forms of obstruction of the nose. Among other points, he stated his preference for the galvano-cautery over chromic acid for inferior turbinated hypertrophies, because of the rapidity with which the former does its work without injury to the overlying ciliated epithelium (which it is so important to preserve), provided the platinum point is plunged into the hypertrophy and run along it under the mucous membrane. For middle turbinated hypertrophies he prefers chromic acid applied, on a platinum carrier and under a good illumination, to the exact spot to be reduced, his preference being based on the immediate shrinking properties of the acid on the tissues diminishing the risk of abnormal adhesions forming between adjacent parts. He specially insisted on the importance of systematic after-treatment of parts exposed by the removal of nasal polypi, to diminish or prevent the chance of their recurrence. He advocates for polypi the cold wire snare, and condemns the forceps as wanting in precision, painful, and dangerous. The necessity of removing the fetid adherent crusts which obstruct the upper channels and sinuses in ozæna before any real improvement could be expected was pointed out ; for if not removed, the usual applications of douches, etc., never reach the diseased sinuses and cells. These can be kept clear only by systematic rhinoscopy and detachment, with delicate crocodile-mouth forceps, of tenacious crusts. The treatment of bony and cartilaginous outgrowths of the septum by the electro-motor trephine was described and the apparatus demonstrated. Trephining of these spurs was stated to be the most painless, the quickest, safest, cleanest, and most effectual way of removing them, so long the bugbear of rhinologists.

Cases were referred to in which deafness, tinnitus, loss of smell, insomnia, snoring, nasal voice, etc., speedily disappeared after the removal of obstructing spurs from the nostrils. In considering the treatment of post-nasal adenoid vegetations, the author said he always prefers when possible to clear out the growths at one operation by Löwenberg's forceps, the patient being anæsthetized. The paper concluded with a strong plea for a more general examination of the nose, and treatment of its morbid states by the numerous delicate, efficient, and satisfactory methods now available.

Mr. Frankish asked for the theory upon which was based the idea that nasal obstruction causes interference with nervous processes.

Dr. Hill commented upon the frequency of nasal obstruction in those suffering from sore throat. He has seen many operations performed upon the nose under the influence of cocaine, without much pain being experienced. He thought chromic acid of more use than Dr. Spicer was inclined to admit.

Dr. Spicer said that aprosexia resulted from a blockage of the communication which existed between the lymphatics of the dura mater and cranial cavity and those of the turbinated bones.—*British Med. Journal*, Feb. 9, 1889.

———◆◆◆———

—Dr. George Johnson has been appointed one of the Physicians Extraordinary to Queen Victoria, in the room of the late Dr. C. J. B. Williams.

—It is reported that a family in London has been poisoned by the fumes from a number of green candles, which were found upon analysis to contain arsenic.

THE
MEDICAL AND SURGICAL
REPORTER.

ISSUED EVERY SATURDAY.

CHARLES W. DULLES, M.D.,
EDITOR AND PUBLISHER.

The Terms of Subscription to the publications of this office are as follows, payable in advance:
Med. and Surg. Reporter (weekly), a year, $5.00
Physician's Daily Pocket Record, - - - 1.00
Reporter and Pocket Record, - - - - 6.00
All checks and postal orders should be drawn to order of
CHARLES W. DULLES,
N. E. Cor. 13th and Walnut Streets,
P. O. Box 843.   Philadelphia, Pa.

TREATMENT OF PUERPERAL ENDO-METRITIS.

With the increase of knowledge concerning the nature and etiology of puerperal septic processes, and the methods of preventing infection, there has been a corresponding decrease in the percentage of cases of puerperal sepsis. This is especially true in well conducted hospitals. Whereas formerly the mortality from septic processes varied in maternity hospitals from three to twenty or more per cent., now, through the beneficent influence of antiseptic midwifery, the mortality from this cause is perhaps less than one per cent. And what is almost equally important, the percentage of morbidity has correspondingly decreased. Still, with the best of care, cases of sepsis do occur, and the practitioner must then face the problems of treatment rather than those of prophylaxis. Removal of particles of secudines, clots, and septic discharges, with the finger and disinfectant douche, together with the use of iodoform locally, and the administration of proper food and constitutional remedies are usually sufficient to arrest promptly the septic process and bring about a cure—especially in the hands of careful men who institute treatment early. But when cases are seen late and marked septic endometritis is present, or when the latter is present in spite of early treatment, the methods of treatment already mentioned are often ineffectual; salpingitis and peritonitis, or cellulitis and true pelvic abscess, or grave constitutional infection frequently follows, resulting in death, or more or less complete invalidism.

When septic endometritis occurs, the process of involution is arrested. The fatty metamorphosis in the layer of the decidua which remains attached to the uterus after labor is changed into a condition of necrosis. This layer of detritus and pus cells forms a favorable nidus for the multiplication of such microörganisms as have gained access to the cavity of the uterus, and thus favors infection of the muscularis and contiguous structures; in addition, the absorption of ptomaines, which result from the putrefaction of this material, causes grave constitutional poisoning. When the process has advanced so far as this, many obstetricians question the advisability of trusting to irrigation to remove this detritus, and assert, with apparent justice, that the irrigation removes only such matter as is free in the cavity of the uterus. They advocate, instead of repeated and continued douches, the thorough scraping of the uterus with the dull curette, whereby the necrosed decidua is thoroughly removed; and they declare that when the use of the curette is followed by a thorough irrigation, the cavity of the uterus is left in a relatively aseptic condition, and thus the course of the disease is much shortened and the necessity for repeated douching avoided.

Among others, Dr. Grandin, of New York, has recently advocated this method of treatment in a communication in the *New York Medical Journal*, Feby. 16, 1889. He states that as soon as fetor of the lochia appears he proceeds to find out its source. He considers that a thorough vaginal douche of boiled water or of some antiseptic solution will cause this fetor to disappear, if it be due to decomposition of the lochia or a clot in the vagina. Should the fetor reappear after the lapse of a few hours, an intra-uterine douche is administered, as the cause may be the retention *in utero* of a clot or of loosened *débris*. If, notwithstanding this douche, the fetor reappears Dr. Grandin believes that the time for active treatment has come. The position of the uterus is determined by bi-manual examination, the patient is put in Sims's position, a tenaculum is hooked into the anterior lip of the cervix to steady the uterus, and a properly curved curette is inserted into the uterine cavity. Then the entire endometrium is thoroughly scraped. In this way Dr. Grandin says that he has literally removed handfuls of degenerated *débris*. When the curetting is done the patient is turned on her back and the uterus thoroughly washed out. Dr. Grandin asserts further that in his experience it has never been necessary to repeat the curetting, and rarely has an additional douching been called for. He moreover affirms that in certain aggravated cases of septic endometritis which he has seen, in which the fetor was intense, the pulse rapid, and the aspect bad, there has been such a marked improvement within twenty-four hours after the removal of the putrid products that it was difficult to realize that he was dealing with the same patient.

There are fashions in medicine as well as in dress, and just now it is becoming the fashion to advocate the use of the curette in cases of septic endometritis after labor. The method of treatment outlined in the first part of this article has been thoroughly tested, and when it has been instituted early the result usually has been good. Hence we believe that the cases are exceptional in which the use of the curette is necessary—those in which the usual treatment has proved ineffectual, and those seen late. In these proper cases, we believe that the use of the curette is clearly indicated, and that it will yield prompt results, especially when the exploring finger is also employed to determine that the uterine cavity is thoroughly emptied. An indication for the employment of the utmost care is the co-existence of parametritis, salpingitis or peritonitis; and interference is positively contra-indicated unless it be certain that a centre of infection is located within the cavity of the uterus.

THE HOUR OF DEATH.

There is a wide-spread popular impression that a very large proportion of deaths from disease take place in the early morning hours—between four and six o'clock. That this is an error is well known to most medical men. From time to time careful observations have been made in hospitals which have resulted in showing that the act of death takes place with fairly equal frequency during the whole twenty-four hours of the day.

Very recently, as reported in the *Journal de Médecine* of Paris, March 24, 1889, an investigation has been made, which showed that there was a certain falling off of the number of deaths between seven and eleven o'clock in the evening, but that, with this exception, the proportion of deaths is about even.

We refer to the matter because some of our readers may be glad to have authority for correcting a misapprehension which is of no very great importance, it is true, but which is held with great tenacity by persons who are hard to convince of error.

THE RESULT OF PASTEUR'S TREATMENT OF HYDROPHOBIA.

The effect of the attention attracted to hydrophobia in France and certain other parts of Europe by the discussion and practice of Pasteur's method of treating persons bitten by animals supposed to be rabid, has been to increase the mortality from what is called hydrophobia. In France the number of deaths has increased so much since this "infallible" method has been in use that in the Department of the Seine—which includes Paris, the centre of Pasteur's operations—there were nineteen deaths attributed to hydrophobia last year. The partisans of Pasteur's method ingeniously manipulate the statistics, so as to make it appear that this is not due to any defect in the method, but they appear to be blind to the obvious inference to be drawn from the fact that in France hydrophobia seems to be on the increase, while in Germany, where Pasteur's methods have never been approved or adopted, hydrophobia has almost utterly disappeared.

Another interesting point in regard to this matter is the fact that Pasteur several years ago announced that he had discovered a method by which dogs, to any number, could be rendered "refractory" to rabies, and yet there is no evidence that he has ever applied this merciful discovery; so that in France dogs "go mad" as much as ever, and all the energy of Pasteur and his followers is directed toward a malady which would be unknown if his method for dogs were really trustworthy and if it were put in practice as it ought to be. Meanwhile good laws for the management of dogs, and good sense on the part of medical men, have reduced rabies almost to an unknown quantity in Germany.

The facts indicate the danger of following an *ignis fatuus*, and may support the conviction of Americans who have never consented to importing into this country a theory and a practice which has worked so poorly in France.

AMERICAN PUBLIC HEALTH ASSOCIATION. —The American Public Health Association will hold its seventeenth annual meeting at Brooklyn, N. Y., Tuesday, Wednesday, Thursday and Friday, October 22-25, 1889. A preliminary announcement, containing a list of the topics for consideration at the meeting, has been issued by the Secretary, Dr. Irving A. Watson, of Concord, N. H.

BOOK REVIEWS.

[Any book reviewed in these columns may be obtained upon receipt of price, from the office of the REPORTER.]

A MANUAL OF INSTRUCTION IN THE PRINCIPLES OF PROMPT AID TO THE INJURED. DESIGNED FOR MILITARY AND CIVIL USE. By ALVAH H. DOTY, M.D., Major and Surgeon, Ninth Regiment, N. G. S. N. Y., etc. Small 8vo, pp. xiii, 224. New York: D. Appleton and Company, 1889. Price, $1.25.

This book contains a great deal of valuable instruction in regard to the management of a variety of accidents and emergencies, and is very abundantly and handsomely illustrated. From our point of view it contains also a great deal which has no special bearing on the subject. The sixty-seven pages devoted to anatomy and physiology are interesting, but, in our opinion rather an encumbrance to a book apparently intended for the laity. If the book is meant for the instruction of hospital stewards, in the army, this will probably be no objection to it.

The general teaching of the book is excellent; but we regret to see the old and widespread error in regard to the treatment of frozen persons repeated and endorsed by the author, and also that the "triangular bandage" of Esmarch is spoken of in a way which shows no knowledge of the fact that it is but a part of the admirable "handkerchief system" of M. Mayor, which has been before the profession for fifty years.

TREATISE ON DISEASES OF THE TESTICLE AND ITS ADNEXA. TRAITÉ DES MALADIES DU TESTICULE ET DE SES ANNEXES, par CH. MONOD, professeur agrégé à la Faculté de médecine de Paris, chirurgien de l'hôpital Saint-Antoine, etc., et O. TERRILLON, professeur agrégé à la Faculté de médecine de Paris, chirurgien de la Salpêtrière, etc. 1 vol. in-8° avec 92 fig. dans le texte. 16 fr.

8vo, pp. xi, 806, with 92 illustrations. Paris: G. Masson, 1889. Price, 16 francs.

This is a magnificent book, on a subject which has not been so fully discussed by any author before Drs. Monod and Terrillon took it up. They have gone at it with a thoroughness, and have concluded it with a finish, which would hardly be possible in any country outside of France. The result is a work which will be classic, a work in which large acquaintance with the subject in hand, great clearness of style, and abundance of admirable illustrations combine to make a book indispensable to the specialist in genito-urinary surgery and of great value to every studious surgeon. We can heartily recommend it to the attention of those of our readers who read the French language, and regret that more of them cannot do so.

In preparing the book before us, the publisher has ably seconded the endeavor of the authors to make it a credit to the country from which it comes.

PAMPHLET NOTICES.

[Any reader of the REPORTER who desires a copy of a pamphlet noticed in these columns will doubtless secure it by addressing the author with a request stating where the notice was seen and *enclosing a postage-stamp.*]

280. DISEASES OF THE SKIN ASSOCIATED WITH DISORDERS OF THE FEMALE SEXUAL ORGANS. BY GEORGE H. ROHÉ, M.D., Baltimore. From the *Buffalo Med. and Surg. Journal*, February, 1889. 13 pages.

281. SECOND ANNUAL REPORT OF THE OPHTHALMOLOGICAL DEPARTMENT OF THE STATE HOSPITAL AT NORRISTOWN, PA., FOR THE YEAR 1887. BY CHARLES A. OLIVER, M.D., Philadelphia. 7 pages.

282. DISCUSSION ON THE NEW CÆSAREAN SECTION. BY HOWARD A. KELLY, M.D., Philadelphia. From the *Transactions of the American Gynæcological Society*, 1888. 8 pages.

283. EXAMINATION OF THE URETERS. BY HOWARD A. KELLY, Philadelphia. From the *Transactions of the Amer. Gynæcological Society*, 1888. 14 pages.

284. CONTRIBUTIONS TO THE HISTORY OF DEVELOPMENT OF THE TEETH. BY CARL HEITZMANN, M.D., and C. F. W. BÖDECKER, D.D.S., New York. From the *Independent Practitioner*, vols. viii and ix. 98 pages.

285. CHRONIC INTERSTITIAL NEPHRITIS, ETC. BY JAMES TYSON, M.D., Philadelphia. From the *University Medical Magazine*. 8 pages.

286. EPIDEMIC CEREBRO-SPINAL MENINGITIS. BY JAMES TYSON, M.D., Philadelphia. From the *Philadelphia Medical Times*, Nov. 15, 1888. 12 pages.

287. THE RELATION OF ALBUMINURIA TO LIFE ASSURANCE. BY JAMES TYSON, M.D., Philadelphia. From the *Medical News*, November 17, 1888. 14 pages.

288. SOME GENERAL REMARKS ON BLOOD-LETTING. BY G. MAXWELL CHRISTINE, M.D., Philadelphia. 12 pages.

280. Dr. Rohé, in this paper, has collated a number of cases in which various skin-diseases have been observed associated with diseases of the sexual organs of women, as well as with certain physiological processes like lactation. It is an interesting and suggestive pamphlet.

281. This pamphlet is one of the indices of the careful work which is done in studying the condition of the insane at the Norristown Hospital. The conclusions of Dr. Oliver are valuable in filling out an obscure part of a picture which still lacks much of being complete.

282. Dr. Kelly, in this pamphlet, describes briefly two cases in which he performed Cæsarean section successfully, and the details of the method which modern experience has shown to be most calculated to secure a good result.

283. In this paper Dr. Kelly describes the methods of examining the ureters in women by means of the catheter and by palpation. These open up a wide field of investigation to the gynecologist, and ought to be understood by all surgeons. As described by Dr. Kelly they are not very difficult

to carry out, and they are capable of affording very useful information [in the treatment of certain diseases of women.

284. The monograph of Drs. Heitzmann and Bödecker contains an exceedingly interesting and thorough study of the histology of the teeth during the period of development. It is illustrated by a large number of admirable engravings of the microscopic appearance of sections of fetal teeth and of their surrounding parts. As a whole the paper is an unusually valuable contribution to the literature of the subject, and might well be in the hands of all intelligent dentists as well as all physicians interested in the fascinating theme of which it treats.

285. Dr. Tyson's paper contains a careful study of the histology of the chronically contracted kidney, in which he supports the theory that thickening of the walls of the arterioles in the kidney, and elsewhere in the body, is an important and perhaps constant factor of the disease. He dissents from the views expressed by Dr. Arthur Meigs, in his paper noticed in these columns Nov. 10, 1888 (Pamphlet notice No. 145). His paper contains, also, an interesting statement of the treatment proper for cases of chronic contracted kidney.

286. This is a clinical lecture by Dr. Tyson, delivered at the Philadelphia Hospital last November, and discusses the symptoms, morbid anatomy, and treatment of cerebro-spinal meningitis.

287. In this paper, which was read before the *Association of American Physicians* last year, Dr. Tyson opposes, with the authority of his long study and large experience in diseases of the kidneys, the view that mere albuminuria should be regarded as an insurmountable bar to life insurance, and gives the points which ought to be considered by medical examiners before accepting or rejecting an applicant who at times has albumin in his urine.

288. "Saul is found among the prophets" so often nowadays, that it excites little surprise to find a homœopathic physician, like Dr. Christine, advocating the practice of such an un-homœopathic procedure as blood-letting, and defending his course theoretically by quotations from homœopathic writers, while demonstrating its soundness by quoting from the most orthodox of the old school. The whole of the practical part of this interesting paper is founded upon citations from Wyeth, Agnew, Quain's Dictionary, and Sir Thomas Watson, and the experience of the author, who has learned that the homœopathic law is not one of universal applicability.

—For the effectual protection of woolen goods against moths the use of cedar-wood boxes and closets is insufficient, and it is stated that there is no other means of protection against the ravages of the insect but perfectly to inclose the woolens in material which is not attacked by the moth, such as cotton cloth. Woolen goods brushed clean from dust, folded together and put into cotton bags, which were well tied, have been found perfectly intact when taken out at the change of the season. The important point, of course, is to see that the clothing is free from moths when first put away.

CORRESPONDENCE.

Congenital Absence of Fingers.

To THE EDITOR.

Sir: I was called May 8, 1889, to Mrs. X., in labor with her third child. The labor was normal, and the child weighed eight pounds and was well developed, except the left hand, in which development was arrested at the carpal and metacarpal articulation. The stump was soft and there was no cicatrix. There were five small tubercles on the end of the stump, corresponding with the fingers and thumb from ulna to radius. The smallest tubercle, on the ulner side, was about the size of a bird-shot; the largest, on the radial side, was about the size of a small pea. The carpus can be flexed and extended; the radius and ulna are of the same length as the bones in the right arm.

If you think this case of sufficient interest to be placed on record, please give it space in the MEDICAL AND SURGICAL REPORTER.

Yours truly,
ORSON HOUGH, M.D.
Conneautville, Pa.,
May 29, 1889.

Midwives in West Virginia.

To THE EDITOR.

Sir: As the MEDICAL AND SURGICAL REPORTER is taken by many of the physicians of my State—West Virginia—I wish to take up a small amount of your space, and write on the subject of "Midwives," or, I should say, those pretending to be such. Since living in this State, I have found to my surprise that the laws are peculiar here, in regard to the practice of midwifery. I am told that these women, often without any education and with little practical sense, may, according to the laws of the State, practise without a license, or certificate, or any examination whatever. A midwife may register at the Clerk's Office, but is not compelled to do so.

Is not child-birth of more importance than that? Does not this belong to the practice of medicine as much as giving powders and looking at tongues? I cannot understand how any State can be so careful that the young physician should have his diploma from the best schools of our land, and see that he has a State certificate to practise his profession, while it permits any woman, who wishes to do so, to practise midwifery. The result of this plan is, that the practice of educated physicians is interfered with, while the lives of women are sacrificed to the ignorance of their attendants. This I find is the observation of my fellow-practitioners, as well as mine; and I call attention to it, in the hope that a more sensible way may be adopted by the authorities of this State.

Yours truly,
MEDICUS.
May 22, 1888.

NOTES AND COMMENTS.

Condition of Physicians in Johnstown.

Dr. C. K. Mills and Dr. Thomas Mays arrived at Johnstown on June 10th, representing the joint committee of the College of Physicians of Philadelphia and the Philadelphia County Medical Society, to bring relief to medical practitioners and their families suffering from the flood. Six physicians were drowned and 21 lost all they had. The number to be cared for is about 20. It is said that about $2000 will be immediately expended in the work, more money being ready to continue it.

The Pennsylvania Medical Society and the Sufferers by the Flood.

The Pennsylvania Medical Society which convened in Pittsburgh on Tuesday, June 4, after passing appropriate resolutions of sympathy with our brethren and the families of those who are lost in the recent floods in Pennsylvania appropriated $1000 for their relief, and adjourned to September 3d. All County Societies were urged to take immediate steps to render aid through the Cambria County Medical Society, of which Dr. F. Shill, of Johnstown, is Treasurer.

Philadelphia Medical Societies and the Sufferers from the Flood.

At a special meeting of the Philadelphia County Medical Society, held June 6, 1889, the following Minute and Resolutions were unanimously adopted:—The members of the Philadelphia County Medical Society, in common with their fellow men and women of all pursuits, have been deeply moved by the loss of life and suffering caused by the recent terrible floods; especially at Johnstown and other places in the Conemaugh Valley. As individual men and women they have felt it their duty to contribute, with the rest of the community and to the very best of their ability, to one or other of the funds collected under various auspices and intended to be disbursed by the Citizens' Committee, for the relief of suffering men and women without distinction. But as an association of physicians, we have felt that our duty did not end here. Realizing as we do the hardships and struggles, and, at best, limited pecuniary rewards of the practice of the profession peculiarly devoted to the relief of human suffering, and having learned that the surviving members of that profession residing in the flooded districts have lost everything they possessed—some of them thus left destitute in old age, after years of faithful endeavor ; we feel an additional responsibility resting upon us for the assistance of these, our brethren ; that they may be enabled as soon as possible to resume the laborious duties of the practice of the sacred profession of medicine.

This meeting is therefore called to give practical expression to our sympathy with the physicians of the storm-stricken region ; and to devise a plan whereby this Society in conjunction with other medical associations of this city, of the state, and of the United States, may collect and wisely disburse, after conference with the general committee and with our distressed colleagues, an amount of money commensurate with the responsibilities of the occasion and adequate to its needs.

Resolved, that the Philadelphia County Medical Society sends its earnest sympathy to the physicians of Johnstown and other flooded places, and pledges itself to aid them to the extent of its ability.

Resolved that a committee of three be appointed to act with the committee of the College of Physicians and with committees that may be appointed for the same purpose by other medical organizations of the city, state, and country, to collect funds for the assistance of physicians and their families, and to disburse same in such manner as may be deemed most advisable after conference with the physicians of the flooded districts and with the general relief committee.

Resolved that the committees of this Society and of the College of Physicians be requested to meet at once and to report to this meeting a list of two or more physicians in each ward of this city, to act as subcommittees for the collection of funds from physicians in their respective districts.

The following Committee was then appointed to act for the Philadelphia County Medical Society: Drs. T. J. Mays, H. Augustus Wilson and S. Solis-Cohen.

The Committee of the College of Physicians consists of Dr. J. Ewing Mears, Charles K. Mills, and Harrison Allen.

The Sanitary Conditions at Johnstown.

Dr. John B. Hamilton, Surgeon General of the Marine Hospital Service, has made a report to the President in regard to the situation of affairs at Johnstown, Pa.

Dr. Hamilton says that the work of clearing up the surface débris was going on well, and, in his judgment, ten days more of the same systematic work would suffice to clear the surface of the main portion of the late city. "The sick and wounded are now mainly confined to those persons working as laborers, and in the various relief organizations outside of the laborers there are few citizens left. Many are lost and many are gone away from the scene of their great calamity. There are some twenty physicians, ten of whom are able to work, but no more are needed, and it would be a great relief if many of those from a distance would go away.

"The water supply of Johnstown is from Stony creek, some miles above the scene of disaster, and is pure, wholesome water. There is little danger of an epidemic among the inhabitants of Johnstown. The danger point, from a sanitary point of view, is the drift at the bridge, and this danger is not to the inhabitants of Johnstown, but to those people depending on the lower river for their water supply. This water, if boiled before drinking, will not be unhealthy, but the thought of drinking water contaminated by dead bodies of human beings and animals is revolting."

The report is confined to the portion covered by Johnstown proper. No attempt has been made to touch upon the general condition of the outlying villages which also suffered from the calamity.

Dr. Groff, a member of the State Board of Health, in charge of the Sanitary Corps, issued the following bulletin on June 10: "The favorable condition stated in the first report continues. No contagious disease of any kind prevails. There are a few cases of a mild type of measles. No signs of any epidemic are manifest. The State Board of Health is fully prepared to meet all emergencies as they arise. As a precautionary measure a hospital for contagious diseases has been established, and if any cases appear they will be promptly met. The air continues pure and wholesome, the water pure. The bodies still in the wreck are so covered with earth as not to be dangerous to health. There is every precaution being taken to prevent contamination of the water supply for the towns below Johnstown. There is no ground whatever for alarm in this matter at present. The bodies in the river are covered with mud and earth, so as not to be dangerous to health. The weather is cool and most favorable. Though the destruction of life has been appalling, there is at present every reason to be encouraged.''

Case of Poisoning with Antifebrin.

Dr. E. Fürth communicates an account of a case of poisoning with antifebrin to the *Wiener med. Presse,* April 21, 1889. A girl suffering with violent hemicrania took sixty grains of antifebrin. Shortly after taking it nausea, eructations and a tendency to vomit occurred. Milk was given her as an antidote by the by-standers, but was immediately vomited. When Dr. Fürth saw the patient, about two hours after the poisoning, he found her deeply unconscious, emitting repeatedly cries of pain and complaining loudly of pains in the epigastrium. The face, with exception of the lips, which were somewhat cyanotic, was deadly pale. The skin felt icy cold; the pulse was 140, weak, scarcely to be felt; respiration was superficial and somewhat quickened. Stimulants were vomited, as the milk had been. Altogether the patient vomited fifteen times, a greenish-watery fluid. One hour later cyanosis spread to the face, so that four hours after the antifebrin was taken the face was reddish blue. The hands also and the feet were deeply cyanosed, especially the fingers; the rest of the body remained pale. In addition there were symptoms of brain irritation: dilated pupils, spasms of the face, gnashing of the teeth, immobility of the upper and lower extremities, lively delirium, which lasted only a short time but was repeated many times. The patient then sank into deep coma, from which she only gradually aroused after the lapse of three hours.

Eight hours after the poisoning, the patient had become again entirely conscious and complained simply of pain in the stomach and of a feeling of dizziness. The pulse was 84, moderately strong; respiration quiet; temperature somewhat below normal. The cyanosis disappeared first after the lapse of twenty-four hours, fading first from the extremities and last from the lips. The patient was able to leave bed in two days.

Sanitary Condition of Paris.

Now that the Paris Exposition is attracting a great crowd of strangers to Paris, it is not without interest to note the excellent sanitary condition of that city. The mortality has at no time this year reached so small a figure as in the week ending May 4. The average for this week in the past five years has been 1,122. This year the mortality was only 984; and in the week following, it fell to 951. Typhoid fever especially has shown, since 1888, a constant decrease. More than all others, this affection belongs to the list of diseases which may be avoided; and it is only necessary that there should be due energy on the part of the public authorities to reduce its frequency in a notable proportion. While typhoid fever and varioloid have decreased, it is unfortunate to note that this is not true of measles and of diphtheria. This results, no doubt, from the fact that the measures which can stay the progress of these diseases depend more upon individual initiative than on public measures. Among the causes which may explain the improved health of Paris may be noted the increased use of the conveyances which are placed by the police at the disposal of those wishing to transport persons suspected of being affected with contagious diseases. In 1886 these carriages were called for only at the rate of thirty to forty per month. In 1888, in the month of April, this number had increased to 211; and in the April just passed, to 231. Another cause acting beneficially is doubtless the improvement in the quality of milk—an improvement due to the constant control exercised by the city laboratory.—*Science,* May 31, 1889.

Immediate Relief of Hoarseness.

The first Napoleon is said to have been subject to sudden attacks of severe hoarseness, for the immediate relief of which his physician was in the habit of prescribing the following, known as Foreau's syrup:

 R Liquor. Ammoniæ fortioris . ♏x
   Syrupi Erysemi . . . . . f℥iss
   Infusionis Tiliæ Florum . . . f℥iiss
 M. To be taken at one dose.

Erysemum officinale (*sisymbrium offic.*) or hedge-mustard is no longer official, but is easily obtained. It is a small annual, growing almost everywhere in the United States and Canada, as well as in Europe. The infusion of linden (tilia) is used simply as an agreeable vehicle, and may be dispensed with or supplanted by any other pleasant vehicle.—*St. Louis Med. and Surg. Journal,* May, 1889.

Simulo as a Remedy in Epilepsy.

Dr. M. Allen Starr, Clinical Professor of Diseases of the Mind and Nervous System in the College of Physicians and Surgeons, New York City, has a communication on Simulo as a Remedy in Epilepsy in the New York *Medical Record*, May 11, 1889. He reports seven cases in which it was used and concludes that simulo has no effect upon attacks of hystero-epilepsy or upon the hysterical state. It has also no effect in modifying the frequency or severity of attacks of *petit mal*, or of procursive epilepsy. It has some effect in modifying the frequency and severity of attacks of *grand mal*, but is inferior in this respect to the bromides. In cases in which for any reason it is deemed necessary to suspend the bromides, he says it would be well to substitute simulo for them.

There seem to be no ill effects from the use of the drug. He found no evidence of change in the rate or character of the pulse or respiration, no dilatation or contraction of the pupils, no muscular weakness, no mental depression or excitement, and no disturbance of the digestion in the doses in which it was used. The suggestion made by Eulenburg, that it would be well to obtain the active principle of the drug, is worthy of consideration. And Dr. Starr thinks it would be well to increase the dose progressively until one or even two ounces are used daily. The chief objection to its use at present is its costliness, the price being twenty-five cents an ounce.

The preparation used by Dr. Starr was the tincture, which is of a yellowish-brown color, and has an aromatic taste, reminding one slightly of sherry. The usual dose was two fluid drachms, three times a day.

Danger of the Suspension Treatment of Locomotor Ataxia.

Dr. Vincent, of Clifton Springs Sanitarium, recently hanged himself unintentionally while experimenting with the Sayre suspension apparatus, which many physicians are now making trial of in the treatment of locomotor ataxia. This unfortunate accident is not the only one, for word comes from France that a man living in the Department of the Dordogne, who was suffering with locomotor ataxia, met his death in the same way. Both these deaths occurred while the persons were alone. The apparatus appears to be free from danger when it is employed under the watchful eye of the physician or in the presence of a skillful attendant.

The New Quarantine Station at the Entrance to Delaware Bay.

It will be remembered that Congress at its last session appropriated a considerable amount of money for the equipment of seven quarantine stations, five for the Atlantic Coast and two for the Pacific. Of this appropriation about $75,000 was assigned for the establishment of a thoroughly-equipped station for the protection of the Delaware Bay and River. Heretofore the only safeguard against the introduction of contagion below the Lazaretto has been the little Hospital of the United States Marine Hospital Service, near Lewes, which was designed simply for the treatment of sick or wounded seamen, with no adequate provision for the isolation of those suffering from infectious diseases. So well has this service been administered, however, that it has on several occasions detained and disinfected pest-laden vessels and their crews, and thus stayed at the threshold diseases which might have led to disastrous epidemics had they gained admission. At or near this point, the Legislature of Delaware has offered to cede to the United States the land necessary for the proposed buildings and appurtenances. The Secretary of the State Board of Health of Pennsylvania, Dr. Benjamin Lee, has been designated a Commissioner on the part of the United States to meet Commissioners appointed by the State of Delaware, and, in conjunction with them to locate and fix the boundaries of this grant. This preliminary will be speedily settled, and work will be begun on the station at an early date. The fumigating steamer for the station is now in process of construction, at Wilmington, Delaware.

A Hospital for Dartmouth.

Mr. Hiram Hitchcock has given to Dartmouth College a hospital, which is to be attached to the Medical School of that institution. The plans for the new building are still in the hands of the architect, but it is expected that the structure will be completed within a year. The ground has been purchased in Hanover, and everything is now in readiness to proceed with the work as soon as the plans shall have been approved. Mr. Hitchcock was led to make this gift by an appreciation of its necessity and by a desire to establish a fitting memorial to his late wife. It will be the handsomest and best equipped institution of the kind in Northern New England.—*Medical Record*, June 8, 1889.

Over-pressure in Schools.

Dr. James Simpson, President of the California State Medical Society, in his annual address before the Society, in April, 1889, speaks as follows concerning over-pressure in schools (*Occidental Medical Times*, May, 1889):

"A diligent search, from the physician's standpoint, into the workings of the modern educational system has led me to regard it with trust and admiration, and has taught me that much of the cry about over-pressure is pure sensationalism. Those who repeat that cry are perhaps sincere, but they often do so without a practical knowledge of the subject, stirred by the hasty fervor that seizes us when we discover a wrong that wants righting. The public look to us for carefully balanced and sifted statements on these questions of general import, and it is regrettable that physicians who have been held up as authorities have solemnly warned them that, in such healthful exercise of the mental cortex of our youth as is provided in school discipline, danger and destruction lurk. Let us be sure we are right before sounding the note of alarm. With the pleasing methods of teaching now in vogue, with the ever-advancing observance of the laws of cerebral hygiene, and with the better provisions for the health and comfort of scholars, most children are better situated in the school-room than at home. Let the contrast be made, as it often must be, between the clean, pleasant class-room on the one hand, and the foul atmosphere, actual or moral, of an ill-kept home on the other. The school-house of to-day, conducted by the teacher of to-day, is the best possible nursing place for strong, broad-minded, intelligent American citizens."

Antiseptic Power of Salol.

At the meeting of the Hunterian Society of London, April 10, Mr. Corner introduced a series of cases illustrative of the antiseptic power of salol (salicylate of phenol) as a dressing for wounds, after the part had been rendered aseptic by a 1 in 20 solution of carbolic acid. He did not claim for it greater power than iodoform, and probably other antiseptics have, but he says it has advantages over some. It possesses a pleasant aromatic odor, can be used freely without fear of irritation or poisoning, is absorbent of moisture, which drying forms a hard but friable covering. It will prevent putrefaction ; it will not destroy it when once established. It has been used in increasing frequency for several years at the Poplar Hospital, and with excellent results, in compound fractures and dislocations, also as a dressing in amputations, minor and major, and in compound comminuted and depressed fractures of the skull. The first case shown by Dr. Corner was a compound comminuted depressed fracture of the frontal bone, in which the bone was elevated and some spicules removed. Afterward the wound was washed with a solution of carbolic acid (1 in 20), the opening filled with salol, and a drainage-tube inserted. The dressing was undisturbed for fourteen days, remained sweet, and healed on the twenty-sixth day. His temperature remained from the first under 100°. A second case, treated in January, 1889, was a compound fracture of the olecranon, head of radius, and humerus, opening the elbow-joint, with considerable damage to the soft parts, the elbow having been crushed by the passage of a railway engine over it. The olecranon was splintered and drawn up, causing serious tension of the skin and necessitating removal of both portions. The antiseptic treatment and dressing were the same as in the previous case, but required changing after four hours and again next day, in consequence of oozing of secretions through the dressing. The parts were then left untouched for thirty days. The temperature went up the day after the injury, and remained about 101° for three days, 100° for two days, and then fell to normal. Two other cases were shown : one a crushed compound fractured finger, dressed twenty-one days before, and not exposed since, there having been neither pain nor elevation of temperature ; the other was a compound fracture of the first phalanx of the finger, only dressed at the time of the accident, and left undisturbed for a month, when it was found perfectly healed. Dr. Corner pointed out that this was the common experience in such cases, and that even if gangrene followed the parts remained sweet. —*Lancet*, May 4, 1889.

Cotton Impregnated with Biniodide of Mercury.

The following formula is given in several foreign journals for the preparation of antiseptic cotton:

Biniodide of mercury .	8 parts ;
Iodide of potassium . .	3 "
Glycerin	120 "
Distilled water . . . to 2,400 "

Absorbent cotton is to be soaked in the solution and then dried.

NEWS.

—Mrs. Jane C. Stormont, the widow of Dr. D. W. Stormont, has given $10,000 to the Kansas Medical Society.

—The American International Congress of Medical Jurisprudence held its first meeting in New York City, June 4.

—On June 4, 1889, the trustees of the University of Pennsylvania elected Dr. John H. Musser Assistant Professor of Clinical Medicine.

—Dr. George H. Makuen, of the staff of Cooper Hospital, Camden, has been appointed Assistant Demonstrator of Anatomy in the Jefferson Medical College.

—It is reported that the City Council of Newport, Rhode Island, has appropriated $300 for the entertainment of the American Medical Association, at its meeting there this month.

—Dr. A. B. Ashworth, the business manager of the *Atlanta Med. and Surg. Journal,* died suddenly in Atlanta on May 18. Dr. Ashworth was graduated from the Atlanta Medical College in 1886.

—At the fortieth annual meeting of the Medical Society of Northampton County, a dinner will be given in honor of Dr. Traill Green, of Easton, Pa., at the Paxinosa Inn, Thursday evening, June 20.

—Dr. Roswell Park, of Buffalo, has been invited to deliver the Mütter lectures on "Some Point or Points connected with Surgical Pathology," before the College of Physicians of Philadelphia, during the winter of 1890–91.

—The grand jury in New York has found indictments for violation of the sanitary law against Doctors Irwin, Ferguson and Hance, the physicians who performed the autopsy on the body of Washington Irving Bishop, the mind reader.

—The Warren Triennial Prize of the Massachusetts General Hospital, amounting to $500, has been awarded to Dr. H. A. Hare and Dr. Edward Martin, of Philadelphia, for an essay on "Some New Studies on the Phrenic Nerve and Artificial Respiration."

—The *American Lancet*, June, 1889, says: The medical profession of Michigan are almost unanimous in the desire that the Medical Department of the Michigan University should be removed to Detroit. But they are not unanimous as to the means by which this end can be accomplished. The most important obstacle is the lack of about a half a million of dollars with which to erect and put in order a plant for its use in Detroit. Possibly a couple hundred thousand dollars less might accomplish the end, but an additional quarter of a million would be far better.

HUMOR.

Fogg says that some of the people on the theatrical stage remind him of his liver, because they don't act worth a cent.—*Boston Transcript.*

A Southern hotel advertises among its attractions a "parlor for ladies 35 feet wide." We trust this paragraph will catch the eye of the woman who occupies three seats in a crowded car.—*Yonkers Statesman.*

A Professional Failure.—"Can you recommend something as a spring tonic?" inquired a sallow dyspeptic, stepping listlessly into an aromatic pharmacy. "Yes," replied the druggist, "I have a number of excellent preparations. What is your line of business?" "I am a professional Faith Curer."—*The Epoch.*

A Remarkable Child.—Caller (*to fond mother*).—"Isn't it somewhat remarkable and wonderful, Mrs. Hobson, that your little boy Frank, though eight years old, can neither read nor write?" Fond Mother.—"Oh yes, I think so. The dear little fellow always was a remarkable and wonderful child."—*Harper's Magazine.*

Dividing the Responsibility.—Doctor—"Yes, you have a tremendous fever. Burning thirst, I suppose?" Patient—"Yes, terrific." Doctor—"Ah, I'll send you round something to relieve that." Patient—"Never mind about the thirst, Doctor. You look after the fever; I'll attend to the thirst myself."—*London Pick-Me-Up.*

OBITUARY.

SAMUEL G. LANE, M.D.

Dr. Samuel G. Lane, a well-known physician of Chambersburg, Pennsylvania, died there June 4, of apoplexy, after a brief illness. Dr. Lane was 62 years old, and was graduated from the Medical Department of the University of Pennsylvania in 1849. He was a member of the Local Board of Pension Examiners, and a trustee of the Pennsylvania State Hospital for the Insane. He was a writer of much ability, and was a frequent contributor to the medical and historical journals.

MEDICAL AND SURGICAL REPORTER

No. 1686.   PHILADELPHIA, JUNE 22, 1889.   VOL. LX.—No. 25.

CONTENTS:

COMMUNICATIONS.

THE FATALITY OF CARDIAC INJURIES.

BY H. A. HARE, M.D. (UNIV. OF PA.),

DEMONSTRATOR OF THERAPEUTICS AND INSTRUCTOR IN PHYSICAL DIAGNOSIS IN THE MEDICAL DEPARTMENT AND IN PHYSIOLOGY IN THE BIOLOGICAL DEPARTMENT, UNIVERSITY OF PENNSYLVANIA.

The question as to how long a human being can live after an injury to the most vital portion of his body is of the greatest importance from several aspects. In the first place there are a large number of medico-legal points of the most important character involved, not only as to circumstantial evidence in criminal cases, but also as to survivorship, and the ability to perform certain conscious acts after the reception of the wound, such as the signing or destroying of any paper, or the infliction of injuries by way of retaliation by the primarily injured party.

My attention has been called to this matter to a considerable extent of late and particularly by the article published in *Lo Sperimentale*, March, 1889, by Cristiani, Assistant Professor of Forensic Medicine in the University of Pisa, the drift of which is, briefly, as follows: A man aged twenty-five was stabbed, in a brawl, in several places. One wound was in the fifth interspace on the left side, near the anterior axillary line. There was a second wound in the eighth interspace on the same side, extending from the posterior border of the axilla toward the shoulder blade. There was also a stab of the left hip and several stabs on the right arm. After the second wound was received—the one near the præcordia—the man fell, but retained consciousness. After being taken home he was seen by a physician, who found him still conscious, with respirations at fifty a minute and pressing dyspnœa. This state lasted for eight or ten days. The wound over the heart healed in seven days, and that in the eighth interspace in eight days. On the eighteenth day the patient got up, though still weak, and on the thirty-seventh day, while yet feeling ill; he walked to Pisa and back—a distance of six miles and a quarter. This was done in the morning; in the afternoon of the same day he walked nearly two miles, climbed a tree after a bird's nest, and fell to the ground, dying ten minutes later.

At the autopsy it was found that the wound in the fifth interspace had penetrated the pericardium and deeply wounded the wall of the left ventricle at a distance of three and a half centimeters from the apex, but had not actually entered the ventricle. The mouth of this wound was filled with a soft clot, which was removed and a mass of organized blood-clot was found below it. This mass had ruptured by reason of the increased strain, so that there was an opening into the ventricle through which the fatal hemorrhage took place.

In the same article is a report by Messeri, of Florence, relating the case of a man, thirty years old, who was stabbed in the fourth interspace a half inch to the left of the sternum. When admitted to the hospital he was apparently dying, but he soon recovered, and his wound healed rapidly. Twenty-one days later he asked to be discharged, and when this was refused fell into a rage, stepped into the garden and dropped dead almost at once, with cyanosis and dyspnœa as prominent symptoms. The thorax contained much blood and an opened wound was found in the right ventricle near the sulcus and also a wound of the septum. Messeri also refers to statistics collected by Zanetti, who finds that, in one hundred and fifty-nine cases of wound of the heart, in only ten was the septum injured, and that in seven of these death occurred at once, in one it took place in an hour and a quarter, in another in two hours, while the other patient lived twenty days.

Having recently had occasion to look into this matter myself, I have found in medical literature a number of cases recorded where similar survival after severe injury occurred. Thus, Fischer[1] has collected no less than four hundred and fifty-two cases of injury to the heart and pericardium, in no less than seventy-two of which the patient recovered, while in two hundred and seventy-six death took place at periods varying from one hour to nine months. Death was immediate in one hundred and four cases. Of the seventy-two recoveries, examinations, made long after, in thirty-six of the cases, proved the diagnosis to be absolutely correct. Of

these seventy-two cases, ten were punctured wounds, forty-three incised, twelve gunshot, and seven lacerated; fifty were wounds of the heart, and twenty-two of the pericardium.

Purple[1] also records forty-two cases of wounds of the heart in which death did not come on immediately. Randalls records a case of a colored boy who lived sixty-seven days with a number of shot in the heart-muscle, and Ferrus a case in which the patient lived twenty-one days with the heart *transfixed with a skewer*.

It is apparent, therefore, that all wounds of the heart do not cause instant death, or even any lethal ending. Further than this Heil[2] records an instance in which the patient survived a year, and died of another disease, the post-mortem disclosing a cicatrix in the walls of the aorta. Again, in the *Lancet*, 1887, a case is recorded in which a man, 77 years old, made nine punctures with a darning needle in different parts of his body, one of them penetrating the heart. He lived "an hour or more" after the cardiac injury. Wharton and Stillé record several cases; and at least three instances are on record in this city.

In the *American Journal of the Medical Sciences*, July, 1861, a case is recorded in which a bullet was imbedded in the heart for 20 years; and as long ago as 1829 Dr. Redman Coxe contributed a paper on this subject to the journal just named. Lamballe, in the *Archives Gén. de Méd.* for September, 1839, has also contributed a valuable paper upon this question.

Ollivier and Lawson[3] have collected 29 instances of penetrating heart wounds, of which only two proved fatal within 48 hours; the rest of the subjects died in from four to twenty-eight days after receiving the injury. The Duc de Berri lived eight hours after a wound of the left ventricle; and Watson saw a case in which a man ran eighteen yards after such a wound. Those who are interested as to further discussion of this subject I may refer to the paper of Mesbrenier in the *Annales d'Hygiene*, 1879, i, p. 257.

These observations and reports are of sufficient interest to show that careful statements should be made by physicians when called to the witness-stand, and to make it evident that a wound of the heart is in itself not necessarily fatal, and that the fatality of such a wound depends upon

---

[1] *Arch. für klin. Chir.* von Langenbeck; Bd. IX. s. 571, 1868.

[1] *New York Med. Journal*, May, 1855.

[2] Henke Zeitschrift, 1847.

[3] *Devergie*, Méd. Légale, vol. ii, p. 253.

the hemorrhage which ensues from a complete solution of continuity of the heart wall or an involvement of the nervous ganglia in the heart substance.

This communication has been made by me rather in the sense of a preliminary note, and I am now carrying out a series of experiments on the heart of the lower animals, with the object of obtaining material for practical deductions, both medico-legal and surgical, and which I hope to place on record before the lapse of many weeks.

117 S. 22d street, Philadelphia.

THE VENTILATION OF CITIES, OR THE SANITARY VALUE OF INTERIOR OPEN SPACES.[1]

BY J. M. ANDERS, M.D.,
PHILADELPHIA.

Large cities cannot afford to be systematically neglectful in regard to sanitary matters. Human life and public health are too valuable to be estimated in dollars and cents. Wherever human beings congregate, a plentiful supply of fresh pure air in constant movement is necessary to the preservation of sound health. A stagnant air is slowly but surely mortal. Among the sanitary needs of a city, good ventilation ranks second to none. In this connection, the question of open spaces in cities is far-reaching in its relation to the cause of many of the more commonly prevailing as well as most fatal diseases; and it also involves a consideration of the ill effects of overcrowding, which is caused largely by the tenement system of building houses, by high buildings, narrow streets, and by small counting-rooms.

It is to be noted that the rate of increase in population of cities and their growth in area are not, as a rule, in equal ratio. As pointed out by Professor E. R. L. Gould,[2] "they grow rapidly in height, but not so fast in length or breadth." The comparative growth of urban and non-urban populations during thirty years is also mentioned by Gould, who writes: "In the United States, in 1850, the inhabitants amounted to 12.5 in each 100 of the total population; in 1880 the number had advanced to 22.5, an increase of 80 per cent."

For the last quarter of a century there has been observed an increasing popular sentiment in favor of small parks. This favorable change of public opinion is due largely to the fact that, wherever open spaces have been created in populous centres, they have proved of incalculable benefit in a great variety of ways.

No member of the medical profession, knowing the importance to sound health of pure fresh air and sunlight, can reflect upon the unfortunate state of society as met with in some of the worst quarters of large cities, where persons are often packed together without the slightest regard to the proper cubic air-space per head, and escape the conviction that something ought to be done speedily to bring relief to all who are exposed to these pernicious influences. That the powers of the human system are intolerant of the baneful effects of overcrowding is no new fact in medical science. Massing a population unduly lowers the general vitality and favors the development of such diseases as rickets, anæmia, phthisis, and others. There is also a group of infectious and contagious diseases—more especially measles, scarlatina, diphtheria and typhoid fever—for whose propagation densely populated districts, where natural ventilation is defective, furnish a good breeding-ground.

All sanitary authorities agree that the cubic air-space per head should not be less than one thousand cubic feet, and that the air of this space should be thrice renewed every hour, if we would prevent undue accumulation of noxious organic substances which are given off in respiration and by the skin. Perhaps all except our best homes fall short of this hygienic requirement; and certain it is that in the homes of the poor the average cubic space per head is reduced to less than one-third of that mentioned as necessary.

Wilson,[1] speaking with special reference to society as found in European cities, states that among the poorer classes the cubic space for each person, instead of approaching to one thousand feet, in numbers of cases does not amount to two hundred feet. In the tenement houses of New York City and Brooklyn we have the most impressive example of the evil consequences of the massing of a population to be found in the United States. One of the wards in New York City has over 290,000 persons to the square mile, and several have a population of 200,000 to the same area. One-half of the whole population, indeed, lives in these houses, while more than seventy-five per

---

[1] Intended to be read before the Medical Society of the State of Pennsylvania, June 5, 1889.

[2] Open Spaces in Cities.

[1] Text-Book of Hygiene, p. 252.

cent. of all deaths occur here. In view of the hygienic truth that the mortality rate increases with the density of the population, the fact that not many years since the death rate in New York City was 28 in 1000 per annum will excite no surprise. And we need not wonder at the declaration of an eminent authority when he states that there is no third generation in many New York tenement houses.

Time was when the chances of life were twice as good in the rural districts of England as in Liverpool and Manchester,[1] and less than half a century ago the mortality rate of nearly all great cities bore to sparsely populated rural districts about the same ratio.

Within the last twenty-five years, however, all this has been greatly changed; the annual average death rate in many of the older cities has already been reduced by nearly one-half. To some extent this has been occasioned by the enforcement of better sanitary rules and regulations, more especially such as pertain to the drainage, on the part of local and state boards of health, and also by a better knowledge of hygienic principles and the spreading of that knowledge among the people. But it has been clearly observed that, in consequence of having created new interior open spaces and public parks and having widened their thoroughfares, thereby securing a better system of outdoor ventilation for the people, many of the older European cities have greatly assisted in lowering their mortality rate.

The sanitary importance of ventilating the home is universally acknowledged. But a perfect system of ventilation implies that the air admitted to our dwellings shall be pure. Now this cannot be the case in districts where the buildings are high, the streets narrow and tortuous, often near alleys and occupied by a dense population, and with light and fresh air practically excluded. Surely under these conditions foul air is abundantly generated and filth especially accumulates. In cities, an efficient system of indoor ventilation must go hand in hand with an efficient system of outdoor ventilation, the one always implying the other. In order to secure a proper air movement and a plentiful supply of fresh air, the streets should be wide, and frequently recurring small breathing spaces should be introduced, especially in over-crowded parts; thus to some extent scattering the population, on the one hand,

and admitting sunlight and fresh air on the other.

Open spaces act as powerful ventilators of large cities, not only by diluting any impurities that may be present, but also by their favorable influence in promoting mild wind-currents. This is especially true where public squares communicate with wide avenues or streets open at each end. With a view of showing the great importance of interior open spaces to the best interests of the inhabitants of large cities, we have the testimony of Dr. T. Newell.[1] This author, speaking with reference to London, a city liberally provided with park areas, says: "Reckoning the population of London at 4,100,000, the reduction in the death rate during the last two hundred years shows a saving of 91,020 lives for the year 1886, more than two-thirds of the population of Providence. The extravagant employment of 'fresh air' and 'elbow room' has doubtless been the most important factor in bringing about this desirable change."

As showing the favorable influence of wide streets over the prevalence of phthisis, we also have the results of the very interesting observations by Dr. Arthur Ransome upon the causes of this disease, in Manchester, England. He writes: "The longest and widest streets in the district were Jersey Street, with ten deaths, and George Street, with eight deaths; but the number in these streets is approached by the mortality of eight deaths in Hood Street, which is only half its length, but which is a mere lane, blocked at each end, so as to obstruct free ventilation. Again, Henry Street, which is a long thoroughfare, has only four such deaths, while Boord Street, a narrow *cul-de-sac*, only a quarter its length, has seven." Dr. Ransome's investigations furnish fresh evidence of the fact that some of the most fatal as well as most prevalent diseases are to a great extent within human control, and that these would lose much of their terror if more decided measures were adopted to prevent them.

So much for the sanitary effects of city air-holes as mere open spaces; much might be said concerning their hygienic value when treated of as spaces filled with growing vegetation. The salutary influence of living plants upon the air, however, having received a good deal of attention during the last decade, will here be dismissed with the mere enumeration of a few well-established facts. The effect of a space filled with growing trees and shrubbery is to

---

[1] Twenty-fifth Report of the Registrar General.

[1] Interior Open Spaces in Cities, 1889.

increase slightly the local degree of saturation and to maintain its equability; to increase the ozonizing power of the atmosphere, thus rendering it safer and purer; to furnish grateful shade, which also has a cooling effect upon the air in summer, and to exercise a well-known moral or æsthetic influence.

This question also has its humanitarian aspects. Every large city has its toiling multitude, which cannot get a change of air during the heated term—cannot even, for want of means and time, reach the larger parks and pleasure grounds, which may be but a few miles distant from the scenes of their daily labor. For this large class, as well as the sick children of workingmen, numerous open spaces, at short distances from each other, though they are small, would, as before stated, be of incalculable benefit as places in which to spend a brief period for refreshing and healthful recreation.

The members of this Society may be interested in knowing what provision has been made by certain leading foreign and American cities in the direction of public parks for the people. The subjoined tables show the park acreage as well as the proportionate population per acre.[1]

PARK ACREAGE OF CITIES OF THE UNITED STATES.

	Population.	Park Acreage.	Population per Acre.
Providence	123,000	123	1,000
Boston	400,000	2,000	200
New York	1,839,000	4,902	375
Philadelphia	971,363	3,000	323
Brooklyn	665,600	940	639
Chicago	704,000	3,000	234
St. Louis	400,000	2,232	179
Washington	205,000	1,000	205
Baltimore	355,000	832	439
Cincinnati	325,000	539	603
San Francisco . . .	270,000	1,181	211
Buffalo	202,000	620	326
Detroit	175,000	740	204
Minneapolis	129,200	808	159
Savannah	33,000	60	550
New Haven	80,000	384	208
Bridgeport	40,000	240	170
Worcester	68,000	280	243
Pittsburgh	156,389	1.25	120,299

FOREIGN CITIES.

	Population.	Park Acreage.	Population per Acre.
London	3,832,000	22,000	174
Paris	2,270,000	58,000	37
Berlin	1,122,000	5,000	229
Vienna	1,103,000	8,000	138
Brussels	380,000	1,000	380
Amsterdam	350,000	800	437
Dublin	250,000	1,900	131
Montreal	120,000	550	218

[1] Dr. T. Newell, Interior Open Spaces.

From a glance at the foregoing tables it is seen that there is great diversity in the extent of the park area in proportion to the population. Among the cities having the smallest park surface are Providence, Brooklyn, Cincinnati, Savannah, and Pittsburgh, the last named having only one and one-third acres, and, although it may appear strange, this small open space is said to be difficult to locate. I may be excused for stating that it is a disgrace to Pittsburgh that it cannot afford more play-grounds for the children and breathing-spaces for their parents. The inhabitants of this enterprising city should remember that to continue to disbelieve in fresh air will inevitably lead to physical degeneration.

Dr. Gould,[1] in a recent article, has formulated a table giving a classification of open spaces as to size, together with the largest open space in acres for certain American cities. What will strike the reader of this table most is the tendency in cities to large parks and the absence of a liberal number of small open spaces in the squalid portions in which the population is densely herded together, and where light and air are most needed.

In conclusion, it should be pointed out that some of our leading American cities are making provision for new open spaces. Indeed, there is scarcely a representative city—excepting Pittsburgh, of course—in the Union which is not to-day bestowing some attention upon the subject of its interior adornment by means of parks and other open spaces, as well as wide and long park-ways; and this is not a question demanding the attention merely of physicians and leaders in social reform, but of all citizens also.

Washington can boast of an ideal park system, with which that of no other city can be compared. In 1866, Chicago began to take decided steps toward creating public parks, and it now ranks next to Washington in point of desirable features in the arrangement of its interior open spaces. In Boston the subject has been before the people for many years, and the excellent results accomplished there are well known to students of municipal history; and the same thing is true of St. Paul, Minneapolis, and of Providence. In New York the movement began in 1881, and already much has been done in the direction of opening up new pleasure grounds. As late as May, 1888, Philadel-

[1] Park Areas and Open Spaces in American and European Cities. Reprint from publications of the American Statistical Association.

phia was awakened to the necessity of creating additional park areas through the influence of a few public-spirited men and women, who about the same time formed the "City Parks Association." This is an active organization which has already achieved excellent results and has been the means of giving Philadelphia five new and valuable public parks.

ANTISEPTICS IN NORMAL LABOR.[1]

BY G. W. H. KEMPER, M.D.,
MUNCIE, IND.

I have practised medicine in civil life twenty-four years, and during that time have attended nine hundred cases of labor, recording a concise history of each case. This number does not include cases I have seen in consultation. In none of the nine hundred cases have I used a single antiseptic measure—in the sense that we apply that term at the present day. I have refused to attend obstetrical cases when I was treating bad cases of erysipelas and scarlet fever, although I have attended a woman and performed version, while her husband was lying in an adjoining room with facial erysipelas. I have, also, attended a woman in confinement who was suffering with phlegmonous erysipelas at the time; and yet, fortunately, no untoward results occurred. I have tried to prevent myself from becoming a "walking pestilence," and aimed to go to every case with "clean hands." I have, when consulted, given proper advice to women in their approaching confinement; but I have never administered, nor caused to be administered, to any woman, any of the popular antiseptic remedies before or after parturition.

Of my nine hundred cases, two of the women died. The first one died as the result of puerperal convulsions, on the seventh day after her confinement, and the second died of acute pneumonia, on the ninth day after her confinement, the iniatory chill having occurred the day preceding the labor. Both women were primiparæ. I have met with no severe case of puerperal fever among my nine hundred cases. To prove that my cases were of the average gravity, I will add the following statistics: of the 900 cases, 299 were primiparæ, and 601 multiparæ. There were 13 cases of twins, and 887 single births; so that 913 children were born. Of these, 874 pre-

[1] Read at the meeting of the Indiana State Medical Society, May 2, 1889.

sented by one of the several head presentations; 36 were breech or footling, and 3 were shoulder presentations. I had 8 cases of puerperal convulsions; 9 cases of *post-partum* hemorrhage; 8 cases of adhesion of placenta, and 4 cases of placenta prævia. I performed version three times, and cephalic version once. In one case inversion of the uterus followed the expulsion of the placenta, and was corrected at once. Finally, I used the forceps 27 times.

My practice reaches back to a period antecedent to the days of Listerism—to days when we had not heard of the new "Gospel of Antiseptics." Prior to that time, I met with cases that would properly have been treated by this class of agents. For instance, I reported a case to this Society in which a dead fetus was carried in the uterus for four or five months, to the great detriment of the mother; and I have met with a few other instances in which the fetus had been dead for a shorter period. In all of these cases, with no vaginal irrigations, the patients made a good and speedy recovery. Suppose that in all these cases I had used medicated injections into the uterus, and applied pads to the vulva; what valuable encomiums I could bestow upon the practice—the *post hoc ergo propter hoc* error.

In presenting my views upon this subject, I am quite aware that I shall antagonize the opinion of gentlemen who hear me. At the meeting of the Indiana State Medical Society last year, when my friend, Dr. L. N. Davis, read his paper on the "Progress, Practice and Obstetrical Record of the Country Doctor," it was apparent that some of his statistics were disbelieved. He stated the mortality of several country practitioners, residing in his locality, as follows:

Dr. J. T. Chenoweth,	1600 labors.	1 death.
" Thomas Botkin,	525 "	5 deaths.
" N. T. Chenoweth,	708 "	2 "
" A. H. Farquhar,	500 "	2 "
" J. S. Blair, . .	419 "	2 "
Total, . .	3752	12

No antiseptic precautions had been taken in the practice of these five physicians, and yet the total rate of mortality to mothers, in 3,752 labors, was 12, or one in every 312. I have the honor of a personal acquaintance with the physicians just mentioned, and, when they furnish obstetrical statistics, I trust them as implicitly as I do statistics furnished by physicians in lying-in hospitals. I am not aware that a country practitioner is more prone to exaggeration than his city brother, nor have I understood veracity to be an exclusively urban product, or that falsity was indigenous to rural localities. Who furnished the wonderful obstetrical statistics collated by Churchill? Were they not masters in lying-in hospitals? And so our statistics at the present day are largely compiled from hospital records. For this reason, when statistics are furnished by men who practise in healthy, rural districts and the mortality is shown to be light, skeptics are disposed to charge a *suppressio veri.*

A class of recent converts to antiseptic measures has sprung up in this country and has introduced the practice into lying-in hospitals. Great success has attended their labors, and they are deserving of praise; for the death-rate has been very materially lessened. In their great zeal in this good work they blindly accuse all who do not avail themselves of these aids, of criminal negligence. A striking example of this indiscriminate accusation is found in the "American System of Obstetrics." Dr. George J. Engelmann contributes an article to the first volume, on the "History of Obstetrics"; and, on page 64, in speaking of antiseptics, uses this extravagant language: "Such is the perfection of obstetric art in the hands of the masters of the art, and in lying-in institutions; whilst in private practice, in the homes of comfort, with the attendance of the best practitioners and the care of good nurses, many a young mother yields her life to the dangers which still accompany home confinement. We are told that the records of a prominent insurance company reveal a mortality of 17 *per cent.* in private practice, and that among the better classes." It is remarkable that Dr. Engelmann should allow the statement that "the records of a prominent life insurance company reveal a mortality of 17 per cent. in private practice, and that among the better classes," to pass unchallenged. In a foot-note, the Editor, Dr. Hirst, corrects the error, and says: "Extensive investigation has shown the mortality of confinement cases in general practice to be about 1 *per cent.*" If Dr. Engelmann and Dr. Hirst design these figures to indicate the mortality of child-birth in the cities, I have no facts bearing upon the question either for proof or for disproof. The statistics I have furnished to-day show that even the ratio of 1 *per cent.* is entirely too high for our country practice. Dr. Bradbury, Health Officer of Delaware County, in which I reside, informs me that during a

period of six years and eight months, in which records have been kept in that county, 4,444 women have been delivered, and of that number 34 died—a ratio of about seven and a half deaths to 1000. This mortality represents the practice of all kinds and qualities of practitioners, including midwives. Ten of the thirty-four women died from accidents which were not amenable in the least degree to antiseptic precautions. Hence our country practice, in the hands of promiscuous practitioners, without antiseptics, presents a more favorable aspect than does the hospital practice in large cities, with antiseptic precautions.

Probably Dr. H. J. Garrigues, of New York, is one of the most ardent, if not the greatest, advocate of antiseptic midwifery in this country, as shown by his work on that subject, which was published last year. I quote from his book: "I believe that by far the greatest number of general practitioners yet conduct their deliveries in the same way that they learned at college many years ago, and which they have been accustomed to follow since they began to practice.

"Some tell us, when the question is discussed in our public societies, that they have delivered so and so many thousand women, and never lost one of puerperal fever, and they have never used other precautions than common cleanliness. Either their memory fails them, or they have a convenient definition of puerperal fever; in consequence of which puerperæ die of peritonitis, metritis, pneumonia, pleurisy, heart disease, liver complaint, kidney trouble, meningitis, typhoid fever, etc., but never of a disease the mere mention of which, septicæmia, would teach the propriety of adopting the antiseptic treatment. To this class I would say, that, if they keep notes of their cases, and will study them in the light of our modern experience, they will find that after all they have not lost so very few patients in child-bed—probably not less than one in a hundred, and that all those diseases of which they have died are precisely the same as those of which our patients used to die in lying-in asylums."

"General practitioners," who "conduct their deliveries in the same way that they learned at college many years ago," may not feel complimented at being told they have learned nothing new since they began to practise midwifery; but they will feel some degree of compensation in learning that a teacher like Dr. Garrigues has made progress and no longer confounds "pneumonia, heart disease, liver complaint, kidney troubles, meningitis, and typhoid fever" with puerperal septicæmia! If Dr. Garrigues will take the pains to examine the records of competent general practitioners, he will find that the mortality of lying-in women is not so great as he imagines, and that antiseptics are not a panacea for the mistakes and ignorance of incompetent practitioners. The paraphernalia and details of antiseptic midwifery, as laid down by Thomas, Garrigues, and some other writers, is expensive and tiresome. In hospitals and cities, where the services of trained nurses can be secured, the system can be practised. In the country, as a rule, women are not visited at all after confinement by the attending physician, or only once or twice. In many instances they are left to the care of a member of the family, or more commonly to the care of a servant-girl, who fills, at one and the same time, the responsible positions of nurse, cook, and chambermaid. In cities it is the rule to engage physician and nurse for the lying-in, and needed preparations are made. The reverse is the rule in the country. I have been called to strange homes and greeted at the threshhold with such words as: "Hurry in here, Doctor; this woman needs you quick." And I have, without even the formality of an introduction, witnessed a number of deliveries within five minutes after my entry into the house. In such cases the time for the ante-preparatory, antiseptic treatment of Prof. Thomas would not equal that for the death-bed repentance of a subject of Judge Lynch.

I make no war on antiseptics in general. In surgical practice I observe the rules of our modern teachers and text-books as regards their use. In obstetrical practice I am particular to clean every instrument, by immersing it in boiling water. If the lochia are offensive, I use disinfecting injections; if the perineum be torn, I would sew it under antiseptic precautions. While I would do all this, and even concede more, if necessity would seem to demand it, I do not feel it is necessary in every case of normal labor, when my patient is surrounded by healthy environments, to attempt to carry out a complicated routine of practice which my experience teaches me is unnecessary.

While preparing this paper, I met with an abstract in the *Journal of the American Medical Association*, April 15, 1889, from a letter written by Dr. Robert Barnes to the *British Medical Journal*, that covers the ground of extremists so thoroughly that I will make short quotation from the paper:

"To see in septicæmia the only evil is to fix all therapeutical energy upon what is commonly understood as antiseptic treatment. This is the course advocated by the more earnest of the septicæmic school. Without affirming that they recognize no other remedies, it is not too much to say that they carry the practice of antiseptic irrigations to an irrational extreme and to the comparative neglect of other important indications. They assume on the other hand that those who deny the exclusive dogma of septicæmia are stricken with therapeutical impotence. 'The doctrine of autogenesis,' exclaims Parvin, 'is a confession of ignorance, the creed of fatalism, the cry of despair . . . the very pessimism of obstetric medicine.' Big words, full of sound, and little else. The truth is that those who take a broad, comprehensive, catholic view of the many factors in the etiology and constitution of puerperal fevers take also a broader, more philosophical, and more rational grasp of the principles of treatment and especially of prophylaxis. . . . The essential thing is to take such a large view of the physiological and pathological processes as will give the right indications to call upon each and all of the therapeutical agents at our command. To fix the mind too intently upon any one of these agents is to incur the danger of neglecting others, and of losing sight of the principles which ought to guide the applications of all as one force directed to one end."

In conclusion I beg leave to submit the following aphorisms:

1. The history of obstetrical practice teaches us that the lying-in hospital has always been a place of danger and mortality; therefore, it is obligatory upon those who have charge of these institutions to utilize every antiseptic measure known to the profession in order to save life.

2. The experience of country practitioners teaches us that women who are confined in healthy, isolated, rural homes are not subject to the contaminating influences of an ochlesis, and consequently do not require all the precautions of those exposed to hospitals, or even to the atmosphere of city life.

3. Country practitioners of medicine will generally show a lower rate of mortality in obstetrical cases than city practitioners, simply for the reason that they practise in

healthier localities, are less exposed to contagious influences, and, possibly, have a healthier class of patients.

4. The insinuations of a number of late writers on antiseptic midwifery, that the death-rate in obstetrical practice of country practitioners is high, are not true, as is shown by statistics.

THE VALUE OF CHLORAL HYDRATE.

BY JEROME HARDCASTLE, M.D.,
CECILTON, MD.

The following cases, occurring in my practice, have made such an impression on my mind in regard to the value of chloral hydrate in the treatment of a variety of conditions requiring a calmative, that I have thought it might be worth while to describe them briefly to my professional brethren.

CASE I. *Puerperal Eclampsia.*—Mrs. N.; aet. 19; primipara; after eight hours' normal labor was delivered of a ten pound boy. For two hours previous to her delivery she had complained of intense cephalalgia; about half an hour after delivery convulsions came on and the patient had two within about half hour. I gave an enema of chloral hydrat, gr. xc, to aq. tepid f ʒ ij, and applied a napkin to the anus, to retain it. The woman had one slight convulsion soon after, and, in one hour from the time of giving the first enema, I repeated it, when a quiet and refreshing sleep of four hours was followed by satisfactory convalescence.

CASE II. *Puerperal Eclampsia.*—Julia, colored; aet. 28; multipara; had suffered from cephalalgia from the beginning of labor. In about four hours convulsions set in, and during the fifth one a girl child was expelled. After a short interval, the convulsions returned. I then gave an enema of chloral and she had no further trouble.

CASE III. *Threatened Miscarriage.*—Mrs. S.; aet. 20; primipara; 7 months advanced; on going out the door fell upon her abdomen. Expulsive pains and uterine hemorrhage ensued. Arriving about one hour after the accident, I found the bed and her clothing saturated, the amniotic membranes distended and protruding through the os uteri, which was dilated to about the size of a walnut. I gave an enema containing 90 grains of chloral and applied cold cloths. In about an hour I used 60 grains more. The pains and hemorrhage then soon ceased, and the patient slept several hours. Three days after she was up and at work. At the expiration of nine months she was delivered of a girl. The child was anemic and fainted from slight causes during the first three years of its life; since which time (the parents having removed) I have not been able to trace its further history.

CASE IV. *Threatened Miscarriage.*—Mrs. H.; aet. 25; multipara; six months advanced; two weeks previous to my visit fell upon her abdomen and had slight pains, which lasted several hours. Upon seeing her I found that the pains had begun three hours before and recurred about every seven minutes. There was no hemorrhage and no perceptible dilatation of the os. I gave 90 grains of chloral by enema, and as the pains did not cease entirely in one hour I gave 60 grs. more. In half an hour she was sleeping quietly. She remained in her room three days, and then resumed her duties, and now, nearly four weeks having elapsed, I find her doing well.

CASE V. *Epilepsy.*—Jim; colored; aet. 8; birth had been effected by forceps; convulsions began to occur soon after and continued about five years, with increasing frequency. His treatment had been with bromides, etc. When called to see him, three years ago, I found that he had been having convulsions about every week, and from six to thirty or more during the day and night. I gave an enema containing ten grains of chloral *hourly* till relieved. Improvement was very marked. Intervals of a month or more came between the attacks, and there were only from two to four. For the past one and a half years the boy has had only one convulsion every three months (*or four a year*), his general health is good, his memory is much better, and his previously quarrelsome disposition has almost deserted him.

CASE VI. *Eclampsia from Dentition.*—Child; aet. 18 months; suffered with convulsions several hours before I saw it. I gave an enema containing eight grains of chloral, and scarified the gums. Two slight tremors occurred afterward, and the child went to sleep and awoke in about six hours as bright as a dollar.

CASE VII. *Eclampsia from Ascarides.*—Child; aet. 3. I gave fifteen grains of chloral by enema and applied a cold cloth to the head and gave a hot mustard footbath. During an hour the child had two more convulsions. At the expiration of this time, I gave ten grains more, and sleep followed for four hours. I then ordered a powder containing calomel, santonin and soda, every two hours until four were taken, and the next morning ol. ricini f ℥ss; spir. terebinth. gtt. xxx. During the following day the child passed a number of worms, and made a good recovery.

As an anti-convulsive I know of no remedy that equals chloral used in the manner above described. It is often impossible to give it by the mouth, and when it can be given so, its effects are much slower, and it is frequently rejected. I do not think it safe to exhibit chloroform or ether by inhalation, and chloral by the mouth at the same time, as I know of two cases—one surgical, the other obstetrical—in which in the former the patient suddenly expired while being prepared for the operation, and in the latter prompt and energetic measures alone saved her. In the case of Mrs. N. (puerperal eclampsia), mentioned above, I used chloroform inhalations freely and chloral *by enema*, and had no untoward symptoms.

SOCIETY REPORTS.

MEDICAL SOCIETY OF THE COUNTY OF NEW YORK.

Stated Meeting, May 27, 1889.

The President, ALEXANDER S. HUNTER, M.D., in the Chair.

DR. A. JACOBI read a paper on

Rheumatism in Infancy and Childhood.

He first alluded to the limited bibliography of rheumatism in infancy and childhood. It began with theses on the subject by two of Roger's pupils, written in 1864 and 1865, and with a paper by Roger himself, in 1867; between this time and 1875, when Dr. Jacobi wrote on the subject in this country, about half a dozen other papers had appeared. In 1885, the study was renewed. Dr. Jacobi, on the present occasion, chiefly considered the question of therapeutics of rheumatism in infancy and childhood, although he spoke briefly of some other points. Since he made the statement, fourteen years ago, that these cases occur frequently, only a few have come to recognize the truth which it contains. He thinks the frequent presence of cardiac disease in childhood sufficient proof of the common enough existence of rheumatism. Then there are also cases of rheumatism at this period which manifest no cardiac disease whatever. Wherever there is any doubt or suspicion of its existence, the heart should be carefully examined; for often the cardiac affection appears to be the first, and perhaps the only clear, symptom of rheumatism. The presence of chorea minor should also lead to a careful examination of the heart and joints, for in not a few cases it is seen at even the very beginning of rheumatism.

The diagnosis in many cases is quite difficult. Fever is a common symptom, but it is also common in any physical disturbance in children. The temperature is sometimes only slightly elevated, and sometimes rises at irregular intervals. The swelling of the joint is apt to be only trifling; and the pain, either arising from pressure or spontaneously, may simulate that due to fatigue, syphilitic disease, etc. The diagnosis is more difficult when only one joint is affected, especially if it is the knee- or hip-joint, which is also often the seat of traumatism and tubercular inflammation. Rheumatism also frequently fails to be recognized because the pains are called "growing pains," a term which should have been dropped long since. Epiphysitis has likewise been confounded with rheumatism.

Turning to the subject of therapeutics, Dr. Jacobi said it has been quite unsatisfactory until modern times. A few indications are furnished by the actual or alleged causes of the disease. For instance, it seems sometimes to be endemic, and when it is so, it is well to remove the child to another locality. It occurs frequently after typhoid fever, diphtheria, scarlet fever, and other infectious diseases; and one should avail himself of this knowledge in prophylaxis. The blood has been found changed in rheumatic fever, being less alkaline; and while this fact is not peculiar to this disease, yet it affords an indication for alkalies, and experience has shown that they are beneficial.

Sudden changes of temperature and of moisture certainly favor the development of rheumatism, especially in those of inherited predisposition. The tendency to be influenced by atmospheric conditions can be modified by the systematic use of cold water. Warm clothing and bedding are called for, as nothing can be more injurious to these patients than exposure to wind and rain.

The swollen and painful joints must be protected against the pressure of blankets by raising the bed-clothing from the limbs, as by inserting the limb through a wastebasket. A wet bandage or pack around the joint is often borne well and is grateful. It should be changed every hour or half hour.

Anæmic children require hot applications, perhaps dry. In very severe cases Dr. Jacobi has sometimes been compelled to administer a few drops of a solution of morphine hypodermically; but as a rule an anodyne applied around the joint, and covered with oiled silk, gives relief from pain. Swelling during convalescence may call for pressure, which can be exerted by means of bandages or collodion, absorption being hastened by gentle massage and the galvanic current, and by the internal administration of iodide of potassium or sodium. He brushes copiously over the swollen part iodoform in collodion. Very old cases with chronic effusion into the joint require aspiration and washing out of the joint.

Endocarditis demands for its treatment absolute rest of the heart and body. For that reason an occasional dose of the bromides or of opium may be beneficial. The ice bag to the præcordial region, or, if that be too heavy, the ice cloth, will do good. It should be remembered, however, that not every murmur indicates endocarditis.

The temperature is rarely high, but there are some cases in which it rises to 104°, or even 107° or more; and in this class occur delirium and other nervous symptoms. The most effective means of reducing the temperature is by the cold pack. Antifebrin, antipyrin, and phenacetine may here be called for. As a rule, salicylate of sodium mitigates the pain, etc., in a short time; but if it produces no effect within from three to five days it should be discontinued. As already stated, alkalies are indicated, and may be administered in the form of bicarbonate of sodium, or of the nitrates, or of the mineral waters. Vegetable acids have been warmly recommended by some. Iodide of potassium and sodium have been justly commended highly, especially where the case shows a tendency to chronicity.

Gonorrhœal rheumatism is sometimes seen in children. It is for the most part confined to one or two joints, as the ankle or shoulder, and is of a subacute nature. The effusion is likely to be excessive, often purulent, and suggests a relationship with pyæmia. A puncture may be made for the purpose of ascertaining the nature of the effusion, and if pus be discovered it should be removed and the cavity thoroughly disinfected. Salicylate of sodium or iodide of potassium and sodium should be continued a long time in these cases. In some cases, during and after an attack of acute rheumatism, small nodes develop in the fascia and periosteum, consisting of young connective tissue, which are tender, and last from a few days to several months. In a few cases there are hemorrhagic spots. Salicylate of sodium tends rather to promote hemorrhage.

Chronic articular rheumatism is rare in childhood. The treatment is about the same as that of the same disease in adults. Salicylate of sodium is to be administered in these cases only when there is an acute exacerbation. The so-called hydropathic treatment is beneficial. Alkaline waters are necessary, and Dr. Jacobi strongly recommends lithia water to which bicarbonate of sodium has been added.

Muscular rheumatism can be diagnosticated occasionally in very young children; but in children from six to twelve years of age it is not very rare. The neck, back and shoulders are most affected. The best preventive measure is the habitual use of cold water.

DR. WILLIAM H. THOMSON said his attention has long ago been called to the influence of climate. It has been said that a cause of rheumatism is cold and moisture; yet it is a common disease among the Arabs and inhabitants of the Desert of Syria, where the climate is very dry and hot during the day. There is one condition, however, to which these people are exposed in common with the inhabitants of cold and moist countries, namely, that the moist skin suddenly becomes cooled during the night following the hot days. This he regards as an important etiological fact. It is an important one also in the differential diagnosis between rheumatism and gout. The latter affection is seen only among persons who use alcoholic drinks, and is due to some error in assimilation. The character of the pulse will distinguish the one affection from the other, it being incompressible and hard in gout, and soft and compressible in rheumatism. Dr. Thomson is disposed to think that in scarlatinal rheumatism there is an approach to a pyæmic condition. He has also in a certain number of cases found an invariable association of acute articular rheumatism and quinsy.

In therapeutics he has a great fondness for the continued use of the warm bath. Among other effects, it is anæsthetic and also renders the urine alkaline. The rheumatic should always wear flannel next the skin. As a further prophylactic he has these subjects use inunctions, especially on the back of the neck and shoulders. He also administers cod-liver oil in chronic rheumatism. He emphasizes the necessity for giving attention to rheumatism in children on account of the injurious consequences of heart complication. There is no doubt in his mind that a relation exists between chorea and rheumatism. Chorea, so to speak, is a result of the rheumatic poison. In treating endocarditis, he places no reliance upon salicylate of sodium for the treatment of the disease, but like all others he administers it for the joint affection. To slow the heart's action, he gives full doses of aconite. At the same time he renders the blood alkaline. The chest should be protected absolutely against drafts, and for that reason he does not allow it to remain bare under any circumstances.

Dr. J. Lewis Smith gave the results of his experience at the Out-door Department of Bellevue Hospital during the past fifteen years. In this time he has made the diagnosis of rheumatism in seventy-eight patients under fifteen years of age, nearly all of them under twelve, the majority about the age of eight years. Most of the children did not have rheumatism when brought to the clinic, but the presence of cardiac disease and the past history in many cases formed the basis of the diagnosis. He has seen a number of cases in private practice also, but has not the records. In general, rheumatism in children under two years of age is accompanied by little swelling, and the diagnosis is difficult. In the majority of cases the disease manifests itself in the lower extremities. Parents are apt to call the trouble "growing pains." Of his seventy-eight cases, forty-nine had distinct cardiac murmurs. As to chorea minor, during the same period he has records of sixty-seven cases, in forty-seven of which rheumatism could be excluded. He has been in the habit of using salicylate of sodium or salicylic acid in the rheumatism of children. It is important to stop the disease and prevent endocarditis.

——————◆◆◆——————

—The Philadelphia *Telegraph*, May 3, says that Dr. Joseph Rogers, whose death was recently announced, was a native of Westmeon, Petersfield, Hants, England, where his great-grandfather, grandfather, father, and brother practised medicine for a century and a quarter. He was the thirteenth of sixteen children, of whom five became doctors. One of his brothers is Professor Thorold Rogers. He was the founder of the Anti-Interment in Towns Association, and for many years was foremost among the sanitary reformers of England.

HOSPITAL NOTES.

——————

CANTON HOSPITAL, CANTON, CHINA.

SERVICE OF J. M. SWAN, M.D.

Opium Poisoning Treated with Atropia Sulphate.

Case I.—April 2, 1889, at four o'clock P. M., I was called into the city to see a Manchu, aged thirty-six years; occupation soldier; married; his family consisting of a wife and three children. About three hours before the time I saw him, he had swallowed a quantity of opium, with the intention of committing suicide. The amount was estimated at about an ounce and a half of the native prepared, watery extract of opium, which is used in smoking. I found his respirations eight to ten per minute; his pulse 80, full and strong; his pupils contracted to the size of a pin head; and, with considerable difficulty, he could be roused, but not to full consciousness. One twenty-fourth of a grain of atropia sulph. was administered hypodermically, and the stomach-pump was at once introduced, and the stomach thoroughly washed out. There was a strong odor of opium given off from the contents withdrawn from the stomach, but no opium was discovered. A dram of brandy in hot water was administered by the mouth, the hypodermic injections of atropia being continued every ten or fifteen minutes.

At first the patient seemed to improve; but soon the narcosis became deeper. As I worked at great disadvantage and with poor assistants, I had the patient placed in a Sedan chair and rapidly conveyed to the hospital. This consumed about twenty minutes, and when the man was brought into the hospital ward his respirations were not over three per minute; there was no radial pulse; his heart sounds were distinctly audible, but feeble; and deep cyanosis was present. One-twelfth of a grain of atropine was at once given hypodermically, his feet and legs were plunged into hot water up to his knees, and artificial respiration was begun. In ten minutes the second one-twelfth grain of atropine was given, the foot-bath being kept as hot as was at all safe without danger of scalding. Very shortly after a third one-twelfth grain dose of atropia was given, the character of the respirations changed. The inspiration became deeper and spasmodic or catching in character, showing a marked stimulus of the respiratory centre. The respirations were now five or six per minute, and the pupils partly dilated. Hypodermic injections of brandy were administered three or four times during the evening. The respirations and the pulse slowly but gradually improved, and the stimulated respirations were quite marked during the greater part of the night.

The next morning the patient, though still rather drowsy and depressed, was able to take some nourishment, and by ten o'clock A. M. he was able to sit alone on his bed. Late in the afternoon of the same day he was quite himself again.

There is a diversity of opinion as to the real value of belladonna, or its alkaloid, in cases of opium poisoning. From a physiological point of view we certainly have a strong argument in favor of its use. The best proof of its efficiency is in the practical test. In the case reported above, the physiological effects of the drug were well marked, but not until about *three-fourths of a grain* had been administered. I believe its free use saved the life of the patient. This opinion is not based on my experience in this case alone, but also on my past experience; for, in two cases, in particular, of opium poisoning did I attribute success in treatment to the use of atropine.

Cases of opium poisoning are quite commonly met with among the Chinese, and it is the usual means by which they often commit suicide.

Dentigerous Cyst of the Antrum of Highmore—Operation.

Case II.—March 12, 1889, Mr. Tsing Chan, aged 20, unmarried, by occupation a farmer, presented himself for the removal of a growth situated on the right side of the face. It had been present for three years, and had been gradually increasing in size. It involved the outer surface of the right superior maxillary bone from the insertion of the lateral incisor tooth to that of the first molar, the facial surface of the bone having been pushed outward and upward. Part of the teeth were loosened but none were thrown out of line. Over a small area external to the alveolar process, and at a point over the orbital, there was distinct fluctuation. The roof of the mouth was undisturbed. There was no history of pain having been present to any marked degree, and the man's general condition was fairly good, though he did not present a very robust appearance.

March 19, the patient was operated upon.

A trochar was first introduced at the lower point of fluctuation, and about two ounces of a thin brownish serous fluid were drawn off. An incision was made extending from a point on the upper lip one inch to the right of the median line, upward and outward external to the infra-orbital foramen, thus avoiding the trunks of the infra-orbital artery and nerve, the incision being fully three inches in length. The teeth involved were extracted, and the facial surface of the bone lying beneath the floor of the sac of the tumor, thus exposing the antrum, which was greatly enlarged and lined with the sac. In the posterior part of the cavity there was a fully developed tooth, corresponding in appearance to a lateral incisor, firmly inserted into that portion of the bone lying beneath the floor of the orbit; and from its length it must have reached very nearly through the floor of the orbit. This tooth having been extracted, the entire sac was easily removed, it being but loosely adherent to the bony walls of the cavity. The sac presented a peculiar velvety appearance, and was one-fourth inch in thickness and exceedingly tenacious. The cavity was filled with absorbent lint and the incision carefully closed, an aperature being left external to the alveolar process, for the purpose of dressing and the daily injection of a ten per cent. solution of boracic acid.

The external incision united by first intention, and at this date—twenty-two days after the operation—the cavity is almost closed, and scarcely any deformity is noticed.

Doubt was entertained as to the correctness of the diagnosis in this case, as the signs very strongly indicated disease of the superior maxillary bone, and as the roof of the mouth was not in any way affected. The result showed that the method sometimes used, of evacuating the sac and injecting a strong solution of carbolic acid or iodine would have proved futile. The question arises whether or not this tumor might be called a dentigerous cyst. Usually such a term is applied only to those cysts connected with the normal teeth. In the above case the sac was closely adherent to the abnormal tooth, and on extraction of the same quite a portion remained attached to the tooth.

—The French Ministry of Marine has decided that on and after January 1, 1890, wine furnished to the naval service must not contain more than thirty grains of sulphate of potassium to each quart.

PERISCOPE.

The Severe Vomiting of Pregnancy.

At the meeting of the American Gynecological Society, at Washington, Sept., 1888, Dr. Graily Hewitt, of London, in a paper with this title, said that the difference between the slight and severe vomiting of pregnancy is only one of degree. Many practitioners seem to be able to find no resource in these cases except the induction of premature labor. Severe vomiting may be due to several different causes. These may be classed as non-uterine and uterine. Among the reported fatal causes of the former class are disease of the stomach, liver, and intestines. Mathews Duncan has described a fatal case of "icterus gravis" during pregnancy; Lomer has recently written a paper on the same subject. The second class of causes are due to abnormal conditions of the uterus—such as anteversions and retroversions or flexions, induration of the cervix, and endometritis. Retroflexion of the gravid uterus does not always cause severe vomiting. On the other hand, retroflexion of the non-gravid uterus sometimes gives rise to vomiting. Several cases of impaction of the anteflexed gravid uterus have been reported; this impaction is due to the unyielding character of the uterine tissue. By dilating the cervix in cases of vomiting we overcome the tension in the neighborhood of the os internum. As regards treatment, most cases are cured by reducing the displacement, or sometimes by simply supporting the uterus. Severe vomiting may be of reflex origin, due to distension of the uterus. Some observers think that the nerves around the os internum are primarily irritated. There is a close parallel between cases of vomiting in flexions of the gravid and of the non-gravid uterus.

Dr. Fordyce Barker, of New York, said that the subject of the paper was one of great interest, and that the profession was already deeply indebted to Dr. Hewitt for former papers on it. The speaker believes that vomiting during pregnancy is largely influenced by the constitution of the patient. Some individuals can not even ride in a railroad car without feeling nauseated, while others are never affected. It is not strange that a constitutional tendency of this nature is apt to be exaggerated during the period of gestation when there is such a total change in the system. He does not believe that anteflexion of the uterus is a potent factor in causing vomiting, and he cited, in support of this opinion, a case of marked anteflexion in which the patient became pregnant and passed through the entire period without experiencing the least nausea. The flexion was not cured by gestation, but recurred after delivery. In another case there was marked retroflexion with absence of vomiting. However, he has seen cases in which vomiting was associated with flexions. He has seen in consultation no less than ten patients who were *in extremis* from severe vomiting, the question of inducing labor having been entertained too late. He has never been obliged to induce labor for this cause, having succeeded in curing the patients without it. There are many methods of treatment, some of them apparently contradictory. Sometimes it is wisest to give the patient what she craves most, as in a case in which he allowed a woman, who had been able to retain nothing whatever, to eat lobster salad, for which she had a longing. The speaker referred to Copeman's method of dilating the cervix, which he had frequently found of value.

Hemorrhage from the Bowel in Typhoid Fever.

Dr. J. A. Lindsay, Physician to Belfast Royal Hospital, in a communication in the *Dublin Journal of Medical Science*, April, 1889, reports two cases of hemorrhage from the bowel occurring in typhoid fever.

In the first case the hemorrhage supervened upon a sharp case of typhoid fever, attended by severe diarrhœa and an unusually high and continuous range of temperature. The hemorrhage, he says, undoubtedly aggravated the case enormously, and death was for some days imminent. In the second case the hemorrhage probably resulted from the patient's continuing to go about and to partake of unsuitable food. It evidently aggravated a case that was already grave through neglect, and was the beginning of the end.

Dr. Lindsay has made an analysis of all the cases of typhoid fever which have occurred at the Royal Hospital during the past twelve months, and thinks the result will throw some light upon the frequency and gravity of intestinal hemorrhage. Including the two cases referred to, the cases number 30. Hemorrhage took place in six instances (20 per cent.), and in two it proved fatal. The remaining patients who had no hemorrhage—24 in number—all recovered. These figures, he remarks, are somewhat unusual. They show 30 cases treated, with 2 deaths—a mortality-rate of less than 7 per cent. The mortality from typhoid fever varies considerably; but taking Ireland as a whole, he thinks it is certainly not less than 15 per cent. The death-rate at the Royal Hospital during the past year has, therefore, been rather less than half the average. This record, he says, becomes still more remarkable when it is noted that both fatal cases were instances of relapse, and that the patients did not come into hospital sooner than the ninth or tenth week. Intestinal hemorrhage occurred in 6 out of the 30 cases—a somewhat large proportion. Louis records 134 cases, with hemorrhage in 8 only, and Murchison calculates that it occurs to an appreciable extent only in from 3 to 4 per cent. of cases. All Dr. Lindsay's cases in which hemorrhage occurred were of unusual severity. Of the six, two patients died, two recovered after hope had been almost abandoned, and the remaining two had very sharp attacks. These facts show (as far as they go) that hemorrhage is a very serious symptom, that it is not infrequently fatal, but that the most desperate cases may rally and make a perfect recovery.

As to the class of cases in which hemorrhage occurred, and the stage of the attack, Dr. Lindsay states that his cases support Murchison's statement that hemorrhage is rare in childhood: The six cases were aged respectively 27, 34, 19, 29, 28, 26. Thus, the average age at which hemorrhage occurred was 27, while the average age of the 24 cases in which there was no hemorrhage was 18½ years. As regards the period at which the hemorrhage occurred, the earliest was on the fourteenth day; in two others it occurred for the first time upon the nineteenth day, in a fourth case upon the twentieth day, and in the two remaining cases in the ninth or tenth week. It would appear that the later the hemorrhage the more serious the prognosis. Thus the four cases in which the hemorrhage occurred before the expiration of the third week all recovered, while in the two remaining cases in which it occurred in the ninth or tenth week both patients died.

With regard to his treatment of intestinal hemorrhage, Dr. Lindsay says he has always been accustomed to follow Murchison's instructions, and has given tannic acid, laudanum, and turpentine, with ice externally and ergotin by hypodermic injection. In one of his cases he gave laudanum pretty freely, in spite of the presence of albumin in the urine, and with good results—no sign of narcotism appearing. He is disposed to think that in intestinal hemorrhage, as in hematocele and other forms of internal bleeding, opium may be given fearlessly, and pushed even to heroic doses. Stimulants are certainly required in some cases, but must be regulated with much caution.

In conclusion, he says that, while intestinal hemorrhage in typhoid fever is a serious symptom, it is by no means usually fatal, and prompt and decisive treatment is called for, and will often prove effectual.

The Significance of a Fœtal Cardiac Rhythm.

M. Huchard has pointed out at the Paris Hospitals Medical Society (*La France Médicale*, No. 46) that the association of tachycardia (great rapidity of heart's beat) with equalization of the two silent periods and similarity of the two sounds is of more serious omen than simple tachycardia. It is found with weakening of cardiac contractility due to degeneration of the heart muscle and extreme lowering of arterial pressure from vascular paresis. Such a condition, therefore, is of grave augury, and the therapeutic indications are to restore the contractile power of the heart by hypodermic injections of caffeine, and that of the vessels by ergotin. He suggests the term "embryocardia," as descriptive of the condition that recalls the rhythm of the fœtal heart. In the discussion, M. Labbé demurred to the term, and expressed surprise at the results obtained by caffeine, doubting if it was absorbed, and fearing that it might be injurious in the large doses proposed by M. Huchard. M. Hallopeau thought the diminution of arterial pressure to be the result of the cardiac enfeeblement, and that cardiac rather than vascular tonics were indicated. Ergot of rye is a cardiac tonic. M. Huchard, in reply, said that he employed the term "embryocardia" because it is short and expressive. He asserts that it is safer to give caffeine (in the amount necessary in such cases) subcutaneously than by the mouth, and said the local inconveniencies at the seat of a hypodermic puncture can not be counted as against the relief afforded to the grave symptoms of the condition in which he employed it (M. Huchard's prescription was fifteen to thirty grains daily, in from four to ten hypodermic injections). Ergot of rye, he said, acts primarily upon the arterial system, and secondarily on the heart. —*Lancet*, April 27, 1889.

Mr. Stanley on Arrow Poison.

The *Lancet*, April 13, 1889, says that the letter from Mr. H. M. Stanley, which was read at a recent meeting of the Royal Geographical Society, contained an extremely interesting reference to the arrow poison employed by the natives of the Lower Congo district, and it afforded a curious insight into the strange perversions of knowledge by which the advances of civilization are retarded. Mr. Stanley says they were much exercised as to what might be the poison on the heads of the arrows by which Lieutenant Stairs and several others were wounded, and from the effects of which four persons died almost directly. The mystery was solved by finding at Arisibba several packets of dried red ants. The bodies of these insects were dried, ground into powder, cooked in palm oil, and smeared on the points of arrows. It is well known that formic acid exists in the free state in red ants, as well as in stinging nettles, and in several species of caterpillars. This acid is, in the pure state, so corrosive that it produces blisters on the skin, and hence there is little ground for doubting that it was the "deadly irritant by which so many men had been lost with such terrible suffering." The multitude of curious insects encountered, which rendered their lives "as miserable as they could well be," bears out Mr. Stanley's idea that many similar poisons can be prepared from insects.

The Bacteriology of Tetanus.

Professor Bizzozero has just submitted to the Royal Medical Academy of Turin the results obtained by Professor Tizzoni, of Bologna, and Signora Giuseppina Cattani on the bacillus tetani. These investigators took their material from a patient in the surgical wards, the victim of a fracture the seat of which had been contaminated by soil from the ground on which he had fallen. Traumatic tetanus of the most characteristic kind had ensued. Experiments made with the living blood in great quantity, with the median nerve and medulla of the bone taken a little above the point of fracture immediately after amputation of the limb, and also with the brain and spleen after death, yielded negative results, both with the cultures and the experiments themselves. From the material taken from the osseous surfaces of the fracture and from the soft parts immediately contiguous, there were obtained other microörganisms and the "bacilli

spilliformes" of Nicolaier. These latter, inoculated in animals, produced tetanus, followed by death after twenty-four or forty hours. Left to themselves for three months in blood serum slightly solidified at a low temperature, there was again obtained from their inoculation distinct tetanus. Cultures of this liquid yielded a coccus, a short bacillus, and the bacillus of Nicolaier. Such colonies become so intimately fused with others that not seldom the transplantings from them turn out impure. This result probably accounts for the findings of Drs. Belfanti and Pescarolo. In any case Drs. Tizzoni and Cattani are the first, according to Professor Bizzozero, who have obtained a pure culture of the bacillus tetani, and who have kept it such throughout successive transplantings. The sequel of their researches will be awaited with special interest.—*Lancet*, April 20, 1889.

Professor Kremianski on Tubercle Bacilli.

Professor Kremianski, of Kharkoff, whose name is known in connection with the so-called aniline treatment of phthisis, has just published, in conjunction with Dr. Tseslinski, an article in the *Meditsinskoë Obozrênie*, or the importance of frequent microscopical examination of the sputum both for diagnostic and for therapeutic purposes, in cases in which phthisis is or may be present. The patients examined amounted to 931, and they were most of them seen in Professor Kremianski's polyclinic or out-patient department, something like 10,000 microscopical observations having been made during the course of the last two years. In addition, very thorough physical examinations were carried out, not merely by means of the stethoscope, but with the help of the spirometer, manometer, thoracometer, thermometer, and weighing machine. As far as possible, too, very complete notes were taken of the effects of different remedies. Of the 931 cases, tubercle bacilli were found in 570, or in 61 per cent., including cases of the most diverse description, some having cavities, some apex consolidation, and some merely signs of bronchitis or broncho-pleuritis. Thus, of the 570 cases presenting bacilli 220 patients, or 38 per cent., had cavities; 229, or 40 per cent., had apex consolidation; 19, or 3 per cent., had simple "bronchitis"; and 5, or 0.8 per cent., had "broncho-pleuritis." A considerable number (97) of the cases were sent by medical men to have the sputum examined for the purpose of diagnosis. It was by no means uncommon to find a complete absence of bacilli in the sputum of patients presenting the clearest physical signs of phthisis—consolidation and even cavities. Of 238 patients with cavities, bacilli were absent in 18, or in 7 per cent. Of 419 cases of consolidation, bacilli were absent in 190, or in 45 per cent. Of 54 cases of "bronchitis" they were only absent in 35, or in 65 per cent. Bacilli were never found in cases of uncomplicated emphysema—*i.e.*, where there were no cavities or consolidation in addition. With regard to Professor Kremianski's special method of treatment, while it was only successful in entirely arresting the development of bacilli in about 30 cases, it produced a cessation of the ordinary symptoms of phthisis—cough, debility, fever, sweats, etc.—in about 300 cases.—*Lancet*, April 27, 1889.

Incurability of Syphilis.

Dr. W. R. Gowers, in the concluding Lettsomian lecture upon syphilis and the nervous system (*British Med. Journal*, Feb. 16, 1889) says: "I believe it is literally correct to say that we have no evidence that syphilis ever is, or ever has been, cured." Again he says: "The conclusion that the essential element in the disease resists treatment, and runs its course uninfluenced by our efforts, is in harmony with what we know of other specific diseases due to a poison introduced from without, and communicable from one person to another. There is not any fact whatever to show that a single disease of this kind can be cut short. The course of the acute exanthemata cannot be arrested by any means at our disposal at any stage of their course, and the same seems true of this chronic exanthematous disease. This is eminently true, also, of the disease that stands perhaps nearer to syphilis than any other known malady—leprosy."

With regard to the methods of administration of mercury, he says: "The old method of inunction seems to me to bring the patient under the influence of the drug as speedily as it can be done with safety, and with a certainty incomparably greater than the administration by the mouth. I have been deterred from a trial by the hypodermic method because the published evidence seemed to me not to afford any satisfactory proof of superiority, being destitute of the element of comparison essential to such proof, and because this method seems to afford an opportunity for psychical influence not free from risk of that which is undesirable. But I would not for one moment suggest that such an influence has entered into the motives or action of those who have used this method." Dr. Gowers believes that full doses of mercury and iodide of potash for from six to ten weeks will effect all that can be achieved in the removal of the syphilitic process. They should be continued only a little longer than is necessary to remove the lesion, being repeated, it may be, after an interval occupied by tonic treatment or by the other of the two chief drugs.

With reference to the consequences of the belief in the incurability of syphilis, he says: "If it is true that we cannot cure syphilis, it is most important to consider how it can best be kept in check. This is why the fact of incurability, if true, is so important. A mistaken belief in curability may dangerously hinder attempts at prevention. If no present treatment can prevent future developments, then it is wise, whether these come or not, to anticipate them. I think a custom, sometimes recommended, is prudent, that every syphilitic subject, for at least five years after the date of his last symptoms, should have a three weeks' course of treatment twice every year, taking, for that time, twenty or thirty grains of iodide a day. If this practice were adopted generally, is it not reasonable to anticipate grave lesions would be much more rare?"

Ectopic Testicle.

Charles Monod and G. Arthaud (*Archiv Gén. de Méd.*, Dec., 1887, say: Ectopic testicle is almost always accompanied by a progressive atrophy of the gland. Three stages of this condition are to be discriminated: 1. The spermatic function may still be preserved. 2. With preservation of the function, perivascular sclerosis and induration of the corpus Highmorianum occur, restraining secretions and producing sterility without atrophy. 3. Finally, atrophy of the gland occurs through connective tissue hypertrophy and disappearance of the epithelium.

They sum up as follows: 1. In almost all cases of ectopic testicle the gland atrophies. 2. No disturbance of function occurs in the beginning; later on, gradual impairment of function occurs. 3. Under the influence of external injuries and age, mechanical restraints to secretion and sterility develop. 4. Progressive sclerosis imparts to the ectopic testicle the conditions of senility.—*Brooklyn Medical Journal*, May, 1889.

Splenectomy for Floating Spleen with Strangulated Pedicle.

Dr. Y. H. Bond communicates to the *Weekly Medical Review*, April 13, an account of a very rare case in which he had performed splenectomy to relieve grave symptoms caused by twisting of the afferent and efferent vessels of the spleen. The patient was a woman, of good health, who had had four healthy children at full term, with no miscarriage, and was five months' pregnant with her fifth child. The symptoms were acute abdominal pain, vomiting, constipation, meteorism, and there was a history of the existence for about four years of a small, hard, movable tumor, about the size of a lemon, in the right iliac fossa. When admitted to hospital the patient was almost in collapse. Exploratory laparotomy was performed March 22, and the condition of the spleen already mentioned was found. The spleen when removed weighed 48 ounces and was 5½ inches wide, 3½ inches thick and 8½ inches long.

The contents of the uterus were expelled early on the morning following the operation. The patient died March 24. The *post-mortem* examination does not seem to have disclosed anything abnormal except general peritonitis.

An Epidemic of Parotitis.

Demme communicates an account of an epidemic of parotitis to the *Wiener med.-chirurg. Centralb.*, vol. xxiv., No. 5. The parotitis of this epidemic was very contagious, and usually affected all children exposed to it except those who were protected by a former attack. The average period of incubation was 8 to 15 days, but one boy, who was brought to the ward from a district in which no cases of mumps had appeared, took the complaint in three days. The duration of the invasion stage was 36 to 52 hours; the symptoms were restlessness and loss of appetite in mild cases, but in severe cases there were intense headache, vomiting, alternate restlessness and somnolence, and even delirium and convulsions. The temperature of this stage was 100° to 101° in mild cases, and 101° to 104° or more in severe cases. The swelling of and around the gland sometimes developed very rapidly—in 4 to 24 hours; in other cases it was so slow that it reached its maximum only in from 5 to 8 days. As a rule, the hardness was limited to the swelling of the gland itself, the surrounding swelling being of an œdematous character. In the majority of instances both glands were affected, though not in an equal degree. In a limited number the submaxillary and sublingual glands were also involved. The secretion of saliva at the beginning and at the height of the disease, was in a few cases diminished. The lymphatic glands behind and below the jaw were nearly always enlarged, and in anæmic individuals this swelling persisted. The enlargement of the parotid lasted usually from 8 to 14 days. The youngest patient was only 3 weeks old, but the commonest age was from 3 to 7 years. The cases occurred between June 1887 and May 1888, and their total number was 117. Eight were of a severe character, two ending in suppuration of the parotid, while two patients developed acute nephritis, and one suppurating otitis media. Two patients, a boy, three and a half years old, and a girl 7 years old, died in consequence of gangrene setting in. The course was much the same in both cases. When the parotid swelling was at its height a dirty greenish-brown vesicle appeared on the skin; this and its dark blue areola rapidly increased in size and soon developed into an ulcer with a dirty offensive discharge. Progress was very rapid. In the boy, 16 days after the appearance of the vesicle, almost the whole of the parotid gland was eaten away, and the nerves and blood-vessels dissected out. In the girl, the course of the gangrene was not quite so rapid, but there was no other essential difference between them. The gangrene was accompanied by extreme prostration, somnolence, cyanosis, cold extremities, epistaxis, and diarrhœa. The temperature gradually became subnormal.— *London Medical Recorder*, April, 1889.

Harmlessness of Saccharin.

The *London Medical Recorder*, April, 1889, says, with reference to the generally current idea that the use of saccharin is injurious, the following report has been published by Dr. Thomas Stevenson, official analyst of the Home Office:—1. Saccharin is quite innocuous when taken in quantities largely exceeding what would be taken in any ordinary dietary. 2. Saccharin does not interfere with or impede the digestive processes when taken in any practicable quantity. 3. His personal experience is that saccharin may be taken for an extended period without interfering with the digestive and other bodily functions; hence there is no reason to think that its continued use is in any way harmful.

THE
MEDICAL AND SURGICAL
REPORTER.

ISSUED EVERY SATURDAY.

CHARLES W. DULLES, M.D.,
EDITOR AND PUBLISHER.

The Terms of Subscription to the publications of this office are as follows, payable in advance :

Med. and Surg. Reporter (weekly), a year, $5.00
Physician's Daily Pocket Record, - - - 1.00
Reporter and Pocket Record, - - - - 6.00

All checks and postal orders should be drawn to order of
CHARLES W. DULLES,
N. E. Cor. 13th and Walnut Streets,
P. O. Box 843. Philadelphia, Pa.

☞ SUGGESTIONS TO SUBSCRIBERS :
See that your address-label gives the date to which your subscription is paid.
In requesting a change of address, give the old address as well as the new one.
If your REPORTER does not reach you promptly and regularly, notify the publisher *at once*, so that the cause may be discovered and corrected.

☞ SUGGESTIONS TO CONTRIBUTORS AND CORRESPONDENTS :
Write in ink.
Write on one side of paper only.
Write on paper of the size usually used for letters.
Make as few paragraphs as possible. Punctuate carefully. Do not abbreviate, or omit words like "the," and "a," or "an."
Make communications as short as possible.
NEVER ROLL A MANUSCRIPT ! Try to get an envelope or wrapper which will fit it.
When it is desired to call our attention to something in a newspaper, mark the passage boldly with a colored pencil, and write on the wrapper "Marked copy." Unless this is done, newspapers are not looked at.
The Editor will be glad to get medical news, but it is important that brevity and actual interest shall characterize communications intended for publication.

A NEW TREATMENT FOR CHRONIC RINGWORM OF THE SCALP.

Only those who have attempted to cure a group of cases of chronic ringworm of the scalp can appreciate the disheartening obstinacy of the affection. Ringworm of the body is easily cured by a few applications of tincture of iodine, and so usually is ringworm of the scalp, when treatment is begun soon after infection has occurred. But when the fungus has once penetrated into the interior of the hairs and hair follicles it is sometimes almost impossible to eradicate it, and the longer the affection has lasted in any case, the more rebellious to treatment does it become. The fungus, so far as we know, does not cease to be suscepti-ble to parasiticides, but the reason why the latter are so slow in acting is that they can not be brought into contact with the fungus, situated as it is deeply beneath the surface of the scalp. One of the most useful suggestions that has hitherto been made, with the view of obviating this difficulty, is that of Mr. A. J. Harrison, of Bristol, England. The results obtained in Philadelphia by the application of Mr. Harrison's method were communicated to the REPORTER, June 23, 1887, in an article by Dr. Herman B. Allyn. Without rehearsing Mr. Harrison's method, suffice it to say, that he employed a solution of caustic potash to soften the hairs and scalp tissues, and when this end was reached, the parasiticide was applied. Two solutions were thus used.

In a communication published in the *British Medical Journal*, March 2, 1889, Mr. Harrison gives what he believes, after considerable experiment and an experience with one hundred cases in two years, is an improvement upon that which has itself produced most excellent results. The author combines the remedies in an ointment composed of: caustic potash, nine grains ; carbolic acid, twenty-four grains ; lanolin and cocoanut oil, of each one-half an ounce. This ointment may be scented with some suitable oil, and a small portion of it should be rubbed into the affected parts night and morning. The caustic potash contained in it acts upon and softens the hair-matter, and in this way allows the carbolic acid to have free access to the fungus and its hosts of spores. The author thinks there is a decided advantage in leaving, when it can be done, as much as a quarter of an inch of hair ; the ointment seems to have better play, and is kept on the part affected.

Those who have tried Mr. Harrison's former plan of treatment will receive his latest suggestion on the subject with great confidence, and will also be glad to learn that shaving of the head and still more, epilation, which is painful to the little patient and extremely trying to the perseverance of the physician, are both unnecessary and even unadvisable. Carbolic acid is, of course, the parasiticide, and as it is not really an acid, there is, of course, no impropriety in combining it with an alkali.

Ringworm of the scalp is such a dreadful scourge that it may be worth while to mention in this connection the means employed by Mr. Harrison to prevent infection. He applies to the heads of children liable to be infected, an ointment composed of boracic acid and oil of eucalyptus, of each two ounces; oil of cloves, one-half a fluid drachm; and oil of cocoa-nut, sufficient to make six ounces. This makes an elegant prophylactic pomade.

TREATMENT OF CANCER BY ELECTRICITY.

The idea of attempting to limit the advance of malignant growths by means of electricity is not a new one. From time to time powerful electrical currents have been passed through morbid structures, in the hope that their physiological or pathological functions would be so altered thereby as to lead to their disappearance. Thus far these attempts have never led to any great success. Very recently, however, Dr. J. Inglis Parsons, of the Chelsea Hospital, London, has made some new experiments in this direction, and has reported their results in the *British Med. Journal*, April 27, 1889. In this report, which is characterized by a tone which, under the circumstances, is remarkably temperate, Dr. Parsons gives an account of the histories of four cases, in which he applied the Voltaic current, as high as 600 *milliampères*, at intervals, with what he believes to have been an effect calculated to encourage the profession to a further trial of this agent for the treatment of cancer.

It would be a good thing, if the hopes suggested by Dr. Parsons could be realized. But, unfortunately, we see little in his report to warrant them. Although he himself does not press any claim to the establishment of a method of treatment, and reports his cases in a manner wholly free from exaggeration or over confidence, still they must not be taken without careful and critical investigation. When these are applied to them, we find that they are not of a character to justify any positive conclusions in regard to the influence of electricity upon cancer. This, because some of the four cases are of doubtful diagnosis, and in some the evidence of improvement is so slight that it requires a decided bias to believe that there was anything in them different from what is often observed in others in which there is no treatment at all, and which eventually end in death.

The theoretical explanation of the influence of the Voltaic current on cancer cells offered by Dr. Parsons is interesting; but it must not be overlooked that it is altogether theoretical, and that it is so far entirely unsupported by any reliable observation.

We have devoted this much space to the matter under discussion, because there are some things in the report which are calculated to incline the reader very favorably to whatever the writer may advocate, and there seems to be some danger that this inclination may lead to too ready an acceptance of a very attractive and tempting hypothesis, which is as yet utterly an hypothesis.

FLUORINE AS A REMEDIAL AGENT.

In addition to the Editorial on fluorine in the REPORTER, Jan. 12, 1889, it will doubtless interest our readers to know that Dr. Ludwig Polyák, of Görbersdorf, has recently made a careful study of the evidence in regard to the effect of inhalations of hydrofluoric acid in phthisis, and concludes that, so far from being of value, they are absolutely injurious.

His report is contained in the *Wiener med. Presse*, Nos. 6 and 7, 1889, and is of the most conclusive sort. It seems clear, on reading it, that nothing as yet points to a method of utilizing the properties of this important chemical agent in the treatment of pulmonary phthisis.

PATHOLOGICAL ANATOMY OF ESSEN-TIAL EPILEPSY.

The exact pathological anatomy of idiopathic or essential epilepsy is still very obscure, so that some recent statements by M. Chaslin before the Biological Society of Paris, at its meeting on March 2, are interesting and may perhaps throw new light on the subject. According to the *Bulletin Médical*, March 6, 1889, M. Chaslin has had occasion to study the brains of several epileptics, and his study has led him to the conclusion that certain lesions, described under the name "cerebral sclerosis," are due to a proliferation of the cells of the neurolgia. He proposes for this process the name "neuroglic sclerosis." Further, he believes the induration at certain points, especially in the horns of the hippocampi majores or in the olivary bodies—which has been long noted in cases of epilepsy—is the external sign of the hidden proliferation of the neuroglia.

According to this view, idiopathic epilepsy would in some cases be due to an excess of development of the connective tissue of the nerve fibres, which Chaslin thinks should be attributed to a lesion received during embryonic life.

IDLENESS AND INSANITY.

The enforced idleness of the male prisoners in the State's prisons of New York, brought about by "the friends of labor," has proved a great misfortune to the convicts. Labor is just as essential to their well being as it is to that of the citizen at large, if not more so. The increase of sickness, and especially of insanity, has been very marked since their regular employment was legislated away from them. The wardens have noticed, and reported, a falling off in their physical strength, while the medical attendants have found mental derangement and sexual perversion result from the idleness and solitary confinement. One of the surgeons resigned lately, and took occasion to express his conviction that a condition of misery would soon follow with which he would be powerless to cope; that, whereas formerly few of the convicts became sick, and rarely did one go insane, lately the hospital has been kept full, and as many as two and three have become fit subjects for transfer to the State asylums. Furthermore, as the prisoners are almost constantly going crazy and becoming more or less violent, in consequence, the danger to the physicians, attendants and their fellow prisoners was vastly increased.

CONSOLIDATION OF MEDICAL JOURNALS.

One of the most interesting signs of the times is to be found in the practical application of the belief that there are in this country altogether too many medical journals. One who is in a position to see how many useless and relatively worthless medical journals start into existence, from time to time, finds it not unnatural to regard with a sense of satisfaction the high rate of mortality that prevails among them. On the other hand, many journals which have already obtained a certain recognition by the profession, though unworthy representatives, from time to time succumb. In addition to this—a much more rare occurrence—once in a while worthy periodicals, which have existed as rivals in the same field, come together as allies, and continue the work which they have begun, with united force and with improved prospects of success.

An occasion of the latter kind is found in the combination of the *Medical Press of Western New York*, and the *Buffalo Medical and Surgical Journal*. The number of the *Medical Press* for June, 1889, contains an exceedingly interesting valedictory editorial, in which Dr. Roswell Parke explains the excellent reasons for which the combination has been made. The result of this combination cannot, we think, fail to be advantageous to the medical profession of Western New York, which has already been ably represented in the two journals, but which must be better represented when all appearances of rivalry between them have disappeared.

The high character of both of these periodicals has always made them welcome visitors to the tables of their contemporaries, and it is a great satisfaction to know that their excellent qualities will hereafter be united in one journal which must be stronger and better than either could be alone.

BOOK REVIEWS.

[Any book reviewed in these columns may be obtained upon receipt of price, from the office of the REPORTER.]

THE PSYCHIC LIFE OF MICRO-ORGANISMS. A STUDY IN EXPERIMENTAL PSYCHOLOGY. By ALFRED BINET. Translated from the French by Thomas McCormack. Small 8vo, pp. xii, 121. Chicago: Open Court Publishing Company, 1889. Price, 75 cents.

This is one of the most interesting books which have come to our table for a long time. The author traces the manifestation of mental activity down into the very lowest forms of animal, and even to those of vegetable life. As an illustration, he says of the hunter Infusoria, that they are constantly running about in quest of prey; but this constant pursuit is not directed toward one object any more than another. They move rapidly hither and thither, changing their direction every moment, with the part of the body bearing the battery of trichocysts held in advance. When chance has brought them in contact with a victim, they let fly their darts and crush it; at this point of the action they go through certain manœuvres that are prompted by a guiding will. It very seldom happens that the shattered victim remains motionless after direct collision with the mouth of its assailant. The hunter, accordingly, slowly makes his way about the scene of action, turning both right and left in search of his lifeless prey. This search lasts a minute at the most, after which, if not successful in finding his victim, he starts off once more to the chase and resumes his irregular and roving course.

In like manner the author discusses a variety of phenomena which indicate purposive actions in protozoans and microphytes. His book is admirably conceived, and excellently written, and cannot fail to interest those who have any inclination to study the powers and possibilities of beings below us in the scale of life.

LITERARY NOTES.

—The *Weekly Medical Review*, of St. Louis, Mo., announces that beginning with the first issue in July it will appear in a new dress, and be enlarged to the size of the *New York Medical Journal*. The subscription price will remain unchanged.

—William Blaikie, author of "How to Get Strong, and How to Stay So," and "Sound Bodies for our Boys and Girls," will write, in *Harper's Magazine* for July, upon the question: "Is American Stamina Declining?" and will make a number of practical suggestions for reforming our system of education in the direction of physical training.

NOTES AND COMMENTS. ¶

The Purification of Sewage.

Science, April 12, 1889, says the plan proposed by Mr. W. Webster, for the purification of sewage by electrolytic methods, has been tried on a large scale, and with encouraging results. The process is very simple, and is described by the *London Electrician* as follows: "The color, density, and constitution of the London sewage varies from hour to hour in the most extraordinary manner; but the first sample to be dealt with was of a light-yellow color, looking something like weak tea with a little milk in it, but, so far as could be seen, it contained very little solid matter in mechanical suspension. This having been poured into a test-jar, a current was passed through it between a pair of iron electrodes, with about six volts electro-motive force. An extremely rapid effect was produced. In less than two minutes the jar was seen to be filled with a flocculent precipitate, which was gradually carried upward by the bubbles of liberated hydrogen. After about three minutes, the electrodes were withdrawn, and the precipitate left to collect at the top. In actual practice, after the effluent has passed into the settling-tank, the precipitate, in the course of about two hours, loses the whole of the entangled hydrogen; it then sinks to the bottom of the tank. The sludge thus formed is similar to that produced by the chemical processes now in use, except that the electrical method possesses the obvious advantage that the total quantity of material has not been increased by the addition of chemicals." But, besides this precipitation, there is an action on the organic matters in solution which robs them of their unpleasant and harmful properties. In the larger experiments, carried on at Crossness, two 20-horse-power engines are used, with an Edison-Hopkinson dynamo. Iron plates are placed in the shoot through which the sewage is discharged. In travelling along the shoot, every particle of the sewage comes in contact with the plates, and finally the whole is received into the settling-tanks. With 27 horse-power, it is possible to treat a million gallons of sewage in twenty-four hours. The consumption of iron in actual working is about two grains per gallon. Taking a town with a daily flow of ten million gallons of sewage a day—corresponding to a population of about 300,000—the consumption of iron should not exceed 304 tons per annum, and the steam-plant required would be about 250. This plant takes the place of the mixing-tanks, machinery, and chemicals employed in the chemical process for the purification of sewage; and, if such electrical plant is designed to meet the peculiar requirements of the district, it should cost less than any other method, besides precipitating and purifying in one operation.

Bicarbonate of Sodium and Bichloride of Mercury in the Treatment of Yellow Fever.

In the *Therapeutic Gazette*, August 15, 1888, Dr. George M. Sternberg suggested the use of bicarbonate of sodium and bichloride of mercury in the treatment of yellow fever. At Decatur, Florida, in the following October, the yellow fever prevailing was of a most malignant type: of 10 physicians practising in the infected area, 9 had yellow fever and 5 died. The treatment referred to was then tried. In the *Gazette* for May 15, 1889, Dr. Sternberg states that 32 white and 32 colored patients were subjected to the treatment by four physicians; of this number, only 4 died—all white. Dr. Mitchell writes from Jacksonville that he treated in all 216 cases of yellow fever, and that the mercury and soda gave the best results. As the result of experience with the bichloride and alkaline treatment, Dr. Sternberg suggests for further trial the following formula, which is a modification of the one first suggested:

    Sodii bicarb. . . . . ʒ iv
    Hydrarg. chlor. corros. . . . gr. ss
    Aquæ puræ . . . . Oii
    M. Sig. One and three-fourths ounces every hour; to be given *ice cold*.

Important Notice to the Medical Profession.

The Department of the Interior, Census Office, at Washington, has just issued a circular calling attention to the fact that Dr. John S. Billings, Surgeon U. S. Army, has consented to take charge of the Report on the Mortality and Vital Statistics of the United States as returned by the Eleventh Census.

As the United States has no system of registration of vital statistics, such as is relied upon by other civilized nations for the purpose of ascertaining the actual movement of population, our census affords the only opportunity of obtaining even an approximate estimate of the birth and death rates of much the larger part of the country, which is entirely unprovided with any satisfactory system of State and municipal registration.

In view of this, the Census Office, during the month of May, 1889, will issue to the medical profession throughout the country "Physician's Registers" for the purpose of obtaining more accurate returns of deaths than it is possible for the enumerators to make. It is earnestly hoped that physicians in every part of the country will co-operate with the Census Office in this important work. The record should be kept *from June 1, 1889, to May 31, 1890*. Nearly 26,000 of these registration books were filled up and returned to the office in 1880, and nearly all of them were used for statistical purposes. It is hoped that double this number will be obtained for the Eleventh Census.

Physicians not receiving Registers can obtain them by sending their names and addresses to the "*Census* Office," Washington, D. C., and, with the Register, an official envelope which requires no stamp will be provided for their return to Washington.

If all medical and surgical practitioners throughout the country will lend their aid, the mortality and vital statistics of the Eleventh Census will be more comprehensive and complete than they have ever been. Every physician should take a personal pride in having this report as full and accurate as it is possible to make it. It is promised that all information obtained through this source shall be held strictly confidential.

Quinine Rash.

At the meeting of the Clinical Society of London, March 8, 1889, Dr. Burney Yeo gave an account of several attacks of a quinine rash which he had personally experienced. The first attack occurred in August, 1887, while he was taking two grains of quinine three times a day for a cold in the head; the second about two months afterward, when taking quinine in the same doses for the same purpose; the third, in Rome, in January, 1888, after a single dose of three grains. The true nature of the eruption was not suspected in the first attack, and doubted in the second, as the author had repeatedly taken quinine during former attacks of coryza without any such manifestations. Thinking there might be some impurity in the quinine, the author in May last obtained a different sample, the purity of which was vouched for, and, after taking two doses of three grains each, the rash shortly made its appearance as before.

Some time afterward he again tested himself by a very small dose, hoping thereby to establish a tolerance of the drug, but a single dose of a quarter of a grain was rapidly followed by precisely the same cutaneous manifestations. The eruption, which the author fully described, assumed the same character and distribution on each occasion, and was of an erythematous nature, in patches of various sizes and forms, most of them a little raised above the surface. A remarkable fact was that on every occasion it was strictly limited to the lower extremities, extending up to the groins, but never passing beyond that limit. There was no constitutional disturbance. The author having referred briefly to the history of quinine rashes, concluded the paper with some interesting reflections and inferences on the remarkable fact that a drug which had been for years, and quite recently, perfectly tolerated, should suddenly in the same person cause such decided cutaneous disorder, and in such minute doses. In answer to a question by Dr. Powell, whether any actual febrile phenomena attended the rash, Dr. Yeo stated that no febrile phenomena had accompanied the appearance of the rash; and that he had experienced no other symptoms of quinine poisoning, and no tenderness of the skin. The eruption was disagreeable at night. He mentioned a case in which similar symptoms had followed the ingestion of a dose of salicylate of soda. He pointed out that the effects of quinine varied very much according to the form in which it was given. When given in the solid form it sometimes proved unsuccessful, while it gave excellent results when administered in the form of an effervescing draught.—*British Med. Journal*, March 16, 1889.

Ice-bags in the Night-Sweats of Phthisis.

Prof. Rosenbach, of Breslau, recommends in the *Berliner klin. Wochenschrift*, No. 15, 1889, the use of ice-bags for the night-sweats of phthisical patients. These bags, moderately filled, are laid during several hours of the night upon the abdomens of the patients. This remedy, he says, is generally well borne, especially by those patients who have a rise of temperature in the evening, and is of service in many cases in which atropine and the dusting of the body with powdered salicylic acid have failed. The bags, he says, can be used for many nights without harm to the patient.

Execution by Electricity.

The Philadelphia *Evening Telegraph*, June 10, says: The appeal made by Kemmler's counsel from the decision of the Buffalo Courts, on the ground that electric execution is "cruel and unusual," will be supported by many electricians of this city, some of whom, it was rumored to-day, are so opposed to the new method of execution that they have opened their purses to pay counsel fees to the condemned man's lawyers. A large number of electricians were interviewed this morning on the main feature of the appeal, namely, that "electrocution is cruel." Every one of them said that the new method is not only cruel, but extremely uncertain. Ralph W. Pope, Secretary of the American Institute of Electrical Engineers, said: "This killing by electricity will prove to be more cruel than hanging, shooting, beheading, or any modern civilized method of execution, because it is the most uncertain, and the criminal must undergo more protracted mental agony during the preparations. We do not know yet just what amount of electricity will kill a subject. Different individuals have different powers of resistance, and not only that, but the power of resistance in the same man may vary very greatly within half an hour or less. Take Kemmler, for instance. A half hour before turning on the presumably fatal current he is 'tested.' There is no assurance of the correctness of this test.

"Of course the sure method would be to apply tremendous pressure, 5,000 volts or more. But then it is extremely possible that the body would be horribly mutilated in that case. It is not difficult to imagine the preliminary sufferings of the man. He must sit in the chair in an agony of expectation, while the executioner and his assistants are running about for an hour or more preparing the apparatus, he not knowing at what moment the current might be turned on; and then suppose, as may happen, that the shock should not prove fatal."

Creosote Pills.

In the *Gazette Hebdomadaire*, May 10, 1889, Dr. Charles Éloy gives the following formula for making creosote pills, which are useful especially when cough and diarrhœa exist:

Creosote . . . . gr. xxx
Acetate of lead . . . . . . gr. iv
Extract of opium . . . . . . gr. iii
Syrup
Gum arabic āā q.s. ad faciendas pil. No. c.

Administration of Belladonna in Whooping-Cough.

Dr. Éloy writes in the *Gazette Hebdomadaire*, May 3, 1889, that belladonna may be administered during the catarrhal period, during the spasmodic stage, and in the decline of whooping-cough.

In the catarrhal period it is useful to combine with it other calmatives. Simon recommends the following formula :

```
Tincture of belladonna
Tincture of aconite root . . . . āā gtt. x
Cherry laurel water  . . . . . f ℥ iiss
Lime (fruit) water     . .      f ℥ iii
Syrup of lettuce . .    . . . . f ℥ i
M.  Sig.  Spoonful every three hours.
```

In the spasmodic stage, following Hufeland and Trousseau, Vienna physicians prescribe the powder of belladonna.

For small children, Bamberger gives morning and evening one of the following powders :

```
Powder of belladonna root . . . . gr. iss
White sugar . . . . . . . . . . gr. lxxv
M.  Div. in pulv. No. x.
```

To older children, Monti administers two or three times a day one of the following powders :

```
Belladonna root . . . . . . . gr. iss
Bicarbonate of soda
Pulverized white sugar . . . āā gr. xxiii
M.  Div. in pulv. No. x.
```

Belladonna may also, as suggested by Monti, be combined in a powder with quinine, of which he gives two or three a day :

```
Powdered belladonna root . . . gr. iss
Sulphate of quinine  .    . . gr. viiss
Powdered white sugar . . .  gr. xxx
M.  Div. in pulv. No. x.
```

The tincture of belladonna may be administered pure—following the example of Bamberger and giving from two to fifteen drops a day, in three or four doses according to the age of the patient, watching the state of the pupil and for symptoms of poisoning—or in the following draught :

```
Tincture of belladonna . . . . gtt. ii–vi
Gum julep . . . . . . . f ℥ ii
M.  A coffeespoonful every two hours.
```

In the intense form, Ellis recommends extract of belladonna, and especially the following mixture :

```
Extract of belladonna . . . . . gr. ⅓
Bromide of potash . . . . . gr. ⅚
Syrup of poppy . . . . .  . gtt. xv
Water . . . . . . . . . ♍ lxxv .
M.  For one dose.
```

This dose is increased, if necessary, up to five-sixths of a grain of the extract a day, if it is well borne, watching closely the action of the remedy.

In the period of decline, it is still proper to prescribe belladonna, according to M. Simon, but in association with tonics—cod liver oil, iodide of iron, and quinine.

Some Abuses of Etherization.

In a paper on this subject in the New York *Medical Record*, Feb. 23, 1889, Dr. George F. Shrady recommends the following precautions in order to avoid many of the abuses of anæsthesia:

1. In commencing the administration of ether the gradual method is to be preferred.

2. Its employment allows the lungs to empty themselves of residual air, prevents coughing and struggling, and places the organs in the best possible condition to receive and rapidly utilize the ether vapor.

3. After the stage of primary anæsthesia is reached, the more pure ether vapor the patient breathes the better.

4. The shorter the time of anæsthesia, and the smaller the amount of ether used, the less likely are the unpleasant sequelæ to occur.

5. The more evenly it is administered the less shock to the patient.

6. Anæsthesia should be entrusted to experienced administrators only.

7. Many of the fashionable efforts to resuscitate patients are not only useless but harmful.

8. The minimum amount of force should be employed to restrain the muscular movements of the patient.

9. Mixed narcosis is often advisable for prolonged operations.

10. The utility of the galvanic battery, in threatened death, is yet to be proven.

11. The most trustworthy means of resuscitating desperate cases are artificial respiration, hypodermic stimulation, inhalation of nitrite of amyl, and inversion of the body.

Strophanthus for Dyspnœa.

Demme, according to the *Deutsche med. Wochenschrift*, April 11, 1889, has recommended the use of strophanthus in the case of children affected with dyspnœa in the course of chronic nephritis, in bronchial asthma, and in whooping cough, and also to obviate dropsy in conditions of low blood pressure. He gives three drops (of the tincture) four or five times a day, and says that as a rule strophanthus should not be given to children under five years of age.

Bichloride of Mercury in Anæmia.

Dr. A. M. Cartledge, Demonstrator of Anatomy in the Kentucky School of Medicine, contributes a paper on bichloride of mercury in anæmia to the *American Practitioner and News*, May 11, 1889. He believes mercury has the power of causing absorption of lymph deposits and of relieving glandular engorgement.

In the anæmia of women the subject of disease connected with the organs of generation, he says he knows of no one constitutional remedy the equal of mercury. Nearly all of these cases are the subject of lymph deposits and ovarian congestion, which is best met by an agent which so decidedly facilitates healthy gland action. In the chlorosis which is so often a manifestation of struma, he says the bichloride of mercury with iron will often effect a cure where iron alone fails. The great good mercury does, especially as calomel, in relieving acute glandular engorgement, is appreciated. What he thinks we need most to be impressed with is its great virtue in relieving those often obscure and chronic obstructions to gland action which exert so potent an influence for evil in the economy.

Treatment of Rheumatism.

At the meeting of the Clinical Society of London, April 16, 1889, Dr. W. N. Maccall read a paper upon the treatment of the various forms of rheumatism. After reviewing the previous treatment of acute rheumatism, during the last twenty-five years, Dr. Maccall considered the value of the present routine treatment by salicylic acid and its allies or derivatives under the following headings: 1. In relieving pain and lessening fever in acute rheumatism, the salicyl treatment is undoubtedly the most effective known. 2. The salicylates do not prevent the rare complication of hyperpyrexia, and are absolutely useless in its treatment. 3. It is doubtful if they prevent endocardial or pericardial troubles, the percentage remaining about the same (50 per cent.) since the salicyl treatment as before. They seem to have no influence in curing these troubles when they do occur. 4. There is no proof that the salicylates prevent relapse. 5. It is not proved that the salicylates lessen the duration of the disease, nor that they prevent anæmia. With regard to the particular form of the remedy, most writers recommend, and Dr. Maccall agrees with them, salicylate of soda in twenty-grain doses, at first every hour for three or four hours, according to circumstances. It should be continued in diminishing doses for at least eight or ten days after all pain and pyrexia have ceased, and in most cases should be followed by iron. Salicylic acid, salicin, and salol may be tried in exceptional cases where the soda salt is not well borne. In young children, antipyrin may be substituted with advantage. In convalescence, Sir A. Garrod's alkaline mixture followed by iron was recommended; and if any joint remain stiff or swollen, blistering or painting with iodine is useful.—*British Med. Journal*, May 4, 1889.

Abortive Treatment of Gonorrhœa after Cocaine Anæsthesia.

A member of the Society of Medicine and Pharmacy of Isère treats gonorrhœa in the following way (*Jour. de la Soc. de Méd. et de Phar. de l'Isère*, Dec., 1888): He first washes out the urethra with a large amount of aseptic water, and then fills it with a ten-per-cent. cocaine solution. After leaving this injection in for about five minutes it is allowed to escape, and what remains is washed out with more sterilized water.

The urethra now being anæsthetized, an aqueous solution of silver nitrate, of the strength of 1 to 25, is injected into the urethra as far as any inflammation is supposed to exist. This application, he says, neither produces nor is followed by any pain.

The complete removal of the cocaine solution is necessary, because of the incompatibility between the silver solution and the hydrochlorate.

As the discharge lessens, a sulphate of zinc solution, 1 to 500, is generally indicated.—*Medical Analectic*, February 21, 1889.

A Large Bill.

A New York paper states that the estate of a late eminent statesman and lawyer is about to be sued for a bill of medical attendance covering visits over 2,200 in number, the value of which is placed at $143,350. If the question of overdue interest does not enter into the account, the average value of these services would be about $65.10 per visit. During a part of the time, however, the physician was in constant attendance upon his illustrious patient, and there is a strong presumption that he will be able to prove his case and win his bill.

Salicylates in Pruritus Senilis.

In one of his recent lectures, according to the *Wiener med. Presse*, May 5, 1889, Besnier recommended the treatment of pruritus senilis with the salicylates. In addition to bran baths, Besnier recommends washing of the body every evening with water to which two tablespoonfuls of the following solution have been added :

Carbolic acid . . . . ʒi
Aromatic vinegar . . . . . . f℥vi

Then the following powder is dusted on :

Salicylate of bismuth . . . . . ʒv
Starch . . . . ℥ii ʒviss

or :

Finely powdered salicylic acid . gr. cl
Starch . . . . ℥ii ʒviss

Treatment of Typhlitis.

Prof. Bouchard, according to the *Bulletin Médical*, April 24, 1889, says the indications are as follows: (1) to allay the pain; (2) to put the intestine at rest and reduce digestive fermentation to the minimum; (3) to ensure asepsis of the large intestine. The following are the proper procedures to fulfil these indications: 1. To allay pain, apply cataplasms, use mercurial and belladonna inunctions, and administer hypodermic injections of morphine. 2. For nourishment, use milk with an alkaline water or with the addition of yolk of egg; avoid solid or easily fermentible substances. As a laxative, to keep the intestine free, give a teaspoonful of magnesia in sweetened water, or a teaspoonful to a dessertspoonful of castor oil, avoiding violent purgatives. 3. To ensure asepsis of the intestines, wash out the large intestine twice a day with a quart of the following solution, heated to a temperature of 100° Fahr. :

Water . . . . f℥xxx
Borate of soda . . . . gr. lxxx
Tincture of benzoin,
Camphorated alcohol . . . . . āā ℳ lxxx

Fatal Injury from Base-ball.

At Dundee, Indiana, two base-ball players came into violent collision, and one of them received injuries which were fatal. It has long been an opprobrium of the English game of foot-ball that so grave—even fatal—injuries frequently result from the misdirected energies of its players; and now to have the American game brought into the same category would be little short of a calamity. The game is universally popular, has much in its favor as an athletic pastime, and is deserving of being so regulated as to be made free from danger to life and limb.

NEWS.

—It is reported that yellow fever exists at Vera Cruz.

—The German Anatomical Society will hold its third meeting in Berlin early in October, 1889.

—Professor Virchow is reported to be engaged in rewriting his great work on Cellular Pathology.

—Prof. Wilhelm Bunsen has resigned his position as Professor of Chemistry in the University of Heidelberg.

—The New York *Medical Record*, June 8, 1889, says that a new case of leprosy is reported to be at the Harlem Hospital.

—The death is reported of Dr. R. Ultzmann, Extraordinary Professor of Diseases of the Urinary Organs in the University of Vienna.

—A man named Hughes, who visited the scene of the disaster at Armagh, Ireland, was so horrified at the sight that he died on the spot.

—Dr. John W. Pearce, of Oxford, Ala., died May 26, at the age of 62 years. He was graduated at the Georgia Medical College in 1857.

—Professor Breisky, of Vienna, the well-known obstetrician, died recently of carcinoma of the sigmoid flexure of the colon. He was fifty-seven years old.

—Dr. J. E. Kunkler, of San Francisco, died in that city May 10, of cancer of the throat. Dr. Kunkler was graduated from the University of the Pacific, now Cooper Medical College, in 1863.

—Professors Virchow, von Bergmann and Waldeyer, the committee entrusted with making arrangements for the International Medical Congress, which meets in Berlin next year, have already held a preliminary meeting.

—Dr. James F. Foulkes died in Oakland, California, May 22, 1889, of diabetes mellitus. Dr. Foulkes studied at Princeton College, New Jersey, and was graduated in medicine from the Jefferson Medical College, in 1852.

—Dr. Lindley, one of the Editors of the *Southern California Practitioner*, has been sued for $20,000 on account of alleged malpractice. The complaint states that in an obstetrical case (one of version) an assistant of the Doctor's, in moving the patient on the bed, dislocated her shoulder.

HUMOR.

"THERE IS SUCH A THING as carrying a choke too far," as a Colorado horse-thief remarked at a neck-tie social.—*Drake's Magazine.*

PROUD FATHER (showing off his boy before company)—"My son, which would you rather be, Shakespeare or Edison?" Little Son (after meditation)—"I'd rather be Edison." "Yes? Why?" "'Cause he ain't dead."—*New York Weekly.*

PLAYWRIGHT—"It seems to me that if I had a better title for my drama it would have more success." His Friend—"Call it 'Anti-Fat.'" Playwright—"Why so?" Friend—"I see it has reduced the audience more than one-half in less than an hour."—*Terre Haute Express.*

TO BUILD UP HIS SYSTEM.—Dr. Schmerz.—"The trouble, Mr. Tyers, is that you don't take enough exercise." Mr. E. Z. Tyers. "Aw, I confess I don't go in vewy heavy on athletics, doctaw. What could you wecommend as a mild exercise to begin on?" Dr. Schmerz. "H'm! You might stretch your arms over your head when you yawn!"—*Puck.*

———◆●◆———

OBITUARY.

JAMES ETHELBERT MORGAN, M.D.

Doctor J. E. Morgan, of Washington, D. C., died at his residence, on the morning of June 2, of Bright's disease. Dr. Morgan was born in St. Mary's County, Maryland, September 25, 1822. He was a descendant of the Morgan and the Cecil families of England. His collegiate education was received at St. John's College, Md. He was graduated in medicine at the Medical Department of the Columbian University, Washington, in 1845, and immediately entered into active practice. Shortly after graduation he was appointed Demonstrator and Assistant to the Professor of Anatomy in the University. In 1852, Dr. Morgan was selected as Professor of Physiology in the Medical Department of the University of Georgetown. This position he resigned in 1858, and, at the earnest solicitation of the Faculty, he accepted the chair of Materia Medica and Medical Jurisprudence, which he held until the re-organization of the Faculty in 1876, when, with Drs. Noble Young, Johnson Eliot and Flodoardo Howard, he retired from active participation in the College duties to become Emeritus Professor.

As a lecturer, Dr. Morgan was clear and forcible, and is affectionately remembered by the hundreds of students who graduated under his teachings. Among the official positions he has held may be mentioned, those of Physician to the Washington Asylum and Small-pox Hospital; member of the Board of Aldermen; member of the Board of Health of the District of Columbia; trustee of the Public Schools; Surgeon-in-charge of the Soldiers' Rest; Surgeon-in-Chief to the Quartermaster's Hospital, Washington, from 1861 to 1865. At the breaking out of the war he was appointed Colonel of the 4th Regiment, D. C. Vols. Dr. Morgan was a member of the Medical Association and of the Medical Society, D. C., and of the American Medical Association, having held various offices in each of them.

In 1854, he married Nora, the daughter of William Dudley Diggs, of Maryland, who, with six children, survives him.

Dr. Morgan's published papers are few, and consist for the most part of addresses before the College to which he was attached, and at the medical societies of which he was a member. He retired from active practice some time ago, but was very frequently sought in consultation, especially by the younger members of the profession, to whom he freely gave the results of his ripe experience. Dr. Morgan possessed a large frame and a vigorous constitution, and only a few weeks ago was apparently a well and hearty man.

His death adds another name to the already long list of losses which have befallen the medical profession of Washington. L. E.

———

JAMES B. HUNTER, M.D.

Dr. James B. Hunter, the well-known surgeon, died at his home in New York, June 10, after an illness of six weeks. Dr. Hunter occupied several prominent positions, having been Attending Surgeon to the Woman's Hospital, Surgeon to the New York Cancer Hospital, of which he was one of the founders, Consulting Surgeon to the New York Infirmary for Women and Children, and Professor of Diseases of Women at the New York Polyclinic. He was a member of various medical societies, and made numerous valuable contributions to current medical literature.

MEDICAL AND SURGICAL
REPORTER

No. 1687. PHILADELPHIA, JUNE 29, 1889. VOL. LX.—No. 26.

CONTENTS:

COMMUNICATIONS.

REPORT OF A CASE OF STRICTURE OF THE RECTUM, THE PROBABLE RESULT OF A SPECIFIC VAGINITIS.

BY LEWIS H. ADLER, JR., M.D.,
LATE RESIDENT PHYSICIAN, UNIVERSITY HOSPITAL,
PHILADELPHIA, PENNA.

The usual causes of stricture of the rectum —when not carcinomatous in nature—are: syphilitic infection; traumatism, in the shape of the introduction of foreign bodies; the careless use of clyster-pipes; and the various operations upon the mucous coat of the bowel, as well as any inflammation or ulceration arising in other ways. *Both gonorrhœal* and *leucorrhœal* discharges may become potent factors in producing this painful affection. Such was the only assignable cause of the stricture in the following case, which I wish to record :—

Mrs. S. H. M.; aet 27; white; a widow, whose occupation was that of a housekeeper, was admitted into the University Hospital in November, 1888, suffering, as she stated, with a lacerated perineum and some rectal trouble, which gave her intense pain every time she had a movement of the bowel. Her family history was good, and showed no evidence of malignant disease, either of the rectum or elsewhere. As a child, she had the various diseases of childhood ; otherwise she was healthy. She first menstruated at 13, and was always regular—she was married at 16, and two years later left her husband, owing to family trouble. Two children were the result of this union. The last child was born in the early part of 1879. Both labors were difficult. Instruments were resorted to in the delivery of the first child. Both children presented by the head. It was in the first labor that she was torn, and she thinks the tear was increased at the birth of the last child.

She suffered more or less from this trouble, owing to the loss of control over the contents of the bowels; but by means of anodynes and careful diet she managed to keep costive. Every two or three weeks she would take an aperient. She was advised to have an operation performed, but refused. Such was her condition up to three years before her admittance into the hospital, under the care of Professor Wm. Goodell.

Her present trouble began in 1885. At the solicitation of a man in the town in which she lived, she had sexual intercourse with him, which resulted in a violent attack of specific vaginitis. Not long after this trouble began, the movements of her bowels caused more pain than ever—so much so, that the thought of going to stool would drive her wild with fear. Instead of resorting now to anodynes, and a diet that would produce hardened feces, she did all in her power to render them easy of passage.

She grew steadily worse, and, though advised to come to the city and undergo an operation, she steadfastly refused. Her stools were now typical of stricture of the rectum. It was not until the end of 1888, when life had become more than a burden, that she consented to come to the city and have Dr. Goodell examine her. An examination made at this time revealed a complete tear of the perineum through the sphincter ani muscle, and a stricture of the rectum of moderate width near the anus. Its lumen was very much contracted, barely admitting the end of a finger. From the dense, fibrous feel of the stricture, it evidently involved all three coats of the intestine.

The treatment in this case was general, as well as local. The pain from the stricture was allayed, in a measure, by cocaine which was used most efficaciously in the form of a suppository, and the bowels were kept in a soluble condition by regulating the diet, and by the administration from time to time of enemata or of mild laxatives. Medicines of a tonic character were freely exhibited.

After one week's stay in the hospital the woman was etherized, and the stricture was forcibly dilated by means of fingers, by Dr. Goodell. An opium suppository was inserted, to allay pain after the stretching had been completed.

The treatment now resorted to in order to restore the part to its normal calibre was the introduction of well oiled bougies every second or third day and finally every day. Previous to their use, a suppository of cocaine was inserted in the rectum, and this did much to prevent pain, though it did not entirely stop it. The cocaine was also used before and after each movement of the bowels. Iodoform suppositories, containing 2½ grains each, were ordered to be inserted both night and morning, in order to disinfect the parts as much as possible.

Not quite a month after the forcible dilation of the stricture, under ether, the patient was discharged and advised to continue the above treatment and come back to the hospital in the course of a month or so. At that time she was able to have a stool

with comparative comfort; the feces passed being nearly of normal calibre.

Dr. Goodell does not intend to operate upon the tear of the perineum until the stricture is fully dilated. At the present writing the woman has not presented herself at the hospital, but when last heard from through her family physician, she was doing well.

It is true that hardened feces may occasion stricture; but the history of this woman, whose bowels of necessity had been kept costive ever since her first child was born—that is for over eight years before the stricture appeared—seems to show that this is not necessarily the case. It is equally true, that a stricture may exist for months and years, without causing a patient any uneasiness,[1] but this is the exception to the rule; and I, therefore, take it that, in the case just described, the evidence points to a specific origin of the stricture.

41 N. Twelfth St.

VALVULAR INCOMPETENCY DUE TO BLOOD STATE AND SIMULATING UNCOMPENSATED ORGANIC DISEASE; DISAPPEARING UNDER IRON AND ARSENIC.

BY FRED. JENNER HODGES, B.Sc., M.D.,

HOUSE PHYSICIAN, COOK COUNTY HOSPITAL, CHICAGO.

History.—On May 5, 1889, William Zellar, a German laborer, single, aged 45, was admitted to the Cook County Hospital, suffering from chronic diarrhœa and marked anæmia. His mother died of cancer of the uterus; his further family history was negative. The patient states that he usually drinks a pint of beer daily, but denies having had any venereal disease, although he has had sore throat at various times. At the age of 12, his spine gradually became curved, forming a marked scoliosis, with the convexity to the left. The curvature begins at about the third and terminates with the eleventh or twelfth dorsal vertebra, and at the point of its greatest deviation is about four inches from the median line. The sternum is also deflected to the left. The curvature never caused pain, and soon became—as it has since remained—stationary.

Present Illness.—Some time before last Christmas the patient began to have a rather profuse diarrhœa; often having from three

[1] Thos G. Morton, M.D., and Henry M. Wetherill, M.D., Pepper's System of Medicine, Vol. II., p. 886.

to six or more, thin yellowish or brownish passages a day, and this condition continued up to the time of his admission. At about the same time he began to be troubled with dyspnœa on the slightest exertion, and had a heavy sensation in the epigastrium, aggravated by taking food. For two weeks he has been unable to retain solid food, and has noticed that his feet have been swollen at night.

Examination.—Temp. 97.8°; pulse 96°, abrupt but compressible; respiration . 20 per minute, with some orthopnœa. Patient complains of little or no pain; has no cough; passes urine easily and in fair quantity; but cannot sleep on account—as he says—of nervousness. To the eye the patient presents the familiar picture suggested by the word,—"cachectic." He has little or no adipose tissue, and but slight muscular development; he has pallid or blueish mucous membranes, and a tawny, yellowish skin, but no discoloration of the conjunctivæ. His respiratory sounds are weak; otherwise the examination of his lungs is negative. The splenic area is enlarged. Firm pressure over liver causes some pain.

At the apex of the heart a systolic blowing murmur can readily be recognized, and less easily a presystolic murmur. At the base, along the left side of the sternum, the systolic murmur may be recognized as well as a marked accentuation of the second sound, with some roughening. Over the arteries of the neck a short distinctly double second sound is heard, while the veins give a pronounced hum. Compression of the veins causes, on the proximal side of the compressing finger, a marked accumulation of blood, pulsating strongly.

Microscopic examination of the blood shows a marked relative increase [1] of white corpuscles. The red corpuscles are very irregular in shape and size, the round form being the exception, while the majority are oval, and not a few have irregular prolongations. As to size, the majority are—as compared with specimens from a half dozen other sources—nearly a fourth larger than normal.

Treatment.—Two or three drachm doses of bismuth subnitrate, given in milk, sufficed to check completely the diarrhœa of five months' standing, and the patient was, at the same time, put upon moderate doses of digitalis for two days, to make possible a more satisfactory examination of the heart. This examination however only served to

[1] Actual proportion could not be determined from lack of proper instruments.

confirm the results of the former one. Anæmia being so marked a feature of the case, the digitalis was replaced by a mixture containing ten drops of Fowler's solution, and two and one-half grains of Valet's mass, given after meals. The patient had before complained of dizziness upon attempting to stand, and, as such attacks began to recur, he received drachm doses of the fluid extract of ergot every four hours for a few days, with considerable benefit. The iron and arsenic were continued, however, with such intermissions as were necessary, for four weeks, with an obvious and continued improvement as regards the œdema, color and digestive symptoms. Having occasion at this time to examine the heart, I was not less gratified than surprised to find the sounds entirely normal, and that, where formally compression of the superficial cervical veins caused a proximal accumulation, showing pulsation, the accumulation now occurred on the distal side of the compressing finger, and of course exhibited no pulsation.

The patient has remained under observation up to the present time (June 12, 1889), but without the slightest abnormality of the heart sounds or any of the symptoms of an uncompensated heart lesion, which were so prominent upon his admission.

AN IMAGINARY TÆNIA.

BY SOLOMON SOLIS-COHEN, M.D.,
PHILADELPHIA.

Dr. J. Solis Cohen, in his work on Diseases of the Throat and Nasal Passages, published in 1879, records a case of hysteria, in which the epiglottis had been mistaken for a water-snake living in the œsophagus and paying an occasional visit to the mouth, physicians having sat by the patient for hours at a time, to watch it and try to catch it with forceps.

On May 25, 1889, Miss K. W., an hysterical patient, under my care for gouty kidney, called and informed me, with great seriousness, that the diet of milk and under done meat upon which she had been placed had given her a tape-worm; and that it came up in her throat and choked her; and she could feel it when she put her finger back. It felt broad and hard. On one occasion the finger came out bloody; and she was convinced that the worm had bitten her!

Laryngoscopic examination showed that the epiglottis was rather long, and that it had been subjected to a great deal of irritation, probably from the finger. Cocaine was applied, and the patient was assured that what she had felt belonged in her throat. In addition, appropriate treatment for globus hystericus was instituted.

SOME NEW INSTRUMENTS.

BY WM. S. FORBES, M.D.,

PROFESSOR OF ANATOMY AND OF CLINICAL SURGERY, IN THE JEFFERSON MEDICAL COLLEGE, PHILADELPHIA.

These instruments I placed before the Philadelphia County Medical Society at one of its meetings of late.

The forceps is represented about two-thirds actual size in Fig. A, 1. When applied to the severed extremity of a blood vessel, large or small, it arrests the flow of blood at once. The operator, leaving the forceps *in situ*, can proceed with his operation, undisturbed by hemorrhage, until he has completed his work, when he can apply a ligature more easily, safely and rapidly over the arched beak of the forceps than he can over the tenaculum or any other instrument I have ever used.

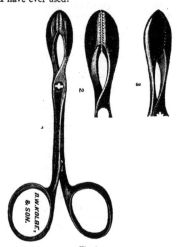

Fig A.

The surface on the curved beak of the forceps—represented at Fig. A, 2 & 3 of actual size, and in two different positions—over which the ligature glides to its destination on the vessel, has just the same curvature the tenaculum has where it penetrates the vessel and neighboring tissue, with its

point sticking up to wound the operator's fingers, while he is sending the knot home, and while the blood is still escaping.

The commonly used duck-bill forceps does not permit the ligature to glide over its extremity.

What time is lost in endeavoring to escape the extremity of the duck-bill forceps and place the ligature on the artery? How often does the assistant find his ligature on the extremity of the duck-bill forceps, and not on the artery?

I have used these forceps now, for some time, in abdominal work as well as in general surgical work, and I know of no other instrument that accomplishes so well the important object in view, of completely arresting hemorrhage and, at the same time, of allowing a ligature to be safely and rapidly applied.

Their smaller size, their lighter weight, and the exactness with which they can be applied to a bleeding point and allow a ligature to be easily placed, make them useful.

The saw which is represented at Fig. B, I devised for opening the vertebral canal

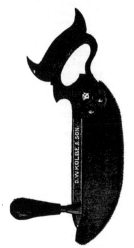

Fig. B.

throughout its entire extent, from the occiput down, in order to examine, *post mortem*, the spinal cord and its meninges.

I have found it to work easily and perfectly well.

1704 Walnut Street, Philadelphia.

SOCIETY REPORTS.

PHILADELPHIA NEUROLOGICAL SOCIETY.

Stated Meeting, April 22, 1889.

Held at the Hall of the College of Physicians. DR. WHARTON SINKLER, Vice-President, in the Chair.

Apparatus for Suspension for Spinal Disease.

DR. J. MADISON TAYLOR exhibited the apparatus devised by Dr. S. Weir Mitchell and used at the Infirmary for Nervous Disease in the treatment by suspension. In all the older forms of sling used in the treatment by suspension, the weight of the body rests chiefly on a support placed under the arm-pit. It is only possible to allow a very moderate amount of pull upon the head. The increasing pressure upon the axillary tissues so affects the bloodvessels of the arms as practically to cut off the pulse at the wrist, and the larger nerve trunks are very seriously affected. In the case of very heavy people, it is found that this becomes so grave a matter that the needed extension of the trunk is limited by the amount of their endurance of the pressure pain. Observing this, it occurred to Dr. Mitchell to apply the support under the elbows—a vastly more comfortable plan.

With this modification it has been found possible to extend the *séance* indefinitely— in certain instances to ten or even twenty minutes.

The adjustment of the head-support is made after the patient has been hoisted by the elbows. This is effected by one of the two plans described in the *Medical News*, April 13, 1889. We use more frequently the device which you see here. To the cheek piece, on each side of the head, a cord is attached which passes over hooks about fourteen inches apart and depends from the transverse bar, and thence passes downward and backward to the rear of each elbow-leather, and there is adjusted by a strap and buckle.

This mechanism may be very readily used in applying plaster jackets, by omitting to use the lower of the two encircling straps.

DR. J. P. C. GRIFFITH: There is a modification in this apparatus which I do not like. In the original form as adopted by Charcot, and described and illustrated in a recent number of *Le Progrès Médical*, the bar from which the straps are suspended is straight; not curved, as in the one here exhibited. This rod is provided with notches, and the tension of the head piece can be nicely graduated, by sliding the rings from one notch to another. The straps and buckles are serviceable for adjusting approximately the suspension of the head. A most delicate and accurate adjustment can then be procured by using the notches. Time is also saved in this way, where a number of cases have each day to be suspended from the same apparatus.

DR. TAYLOR, in reply to Dr. Griffith, said: I do not think that Dr. Griffith would like that method of elevating the head piece by means of sliding the rings over notches so well as this I have described, if he had any practical experience in using both. We have, and find this infinitely more comfortable. Also, if he had seen the second cross-bar and pulley attachment used, he would find it very nice to adjust and agreeable to the subject.

Exhibition of a Tumor of the Brain.

DR. JAMES HENDRIE LLOYD, said: I have here an interesting specimen of brain-tumor, for the opportunity of exhibiting which I am indebted to Dr. S. S. Stryker, of West Philadelphia. I never saw the patient in life. The autopsy was made by Dr. William E. Hughes. The history which I have gathered is as follows. The woman was 63 years of age, and twenty-five years ago had her first epileptic fit. This came on at the close of a period of great mental strain and physical effort in nursing her sick children, one of whom died. It was decided that she and a remaining child should go into the country for rest. At the end of a ride of twenty miles, on a hot summer day, she had her first fit. She was then about forty years of age. Since then she had more or less frequently repeated epileptic seizures. Dr. Stryker has had the case under observation since 1871. The case was regarded as one of epilepsy with more or less mental deterioration. Within the last year it was noted that there was some increase in the size of the head. The right side especially was bulging. The right eye was a little more prominent than the left. One week ago, she was taken with right sided hemiplegia which was spastic in character. The arm was kept tightly across the chest, and it was with difficulty that it could be straightened out.

At the autopsy, which was made to-day, we found that there was great thickening of the skull. I have here a section of the bone, which is fifteen-sixteenths of an inch in thickness. In some parts, the skull cut like cheese, and the bone was of a blueish color. A large tumor was found on the left side, between the temporo-sphenoidal and the under part of the frontal lobe. It is apparently sarcomatous in character. It has a gritty feeling, as though it contained sandy deposits. The neighboring convolutions have been hollowed out by the tumor. The upper surface of the left hemisphere was covered with dark coagulated blood, the immediate cause of death being sub-dural hemorrhage.

An interesting point about this case is that for twenty-five years this woman has been a confirmed epileptic, and has had gradually developing secondary changes in the skull. There is in this brain no evidences of pachymeningitis hemorrhagica. There is simply this history of epilepsy, with gradual failure of mental power, and gradual increase in the thickness of the skull. This case has not been studied with the view of localizing the growth. Dr. Stryker's diagnosis was a tumor of the brain, but he did not attempt to determine its situation. It is not possible, of course, to tell the structure of this tumor before a microscopic study of it is made. The long duration of the case is, to me, one of its remarkable features. Epilepsy coming on in middle life, as in this case, is usually due to some structural changes, as trauma, neoplasm, or degenerative processes. Can it be possible that this tumor, slowly growing, has been the cause of epileptic seizures for twenty-five years? In a table of one hundred cases of brain tumor appended to the paper on brain-tumor by Dr. Mills and myself, in the Am. Syst. of Medicine, the longest duration authentically reported was three years.

———●●●———

—Carpenter recently exhibited to the Hunterian Society of London a child three years old, born without an iris, and having very pronounced nystagmus. The eye was otherwise normal. The child presented another deformities consisting of a congenital pes equino-varus, which was operated on soon after birth. The mother had left internal strabismus, nystagmus, and complete absence of the iris. The mother and sister of the child are healthy, and the deformity is not present in either maternal or paternal grandparents.

NEW YORK ACADEMY OF MEDICINE.

Stated Meeting, June 6, 1889.

The President, ALFRED L. LOOMIS, M.D., in the Chair.

DR. P. A. MORROW read a paper on

Personal Observations of Leprosy in Mexico and the Sandwich Islands.

He began his remarks by saying that leprosy, to the majority of persons, possesses an historical interest only. They place it in the category of pestilences and plagues, which formerly devastated countries but which are now extinct. Unfortunately, however, leprosy can not fairly be thus regarded, for it is a living reality. In extent it embraces fully one third of the earth, and all varieties of climate and soil; it is present in India, China, Japan, Egypt and elsewhere in Africa, in South America, and in the islands of the Pacific, etc. Whenever it makes its appearance in a new country it can be traced to a human agent; it never originates spontaneously. It was, for instance, introduced into the Northwestern States by the Scandinavians, into California by the Chinese, into other places by the French. Dr. Morrow has learned, during his voyage of study, that there are also cases in Salt Lake City, which were brought by Mormon converts from the Sandwich Islands. Dr. Morrow saw a number of cases in Mexico, and half a dozen in the pest house at San Francisco; but the best place for studying the disease is in the Sandwich Islands. There it has been of comparatively recent introduction. There are many cases in the leper settlements, which afford a good opportunity for investigating the questions of heredity, contagion, etc.

The greatest advances in the study of the disease have been made in the past twenty-five years by modern methods. Our positive knowledge of it may be formulated as follows: It is a parasitic disease; the leper bacillus presents certain analogies with that of tuberculosis. Like the latter, it is endowed with remarkable vitality; like all specific microbes, it shows an affinity for certain fluids and solids of the human organism. It is found both in diffused and also in nodular infiltrations upon the skin and mucous membrane; it is abundant in the lymphatic glands and spaces; it is present in the liver, spleen, and testicles, and is abundant in the connective tissue and peripheral nerves. It is absent from the blood, the urine, and physiological secretions. It is present in vaccine pustules. The author said it originates only from persons affected with leprosy, and does not attach itself to the soil, water, air, or food. Leprosy has a more or less prolonged stage of incubation, varying from three to four years; and in some instances the stage is supposed to be prolonged twelve or fifteen years. It is slow and irregular in course, and progresses almost invariably to a fatal termination.

Belief in the contagiousness of leprosy was almost universal until, in 1867, the Royal College of Physicians of London expressed the view that it is not contagious; their dogma was very commonly accepted in Europe until recent years. In America, however, leading dermatologists do not accept the heresy of non-contagion. The history of its development in the Sandwich Islands affords the most striking evidence of contagion. Dr. Morrow has had an opportunity to examine a great many cases there, and his experience is like that of most others, namely, that in almost every instance one can get a history of exposure, either in sexual relations or by prolonged intimate contact. A fact of note is, that many of the helpers, usually relatives or friends of the afflicted, sent to the settlements and well when they went there, become lepers themselves after a time. Then there are foreigners who become lepers after a stay in the Sandwich Islands, although the disease is unknown in the country whence they come. The majority of cases probably develop from sexual contact; but in some instances it is due to contact with an abrasion of the skin or mucous membrane. One patient told Dr. Morrow that he had acquired leprosy from the bite of a leper; another said he had acquired it from sticking into his skin a pin which a leper had used in the same way. It seems to have been spread at points in the islands by vaccination with virus obtained probably from lepers. Dr. Morrow has had an opportunity to examine the criminal who had been condemned to death, and given a choice between the death penalty, and inoculation with leprosy virus and imprisonment for life. He chose the latter, was vaccinated in 1884, and for some time his case was thought to be negative; but now there are, to Dr. Morrow's mind, undoubted signs of leprosy; and he found the bacillus of leprosy in the tissues at the former seat of inoculation.

The speaker does not believe leprosy is directly hereditary in the sense that the bacillus is transmitted from parent to offspring; but he thinks a predisposition to the disease may be transmitted, just as in tuberculosis. There is no record of a case of congenital leprosy. The disease never manifests itself before the third or fourth year; the majority of cases develop between the thirtieth and fiftieth years. The disease shows a certain analogy to late hereditary syphilis. He believes that in nearly all cases of so-called hereditary leprosy a careful investigation will reveal contagion through intimate relations with the diseased after the child's birth.

Dr. Morrow threw on the screen photographs of individuals and groups of individuals affected with leprosy, whom he had seen in California and the Sandwich Islands. In one instance the tubercular infiltration involved the skin of the penis, a place in which it has been supposed never to manifest itself. Some of the patients had the tubercular, others the anæsthetic, and others mixed forms of the disease. Dr. Morrow thinks the anæsthetic form is slightly if at all contagious; and this fact accounts in part for the slight spread of leprosy in some communities in which it has gained an entrance. In some places the tubercular form predominates, in others the anæsthetic; but there are always a sufficient number of the tubercular or mixed varieties to keep up the contagion.

The Danger of the Spread of Leprosy in the United States.

This was the subject for general discussion, which was participated in by Drs. C. W. Allen, L. D. Bulkley, G. H. Fox, H. C. Piffard, R. W. Taylor, and P. A. Morrow. Drs. Allen, Piffard, and Morrow thought legislative action should be taken to prevent the entrance of lepers into the United States, and to cause segregation of those already here. Dr. Piffard thought quarantine laws should prevent their further admission, and that the general government might establish a hospital where such as chose could enter without cost; while enforced segregation, if necessary, could be carried out by the States. All the speakers admitted the contagiousness of the disease, but some thought the immediate danger not very great, and Dr. Fox expressed himself as decidedly opposed to creating any alarm. Leprosy, he said, does not spread in civilized countries; there are few cases here, the contagious element is very weak. We assume many other dangers of much greater gravity without any necessity for doing so; we are ten times as likely to get syphilis, and about as likely to get hydrophobia on account of the presence of dogs in our midst; yet that danger does not lead people to kill off all the dogs.

DR. MORROW said in reply to Dr. Fox that the Sandwich Islanders could no longer be regarded as barbarians; they are cleanly, and much less filthy and crowded than people in the New York tenements; yet leprosy prevails to an alarming degree there.

FOREIGN CORRESPONDENCE.

LETTER FROM BERLIN.

(FROM OUR SPECIAL CORRESPONDENT.)

On Hydracetin, the new Antipyretic and Analgesic.—Bronze Coloration in Miliary Tuberculosis.—The Latest Regarding Tuberculosis.—Singular Tolerance of Iodide of Potassium.

BERLIN, May 17, 1889.

In the last meeting of the Berliner Medicinische Gesellschaft, Dr. Guttmann read a highly interesting paper on *hydracetin*, the new antipyretic and analgesic. The drug is, chemically speaking, an acetylphenylhydracin, but as the mere enunciation of this appalling word might produce disastrous consequences in typhoid fever or neurotic disorders, hydracetin will do well enough. A still more felicitous designation for the new drug is the one adopted by English chemists, viz.: pyrodin. The drug, as presented by Dr. Guttmann to the Society, was a white crystalline powder, without taste and odor, soluble in water in the proportion of one to fifty, but easily soluble in acetic acid. . Experiments made on various animals show the toxicity of the drug even in small doses. Rabbits receiving 7 or 8 grains by the mouth, or injected into the peritoneum, perish in a day; in a single case even 4 grains proved fatal. A *post-mortem* examination made by Guttmann on five animals, revealed the following: Liver, spleen, and lungs were of a brown-red color; blood was present in the heart and in the vena cava, and the coloring matter of the blood, but no blood corpuscles, in the bladder. Microscopic sections of the kidneys and the liver showed a brown detritus in the vessels and urinary tubules, evidently the result of decomposition of red-blood corpuscles. The same toxic action results from the direct appli-

cation of the drug to the heart. The new chemical is a reducing agent, and its action is the result of its power to absorb oxygen.

Hydracetin shows even in small doses a powerful antipyretic action, as has been found by Guttmann in 8 cases of typhoid fever, 3 of consumption, 2 of scarlet fever, 1 each of erysipelas, acute miliary tuberculosis, and septicæmia. The average dose of the drug is two to three grains, though five grain doses have also been exhibited by Guttmann. All measurements of temperature on patients under the influence of hydracetin were made in the hours from 10 A.M. to 12 M., when no spontaneous fall of the fever was looked for. If two grains of the drug are given at about 10 o'clock in the morning and one and a half grains an hour later, the temperature begins to fall half an hour after the administration of the drug, and reaches its lowest level in two or three hours. The fall amounts to two or three degrees Centigrade—in some cases even to three or four degrees. The period of apyrexia lasts, however, but a short time, the temperature rising again with moderate slowness and regaining its former height in three to five hours. Perspiration sets in during the fall of temperature, as is the case with all other antipyretics, but disappears as soon as the lowest level has been reached. The frequency of pulse and respiration is lowered simultaneously with the fall of temperature. Regarding the affections themselves, the drug of course showed no influence whatever.

The action of hydracetin in acute articular rheumatism, as tested by Guttmann in eight typical cases, deserves the practitioner's special attention. A two-grain dose affords a distinct remission of pain, beginning one-half to one hour after the administration of the remedy, and lasting for several hours. A two-grain dose, given both in the forenoon and in the afternoon, suffices to remove the pain completely or, at least, to alleviate its severity. The analgesic action of hydracetin was found to be a constant one and did not fail in a single instance. This feature of promptness and reliability of course materially enhances the therapeutic value of the drug. Both its antipyretic and its analgesic action are to be ascribed to its reducing power. Guttmann then showed some interesting color reactions of the drug. Hydracetin, added to an alkaline solution of copper, precipitates the red suboxide of copper and when added to an alkaline solution of silver, precipitates metallic silver. If the crystals of hydracetin are dissolved in

$H_2SO_4 + HNO_3$ (sulphuric plus nitric acid) in the proportion of eight parts of the former to two of the latter, a beautiful red coloration appears immediately. In the urine of a person who had taken the drug for some time, only small quantities of reducing agents could be detected.

Guttmann obtained also gratifying results with the new remedy in two cases of psoriasis, employing a lanolin salve containing 10 per cent. of hydracetin. The first case was only of five days' standing, and was cured in seven days, inunctions having been used daily. Equally beneficial results were obtained in two cases of sciatica, where the analgesic action of the drug was found to be wonderfully prompt. Guttmann, in concluding his remarks, advocated further trials with this promising remedy; but he advised some caution in its internal exhibition, as he had noted in three cases pallor of the face after four-grain doses. This symptom—which, however, soon disappeared—Guttmann ascribes to the dissolution of the blood, produced by the drug, as proven by his experiments. In two-grain doses hydracetin is, in the author's opinion, a safe and welcome remedy for fevers, acute articular rheumatism, and neuralgia.

At the same meeting of the Society, Dr. Lehfeld showed interesting specimens of bronze coloration of the skin, occurring in connection with general miliary tuberculosis. The clinical history of the subject from whom the specimens were taken gives the following points: A young man, 18 years old, four weeks before his death, had loss of appetite, diarrhœa, fever, great emaciation, and an intense bronze coloration, especially noticeable on the extremities. The temperature and pulse were normal. The diagnosis was: Bronze coloration and intestinal tuberculosis. On the next day, the patient had intestinal cramps, became collapsed, and died on the following day. The autopsy showed that the heart was normal; in the superior anterior part of the right lung was an old cheesy focus, besides tubercular tracheitis. The abdominal organs showed miliary tuberculosis, the liver and kidneys being crowded with tubercles. The interior of the intestines showed follicular swelling, and the suprarenal capsule a complete cheesy degeneration.

The recent investigations of Dr. Cornet and Koch, of the Berlin Hygienic Institute, on the mode of propagation of the bacillus tuberculosis, followed by stringent police regulations concerning the treatment of consumptives and their sputa, have revived the interest in the therapeutics of consumption. This interest, though at no time extinct, has always had its periods of greater or less activity, in accordance with various accidental events. It will be opportune, therefore, to review at present the latest researches on this subject, as recorded in European journals. In the *Centralblatt für Bakteriologie*, No. 8, 1889, we find the experiments of Grancher and Gennes on the disinfection of the tubercle bacilli. These observers confirm the assertion of Petri, that the expired air of consumptives is not contagious. A one per cent. solution of corrosive sublimate produces a thorough disinfection of the sputa in twenty-four hours. The best and cheapest apparatus for the disinfection of spittoons, is that of Geneste and Herscher, which disinfects twenty-four spittoons in an hour by means of steam.

Of considerable interest is a recently published pamphlet of Dr. Petrescu, of Budapest, on the prevention of the contagiousness of consumptives. The author uses a Drechsel bottle (such as is used in chemical laboratories for the washing of gases), which he has transformed into an inhalator for volatile substances. The principle of this apparatus is the same as that of the Turkish Nargileh, or water smoking-pipe. Air having passed through sterilized cotton and the antiseptic contents of the bottle, is sucked up by means of an India-rubber tube. As contents of the bottle, Petrescu orders usually:

℞ Iodoform . . . . gr. xv
Eucalyptol,
Creasote,
Turpentine . . . . āā ℳxxx
Distilled water . . . . . . f℥iii
Sig. For two days' inhalation.

The idea of the author is to produce, by the prolonged antiseptic inhalations—extended over months and years—a saturation of the organism with microbicide substances, and thus to render the former an unfavorable soil for the development of the bacillus tuberculosis. In this manner he thought of exercising not only a prophylactic but also a curative influence over the tubercular process. But, unfortunately, such an assumption is an erroneous one, as real disinfection of the organism can never be attained by minimal doses of volatile agents, this bacillus having an extremely tenacious life. His apparatus, nevertheless, answers very well as an inhalator. Far more convenient, however, for obtaining the same result are the so-called "nasal capsules" of Feldbausch. The present desideratum in the therapeutics of tuberculosis is evidently not the prevention of the contagiousness of the sputum previous to expectoration, but after it. To effect this, however, stringent police regulations are a *conditio sine qua non.*

Of equal interest are the experiments of Prof. de Renzi, on the treatment of tuberculosis with hot air. He has formulated his results, obtained in eight cases 'of tuberculosis, as follows: 1. To produce beneficial effects the air must be of a temperature of 140° C. (284° F.). 2. The inhalations must be continued for one-quarter to one-half an hour. 3. The inhalations improve the general feeling, appetite, and innervation of the patients. 4. They also increase their bodily weight. 5. They are invariably well borne.

Prof. Mangardi has again taken up hydrofluoric acid as a remedy in tuberculosis, and publishes in some Italian journal very favorable results from its use.

The following note of a German military surgeon illustrates the great tolerance by some persons of iodide of potassium: A soldier emptied in 12 hours a bottle containing a solution of three hundred grains of iodide of potassium in eight fluid ounces of water, without experiencing any deleterious effects.

PERISCOPE.

Origin of the Yellow Fever on the "Boston" and "Yantic."

Dr. William M. Smith, the Health Officer of New York City, in his annual report to the Board of Commissioners of Quarantine, gives in some detail the history of the occurrence of yellow fever on the U. S. cruiser "Boston" and on the U. S. sloop-of-war "Yantic." Dr. Smith says that neither the "Boston" nor the "Yantic" received anything on board from the shore while at Port-au-Prince, except meal and fruit. The fruit, consisting of bananas and oranges, was taken to the vessels by natives, in what is called "bumboats," and sold to those on board. The main decks of the "Boston" and "Yantic" are so low, that communication between those on them and the "bumboats" was easy, and doubtless frequent, while the natives were vending their fruit. The wet, dirty, and sun-heated bottoms and timbers of the boats of the natives, exposed, as they must be at all times when at the shores or wharves, to an infected atmosphere as well as to the infected filth of the gutters that drain into the bay, certainly supply all the conditions necessary for the propagation of the infection. It would be rather a matter of surprise than otherwise, if the boats of the natives were not impregnated with the infection of yellow fever when it prevails at Port-au-Prince. The history of the disease on the "Boston" and the "Yantic" affords satisfactory evidence to Dr. Smith that the persons who suffered from it contracted the infection while at Port-au-Prince, and that the infection did not infect either vessel; in other words, that the infection was limited to the individuals who contracted the infection at that port.—*Science*, April 19, 1889.

Large Gumma in the Nostril.

Dr. S. G. Dabney reports the following case in the *American Practitioner and News*, Feb. 16, 1889:

Mr. B. was referred to me by Dr. A. M. Cartledge on the 10th of last November. He gave this history: was twenty-eight years old, married, and the father of several healthy children; he denied having had syphilis. Four or five weeks previous to his visit to me he noticed an obstruction in his right nostril; this had rapidly increased, until respiration through that side was prevented; there was sharp pain in the nose and over the whole of that side of the head. On examination I found a growth over the lower left turbinated bone, occluding that nostril and pressing against the septum. The growth was hard and sensitive to pressure; the surface toward the septum was ulcerated; the corresponding ala of the nose bulged outward. The lymphatic glands at the angle of the lower jaw and in the neck of the same side were enlarged, but no involvement was to be detected elsewhere. From the rapid growth, sharp pain, and implication of the neighboring glands, a malignant tumor seemed probable, all the more so, as the patient denied any taint of syphilis. Notwithstanding this, however, I prescribed fifteen grains of iodide of potassium three times a day, and soon increased the dose to thirty grains. No symptoms of iodism were produced, and the growth very rapidly disappeared; it seemed almost to melt away, thus establishing its syphilitic nature. The man afterward confessed that he had had a sore on his penis ten years before, and had taken some medicine which a doctor prescribed for him, but gave no further history of constitutional syphilis.

THE
MEDICAL AND SURGICAL
REPORTER.

ISSUED EVERY SATURDAY.

CHARLES W. DULLES, M.D.,
EDITOR AND PUBLISHER.

The Terms of Subscription to the publications of this office are as follows, payable in advance:

Med. and Surg. Reporter (weekly), a year, **$5.00**
Physician's Daily Pocket Record, - - 1.00
Reporter and Pocket Record, - - - - 6.00

All checks and postal orders should be drawn to order of

CHARLES W. DULLES,
N. E. Cor. 13th and Walnut Streets,
P. O. Box 843. Philadelphia, Pa.

☞SUGGESTIONS TO SUBSCRIBERS:
See that your address-label gives the date to which your subscription is paid.
In requesting a change of address, give the old address as well as the new one.
If your REPORTER does not reach you promptly and regularly, notify the publisher *at once*, so that the cause may be discovered and corrected.

☞SUGGESTIONS TO CONTRIBUTORS AND CORRESPONDENTS:
Write in ink.
Write on one side of paper only.
Write on paper of the size usually used for letters.
Make as few paragraphs as possible. Punctuate carefully. Do not abbreviate, or omit words like "the," and "a," or "an."
Make communications as short as possible.
NEVER ROLL A MANUSCRIPT! Try to get an envelope or wrapper which will fit it.
When it is desired to call our attention to something in a newspaper, mark the passage boldly with a colored pencil, and write on the wrapper "Marked copy." Unless this is done, newspapers are not looked at.
The Editor will be glad to get medical news, but it is important that brevity and actual interest shall characterize communications intended for publication.

THE MEETING OF THE AMERICAN MEDICAL ASSOCIATION.

The meeting of the American Medical Association, held in Newport this week, was attended by about seven hundred delegates and members. Owing to the fact that the place of meeting was so far in the East, the attendance included many physicians living east of the Allegheny Mountains, but there was a large number of western and southern men present.

One of the most interesting questions which came up for decision referred to the choice of an Editor for the *Journal* of the Association. This came directly before the Trustees; but the members of the Association—who are so deeply interested in the matter—did not leave the Trustees without such suggestions as might indicate their views as to the principles upon which a choice should be made. No Editor, however, was selected, and no change was announced in the editorial management. For Trustees of the *Journal*, the present incumbents were continued, with the exception of Dr. Hamilton and Dr. Moore, in whose stead Dr. W. W. Dawson, of Cincinnati, and Dr. I. N. Love, of St. Louis, were chosen.

Another interesting question related to the place for the next meeting. There was a general understanding that Philadelphia might be considered, if this would be agreeable to the profession in that city; but on mature consideration it was decided to meet in 1890 at Nashville, Tennessee.

Important amendments to the fundamental laws of the Association came before the meeting. The most important was that substituting for the Nominating Committee a "General Committee," composed of two members from each State and the Army, Navy and Marine Hospital Service, one to be elected to serve for two years each alternate year. None of the amendments was adopted.

A few modifications—elsewhere recorded—were made in regard to the name and scope of the sections.

The entertainments provided for the pleasure of the members of the Association were excellently arranged, and the social features of the meeting were very agreeable.

The meeting was successful in a scientific sense, the papers being numerous and valuable, and the discussions thorough and instructive. It will be remembered as one at which much good work was done, and much was accomplished to strengthen the bond of kindly feeling between the members of the medical profession in all parts of the broad territory of the United States.

RAILWAY SPINE.

One of the most curious developments of modern medical study, and one with an extremely important practical bearing, relates to a form of disorder following railway accidents, which is known by the name of "railway spine."

To those unfamiliar with the manifestations of this disorder, it would appear almost incredible that it should play so serious a *rôle* in the lives of persons who have received injuries which often seem far from severe, and be so often the occasion of protracted medico-legal contests. But one who has studied its phases, under circumstances favorable to a just discrimination between actual morbid phenomena and the simulations which are sometimes practised in order to wring money from a rich corporation, will not wonder that it is regarded as a very grave matter by medical experts, and that they warmly resent the common impression that it is frequently only a form of malingering.

There can be no doubt that instances occur, in which an avaricious patient and a willing or pliable physician unite to over-estimate the damage done by a railway accident; but these cases are far more rare than is often supposed, and there is, on the whole, more danger of error in being too skeptical of the real existence of a condition for which no better name has yet been suggested than "railway spine," than there is in recognizing it and endeavoring to estimate it justly.

The cases which give most trouble are those in which there are few or no evidences of gross lesions in the spinal cord or its surrounding hard and soft parts, but in which there are manifestations of nervous disorder, following an accident and attributed to it, which may be deliberately affected from motives of cupidity. To discriminate between sufferers and pretenders, under these circumstances, is by no means an easy or a pleasant task for most medical men. But much help may be gained for the task by a study of what has been written by men of experience in such cases. A valuable paper on the subject, by Dr. Dercum, of Philadelphia, is in the Department of the REPORTER for Pamphlet Notices, No. 296. In this pamphlet Dr. Dercum describes the classes of injury which are likely to follow blows or falls upon the region of the spinal column, and gives a very instructive review of the principles which should guide a medical witness in deciding upon the actual condition of a person who claims damages for such injuries. We cannot repeat, or even summarize, his conclusions; but would call attention to one point in particular in regard "railway spine," and this is, that there are not a few cases in which, with no gross lesions whatever, a person who has never been nervous, or timid, or hypochondriacal, develops all these characteristics after a railway injury. In women—as Dr. Dercum points out—this alteration of character sometimes takes the form of hysteria, while in the case of men precisely the same condition sometimes follows participation in a railway accident. To give the condition the name of hysteria may be—except for the etymological error of the term—scientifically correct; but to permit this to blind one to the realness of the misfortune would be a grave injustice to the subject of it.

Here is the most delicate question which can arise in the mind of a medical witness; and we believe that it is not untimely to say this word, to fortify any of our readers who may find it hard to meet the objections of counsel for railroad companies, who often honestly think medical men too prone to testify to the existence of evils which are not actually present. The medical witness ought not to ignore the possibility that a claimant for damages may be assuming or exaggerating the appearances of real nervous disorders; but no more ought he to permit himself to be deterred from doing justice to the victim of a railway accident, because there is a natural prejudice against charging whatever follows such an accident to it.

PAMPHLET NOTICES.

[Any reader of the REPORTER who desires a copy of a pamphlet noticed in these columns will doubtless secure it by addressing the author with a request stating where the notice was seen and *enclosing a postage-stamp.*]

289. DISEASED CONDITIONS FOR WHICH SEA AIR IS OF DOUBTFUL BENEFIT. From the *Trans. of the American Climatological Association.* And, THE RESTORATIVE TREATMENT OF SLEEPLESSNESS FROM BRAIN EXHAUSTION. From the *Journal of the American Medical Association.* BY BOARDMAN REED, M.D., Atlantic City, N. J. 8 pages.

290. NOTE ON RUMBOLD'S METHOD OF TREATMENT OF CATARRHAL INFLAMMATIONS OF THE UPPER AIR PASSAGES. BY ELY McCLELLAN, M.D., Surgeon U. S Army. From the *Journal of the Amer. Med. Association,* Jan. 5, 1889. 16 pages.

291. THE MEDICAL JURISPRUDENCE OF INEBRIETY. BY JOSEPH PARRISH, M.D., Burlington, N. J. From the *Journal of Inebriety,* January, 1888. 7 pages.

292. DAS HÖHENKLIMA, IN METEOROLOGISCHER, PHYSIOLOGISCHER UND THERAPEUTISCHER BEZIEHUNG. VON DR. AUGUST LADENDORF, St. Andreasberg. From the *Deutsche Medizinal-Zeitung.* Erster Theil. 70 pages.

293. THERAPEUTICS CAN BECOME A SCIENCE. BY WILLIAM SHARP, M.D., Rugby, England. 33 pages.

294. ON THE RELATION BETWEEN THE GENERAL PRACTITIONER AND THE CONSULTANT OR SPECIALIST. BY L. DUNCAN BULKLEY, M.D., New York. From the *Journal of the Amer. Med. Ass'n,* Feb. 2, 1889. 12 pages.

289. Dr. Reed calls attention to imprudences which sometimes prevent the sea air from doing good to invalids, and also the fact that sea air is not a cure-all, but even seems to act injuriously upon patients affected with certain diseases. In the second half of his pamphlet he impresses the importance of recognizing the fact that sleeplessness is often a manifestation of brain exhaustion and to be treated with tonics and a stimulating hygiene rather than with hypnotics.

290. This pamphlet contains a clear and concise description of the method employed by the author in the treatment of nasal and naso-pharyngeal catarrh, and which has yielded most satisfactory results in his hands. His pamphlet contains illustrations which make the meaning of the text perfectly plain, and it can be recommended to the thoughtful consideration of our readers.

291. The pamphlet advocates the view that the tendency to the intemperate use of alcoholic stimulants is a disease, and cites several interesting cases as evidence of the mental state into which inebriates sometimes fall. Some of these stories sound rather strained, and give the impression that one would need the glasses of the alcoholism specialist to see them in just the same light.

292. A learned study of the conditions of weather, rainfall, sunshine, etc., found at high altitudes in different parts of the world, with a certain amount of allusion to their effect upon the human system in health and disease.

293. This Essay is dated on the author's 84th birthday and indicates that, at this age, he retains a warm interest in theoretical and practical medical questions. The practice recommended covers features which appear not unlike homœopathy and others which are heroic enough for any one. It is interesting reading, though parts of it sound like hobbies rather than scientific theories.

294. Dr. Bulkley's pamphlet contains sound and conservative rules for the guidance of specialists and general practitioners in regard to patients common to both.

LITERARY NOTES.

—Dr. Byrom Bramwell, one of the most enterprising clinical teachers of the Edinburgh School of Medicine, has begun the publication of a new semi-monthly magazine, entitled : " *Studies in Clinical Medicine.*" The object of this new venture in British journalism is to bring to the notice of a large number of persons the results of Dr. Bramwell's examinations of patients who present themselves at his clinic, and to give in an informal manner his remarks—which are taken down in short-hand—upon the treatment of the cases.

NOTES AND COMMENTS.

New Jersey State Medical Society.

The one hundred and twenty-third annual meeting of the New Jersey State Medical Society was held at Asbury Park, June 18 and 19, 1889. The following officers were elected for the ensuing year : *President,* B. A. Watson, M.D., Jersey City ; *First Vice-President,* James S. Green, M.D., Elizabeth ; *Second Vice-President,* E. J. Marsh, M.D., Paterson ; *Third Vice-President,* George T. Welch, M.D., of Key Port ; *Corresponding Secretary,* William Elmer, Jr., M.D., Trenton ; *Recording Secretary,* William Pierson, M.D., Orange ; *Treasurer,* W. W. L. Phillips, M.D., Trenton. *Standing Committee,* T. J. Smith, M.D., Bridgeton ; D. C. English, M.D., New Brunswick ; J. G. Ryerson, M.D., Boonton. The meeting adjourned to meet in June, 1890, at Schooley's Mountain.

The Cook County Asylum.

In the REPORTER, June 1, reference was made to the disgraceful condition of affairs existing in the Cook County Asylum for the Insane. On June 19, Judge Prendergast, of Chicago, rendered his decision in the matter of the investigation into the management of the Asylum. The decision is a long one, but the central idea is explained in the Judge's reference to the political influences which were allowed to control the Asylum. The institution, he says, must be removed from the influences of partisanship in order that the "sweet waters of charity may not be polluted by politics." The Judge recommends that the Asylum be removed from its present site, and that a special session of the State Legislature be called to attend to the matter.

College of Physicians and Surgeons, New York.

At the last meeting of the Faculty of this institution, Dr. James W. McLane was elected to the position of President to fill the place of the late Dr. John C. Dalton. Dr. Markoe was re-elected Vice-President and Dr. Curtis, Secretary. One change only has taken place in the teaching Faculty. Dr. Richard John Hall resigns the chair of anatomy because of ill health. The vacancy will not be permanently filled this year. The graduating class this year was the largest yet sent forth by this college; numbering 167.

The Woman's Medical College of Baltimore.

At the annual meeting of the Faculty and Trustees of the Woman's Medical College of Baltimore, held May 1, the clause allowing " one year's study under a preceptor " to stand for one course of lectures was abolished, so that this institution now places itself squarely among the schools having a three-year compulsory course. The sessions are seven months long, and the instruction is graded with written and oral examinations at the end of each year. There has been a preliminary examination (in English only) since 1883. An average of 70 out of 100 is required for graduation.—*Maryland Medical Journal*, June 15, 1889.

Sanitary Condition of Johnstown.

Dr. Benjamin Lee, executive officer of the State Board of Health of Pennsylvania issued a bulletin on June 17, in which the sanitary condition of Johnstown and surrounding boroughs is reported to be excellent, in view of existing circumstances.

Dr. Lee says there has been a gradual improvement in the health of the boroughs. Coopersdale is somewhat inaccessible owing to high water in the Conemaugh, and there are some cases of gastric disorders in consequence of poor food. There have been no cases of contagious disease at the general hospital, and only one fatal case of diph-

theria at the Red Cross Hospital and one other case. Among the soldiery there is not a single hospital case. The number of cases of measles is diminishing. Gangs are engaged in collecting the carcasses of dead animals along the different streams and are burning them.

Formula for a Mucilaginous Ointment.

Vigier suggests the following formula in the *Gazette Hebdomadaire*, May 3, 1889 :

Vaseline	℥i
Oxide of zinc	℥i
Powdered gum tragacanth	℥ss
Distilled Water	f℥ iiss
Tincture of benzoin	gtt. xxx
Soap powder	gr. vi

Mix the oxide of zinc and vaseline in a mortar and add a little of the mucilage prepared in another ; then add the soap powder and finally the tincture. Mix carefully and preserve in a tight box.

OBITUARY.

J. W. KERR, M.D.

Dr. J. W. Kerr, a venerable and widely-known physician of York, Pennsylvania, died at his residence, June 11, after an illness of two weeks. He was a native of Lancaster County, and was born September 19, 1813. He was graduated from Jefferson College in 1834, and from the University of Pennsylvania in 1839. In the same year he came to York and began the practice of medicine, which he continued without intermission until his death. In 1844 he was married to Miss Jane McIlvain, a native of York. Of three children born, only one survives, Mrs. Dr. W. F. Bacon.

DR. DANIEL W. HAND, M.D.

Dr. Daniel W. Hand died at St. Paul, Minnesota, recently. Dr. Hand was born at Cape May Court House, New Jersey, in 1834. He was graduated at the University of Pennsylvania in 1856, and went to St. Paul in 1857. At the outbreak of the late war, he was commissioned Assistant Surgeon of the First Minnesota Regiment, and was soon promoted to Brigade-Surgeon. He was stationed at Plymouth, N. C., when the yellow fever broke out and remained there through the entire time, nearly one-half the population having died of the fever. Dr. Hand enjoyed the reputation of being one of the ablest physicians of the Northwest. At the time of his death he was Surgeon-General of the State Militia of Minnesota.

Lightning Source UK Ltd.
Milton Keynes UK
UKHW020656211218
334381UK00011B/618/P